Crohn's Disease and Ulcerative Colitis

Daniel C. Baumgart
Editor

Crohn's Disease and Ulcerative Colitis

From Epidemiology and Immunobiology to a Rational Diagnostic and Therapeutic Approach

Second Edition

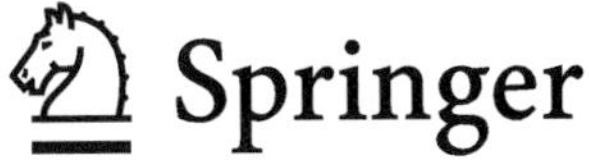

Editor
Daniel C. Baumgart
Inflammatory Bowel Disease Center
Department of Gastroenterology and Hepatology
Charité Medical School—Humboldt-University of Berlin
Berlin, Germany

ISBN 978-3-319-33701-2 ISBN 978-3-319-33703-6 (eBook)
DOI 10.1007/978-3-319-33703-6

Library of Congress Control Number: 2016959449

Printed on acid-free paper

This Springer imprint is published by Springer Nature
The registered company is Springer International Publishing AG Switzerland
The registered company address is: Gewerbestrasse 11, 6330 Cham, Switzerland

Foreword

The clinical features of the major forms of Inflammatory Bowel Disease, Crohn's disease and ulcerative colitis, have been generally well known for decades. After a long period in which advances in our understanding of the causation and pathogenesis of inflammatory bowel diseases remained painfully slow and, in parallel, improvements in management were at best incremental, the momentum of progress has accelerated over the past several years, making a textbook that draws together the full continuum of these advances timely.

The recent pace of progress in understanding the underlying pathogenesis has been especially remarkable. This has been possible because of more powerful methodological approaches as well as a growing community of investigators focused on these disorders and the basic processes associated with them. Progress in recent years has been rapid along a number of fronts, and a general paradigm has emerged to suggest that these disorders result from alterations in the host response to the microflora present within the GI tract. These host responses comprise the collective functional integrity of the mucosal epithelium and the complex set of innate and adaptive immune responses. While many details remain to be fleshed out, molecular pathways intrinsic to the interactions and functional regulation of these responses have been identified and it is clear that for many the "set point" is determined by the genotypic variations at dozens of susceptibility genes. Undoubtedly surprises remain. History suggests the skeptic of any entrenched dogma has a good likelihood of eventually being proven right. However, this paradigm or model has proven a powerful context to ask better questions that should eventuate in more complete answers about the causation and pathogenesis of inflammatory bowel diseases. Progress in understanding of the basic processes underlying the development of inflammatory bowel diseases should be an engine for still more effective therapies as well as diagnostic tools to facilitate management.

On the clinical front, the global epidemiology of inflammatory bowel diseases continues to evolve. While incidence and prevalence plateaued after a long period of steady rise in those regions that remain highest, Europe and North America, other areas of the world are seeing a characteristic pattern of increases in the frequency of ulcerative colitis followed *pari passu* by increases in Crohn's disease. Clinicians caring for these patients cannot be complacent. There is more information that needs to be incorporated into management decisions and, most importantly, much more to offer patients. Improvements in management include evolving surgical approaches and, in some instances, alternative interventions via endoscopy offering efficacy with less morbidity. Advances in nonsurgical medical therapy have had an even greater impact on treatment of IBD patients. These include categorically new agents, which have been developed on the basis of advances in our understanding of mechanisms relevant to the pathogenesis of these disorders. As exemplified by anti-TNF agents, the age of biologics has arrived. Given that understanding of pathogenesis is still progressing rapidly, one can anticipate that more and more effective agents will yet be forthcoming.

These advances have resulted in greater complexity in good decision-making. Those caring for these patients should welcome this complexity in so far as it reflects the possibility of finding management strategies better tailored to the specific needs of an individual patient. The opportunities to make more confident management decisions, if not initial diagnosis as well, have also become both more complicated and more promising with the advent of new imaging modalities (both "radiologic" and "endoscopic") as well as various biomarkers. While it is not yet clear how specific susceptibility genotypes might be best used clinically there is, in concept, the possibility of more definitive diagnosis after decades in which diagnosis has remained, in the final analysis, an empiric process.

In these general reflections on recent progress are clear indications of the timeliness for a textbook that endeavors to bring these new advances into better focus. The editors have embraced this ambitious goal and assembled an outstanding group of authors who have been at the forefront of much of this progress. This volume provides both the clinician and the scientist with an understanding of the most recent advances as well as the context for each of them to be pursuing their mission of caring for patients and advancing our knowledge, respectively. However, these general reflections also come with an embedded caution. Clinicians will recognize that even with this progress, unmet needs persist and there remain many patients for whom current approaches are simply not good enough. The scientist will recognize how still incomplete our understanding of these diseases remains. So, this textbook provides a powerful tool to ensure that clinicians can provide today's best care and scientists can pose today's best questions. One can only hope that within a few years the next volume will be ready to be written.

Professor of Medicine Daniel K. Podolsky
President of the University of Texas Southwestern Medical Center
Dallas, TX, USA

Preface to the Second Edition

Crohn's disease and ulcerative colitis—two chronic inflammatory diseases (IBD) on the rise—result from an inappropriate immune response, in genetically susceptible individuals, to microbial antigens of commensal microorganisms. This inappropriate response is promoted by certain environmental factors including Western life style, explaining their globally increasing incidence. As a systemic disorder of the immune system, IBD manifest itself primarily in the gastrointestinal tract but can affect all of the organ systems of the human body. Thus, not only gastroenterologist, but many other clinicians are confronted with IBD.

On the other hand IBD is an excellent example of how the exponential growth of knowledge in biomedical science can make a remarkable impact on clinical practice and patient's quality of life. The number of novel and targeted treatments is growing rapidly. They are continuously being refined to treat not only the two original conditions of the gut but also the variety of associated immune disorders. New therapies are sometimes complex and associated with important risks requiring a deeper understanding of their molecular principles from clinicians.

This book continues to serve as a unique combined resource for physicians and scientists addressing the needs of both groups. It is meant to help stimulate exchange and collaboration, shorten the path between discovery and clinical application, and also help clinicians understand new therapeutic concepts from their origins.

The great success of the first edition confirms our concept. It encouraged us to not only bring all chapters up to date but also include new scientific and clinical trends in new chapters.

I'm grateful to my colleagues from all over the world who took out time out of their busy days to contribute new and updated chapters in their respective fields of expertise to make accomplishing the goals of this book possible.

Berlin, Germany

Daniel C. Baumgart

Preface

Crohn's disease and ulcerative colitis—two chronic inflammatory diseases (IBD) on the rise—result from an inappropriate immune response, in genetically susceptible individuals, to microbial antigens of commensal microorganisms. This inappropriate response is promoted by certain environmental factors including Western life style, explaining their globally increasing incidence. As a systemic disorder of the immune system, IBD manifest itself primarily in the gastrointestinal tract but can affect all of the organ systems of the human body. Thus, not only gastroenterologist, but many other clinicians are confronted with IBD.

On the other hand IBD is an excellent example of how the exponential growth of knowledge in biomedical science can make a remarkable impact on clinical practice and patient's quality of life. It has led to the development of a number of novel targeted and tailored treatments. These are continuously being refined to treat not only the two original conditions in the gut but also the variety of associated immune disorders. New therapies are sometimes complex and associated with important risks requiring a deeper understanding of their molecular principles from clinicians.

This book is intended to serve as a unique combined resource for physicians and scientists addressing the needs of both groups. It is meant to help stimulate exchange and collaboration and shorten the path between discovery and application of new knowledge and also help clinicians understand new therapeutic concepts from their origins.

I'm grateful to my colleagues from all over the world who contributed chapters in their respective fields of expertise and made accomplishing the goals of this book possible.

Berlin, Germany — Daniel C. Baumgart

Contents

Part VI Extraintestinal Manifestations

Part VII Nutrition

Part VIII Pregnancy, Family Planning and Pediatric Aspects

Part IX Surveillance and Prevention

Part X Patient Perspective and Resources

Contributors

C. Agné, M.D. Department of Gastroenterology, Hepatology and Endocrinology, Hannover Medical School, Hannover, Germany

Caroline P. Allen Department of Dermatology, Oxford University Hospitals NHS Trust, Oxford, UK

Alessandro Armuzzi, M.D., Ph.D. IBD Unit, Complesso Integrato Columbus, Gemelli Hospital, Catholic University Foundation, Rome, Italy

Daniel C. Baumgart Department of Gastroenterology and Hepatology, Inflammatory Bowel Disease Center, Charité Medical Center—Virchow Hospital, Medical School of the Humboldt University of Berlin, Berlin, Germany

Charles N. Bernstein, M.D. University of Manitoba IBD Clinical and Research Centre, Winnipeg, MB, Canada

Charles L. Bevins, M.D., Ph.D. Department of Microbiology and Immunology, University of California Davis School of Medicine, Davis, CA, USA

Atul K. Bhan, M.B.B.S., M.D. Department of Pathology, Massachusetts General Hospital, Harvard Medical School, Boston, MA, USA

Paolo Biancheri, M.D., Ph.D. Centre for Immunobiology, Barts and The London School of Medicine and Dentistry, Queen Mary University of London, London, UK

A. Biswas Division of Gastroenterology, Hepatology and Nutrition, Boston Children's Hospital, Boston, MA, USA

Brendan Boyle Division of Pediatric Gastroenterology, Hepatology, and Nutrition, Nationwide Children's Hospital, The Ohio State University, College of Medicine and Public Health, Columbus, OH, USA

Per Brandtzaeg, M.D., Ph.D. Centre for Immune Regulation (CIR), University of Oslo, Oslo, Norway

Laboratory for Immunohistochemistry and Immunopathology (LIIPAT), Department of Pathology, Oslo University Hospital—Rikshospitalet, Nydalen, Oslo, Norway

Brian Bressler Division of Gastroenterology, University of British Columbia, Vancouver, BC, Canada

Alan L. Buchman, M.D., M.S.P.H. Department of Surgery, University of Illinois at Chicago, Glencoe, IL, USA

Susan M. Burge, B.Sc., D.M., F.R.C.P. Department of Dermatology, Oxford University Hospitals NHS Trust, Oxford, UK

Johan Burisch, M.D., Ph.D. Danish Centre for eHealth & Epidemiology, Department of Gastroenterology, North Zealand Hospital, Frederikssund, Denmark

Ludovica F. Buttó, Ph.D. Chair of Nutrition and Immunology, Technische Universität München, Freising-Weihenstephan, Germany

Eduard Cabré, M.D., Ph.D. IBD/G-I Unit, Department of Gastroenterology, Hospital Universitari Germans Trias i Pujol, Badalona, Catalonia, Spain

CIBERehd, Barcelona, Catalonia, Spain

Carlo Calabrese Department of Medical and Surgical Sciences (DIMEC), University of Bologna, Bologna, Italy

Andrea Calafiore Department of Medical and Surgical Sciences (DIMEC), University of Bologna, Bologna, Italy

Eric L. Campbell, Ph.D. Department of Medicine and the Mucosal Inflammation Program, University of Colorado School of Medicine, Aurora, CO, USA

Katrine Carlsen Department of Pediatrics, Hvidovre Hospital, Hvidovre, Denmark

Roger W. Chapman Department of Translational Gastroenterology, John Radcliffe, Oxford, UK

Britt Christensen Department of Medicine, University of Chicago Medicine, Inflammatory Bowel Disease Center, Chicago, IL, USA

Department of Gastroenterology, Alfred Hospital and Monash University, Melbourne, Australia

Robert R. Cima, M.D., M.A. Division of Colon and Rectal Surgery, Mayo Clinic College of Medicine, Rochester, MN, USA

Sean P. Colgan, Ph.D. Department of Medicine and the Mucosal Inflammation Program, University of Colorado School of Medicine, Aurora, CO, USA

Jacques Cosnes, M.D. Service de Gastroentérologie et Nutrition, Hôpital St-Antoine (APHP) and Pierre-et-Marie Curie University (Paris VI), Paris, France

Nigel Crawford Department of General Medicine, Royal Children's Hospital Melbourne, Parkville, VIC, Australia

Geert D'Haens Department of Gastroenterology, Academic Medical Centre, Amsterdam, The Netherlands

Laurence Egan, M.D., F.R.C.P.I. Clinical Science Institute, University Hospital Galway, Galway, Ireland

Rami Eliakim, M.D. Department of Gastroenterology, Chaim Sheba Medical Center, Sackler School of Medicine, Tel-Aviv University, Tel Aviv, Israel

Francis A. Farraye, M.D., M.Sc. Department of Gastroenterology, Boston Medical Center, Boston University School of Medicine, Boston, MA, USA

Brian G. Feagan, M.D. Robarts Clinical Trials, University of Western Ontario, London, ON, Canada

Division of Gastroenterology, Department of Medicine, University of Western Ontario, London, ON, Canada

Department of Epidemiology and Biostatistics, University of Western Ontario, London, ON, Canada

Richard N. Fedorak, M.D., F.R.C.P.C., F.R.S.C. Department of Medicine, Zeidler Ledcor Centre, University of Alberta, Edmonton, Canada

Andreas Fischer Department of Gastroenterology and Hepatology, Inflammatory Bowel Disease Center, Charité Medical Center—Virchow Hospital, Medical School of the Humboldt University of Berlin, Berlin, Germany

M. Flamant Institut des Maladies de l'Appareil Digestif (IMAD), Hotel Dieu, Nantes, Cedex, France

J.G. Fletcher Mayo Clinic, Rochester, MN, USA

Miquel A. Gassull, M.D., Ph.D. Health Science Research Institute, Germans Trias i Pujol Foundation, Badalona, Catalonia, Spain

Gastroenterology and Hepatology Department, Germans Trias I, Pujol University Hospital, Badalona, Catalonia, Spain

M. Gebel, M.D. Department of Gastroenterology, Hepatology and Endocrinology, Hannover Medical School, Hannover, Germany

Peter R. Gibson, M.D., F.R.A.C.P. Department of Gastroenterology, The Alfred Hospital and Monash University, Melbourne, VIC, Australia

Paolo Gionchetti, M.D. Department of Medical and Surgical Sciences (DIMEC), University of Bologna, Bologna, Italy

D. Neil Granger, Ph.D. Department of Molecular & Cellular Physiology, Louisiana State University Health Sciences Center—Shreveport, Shreveport, LA, USA

Marco Greco, Ph.D. European Federation of Crohn's and Ulcerative Colitis Associations (EFCCA), Brussels, Belgium

European Patients' Forum (EPF), Brussels, Belgium

Matthew B. Grisham, Ph.D. Department of Immunology and Molecular Microbiology, Texas Tech University Health Sciences Center, Lubbock, TX, USA

Luís Guimarães Department of Medical Imaging, Princess Margaret Hospital, Toronto, ON, Canada

Dirk Haller, Ph.D. Chair of Nutrition and Immunology, Technische Universität München, Freising-Weihenstephan, Germany

Grace Harkin, M.B., M.R.C.P.I. Clinical Science Institute, University Hospital Galway, Galway, Ireland

Norman R. Harris, Ph.D. Department of Molecular & Cellular Physiology, Louisiana State University Health Sciences Center—Shreveport, Shreveport, LA, USA

Pieter Hindryckx Department of Gastroenterology, University Hospital of Ghent, Ghent, Belgium

Daniel W. Hommes Division of Medicine, Gastroenterology, Department of Medicine, Ronald Reagan UCLA Medical Center, Los Angeles, CA, USA

Vivian W. Huang Department of Medicine, Zeidler Ledcor Centre, University of Alberta, Edmonton, AB, Canada

Jeffrey S. Hyams, M.D. Division of Digestive Diseases, Hepatology, and Nutrition, Connecticut Children's Medical Center, Hartford, CT, USA

University of Connecticut School of Medicine, Hartford, CT, USA

Peter M. Irving Department of Gastroenterology, Guy's and St Thomas' Hospital, London, UK

Hanna Johnsson Institute of Infection, Immunity and Inflammation, College of MVLS, University of Glasgow, Glasgow, UK

Nora E. Joseph Department of Pathology and Laboratory Medicine, NorthShore University Health System, Evanston, IL, USA

Terumi Kamisawa, M.D., Ph.D. Department of Internal Medicine, Tokyo Metropolitan Komagome Hospital, Tokyo, Japan

Takanori Kanai, M.D. Division of Gastroenterology and Hepatology, Department of Internal Medicine, Keio University School of Medicine, Tokyo, Japan

Arthur Kaser Division of Gastroenterology and Hepatology, Department of Medicine, Addenbrooke's Hospital, University of Cambridge, Cambridge, UK

Catherine Van Kemseke Department of Gastroenterology, University Hospital CHU of Liège, Liège, Belgium

Reena Khanna Robarts Clinical Trials, University of Western Ontario, London, ON, Canada

Department of Medicine, Division of Gastroenterology, University of Western Ontario, London, ON, Canada

R. Kiesslich Klinik für Innere Medizin II (ZIM II), HELIOS Dr. Horst Schmidt Kliniken Wiesbaden, Wiesbaden, Germany

Jan-Michael A. Klapproth Division of Gastroenterology, Department of Medicine, University of Pennsylvania, Philadelphia, PA, USA

Go Kuwata, M.D. Department of Internal Medicine, Tokyo Metropolitan Komagome Hospital, Tokyo, Japan

Adi Lahat, M.D. Department of Gastroenterology, Chaim Sheba Medical Center, Sackler School of Medicine, Tel-Aviv University, Tel Aviv, Israel

Mindy Lam Division of Gastroenterology, University of British Columbia, Vancouver, BC, Canada

Barrett G. Levesque Division of Gastroenterology, University of California San Diego, La Jolla, CA, USA

Gary R. Lichtenstein, M.D. Division of Gastroenterology, Department of Medicine, University of Pennsylvania, Philadelphia, PA, USA

Jimmy K. Limdi Division of Gastroenterology, The Pennine Acute Hospitals NHS Trust, Manchester, UK

Institute of Inflammation and Repair, University of Manchester, Manchester, UK

Edward V. Loftus Jr. , M.D. Division of Gastroenterology & Hepatology, Mayo Clinic, Rochester, MN, USA

Sanna Lönnfors, M.Sc.P.H., M.A. European Federation of Crohn's and Ulcerative Colitis Associations (EFCCA), Brussels, Belgium

Edouard Louis Department of Gastroenterology, University Hospital CHU of Liège, Liège, Belgium

Kristine Macartney, M.D., F.R.A.C.P. The Children's Hospital of Westmead, The National Centre for Immunisation Research and Surveillance, Westmead, NSW, Australia

Thomas T. MacDonald, Ph.D., F.R.C.Path., F.Med.Sci. Centre for Immunobiology, Barts and The London School of Medicine and Dentistry, Queen Mary University of London, London, UK

Uma Mahadevan, M.D. UCSF Center for Colitis and Crohn's Disease, San Francisco, CA, USA

Peter Mannon Professor of Medicine and Microbiology, University of Alabama at Birmingham, Birmingham, AL, USA

Michael P. Manns, M.D. Department of Gastroenterology, Hepatology and Endocrinology, Hannover Medical School, Hannover, Germany

John K. Marshall, M.D., M.Sc., F.R.C.P.C. Department of Medicine, Farncombe Family Digestive Health Research Institute, McMaster University, Hamilton, ON, Canada

Division of Gastroenterology (2F59), McMaster University Medical Centre, Hamilton, ON, Canada

Rebecca Matro Oregon Health and Sciences University, Portland, OR, USA

Iain B. McInnes Institute of Infection, Immunity and Inflammation, College of MVLS, University of Glasgow, Glasgow, UK

Marjorie Merrick, M.A. Research and Scientific Programs, Crohn's & Colitis Foundation of America, New York, NY, USA

Atsushi Mizoguchi Department of Immunology, Kurume University School of Medicine, Fukuoka, Japan

Jorge O. Múnera Division of Developmental Biology, Cincinnati Children's Hospital Research Foundation, Cincinnati, OH, USA

Pia Munkholm, M.D. Danish Centre for eHealth & Epidemiology, Department of Gastroenterology, North Zealand Hospital, Frederikssund, Denmark

Takashi Nagaishi, M.D., Ph.D. Department of Gastroenterology, Tokyo Medical and Dental University, Tokyo, Japan

D. Nguyen Division of Gastroenterology, Hepatology and Nutrition, Boston Children's Hospital, Boston, MA, USA

Matthew A. Odenwald, Ph.D. Department of Pathology, The University of Chicago, Chicago, IL, USA

Remo Panaccione, M.D., F.R.C.P.C. Inflammatory Bowel Disease Clinic, Professor of Medicine, University of Calgary, Calgary, Canada

Farhad Peerani Division of Gastroenterology, Department of Medicine, University of Alberta, Zeidler Ledcor Centre, Edmonton, AB, Canada

John H. Pemberton, M.D. Division of Colon and Rectal Surgery, Mayo Clinic College of Medicine, Rochester, MN, USA

A. Potthoff, M.D. Department of Gastroenterology, Hepatology and Endocrinology, Hannover Medical School, Hannover, Germany

Daniela Pugliese IBD Unit, Complesso Integrato Columbus, Gemelli Hospital Catholic University Foundation, Rome, Italy

Catherine Reenaers Department of Gastroenterology, University Hospital CHU of Liège, Liège, Belgium

Walter Reinisch Division of Gastroenterology, Department of Medicine, McMaster University, Hamilton, ON, Canada

Fernando Rizzello Department of Medical and Surgical Sciences (DIMEC), University of Bologna, Bologna, Italy

X. Roblin Service de Gastroentérologie, CHU de Saint Etienne, Hopital Nord, Saint-Priest-en-Jarez, France

Patrik Rogalla, BS, MD Department of Medical Imaging, Princess Margaret Hospital, Toronto, ON, Canada

Gerhard Rogler Division of Gastroenterology and Hepatology, University Hospital of Zürich, Zürich, Switzerland

David T. Rubin, M.D. Department of Medicine, University of Chicago Medicine Inflammatory Bowel Disease Center, Chicago, IL, USA

Mark A. Samaan Department of Gastroenterology, Guy's and St Thomas' Hospital, London, UK

Bruce E. Sands, M.D., M.S. Dr. Henry D. Janowitz Division of Gastroenterology and Department of Medicine, Icahn School of Medicine at Mount Sinai, New York, NY, USA

Nora Schweitzer, M.D. Department of Gastroenterology, Hepatology and Endocrinology, Hannover Medical School, Hannover, Germany

S. Snapper Division of Gastroenterology, Hepatology and Nutrition, Boston Children's Hospital, Boston, MA, USA

Division of Gastroenterology, Brigham and Women's Hospital, Boston, MA, USA

Harry Sokol, M.D., Ph.D. Service de Gastroentérologie et Nutrition, Hôpital St-Antoine (APHP) and Pierre-et-Marie Curie University (Paris VI), Paris, France

A. Hillary Steinhart, M.D., M.Sc., F.R.C.P.(C) IBD Centre, Mount Sinai Hospital and Department of Medicine, University of Toronto, Toronto, ON, Canada

Kirstin Taylor Department of Gastroenterology, The Alfred Hospital and Monash University, Melbourne, VIC, Australia

Alistair Tindell Institute of Infection, Immunity and Inflammation, College of MVLS, University of Glasgow, Glasgow, UK

Jerrold R. Turner, M.D., Ph.D. Department of Pathology, The University of Chicago, Chicago, IL, USA

Departments of Pathology and Medicine (GI), Brigham and Women's Hospital and Harvard Medical School, Boston, MA, USA

Morten H. Vatn, M.D., Ph.D. Section of Gastroenterology, Oslo University Hospital, Nydalen, Oslo, Norway

Akershus University Hospital, Institute of Clinical Medicine, University of Oslo, Nordbyhagen, Akershus, Norway

Severine Vermeire, M.D., Ph.D. Department of Gastroenterology, University Hospitals Leuven, Leuven, Belgium

Mamoru Watanabe, M.D., Ph.D. Department of Gastroenterology, Tokyo Medical and Dental University, Tokyo, Japan

Cynthia Reinoso Webb, B.S., M(ASCP) Department of Immunology and Molecular Microbiology, Texas Tech University Health Sciences Center, Lubbock, TX, USA

Christopher R. Weber, M.D., Ph.D. Department of Pathology, The University of Chicago, Chicago, IL, USA

James M. Wells, Ph.D. Division of Developmental Biology, Cincinnati Children's Hospital Research Foundation, Cincinnati, OH, USA

Ayesha Williams IBD Help Center, Crohn's & Colitis Foundation of America, New York, NY, USA

Kate D. Williamson Department of Translational Gastroenterology, John Radcliffe, Oxford, UK

Christine Y. Yu, M.D. GI fellow, University of California, Los Angeles, USA

Part I

Epidemiology

Environmental Factors in the Epidemiology of Inflammatory Bowel Disease

1

Morten H. Vatn

Introduction

The occurrence of IBD has been increasing in Western Europe and North America [1, 2] over several decades after the Second World War. It has been assumed that socioeconomic factors represent the most important explanation for this increase [3]. A part of this increase may have been related to more awareness and recognition of the diseases, as well as generally better registration in all countries.

It is important to realize that the general acceptance of endoscopy as the main internationally accepted diagnostic procedure is quite young, and that we may divide the history into a pre-endoscopic area before 1970, an early endoscopic period between 1970 and 1990 characterized by a relatively large heterogeneity among studies, and a post-endoscopic period from around 1990, whereafter a widespread distribution of equipment and skills of endoscopy enabled all countries to perform uniform diagnostic procedures (Table 1.1). Moreover, after this point in time, most international studies have been performed according to generally accepted definitions and criteria of diagnosis [4].

However, even if we generally include only endoscopy-based studies, the heterogeneity of even the Western materials is striking and difficult to compare, regarding incidence, prevalence, and subtypes. One important reason for this is the selection of cohorts in the different countries. In most centers, the registration of IBD has been hospital based, by which the type of recorded patients were depending on the level of each hospital in the health-care system of each country, including access to health care. Additionally, great variations exist in the recording systems, both between hospitals and between countries, and in how well the patients were characterized on the basis of first or later admissions [4, 5]. The centers which have achieved most experience in IBD are second or third line hospitals with large databases, including patients with relatively more complicated disease [6–8].

In population-based studies, in which the cohorts better represent the total number of patients with IBD in an area, increased number of patients are recorded with light to moderate disease and less complications, and with a relatively higher age at diagnosis [8–14].

In spite of the variation in incidence and prevalence of IBD between the Western countries, the recognition of increased occurrence has been a common feature (Figs. 1.1 and 1.2). Although follow-up studies have given increased knowledge of outcome of disease, repeated prospective studies on incidence have only recently been performed [9], and mostly in children (Figs. 1.3 and 1.4; Tables 1.2 and 1.3) [15, 16]. These studies tend to suggest that the incidence of CD may still be increasing in the Western world, despite signs of a stable frequency of UC in the same cohorts [15–17]. In spite of the reported higher incidence rates of CD than of UC from Canada and the middle of Europe, UC is the predominant phenotype of IBD in the rest of Europe. Moreover, studies from certain areas of Northern [18, 19] and Eastern Europe [20], as well as New Zealand [21], may suggest that UC is still increasing among adults.

When looking for a cause relationship behind CD and UC, the environmental factors of importance mainly seem to be related to the Western lifestyle. Nevertheless, the variation in lifestyle, between countries and areas within countries, is great. Additionally, the emerging increase in prevalence reported from outside the Western countries, makes the focus on environmental factors even more important. A burning question is therefore, whether certain specific risk factors for the development of IBD are related to increased socioeconomic status, regardless of geography, and in addition to public awareness and access to health care? Additionally, we have to bear in mind that in diseases like IBD, with a multifactorial etiology, different risk factors

M.H. Vatn, M.D., Ph.D. (✉)
Section of Gastroenterology, Oslo University Hospital, Nydalen, P.O. Box 4959, 0424 Oslo, Norway

Akershus University Hospital, Institute of Clinical Medicine, University of Oslo, 1474 Nordbyhagen, Akershus, Norway
e-mail: m.h.vatn@medisin.uio.no

D.C. Baumgart (ed.), *Crohn's Disease and Ulcerative Colitis*, DOI 10.1007/978-3-319-33703-6_1

Table 1.1 Registration of IBD

Possible causes for change over time
• Before 1970
– Retrospective data
– Hospital based
– Cross-sectional studies
– Unclear definitions
– Pre-endoscopic period
• After 1970
– Early endoscopic period
– Defined populations
– Prospective registration
– GP/hospital based
• After 1990
– Endoscopy-based diagnosis
– International criteria
– Subgroups: proctitis/indeterminate
– Controlled on specialist level
– Follow-up controls
– Possibility for "case–control" studies

may cause imbalance of the environmental–host relationship in different parts of the world. Suspected consequences of industrialization might not necessarily be relevant for disease development in different geographic regions, although our traditional reductionism of logic thinking tends to look for a simplified explanation for cause relationships.

In the following, it seems necessary to relate environmental factors to the reported occurrence of IBD in the different geographic areas, and thereafter discuss the degree of potential risk factors of disease present in each specific region, to the best of our present knowledge.

Geography

Variation Between Countries

The fact that IBD occurs with the highest frequency in the Western world is undisputable, and the experience is based on hospital materials from the large centers in Europe and North America. These areas also have in common that remarkable increasing prevalence rates have been recorded during the second half of the twentieth century [1, 2] (Figs. 1.1 and 1.2).

In addition to that, differences between regions of Europe and North America have been recorded. In Europe, a North–South gradient for incidence rate, phenotype, and recurrence, has been demonstrated [10, 22, 23] based on modern diagnostic procedures and prospective follow up.

Interestingly, the highest incidence rates of both the North and South of Europe have been demonstrated in the islands of Iceland and Faroe Islands [10], and the islands of Crete and Sicily and Mallorca [10], respectively (Fig. 1.5). This might raise interesting questions regarding both genetic and environmental explanations. Recently, also high incidence rates of IBD have been reported from New Zealand and Australia (Wilson J, Hair C, Knight R. High incidence of inflammatory bowel disease in Australia: a prospective population-based Australian incidence study. Inflamm Bowel Dis 2010;16:1550–6), which may contribute to this discussion. In Japan, most of the experience in IBD is based on the reports from large hospital-based centers, all reporting on increased prevalence rates, although definitively much lower than in the Western world [24]. Some reports have also come from South America [25].

Racial differences of IBD prevalence rates have been reported from North America [26], showing much lower rates among Hispanic and Asian people compared to whites and African Americans. High prevalence rates for Crohn's disease and ulcerative colitis have also been shown for North American Ashkenazi and Israeli Jews [27, 28]. The suggested effect of ethnicity on disease location, complications, and anticipation may be partly explained by genetic and environmental factors [25–27].

Developing regions have traditionally reported lower prevalence of IBD, which seems to increase, probably as a consequence of a rising incidence of IBD in many of these nations, such as India and China, as they have become industrialized [29, 30].

Furthermore, migrant studies have demonstrated that individuals immigrating from regions with low prevalence to countries with higher prevalence rates are at an increased risk for developing IBD, particularly among first and second generation children [30, 31].

In the USA, also, a North–South gradient has been shown by hospital-based registrations [6, 32, 33], whereas in Canada, an East–West gradient has been demonstrated in a nationwide comparison [13] (Fig. 1.6). Moreover, the population-based registry of Manitoba, Canada [13] has demonstrated some of the highest incidence rates of IBD in the world.

In the population based ECCO-Epicom study (Burisch J, Pedersen N, Cukovic-Lavka S, et al. East-West gradient in the incidence of inflammatory bowel disease in Europe: the Ecco-Epicom inception cohort. Gut 2014;63:588–97), an east–west ratio was demonstrated for Europe, with the highest incidence rate in Western Europe. Recent review articles have reported on global variability in IBD and environmental risk factors in adults (Ng SC, Bernstein CN, Vatn MH, et al. Geographic variability and environmental risk factors in inflammatory bowel disease. Gut 2013;62:630–49; Moledecky NA, Soon IS, Rabi DM, et al. Increasing incidence and prevalence of inflammatory bowel disease with time, based on systematic review. Gastroenterology 2012;142:46–54) and children (Benchimol EI, Fortinsky KJ, Gozdyra P, et al. Epidemiology of pediatric inflammatory bowel disease: a systematic review of international trends. Inflamm Bowel Dis 2011;17:423–39).

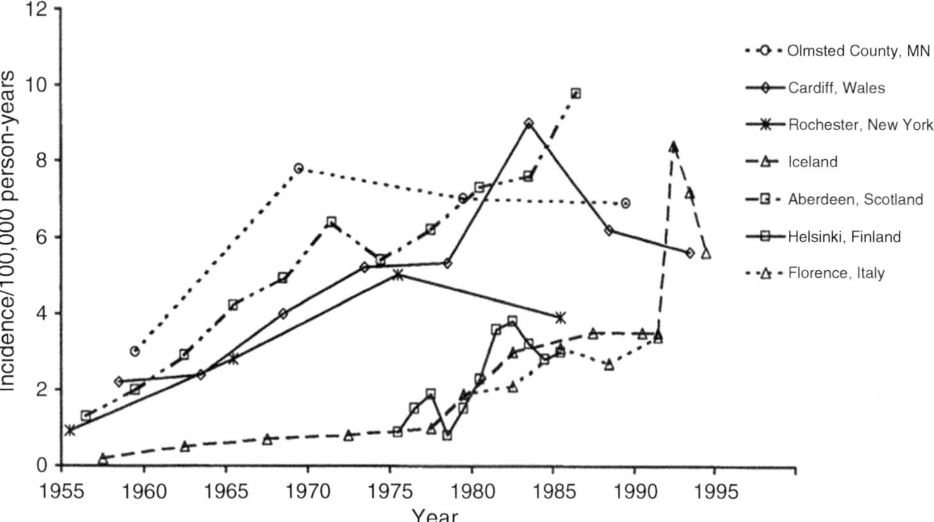

Fig. 1.1 Temporal trends in incidence rates (cases per 100,000 person-years) of Crohn's disease in selected areas (Olmsted County, Minnesota; Cardiff, Wales, UK; Rochester, New York; Iceland; Aberdeen, Scotland, UK; Helsinki, Finland; and Florence, Italy). [Reprinted from Gastroenterology; 126(6). Loftus E. Clinical epidemiology of inflammatory bowel disease: incidence, prevalence, and environmental influences: 1504–17. ©2004 with permission from Elsevier]

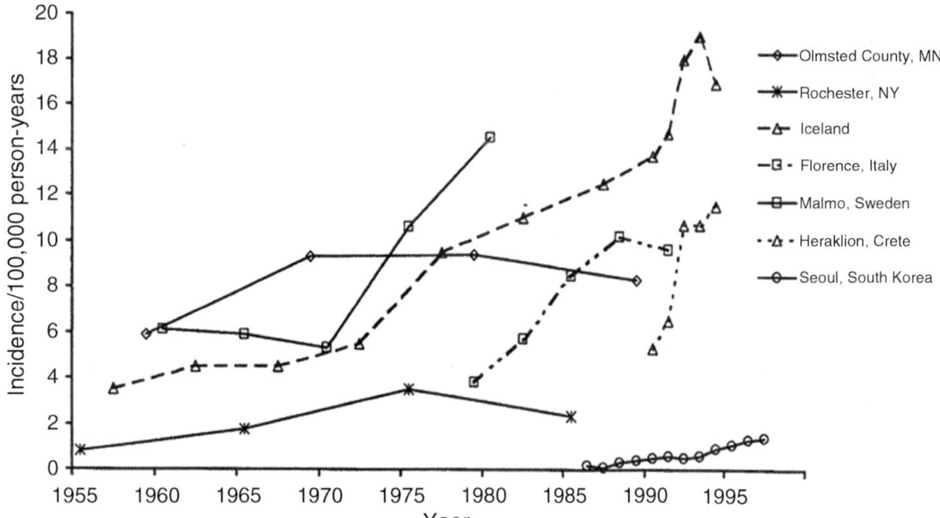

Fig. 1.2 Temporal trends in incidence rates (cases per 100,000 person-years) of ulcerative colitis in selected geographic regions (Olmsted County, Minnesota; Rochester, New York; Iceland; Florence, Italy; Malmo, Sweden; Heraklion, Crete, Greece; and Seoul, South Korea). [Reprinted from Gastroenterology; 126(6). Loftus E. Clinical epidemiology of inflammatory bowel disease: incidence, prevalence, and environmental influences: 1504–17. ©2004 with permission from Elsevier]

Variations Within European Countries: Population-Based Studies (Fig. 1.7)

In Europe, great differences have been reported regarding variation in frequency of IBD between centers within countries. In Greece, the island of Crete showed a markedly higher incidence of IBD compared to Joannina in the North [10] similar to a higher incidence in Sicily compared to the North of Italy [10]. Based on comparisons on the Italian continent, also a North–South gradient is indicated, similar to a North–South gradient in Portugal and Spain [10].

In France, a higher incidence and prevalence in the North compared to the South has been reported, based on a partly hospital-based Nationwide registry [34].

Within Germany, Spain, and the UK, national variations based on direct comparisons have not been reported, although variations between single center studies are obvious within countries. High incidence rates have been reported from Ireland, Scotland, and the Netherlands compared to the UK and Western Germany [10]. Many of these differences, however, might be explained by variation in type of cohorts and organization of health care.

From Denmark and Norway, generally high incidence rates have been reported in population-based studies [1, 10–12]. In Norway, similar incidence rates have been shown between the Northern [35], Western [36], and the South-Eastern part [12], whereas great differences were shown between counties for the two latter areas compared to a more even distribution within the former [35]. This could be

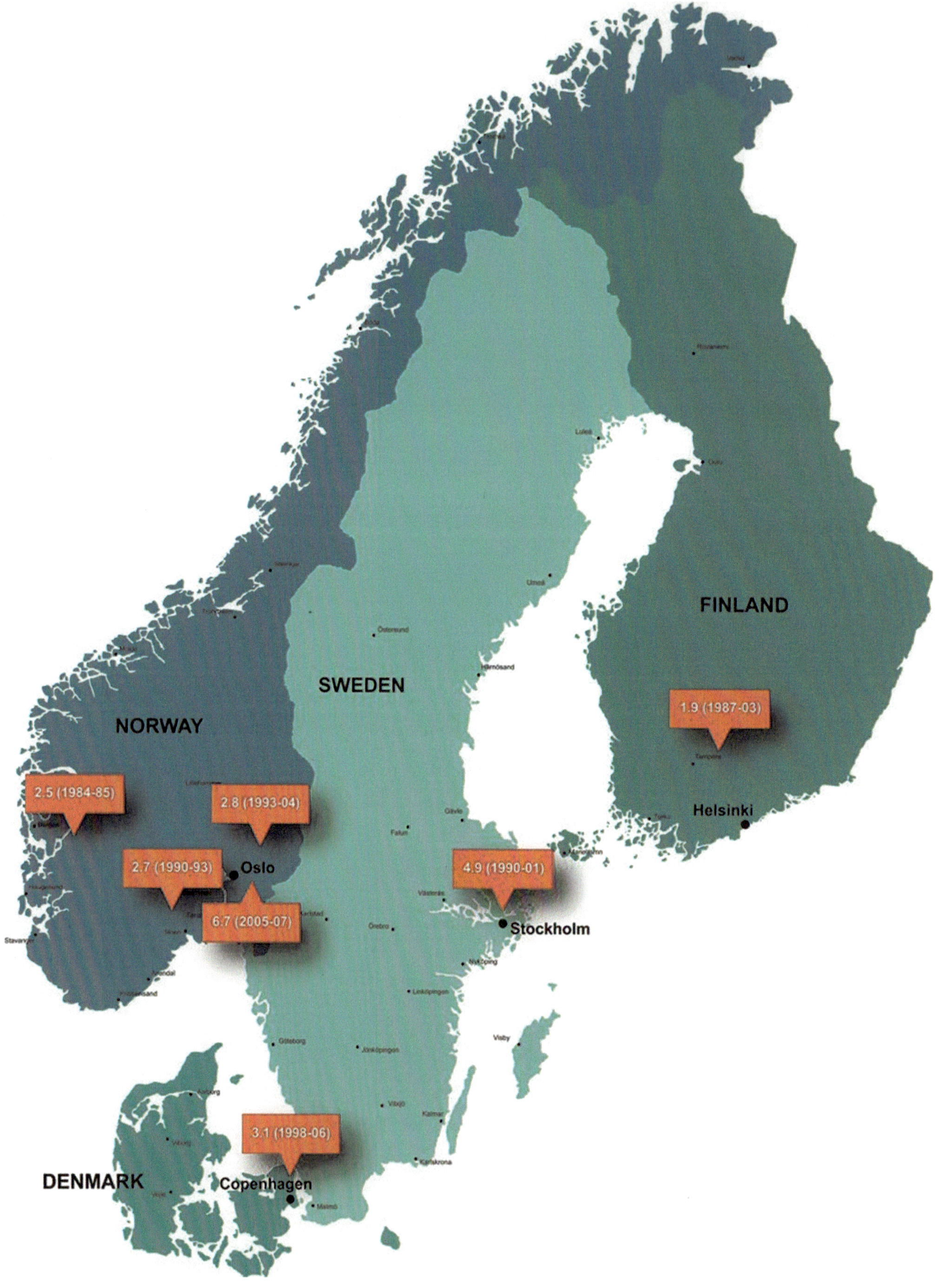

Fig. 1.3 Incidence of CD in children (Table 1.2)

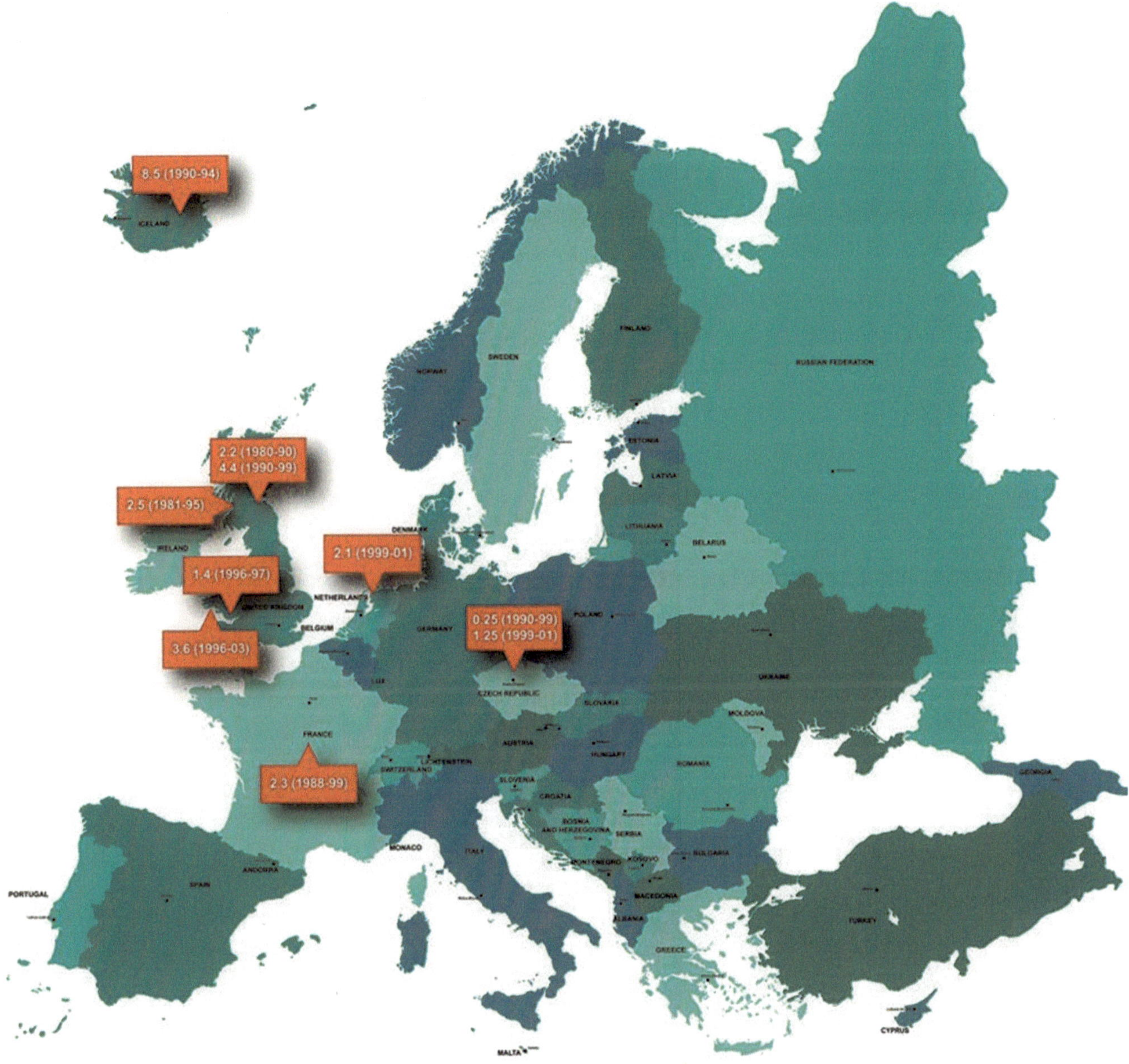

Fig. 1.4 Incidence of CD in children (Table 1.3)

Table 1.2 Incidence of pediatric IBD in the Nordic countries

Country	Year	Incidence of CD	Incidence of UC	*N*
Norway (IBSEN)	1990–1993	2.7	2.0	29 <16 years
Norway (AHUS)	1993–2004	2.8	3.9	49 <16 years
Norway (IBSEN II)	2005–2007	6.7	3.9	48 <16 years
West Norway	1984–1985	2.5	4.3	27 <16 years
Denmark	1998–2006	3.1	1.6	50 <15 years
Sweden	1990–2001	4.9	2.5	152 <16 years
Finland	1987–2003	1.9	3.9	604 <18 years

Table 1.3 Incidence of pediatric IBD in Europe

Country	Year	Incidence of CD	Incidence of UC	*N*
Scotland	1981–1995	2.5	3.8	665 <16 years
	1980–1990	2.2		107 <16 years
	1990–1999	4.4		107 <16 years
Iceland	1990–1994	8.5		
Wales	1996–1997	1.36	2.6	38 <16 years
	1996–2003	3.6	5.4	39 <16 years
England	1998–1999	3.1	5.2	739 <16 years
Czechoslovakia	1990–1999	1.25		470 <15 years
	1999–2001			
North France	1988–1999	2.3	3.1	509 <17 years
Netherlands	1999–2001	2.1	7.3	220 <18 years

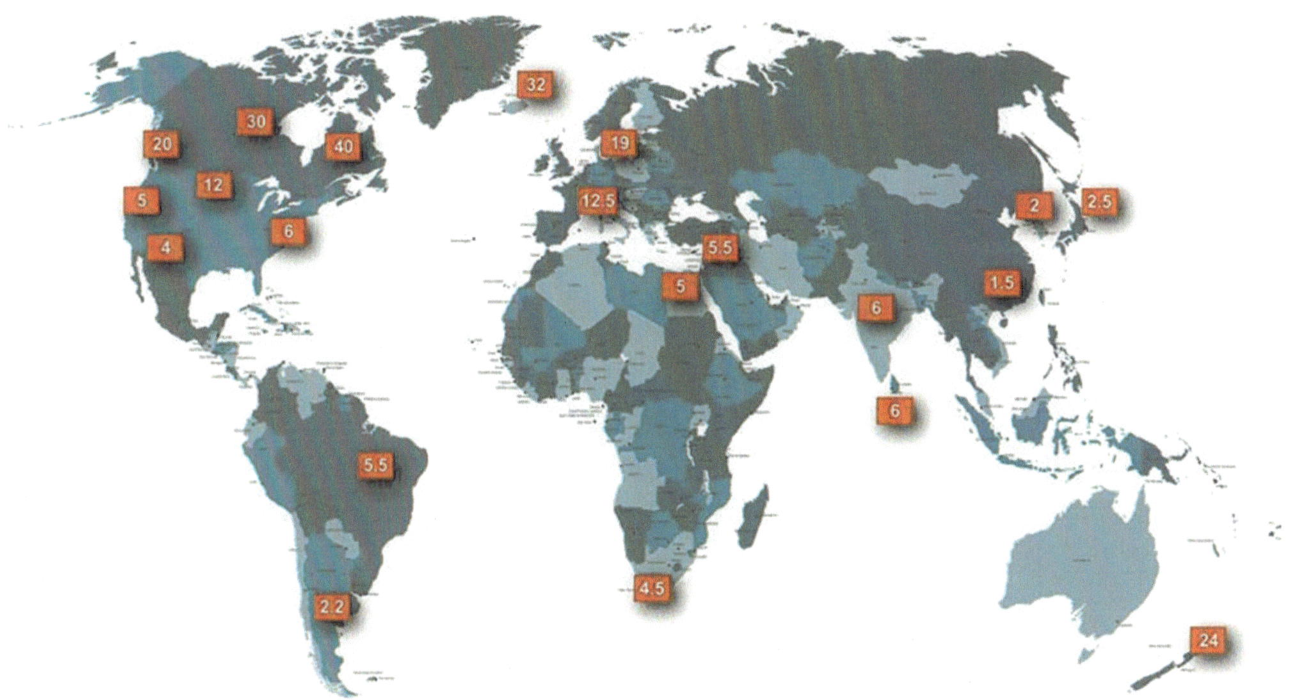

Fig. 1.5 Global incidence of IBD

explained by a generally mixed urban rural population in the North and a better separation between urban and rural areas in the two others. Both the Western and South-Eastern part showed a generally higher incidence rate in the scattered rural populations, opposite to previous international experience, in which urban areas have been considered to be areas of increased risk of IBD.

An explanation for this discrepancy within the literature might be that different risk factors are acting concomitantly within an area in addition to the existence of different risk factors between areas. One should not, however rule out the possibility of variations in efficiency and quality of registration between areas.

In Norway, the counties with most scattered and rural populations were also the areas with only one hospital, in contrast to the many recording hospitals and multidisciplinary doctors in the cities. This gave a variation in incidence rate between 17/100,000 in Oslo and 28/100,000 in the scattered populated area of Aust Agder, with one hospital in the only city of the county.

These data may provide evidence for the importance of access to health care and awareness of the population under examination. To increase the understanding of the complexity of this problem, one might add, that the area with the highest incidence of IBD, had the highest increase in socioeconomic status during the decade prior to the incidence

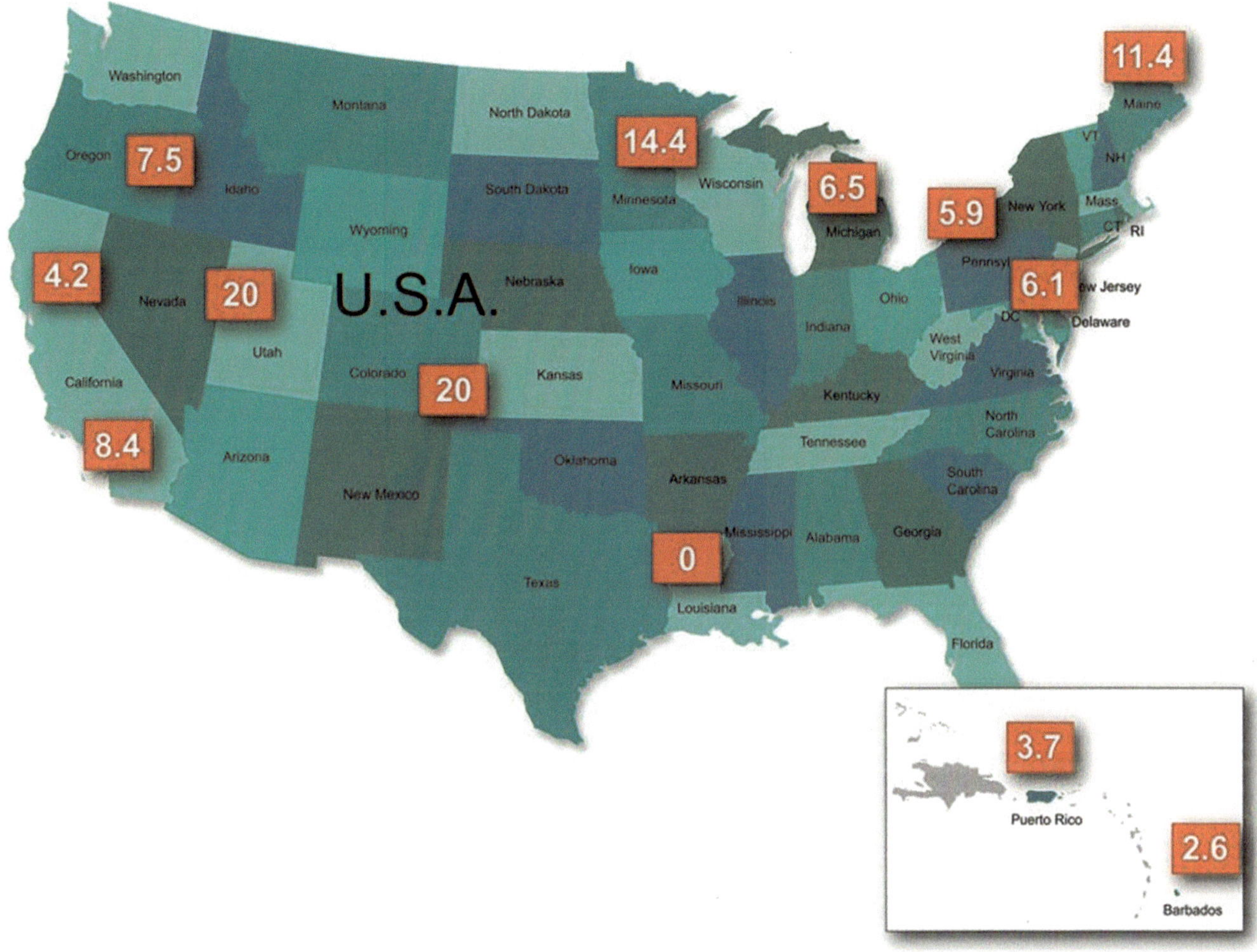

Fig. 1.6 Incidence of IBD in the USA

study, as measured by the number of individuals obtaining higher education. Although a much higher level of education was seen for Oslo, this level had been stable during the previous decades. With this respect, a factor that might be of importance in the Western societies is the increasing rate of immigration. Recent reports from the UK, reported on an unexpected high prevalence rate of IBD among immigrants from Southeastern Asia [37].

Relationship Between UC and CD

Although a change in socioeconomic level seems to be a common risk factor for UC and CD, it is important to note that these diseases may react quite differently, not only genetically, but also to environmental risk factors. A solid background of geographic examinations is therefore important.

In addition to variations between countries and regions regarding incidence and prevalence of IBD in general, the ratio between UC and CD has also shown geographic variations. A generally higher incidence rate for UC than for CD has been shown both in the North, East and the South of Europe, but with a smaller difference in the South [9]. In Canada and the USA, however, CD seems to occur with a higher frequency than UC [13], similar to Northern France [10]. Since this now also seems to be the case for Southern Germany [38] and parts of Eastern Europe [20] (Sjucic BM, Vuculic B, Persic M, et al. Incidence of inflammatory bowel disease in Primorsko-Gromska county, Croatia, 2002–2004: a prospective population based study. Scand J Gastroenterol 2006;41:437–44), we may no longer describe this as a French enigma, but rather as a tendency for middle Europe. The variation in ratios of UC/CD between countries and areas might reflect differences in environmental risk factors, although genetic predispositions may occur. It might be interesting to note that in Europe, the incidence of NOD2 mutations seems to be highest in the middle part, corresponding to the region with an increased CD to UC ratio.

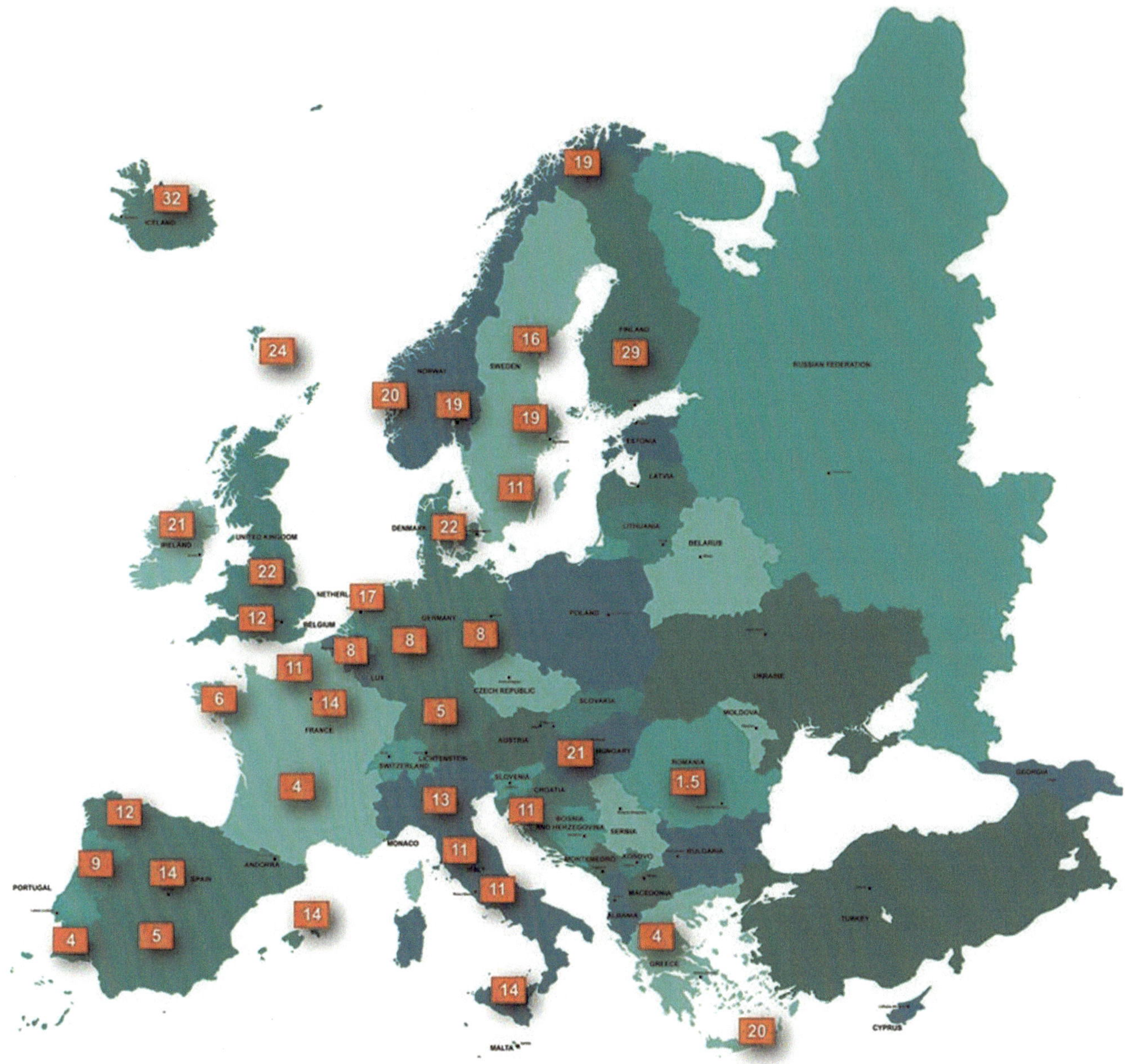

Fig. 1.7 Incidence of IBD in Europe—adults

Although unsolved questions exist regarding patterns of IBD in Europe, the risk factors and frequency of IBD in Eastern Europe must principally be regarded as related to the same socioeconomic trends as the rest of the continent and North America, in contrast to the developing countries. It is, therefore, relevant to discuss the environmental risk factors of IBD generally for the whole Europe as one area.

The question if the incidence and prevalence rates of IBD still are increasing is generally an unsolved question in most parts of the world. The reasons for this are different in the Western world compared to the developing countries. In the USA and Europe, few data exist based on comparable prospective studies performed during different time periods within the same area. A study from Copenhagen may suggest that the incidence of CD in adults is still increasing during the last decade [9]. In children, however, studies from several countries have suggested that the incidence still is increasing for CD but not for UC [15, 16]. The relationship between this increase and immigration is unclear, but studies on the risk of acquiring IBD among first-generation immigrants are underway. In a recent study from Oslo [17], the incident cases of CD representing first-degree immigrants from developing countries were partly responsible for the 100 % increase in incidence of CD over the last decade. To what extent the shift of environment has an impact on the development of IBD will have to be focused in the future.

The geographic difference between the North and South of Europe was the same for UC as for CD [10, 22, 23], also with regard to outcome and complications. For the above-mentioned reasons, it is not quite clear if the incidence of UC has stabilized or in some areas still is changing. A recent study from Finland indicates a dramatic increase in UC, based on partly population-based data from a regional registry. For all registry-derived data, some uncertainty exists, regarding reliability of the recording system over time. On the other hand, since recently also an increase of UC has been suggested in Hungary, a combined causality of environmental factors and ethnicity could explain a parallel increase in Finland and Hungary.

Reports from developing countries on the incidence and prevalence of IBD are still missing as regards population-based studies. Regional studies from India [24], may, however, suggest an increase over time in well-defined regions. Documented increase of incidence or prevalence in Japan would, however, be of particular interest, since Japan may be the only country in Asia with stable socioeconomic conditions over several decades. An eventual increase in frequency of IBD would then have to be related to other than direct socioeconomic factors, and rather to other changes in the environment or lifestyle, such as dietary habits.

Environmental Factors

Relationship to Microbiology

Today, the most important environmental factor, with a cause relationship to the development of IBD, is considered to be related to an imbalance in the microbial–host relationship with mucosal barrier dysfunction and reduced microbial diversity [39]. Resent publications have further developed our understanding of the changed bacterial composition in IBD (Manishanh C, Bourruel N, Casellas F, Guarner F. The gut microbiota in IBD. Nat Rev Gastroenterol Hepatol 2012;9:599–608; Hold GL, Smith M,, Grange C, et al. Role of gut microbiota in inflammatory bowel disease pathogenesis: what have we learned in the past 10 years? World J Gastroenterol 2014;20:1192–1210; Sartor RB, Mazmanian SK. Intestinal microbes in inflammatory bowel diseases. Am J Gastroenterol Suppl 2012;1:15–21; Matsuoka K, Kanai T. The gut microbiota and inflammatory bowel disease. Semin Immunopathol 2015;37:47–55) The hygiene hypothesis is an attempt to explain why improvement of hygienic conditions may result in intestinal dysbiosis as a primary event, resulting in IBD among genetically predisposed individuals. This hypothesis implies that the rising frequency of immunologic disorders can be attributed to lack of childhood exposure to enteric pathogens. This dysbiosis may on the one hand be characterized by an imbalance between commensal bacteria, and on the other hand, by secondary development of pathogens, which by omitting the immunocompromised cells of the different barrier systems, may lead to chronic inflammation. The suggested "Cold chain hypothesis" represents a more direct explanation of a cause relationship between specific bacteria and the immunocompromised host, from a molecular perspective, postulating that CD is a result of a defect in the host recognition of pathogenic bacterial components that usually escape the immune response (e.g., Yop molecules), leading to an excessive host response to bacteria, such as *Yersinia* spp. and *Listeria* spp., which can survive refrigerator temperature [40]. The definition relies on the introduction of refrigeration in society, which was related to the time of increased prevalence of CD. A support for this hypothesis has been reported in case–control studies, partly in combination with other socioeconomic risk factors [41, 42].

In support of the hygiene hypothesis are the generally negative association to the epidemiology of *Helicobacter pylori* [43] and the inverse association to the prevalence of helminthic colonization [44, 45].

It is still an issue if primary pathogens like *Mycobacterium avium paraturbeculosis* (MAP), Johne's disease [46], may be an etiologic factor, but problems related to the biologic methodology has been a major concern, and further studies are expected in the years to come. Clinical studies up to now have been inconclusive with regard to the impact of MAP in IBD, and a study of seropositivity showed a high prevalence for IBD, but failed to demonstrate a difference between CD, UC, and controls [47].

Several studies, however, have detected a high prevalence rate of MAP in CD patients, and a meta-analysis of 28 case–control studies showed a positive association, both for enzyme-linked immunosorbent assay (ELISA) and PCR [48].

A recent examination [49], however, performed with highly sensitive methods in intestinal mucosa, could not detect the presence of MAP in newly diagnosed, treatment naïve cases, in contrast to many affected cases among hospitalized CD patients on treatment, in the same catchment area. MAP was not found among patients with long-standing UC. According to these results, MAP is probably not an etiologic factor, but a bystander appearing during the course of disease and appearing in patients on treatment. Another interpretation could be that MAP remains elusive to detection during the early phase of disease, and that a longer duration of immune decompensation is needed for diagnosis by the present methods.

The high prevalence of adherent-invasive *Escherichia coli* spp. associated to ileal CD may represent another primary pathogenic strain of bacteria, which is able to adhere to intestinal epithelial cells, to invade epithelial cells via a mechanism involving actin polymerization and microtubules, and to survive and replicate within macrophages [50].

Other hospital-based studies have demonstrated a geographic covariation related to hospitalization and mortality for IBD and *Clostridium difficile* [51].

Since IBD is most common in the northern hemisphere, most studies with regard to microbial risk factors have been performed in this region. As, on the one hand, one might speculate that improvement in sanitary conditions is responsible for reduced microbial diversity, industrial pollution in society might serve as another explanation for changed environment. It is probably unlikely that the exogenous predisposition for IBD can be explained by one single environmental factor. At the moment, our knowledge regarding possible risk factors derived from industrialization must be divided mainly into primary direct effects of endogenous dysbiosis and secondary effects on this microbial imbalance. The latter explanation will include all the risk factors that will either increase the microbial instability or increase the vulnerability of the host organism.

For testing of dysbiosis, a genetic test applied on human feces has been published recently, comparing IBD with IBS and controls. Such comparisons need to be performed globally to be relevant to all populations (Casén C, Vebo H, Sekelja M, et al. Deviations in human gut microbiota: determining dysbiosis in a diagnostic setting in IBS and IBD patients. Aliment Pharmacol Ther 2015).

Relationship Between Environment and Geography

Of factors that may act on the intestinal microbial composition, geography may represent a risk in addition to socioeconomic development. Living on the northern hemisphere may therefore explain the increased incidence of IBD, only based on this single factor, which might be explained by increasing intestinal dysbiosis. It has been suggested that this risk increases with increasing latitude from the Equator to the North Pole [52]. This explanation needs support from more comparable studies, which need to be performed by standardized examinations on preferentially unselected materials.

Although latitude alone may represent a risk for development of IBD, the reports from Canada, showing a marked East–West gradient, which at least up to now, might have been the case also for Europe, seems to indicate that contemporary differences within a society or within a region over time, represent the most important risk factors. These two examples of East–West gradients may therefore strengthen the argumentation for industrialization as a main causative factor for IBD. The North–South gradient in Europe does not necessarily depend on the same differences, because industrialization and socioeconomic growth patterns have in part ran more parallel in the North and South of Europe.

Other environmental factors, such as water supply, may act in addition to, or increase, the instability, primarily caused by the dysbiotic intestine. In a recent study, a strong association between iron concentration in the sources of drinking water and the community incidence of IBD, both CD and UC, was found [53]. Other metals showed no association to IBD, opposed to the proposed focus on aluminum as a risk factor [54]. One explanation why inorganic iron might be a risk factor is its known ability to cause oxidative stress, whereas another might be its effect on bacterial growth. The results might generally agree with a role for oxygen radicals in animals and humans [55].

Relationship to latitude might also be explained by changes in sun exposure and vitamin D [56] Geographic patterns related to IBD seem to involve complex interactions between genetics and sun exposure, both related to latitude (Scilagyi A, Leighton H, Burstein B, Xiaoquing Xue. Latidude, sunshine, human lactase phenotype distributions may contribute to geographic patterns of modern disease: the inflammatory bowel disease model. Clinical Epidemiology 2014;6:183–98).

Socioeconomic Factors

One might speculate that the role of latitude is part of the North–South gradient in Europe, although other environmental factors, such as diet or socioeconomics, may be responsible for the variation in the occurrence of IBD.

Several studies have reported on increased incidence of both UC and CD in more densely populated areas [57–61]. Both family size and number of older siblings, as well as birth order, have been related to increased risk of UC, and with smaller families and few older siblings related to CD [62], which might be a sign that UC is more directly affected by environmental factors than CD. This explanation was also supported by a shorter interval between first-degree relatives acquiring UC compared to CD [63]. The relationships between these diseases and other household-related conditions, such as pets, are unclear [64–67].

It has previously been reported that both UC and CD are affecting white collar more than blue collar employees [68]. Further studies among German employees suggested that work in the open air and physical exercise were protective, while being exposed to air conditioned, artificial working conditions or extending and irregular shift working increased the risk of IBD [69]. In population-based studies in Norway, the incidence of IBD was higher in rural areas with a recent increase in socioeconomic status, based on years of education, compared to urban areas with a stable high socioeconomic level [12, 36].

Other factors which might be related to socioeconomics are sanitary conditions, which actually formed the basis for the hygiene hypothesis. In an epidemiological study in the UK, the availability of a fixed hot water supply in childhood before the age of 11 was associated with Crohn's disease [3].

As socioeconomic differences within each of the Western countries have been reduced, the relationship to IBD seems somewhat unclear, however, on a global level these differences are obvious. For future examinations, the factors of importance will have to be clearly defined for each country under study.

Smoking

Smoking has generally been accepted as a risk factor in Crohn's disease, for worsening of the disease course, such as reduced response to treatment, increased relapse rate, and complications [70], whereas in UC, smoking has a protective effect against the same outcomes of disease [23].

Regarding onset of disease, the connection to smoking is less clear, but a meta-analysis showed an OR of 0.58 for UC and 1.76 for CD among smokers [71] in the general population which could implicate that smoking is a part of a primary event, and not only as a secondary factor influencing the course of disease. Passive exposure to smoking during childhood has also been shown to influence the risk of IBD [72]. A possible relationship between age at diagnosis and smoking has also been suggested [73].

No single explanation for the mechanism behind smoking and the onset of IBD has been postulated, but among siblings discordant for smoking, smokers tended to develop CD, whereas nonsmokers tended to develop UC [74]. This may suggest an interaction between smoking and genetic susceptibility. In UC, the significantly reduced frequency of pANCA positivity among smokers, and a tendency of increased frequency of ASCA positivity, may either be supportive of such a mechanism or may be explained by other mechanisms, such as direct reaction to yeast, a result of disease activity or exposure to treatment [23].

A meta-analysis of 245 articles [71] reported on evidence for an association between current smoking and CD (OR, 1.76) and former smoking and UC (OR). Current smoking had a protective effect on the development of UC when compared with controls (OR, 0.58). These results confirmed that smoking is an important environmental factor in IBD with differing effects in UC and CD.

In a global perspective, a high occurrence of smoking is reported from many countries with a low frequency of IBD. Future studies will show if this inverse relationship still is present for populations with increasing incidence of IBD, and especially among immigrants to Western societies.

Nutrition and Diet

Considerable efforts have been made in the search for nutritional factors related to, and maybe even responsible for the development of IBD. The methodology of this research has been hampered by the problems of confounding factors and the fact that many patients will change their nutritional habits as a consequence of the disease. There are many studies in small cohorts of patients, who claim that intake of certain diet constituents like fat, refined sugar, fruits, vegetables, and fiber affect the expression of IBD. These studies do not provide unequivocal evidence to incriminate any particular dietary factor. A recent survey of Medline and the Cochrane database concluded that, based on the current levels of knowledge concerning dietary risk factors for IBD and the therapeutic efficacy of dietary and nutritional interventions, the results need to be supported by well-designed trials in large cohorts of patients [75].

A multitude of factors, including drug–nutrient interactions, disease location, symptoms, and dietary restrictions can lead to protein energy malnutrition and specific nutritional deficiencies.

Studies have revealed that nutritional deficiencies are relatively common in IBD, both regarding reduced intake of food and vitamin and mineral deficiencies. It is estimated that up to 85% of hospitalized IBD patients have protein energy malnutrition, based on abnormal anthropometric and biochemical parameters [76, 77].

It is clear that nutrition plays an important role in the management of patients with IBD. The need and advice for nutritional therapy is, due to the heterogeneity of the diseases, quite variable and based on the individual subtype of disease, disease stage, and the patients' total situation. Consequently, there are no specific nutritional therapies that may be recommended to all patients.

Attention to weight changes, to eating habits, and to GI symptoms are the best guides for the clinician. Any abnormality, regarding general health, clinical, or biochemical measurements, must be considered as risk factors regarding disease outcome. Nutritional factors of importance for the outcome of IBD represent the basis for prophylaxis against complicated disease and malnutrition. Specific dietary therapy to avoid symptoms and supplements to meet nutritional depletion are active measures to avoid complications to disease. Metabolic dysfunction and secondary osteoporosis and osteomalacia are serious complications related to malabsorption in CD.

Regarding primary risk factors for development of disease, studies have focused on preventive measures and potential risk factors.

In a relatively large surveillance of patients with UC and CD in Italy [78], in addition to the previously documented relationships between these diseases and smoking, the study reported that lack of breast feeding was associated with increased risk of both UC (OR 1.5) and CD (OR 1.9). A meta-analysis of 14 case–control studies reported on a protective role for breastfeeding in both CD and UC [79].

In a French case–control study of incident cases with CD and UC occurring before 17 years of age, performed between January 1988 and December 1997, 140 variables covering familial history of IBD, events during the perinatal period, infant and child diet, vaccinations, childhood diseases, household amenities, and family socioeconomic status were recorded. Among nutritional factors, regular drinking of tap water was protective against IBD, whereas breast feeding was a risk factor [80], opposite to the previously mentioned report [79]. The preponderance of evidence suggests that breastfeeding is a protective factor for IBD, with a greater effect for CD than UC, based on a recent meta-analysis [81].

The role of dietary macronutrients in the etiology of IBD was recently examined in a large prospective cohort of women living in France, aged 40–65 years. Based on questionnaires on disease occurrence and lifestyle factors that were completed every 24 months, high total protein intake, specifically animal protein, was associated with a significantly increased risk of IBD [82]. This could fit well with the previously reported association with consumption of fast food for both UC (OR 3.4, 1.3–3.9) and CD (OR 3.9, 1.4–10.6) in a population-based incidence study in Sweden. The study, performed by a questionnaire, covered retrospectively the 5 years prior to diagnosis of IBD [83].

Another study showed that total fat and intake of monounsaturated and polyunsaturated fats, as well as intake of vitamin B6, were related to UC, whereas a negative association was found for carbohydrates [84]. A relationship to fat consumption was also found in another study, for UC [75], whereas intake of dietary fiber, fruit, and vegetables was reported to be protective for both [85, 86].

In another prospective controlled study of pre-illness changes in IBD, approximately one-third of patients changed their diet prior to the diagnosis of IBD due to nonspecific symptoms. Of the patients not changing their diet, moderate and high consumption of margarine (OR = 11.8 and OR = 21.37) was associated with ulcerative colitis, while high consumption of red meat (OR = 7.8) and high intake of cheese were associated with Crohn's disease [87].

In a retrospective study performed within 3 years after diagnosis, the results also showed different, but significant associations for both UC and CD with regard to food consumption [86].

Especially, the French study [82], being the first large-scale prospectively performed study of diet recorded before the onset of disease, lends strong support to fat and meat consumptions as risk factors of IBD. Especially, the animal proteins from meat and fish represented a risk factor, whereas dairy and vegetable proteins did not. Again the risks were increased for both UC and CD; however, the study was limited to middle aged females. Nevertheless, the study partly supported the previous findings from Japan, where the reported increase of CD during the period 1966–1985 was strongly associated to increased intake of animal protein and somewhat less to increased $n-6/n-3$ polyunsaturated fatty acid ratio [88], by multivariate analysis.

A nested case–control study of a prospective cohort study within seven regions in Europe, identified linoleic acid, in contrast to docosahexaenoic acid, as a significant risk factor for the development of UC [89], however, failed to find a significant association between micronutrients or macronutrients and disease, based on data from partly the same regions [90]. The evidence for these dietary risk factors in IBD, therefore, has to await further documentation from different populations and subgroups of patients in the future.

A recent systematic review of pre-illness intake of nutrients based on 2609 IBD patients concluded that high intake of total fats, PUFA's, omega-6 fatty acids, and meat were associated with an increased risk of CD and UC. High fiber and fruit intakes were associated with decreased CD risk, and high vegetable intake was associated with a decreased risk of UC (Hou JK, Abraham B, El-Seraq H. Dietary intake and risk of developing inflammatory bowel disease: a systematic review of the literature. Am J Gastroenterol 2011;106:563–73).

Based on epidemiological data, case–control studies, and search in Medline, it has been speculated that the reported relationships between changes in food consumption would fit, in a timely manner, with a change of intestinal microbes associated to IBD [91]. A time relationship between IBD and change in dietary consumption has also been reported for intake of carbohydrates.

Case–control studies from Germany [92] and the UK [93] demonstrated an association between intake of sugar and CD. Another case–control study from the UK showed that intake of sugar and smoking were separate but interactive risk factors [94]. The association between both monosaccharides and disaccharides and CD was also shown in Israel [95], Japan [96], and Italy [97]. The general question regarding the carbohydrate hypothesis is, to what extent reporting of increased consumption is related to early change of diet due to onset of disease, or if it represents an etiologic factor. This question may also be raised regarding the increased frequency of bran eaters among patients with CD [98].

Another factor of increasing interest is the host response to yeast. Several studies have shown increased IgG and IgA antibodies to baker's yeast (*Saccharomyces cerevisiae*) in patients with CD but not UC [99, 100] as a consequence of intake of wheat. A recent report from studies in twins, however, suggested ASCA to be a marker of shared environment but with a genetic susceptibility, other than NOD2/Card15, as regards the titer level [101].

Recent reports have focused on the possibility of a nutrient–gene interaction, which might be a part of an individualized immunogenic therapy in the future [102].

Mechanisms by way of food consumption might also be further elucidated by studies on the role of epigenetic factors for the development of IBD in the future [103, 104].

Microparticles and Pollution

Both in food and water supply, metals and minerals, as well as other microparticles, are abundant, and as such more common as part of pollution in industrialized areas. These particles may act in different ways with the immune system, causing primary or secondary effects. It has been suggested that exposure to xenobiotic-like metals may induce immune responses in autoimmune diseases. Such reactions have been related to effects of mercury [105], cobalt, zirconium, beryllium, silver, and aluminum [54]. Especially aluminum is ubiquitous in the Western culture and represents the most widely used trace element in food, water, soil, and pharmaceutical agents. Moreover, food additives and processed foods, such as cheese, baked goods, grain products, cake, and pancake mixes, vending machine powdery, milk, cream powder substitute, and soy-based milk formulae, sugar and frozen dough, add substantial amount to Al intake. Additionally, different substances, when added to water and even water purification procedures, may increase the bioavailability and toxicity in aqueous organisms resulting in facilitating Al entry into the food chain. On these grounds, a hypothesis of a bacterial–metal interaction was put forward as a factor in CD induction [106].

In line with this, the recently reported strong association between iron concentration in the sources of drinking water and the community incidence of IBD, both CD and UC, may support a bacterial–metal interaction [53]. In this study, however, other metals showed no association to IBD, opposed to the proposed focus on aluminum as a risk factor in IBD. Interactions between microparticles and the immune system, possibly by accumulation in macrophages, has also been postulated as a basis for the use of low microparticle diets in the treatment of IBD [107].

There is an increasing evidence for a role of air pollution as a risk factor for CD, supported by a proinflammatory effect of pollutants in animal studies (Beamish LA, Osornio-Vargas AR, Wine E. Air pollution: an environmental factor contributing to intestinal disease. J Chron Colitis 2011;5:279–86). Nitrogen dioxide has been associated with early onset CD (Kaplan GG, Hubbard J, Korzenik J, et al. The inflammatory bowel diseases and ambient pollution: a novel association. Am J Gastroenterol 2010;105:2412–19). Moreover, a correlation was found between air pollution and the rate of IBD hospitalizations (Ananthakrisnan AN, McGinley EL, Binion DG, Saeian K. Ambient air pollution correlates with hospitalization for inflammatory bowel disease: An ecologic analysis. Inflamm Bowel Dis 2011;17:1138–45).

Nonsteroidal Anti-inflammatory Drugs

Nonsteroid anti-inflammatory drugs have been considered as a potential risk factor for outbreak of inflammation, relapse, and increased activity of established IBD.

Several hypotheses have been put forward on the pathophysiology of intestinal damage by NSAIDs [108], such as enhanced intestinal permeability, inhibition of cyclooxygenase (COX), enterohepatic recirculation, and formation of adducts. The effects of COX-2 selective inhibitors, which appear to have better gastric tolerability when compared to nonselective NSAIDs, on normal and inflamed intestinal mucosa, as in Crohn's disease or ulcerative colitis, are still largely unexplored. If COX-2 inhibition plays a key role in suppressing the inflammatory process, recent evidence suggests that COX-2 products are involved in maintaining the integrity of intestinal mucosa, in the healing of gastrointestinal ulcers and in the modulation of inflammatory bowel disease (IBD). Animal models of intestinal inflammation have so far yielded conflicting results on the effects of COX-2 selective inhibitors on the intestinal mucosa. It is now clear that NSAIDs do not act through cyclooxygenase inhibition alone, but also have different effects on targets, such as nuclear factor-kappaB and/or on peroxisome proliferator-activated receptors (PPAR). The peculiar pharmacological profile of each compound may help to explain the different impact of each NSAID on the inflammatory process and on IBD. Notably, the salicylic acid derivative 5-ASA is widely used in the treatment of IBD and is believed to act through nuclear factor-kappaB interaction. Although the use of COX-2 selective inhibitors remains contraindicated in patients with IBD, studying their effects on intestinal mucosa may offer new insights into their subcellular mechanisms of action and open new avenues for the development of novel therapies for IBD.

The general agreement that NSAIDs increase intestinal permeability still makes these drugs a potential risk factor for exacerbation of disease, relapse rate, and increased activity [109].

Recent studies of tolerability of selective Cox-2 inhibitors have demonstrated that these drugs are safe and beneficial in most patients with IBD and not associated with exacerbation of the underlying IBD- and GI-related complications [110].

Oral Contraceptives

Several studies have reported an increased risk of IBD following the use of oral contraception [111]. The association has been shown especially for Crohn's disease, in contrast to ulcerative colitis, and an interaction has been shown for current smoking [111]. This risk was also shown in a population-based case–control study from the USA. Women who reported oral contraceptive use within 6 months before disease onset were at increased risk for both diseases compared with never users. Women who had used oral contraceptives for more than 6 years had the highest risk of Crohn's disease (RR = 5.1, 95% CI 1.8–14.3). In contrast, increased duration of use was not associated with increased risk of ulcerative colitis.

There has been a concern that females on contraceptives are at increased risk of disease relapse and other adverse events, such as thrombosis [112]. In this research of 207 articles in PubMed, results gave little evidence to suggest an increased risk of disease relapse among women with IBD who use oral contraceptives, and there seemed to be no differences in the absorption of higher-dose combined oral contraceptives, between women with mild ulcerative colitis or small ileal resections and healthy women.

A recent meta-analysis reported on a positive association for use of oral contraceptives and both UC and CD [113], with a reduced effect upon discontinuation. The study was not able to show an effect of dose reduction.

Strong confirmatory evidence for oral contraceptives as risk factors of IBD has recently been published in two prospective cohort studies, Nurses Health study I and II, based on 117,375 women enrolled since 1976, and 115,077 enrolled since 1989. The use of oral contraceptives was associated with a risk of CD. The association to UC was limited to women with a history of smoking (Khalili H, Higuchi LM, Ananthakrishnan AN, et al. Gut 2012; doi:10.1136/GutJNL-2012-30.2362).

Although most of the literature recommends oral contraceptives in IBD, monitoring for thromboembolic events has also been recommended [114].

Seasonal Variability

It has been speculated that the reported seasonal variations of relapse rate in ulcerative colitis [115] or incidence in UC [116] may be explained by change in environmental risk factors throughout the year. In the Swedish cohort study [115], a significantly higher relapse rate was found during the summer, whereas a significantly increased incidence rate of IBD was found during the early winter months of December and January in the Norwegian population-based incidence study. A recent controlled cohort study based on the Hospital Episode statistics (HES) in the UK of all admitted IBD patients between 1997 and 2006 did not show a seasonal birth pattern [117]. By monthly comparison year by year, different fluctuations were found for CD and UC, with a weak but significant correlation (0.078, $p=0.018$). A slight trend for stronger correlation occurred during the later decades. Nevertheless, the author concluded that patterns of birth dates among IBD patients do not support the contention that seasonally or monthly varying environmental factors during early childhood shape the subsequent risk of developing IBD.

In a study from the USA, norovirus was associated to exacerbation of both UC and CD in pediatric patients, in all cases associated with bloody diarrhea, and with demand for hospitalization. This was in contrast to diarrhea without hematochezia when the infection occurs in the absence of IBD [118].

Based on these observations, the relationship between seasonal environmental risk factors may affect the outbreak of IBD differently according to the occurrence of risk factors around the world. One cannot rule out the possibility that also perinatal risk factors might be of importance at the presents of combination of risk factors, such as in selected areas or individual groups. Large nationwide studies might dilute important local variations, which might seem negligible when the results are not broken down into smaller regions, such as communities [119].

Appendectomy and Tonsillectomy

The inverse relationship between previous appendectomy and ulcerative colitis has been confirmed in several studies. In a study including 213 patients with UC, 110 with CD and 337 controls, a highly significant association to appendectomy was found for UC (OR 0.20), and even higher when the operation was performed before the age of 20 (OR 0.14). No association was found for CD, and no association for tonsillectomy for either disease [120]. Moreover, the study from Spain also showed that appendectomy was less frequent, not only among UC and CD patients, but also among their relatives [120], compared to the general population. A case–control study from Iran confirmed the inverse relationship between appendectomy and UC in contrast to Crohn's disease [121]. A population-based study from New Zealand reported that not only appendectomy, but also tonsillectomy, infectious mononucleosis, and asthma were more common in CD patients than controls [122]. Another case–control study from Spain [123] showed that both appendectomy and current smoking were protective for UC. Additionally, this study showed that better living conditions during childhood were associated to increased risk for IBD. A case–control study from Greece [124] could neither confirm a significantly inverse relationship to UC (OR 0.6) nor a significant association to CD (OR 2.2), although well-known risk factors such as family history and smoking were confirmed. A multivariate regression analysis, however, showed positive associations between appendectomy and tonsillectomy for CD, but no independent inverse association to UC.

A meta-analysis in 2008 showed great heterogeneity among the studies. The risk of CD was largely increased in the first year after appendectomy, and was no longer significant after 5 years (Kaplan GG, Jackson T, Sands BE, et al. The risk of developing Crohn's disease after an appendectomy: a meta-analysis. Am J Gastroenterol 2008;103:2925–31).

With some variation in results, however, the literature shows strong relationships between previous appendectomy and the development of CD, and inversely to UC, which again might indirectly support the impact of the hygiene hypothesis as an explanation for the importance of socioeconomic conditions in the development of IBD.

General Remarks and Future Aspects Regarding Global Environmental Risk Factors in IBD

The evidence for increased frequency of IBD in the industrialized parts of the world is strong and is mainly explained by environmental risk factors. Of all the identified risk factors, not a single one alone may, up to now, totally explain the increasing incidence in any part of the world. This might be explained by a multiplicity of potential routes for disturbances of the microbial–host interactions. It is also possible that the strength of influence by risk factors or lack of protective factors in a society is different, depending on geography or urbanization.

It is still possible that a common single explanation for the microbial–host imbalance will be found in the future, based on an explanation which up to now has been too difficult to grasp. A model has been suggested for changes in human adaption to the socioeconomic burden, related to endogenous changes, caused by individually based stressors of psychoimmunological origin (Ananthakrishnan AN, Khalidi H, Pan A, et al. Association between depressive symptoms and incidence of Crohn's disease and ulcerative colitis: results from the Nurses Health study. Clin Gastroenterol hepatol 2013;11:57–62; Bitton A, Dobkin PL, Edwardes MD et al. Predicting relapse in Crohn's disease: a biopsychological model. Gut 2008;57:1386–92). Such a model will have to be tested prospectively in different populations. If any one new single explanation for the microbial–host imbalance is found, it might leave several of our present risk factors as confounders.

Nevertheless, the increased molecular understanding of disease development in IBD during the last few decades must be expected to reveal new and important contributions, and also lead to the evaluation of the different environmental risk factors, together with geographic and individual susceptibility of the person at risk.

References

1. Munkholm P, Langholz E, Nielsen OH, et al. Incidence and prevalence of Crohn's disease in the county of Copenhagen, 1962–87: a sixfold increase in incidence. Scand J Gastroenterol. 1992;27: 609–14.
2. Lofthus EV. Clinical epidemiology of inflammatory bowel disease: incidence, prevalence, and environmental influences. Gastroenterology. 2004;126:1504–17.
3. Duggan AE, Usmani I, Neal KR, Logan RFA. Appendicectomy, childhood hygiene, Helicobacter pylori status, and risk of inflammatory bowel disease: a case control study. Gut. 1998;43:494–8.
4. Lennard-Jones JE. Classification of inflammatory bowel disease. Scand J Gastroenterol. 1989;24 Suppl 170:2–6.
5. Logan RFA. Inflammatory bowel disease incidence: up, down or unchanged? Gut. 1998;42:309–11.
6. Sonnenberg A, McCarty DJ, Jacobsen SJ. Geographic variation in the incidence of and mortality from inflammatory bowel disease. Dis Colon Rectum. 1986;29:854–61.
7. Primatesta P, Goldacre MJ. Crohn's disease and ulcerative colitis in England and the Oxford Record linkeage study area: a profile of hospitalized morbidity. Int J Epidemiol. 1995;24:922–8.
8. Cosnes J, Cattan S, Blain A, et al. Long-term evolution of disease behavior of Crohn's disease. Inflamm Bowel Dis. 2002;8:244–50.
9. Vind I, Riis L, Knudsen E, et al. Increasing incidences of inflammatory bowel disease and decreasing surgery rates in Copenhagen city and county, 2003–2005: a population based study from the Danish Crohn colitis database. Am J Gastroenterol. 2006;101: 1274–82.
10. Shivananda S, Lennard-Jones J, Logan RFA, et al. Incidence of inflammatory bowel disease across Europe: is there a difference between north and south? Results of the European collaborative study on inflammatory bowel disease (EC-IBD). Gut. 1996;39: 690–7.
11. Moum B, Vatn MH, Ekbom A, et al. Incidence of ulcerative colitis and indeterminate colitis in four counties of south-eastern Norway 1990–1993. A large prospective population-based study. Scand J Gastroenterol. 1996;31:356–60.
12. Moum B, Vatn MH, Ekbom A, et al. Incidence of Crohn's disease in four counties of south-eastern Norway 1990–1993. A large prospective population-based study. Scand J Gastroenterol. 1996;31: 350–4.
13. Bernstein CN, Wajda A, Svenson LW, et al. The epidemiology of inflammatory bowel disease in Canada: a population based study. Am J Gastroenterol. 2006;101:1559–68.
14. Jess T, Lofthus Jr EV, Velayos FS, et al. Incidence and prognosis of colorectal dysplasia in inflammatory bowel disease: a population-based study from Olmsted County, Minnesota. Inflamm Bowel Dis. 2006;12:669–76.
15. Hildebrand H, Finkel Y, Grahnquist L, et al. Changing pattern of paediatric inflammatory bowel disease in northern Stockholm 1990–2001. Gut. 2003;52:1432–4.
16. Perminow G, Frigessi A, Rydning A, et al. Incidence and clinical presentation of IBD in children: comparison between prospective and retrospective data in a selected Norwegian population. Scand J Gastroenterol. 2006;41:1433–9.
17. Perminow G, Brackmann S, Lyckander LG, et al. Characterization in childhood inflammatory bowel disease. A new population-based inception cohort from South-Eastern Norway, 2005–07, showing increased incidence in Crohn's disease. Scand J Gastroenterol. 2008;43:1–11.
18. Lehtinen P, Ashorn M, Iltanen S, et al. Incidence trends of pediatric inflammatory bowel disease in Finland, 1987–2003, a nation-wide study. Inflamm Bowel Dis. 2010 [Epub ahead of print]. PMID: 21080459
19. Manninen P, Karvonen A-L, Huhtala H, et al. The epidemiology of inflammatory bowel diseases in Finland. Scand J Gastroenterol. 2010;45:1063–7.
20. Lakatos L, Lakatos PL. Changes in the epidemiology of inflammatory bowel diseases. Orv Hetil. 2007;148:223–8.
21. Gearry RB, Richardson AK, Frampton CM, Dodgshun AJ, Barclay ML. Population-based cases control study of inflammatory bowel disease risk factors. J Gastroenterol Hepatol. 2010;25:325–33.
22. Wolthers F, Russel MG, Sijbrandij J, et al. Phenotype at diagnosis predicts recurrence rates in Crohn's disease. Gut. 2006;55:1124–30.
23. Hoie O, Wolters F, Riis L, et al. Ulcerative colitis: patients characteristics may predict 10-years disease recurrence in a European-wide population based cohort. Am J Gastroenterol. 2007;102: 1692–701.
24. Goh KL, Xiao S-D. Inflammatory bowel disease: a survey of the epidemiology in Asia. J Dig Dis. 2010;10:1–6.

25. Victoria CR, Sassak LY, Nunes HR. Incidence and prevalence rates of IBDs in midwestern of Sao Paulo State, Brazil. Arq Gastroenterol. 2009;46:20–5.
26. Kurata JH, Kantor-Fish S, Frankl H, et al. Crohn's disease among ethnic groups in a large health maintenance organization. Gastroenterology. 1992;102:1940–8.
27. Heresbach D, Gulwani-Alkolkar B, Lesser M, et al. Anticipation in Crohn's disease may be influenced by gender and ethnicity of the transmitting parent. Am J Gastroenterol. 1998;93:2368–72.
28. Niv Y, Abuksis G, Fraser GM. Epidemiology of ulcerative colitis in Israel: a survey of Israeli kibbutz settlements. Am J Gastroenterol. 2000;95:693–8.
29. Zheng JJ, Zhu XS, Huangfu Z, Gao ZX, Guo ZR, Wang Z. Crohn's disease in mainland China: a systematic analysis of 50 years of research. Chin J Dig Dis. 2005;6:175–81.
30. Desai HG, Gupte PA. Increasing incidence of Crohn's disease in India: is it related to improved sanitation? Indian J Gastroenterol. 2005;24:23–4.
31. Bernstein CN, Shanahan F. Disorders of a modern lifestyle: reconciling the epidemiology of inflammatory bowel diseases. Gut. 2008;57:1185–91.
32. Calkins BM, Lilienfeld AM, Garland CF, et al. Trends and incidence rates of ulcerative colitis and Crohn's disease. Dig Dis Sci. 1984;29:913–20.
33. Garland CF, Lilienfield AM, Mendeloff AI, et al. Incidence rates of ulcerative colitis and Crohn's disease in fifteen areas of the United States. Gastroenterology. 1981;81:1115–24.
34. Nerich V, Monnet E, Etienne OA, et al. Geographical variations of inflammatory bowel disease in France: a study based on national health insurance data. Inflamm Bowel Dis. 2006;12:218–26.
35. Kiledebo S, Breckan R, Norgaard K, et al. The incidence of Crohn's disease in northern Norway from 1983 to 1986. Scand J Gastroenterol. 1989;24:1265–70.
36. Haug K, Schrumpf E, Halvorsen JF, et al. Epidemiology of Crohn's disease in Western Norway. Scand J Gastroenterol. 1989;24:1271–5.
37. Smith LA, Rameshanker R, Healy J, et al. An unusual prevalence of inflammatory bowel disease in a multiethnic population-single centre UK data. Gut. 2010;59(Suppl III):A181.
38. Ott C, Obermaier F, Thieler S, et al. The incidence of inflammatory bowel disease in a rural region of southern Germany: a prospective population based study. Eur J Gastroenterol Hepatol. 2008;20:917–23.
39. Frank DNA, St Amand AL, Feldman RA, et al. Molecular-phylogenetic characterization of microbial community imbalances in human inflammatory bowel diseases. Proc Natl Acad Sci U S A. 2007;104:13780–8.
40. Hugot J-P, Alberti C, Berrebi D, Bingen E, Cezard J-P. Crohn's disease: the cold chain hypothesis. Lancet. 2003;362:2012–5.
41. Forbes A, Kalantzis T. Crohn's disease: the cold chain hypothesis. Int J Colorectal Dis. 2006;21:399–401.
42. Malekzadeh F, Alberti C, Nouraei M, et al. Crohn's disease and early exposure to domestic refrigeration. PLoS ONE. 2009;4(1):e4288.
43. Luther J, Dave M, Higgins PDR, Kao JY. Association between Helicobacter pylori infection and inflammatory bowel disease: a meta-analysis and systematic review of the literature. Inflamm Bowel Dis. 2009;16:1077–84.
44. Koloski N-A, Bret L, Radford-Smith G. Hygiene hypothesis in inflammatory bowel disease: a critical review of the literature. World J Gastroenterol. 2008;14:165–73.
45. Korzenik JR. Past and current theories of etiology of IBD: toothpaste, worms, and refrigerators. J Clin Gastroenterol. 2005;39(4 Suppl 2):S59–65.
46. Chacon O, Bermudez LE, Barletta RG. Johne's disease, inflammatory bowel disease, and Mycobacterium paratuberculosis. Annu Rev Microbiol. 2004;58:329–63.
47. Bernstein CN, Blanchard JF, Rawsthorne P, Collins MT. Population-based case control study of seroprevalence of Mycobacterium paratuberculosis in patients with Crohn's disease and ulcerative colitis. J Clin Microbiol. 2004;42:1129–35.
48. Feller M, Huwiler K, Stephan R, et al. Mycobacterium avium subspecies paratuberculosis and Crohn's disease: a systematic review and meta-analysis. Lancet Infect Dis. 2007;7:607–13.
49. Ricanek P, Lothe SM, Szpinda I, et al. Paucity of mycobacteria in mucosal bowel biopsies from adults and children with early inflammatory bowel disease. J Crohn's Colitis. 2010;4:561–6.
50. Darfeuille-Michaud A, Boudeau J, Bulois P, et al. High prevalence of adherent-invasive Escherichia coli associated with ileal mucosa in Crohn's disease. Gastroenterology. 2004;127:412–21.
51. Sonnenberg A. Similar geographic variations of mortality and hospitalization associated with IBD and Clostridium difficile colitis. Inflamm Bowel Dis. 2010;16:487–93.
52. Hildebrand H. On the generality of the latitudinal diversity gradient. Am Nat. 2004;163:192–211.
53. Aamodt G, Bukholm G, Jahnsen J, et al. The association between water supply and inflammatory bowel disease based on a 1990–1993 cohort study in southeastern Norway. Am J Epidemiol. 2008;168:1065–72.
54. Lerner A. Aluminum is a potential environmental factor for Crohn's disease induction. Extended hypothesis. Ann N Y Acad Sci. 2007;1107:329–45.
55. Rezaie A, Parker RD, Abdollahi M. Oxidative stress and pathogenesis of inflammatory bowel disease: an epi-phenomenon or the cause? Dig Dis Sci. 2007;52:2015–21.
56. Hayes CE, Nashold FE, Froicu M, et al. The immunological functions of the vitamin D endocrine system. Cell Mol Biol (Noisy-le-Grand). 2003;49:277–300.
57. Ekbom A, Adami HO, Helmick CG, Jonzon A, Zack MM. Perinatal risk factors for inflammatory bowel disease: a case-control study. Am J Epidemiol. 1990;132:1111–9.
58. Klement E, Lysy J, Hoshen M, Avitan M, Goldin E, Israeli E. Childhood hygiene is associated with the risk for inflammatory bowel disease: a population-based study. Am J Gastroenterol. 2008;103:1775–82.
59. Radon K. Contact with farm animals in early life and juvenile inflammatory bowel disease: a case-control study. Pediatrics. 2007;120:354–61.
60. Wurzelmann JI, Lyles CM, Sandler RS. Childhood infections and the risk of inflammatory bowel disease. Dig Dis Sci. 1994;39: 555–60.
61. Green C, Elliott L, Beaudoin C, Bernstein CN. A population-based ecologic study of inflammatory bowel disease: searching for etiologic clues. Am J Epidemiol. 2006;164:615–23. discussion 624–28.
62. Montgomery SM, Lambe M, Wakefield AJ, Pounder RE, Ekbom A. Siblings and the risk of inflammatory bowel disease. Scand J Gastroenterol. 2002;37:1301–8.
63. Bengtson M-B, Solberg C, Aamodt G, et al. Clustering in time of familial IBD separates ulcerative colitis and Crohn's disease. Inflamm Bowel Dis. 2009;15:1867–74.
64. Lashner BA, Loftus Jr EV. True or false? The hygiene hypothesis for Crohn's disease. Am J Gastroenterol. 2006;101:1003–4.
65. Amre DK, Lambrette P, Law L, et al. Investigating the hygiene hypothesis as a risk factor in pediatric onset Crohn's disease: a case-control study. Am J Gastroenterol. 2006;101:1005–11.
66. Bernstein CN, Rawsthorne P, Cheang M, Blanchard JF. A population-based case control study of potential risk factors for IBD. Am J Gastroenterol. 2006;101:993–1002.
67. Feeney MA, Murphy F, Clegg AJ, Trebble TM, Sharer NM, Snook JA. A case-control study of childhood environmental risk factors for the development of inflammatory bowel disease. Eur J Gastroenterol Hepatol. 2002;14:529–34.

68. Sonnenberg A. Disability from inflammatory bowel disease among employees in West Germany. Gut. 1989;30:367–70.
69. Sonnenberg A. Occupational distribution of inflammatory bowel disease among German employees. Gut. 1990;31:1037–40.
70. Solberg IC, Vatn MH, Hoie O, et al. Clinical course in Crohn's disease: results of a population based ten-year follow-up study. Clin Gastroenterol Hepatol. 2007;5:1430–8.
71. Mahid SS, Minor KS, Soto RE, et al. Smoking and inflammatory bowel disease: a meta analysis. Mayo Clin Proc. 2006;81:1462–71.
72. Russel RK, Farhodi R, Wilson M, et al. Perinatal passive smoke exposure may be more important than childhood exposure in the risk of developing childhood IBD. Gut. 2005;54:1500–1.
73. Regueiro M, Kevin EK, Onki C, et al. Cigarette smoking and age at diagnosis of inflammatory bowel disease. Inflamm Bowel Dis. 2005;11:42–7.
74. Bridger S, Lee JCW, Bjarnason L, et al. Inflammatory bowel disease. In siblings with similar genetic susceptibility for inflammatory bowel disease, smokers tend to develop Crohn's disease and non-smokers develop ulcerative colitis. Gut. 2002;51:21–5.
75. Yamamoto T, Nakahigashi M, Saniabadi AR. Review article: diet and inflammatory bowel disease-epidemiology and treatment. Aliment Pharmacol Ther. 2009;30:99–112.
76. Graham TO, Kandil HM. Nutritional factors in inflammatory bowel disease. Gastroenterol Clin N Am. 2002;31:203–18.
77. Han PD, Burke A, Baldassano N, Rombeau JL, Lichtensein GR. Nutrition and inflammatory bowel disease. Gastroenterol Clin N Am. 1999;28:423–43.
78. Corrao C, Traguone A, Caprilli R, et al. Risk of inflammatory bowel disease attributable to smoking, oral contraception and breast feeding in Italy: a nationwide case-control study. Int J Epidemiol. 1998;27:397–404.
79. Klement E, Cohen RV, Boxman J, Joseph A, Reif S. Breastfeeding and risk of inflammatory bowel disease: a systematic review with meta-analysis. Am J Clin Nutr. 2004;80:1342–52.
80. Baron S, Turck D, Leplat C, et al. Environmental risk factors in paediatric inflammatory bowel diseases: a population based case control study. Gut. 2005;54:357–63.
81. Mikhailov TA, Furner SE. Breastfeeding and genetic factors in the etiology of inflammatory bowel disease in children. World J Gastroenterol. 2009;15:270–9.
82. Jantshou P, Morois S, Clavel-Chapelon F, Boutron-Ruault MC, Carbonell F. Animal protein intake and risk of inflammatory bowel disease: the E3N prospective study. Am J Gastroenterol. 2010;105:2195–201.
83. Persson P-G, Ahlbom A, Hellers G. Diet and inflammatory bowel disease: a case-control study. Epidemiology. 1992;3:47–52.
84. Amre DK, D'Souza S, Morgan K, et al. Imbalances in dietary consumption of fatty acids, vegetables, and fruits are associated with risk for Crohn's disease in children. Am J Gastroenterol. 2007;102:2016–25.
85. Geerling BJ, Dagnelie PC, Badart-Smook A, Russel MG, Stockbrugger RW, Brummer RJ. Diet as a risk factor for the development of ulcerative colitis. Am J Gastroenterol. 2000;95:1008–13.
86. Sakamoto N, Kono S, Wakai K, et al. Dietary risk factors for inflammatory bowel disease: a multicenter case-control study in Japan. Inflamm Bowel Dis. 2005;11:154–63.
87. Maconi G, Ardizzone S, Cucino C, Bezzio C, Russo AG, Bianchi-Porro G. Pre-illness changes in dietary habits and diet as a risk factor for inflammatory bowel disease: a case-control study. World J Gastroenterol. 2010;16:4297–304.
88. Shoda R, Matsueda K, Yamato S, Uemada N. Epidemiologic analysis of Crohn's disease in Japan: increased dietary intake of n-6 polyunsaturated fatty acids and animal protein relates to the increased incidence of Crohn's disease in Japan. Am J Clin Nutr. 1996;63:741–5.
89. Hart AR et al. Linoleic acid, a dietary n-6 polyunsaturated fatty acid, and aetiology of ulcerative colitis: a nested case-control study within a European prospective cohort study. Gut. 2009;58: 1606–11.
90. Hart AR, Luben R, Olsen A, et al. Diet in the aetiology of ulcerative colitis: a European prospective cohort study. Digestion. 2008;77:57–64.
91. Azakura H, Suzuki K, Kitahora T, Morizane T. Is there a link between food and intestinal microbes and the occurrence of Crohn's disease and ulcerative colitis? J Gastroenterol Hepatol. 2008;23:1794–801.
92. Martini GA, Brandes JW. Increased consumption of refined carbohydrates in patients with Crohn's disease. Klin Wschr. 1976;54: 367–71.
93. Penny WJ, Mayberry JF, Aggett PJ, et al. Relationship between trace elements, sugar consumption, and taste in Crohn's disease. Gut. 1983;24:288–92.
94. Katschinski B, Logan RFA, Edmond M, Langman MJS. Smoking and sugar intake are separate but interactive risk factors in Crohn's disease. Gut. 1988;29:1202–6.
95. Silkoff K, Hallak A, Yegena L, et al. Consumption of refined carbohydrate by patients with Crohn's disease in Tel-Aviv-Yafo. Postgrad Med J. 1980;56:842–6.
96. Matsui T, Iida M, Fujishima M, et al. Increased sugar consumption in Japanese patients with Crohn's disease. Gastroenterol Jpn. 1990;25:271.
97. Tragnone A, Valpiani D, Miglio F, et al. Dietary habits as risk factors for inflammatory bowel disease. Eur J Gastroenterol Hepatol. 1995;7:47–51.
98. James AH. Breakfast and Crohn's disease. Br Med J. 1977;1: 943–5.
99. Young CA, Sonnenberg A, Burns EA. Lymphocyte proliferation response to Baker's yeast in Crohn's disease. Digestion. 1994;55:40–3.
100. Mckenzie H, Main J, Pennington CR, Parrat D. Antibody to selected strains of Saccharomyces cervisiae (baker's and brewer's yeast) and candida albicans in Crohn's disease. Gut. 1990;31: 536–8.
101. Halfvarson J, Standaert-Vitse A, Järnerot G, et al. Anti-Saccharomyces cerevisiae antibodies in twins with inflammatory bowel disease. Gut. 2005;54:1237–43.
102. Lee G, Buchman AL. DNA-driven nutritional therapy of inflammatory bowel disease. Nutrition. 2009;25:885–91.
103. Beaudet al. Epigenetics and complex human disease: is there a role in IBD? J Pediatr Gastroenterol Nutr. 2008;46 Suppl 1:E2.
104. Lin Z, Hegarty JP, Cappel J, Yu W, Chen X, Faber P, et al. Identification of disease-associated DNA methylation in intestinal tissues from patients with inflammatory bowel disease. Clin Genet. 2010; doi:10.1111/j.1399-0004.2010.01546.x. [Epub ahead of print]
105. Kosuda LL, Greiner DL, Bigazzi PE. Mercury-induced renal autoimmunity changes in RT6+ T-lymphocytes of susceptible and resistant rats. Environ Health Perspect. 1993;101:178–85.
106. Perl DP, Fogarty U, Harpaz N, et al. Bacterial-metal interactions: the potential role of aluminum and other trace elements in the etiology of Crohn's disease. Inflamm Bowel Dis. 2004;10:881–3.
107. Lomer MCE, Harvey RSJ, Evans SM, et al. Efficacy and tolerability of a low microparticle diet in a double blind, randomized, pilot study in Crohn's disease. Eur J Gastroenterol Hepatol. 2001;13: 101–6.
108. Cipola G, Crema F, Sacco S, Moro E, di Ponti F, Frigo G. Anti-inflammatory drugs and inflammatory bowel disease: current perspectives. Pharmacol Res. 2002;46:1–6.
109. Bjarnason I, Takeutchi K. Intestinal permeability in the pathogenesis of NSAID-induced enteropathy. Scand J Gastroenterol. 2009;44 Suppl 19:23–9.

110. El Miedany Y, Yossef S, Ahmed I, El Gafary M. The gastrointestinal safety and effect on disease activity of etoricoxib, a selective cox-2 inhibitor in inflammatory bowel diseases. Am J Gastroenterol. 2006;101:311–7.
111. Sandler RS, Wurzelmann JI, Lyles CM. Oral contraceptive use and the risk of inflammatory bowel disease. Epidemiology. 1992;3:374–8.
112. Zappata LB, Paulen MB, Cancino C, Marchbanks PA, Curtis KM. Contraceptive use among women with inflammatory bowel disease: a systematic review. Contraception. 2010;82:72–85.
113. Cornish JA, Tan E, Simillis C, Clark SK, Teare J, Tekkis PP. The risk of oral contraceptives in the etiology of inflammatory bowel disease: a meta-analysis. Am J Gastroenterol. 2008;103: 2394–400.
114. Okori NI, Kane SV. Gender-related issues in the female inflammatory bowel disease patient. Expert Rev Gastroenterol Hepatol. 2009;3:145–54.
115. Tysk C, Järnrot G. Seasonal variation in exacerbation of ulcerative colitis. Scand J Gastroenterol. 1993;28:95–6.
116. Moum B, Aadland E, Ekbom A, et al. Seasonal variation in the onset of ulcerative colitis. Gut. 1996;38:376–8.
117. Sonnenberg A. Date of birth in the occurrence of inflammatory bowel disease. Inflamm Bowel Dis. 2009;15:206–11.
118. Kahn RR, Lawson AD, Minnich LL, Martin K, Nasir A, Emmet MK, et al. Gastrointestinal norovirus infection associated with exacerbation of inflammatory bowel disease. J Pediatr Gastroenterol Nutr. 2009;48:328–33.
119. Aamodt G, Jahnsen J, Bengtson MB, et al. Geographic distribution and ecological studies of inflammatory bowel disease in southeastern Norway in 1990–1993. Inflamm Bowel Dis. 2008;14(7):984–91.
120. Lopez RD, Gabriel R, Cantero PJ, Moreno OR, Fernandez BM, Mate JJ. Association of MALTectomy (appendectomy and tonsillectomy) and inflammatory bowel disease: a familial case control study. Rev Esp Enferm Dig. 2001;93:303–14.
121. Firouzi F, Bahari A, Aghazadeh R, Zali MR. Appendectomy, tonsillectomy, and risk of inflammatory bowel disease: a case control study in Iran. Int J Colorectal Dis. 2006;21:155–9.
122. Gearry RB, Richardson AK, Frampton CM, Dodshun AJ, Barclay ML. Population based cases control study of inflammatory bowel disease risk factors. J Gastroenterol Hepatol. 2010;25:227–8.
123. Lopez-Serrano P, Perez-Calle JL, Perez-Fernandez MT, Fernandez-Font JM, Boixeda deMiguel D, Fernandez-Rodriguez CM. Environmental risk factors in inflammatory bowel diseases. Investigating the hygiene hypothesis: a Spanish case control study. Scand J Gastroenterol. 2010;45:1464–71.
124. Kontroubakis IE, Vlachonicolis IG, Kapsoritakis A, et al. Appendectomy, tonsillectomy, and risk of inflammatory bowel disease: a case-controlled study in Crete. Dis Colon Rectum. 1999;42:225–30.

Part II

Immunobiology

Role of the Intestinal Immune System in Health

2

Per Brandtzaeg

Introduction

The pathogenesis of inflammatory bowel disease (IBD) reflects disturbed mucosal immunophysiology. The gut epithelium is monolayered and vulnerable, covering a surface area of perhaps 300 m^2 in adults when villi, microvilli, crypts, and folds are taken into account. It is protected by numerous chemical and physical innate defense mechanisms which cooperate intimately with a local adaptive immune system. The dominating component of the latter is an immunoglobulin A (IgA)-generating B-cell population which provides an anti-inflammatory first-line defense by giving rise to secretory IgA (SIgA) antibodies which perform "immune exclusion" [1, 2]. This term is coined for low- and high-affinity antibody functions at the mucosal surface, aiming to control microbial composition and colonization as well as inhibiting penetration of noxious antigens through the epithelial barrier [3, 4].

The generation of SIgA depends on IgA-producing plasma cells (PCs) and their immediate precursors (plasmablasts) which accumulate in the mucosa by selective homing mechanisms after priming of B cells in gut-associated lymphoid tissue (GALT)—including Peyer's patches, isolated (solitary) lymphoid follicles (ILFs) and the appendix [2, 5]. At least 80 % of the body's Ig-producing cells are located in the intestinal lamina propria, amounting to some 10^{10} PCs per meter of normal adult gut, which thus constitutes the body's largest effector organ of humoral immunity [6]. In addition, hypersensitivity due to excessive penetration of exogenous antigens into the mucosa is normally counteracted by adaptive hyporesponsiveness to innocuous agents. This phenomenon is traditionally referred to as "oral tolerance" when induced via the gut [7]; it counteracts particularly overreaction to dietary proteins and components of the commensal microbiota and depends on T cells (Treg cells) with regulatory functions [8, 9].

The mucosal induction of all these homeostatic mechanisms requires immunological stimuli, and the neonatal period is critical in this respect. The mucosal barrier and its reinforcement by SIgA, as well as the immunoregulatory network, depends on both adaptive and innate induction by antigens or conserved microbe-associated molecular patterns (MAMPs)—the latter activating germ line-encoded cellular pattern recognition receptors (PRRs) [10–12]. This adaptation is remarkably successful in view of the fact that a ton of food may pass through the gut of an adult human being every year, usually without causing adverse reactions. In addition, the healthy gut harbors a number of beneficial bacteria which is some ten times the number of cells in the body, perhaps amounting to 10^{13}–10^{14} microorganisms with a total weight of 1–2 kg [10]. Classical food allergy and IBD apparently reflect lack of this adaptive homeostasis, either due to retarded immunological development and immaturity of the mucosal barrier with its innate defense, abrogation of the epithelial barrier function, or a persistently imbalanced immunoregulatory network—probably on a polygenic susceptibility background.

The mainstream theory explaining the rise of allergies and other immune-mediated disorders such as IBD observed in affluent societies [13] is based on the extended hygiene hypothesis, underscoring an important role of changes in the environmental microbial impact on the immune system [14]. In essence, the idea is that industrialized societies, by modern measures introduced over the last decades, have deprived the infants of adequate immunological stimuli [15]. The relations between a westernized lifestyle and the origins of human disease comprise hygienic, dietary, and medical practices that have altered the pattern of microbial exposure, including the composition of the gut microbiota. Therefore, research on microbial–host interactions aims to reverse hypersensitivity by promoting tolerance [12, 16, 17].

P. Brandtzaeg, M.D., Ph.D. (✉)
Centre for Immune Regulation (CIR), University of Oslo, Oslo, Norway

Laboratory for Immunohistochemistry and Immunopathology (LIIPAT), Department of Pathology, Oslo University Hospital—Rikshospitalet, Nydalen, P.O. Box 4950, 0424 Oslo, Norway
e-mail: per.brandtzaeg@medisin.uio.no

D.C. Baumgart (ed.), *Crohn's Disease and Ulcerative Colitis*, DOI 10.1007/978-3-319-33703-6_2

For effective strategies to prevent immune-mediated diseases it is essential to understand how exogenous variables influence the adaptive immunological programming and how the effector mechanisms are regulated. The scientific basis of such efforts is discussed in this chapter.

Induction and Regulation of Intestinal Immunity

Mechanisms Promoting Homeostasis

Numerous genes regulate both the innate and adaptive arms of the immune system. Human immunogenetics has evolved to identify "danger" under the pressure of a "dirty environment," even long beyond the hunting-gathering period. In this evolutionary process the intestinal immune system has generated its two adaptive anti-inflammatory strategies: immune exclusion performed by SIgA to control surface colonization of microorganisms and inhibits mucosal penetration of potentially dangerous agents; and oral tolerance to avoid local and peripheral hypersensitivity against innocuous antigens which have trespassed the epithelial barrier (Fig. 2.1). Together, the two strategies apparently explain why overt and persistent problems with gut immunopathology are relatively rare. Remarkably, the suppressive mechanisms usually operate successfully in face of the enormous commensal microbiota separated from the internal body milieu only by the monolayered epithelium with its mucus coat [10, 11, 18, 19]. Notably, however, immunoregulatory differences apparently exist between humans and clean laboratory mice due to a stricter shielding of gut bacteria from the systemic immune system in this rodent species [10, 11, 20–22].

Oral tolerance is clearly a robust adaptive immune function because even healthy adult subjects absorb small amounts of intact food antigens, particularly after meals—corresponding to 10^{-5} of the intake and reaching a circulating level of 3–10 ng/ml [23]—as part of the total daily protein uptake of 130–190 g [24]. The epithelial tightness and the immunoregulatory network remain fragile for a variable period after birth [25, 26]. Importantly, animal experiments show that the postnatal development of mucosal homeostasis depends on the establishment of a balanced commensal microbiota as well as on adequate timing and dosing of foreign dietary antigens when first introduced [7, 10, 26, 27].

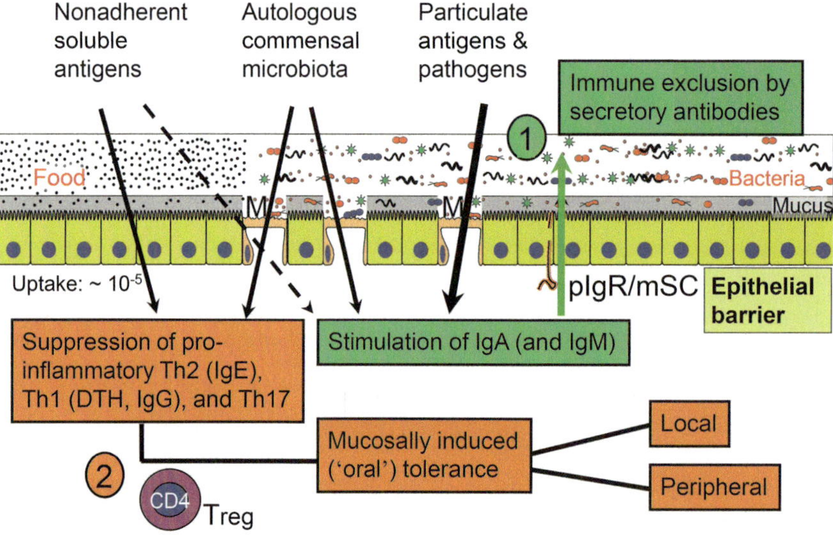

Fig. 2.1 Two-layers of anti-inflammatory mucosal immune defense preserving the integrity of the intestinal epithelial barrier. Depiction of the homeostatic mechanisms: (*1*) Immune exclusion to control epithelial colonization of microorganisms and penetration of exogenous antigens. This first line of defense is principally mediated by secretory antibodies of the IgA (and IgM) class in cooperation with innate protective factors (not shown). The secretory antibodies are actively exported by the epithelial polymeric Ig receptor (pIgR), also called membrane secretory component (mSC). Secretory immunity is preferentially stimulated by particulate antigens such as pathogens taken up through M cells (M) located in the dome epithelium covering gut-associated lymphoid tissue (see Figs. 2.2 and 2.3). (*2*) Innocuous soluble antigens (e.g., food proteins; magnitude of normal uptake indicated) and the commensal microbiota are also stimulatory for secretory immunity (*graded arrows*), but induce additionally suppression of pro-inflammatory Th2-dependent responses (IgE antibodies), Th1-dependent delayed-type hypersensitivity (DTH), IgG antibodies, and Th17-dependent neutrophilic reactions. This homeostatic Th-cell balance is regulated by a complex mucosally induced phenomenon called "oral tolerance." The suppressive effects can be observed both locally and in the periphery, and are mediated by regulatory T (Treg) cells

Inductive Gut-Associated Lymphoid Tissue Structures

It follows from the preceding sections that immune cells are located in three intestinal compartments: GALT, the mucosal lamina propria, and the surface epithelium (Figs. 2.2 and 2.3). GALT structures represent inductive sites for immune responses, while the lamina propria and epithelial compartment principally constitute effector sites but may nevertheless contribute to retention, proliferation, and differentiation of immune cells [2, 28].

The lymphoid structures of Peyer's patches and the draining mesenteric lymph nodes (MLNs) are formed before birth with discrete T- and B-cell areas being apparent after 19 weeks' gestation in humans [25]; but the size of these structures and germinal centers (GCs) of B-cell follicles depend on the postnatal microbial colonization. Also, ILFs cannot be observed until after birth. Cryptopatches are seen only in mice, perhaps depending on the age at tissue sampling, and these structures are believed to develop into ILFs [29] (Fig. 2.2). B cells of GCs in GALT express mainly surface IgA as a result of Ig heavy-chain gene switching in the course of B-cell differentiation to IgA-producing plasmablasts. Notably, IgA induction is much more prominent in GALT than in other structures of mucosa-associated lymphoid tissue (MALT) [2, 28].

It takes some time after birth before the Peyer's patches become activated as signified by GCs, and the induction of ILF organogenesis from cryptopatches as seen in mice depends on postnatal exogenous stimuli [2, 30]. The B-cell follicles of GALT are covered by a specialized follicle-associated epithelium (FAE) containing very thin "microfold" or "membrane" (M) cells which, together with intraepithelial dendritic cells (DCs), transport antigens from the gut lumen into the lymphoid tissue [31].

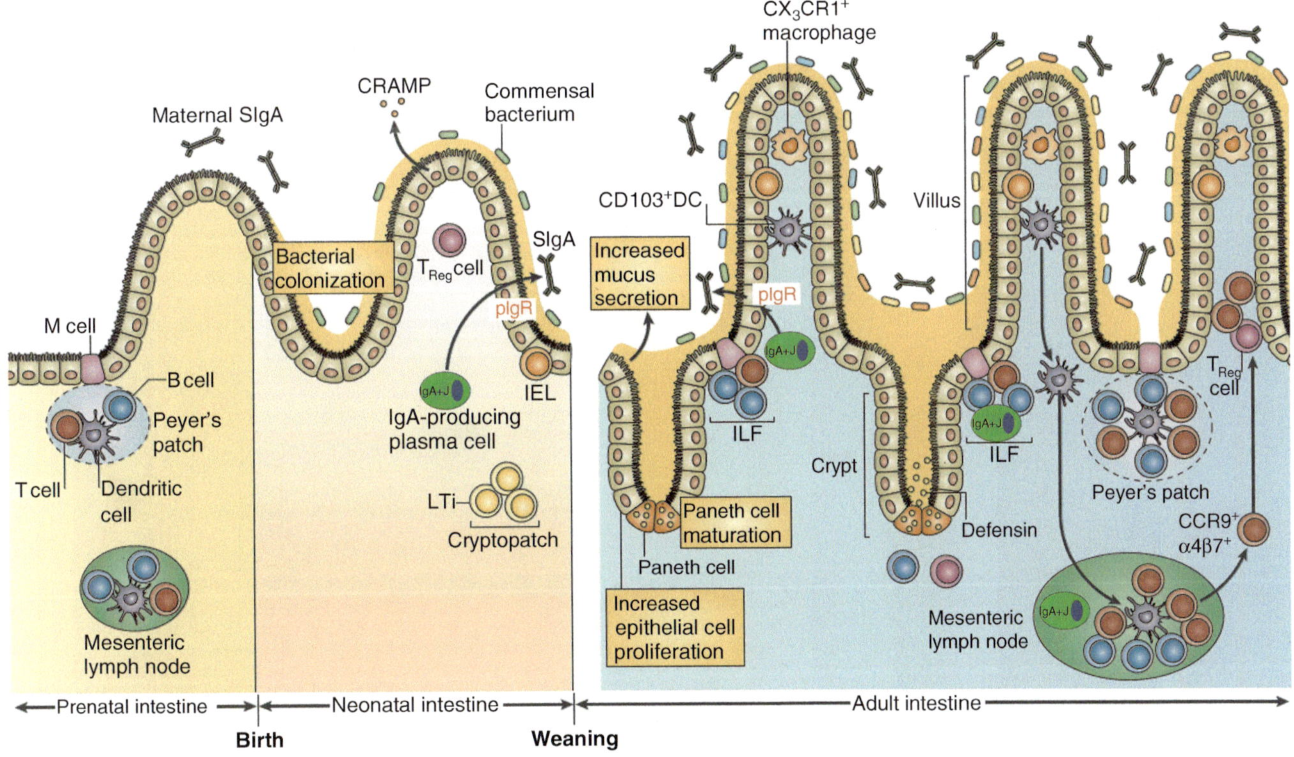

Fig. 2.2 Development of the intestinal immune system. Inherent and environmental signals drive the mucosal changes observed both in mice and humans; the postnatal establishment of an increasingly complex and dense gut microbiota is a decisive variable. The lymphoid structures of Peyer's patches and mesenteric lymph nodes are generated before birth but mature during the postnatal period. By contrast, cryptopatches (seen clearly only in mice) and isolated lymphoid follicles (ILFs) are formed after birth. Specialized antigen-sampling epithelial cells, known as M cells, reside above Peyer's patches and ILFs and facilitate antigen transport from the gut lumen to the underlying lymphoid cells. Simultaneously, innate lymphocytes, such as lymphoid tissue inducer (LTi) cells, as well as adaptive T cells leave the liver and thymus, respectively, and colonize the mucosa, including the epithelium. Intraepithelial lymphocytes (IELs) reside in close proximity to epithelial cells. Also, increasing numbers of CD103$^+$ dendritic cells and CX3CR1$^+$ macrophage-like cells home to the gut mucosa. In contrast to innate lymphocytes, regulatory T (Treg) cells populate the intestinal mucosa in response to bacterial colonization. Although B cells are present in gut tissue during early development, plasma cells producing dimeric IgA are only generated after birth to provide secretory IgA (SIgA) which is transported to the lumen by the polymeric Ig receptor (pIgR). Maternal SIgA is provided by breast milk during the early postnatal period. Modified from Renz et al. [29]

Peyer's patches are defined as at least five aggregated B-cell follicles. These structures resemble lymph nodes with inter-follicular T-cell zones and a variety of antigen-presenting cells (APCs) such as DCs and macrophages, whereas ILFs have a sparser T-cell zone. All GALT structures are devoid of encapsulation and contain no afferent lymphatics [2, 5]; their supply of antigens depends exclusively on sampling directly from the mucosal surface through the FAE. Induction and regulation of mucosal immunity hence takes place primarily in GALT and mucosa-draining lymph nodes, while terminal differentiation of B cells to PCs occurs in the lamina propria (Figs. 2.2 and 2.3) where secondary T-cell signals are generated when antigens are presented by local DCs and macrophages [2, 28]. However, animal experiments have shown that oral tolerance can be induced in the absence of GALT, thus being dependent on antigen transport to mesenteric lymph nodes (MLNs) from gut mucosa through lymph by specialized DCs, as discussed later [32, 33].

Activation and Homing of Intestinal B Cells

Antigens are presented to T cells in GALT and draining lymph nodes by APCs after intracellular processing. The activated helper T (Th) cells release mediators (cytokines), and especially transforming growth factor (TGF)-β induces the switch of B cells from surface membrane expression of IgM to IgA in GCs of GALT [2, 28]. Memory/effector cells migrate rapidly via lymphatics to MLNs where B cells may be further differentiated to plasmablasts, which then reach peripheral blood via the thoracic duct and finally become seeded into secretory effector sites (Fig. 2.3). This homing targets particularly the intestinal lamina propria but to some extent also distant secretory mucosae and glandular sites—notably the lactating mammary glands [2, 34].

The extravasation of plasmablasts at effector sites is facilitated by compartmentalized homing receptors interacting with ligands (addressins) on the microvascular endothelium, while additional fine-tuned navigation is conducted by

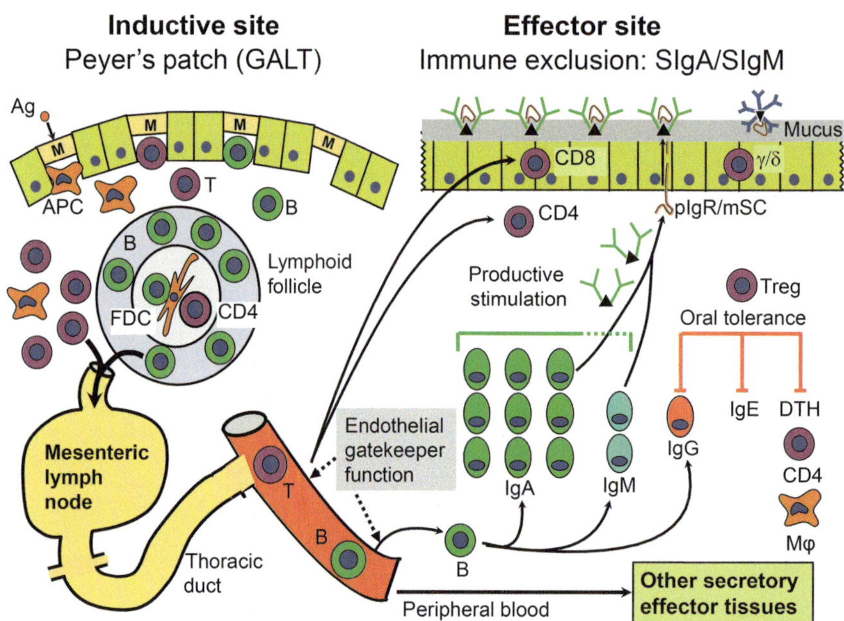

Fig. 2.3 Depiction of the intestinal mucosal immune system. Inductive sites for T and B cells are constituted by gut-associated lymphoid tissue (GALT) such as Peyer's patches with B-cell follicles and M cell (M)-containing follicle-associated epithelium through which exogenous antigens (Ag) are transported to reach antigen-presenting cells (APC), including dendritic cells, macrophages (Mφ), and follicular dendritic cells (FDC). After being primed, naïve T and B cells become memory/effector cells and migrate from GALT to mesenteric lymph nodes via lymph and then via the thoracic duct to peripheral blood for subsequent extravasation at mucosal effector sites. This process is directed by the profile of adhesion molecules and chemokines expressed on the local microvasculature—the endothelial cells thus exerting a "gatekeeper function" for mucosal immunity (see Figs. 2.3 and 2.5). The lamina propria (effector site) is illustrated with its various immune cells, including B cells (B), the approximate proportions of various Ig-producing plasma cells, and $CD4^+$ T cells. The distribution of intraepithelial T lymphocytes (mainly $CD8^+$ with α/β T-cell receptor; some γ/δ) is also depicted. Additional features are the generation of secretory IgA (SIgA) and secretory IgM (SIgM) via pIgR/membrane secretory component (mSC)-mediated epithelial export. The combined effect of oral tolerance mechanisms, mainly the action of regulatory T (Treg) cells, provides a suppressive tone in the gut, normally keeping inflammation driven by IgG and IgE antibodies as well as cell-mediated ($CD4^+$ T cell and Mφ) delayed type hypersensitivity (DTH) under control

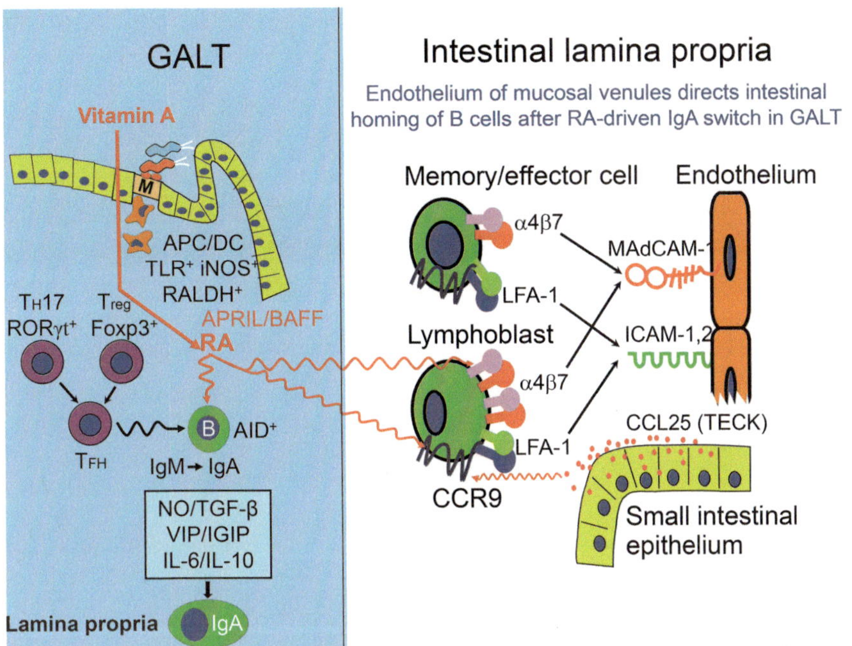

Fig. 2.4 Induction of IgA switch in mucosal B cells (B) and imprinting of their gut-homing molecules α4β7 and CCR9 occurs in gut-associated lymphoid tissue (GALT) and mesenteric lymph nodes (not shown). As described in the text, antigen-presenting cells (APC/DC) in GALT are, through their pattern recognition receptors, activated by commensal bacteria and express iNOS and RALDH. The latter enzyme converts vitamin A from the diet to retinoic acid (RA) which stimulates expression of the heterodimeric integrin α4β7 and the chemokine receptor CCR9—attracting the B cells to their ligands in the small intestinal lamina propria (see Fig. 2.5). The level of α4β7 is particularly high on lymphoblasts, and the B-cell adherence to microvascular endothelium is strengthened by interactions between generalized adhesion molecules such as LFA-1 and ICAM-1/ICAM-2, as indicated. Also the switching from IgM to IgA expression is enhanced by RA in B cells expressing activation-induced cytidine deaminase (AID), and this process is stimulated by follicular helper T (T_{FH}) cells which may be derived from RORγt⁺ Th17 cells or from Foxp3⁺ regulatory T (Treg) cells. Cytokines promoting the IgA development are framed: TGF-β is a switch factor and nitric oxide (NO) may contribute to its activation; IgA-inducing protein (IGIP) is another switch factor whose expression in DCs may be stimulated by vasoactive intestinal polypeptide (VIP); and IL-6 and IL-10 stimulate terminal differentiation to IgA-producing plasma cells. The T cell-independent switch factors APRIL and BAFF are also expressed in GALT, as indicated

chemokines [1, 2]. The extent of B-cell retention and terminal differentiation to PCs in the gut lamina propria (Fig. 2.3) depends on the local intensity of second signals, provided by chemokines and APC-processed antigens via activated CD4⁺ Th cells and their cytokines [2, 28].

Retinoic acid (RA) derived from vitamin A exerts a positive impact both on intestinal differentiation of naïve B cells arriving in GALT and their subsequent migration as precursors for the mucosal IgA-producing PCs [2, 35]. Thus, the heavy chain switching to IgA both in humans and mice is enhanced by RA, and so is the expression of the gut-homing molecules integrin α4β7 and the CC chemokine receptor CCR9 (Figs. 2.4 and 2.5). The phenotype of APCs in GALT, which seems to be imprinted by the action of gut bacteria on cellular PRRs, promotes RA generation by the expression of retinaldehyde dehydrogenase (RALDH); and the expression of inducible nitric oxide synthase (iNOS) enhances, via nitric oxide (NO), the release of innate switch factors which are cytokine members of the tumor necrosis factor (TNF) family, namely APRIL (A Proliferation Inducing Ligand) and BAFF/BlyS (B cell-activating factor of the TNF family/B lymphocyte stimulator), as well as the release of the activated IgA switch factor TGF-β from Th cells [2]. Furthermore, it has been reported that in mice a fraction for these follicular T helper (T_{FH}) cells may be derived from regulatory T (Treg) cells [36]. There may thus be a cellular link between intestinal IgA and mucosal tolerance induction, for which TGF-β is likewise important. Also interleukin (IL)-10 that contributes to terminal differentiation of IgA⁺ PCs together with IL-6 (Fig. 2.4) is an important cytokine in oral tolerance, as discussed later.

However, a more recent study was unable to reproduce these findings and showed, instead, that the T_{FH} cells were derived from Th17 cells [37]. It has been speculated that this disparity might be explained by differences in gut microbiota of the experimental mice [38]. In addition, a proper function of the GCs depends on the presence of follicular Treg (T_{FR}) cells, controlling the proliferative activity of the B cells and the quality of the IgA produced [38].

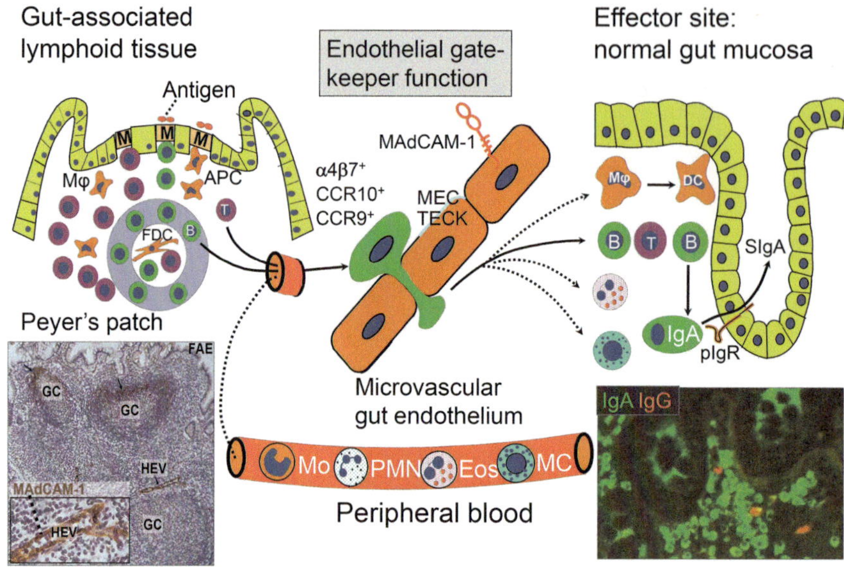

Fig. 2.5 Depiction of homing mechanisms that attract gut-associated lymphoid tissue (GALT)-derived B and T memory/effector cells to the small intestinal lamina propria (to the *right*; see Figs. 2.2 and 2.3). Interactions between the multidomain unmodified (containing no L-selectin-binding O-linked carbohydrates) mucosal addressin cell adhesion molecule (MAdCAM)-1 expressed on ordinary flat lamina propria venules is important as part of the endothelial "gatekeeper function" to direct mucosal α4β7-bearing memory/effector B and T cells to the normal gut mucosa (*solid arrows*). Selectively produced by the epithelium of the small intestine, the chemokine TECK (CCL25) attracts GALT-derived B and T cells expressing CCR9 to this segment of the gut, whereas MEC (CCL28) is a more generalized chemokine interacting with CCR10 on mucosal B cells. A GALT structure with its M cells (M), antigen-presenting cells (APC) such as macrophages (Mφ) and follicular dendritic cells (FDC), is depicted on the *left*. The *bottom left panel* shows immunohistology of a Peyer's patch with lymphoid follicles containing germinal centers (GC); the insert shows that MAdCAM-1 (with L-selectin-binding capacity) is expressed (*brown color*) on high endothelial venules (HEV) to attract naïve lymphocytes for priming. The access to the mucosal effector site is normally limited (*broken arrows*) for circulating proinflammatory cells such as monocyte (Mo)-derived Mφ, polymorphonuclear neutrophils (PMN), eosinophils (Eos) and mast-cell (MC) precursors, whereas the favored GALT-derived B and T cells promote mucosal immunity including polymeric Ig receptor (pIgR)-dependent secretory IgA (SIgA) generation. Mo-derived mucosal dendritic cell (DC) may develop through a transitional Mφ phenotype, as indicated. *Right bottom panel* shows paired immunofluorescence staining for IgA- and IgG-producing plasma cells (see *color key*) in normal colonic human mucosa and crypts with selective transport of IgA to the lumen. Note the negatively stained goblet cells

The long-lasting debate about the role of vasoactive intestinal polypeptide (VIP) in IgA induction seems to be clarified (Fig. 2.4). An IgA-inducing protein (IGIP), first identified in the bovine species, has also been characterized in humans—with somewhat different properties [39]; its CD40L-stimulated expression in DCs was found to be 35-fold enhanced by VIP, and IGIP was directly shown to induce CSR to IgA in naïve (IgM$^+$IgD$^+$) B cells.

However, a problem with all the experimental studies on IgA-promoting factors operating in GALT, such as TGF-β, RA and IGIP, is that they have not been tested for J chain-inducing properties. This small polypeptide is a prerequisite for the production of dimeric IgA and its binding to the epithelial polymeric Ig receptor (pIgR), as discussed later. Although there is considerable information about the regulation of J-chain expression in mice, such knowledge is lacking in humans; and the factors responsible for the high level of J chain in GALT-derived B cells are not known in any species [2, 40].

Regional Intestinal Immune Differences

The effect of the indigenous bacteria on the postnatal development of GALT and intestinal PCs is strikingly revealed in experimental animals colonized with a conventional microbiota after being reared in a germ-free state [41, 42]. Also food proteins contribute [2], as for instance observed in mice reared on a diet containing casein compared with a balanced amino acid-based diet [43]. Whereas MAMPs and small chain fatty acids (SCFAs) such as butyrate from the gut microbiota are abundant as stimulatory factors in the distal gut, this is not the case in the upper small intestine (Fig. 2.6). It may therefore seem surprising that the number of PCs per intestinal length unit is virtually the same in the duodenum as in the colon, and there is a higher proportion of the IgM phenotype in the former (Fig. 2.6). The reason may be the impact of high levels of food antigens and retinoids from bile and vitamin A in the diet [18], and also an involvement of the celiac lymph node complex in the immune induction in that region.

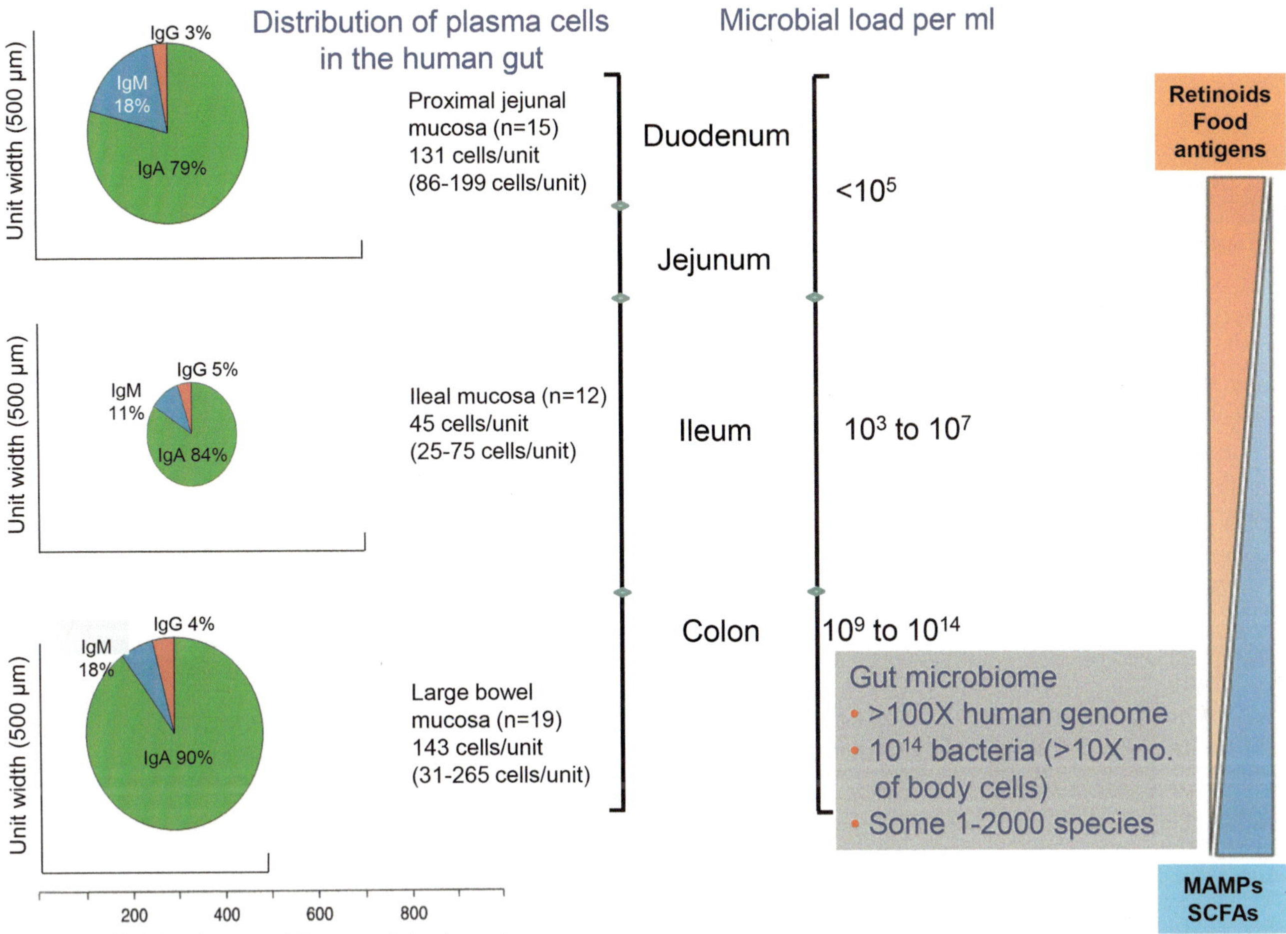

Fig. 2.6 Histomorphometric estimation of the distribution of plasmablast/plasma cell (PC) phenotypes in healthy human intestinal mucosa. A "tissue unit" is defined in a 6-μm thick section prepared for immunohistochemical analysis. The included lamina propria area varies among different specimens depending on the height of the tissue unit; and the total number of PCs per unit is determined by this variable as well as by the actual tissue density of such cells. The pie charts depict the average percentage and numerical distribution of PCs in various segments of the gut, with median numbers (and ranges) per mucosal tissue unit indicated. All units are 500 μm wide (vertical axis), and the median height (horizontal axis) for each specimen category is shown (n = number of subjects). Based on published data from the author's laboratory; see Fig. 20 in Brandtzaeg [2]. The *right part* of the figure is modified from Fig. 2 in Mowat and Agace [18]

The propensity of the mucosal immune system to generate low-affinity cross-reactive antibodies, at least in the distal gut, is probably explained by the extensive innate drive exerted by MAMPs derived from the abundant indigenous microbiota interacting with PRRs, as alluded to above. Thus, experiments have revealed a role of the important PRRs designated Toll-like receptors (TLRs) for B-cell differentiation in GALT [2, 5]. Interestingly, human GALT follicles contain the apparatus to support both T cell-dependent and T cell-independent (not involving CD40–CD40L interactions) class switch recombination (CSR) pathways to IgA (Fig. 2.4). This has been documented by showing GALT-restricted human expression of activation-induced cytidine deaminase (AID)—an essential enzyme for CSR to take place [44, 45]. Also notable, the T cell-independent switch factor APRIL, and its receptors TACI (Transmembrane Activator and CAMEL Interaction) and BCMA (B Cell Maturation Antigen) are expressed both in human GALT and human intestinal mucosa but, importantly, there is no co-expression of these receptors and AID beyond the GALT structures [44].

Thus, previous claims about B-cell switch to IgA in human colonic lamina propria appear questionable, and the same is true for the proposed extrafollicular switch from IgA1 to IgA2 [46]. A recent study showed that if these events occur outside of GALT structures, their biological importance must be negligible [47]. The possibility remains, however, that the unique T cell-independent B1 cell population generated in the mouse omentum [48] may provide a substantial fraction of lamina propria PCs and be subjected to IgA switch either in the peritoneal cavity or in the lamina propria of this species [49, 50]. However, other studies suggest that T cell-independent CSR in the mouse gut does depend on GALT structures although not on GCs [51]. Thus, a likely possibility is that T cell-independent switch to IgA in the mouse mainly takes place in the numerous ILFs present in the distal gut [2, 5, 52], and that APRIL outside of GALT structures both in mice and humans mainly promotes the survival of PCs in the mucosa, similarly to the role of BAFF in the bone marrow [53].

Intestinal Immunity in Infancy

In parallel with the bacterial colonization, the homing of lymphocytes (including IgA$^+$ plasmablasts) to the gut lamina propria seems to follow a defined kinetics—apparently reflecting a series of endogenous and exogenous signals regulating intestinal postnatal immune maturation (Fig. 2.2). Innate cells—such as lymphoid tissue inducer (LTi) cells, natural killer (NK) cells, NK-like NKp46$^+$ cells, and T helper 2 (Th2)-like cells—migrate during the first 4 weeks after birth from the murine fetal liver to the gut mucosa driven by endogenous signals [29]. By contrast, enhanced recruitment of CD8$^+$ intraepithelial lymphocytes (IELs) and forkhead box protein 3 (Foxp3)$^+$ Treg cells to the rodent gut, and also the production of anti-inflammatory IL-10, have been associated with the establishment of the intestinal microbiota [29, 54]. The Treg cells help to keep proinflammatory CD4$^+$ Th cells and cytotoxic CD8$^+$ T cells under control to preserve the epithelial barrier [55].

The delay of the postnatal mucosal immune activation parallels a temporary immaturity of systemic immunity [25]. Very few plasmablasts occur in peripheral blood of newborns [56], but after 1 month those with IgA-producing capacity (presumably GALT-derived) are remarkably increased [57], signifying progressive microbial stimulation. Thus, the number of IgA$^+$ plasmablasts in the blood of newborns is <8 per million mononuclear cells, but is increased to ~600 per million mononuclear cells already after 1 month, apparently reflecting the progressive microbial stimulation of GALT [57]. An initial early elevation of circulating plasmablasts (mainly IgM$^+$) occurs in preterm infants, especially those with intrauterine infections [56]. Thus, mucosal immune cells are competent at least during the final trimester, but APCs need to be activated by microbial factors that enable them to provide appropriate co-stimulatory signals to naïve T cells [58]. The commensals are important to this end as shown by the fact that the number of intestinal IgA$^+$ PCs is normalized 4 weeks after exposure of germ-free mice to a conventional complex gut microbiota [59, 60]. *Bacteroides* and *Escherichia coli* strains seem to be particularly immunostimulatory, but also lactic acid-producing bacteria contribute [61, 62]. A study showed that an optimal stimulatory effect requires a host-specific microbiota, and the same holds true for small-intestinal T-cell activity [63].

In agreement with these observations, only scattered IgM$^+$ (and IgG$^+$) intestinal PCs could be seen in newborns, and IgA$^+$ cells were either absent or extremely rare even at 10 days of age [25]. The numbers of IgM- and IgA-producing cells increased rapidly after 2–4 weeks—the latter becoming predominant at 1–2 months, usually peaking around 12 months. However, in affluent societies it may take several years for the size of the IgA$^+$ PC population to reach that of healthy adults, whereas a fast postnatal increase of SIgA was observed in children living in developing countries with a heavy microbial load [55].

The retarded postnatal activation of GALT parallels the functionally decreased systemic immunocompetence in the newborn period [25, 26, 58, 64]. Thus, peripheral CD4$^+$ Th cells of infants show reduced capacity for cytokine production and B-cell help. One reason may be that there are relatively few circulating memory (CD45R0$^+$) T cells in infancy, although the responsiveness of neonatal naïve (CD45RA$^+$) T cells does not differ significantly from that of virgin counterparts in adults. Indeed, the chief explanation for the immunological immaturity in infancy appears to be a deficient APC function [65]. Interestingly, pioneering studies in mice showed that the microbiota stimulates a self-limiting intestinal SIgA response [66]. Such transient SIgA production is probably necessary to allow access of microbial constituents to GALT. In this manner, it seems that the intestinal IgA response is continuously adapting to the changing microbiota [67], which would be especially relevant in the early postnatal period.

Secretory Immunity and the Epithelial Barrier Function

Formation and Properties of Secretory Antibodies

Most mucosal PCs produce dimers and larger polymers of IgA (collectively called pIgA), which contain a disulfide-linked 15-kDa polypeptide called the "joining" or J chain (Fig. 2.7). The J chain is a prerequisite for active dimerization and the export of pIgA through secretory epithelia such as the intestinal crypts [68, 69]. This transport is mediated by a ~100-kDa glycoprotein called pIgR, which is also known as membrane secretory component (SC) [70]. J chain-containing pentameric IgM is externally transported by the same mechanism (Figs. 2.3 and 2.7) [68, 71], and this peptide is part of the binding site for pIgR/SC independent of its involvement in the polymerization process [72].

Apical proteolytic cleavage of the extracellular portion of pIgR enables release of SIgA and secretory IgM (SIgM) to the lumen. In this manner the ectodomain of pIgR (~80 kDa) is "sacrificed" to become bound SC which stabilizes the qua-

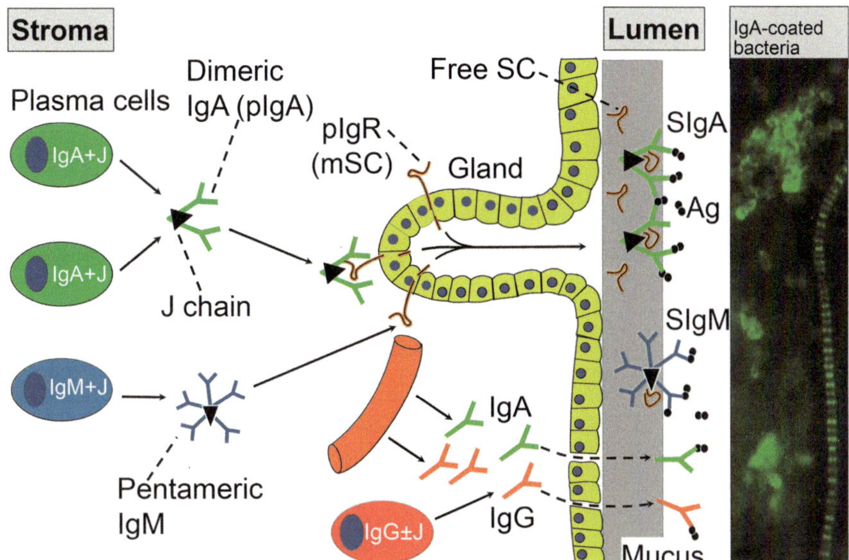

Fig. 2.7 Receptor-mediated export of dimeric IgA and pentameric IgM to provide secretory antibodies (SIgA and SIgM) functioning in immune exclusion of antigen (Ag) at the mucosal surface. Polymeric Ig receptor (pIgR) is expressed basolaterally as membrane secretory component (mSC) on mucosal epithelial cells and mediates transcytosis of dimeric IgA and pentameric IgM, which are produced locally with incorporated J chain (IgA+J and IgM+J) by local plasma cells. Although J chain is often expressed by mucosal IgG plasma cells (70–90 %), it does not combine with this isotype and is therefore degraded intracellularly as denoted (±J). Locally produced (and serum-derived) IgG is therefore not subject to pIgR-mediated transport, but can be transmitted paracellularly to the lumen together with monomeric IgA, as indicated. Free SC (depicted in mucus) is generated when pIgR in its unoccupied state (top basolateral symbol) is cleaved at the apical face of the epithelium like bound SC in SIgA and SIgM. Commensal bacteria in the *right-hand panel* are coated in vivo with SIgA, which aids their containment and thereby promotes microbial–host mutualism. Immunofluorescence illustration from Brandtzaeg et al. [161]

ternary structure of the secretory antibodies, particularly SIgA where a disulfide bridge is formed between the two partners [28]. Unoccupied pIgR (some 50 %) is constitutively exported in the same manner; the cleaved ectodomain is then called free SC [70] and exhibits certain innate immune properties such as affinity for *E. coli* and *Clostridium difficile* toxin [3]. Bound SC confers such properties to SIgA and contributes to its mucus-binding capacity and its property of trapping bacteria in biofilms [73].

Immune exclusion performed by SIgA and SIgM thus depends on an intimate cooperation between the mucosal B-cell system and the pIgR-expressing epithelium (Fig. 2.7). Serum-derived and locally produced IgG antibodies may also to some extent contribute to immune exclusion when reaching the lumen by noninjurious paracellular diffusion [74] or after being transported by the neonatal Fc receptor, FcRn [75]. However, IgG is rapidly degraded in the gut lumen, although the hepatic super antigen (protein Fv) may form large complexes with degraded antibodies of different specificities, thereby reinforcing their immune exclusion function [76].

As alluded to above, only smaller amounts of pentameric IgM are normally exported by the pIgR, and SIgM is not as stable as SIgA because bound SC is covalently stabilized only in the latter [74]. Immune exclusion is therefore normally performed mainly by SIgA (Fig. 2.3) in cooperation with innate defenses such as mucus, defensins, and peristalsis [55]. In newborns and subjects with selective IgA deficiency, however, SIgM antibodies are of greater importance than in healthy adults [25, 28]. Thus, while IgA is generally undetectable in the mucosa before 10 days of age, IgM$^+$ PCs may remain predominant up to 1 month. Thereafter a rapid expansion of IgA$^+$ PCs takes place, and some increase may be seen up to 1 year of age (Fig. 2.8). The epithelial production of pIgR/SC, however, begins in fetal human life around 3–5 months and is constitutively regulated [25]; its expression increases steadily until birth and may be followed by a postnatal peak (Fig. 2.8), which could reflect the microbial encounter. Accordingly, traces of SIgA and SIgM occur in intestinal fluid during the first postnatal period, and some IgG is often present—mainly reflecting passive transmission from the lamina propria which after 34 weeks of gestation contains readily detectable maternal IgG [25].

A much faster establishment of SIgA immunity can be seen in developing countries with a heavy microbial load [77]. Some reports suggest that also probiotic treatment enhances the production of IgA, but this was not confirmed by measuring IgA in saliva [78]. Nevertheless, after a combination of prebiotic and probiotic treatment given perinatally and for the first 6 months of life, infants that showed an early elevation of fecal IgA had reduced risk of allergies before 2 years of age [79]. Also, in another study it was shown that

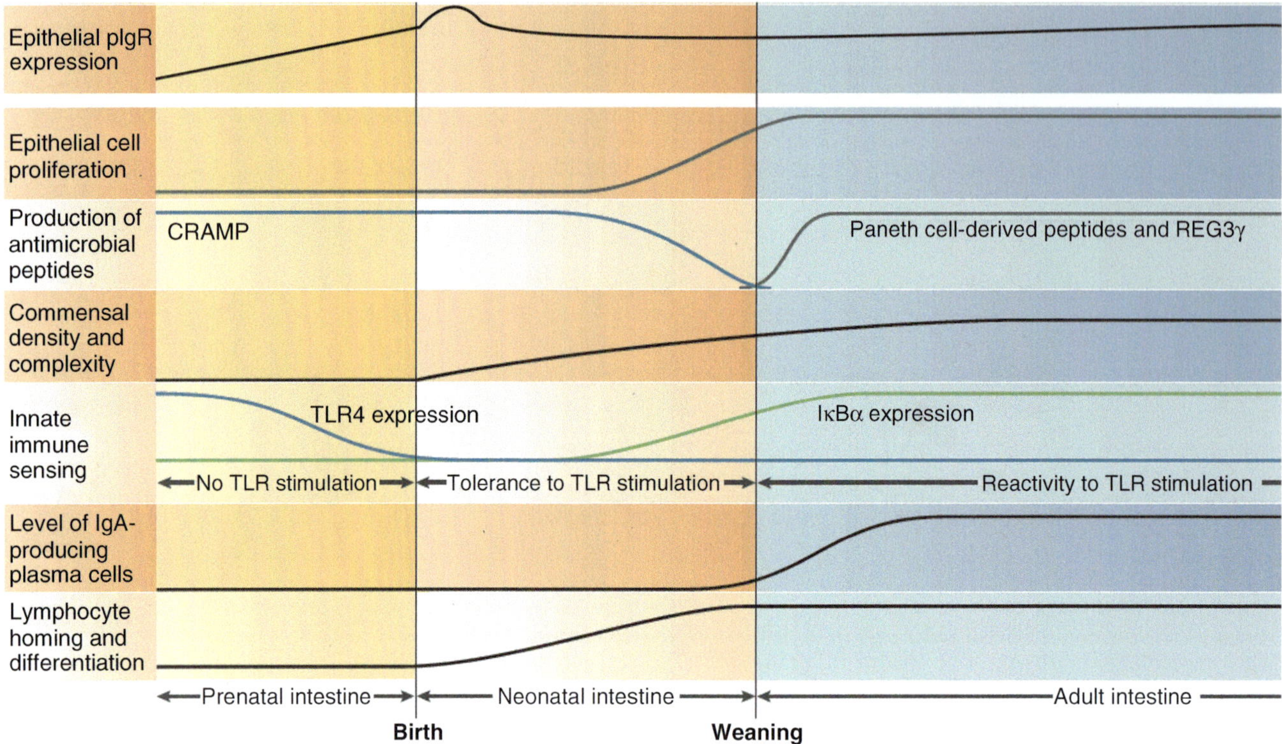

Fig. 2.8 Maturation of the intestinal immune system and the epithelial barrier. The production of the human polymeric Ig receptor (pIgR) begins in fetal life at 3–5 weeks gestation, but the plasma cells producing its ligand dimeric IgA are hardly presence before birth. The murine neonatal mucosa is characterized by little epithelial cell proliferation, absence of developed crypts (intestinal glands) and crypt-based Paneth cells, but marked expression of cathelicidin-related antimicrobial peptide (CRAMP); by contrast, the formation of intestinal crypts late during the second week after birth in mice initiates increased proliferation and rapid epithelial cell renewal, generation of α-defensin-producing Paneth cells, and upregulation of the antibacterial C-type lectin regenerating islet-derived protein 3γ (REG3γ). A decrease in the epithelial expression of Toll-like receptor 4 (TLR4) before birth, and a steady increase in the level of the nuclear factor-kB inhibitor IkBα during the postnatal period reduce the responsiveness to bacterial lipopolysaccharide and other pro-inflammatory stimuli. Such acquisition of epithelial TLR tolerance creates a neonatal period of decreased innate immune responsiveness. Note that the small intestinal epithelium at birth has a more mature phenotype in humans than in mice. Modified from Renz et al. [29]

early intestinal colonization with *Bifidobacterium* species was associated with significantly elevated levels of SIgA in saliva at 6 months of age [80].

The Epithelial Barrier Function

The neonatal gut varies among species in terms of maturity, depending in part on the length of the gestation period. The small intestinal mucosa of newborn humans has a mature crypt–villous architecture, with continuous stem cell proliferation, and epithelial cell migration and differentiation. In mice, small intestinal crypts only develop 10–12 days after birth, accompanied by increased epithelial cell renewal and transcriptional reprogramming of enterocytes, which includes changed expression of genes involved in nutrient transport, metabolism, and cell differentiation [29]. Also, the enteric spectrum of antimicrobial peptides changes significantly during neonatal development in mice (Fig. 2.8). During the first 2 weeks of postnatal life, when mature crypt-based Paneth cells are absent, the mouse intestinal epithelium expresses cathelicidin-related antimicrobial peptide, or CRAMP. The Paneth cells start to produce defensins at weaning, and then the CRAMP expression decreases.

While defensin production by Paneth cells is independent on bacterial colonization, expression of other antimicrobial peptides by epithelial cells—such as the C-type lectin regenerating islet-derived protein 3γ (REG3γ)—requires a microbiota (Fig. 2.8) and is supported by IL-22-producing RORγt^{+}NKp46^{+} lymphocytes [29]. Thus, administration to mice of broad-spectrum antibiotics by gavage has been shown to reduce significantly the colonic epithelial expression of 70 genes; and five of the seven genes that were more than fourfold less active than normal, encoded antimicrobial peptides including Ang4, Pla2g2a, Retnlb, REG3γ, and REG3β [55]. REG3γ has furthermore been detected in murine γδ IELs in response to microbial stimulation of epithelial cell-intrinsic adapter protein MyD88 signaling, probably mediated through TLRs [81, 82]. Also human γδ IELs seem to belong to the first-line innate mucosal defense as

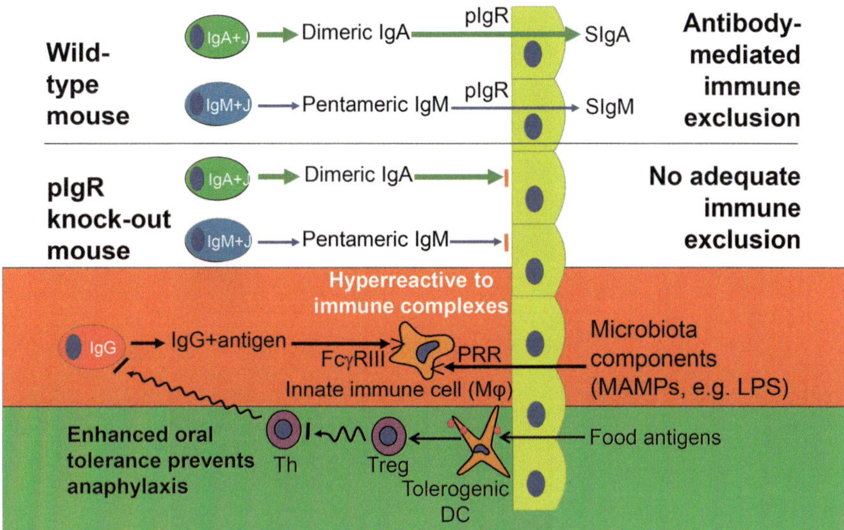

Fig. 2.9 Depiction of experimental model for hypersensitivity and oral tolerance. Lack of secretory antibodies (SIgA and SIgM) in pIgR knockout mice leads to inadequate immune exclusion of bacterial components from the gut microbiota. Such conserved microbe-associated molecular patterns (MAMPs), e.g., lipopolysaccharide (LPS), will interact with pattern recognition receptors (PRRs) on innate immune cells, including macrophages (Mφs), which become hyperreactive. These cells are therefore sensitive to IgG-containing immune complexes interacting with Fc receptors (FcγRIII), which renders the mice predisposed to hypersensitivity (anaphylaxis). The deficient epithelial barrier also allows increased uptake of food antigens from the gut lumen (e.g., fed ovalbumin) which enhances induction of oral tolerance, providing a net anti-inflammatory effect against undue penetration of the same antigen into the body by any route (e.g., dermal). Production of IgG antibodies against this sensitizing antigen will thus be downregulated, and the animal is protected against anaphylaxis and delayed hypersensitivity (not shown) after antigen challenge. Adapted from Karlsson et al. [88]

deemed from their behavior in AIDS patients and lack of response to antiretroviral treatment [83].

Although the so-called "gut closure" normally occurs in humans mainly before birth, the mucosal barrier may be inadequate up to 2 years of age; the mechanisms involved remain poorly defined [84], but the development of secretory immunity is probably one decisive variable. Importantly in this context, pIgR-deficient knockout mice that lack SIgA and SIgM exhibit aberrant mucosal leakiness [85] and have increased uptake of food proteins and commensal bacteria [86]. A thick virtually microbe-devoid inner mucus layer has been revealed at the apical epithelial surface of the normal colon [87]; this protected zone apparently limits direct bacterial contact with host cells, but it may nevertheless be permeable for MAMPs and antigens derived from the abundant microbiota present in the outer mucus layer—particularly when SIgA is absent (see later).

Mice lacking pIgR (knockout mice) show significantly elevated production of IgG antibodies to commensal bacterial antigens but, interestingly, not to food proteins [85, 86]. The undue influx of microbial products causes a generalized hyperreactive state with overactivation of the innate cellular NF-kB transcription pathway, resulting in 50 % liability of these mice to anaphylactic death after systemic antigen sensitization (ovalbumin, OVA) and low-dose intradermal challenge [88]. However, the pIgR-deficient mice exhibit enhanced capacity for induction of oral tolerance, which after OVA feeding was fully able to control IgG1- and T cell-dependent hypersensitivity against the same antigen (Fig. 2.9). This observation might imply that at the same time as an inadequate intestinal barrier in the infant represents a risk for hypersensitivity reactions, it will promote tolerance against cognate antigens when they are continuously present in the gut [12].

The postnatal balance between the epithelial barrier function and oral tolerance thus appears to be critical for the induction of immunological homeostasis. Notably, although the incidence of food allergy (apparently non-IgE-mediated) is increased in children with IgA deficiency, it is not strikingly elevated [89]—perhaps because the induction of Treg cells is enhanced in addition to compensatory SIgM, which in such individuals partially replaces the lacking SIgA in the gut [31, 90]. Also, bacterial overgrowth occurs in the jejunum of vagotomized patients only when IgA deficiency is combined with suboptimal function of innate defenses such as gastric acid and peristalsis [91]. In this context, it is notable that the frequency of selective IgA deficiency among IBD patients in Sweden is significantly increased, especially for those with Crohn's disease (prevalence ratio, 5.7, compared with 3.9 in ulcerative colitis) [92].

AID knockout mice that have SIgA deficiency due to lack of Ig class switching, and also exhibit a defect IgM antibody response, show massive intestinal overgrowth of commensal anaerobic bacteria with a resulting striking hypertrophy of

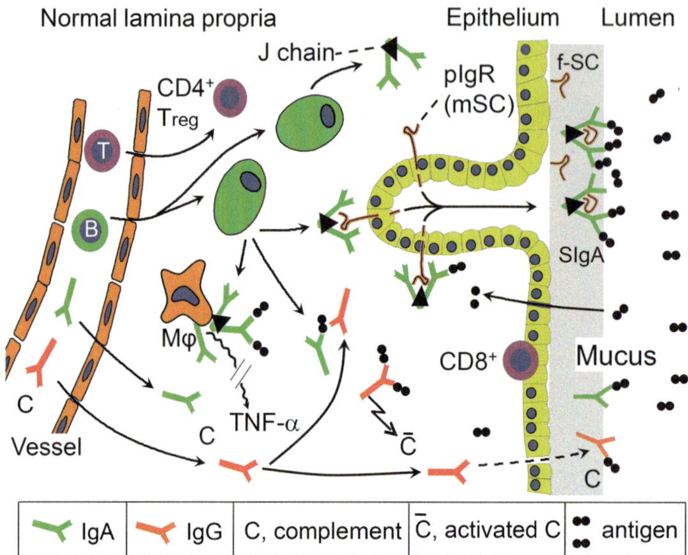

Fig. 2.10 Mucosal homeostasis in the normal gut. Contributing variables are presented as a balance between Ig classes (for simplicity, only IgA and IgG are indicated) and regulatory T (Treg) cells. Secretory IgA (SIgA) is generated from dimeric IgA (with associated J chain) produced by local plasma cells and transported to the lumen by the polymeric Ig receptor (pIgR), also called membrane secretory component (mSC). After apical cleavage, unoccupied receptor is translocated in the same manner and called free SC (f-SC), in contrast to the bound SC in SIgA. The secretory antibodies act in first-line defense by performing antigen exclusion at the mucosal surface (to the *right*). Antigens penetrating the epithelial barrier may meet serum-derived IgG antibodies in the lamina propria. The formed immune complexes can activate complement, and the resulting inflammatory mediators may cause temporarily increased paracellular leakage of IgG antibodies (*broken arrow*). Sustained inflammation is normally inhibited by blocking antibody activities in the lamina propria exerted by serum-derived or locally produced IgA (competition for antigen depicted) and anti-inflammatory Treg cells. Independent of antibody specificity, IgA-containing immune complexes may also inhibit pro-inflammatory mediator release (TNF-α depicted) from activated phagocytic cells such as macrophages (Mφ). Moreover, antigens bound to dimeric IgA may be returned in a non-inflammatory manner to the gut lumen by the pIgR-mediated transport mechanism, as indicated

ILFs over time [93]. This development has some resemblance to the irregular lymphoid aggregates seen in long-standing IBD [94]. In contrast to AID and pIgR knockout mice, however, IgA-deficient mice (like IgA-deficient humans) have compensatory SIgM antibodies in their gut lumen [95]. Interestingly, these mice show no increased susceptibility to various gut infections or to dextran sulfate sodium (DSS)-induced colitis, whereas pIgR deficient mice do—probably because they lack both SIgA and SIgM [95, 96].

It has been suggested that postnatal hyperreactivity of the immune system may also result from intrauterine events, probably causing genetically or epigenetically determined poor Treg-cell function and immunological immaturity [97, 98], as also suggested from cord blood studies [99]. In normal mice it has been shown that neonatal (but not adult) CD4+ T cells are strikingly prone to differentiate into Treg cells upon stimulation [100]. Moreover, the intestinal epithelium itself is equipped with a vast array of features to control immune barrier homeostasis (Fig. 2.8) [101]. These key intrinsic mechanisms have been reviewed and include variables such as secretion of mucins and defensins, inflammasome function, intercellular junctional complex regulation, and PRR signaling [102]. As discussed in a subsequent section, the latter is downregulated in the neonatal gut epithelium to preserve its integrity upon the encounter with the commensal microbiota [103, 104].

Additional IgA Antibody Functions

Antibody production by the numerous intestinal pIgA+ PCs may also be important for homeostasis within the lamina propria as a result of several anti-inflammatory mechanisms. IgA lacks ordinary complement-activating properties [105] and can therefore block nonspecific biological amplification triggered by locally produced or serum-derived IgG antibodies (Fig. 2.10), which may actually increase the penetration of exogenous bystander antigens through the surface epithelium [106]. This is important in view of the fact that immune complexes are probably formed even within the normal lamina propria due to some influx of soluble antigens, particularly following food intake [23]. Also, in vitro and in vivo experiments have suggested that soluble antigens—after pIgA-mediated noninflammatory trapping in immune complexes—may be cleared by the secretory epithelium via pIgR-mediated translocation to the lumen (Fig. 2.10) [3, 4, 107]. Similar experiments have suggested that pIgA antibodies can neutralize lipopolysaccharide (LPS) and viruses within secretory epithelial cells during pIgR-mediated export [3, 4], and thus return harmful microbial components to the gut lumen (Fig. 2.11). Mouse models have confirmed that the latter mechanism contributes to the intestinal defense against rotavirus infection [108], and IgA+ PCs with specificity for rotavirus occur in normal jejunal mucosa of adults with no signs of current infection [109].

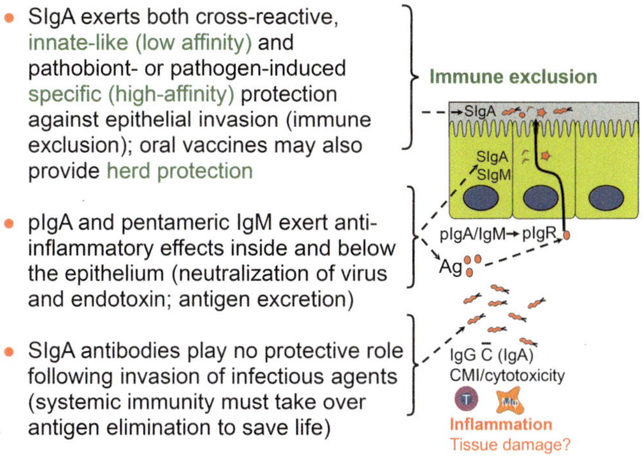

- SIgA exerts both cross-reactive, innate-like (low affinity) and pathobiont- or pathogen-induced specific (high-affinity) protection against epithelial invasion (immune exclusion); oral vaccines may also provide herd protection
- pIgA and pentameric IgM exert anti-inflammatory effects inside and below the epithelium (neutralization of virus and endotoxin; antigen excretion)
- SIgA antibodies play no protective role following invasion of infectious agents (systemic immunity must take over antigen elimination to save life)

Fig. 2.11 Different principles for how secretory antibodies (SIgA and SIgM) may contribute to mucosal homeostasis. In addition to immune exclusion, the pIgR-mediated external transport of dimeric IgA and pentameric IgM (pIgA/IgM) may be exploited for intraepithelial virus and toxin neutralization, as well as non-inflammatory antigen (Ag) excretion from the lamina propria (see Fig. 2.11). However, when infection with invasion occurs, systemic immunity takes over; this involves proinflammatory mechanisms such as activation of complement (Ċ) by IgG antibodies, cell-mediated immunity (CMI), and cytotoxicity—all of which may cause tissue damage. Research forming the basis for the depicted mechanisms is reviewed in more detail elsewhere [4, 5, 40]

The mucosal clearance function exhibited by pIgA (and probably pentameric IgM) antibodies reinforces the immune exclusion mediated by SIgA (and SIgM) with innate-like low-affinity antibody activity generated against commensal bacteria [20, 101], and which to some extent may be cross-reactive (Fig. 2.11). The high-affinity antibodies induced by pathogens or properly adjuvanted oral vaccines may even more efficiently contribute to both immune exclusion and mucosal clearance, as reviewed elsewhere [4].

Locally produced pIgA may further influence homeostasis by interacting with the Fcα receptor (FcαRI, CD89) on leukocytes in the lamina propria. First, on the one hand it has been shown that pIgA-containing immune complexes are able to suppress attraction of neutrophils, eosinophils, and monocytes, thereby reducing their proinflammatory activities. On the other hand, when such complexes interact with CD89 on neutrophils, leukotriene B4 is released as a chemotactic factor attracting more of these cells [111]. Second, IgA can apparently downregulate the secretion of proinflammatory cytokines such as TNF-α from activated monocytes [112]. However, it is uncertain whether this mechanism operates in the normal gut (Fig. 2.10) because mucosal macrophages do not express detectable surface CD89—at least not in the small intestine [113, 114]. Third, neutrophil and monocyte activation that results in generation of reactive oxygen metabolites ("respiratory burst") is reportedly inhibited by IgA [115]. Conversely, pIgA may temporarily trigger monocytes to enhanced activity—including TNF-α secretion [116]—and IgA (particularly SIgA) appears to be a potent activator of eosinophils [117, 118]. Indeed, complexed SIgA induces respiratory burst and degranulation of these cells, while soluble SIgA enhances their survival in vitro [119].

Thus, cross-linking of CD89 during infection with IgA-opsonized pathogens may cause proinflammatory responses, whereas naturally occurring IgA (not complexed) may induce inhibitory signals through CD89, thereby damaging excessive reactions [120]. Together, these results suggest that the participation of pIgA in mucosal homeostasis is quite fine-tuned [121]—perhaps being skewed towards a proinflammatory potential in IBD where there are numerous granulocytes [111] along with recently recruited monocyte-like macrophages which express of the LPS co-receptor CD14 and PRRs such as TLR2 and TLR4 [122, 123].

Initially, the shift from the normal predominance of mucosal pIgA production to IgG and monomeric IgA in IBD lesions [124] may represent a powerful second line of defense because these antibodies may efficiently mediate immune elimination of penetrating bacteria via phagocytosis and antibody-dependent cell-mediated cytotoxicity (Fig. 2.11). Notably, by means of CD89 both neutrophils [111] and liver Kupffer cells [125] may phagocytose translocated gut bacteria opsonized even with serum-type monomeric IgA as alluded to above. Rodent studies suggest that the liver is designed to handle this antigen elimination in a silent manner because of its unique tolerogenic capacity, including induction of Treg cells by plasmacytoid DCs [126]. Antigen elimination within the intestinal lamina propria, however, may more readily cause inflammation and tissue damage when systemic type of immunity is involved; this is a risk the immune system sometimes must take to hinder sepsis and save life (Fig. 2.11). The role of mucosal IgA and oral tolerance is to counteract overactivation of potentially harmful immune reactions.

Effect of Microbial–Host Interactions on Innate and Adaptive Immunity

The Epithelial Barrier and Secretory Immunity

In fetal life, murine gut epithelial cells are sensitive to microbial factors such as LPS (endotoxin) because they highly express intracellularly a PRR for this MAMP, namely TLR4 (Fig. 2.8) [103]. Exposure to LPS in the vaginal tract during birth activates the neonatal gut epithelium via TLR4 and temporarily upregulates microRNA-146a (miR-146a), which leads to degradation of the TLR signaling molecule IL-1R-associated kinase 1 (IRAK1). Such translational repression of IRAK1 protects the epithelium from microbiota-induced damage during transition from a relatively sterile environment [104, 127]. In remarkable contrast, epithelial tolerance to the commensal bacteria does not occur in mice delivered by cesarean section [103]. These experimental observations may be related to the fact that children delivered by cesarean section appear particularly prone to develop food allergy if they have a genetic predisposition for atopy [128, 129].

The epithelial expression of the NF-kB inhibitor IkBα steadily increases during the postnatal period [130]. The combination of decreasing levels of TLR4 and increasing levels of IkBα in the epithelial cells effectively increases the threshold of immune activation in the gut epithelium (Fig. 2.8). Also interestingly, decreased IRAK1 protein expression in mouse neonatal epithelium requires continuous TLR signaling. This facilitates prolonged upregulation of miR-146a expression and simultaneously induces sustained expression of genes supporting cell maturation, survival and nutrient absorption [131]. Innate immune signaling by epithelial cells seems to be essential for immune tolerance, as lack of the proinflammatory signaling molecule TGF-β-activated kinase 1 (TAK1) specifically in the murine intestinal epithelium leads to early inflammation, tissue damage and postnatal mortality [132]. Thus, although inappropriate stimulation of the neonatal innate immune system by the microbiota must be prevented, controlled innate immune activation significantly contributes to nutrient absorption, angiogenesis, epithelial cell differentiation, and barrier reinforcement [133].

Despite the decreased sensitivity of epithelial cells to TLR stimulation in murine neonates, other innate immune signaling pathways remain fully functional. For example, rotavirus infection of the intestinal epithelium in neonatal mice is efficiently sensed by the helicases retinoic acid-inducible gene I (RIG-I) and melanoma differentiation-associated gene 5, or MDA5 [134]. Confronted with the colonization of the gut microbiota, therefore, the neonatal intestinal epithelium seems to calibrate its bacterial sensitivity and modify its signaling pathways after initial stimulation while maintaining antiviral host defenses.

Mouse experiments have thus demonstrated a crucial postnatal role of commensal gut colonization, both in establishing and regulating the epithelial barrier, which also includes upregulation of pIgR expression [133, 135]. Such beneficial effects of microbiota-derived MAMPs appear again to be mediated largely via PRRs, particularly TLRs and similar innate sensors on the epithelial plasma membrane (apically or basolaterally) or on endosomal membranes [101, 136]. Cell culture experiments with the polarized human colon carcinoma cell line HT-29 have shown that ligation of TLR3 and TLR4 with the respective MAMPs (double-stranded RNA and LPS) from the apical side upregulates pIgR expression (Fig. 2.12) [137], which may then increase SIgA (and SIgM) export and thus enhance secretory immunity [138]. Gut bacteria of the family *Enterobacteriaceae* can induce this effect [139].

Vitamin A supports secretory immunity, not only by enhancing IgA switch and homing of mucosal B cells (Fig. 2.4) but also by a positive effect of RA on cytokine-induced pIgR expression in intestinal epithelial cell at the transcriptional level [140, 141]. Several cytokines derived from activated Th cells or APCs may upregulate pIgR expression and thereby increase the export of secretory antibodies in response to microbial stimulation (Fig. 2.12) [40, 138]. A similar pIgR-enhancing effect has been shown for the SCFA butyrate in combination with various cytokines (Fig. 2.12) [142]. Butyrate is an anaerobic microbial fermentation product of oligosaccharides and an important energy source of colonic epithelial cells. Notably, it can increase

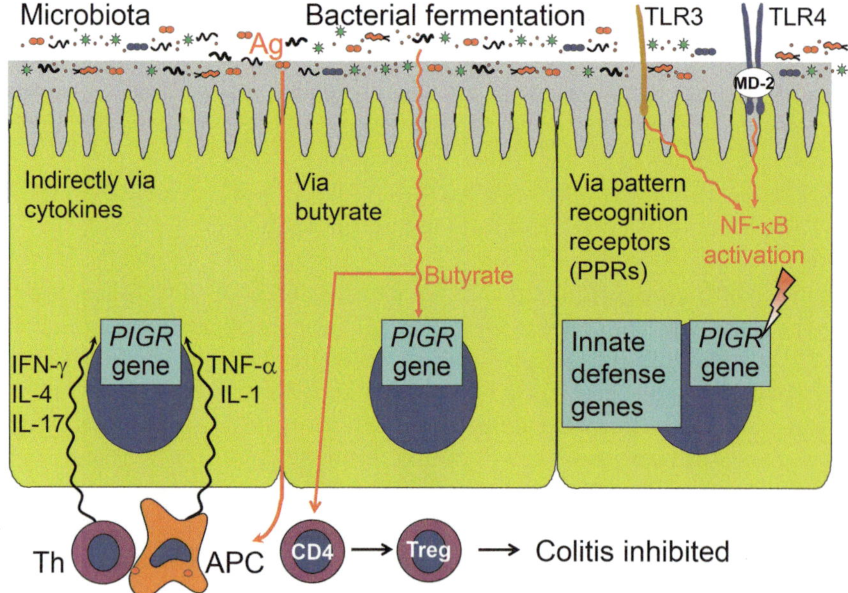

Fig. 2.12 Schematic illustrations of three possible manners in which pIgR expression can be upregulated by activation of its gene locus *PIGR*. The effect of the cytokines interferon (IFN)-γ, interleukin (IL)-4, IL-17, tumor necrosis factor (TNF)-α, and IL-1 can be enhanced by the vitamin A derivative retinoic acid (not shown). The microbial fermentation product butyrate in combination with cytokines also has an enhancing effect on *PIGR*, and butyrate may directly induce regulatory T (Treg) cells that counteract colitis. Activation of epithelial Toll-like receptors (TLR) may not only active *PIGR* but also innate defense genes

gene transcription levels through specific DNA sequences [143]. It has, moreover, been shown in different studies that butyrate can directly induce Treg cells in the gut [144] and thereby inhibit experimental colitis in a mouse model [145].

Altogether, there are many mechanisms by which exogenous variables may maintain the "tone" of intestinal pIgR expression above the constitutive level and thus reinforce immune exclusion. In addition, polarized gut epithelial cells seem to retain their ability to dampen the proinflammatory effect of PRR-mediated signals coming from the luminal side [135, 136, 146]; but after bacterial invasion, PRR signaling from the basolateral side results in NF-kB activation with release of epithelial defensins to join the combat against infection [101, 147]. Accumulating evidence suggests that barrier-related homeostasis depends on "cross talk" between the epithelium (via cytokines and other factors) and lamina propria cells including macrophages, DCs, and T cells [148–151].

Thus, when immune regulation is operating in a healthy manner, the small amounts of MAMPs and exogenous antigen penetrating into the lamina propria seem to be handled in a homeostatic manner by DCs and macrophages, with a balanced cytokine secretion and induction of Treg cells (Fig. 2.13). However, if the influx is excessive or regulatory mechanisms are defect, immune reactions may be driven into hypersensitivity and enter a vicious circle with proinflammatory cytokines and epithelial apoptosis [12, 150–152]. In this manner a "point of no return" may be reached, as seen in IBD with apoptosis-resistant pathogenic T cells and tissue damage (Fig. 2.13). The take-home lesson from most disease models in gene-manipulated animals is that a predilection exists for immunopathology to occur in the distal gut—where most commensals reside—when adaptive immunity is dysregulated and innate immunity or the intestinal barrier function compromised [153, 154].

The Role of Mucus in Intestinal Barrier Function

Goblet cells secrete mucin glycoproteins and MUC2 is the major mucin making up the mucus coat of the intestinal epithelium [87]. This coating is of great importance for the interactions between the microbiota and the immune system [155]. The epithelium of the small intestine is covered by a single loose mucus layer which allows microbial penetration (Fig. 2.14a). Nevertheless, bacteria are normally kept at a certain distance from the epithelial cells because of

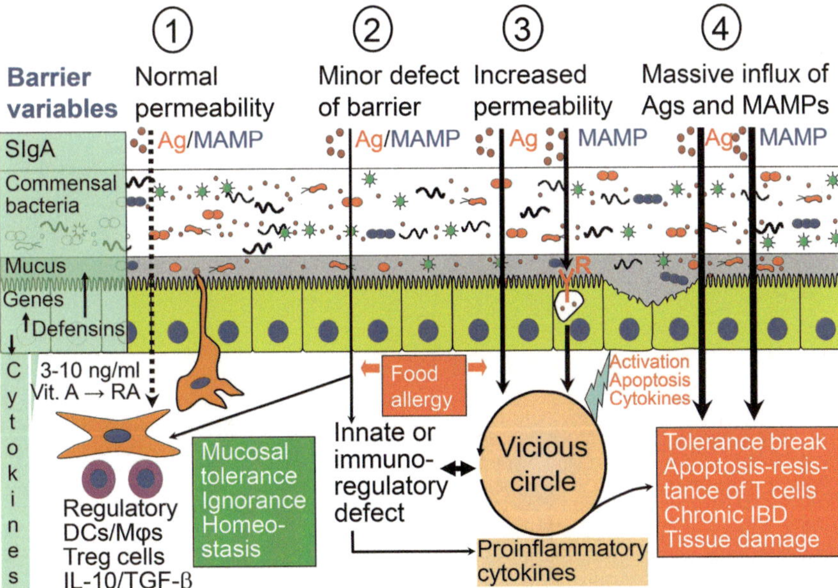

Fig. 2.13 Model for maintenance of mucosal homeostasis in the gut and abrogation of oral tolerance. Epithelial barrier variables, including secretory IgA (SIgA), mucus, defensins, genes (e.g., regulating tight junctions), and cytokines are indicated in the *light green panel* to the *left*. (*1*) Normal permeability of the gut epithelium allows some MAMP (microbe-associated molecular pattern) and exogenous antigen (Ag) uptake (amounts of dietary proteins detected in the circulation after a meal are indicated). (*2*) A minor barrier defect results in increased uptake, but mucosal homeostasis is maintained (*green panel*) when oral tolerance is adequately induced by quiescent dendritic cells (DCs) and macrophages (Mφs), which both can convert dietary vitamin A to retinoic acid (RA) as an aid in their induction of regulatory T (Treg) cells (providing the suppressive cytokines IL-10 and TGF-β). If there is an innate or immunoregulatory defect, a vicious circle will develop which reciprocally acts also on the regulatory network. (*3*) With more skewing towards regulatory dysfunction, the vicious circle will activate the epithelium, and MAMP and Ag uptake is enhanced (*graded vertical arrows*), both by increased permeability and aberrant receptor (R) expression apically on epithelial cells. Food allergy may occur in the dysfunctional, to some extent reversible, zone between *2* and *3*, as indicated. (*4*) The adverse development may finally result in epithelial activation and apoptosis, increased secretion of proinflammatory cytokines, chronic inflammation, apoptosis-resistant effector T cells, chronic inflammatory bowel disease (IBD), and tissue damage (*red panel* to the *right*)

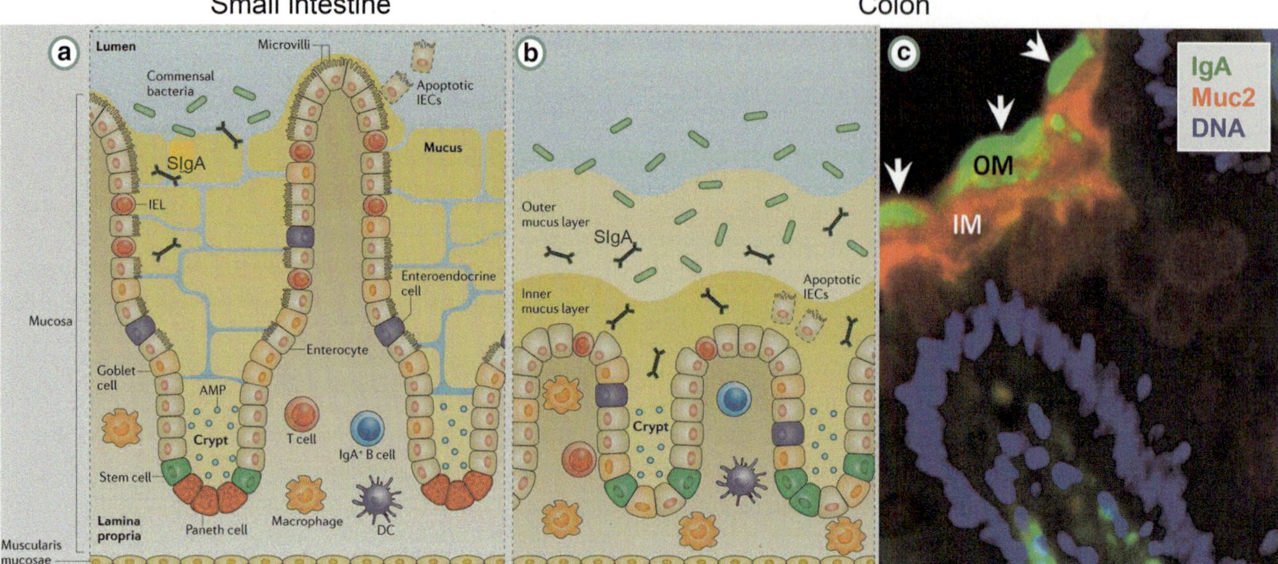

Fig. 2.14 Schematic depiction of the small intestine and colon with the varying distribution of mucus. (**a**, **b**) Intestinal epithelial cells are produced from stem cells near the bottom of the glands (named crypts) and move upwards to replace the loss of apoptotic cells. Stem cells also give rise to mucus-producing goblet cells, and to Paneth cells which move downwards to the bottom of the crypts and produce a variety of antimicrobial peptides (AMP). Intraepithelial lymphocytes (IEL) are more numerous in the small intestine than in the colon. The small intestine is covered by a loose layer of mucus whereas the colon has a compact inner layer and an outer loose layer where bacteria are retained. (**c**) Three-color immunofluorescence of a tissue section from the human colon, showing that IgA is concentrated in the outer mucus layer (OM) but hardly detectable in the inner mucus layer (IM). The cartoon on the *left* is adapted from Fig. 1 in Mowat and Agace [18] while the immunofluorescence illustration on the *right* is from Fig. 6 in Rogier et al. [159]

antimicrobial peptides such as REG3γ (Fig. 2.8) [156]. In the colon, however, the mucus coat is stratified, with a relatively compact inner layer ranging in thickness from 50 μm in the mouse to several hundred microns in humans (Fig. 2.14b) [157]. This layer normally resists microbial penetration although allowing diffusion of structural components of bacteria (e.g., MAMPs) and metabolic products such as SCFAs (Fig. 2.12). The outer mucus layer is much looser and contains a large number of bacteria which are retained there partly because of SIgA antibodies (Fig. 2.14c).

Rogier et al. [158] examined the role of mucus and SIgA in inhibiting translocation of bacteria from the gut lumen by exploiting knockout mice deficient in pIgR. *Pigr+/−* females were crossed with *Pigr−/−* males, and vice versa. Colonic lumens of newborn offspring of *Pigr−/−* dams were devoid of IgA, whereas offspring of *Pigr+/−* dams had abundant IgA in colonic lumens and feces. At weaning these levels dropped, reflecting the loss of maternal SIgA, but then at about 4 weeks began to increase in *Pigr+/−* offspring because of endogenous pIgR-mediated external transport of SIgA. Failure to receive maternal or endogenous SIgA resulted in translocation of aerobic bacteria into MLNs. Early exposure to SIgA in breast milk produced a gene expression pattern of epithelial cells different from that of mice not receiving SIgA, which mimicked that associated with IBD in humans. Also, maternal SIgA reduced colonic damage in a DSS-model of IBD. It was concluded that breastfeeding may promote life-long intestinal homeostasis.

In a different publication [159], the same authors found that SIgA co-localized with gut bacteria in the outer colonic mucus layer. By using mice deficient for pIgR and/or Muc2, they found that Muc2 plays a dominating role in excluding bacteria. Accordingly, mice deficient in Muc2 develop a spontaneous colonic inflammation similar to IBD in humans [160].

Interactions of SIgA with Commensal Bacteria

A great proportion of the commensal bacteria in the healthy human gut or at other mucosal surfaces are coated by IgA [161, 162], probably representing mainly low-affinity SIgA antibodies (Fig. 2.7). Such microbial–host interactions contain commensal bacteria in the mucus without eliminating them (Fig. 2.14). Thus, it has been shown in a murine infection model with *Salmonella typhimurium* that bacteria coated with innate-like, cross-reactive SIgA antibodies showed reduced shedding and less liability to horizontal spreading by the fecal–oral route [95, 110]. Mouse experiments have further documented that a gut IgA response to a single commensal microbial epitope (capsular polysaccharide A, PSA) can be immunomodulatory and protect against pathogen-induced colitis [48]. Germfree mice monocontaminated with the gut commensal *Bacteriodes thetaiotaomicron* demonstrated that specific SIgA antibodies directed against PSA in the gut inhibit activation of innate response markers such as oxidative burst and NFkB, thereby inducing crucial modulation of immune homeostasis as well as antigenic drift [163]. SIgA antibodies can hence control the intestinal microbiota in a non-inflammatory manner, promoting mutualism with the host [164].

Although mucosal IgA responses to commensal bacteria may be multicentered, of low affinity and diverse, oral immunization of mice with a cholera toxin-adjuvanted novel antigen was shown to result in a strong oligoclonal response of affinity-matured IgA$^+$ B cells [165]. Interestingly, it was found that the response was highly synchronized throughout the entire intestine by involving multiple Peyer's patches. Thus, by reutilizing already existing CGs, antigen-specific B cells would be subjected to clonal expansion and somatic hypermutation. This process was shown to require antigen recall by multiple immunizations, and the study helps to clarify mechanisms underlying the functional flexibility of mucosal antimicrobial IgA responses: from "natural" polyreactive (or cross-reactive) low-affinity to a specific high-affinity "classical" response (PB)—a distinction that is a major challenge to mucosal vaccine design [166].

The difficult issue of affinity maturation of mucosal B cells, and how the mucosal immune system can distinguish between the indigenous microbiota and overt exogenous pathogens, has been discussed in several articles [167–171]. The mucosal barrier and its reinforcement by SIgA, as well as the mucosal immunoregulatory network, require both adaptive and innate induction by antigens and conserved MAMPs—the latter activating germ line-encoded cellular PRRs such as TLRs [10, 11]. It is elusive how such receptors would be able to discriminate between signals provided by MAMPs from commensals and MAMPs from pathogens (previously called pathogen-associated molecular patterns, PAMPs); but this distinction is clearly required to elicit tolerogenic versus proinflammatory immune responses needed for protection against invasive infections (Fig. 2.15). Various scenarios may be visualized—the most likely being that overt pathogens, in addition to signaling through PRRs and B-cell receptors, exhibit special danger signals or immune evasion mechanisms related to the pathogenicity—that is, factors determining virulence and invasiveness [172–174], or the so-called effector-triggered immunity [175, 176], while competition for metabolically shared nutrients may also be involved [177, 178].

In human feces, some 40 % of the anaerobic bacteria are normally coated with IgA[162] and this phenomenon can be observed in early childhood [179]. Such IgA containment of commensals, without eliminating them, is probably important for the mutual host–microbe interaction, contributing to sustainable homeostasis by dampening proinflammatory

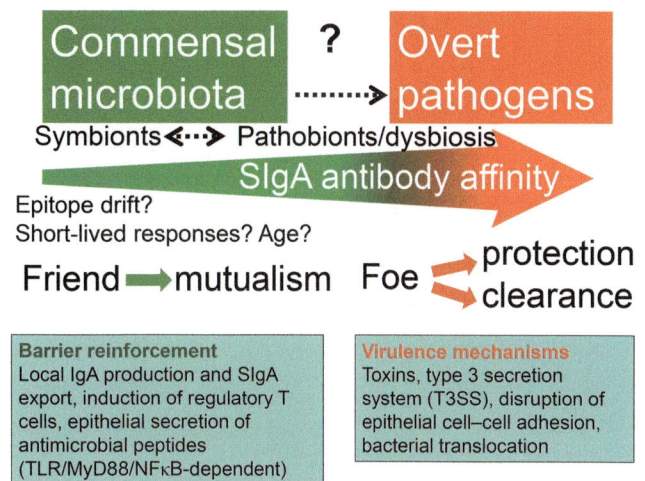

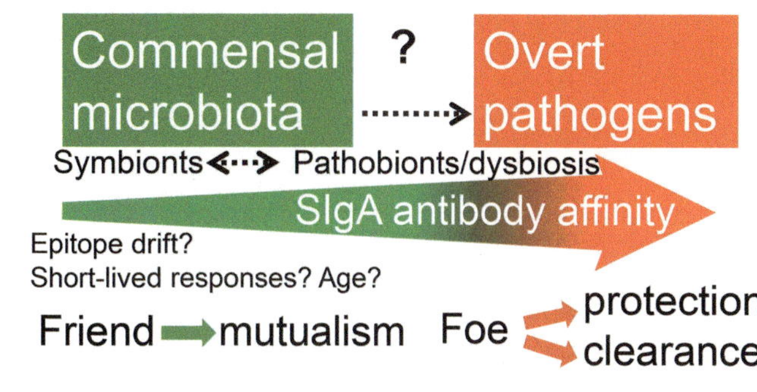

Fig. 2.15 Hypothetical depiction of how the intestinal immune system handles symbionts and potentially pathogenic residents (pathobionts) of the commensal microbiota versus overt exogenous pathogens. Secretory IgA (SIgA) antibody levels against commensal bacteria may go in waves because of epitope drift and shielding of gut-associated lymphoid tissue from antigen uptake. The overall affinity of SIgA antibodies probably increases with age and may be enhanced (or reduced?) against pathobionts during dysbiosis, and particularly raised by persistent stimulation with overt pathogens. One goal of mutualism with commensals is mucosal barrier reinforcement by mechanisms listed such as SIgA export and induction of regulatory T cells and antimicrobial peptides, whereas pathogens as exemplified in the *right panel* exhibit various virulence mechanisms to break the barrier. Adapted from Brandtzaeg [55]

signaling in the host and providing an immune pressure on commensal bacteria [178, 180]. This results in antigenic drift without altered composition of the microbiota, or the so-called dysbiosis [163, 181]. Most likely this IgA coat largely represents "natural" cross-reactive antibodies [20, 60] but may also depend on innate properties of SIgA, as discussed previously [3]. In mouse experiments with *Salmonella typhimurium* infection it was found that bacteria coated with such "natural" IgA showed reduced shedding and less liability to horizontal spreading by the fecal–oral route [110].

The IgA coating of gut bacteria in mice has been shown to be unrelated to the total amount of SIgA exported to the intestinal lumen, supporting that a specific reaction is involved [182]. Also, other mouse experiments demonstrated that the commensal coating with IgA in feces depended on appropriate clonal B-cell selection and affinity maturation in GCs of GALT, and perhaps to some extent also in the lamina propria [181]. This finding showed that the coating to a substantial degree reflects a specific IgA response. It has therefore been speculated that potentially pathogenic commensals (pathobionts) might show increased IgA coating in the gut lumen. This idea is supported by findings in patients with IBD, where there is dysbiosis [178, 183] and the fraction of anaerobic bacteria with IgA is raised to 65 %, with 45 % also

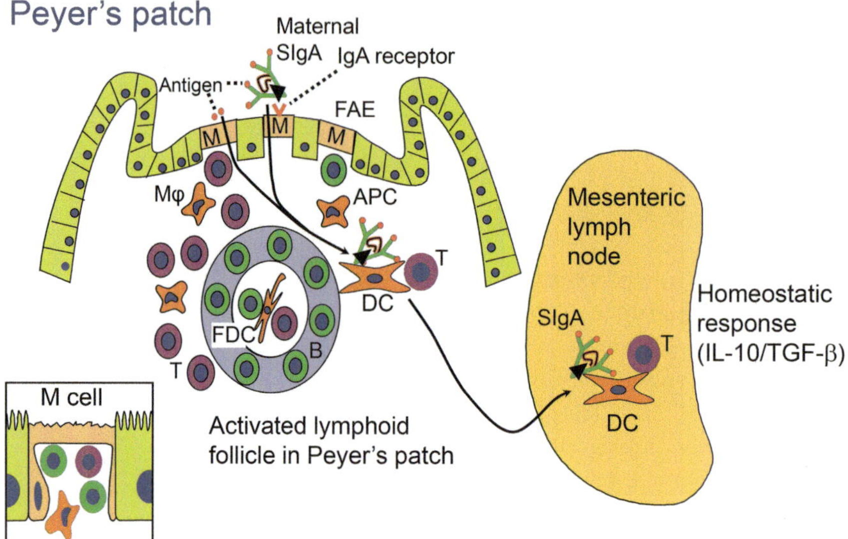

Fig. 2.16 Putative integration of the immune systems of mother and her breast-fed baby via M cell-mediated antigen uptake. Secretory IgA (SIgA) antibodies in breast milk may guide induction of the infant's intestinal immune system because M cells of Peyer's patches express receptor(s) for IgA. This as yet uncharacterized receptor may facilitate uptake of antigens that have formed immune complexes with cognate maternal SIgA antibodies in the gut lumen of the infant. The complexes may be further target to dendritic cells (DC) which carry them to mesenteric lymph nodes where a homeostatic immune response dominated by secretion of TGF-β and IL-10 is induced. Based on experimental data reviewed by Corthésy [3]. Details of M-cell pocket with its cellular content is schematically shown in the panel on the *left*. *FAE* follicle-associated epithelium, *Mφ* macrophage, *APC* antigen-presenting cell, *FDC* follicular DC, *TGF* transforming growth factor, *IL* interleukin

carrying IgG [184]. Thus, increased antibody coating could reflect dysbiosis (Fig. 2.15). However, in celiac disease, where there is also dysbiosis [185], the IgA coating of fecal bacteria is significantly reduced [179]. So the biological significance of this phenomenon remains uncertain, and the degree of IgA coating might reflect a combination of innate and specific bacterial binding properties of SIgA. In a recent study, however, it was suggested that high SIgA coating of certain commensals trapped in the mucus identified colitogenic bacteria able to drive colitis in a mouse model [186].

Altogether, SIgA does not seem to cause clearance of commensal bacteria, but controls in various ways their colonization and inhibits the penetration of agents that could potentially cause hypersensitivity reactions or infection [55]. In the absence of B cells, or when IgA is lacking, the intestinal epithelium of mice will, in response to commensal bacteria, upregulate its innate defense in an NFkB- and interferon-dependent manner [55, 180]; this could be at the expense of expression of genes that regulate fat and carbohydrate metabolism [187]. As a consequence, the epithelial gene signature might correlate with the development of lipid malabsorption [188]. The intestinal epithelial barrier is a cross-road between surface defense and nutrition, and SIgA is apparently essential to keep the balance between these two functions and thus maintain mucosal homeostasis.

Experimental studies have also revealed how intestinal homeostasis is mediated by host–microbe interactions in mice mono-colonized with the *Clostridia*-related segmented filamentous bacterium (SFB) which particularly grows in the distal ileum [189, 190]. SFB adheres to murine GALT structures and stimulate T-cell as well as IgA responses. Here a distinction is needed between murine B1 (T cell-independent) and B2 (T cell-dependent) responses when comparing these structures with the lamina propria; this distinction is as yet not clear [5, 36]. It is also possible that GALT may take up immune complexes containing SIgA bound to commensals via an as yet uncharacterized receptor for IgA on M cells and then induce a homeostatic response (Fig. 2.16). This mechanism was suggested to direct the opportunistic bacterium *Alcaligenes* into murine GALT and thereby make these tissue structures more resistant to pathogen invasion [191]. More recently it has been shown that goblet cells may also be involved in uptake of antigens from the gut lumen [192].

Role of IgA and Breastfeeding in Immune Control

The level of SIgA appears to contribute to an individual's threshold for hypersensitivity reactions to exogenous antigens [12]. Thus, the risk of contracting allergy seems increased when the development of the IgA system is retarded and the SIgA-dependent barrier function insufficient [193]. Minor dysregulations of both innate and adaptive immunity (especially IgA) have been observed in children with multiple food allergies [194]. These clinical observations are in accordance with the hyperreactivity (Fig. 2.9) and sensitivity to DSS-induced colitis seen in pIgR knockout mice [96].

It is therefore not surprising that exclusive breastfeeding up to the age of at least 4 months has an allergy-preventive effect, also in families without atopic heredity [195–197]. Moreover, having been breast-fed for at least 3 months protects against both Crohn's disease and ulcerative colitis in adulthood [198], and probably also against pediatric IBD [199]. Importantly, mothers with IBD receiving anti-inflammatory drugs can in most cases safely breastfeed their babies, and it may even provide a protective effect against disease flare [200–202].

In addition to the remarkable reinforcement of mucosal defense provided by maternal SIgA (and SIgM) antibodies as a natural immunological "substitution therapy," it is important to emphasize the positive nutritional effect of breastfeeding on immune development [193]. Mother's milk also contains a number of immune cells, cytokines, and growth factors that may exert a significant biological effect in the breast-fed infant's gut, apparently enhancing in an indirect way even the subsequent health of the individual [34, 193, 203]. Moreover, its high content of human-specific oligosaccharides serves as a prebiotic promoting the growth of lactic acid-producing bacteria and reducing anaerobic bacteria in the gut of breast-fed infants [193]. Probiotic bacteria can reportedly also occur in breast milk [204], perhaps after being transported to the mammary glands from the gut by DCs [205].

Numerous studies of the effect of breastfeeding on the development of secretory immunity have been performed with salivary IgA measurements as a readout system. Discrepant observations have been made and the influence of contaminating the sample with milk SIgA, shielding of the suckling's mucosal immune system by maternal SIgA antibodies, and altered growth and composition of the infant's gut microbiota have been discussed as possible uncontrollable variables. Moreover, several prospective studies have reported that the postnatal increase of salivary IgA (and IgM) initially is more prominent in formula-fed than in solely breast-fed infants [25].

Nevertheless, evidence suggests that breastfeeding promotes the development of secretory immunity over time [26, 193], apparently even at extraintestinal sites such as the urinary tract [203]. Thus, although breastfeeding initially may reduce the induction of SIgA, it appears later on in infancy (up to 8 months) to boost secretory immunity. As mentioned above, one possibility is that SIgA antibodies in mother's milk guide the uptake of cognate luminal antigens via receptor(s) for IgA on M cells (Fig. 2.16); as suggested by mouse experiments, the antigens may further be targeted to DCs which migrate to MLNs where they induce a homeostatic immune response [3].

Traces of exogenous antigen transferred into the milk of mothers may thus contribute to the induction of oral tolerance in the breast-fed infant; therefore, allergen avoidance during lactation is no longer recommended [12]. Various mouse models have indeed documented that antigen appears in the milk of exposed mothers and that it can induce Treg cells in the suckling neonate, either together with TGF-β or after complexing with IgG antibody and transfer by FcRn into gut mucosa [206, 207]. In human milk, maternal SIgA-containing immune complexes may perform a similar function (Fig. 2.16). Interestingly in this context, a review of TGF-β levels in human milk suggested that this cytokine protects against allergy in the breast-fed infants and young children [208]. It has also been reported that genes modulated during epithelial gut differentiation in the neonate, are differentially expressed in breast-fed and formula-fed infants [209]. It is unknown whether this was a direct effect of milk components or caused by differences in the microbiota of the two feeding groups.

Mucosal Homeostasis Versus Hypersensitivity

Oral Tolerance in Humans

It is believed that oral tolerance is largely explained by different T-cell events such as anergy, clonal deletion, and induction of Treg cells by conditioned APCs, although other regulatory principles may be involved [12, 26, 193, 210–212]. For ethical reasons, the existence of mucosally induced tolerance in human beings is supported mainly by circumstantial evidence. Thus, the gut mucosa of healthy individuals contains virtually no hyperactivated T cells and hardly any proinflammatory IgG production, and their serum levels of IgG antibodies to food antigens are low [193]. Moreover, the systemic IgG response to dietary antigens tends to decrease with increasing age [213, 214], and a hyporesponsive state to bovine serum albumin has been demonstrated by intradermal testing in adults [215]. Interestingly, nasal application or feeding of a novel antigen (keyhole limpet hemocyanin) in healthy people induced peripheral downregulation of T-cell immunity and, less consistently, also suppressed systemic antibody responses to subsequent parenteral immunization [216, 217]. By contrast, oral tolerance could not be induced in patients with IBD where the epithelial barrier is severely deteriorated and the immunogenetics favors mucosal inflammation [218, 219].

Mucosal Tolerance Induction

In healthy human gut mucosa, resident APCs are quite inert in terms of immune-productive stimulatory properties [220], and they hardly express detectable surface levels of TLR2 or TLR4 [221]. Also, only negligible expression of the LPS co-receptor CD14 is normally observed on these cells, and their proinflammatory cytokine response is usually low after LPS stimulation [113, 222]. Nevertheless, the phagocytic and bacteriocidal activity of mucosal macrophages is maintained [223], which would be important for silent clearance of commensal bacteria normally penetrating into the mucosa in small numbers [11, 20, 224].

These observations support the notion that both macrophages and DCs play a central role in oral tolerance [13], and most human intestinal APCs come from a common myeloid progenitor and often show an intermediate phenotype [225, 226]. Heterogeneity of murine lamina propria APCs has also been highlighted [227, 228]. In vivo observations in mice suggest that DC development from monocytes to the phenotype DC-SIGN/CD209$^+$ is a predominant pathway when abundant LPS is available [229], such as in the gut. The subepithelial band of monocyte-derived CD103$^-$CX3CR1$^+$ cells in the murine gut mucosa is indeed macrophage-like [226]. These cells express tight-junction proteins and can extend their dendrites into the lumen to sample antigens.

In a quiescent steady state, however, mucosal CD103$^+$CCR7$^+$ DCs (and possibly macrophages) are migratory and carry penetrating dietary and innocuous microbial antigens away from the gut mucosa after being transferred to them from CX3CR1$^+$ cells through gap junctions [33, 230–232]. This may be particularly relevant for the upper small intestine where the CD103$^+$ DCs end up in lymph nodes whose environment is different from that of MLNs in the more distal gut [18]. In the mucosa-draining lymph nodes a portion of the migrating CD103$^+$ DCs becomes conditioned for tolerance induction and drives the expansion of Treg cells [26]. It has been shown in humans that the tolerogenic properties of these DCs partly depends on expression of indoleamine 2,3-dioxygenase (IDO) [233]—an enzyme known to be involved in DC induction and function [234]. Hyperactivation of effector T cells in the intestinal mucosa with accompanying inflammation can thus be inhibited by this DC-dependent regulatory mechanism, both initially and subsequently. This is so because homeostatic control is also exerted when the generated Treg cells home from the lymph node to the lamina propria [12]—a homing that seems to be particularly active in infancy [235]. In the lamina propria the Treg cells are then expanded by IL-10 derived from macrophages [236].

A dietary effect on the induction of Treg cells is exerted through the conversion of vitamin A to RA by the enzyme RALDH, which is expressed both by intestinal DCs, macrophages, and epithelial cells [37, 227], as well as by MLN stromal cells [237]. In the upper part of the small bowel, retinoids from bile may exert an important enhancing effect [18, 238]. In a recent study RA signaling in B cells was, moreover, shown to be essential for their IgA response and for interacting with the microbiota [239]. The impact of bile retinoids on the mucosa of the upper small intestine may therefore be crucial for immune homeostasis in relation to both dietary and microbial antigens in that region.

Together with IL-2, TGF-β and IL-10, RA can drive induction of Treg cells [240–243]—which in the human periphery are heterogeneous and apparently may differentiate either by conversion from a naive (CD45RA$^+$) phenotype or from rapidly proliferating T cells with a memory/effector (CD45R0$^+$) phenotype with different migratory properties [244, 245]. It is the latter that expresses high levels of the transcription factor Foxp3 and seems to be actively suppressive [246].

Most information about Treg cells is necessarily derived from mouse experiments. Human Treg cells seem to be functionally and phenotypically more diverse than the murine counterparts, including the expression of the activation marker CD25 and the Foxp3 transcription factor [247]. There is also a need for better understanding for the functional stability and plasticity (e.g., acquisition of a Th17 phenotype) of Treg cells [248].

Recognition of Microbial Components

Final cellular conditioning for oral tolerance in MLNs appears to depend on appropriate stimulation of the migrating mucosal APCs by certain MAMPs derived from commensal bacteria (Fig. 2.17), which induce the signaling molecules and transcription factors dictating the differentiation pathways and cytokine profiles of the activated T cells [11, 12, 249]. Components of intestinal parasites such as helminths can exert similar immune modulation [10, 14, 250–252]—apparently to some extent through induction of Treg cells by mimicking the effect of TGF-β by ligation of its receptor [253]. Indeed, helminth-derived immunomodulators may be important in future medication for IBD [254]. Also of note, several studies suggest that LPS plays a central role in the early programing of the immune system [255, 256]; and there is an ongoing search to find out if hypersensitivity to exogenous factors is associated with hereditary single nucleotide mutations (polymorphism) in PRRs recognizing this and other MAMPs, such as CD14, TLR2, TLR4, and NOD [257, 258]. For instance, a proof of principle in Crohn's disease is the dose effect of mutations affecting the intraepithelial PRR function of the NOD2 (CARD15) gene encoded by the IBD susceptibility locus (IBD1) on chromosome 16 [259]. One of several putative pathogenic mechanisms is illustrated (Fig. 2.18) [260].

Altogether, the extended hygiene hypothesis implies that suboptimal PRR stimulation, with delayed maturation of the mucosal immune system with insufficient induction of Treg cells or other components of the mucosal barrier defense, contributes significantly to the increasing incidence of not only allergy—commonly reflecting overactivation of Th2 cells—but also other immune-mediated inflammatory disorders such as IBD—reflecting overactivation of Th1 or Th17 cells (Fig. 2.18). In the perspective of evolution, Th2 cells

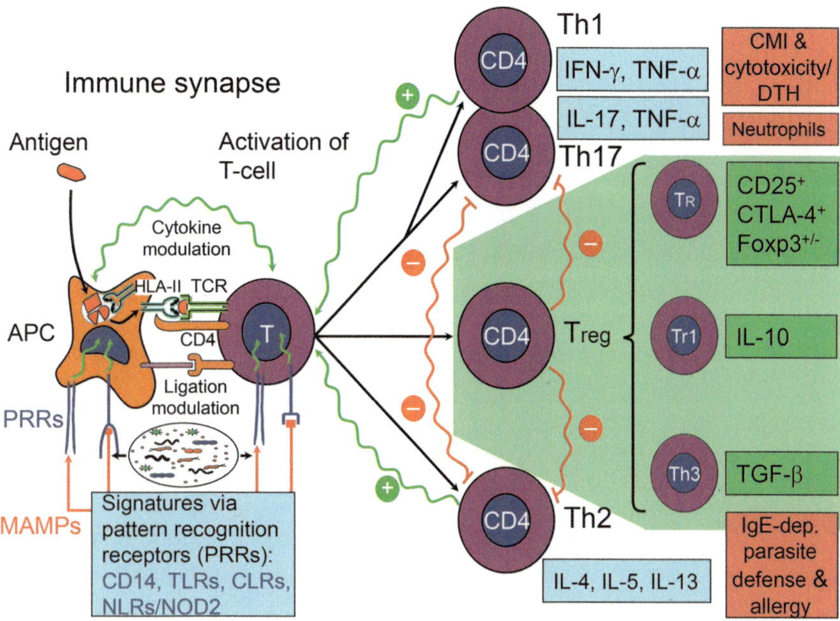

Fig. 2.17 Decision-making in the mucosal immune system is modulated by co-stimulatory signals (cytokines and ligands) operating in the synapse between antigen-presenting cell (APC) and T cell. Activation of CD4⁺ T cells occurs when APC takes up antigen and processes (degrades) it to immunogenic peptides for display to the T-cell receptor (TCR) in the polymorphic grove of HLA class II molecules (HLA-II). The level of co-stimulatory signals determines T-cell modulation (activation and conditioning). When CD4⁺ helper T (Th) cells are primed for productive immunity, they differentiate into Th1, Th17, or Th2 effector cells with polarized cytokine secretion (*blue panels* on the *right*). Such skewing of the adaptive immune response depends on the presence of microenvironmental factors, including cytokines, as well as signals from microbial components. Bacterial endotoxin (lipopolysaccharide), lipoproteins, unmethylated CpG DNA, and other conserved structural motifs are called microbe-associated molecular patterns (MAMPs); they are sensed by cellular pattern-recognition receptors (PRRs) such as CD14, toll-like receptors (TLRs), C-lectin receptors (CLRs), and NOD-like receptors (NLRs), including NOD2. Signaling from PRRs to the nucleus of APCs and T cells stimulates various degrees of activation and functional maturation of APCs and will thereby dictate differential expression of various co-stimulatory signals directing activation of either Th1 or Th17 or Th2 cells. Their cytokines induce various adaptive defense mechanisms or immunopathology (*red panels* on the *right*). The Th cytokine profiles are further promoted by the depicted positive and inhibitory feedback loops. Under certain conditions, rather immature but yet conditioned APCs may induce various subsets of regulatory T (Treg) cells as indicated in the light green area; by their cytokines IL-10 and TGF-β, or by interactions depending on CTLA-4 and the transcription factor Foxp3, the Treg cells can suppress Th1, Th17, and Th2 responses, including pathogenicity with detrimental innate immunity and inflammation (*red panels* on the *right*). CTLA-4, cytotoxic T-lymphocyte antigen 4; IFN, interferon; IL, interleukin; TGF, transforming growth factor; TNF, tumor necrosis factor. *CMI* cell-mediated immunity, *DTH* delayed-type hypersensitivity

have had a crucial role in host defense against parasites [261], whereas Th1 and Th17 cells are normally important for proper defense against infections [10, 14].

This basis for the hygiene hypothesis has been tested in several clinical studies evaluating the beneficial effect on immune homeostasis exerted by probiotic bacterial preparations derived from the commensal intestinal microbiota and eggs of the porcine helminth (whipworm) *Trichuris suis* [14, 252]. In this context, viable strains of lactobacilli and bifidobacteria have been reported to enhance IgA, both in humans and experimental animals, but these responses have not translated convincingly into clinical effects [262, 263]. To select the right probiotic strains, or symbiotic combinations with prebiotics or breast milk, remains a difficult task—and there are safety issues [264, 265]. Experimental studies have indicated that certain probiotic bacterial strains in fact may be proinflammatory while others may induce DCs, directly or via epithelial mediators, to exert anti-inflammatory effects [266].

It is unknown whether probiotics and prebiotics might work mainly through SIgA-mediated reinforcement of the barrier function, expansion of Treg cells, or the involvement of both these anti-inflammatory mechanism—perhaps combined with direct strengthening of epithelial integrity (Figs. 2.13 and 2.18). Notably, the most promising results have been reported for atopic eczema [262]. This skin disease is often seen in patients with IgE-mediated food allergy (20–40 %) and is particularly associated with loss-of-function mutations in the fillagrin gene, which is involved in the epidermal barrier function [267]. Similar mutations appear to predispose for the combination of atopic eczema and asthma [268]. These findings apparently reflect that a leaky surface epithelium anywhere in the body may be a predisposing condition for allergen penetration, and that food allergy could be a consequence rather than a cause of atopic eczema [12]. Therefore, the use of this disorder as a clinical readout of intervention effects on food allergy may not be scientifically acceptable.

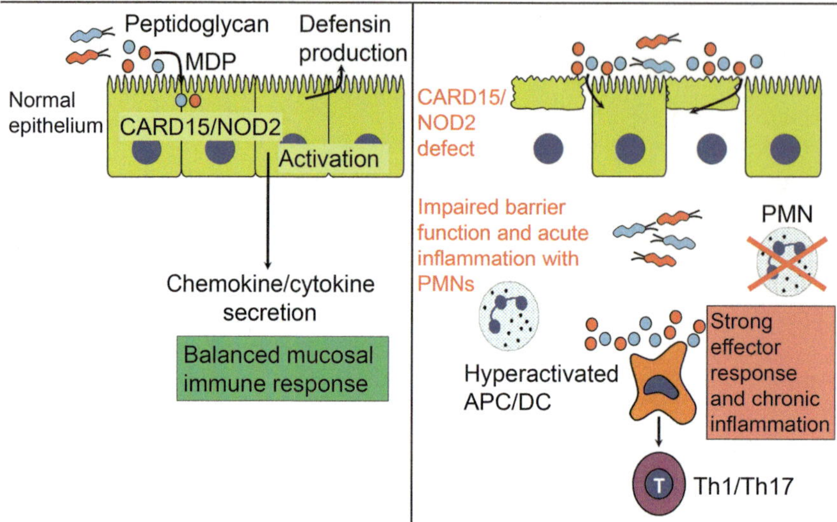

Fig. 2.18 Hypothetical model for the role of NOD2 (CARD15) in maintenance of intestinal mucosal homoeostasis (*left*), and how a defect in this susceptibility gene for Crohn's disease may impair the epithelial barrier function and lead to innate inflammation (*right*). Secretion of antimicrobial peptides, such as defensins from epithelial cells (particularly Paneth cells), depends on intracellular sensing of CARD15/NOD2 ligands, particularly the peptidoglycan muramyl dipeptide (MDP). Certain mutations in CARD15/NOD2 impair this defense function, leading to penetration of luminal antigens and bacteria which will result in acute inflammation with accumulation of polymorphonuclear granulocytes (PMN). However, when this innate response is defect, as seen in Crohn's disease, antigen-presenting cells (APC), such as dendritic cells (DC), will be hyperactivated, leading to a strong chronic effector response with stimulation of pathogenic Th1 and Th17 cells. Model based on an idea proposed by Marks et al. [265]

Innate Signals Dictating Homeostasis

Microorganisms have inhabited Earth for at least 2.5 billion years, and the power of the immune system is a result of coevolution in which especially commensal bacteria have shaped host defense in a state of mutualism [10, 14]. The prevailing mucosal homeostasis in the gut mucosa is indeed remarkable because of the large surface area to be defended—continuously being exposed to at least 1000 different bacterial species (Figs. 2.6 and 2.13). The gut microbiome is perhaps 100 times larger than the human genome [269]. In addition, the human gut harbors an unknown number of viruses [270]. Thus, while the intestine represents the largest exposure to microorganisms, it is also a major route of exposure to exogenous protein antigens (i.e., food) and micronutrients with immunomodulatory properties [12].

The original hygiene hypothesis postulated that the increasing incidence of allergy in westernized societies was explained by reduced or aberrant microbial exposure early in infancy, resulting in too little Th1-cell activity and therefore an insufficient IFN-γ level to downregulate optimally the prenatal Th2-cell responses which apparently can be ascribed to the cytokine thymic stromal lymphopoietin (TSLP) secreted by placental trophoblasts [271]. In this context, an appropriate postnatal encounter with a balanced commensal microbiota and exposure to foodborne and orofecal pathogens probably may exert an important homeostatic impact [272, 273], both by enhancing the SIgA-mediated barrier and promoting oral tolerance through a shift from a predominant Th2-cell activity in the newborn period [274]. The extended hygiene hypothesis postulates that induction of Treg cells is an important part of such microbe-driven homeostasis to avoid both allergy and other immune-mediated inflammatory disorders such as IBD [14].

Naturally occurring Treg cells with suppressive properties are present in large numbers in human fetal MLNs [275], probably as part of a peripheral tolerance to keep autoreactive effector T cells in check to avoid inflammation and tissue damage [243]. These Treg cells are apparently induced in the thymus and expanded in the periphery [276, 277]. After birth, the decision for induction of hyporesponsiveness against innocuous exogenous antigen, versus potentially harmful systemic-type productive immunity, may be largely instructed in mucosa-draining lymph nodes such as MLNs, as discussed above. In the distal part of the gut, the driving force in this homeostatic mechanism appears to be the microbial impact that conditions APCs and T cells for tolerance by balancing polarizing cytokines induced via PRRs (Fig. 2.17).

Thus, MAMPs do directly modulate not only the epithelial barrier function of neonates [103, 104] but also the activation profiles of innate and adaptive immune cells (Fig. 2.13). Appropriate balancing of the immune system appears to depend on a fine-tuned "cross talk" between APCs/innate immunity and T cells/adaptive immunity during certain windows of opportunity, particularly early in the newborn period [12, 14, 26], and probably even late in fetal life [278]. Concepts such as epigenetic programming in utero and subsequent epigenetic regulation are being considered as critical pathways through which environmental changes could alter expression of genes which lead to immune homeostasis or dysregulation [98], apparently also involving Treg cells and the Th1/Th17:Th2 balance [279, 280]. It is possible that opportunities for reprogramming may be a life-long process, thus explaining the late emergence of immune-mediated diseases in some individuals.

Effects of Genes Versus the Environment

The increasing incidence of immune-mediated diseases in affluent societies indicates that susceptibility genes for dysregulation are quite universal, such that they can be induced readily with environmental change. Epigenetics is an active research field providing novel understanding of how the environment can have heritable genomic effects and promote disease [98, 258, 280]. A number of early life exposures, including dietary nutrients and microbial exposure in utero, have been shown to have effects on gene expression with an impact on the clinical phenotype. For instance, mice born to dams exposed to bacteria during pregnancy experienced less allergy than those born to unexposed mothers, and maternal TLR signaling was needed for this transmission of protection [281]. Even the sensitivity of gut epithelial cells to LPS exposure via TLR4 may be subjected to epigenetic regulation [282].

However, the heredity of polygenic diseases is complex and the family history remains the best prediction of both allergy [283] and IBD [284]. Hopefully, the apparently inherent plasticity of the immune system may in the future provide opportunities for reprogramming to facilitate more effective prevention and treatment of these disorders. Thus, even APCs of adults can be conditioned to induce Treg cells by environmental factors such as LPS and cell wall lipids from parasites [285, 286]. Moreover, transient infestation with porcine helminths has been shown to have a beneficial effect on mucosal homeostasis in adult IBD patients [252], and the same has been shown in experimental models of allergy [251].

How Decisive Are Commensal Bacteria?

Commensal gut bacteria play a central role in the extended hygiene hypothesis. Thus, the intestinal microbiota of young children in Sweden was found to contain a relatively large number of *Clostridium* spp., whereas high levels of *Lactobacillus* spp. and *Eubacterium* spp. were detected in an age-matched population from Estonia [287]; this difference might contribute to the lower incidence of allergy in the Baltic countries compared with Scandinavia [288]. A Finnish study likewise reported that allergic infants had more Clostridia and tended to have fewer bifidobacteria in their stools than nonallergic controls [289].

Absence of early postnatal gut colonization with a normal commensal microbiota dominated by lactic acid-producing bacteria might likewise contribute to the increased risk for food allergy generally noted in children delivered by cesarean section, particularly when genetically predisposed [138, 139]. Nevertheless, in clinical studies it has been difficult to reveal a convincing effect on oral tolerance by probiotic perinatal intervention, even in children at high risk for food allergy [262]. The same conclusion was reached with regard to IgE-mediated allergy at the age of 5 years (including food allergy) after extending the postnatal intervention (four probiotic strains combined with prebiotics) until the age of 6 months, as observed in a Finnish study [290]. However, for children delivered by cesarean section a modest but significant allergy reduction was noted when they were randomized to the same regime [290]. Thus, there is hope for clinical benefits by balancing the colonization of the gut microbiota and inducing homeostatic immune regulation [12].

The feeding and treatment conditions (e.g., antibiotics) to which the newborn is subjected, and also the general nutritional state, may have an impact on the indigenous microbiota and on epithelial integrity; such variables may hence modulate the programming of the mucosal immune system [291, 292]. Intestinal colonization of lactobacilli and bifidobacteria is promoted by breast milk because it acts as prebiotics through its large amounts of human oligosaccharides [193, 292], and it may also contain probiotic gut bacteria [204, 293].

Cell culture studies have suggested that probiotics could be directly immunomodulatory by enhancing the Th1 profile via induction of IL-12, IL-18, and IFN-γ secretion [294, 295]. Also notably, *E. coli* is a strong inducer of IL-10 secretion, apparently derived both from APCs and Treg cells [244, 296]. Importantly, Treg cells bear PRRs for several MAMPs [297], and IL-10 is crucial for maintained expression of the Foxp3 transcription factor [298], which contributes significantly to the suppressive function of these cells [243]. IL-10 has been directly shown to be an important suppressive cytokine in the murine gut [299].

The above information collectively implies that the gut microbiota has an impact on mucosal homeostasis beyond that of enhancing the SIgA system, namely by promoting a balanced development of Th1, Th17, Th2, and Treg cells [262, 264]. As mentioned previously, however, the selection of safe and effective probiotic strains remains difficult.

It has been reported that murine colonic Treg cells are largely specific for antigens derived from commensal bacteria, suggesting that the Treg-cell repertoire is shaped significantly by the local antigenic environment in a process of peripheral education of the immune system [300]. Such extrathymic generation of Treg cells has also been observed in the gut of mice fed a soluble protein antigen; and there is apparently a reciprocal effect on preserving the composition of the gut microbiota, probably because the local induction of Treg cells maintains a healthy mucosa [301]. However, it remains unclear how DCs and T cells can integrate stimulation derived through a variety of their PRRs, although it has been shown that C-typ lectins with affinity for microbial or protein-associated carbohydrates may provide signals that skew the immune response towards being anti-inflammatory rather than proinflammatory [302, 303].

A prominent member of the gut microbiota in human infants, *Bifidobacterium infantis*, was after deliberate consumption in mice shown to markedly induce Foxp3$^+$ Treg cells [304]. Notably, neonatal CD4$^+$ T cells in mice are prone to differentiate into Treg cells following stimulation [100], as are human cord blood cells, probably as a result of perinatal exposure to maternal progesterone [305]. Later in development, members of the *Clostridium* cluster IV and XIVa might take over the role of *B. infantis* in promoting the local expansion of Treg cells in the colon [306]. The induced anti-inflammatory response could partially depend on release of TGF-β from IELs [307]. Also *Bacteroides fragilis* seems to have unique Treg cell-inducing and epithelium-associating properties.

Loss of Intestinal Immune Homeostasis in IBD

Alterations of Mucosal IgA and Epithelial Barrier Function

IBD lesions exhibit excessive numbers of IgA$^+$ and IgG$^+$ PCs with a remarkably skewing towards IgG production—depending on the severity of inflammation [308–310]. Initially, this shift from the normal pIgA predominance may be beneficial as a powerful second line of defense because IgG antibodies can efficiently mediate immune elimination of bacteria via phagocytosis and antibody-dependent cell-mediated cytotoxicity (Fig. 2.11). However, the chronicity of IBD signifies that a defective epithelial barrier over time results in severely altered mucosal homeostasis and (Fig. 2.13). Thus, whereas fluorescent in situ hybridization on tissue sections from normal colon reveals no microorganisms, 83 % of ulcerative colitis and 25 % of colonic Crohn's disease specimens show mucosal invasion of commensal bacteria [311]. In ulcerative colitis a proinflammatory antimicrobial response is additionally promoted by a significant shift towards the highly complement-activating IgG1 subclass [312]—apparently reflecting a genetic impact as revealed by comparing identical twins, healthy or afflicted with this IBD [313].

In parallel with the disproportionately increased IgG$^+$ PC subset, the J-chain expression is decreased in IBD lesions [309, 314] and there is a shift from the IgA2 to the less stable IgA1 subclass [309, 315]. Thus, more than 50 % of the IgA1$^+$ PCs are J chain-deficient, therefore producing monomers that cannot be exported by the pIgR [309, 316]. The same is true for a fraction (25–35 %) of the expanded IgA2$^+$ PC subset. These adverse alterations supposedly reflect a less restricted leukocyte extravasation due to a changed profile of adhesion molecules and chemokines on the mucosal microvascular endothelium (Fig. 2.5), allowing B cells expressing characteristics of systemic immunity to enter the lesion [308, 310].

A deficient epithelial barrier in IBD not only promotes bacterial invasion [311] but also increases food-antigen uptake and sensitization after rectal challenge, as shown in Crohn's disease [317]. This finding parallels with the increased mucosal leakiness of pIgR knockout mice (Fig. 2.9) [85, 86]. In addition, natural killer (NK) cells, which may exert cytotoxic and immunoregulatory functions, are located mainly in the epithelium and subepithelial lamina propria. It is known that considerable heterogeneity exists among NK cells, and subsets with variable expression levels of the classical CD56 marker have been identified Immature CD56$^+$ NK cells with abundant production of CXCL8 (IL-8) has also been reported and might depend on a particular maturational stage [318]. The best known function of CXCL8 is chemotactic activity on neutrophils in acute inflammation (Fig. 2.18), but this cytokine could also contribute to the growth of cells belonging to the NK-cell lineage. NK cells may, in addition, produce varying amounts of IL-22—a cytokine thought to be of importance for mucosal homeostasis [319, 320].

Conventional NK cells are now included in a complex group of lymphocytes referred to as innate lymphoid cells (ILCs) which are preferentially located at barrier surfaces and considered to be important for protection against pathogens [321, 322]. These lymphocytes do not rearrange their T-cell receptor, and include cells that behave similarly to Th cells by producing comparable cytokines. Thus, type 1 ILCs react with production of IFN-γ and TNF-α in response to IL-12 and IL-15; type 2 ILCs produce large amounts of IL-5 and IL-13 in response to IL-25 and IL-3, and are important in the protection against helminth infection; and type 3 ILCs are characterized by their abundant IL-22 production [323].

New members of ILCs are emerging. Thus, a novel subset involved in innate immunity against bacterial infections was recently described in mice and humans [324]. It expresses CD8a homodimers and was therefore called innate CD8a (iCD8a) cells. These cells were closely associated with the intestinal epithelium, apparently being involved in innate defense against bacterial infections. Notably, they were depleted in necrotizing enterocolitis of newborns. Moreover, there has been an increased interest in an innate-like T-cell subset referred to as "mucosal-associated invariant" (MAIT) [325]. Although their frequency and role remain largely unknown, MAIT cells accumulate in the intestinal lamina propria where exogenous microbes may gain access to the body.

Antibodies to Commensals and Abrogated Tolerance

Locally produced IgG in IBD lesions has been reported to react with cytoplasmic antigens from a range of gram-positive and gram-negative fecal bacteria, with higher activity in Crohn's disease than in ulcerative colitis, and higher in ulcerative colitis than in other types of intestinal inflammation [326]. Thus, nonspecific mucosal damage and bacterial invasion alone do not seem to explain the intensified local IgG response to commensals. Studies in rodents have shown that indigenous gut bacteria normally are poorly stimulatory for the systemic B-cell system [327, 328]. One explanation might be that the indigenous microbiota, while permanently colonizing the gut, induces waves of SIgA responses performing immune exclusion and thus being self-limiting [66]. Such intermittent immune exclusion could contribute to the hyporesponsiveness or apparent oral tolerance against gut commensals. This mechanism is clearly abrogated in IBD [218, 219], which agrees with several experimental models of intestinal inflammation in rodents [153]. Also, it has been shown that dysfunction in either the adaptive or innate mucosal immune system leads to systemic antibody hyperreactivity to the gut microbiota in mice [85, 86, 88, 329].

In human IBD break of tolerance to the commensal microbiota is suggested by increased in vivo antibody coating of gut bacteria. In healthy controls, approximately 40 % of fecal anaerobic bacteria are coated with IgA, 12 % with IgG and 12 % with IgM [162]. In IBD these figures are raised to 65 %, 45 % and 50 %, respectively [184]. This result parallels the markedly elevated mucosal Ig production in IBD [308, 309]—with the relative average increase being more prominent for IgG (×30) and IgM (×2.5) than for IgA (×1.7–2.0). In fact, adjacent to Crohn's ulcers the number of PCs is increased 100- to 200-fold for the IgG class and 8- to 12-fold for the IgM class, compared with 1.2- to 6.7-fold for the IgA class.

Based on analysis of serum antibodies, however, there seems to be considerable heterogeneity in microbial specificities among IBD patients; rather than a global loss of tolerance against the intestinal microbiota, individual subsets of patients with varying immune responses to selected bacterial antigens has been identified [330]. Whether this is the cause or the effect of a more restricted gut microbiota [164, 185]—with 25 % fewer bacterial genes than normal—is currently unknown [269]. Interestingly in this context, experimental colitis induced in a genetically manipulated mouse model can be transferred to healthy mice by a selected combination of commensal gut bacteria in the setting of a normal microbiota [331]. This result reflects the complexity of the microbial–microbial and the microbial–host interactions directing immune regulation in the gut [332].

Conclusions

A balanced indigenous microbiota is required to drive the normal development of both mucosa-associated lymphoid tissue, the epithelial barrier with its SIgA (and SIgM) system, and mucosally induced tolerance mechanisms—including the generation of Treg cells. Notably, pIgR/SC knockout mice that lack SIgA and SIgM antibodies show reduced epithelial barrier function and increased uptake of antigens from food and commensal bacteria (Fig. 2.9). They therefore have a hyperreactive immune system and show predisposition for systemic anaphylaxis after antigen sensitization; but this untoward development is counteracted by enhanced intestinal induction of cognate oral tolerance as a homeostatic backup mechanism.

A number of biological variables influence SIgA-dependent intestinal immunity and induction of oral tolerance. Increased epithelial permeability for exogenous antigens is clearly an important primary or secondary event in the pathogenesis of IBD (Fig. 2.3). The postnatal mucosal barrier function is determined by the individual's age (e.g., preterm versus term infant), genetics, mucus composition, interactions between mast cells, nerves and neuropeptides, concurrent infection, and the mucosa-shielding effect of SIgA provided by breast milk or produced in the infant's gut. The integrity of the epithelial barrier furthermore depends on homeostatic regulatory mechanisms, including mucosal induction of Treg cells, where commensal microbe–host interactions apparently play decisive roles as well as food antigens and retinoids such as vitamin A.

The incidence of both food allergy and IBD (especially Crohn's disease) is increased in IgA deficiency. As mentioned above, a defect gut barrier due to SIgA/SIgM deficiency leads to systemic hyperreactivity in an experimental mouse model but may at the same time enhance oral tolerance induction by cognate antigen in a delicate balance (Fig. 2.9). Boirivant et al. [333] likewise reported that a mild or transient breaching of zonula occludens in the intestinal epithelium of mice leads to a dominant anti-inflammatory Treg cell response. Also notable, children who have grown out of their cow's milk allergy, as revealed by oral challenge, show expansion of Treg cells in peripheral blood [334], perhaps reflecting that early infancy is the time when oral tolerance is best achieved. The relatively leaky gut epithelium probably promotes tolerance induced by continuous mucosal exposure to small amounts of luminal antigens, and the homeostatic balance might be enhanced by cognate SIgA antibodies (Fig. 2.16). Therefore, it is not surprising that epidemiological reports suggest that breastfeeding protects against food allergy and IBD. The remarkable output of SIgA during feeding represents an optimally targeted passive immunization of the breast-fed infant's gut, and might serve as a positive homeostatic feedback loop [34].

Altogether, the secretory immune system is critical for the mucosal barrier function because SIgA not only forms the first line of defense but also maintains mutualism with the indigenous microbiota. Notably, the epithelial barrier in the distal gut depends on exposure to components from the complex commensal microbiota (MAMPs) and the environment, both by direct interaction with PRRs of the intestinal epithelium (Figs. 2.12 and 2.18) and induction of oral tolerance via mechanisms such as tolerogenic APCs and Treg cells (Figs. 2.13 and 2.17). It has therefore been proposed that the hygiene hypothesis as an explanation of the increase of immune-mediated disease in affluent societies instead should be called the "microbial deprivation hypothesis" [15]. In mouse experiments it has indeed been shown that a single immunomodulatory molecule from a commensal gut bacterium can induce crucial modulation and homeostasis of the host's immune system [163]. This gives hope for future therapeutic manipulation of the intestinal immune system of patients suffering from IBD.

Acknowledgments Hege Eliassen is thanked for excellent secretarial assistance. The author is supported by the Research Council of Norway through its Centers of Excellence funding scheme (Project No. 179573/V40), and by the Department of Pathology, Oslo University Hospital.

References

1. Brandtzaeg P. Mucosal immunity: induction, dissemination, and effector functions. Scand J Immunol. 2009;70:505–15.
2. Brandtzaeg P. The mucosal B-cell system. In: Mestecky J, Strober W, Russell MW, Kelsall BL, Cheroutre H, Lambrecht BN, editors. Mucosal immunology. 4th ed. Amsterdam: Academic Press/Elsevier; 2015. p. 623–81. Chapter 31.
3. Corthésy B. Role of secretory immunoglobulin A and secretory component in the protection of mucosal surfaces. Future Microbiol. 2010;5:817–29.
4. Brandtzaeg P. Induction of secretory immunity and memory at mucosal surfaces. Vaccine. 2007;25:5467–84.
5. Brandtzaeg P. Functions of mucosa-associated lymphoid tissue in antibody formation. Immunol Invest. 2010;39:303–55.
6. Brandtzaeg P, Halstensen TS, Kett K, Krajci P, Kvale D, Rognum TO, et al. Immunobiology and immunopathology of human gut mucosa: humoral immunity and intraepithelial lymphocytes. Gastroenterology. 1989;97:1562–84.
7. Brandtzaeg P. History of oral tolerance and mucosal immunity. Ann N Y Acad Sci. 1996;778:1–27.
8. Turner JR. Intestinal mucosal barrier function in health and disease. Nat Rev Immunol. 2009;9:799–809.
9. Lin X, Chen M, Liu Y, Guo Z, He X, Brand D, et al. Advances in distinguishing natural from induced Foxp3$^+$ regulatory T cells. Int J Clin Exp Pathol. 2013;6:116–23.
10. Neish AS. Microbes in gastrointestinal health and disease. Gastroenterology. 2009;136:65–80.
11. Hooper LV, Macpherson AJ. Immune adaptations that maintain homeostasis with the intestinal microbiota. Nat Rev Immunol. 2010;10:159–69.
12. Brandtzaeg P. Food allergy: separating the science from the mythology. Nat Rev Gastroenterol Hepatol. 2010;7:380–400.
13. Bach JF. The effect of infections on susceptibility to autoimmune and allergic diseases. N Engl J Med. 2002;347:911–20.
14. Guarner F, Bourdet-Sicard R, Brandtzaeg P, Gill HS, McGuirk P, van Eden W, et al. Mechanisms of disease: the hygiene hypothesis revisited. Nat Clin Pract Gastroenterol Hepatol. 2006;3:275–84.
15. Björkstén B. The hygiene hypothesis: do we still believe in it? In: Brandtzaeg P, Isolauri E, Prescott SL, editors. Microbial–host interaction: tolerance versus allergy. Nestlé nutr. workshop ser. pediatr. program, vol 64. Basel: Nestec Ltd., Vevey/S, Karger AG; 2009. p. 11–22.
16. Vickery BP, Burks AW. Immunotherapy in the treatment of food allergy: focus on oral tolerance. Curr Opin Allergy Clin Immunol. 2009;9:364–70.
17. von Hertzen LC, Savolainen J, Hannuksela M, Klaukka T, Lauerma A, Mäkelä MJ, et al. Scientific rationale for the Finnish Allergy Programme 2008–2018: emphasis on prevention and endorsing tolerance. Allergy. 2009;64:678–701.
18. Mowat AM, Agace WW. Regional specialization within the intestinal immune system. Nat Rev Immunol. 2014;14:667–85. doi:10.1038/nri3738.
19. Pelaseyed T, Bergström JH, Gustafsson JK, Ermund A, Birchenough GM, Schütte A, et al. The mucus and mucins of the goblet cells and enterocytes provide the first defense line of the gastrointestinal tract and interact with the immune system. Immunol Rev. 2014;260:8–20. doi:10.1111/imr.12182.
20. Macpherson AJ, Geuking MB, McCoy KD. Immune responses that adapt the intestinal mucosa to commensal intestinal bacteria. Immunology. 2005;115:153–62.
21. Konrad A, Cong Y, Duck W, Borlaza R, Elson CO. Tight mucosal compartmentation of the murine immune response to antigens of the enteric microbiota. Gastroenterology. 2006;130:2050–9.
22. Duerkop BA, Vaishnava S, Hooper LV. Immune responses to the microbiota at the intestinal mucosal surface. Immunity. 2009;31:368–76.
23. Brandtzaeg P. Mechanisms of gastrointestinal reactions to food. Environ Toxicol Pharmacol. 1997;4:9–24.
24. Scurlock AM, Burks AW, Jones SM. Oral immunotherapy for food allergy. Curr Allergy Asthma Rep. 2009;9:186–93.
25. Brandtzaeg P, Nilssen DE, Rognum TO, Thrane PS. Ontogeny of the mucosal immune system and IgA deficiency. Gastroenterol Clin North Am. 1991;20:397–439.
26. Brandtzaeg P. Development and basic mechanisms of human gut immunity. Nutr Rev. 1998;56:S5–18.
27. Neish AS. Mucosal immunity and the microbiome. Ann Am Thorac Soc. 2014;11 Suppl 1:S28–32. doi:10.1513/AnnalsATS.201306-161MG.
28. Brandtzaeg P, Johansen F-E. Mucosal B cells: phenotypic characteristics, transcriptional regulation, and homing properties. Immunol Rev. 2005;206:32–63.
29. Renz H, Brandtzaeg P, Hornef M. The impact of perinatal immune development on mucosal homeostasis and chronic inflammation. Nat Rev Immunol. 2011;12:9–23. doi:10.1038/nri3112.
30. van de Pavert SA, Mebius RE. New insights into the development of lymphoid tissues. Nat Rev Immunol. 2010;10:664–74.
31. Neutra MR, Mantis NJ, Kraehenbuhl JP. Collaboration of epithelial cells with organized mucosal lymphoid tissues. Nat Immunol. 2001;2:1004–9.
32. Kraus TA, Brimnes J, Muong C, Liu JH, Moran TM, Tappenden KA, et al. Induction of mucosal tolerance in Peyer's patch-deficient, ligated small bowel loops. J Clin Invest. 2005;115:2234–43.
33. Worbs T, Bode U, Yan S, Hoffmann MW, Hintzen G, Bernhardt G, et al. Oral tolerance originates in the intestinal immune system and relies on antigen carriage by dendritic cells. J Exp Med. 2006;203:519–27.
34. Brandtzaeg P. The mucosal immune system and its integration of the mammary glands. J Pediatr. 2010;156 Suppl 1:S8–15.

35. Mora JR, Iwata M, von Andrian UH. Vitamin effects on the immune system: vitamins A and D take centre stage. Nat Rev Immunol. 2008;8:685–98.
36. Tsuji M, Komatsu N, Kawamoto S, Suzuki K, Kanagawa O, Honjo T, et al. Preferential generation of follicular B helper T cells from Foxp3+ T cells in gut Peyer's patches. Science. 2009;323:1488–92.
37. Hirota K, Turner JE, Villa M, Duarte JH, Demengeot J, Steinmetz OM, et al. Plasticity of Th17 cells in Peyer's patches is responsible for the induction of T cell-dependent IgA responses. Nat Immunol. 2013;14:372–9. doi:10.1038/ni.2552.
38. Kato LM, Kawamoto S, Maruya M, Fagarasan S. Gut TFH and IgA: key players for regulation of bacterial communities and immune homeostasis. Immunol Cell Biol. 2014;92:49–56. doi:10.1038/icb.2013.54.
39. Endsley MA, Njongmeta LM, Shell E, Ryan MW, Indrikovs AJ, Ulualp S, et al. Human IgA-inducing protein from dendritic cells induces IgA production by naive IgD+ B cells. J Immunol. 2009;182:1854–9.
40. Johansen F-E, Brandtzaeg P. Transcriptional regulation of the mucosal IgA system. Trends Immunol. 2004;25:150–7.
41. Yamanaka T, Helgeland L, Farstad IN, Fukushima H, Midtvedt T, Brandtzaeg P. Microbial colonization drives lymphocyte accumulation and differentiation in the follicle-associated epithelium of Peyer's patches. J Immunol. 2003;170:816–22.
42. Round JL, Mazmanian SK. The gut microbiota shapes intestinal immune responses during health and disease. Nat Rev Immunol. 2009;9:313–23. Erratum in: Nat Rev Immunol. 2009;9:600.
43. Menezes JS, Mucida DS, Cara DC, Alvarez-Leite JI, Russo M, Vaz NM, et al. Stimulation by food proteins plays a critical role in the maturation of the immune system. Int Immunol. 2003;15:447–55.
44. Barone F, Patel P, Sanderson JD, Spencer J. Gut-associated lymphoid tissue contains the molecular machinery to support T-cell-dependent and T-cell-independent class switch recombination. Mucosal Immunol. 2009;2:495–503.
45. Barone F, Vossenkamper A, Boursier L, Su W, Watson A, John S, et al. IgA-producing plasma cells originate from germinal centers that are induced by B-cell receptor engagement in humans. Gastroenterology. 2011;140:947–56. doi:10.1053/j.gastro.2010.12.005.
46. Cerutti A, Rescigno M. The biology of intestinal immunoglobulin A responses. Immunity. 2008;28:740–50.
47. Lin M, Du L, Brandtzaeg P, Pan-Hammarström Q. IgA subclass switch recombination in human mucosal and systemic immune compartments. Mucosal Immunol. 2014;7:511–20. doi:10.1038/mi.2013.68.
48. Rangel-Moreno J, Moyron-Quiroz JE, Carragher DM, Kusser K, Hartson L, Moquin A, et al. Omental milky spots develop in the absence of lymphoid tissue-inducer cells and support B and T cell responses to peritoneal antigens. Immunity. 2009;30:731–43.
49. Brandtzaeg P, Baekkevold ES, Morton HC. From B to A the mucosal way. Nat Immunol. 2001;2:1093–4.
50. Brandtzaeg P, Pabst R. Let's go mucosal: communication on slippery ground. Trends Immunol. 2004;25:570–7.
51. Bergqvist P, Stensson A, Lycke NY, Bemark M. T cell-independent IgA class switch recombination is restricted to the GALT and occurs prior to manifest germinal center formation. J Immunol. 2010;184:3545–53.
52. Tsuji M, Suzuki K, Kitamura H, Maruya M, Kinoshita K, Ivanov II, et al. Requirement for lymphoid tissue-inducer cells in isolated follicle formation and T cell-independent immunoglobulin A generation in the gut. Immunity. 2008;29:261–71.
53. Huard B, McKee T, Bosshard C, Durual S, Matthes T, Myit S, et al. APRIL secreted by neutrophils binds to heparan sulfate proteoglycans to create plasma cell niches in human mucosa. J Clin Invest. 2008;118:2887–95.
54. Brandtzaeg P, Farstad IN, Helgeland L. Phenotypes of T cells in the gut. Chem Immunol. 1998;71:1–26.
55. Brandtzaeg P. Gate-keeper function of the intestinal epithelium. Benef Microbes. 2013;4:67–82. doi:10.3920/BM2012.0024.
56. Stoll BJ, Lee FK, Hale E, Schwartz D, Holmes R, Ashby R, et al. Immunoglobulin secretion by the normal and the infected newborn infant. J Pediatr. 1993;122:780–6.
57. Nahmias A, Stoll B, Hale E, Ibegbu C, Keyserling H, Innis-Whitehouse W, et al. IgA-secreting cells in the blood of premature and term infants: normal development and effect of intrauterine infections. Adv Exp Med Biol. 1991;310:59–69.
58. Siegrist CA, Aspinall R. B-cell responses to vaccination at the extremes of age. Nat Rev Immunol. 2009;9:185–94.
59. Crabbé PA, Nash DR, Bazin H, Eyssen H, Heremans JF. Immunohistochemical observations on lymphoid tissues from conventional and germ-free mice. Lab Invest. 1970;22:448–57.
60. Macpherson AJ, Harris NL. Interactions between commensal intestinal bacteria and the immune system. Nat Rev Immunol. 2004;4:478–85.
61. Lodinová R, Jouja V, Wagner V. Serum immunoglobulins and coproantibody formation in infants after artificial intestinal colonization with *Escherichia coli* 083 and oral lysozyme administration. Pediatr Res. 1973;7:659–69.
62. Moreau MC, Ducluzeau R, Guy-Grand D, Muller MC. Increase in the population of duodenal immunoglobulin A plasmocytes in axenic mice associated with different living or dead bacterial strains of intestinal origin. Infect Immun. 1978;21:532–9.
63. Chung H, Pamp SJ, Hill JA, Surana NK, Edelman SM, Troy EB, et al. Gut immune maturation depends on colonization with a host-specific microbiota. Cell. 2012;149:1578–93. doi:10.1016/j.cell.2012.04.037.
64. Holt PG, Jones CA. The development of the immune system during pregnancy and early life. Allergy. 2000;55:688–97.
65. Ridge JP, Fuchs EJ, Matzinger P. Neonatal tolerance revisited: turning on newborn T cells with dendritic cells. Science. 1996;271:1723–6.
66. Shroff KE, Meslin K, Cebra JJ. Commensal enteric bacteria engender a self-limiting humoral mucosal immune response while permanently colonizing the gut. Infect Immun. 1995;63:3904–13.
67. Hapfelmeier S, Lawson MA, Slack E, Kirundi JK, Stoel M, Heikenwalder M, et al. Reversible microbial colonization of germ-free mice reveals the dynamics of IgA immune responses. Science. 2010;328:1705–9.
68. Brandtzaeg P, Prydz H. Direct evidence for an integrated function of J chain and secretory component in epithelial transport of immunoglobulin. Nature. 1984;311:71–3.
69. Johansen F-E, Braathen R, Brandtzaeg P. The J chain is essential for polymeric Ig receptor-mediated epithelial transport of IgA. J Immunol. 2001;167:5185–92.
70. Brandtzaeg P, Kiyono H, Pabst R, Russell MW. Terminology: nomenclature of mucosa-associated lymphoid tissue. Mucosal Immunol. 2008;1:31–7.
71. Brandtzaeg P. Human secretory immunoglobulin M. An immunochemical and immunohistochemical study. Immunology. 1975;29:559–70.
72. Braathen R, Hohman VS, Brandtzaeg P, Johansen F-E. Secretory antibody formation: conserved binding interactions between J chain and polymeric Ig receptor from humans and amphibians. J Immunol. 2007;178:1589–97.
73. Bollinger RR, Everett ML, Wahl SD, Lee YH, Orndorff PE, Parker W. Secretory IgA and mucin-mediated biofilm formation by environmental strains of *Escherichia coli*: role of type 1 pili. Mol Immunol. 2006;43:378–87.
74. Persson CG, Gustafsson B, Erjefält JS, Sundler F. Mucosal exudation of plasma is a noninjurious intestinal defense mechanism. Allergy. 1993;48:581–6.

75. Kuo TT, Baker K, Yoshida M, Qiao SW, Aveson VG, Lencer WI, et al. Neonatal Fc receptor: from immunity to therapeutics. J Clin Immunol. 2010;30:777–89.
76. Bouvet JP, Pires R, Iscaki S, Pillot J. Nonimmune macromolecular complexes of Ig in human gut lumen. Probable enhancement of antibody functions. J Immunol. 1993;151:2562–71.
77. Mellander L, Carlsson B, Jalil F, Söderström T, Hanson LA, Carlsson B, et al. Secretory IgA antibody response against *Escherichia coli* antigens in infants in relation to exposure. J Pediatr. 1985;107:430–3.
78. Martino DJ, Currie H, Taylor A, Conway P, Prescott SL. Relationship between early intestinal colonization, mucosal immunoglobulin A production and systemic immune development. Clin Exp Allergy. 2008;38:69–78.
79. Kukkonen K, Kuitunen M, Haahtela T, Korpela R, Poussa T, Savilahti E. High intestinal IgA associates with reduced risk of IgE-associated allergic diseases. Pediatr Allergy Immunol. 2010;21(1 Pt 1):67–73.
80. Sjögren YM, Tomicic S, Lundberg A, Böttcher MF, Björkstén B, Sverremark-Ekström E, et al. Influence of early gut microbiota on the maturation of childhood mucosal and systemic immune responses. Clin Exp Allergy. 2009;39:1842–51.
81. Ismail AS, Severson KM, Vaishnava S, Behrendt CL, Yu X, Benjamin JL, et al. Gammadelta intraepithelial lymphocytes are essential mediators of host-microbial homeostasis at the intestinal mucosal surface. Proc Natl Acad Sci U S A. 2011;108:8743–8. doi:10.1073/pnas.1019574108.
82. Smith PM, Garrett WS. The gut microbiota and mucosal T cells. Front Microbiol. 2011;2:111. doi:10.3389/fmicb.2011.00111.
83. Nilssen DE, Brandtzaeg P. Intraepithelial γδ T cells remain increased in the duodenum of AIDS patients despite antiretroviral treatment. PLoS One. 2012;7:e29066. doi:10.1371/journal.pone.0029066.
84. van Elburg RM, Uil JJ, de Monchy JG, Heymans HS. Intestinal permeability in pediatric gastroenterology. Scand J Gastroenterol. 1992;194(Suppl):19–24.
85. Johansen F-E, Pekna M, Norderhaug IN, Haneberg B, Hietala MA, Krajci P, et al. Absence of epithelial immunoglobulin A transport, with increased mucosal leakiness, in polymeric immunoglobulin receptor/secretory component-deficient mice. J Exp Med. 1999;190:915–21.
86. Sait LC, Galic M, Price JD, Simpfendorfer KR, Diavatopoulos DA, Uren TK, et al. Secretory antibodies reduce systemic antibody responses against the gastrointestinal commensal flora. Int Immunol. 2007;19:257–65.
87. Johansson ME, Larsson JM, Hansson GC. The two mucus layers of colon are organized by the MUC2 mucin, whereas the outer layer is a legislator of host-microbial interactions. Proc Natl Acad Sci U S A. 2011;108 Suppl 1:4659–65. doi:10.1073/pnas.1006451107.77.
88. Karlsson MR, Johansen FE, Kahu H, Macpherson A, Brandtzaeg P. Hypersensitivity and oral tolerance in the absence of a secretory immune system. Allergy. 2010;65:561–70.
89. Janzi M, Kull I, Sjöberg R, Wan J, Melén E, Bayat N, et al. Selective IgA deficiency in early life: association to infections and allergic diseases during childhood. Clin Immunol. 2009;133:78–85.
90. Brandtzaeg P, Karlsson G, Hansson G, Petruson B, Björkander J, Hanson LA. The clinical condition of IgA-deficient patients is related to the proportion of IgD- and IgM-producing cells in their nasal mucosa. Clin Exp Immunol. 1987;67:626–36.
91. McLoughlin GA, Hede JE, Temple JG, Bradley J, Chapman DM, McFarland J. The role of IgA in the prevention of bacterial colonization of the jejunum in the vagotomized subject. Br J Surg. 1978;65:435–7.
92. Ludvigsson JF, Neovius M, Hammarström L. Association between IgA deficiency & other autoimmune conditions: a population-based matched cohort study. J Clin Immunol. 2014;34:444–51. doi:10.1007/s10875-014-0009-4.
93. Fagarasan S, Muramatsu M, Suzuki K, et al. Critical roles of activation-induced cytidine deaminase in the homeostasis of gut flora. Science. 2002;298:1424–7.
94. Carlsen HS, Baekkevold ES, Johansen F-E, et al. B cell attracting chemokine 1 (CXCL13) and its receptor CXCR5 are expressed in normal and aberrant gut associated lymphoid tissue. Gut. 2002;51:364–71.
95. Strugnell RA, Wijburg OL. The role of secretory antibodies in infection immunity. Nat Rev Microbiol. 2010;8:656–67.
96. Murthy AK, Dubose CN, Banas JA, et al. Contribution of polymeric immunoglobulin receptor to regulation of intestinal inflammation in dextran sulfate sodium-induced colitis. J Gastroenterol Hepatol. 2006;21:1372–80.
97. Smith M, Tourigny MR, Noakes P, Thornton CA, Tulic MK, Prescott SL. Children with egg allergy have evidence of reduced neonatal $CD4^+CD25^+CD127^{lo/-}$ regulatory T cell function. J Allergy Clin Immunol. 2008;121:1460–6. 466.e1–7.
98. Martino DJ, Prescott SL. Silent mysteries: epigenetic paradigms could hold the key to conquering the epidemic of allergy and immune disease. Allergy. 2009;65:1–15.
99. Haddeland U, Karstensen AB, Farkas L, Bø KO, Pirhonen J, Karlsson M, et al. Putative regulatory T cells are impaired in cord blood from neonates with hereditary allergy risk. Pediatr Allergy Immunol. 2005;16:104–12.
100. Wang G, Miyahara Y, Guo Z, Khattar M, Stepkowski SM, Chen W. "Default" generation of neonatal regulatory T cells. J Immunol. 2010;185:71–8.
101. Artis D. Epithelial-cell recognition of commensal bacteria and maintenance of immune homeostasis in the gut. Nat Rev Immunol. 2008;8:411–20.
102. Cario E. Heads up! How the intestinal epithelium safeguards mucosal barrier immunity through the inflammasome and beyond. Curr Opin Gastroenterol. 2010;26:583–90.
103. Lotz M, Gütle D, Walther S, Ménard S, Bogdan C, Hornef MW. Postnatal acquisition of endotoxin tolerance in intestinal epithelial cells. J Exp Med. 2006;203:973–84.
104. Pott J, Hornef M. Innate immune signalling at the intestinal epithelium in homeostasis and disease. EMBO Rep. 2012;13:684–98. doi:10.1038/embor.2012.96.
105. Russell MW, Reinholdt J, Kilian M. Anti-inflammatory activity of human IgA antibodies and their Fab α fragments: inhibition of IgG-mediated complement activation. Eur J Immunol. 1989;19:2243–9.
106. Brandtzaeg P, Tolo K. Mucosal penetrability enhanced by serum-derived antibodies. Nature. 1977;266:262–3.
107. Mazanec MB, Nedrud JG, Kaetzel CS, et al. A three-tiered view of the role of IgA in mucosal defense. Immunol Today. 1993;14:430–5.
108. Robinson JK, Blanchard TG, Levine AD, et al. A mucosal IgA-mediated excretory immune system in vivo. J Immunol. 2001;166:3688–92.
109. Di Niro R, Mesin L, Raki M, Zheng NY, Lund-Johansen F, Lundin KE, et al. Rapid generation of rotavirus-specific human monoclonal antibodies from small-intestinal mucosa. J Immunol. 2010;185:5377–83.
110. Wijburg OL, Uren TK, Simpfendorfer K, Johansen FE, Brandtzaeg P, Strugnell RA. Innate secretory antibodies protect against natural Salmonella typhimurium infection. J Exp Med. 2006;203:21–6.
111. van der Steen L, Tuk CW, Bakema JE, Kooij G, Reijerkerk A, Vidarsson G, et al. Immunoglobulin A: Fc(alpha)RI interactions induce neutrophil migration through release of leukotriene B4. Gastroenterology. 2009;137:2018–29.e1–3.
112. Wolf HM, Fischer MB, Puhringer H, et al. Human serum IgA downregulates the release of inflammatory cytokines (tumor necrosis factor-α, interleukin-6) in human monocytes. Blood. 1994;83:1278–88.

113. Smith PD, Smythies LE, Mosteller-Barnum M, et al. Intestinal macrophages lack CD14 and CD89 and consequently are down-regulated for LPS- and IgA-mediated activities. J Immunol. 2001;167:2651–6.
114. Hamre R, Farstad IN, Brandtzaeg P, Morton HC. Expression and modulation of the human immunoglobulin A Fc receptor (CD89) and the FcR gamma chain on myeloid cells in blood and tissue. Scand J Immunol. 2003;57:506–16.
115. Wolf HM, Vogel E, Fischer MB, et al. Inhibition of receptor-dependent and receptor-independent generation of the respiratory burst in human neutrophils and monocytes by human serum IgA. Pediatr Res. 1994;36:235–43.
116. Deviere J, Vaerman JP, Content J, et al. IgA triggers tumor necrosis factor α secretion by monocytes: a study in normal subjects and patients with alcoholic cirrhosis. Hepatology. 1991;13:670–5.
117. Lamkhioued B, Gounni AS, Gruart V, et al. Human eosinophils express a receptor for secretory component. Role in secretory IgA-dependent activation. Eur J Immunol. 1995;25:117–25.
118. Motegi Y, Kita H. Interaction with secretory component stimulates effector functions of human eosinophils but not of neutrophils. J Immunol. 1998;161:4340–6.
119. Bartemes KR, Cooper KM, Drain KL, Kita H. Secretory IgA induces antigen-independent eosinophil survival and cytokine production without inducing effector functions. J Allergy Clin Immunol. 2005;116:827–35.
120. Monteiro RC. Immunoglobulin A, as an anti-inflammatory agent. Clin Exp Immunol. 2014;178 Suppl 1:108–10. doi:10.1111/cei.12531.
121. Pasquier B, Launay P, Kanamaru Y, Moura IC, Pfirsch S, Ruffié C, et al. Identification of FcalphaRI as an inhibitory receptor that controls inflammation: dual role of FcRgamma ITAM. Immunity. 2005;22:31–42.
122. Rugtveit J, Bakka A, Brandtzaeg P. Differential distribution of B7.1 (CD80) and B7.2 (CD86) co-stimulatory molecules on mucosal macrophage subsets in human inflammatory bowel disease (IBD). Clin Exp Immunol. 1997;110:104–13.
123. Hausmann M, Rogler G. Immune-non immune networks in intestinal inflammation. Curr Drug Targets. 2008;9:388–94.
124. Brandtzaeg P, Carlsen HS, Halstensen TS. The B-cell system in inflammatory bowel disease. Adv Exp Med Biol. 2006;579:149–67.
125. van Egmond M, van Garderen E, van Spriel AB, Damen CA, van Amersfoort ES, van Zandbergen G, et al. FcalphaRI-positive liver Kupffer cells: reappraisal of the function of immunoglobulin A in immunity. Nat Med. 2000;6:680–5.
126. Thomson AW, Knolle PA. Antigen-presenting cell function in the tolerogenic liver environment. Nat Rev Immunol. 2010;10:753–66.
127. Barbalat R, Barton GM. MicroRNAs and LPS: developing a relationship in the neonatal gut. Cell Host Microbe. 2010;8:303–4.
128. Eggesbø M, Botten G, Stigum H, Nafstad P, Magnus P. Is delivery by cesarean section a risk factor for food allergy? J Allergy Clin Immunol. 2003;112:420–6.
129. Koplin J, Allen K, Gurrin L, Osborne N, Tang ML, Dharmage S. Is caesarean delivery associated with sensitization to food allergens and IgE-mediated food allergy: a systematic review. Pediatr Allergy Immunol. 2008;19:682–7.
130. Claud EC, Lu L, Anton PM, Savidge T, Walker WA, Cherayil BJ. Developmentally regulated IkappaB expression in intestinal epithelium and susceptibility to flagellin-induced inflammation. Proc Natl Acad Sci U S A. 2004;101:7404–8.
131. Chassin C, Kocur M, Pott J, Duerr CU, Gütle D, Lotz M, et al. miR-146a mediates protective innate immune tolerance in the neonate intestine. Cell Host Microbe. 2010;8:358–68. doi:10.1016/j.chom.2010.09.005.
132. Kajino-Sakamoto R, Inagaki M, Lippert E, Akira S, Robine S, Matsumoto K, et al. Enterocyte-derived TAK1 signaling prevents epithelium apoptosis and the development of ileitis and colitis. J Immunol. 2008;181:1143–52.
133. Hooper LV, Wong MH, Thelin A, Hansson L, Falk PG, Gordon JI. Molecular analysis of commensal host-microbial relationships in the intestine. Science. 2001;291:881–4.
134. Broquet AH, Hirata Y, McAllister CS, Kagnoff MF. RIG-I/MDA5/MAVS are required to signal a protective IFN response in rotavirus-infected intestinal epithelium. J Immunol. 2011;186:1618–26. doi:10.4049/jimmunol.1002862.
135. Neish AS, Gewirtz AT, Zeng H, Young AN, Hobert ME, Karmali V, et al. Prokaryotic regulation of epithelial responses by inhibition of IkB-α ubiquitination. Science. 2000;289:1560–3.
136. Lavelle EC, Murphy C, O'Neill LA, Creagh EM. The role of TLRs, NLRs, and RLRs in mucosal innate immunity and homeostasis. Mucosal Immunol. 2010;3:17–28.
137. Schneeman TA, Bruno ME, Schjerven H, Johansen FE, Chady L, Kaetzel CS. Regulation of the polymeric Ig receptor by signaling through TLRs 3 and 4: linking innate and adaptive immune responses. J Immunol. 2005;175:376–84.
138. Brandtzaeg P, Halstensen TS, Huitfeldt HS, Krajci P, Kvale D, Scott H, et al. Epithelial expression of HLA, secretory component (poly-Ig receptor), and adhesion molecules in the human alimentary tract. Ann N Y Acad Sci. 1992;664:157–79.
139. Bruno ME, Rogier EW, Frantz AL, Stefka AT, Thompson SN, Kaetzel CS. Regulation of the polymeric immunoglobulin receptor in intestinal epithelial cells by Enterobacteriaceae: implications for mucosal homeostasis. Immunol Invest. 2010;39:356–82.
140. Sarkar J, Gangopadhyay NN, Moldoveanu Z, Mestecky J, Stephensen CB. Vitamin A is required for regulation of polymeric immunoglobulin receptor (pIgR) expression by interleukin-4 and interferon-gamma in a human intestinal epithelial cell line. J Nutr. 1998;128:1063–9.
141. Takenouchi-Ohkubo N, Asano M, Chihaya H, Chung-Hsuing WU, Ishikasa K, Moro I. Retinoic acid enhances the gene expression of human polymeric immunoglobulin receptor (pIgR) by TNF-alpha. Clin Exp Immunol. 2004;135:448–54.
142. Kvale D, Brandtzaeg P. Constitutive and cytokine induced expression of HLA molecules, secretory component, and intercellular adhesion molecule-1 is modulated by butyrate in the colonic epithelial cell line HT-29. Gut. 1995;36:737–42.
143. Glauber JG, Wandersee NJ, Little JA, Ginder GD. 5′-Flanking sequences mediate butyrate stimulation of embryonic globin gene expression in adult erythroid cells. Mol Cell Biol. 1991;11:4690–7.
144. Arpaia N, Campbell C, Fan X, Dikiy S, van der Veeken J, deRoos P, et al. Rudensky AY Metabolites produced by commensal bacteria promote peripheral regulatory T-cell generation. Nature. 2013;504:451–5. doi:10.1038/nature12726.
145. Furusawa Y, Obata Y, Fukuda S, Endo TA, Nakato G, Takahashi D, et al. Commensal microbe-derived butyrate induces the differentiation of colonic regulatory T cells. Nature. 2013;504:446–50. doi:10.1038/nature12721.
146. Lee J, Mo JH, Katakura K, Alkalay I, Rucker AN, Liu YT, et al. Maintenance of colonic homeostasis by distinctive apical TLR9 signalling in intestinal epithelial cells. Nat Cell Biol. 2006;8:1327–36.
147. Nenci A, Becker C, Wullaert A, Gareus R, van Loo G, Danese S, et al. Epithelial NEMO links innate immunity to chronic intestinal inflammation. Nature. 2007;446:557–61.
148. Rescigno M, Lopatin U, Chieppa M. Interactions among dendritic cells, macrophages, and epithelial cells in the gut: implications for immune tolerance. Curr Opin Immunol. 2008;20:669–75.
149. Iliev ID, Spadoni I, Mileti E, Matteoli G, Sonzogni A, Sampietro GM, et al. Human intestinal epithelial cells promote the differentiation of tolerogenic dendritic cells. Gut. 2009;58:1481–9.
150. Shale M, Ghosh S. How intestinal epithelial cells tolerise dendritic cells and its relevance to inflammatory bowel disease. Gut. 2009;58:1291–9.

151. Abreu MT, Palladino AA, Arnold ET, Kwon RS, McRoberts JA. Modulation of barrier function during Fas-mediated apoptosis in human intestinal epithelial cells. Gastroenterology. 2000;119: 1524–36.
152. Groschwitz KR, Hogan SP. Intestinal barrier function: molecular regulation and disease pathogenesis. J Allergy Clin Immunol. 2009;124:3–20. quiz 21–22.
153. Strober W, Fuss I, Mannon P. The fundamental basis of inflammatory bowel disease. J Clin Invest. 2007;117:514–21.
154. Feng T, Wang L, Schoeb TR, et al. Microbiota innate stimulation is a prerequisite for T cell spontaneous proliferation and induction of experimental colitis. J Exp Med. 2010;207:1321–32.
155. Hooper LV, Littman DR, Macpherson AJ. Interactions between the microbiota and the immune system. Science. 2012;336:1268–73. doi:10.1126/science.1223490.
156. Vaishnava S, Yamamoto M, Severson KM, Ruhn KA, Yu X, Koren O, et al. The antibacterial lectin RegIIIgamma promotes the spatial segregation of microbiota and host in the intestine. Science. 2011;334:255–8. doi:10.1126/science.1209791.
157. Hansson GC. Role of mucus layers in gut infection and inflammation. Curr Opin Microbiol. 2012;15:57–62. doi:10.1016/j.mib.2011.11.002.
158. Rogier EW, Frantz AL, Bruno ME, Wedlund L, Cohen DA, Stromberg AJ, et al. Secretory antibodies in breast milk promote long-term intestinal homeostasis by regulating the gut microbiota and host gene expression. Proc Natl Acad Sci U S A. 2014;111:3074–9. doi:10.1073/pnas.1315792111.
159. Rogier EW, Frantz AL, Bruno ME, Kaetzel CS. Secretory IgA is concentrated in the outer layer of colonic mucus along with gut bacteria. Pathogens. 2014;3:390–403. doi:10.3390/pathogens3020390.
160. Wenzel UA, Magnusson MK, Rydström A, Jonstrand C, Hengst J, Johansson ME, et al. Spontaneous colitis in Muc2-deficient mice reflects clinical and cellular features of active ulcerative colitis. PLoS One. 2014;9:e100217. doi:10.1371/journal.pone.0100217.
161. Brandtzaeg P, Fjellanger I, Gjeruldsen ST. Adsorption of immunoglobulin A onto oral bacteria in vivo. J Bacteriol. 1968;96:242–9.
162. van der Waaij LA, Limburg PC, Mesander G, van der Waaij D. In vivo IgA coating of anaerobic bacteria in human faeces. Gut. 1996;38:348–54.
163. Peterson DA, McNulty NP, Guruge JL, Gordon JI. IgA response to symbiotic bacteria as a mediator of gut homeostasis. Cell Host Microbe. 2007;2:328–39.
164. Hansen J, Gulati A, Sartor RB. The role of mucosal immunity and host genetics in defining intestinal commensal bacteria. Curr Opin Gastroenterol. 2010;26:564–71.
165. Bergqvist P, Stensson A, Hazanov L, Holmberg A, Mattsson J, Mehr R, et al. Re-utilization of germinal centers in multiple Peyer's patches results in highly synchronized, oligoclonal, and affinity-matured gut IgA responses. Mucosal Immunol. 2013;6:122–35. doi:10.1038/mi.2012.56.
166. Spencer J, Klavinskis LS, Fraser LD. The human intestinal IgA response; burning questions. Front Immunol. 2012;3:108. doi:10.3389/fimmu.2012.00108.
167. Lindner C, Wahl B, Föhse L, Suerbaum S, Macpherson AJ, Prinz I, et al. Age, microbiota, and T cells shape diverse individual IgA repertoires in the intestine. J Exp Med. 2012;209:365–77. doi:10.1084/jem.20111980.
168. Pabst O. New concepts in the generation and functions of IgA. Nat Rev Immunol. 2012;12:821–32. doi:10.1038/nri3322.
169. Slack E, Balmer ML, Fritz JH, Hapfelmeier S. Functional flexibility of intestinal IgA—broadening the fine line. Front Immunol. 2012;3:100. doi:10.3389/fimmu.2012.00100.
170. Brandtzaeg P. Secretory IgA: designed for anti-microbial defense. Front Immunol. 2013;4:222. doi:10.3389/fimmu.2013.00222.
171. Macpherson AJ, Köller Y, McCoy KD. The bilateral responsiveness between intestinal microbes and IgA. Trends Immunol. 2015;36:460–70. doi:10.1016/j.it.2015.06.006.
172. Ashida H, Ogawa M, Kim M, Mimuro H, Sasakawa C. Bacteria and host interactions in the gut epithelial barrier. Nat Chem Biol. 2011;8:36–45. doi:10.1038/nchembio.741.
173. Hajishengallis G, Lambris JD. Microbial manipulation of receptor crosstalk in innate immunity. Nat Rev Immunol. 2011;11: 187–200. doi:10.1038/nri2918.
174. Sansonetti PJ. To be or not to be a pathogen: that is the mucosally relevant question. Mucosal Immunol. 2011;4:8–14. doi:10.1038/mi.2010.77.
175. Stuart LM, Paquette N, Boyer L. Effector-triggered versus pattern-triggered immunity: how animals sense pathogens. Nat Rev Immunol. 2013;13:199–206. doi:10.1038/nri3398.
176. Srinivasan N. Telling apart friend from foe: discriminating between commensals and pathogens at mucosal sites. Innate Immun. 2010;16:391–404. doi:10.1177/1753425909357577.
177. Kamada N, Kim YG, Sham HP, Vallance BA, Puente JL, Martens EC, et al. Regulated virulence controls the ability of a pathogen to compete with the gut microbiota. Science. 2012;336:1325–9. doi:10.1126/science.1222195.
178. Kamada N, Seo SU, Chen GY, Núñez G. Role of the gut microbiota in immunity and inflammatory disease. Nat Rev Immunol. 2013;13:321–35. doi:10.1038/nri3430.
179. De Palma G, Nadal I, Medina M, Donat E, Ribes-Koninckx C, Calabuig M, et al. Intestinal dysbiosis and reduced immunoglobulin-coated bacteria associated with coeliac disease in children. BMC Microbiol. 2010;10:63. doi:10.1186/1471-2180-10-63.
180. Reikvam DH, Derrien M, Islam R, Erofeev A, Grcic V, Sandvik A, et al. Epithelial-microbial crosstalk in polymeric Ig receptor deficient mice. Eur J Immunol. 2012;42:2959–70. doi:10.1002/eji.201242543.
181. Kawamoto S, Tran TH, Maruya M, Suzuki K, Doi Y, Tsutsui Y, et al. The inhibitory receptor PD-1 regulates IgA selection and bacterial composition in the gut. Science. 2012;336:485–9. doi:10.1126/science.1217718.
182. Tsuruta T, Inoue R, Nojima I, Tsukahara T, Hara H, Yajima T. The amount of secreted IgA may not determine the secretory IgA coating ratio of gastrointestinal bacteria. FEMS Immunol Med Microbiol. 2009;56:185–9. doi:10.1111/j.1574-695X.2009.00568.x.
183. Robles Alonso V, Guarner F. Linking the gut microbiota to human health. Br J Nutr. 2013;109 Suppl 2:S21–6. doi:10.1017/S0007114512005235.
184. van der Waaij LA, Kroese FG, Visser A, Nelis GF, Westerveld BD, Jansen PL, et al. Immunoglobulin coating of faecal bacteria in inflammatory bowel disease. Eur J Gastroenterol Hepatol. 2004;16:669–74.
185. Carding S, Verbeke K, Vipond DT, Corfe BM, Owen LJ. Dysbiosis of the gut microbiota in disease. Microb Ecol Health Dis. 2015;26:26191. doi:10.3402/mehd.v26.26191.
186. Palm NW, de Zoete MR, Cullen TW, Barry NA, Stefanowski J, Hao L, et al. Immunoglobulin A coating identifies colitogenic bacteria in inflammatory bowel disease. Cell. 2014;158:1000–10. doi:10.1016/j.cell.2014.08.006.
187. Shulzhenko N, Morgun A, Hsiao W, Battle M, Yao M, Gavrilova O, et al. Crosstalk between B lymphocytes, microbiota and the intestinal epithelium governs immunity versus metabolism in the gut. Nat Med. 2011;17:1585–93. doi:10.1038/nm.2505.
188. Chorny A, Cerutti A. A gut triumvirate rules homeostasis. Nat Med. 2011;17:1549–50. doi:10.1038/nm.2592.
189. Gaboriau-Routhiau V, Rakotobe S, Lécuyer E, Mulder I, Lan A, Bridonneau C, et al. The key role of segmented filamentous bacteria in the coordinated maturation of gut helper T cell responses. Immunity. 2009;31:677–89.
190. Ivanov II, Littman DR. Segmented filamentous bacteria take the stage. Mucosal Immunol. 2010;3:209–12.
191. Obata T, Goto Y, Kunisawa J, Sato S, Sakamoto M, Setoyama H, et al. Indigenous opportunistic bacteria inhabit mammalian gut-associated lymphoid tissues and share a mucosal antibody-mediated symbiosis. Proc Natl Acad Sci U S A. 2010;107:7419–24.

192. McDole JR, Wheeler LW, McDonald KG, Wang B, Konjufca V, Knoop KA, et al. Goblet cells deliver luminal antigen to CD103+ dendritic cells in the small intestine. Nature. 2012;483:345–9. doi:10.1038/nature10863.
193. Brandtzaeg P. Mucosal immunity in the healthy gut. In: Calder PC, Yaquob P, editors. Diet, immunity and inflammation. Cambridge: Woodhead Publishing; 2013. p. 34–80. Chapter 2. ISBN 978-0-85709-037-9.
194. Latcham F, Merino F, Lang A, Garvey J, Thomson MA, Walker-Smith JA, et al. A consistent pattern of minor immunodeficiency and subtle enteropathy in children with multiple food allergy. J Pediatr. 2003;143:39–47.
195. van Odijk J, Kull I, Borres MP, Brandtzaeg P, Edberg U, Hanson LA, et al. Breastfeeding and allergic disease: a multidisciplinary review of the literature (1966–2001) on the mode of early feeding in infancy and its impact on later atopic manifestations. Allergy. 2003;58:833–43.
196. U.S. Department of Health. Breastfeeding and maternal and infant health outcomes in developed countries. Agency for Healthcare Research and Quality (AHRQ), Publication No. 07-E007, Evidence Report/Technology Assessment Report No. 153, 2007.
197. Høst A, Halken S, Muraro A, Dreborg S, Niggemann B, Aalberse R, et al. Dietary prevention of allergic diseases in infants and small children. Pediatr Allergy Immunol. 2008;19:1–4.
198. Gearry RB, Richardson AK, Frampton CM, Dodgshun AJ, Barclay ML. Population-based cases control study of inflammatory bowel disease risk factors. J Gastroenterol Hepatol. 2010;25:325–33.
199. Barclay AR, Russell RK, Wilson ML, Gilmour WH, Satsangi J, Wilson DC. Systematic review: the role of breastfeeding in the development of pediatric inflammatory bowel disease. J Pediatr. 2009;155:421–6.
200. Moffatt DC, Ilnyckyj A, Bernstein CN. A population-based study of breastfeeding in inflammatory bowel disease: initiation, duration, and effect on disease in the postpartum period. Am J Gastroenterol. 2009;104:2517–23.
201. Moscandrew M, Kane S. Inflammatory bowel diseases and management considerations: fertility and pregnancy. Curr Gastroenterol Rep. 2009;11:395–9.
202. Collins J. Breastfeeding in inflammatory bowel disease: positive results for mother and child. Inflamm Bowel Dis. 2011;17:663–4. doi:10.1002/ibd.21338.
203. Hanson LA. Session 1: Feeding and infant development breastfeeding and immune function. Proc Nutr Soc. 2007;66:384–96.
204. Abrahamsson TR, Sinkiewicz G, Jakobsson T, Fredrikson M, Björkstén B. Probiotic lactobacilli in breast milk and infant stool in relation to oral intake during the first year of life. J Pediatr Gastroenterol Nutr. 2009;49:349–54.
205. Donnet-Hughes A, Perez PF, Doré J, Leclerc M, Levenez F, Benyacoub J, et al. Potential role of the intestinal microbiota of the mother in neonatal immune education. Proc Nutr Soc. 2010;69:407–15.
206. Verhasselt V, Milcent V, Cazareth J, Kanda A, Fleury S, Dombrowicz D, et al. Breast milk-mediated transfer of an antigen induces tolerance and protection from allergic asthma. Nat Med. 2008;14:170–5.
207. Mosconi E, Rekima A, Seitz-Polski B, Kanda A, Fleury S, Tissandie E, et al. Breast milk immune complexes are potent inducers of oral tolerance in neonates and prevent asthma development. Mucosal Immunol. 2010;3:461–74.
208. Oddy WH, Rosales F. A systematic review of the importance of milk TGF-beta on immunological outcomes in the infant and young child. Pediatr Allergy Immunol. 2010;21(1 Pt 1):47–59.
209. Chapkin RS, Zhao C, Ivanov I, Davidson LA, Goldsby JS, Lupton JR, et al. Noninvasive stool-based detection of infant gastrointestinal development using gene expression profiles from exfoliated epithelial cells. Am J Physiol Gastrointest Liver Physiol. 2010;298:G582–9.
210. Broere F, du Pré MF, van Berkel LA, Garssen J, Schmidt-Weber CB, Lambrecht BN, et al. Cyclooxygenase-2 in mucosal DC mediates induction of regulatory T cells in the intestine through suppression of IL-4. Mucosal Immunol. 2009;2:254–64.
211. Saurer L, Mueller C. T cell-mediated immunoregulation in the gastrointestinal tract. Allergy. 2009;64:505–19.
212. Westendorf AM, Fleissner D, Groebe L, Jung S, Gruber AD, Hansen W, et al. $CD4^+Foxp3^+$ regulatory T cell expansion induced by antigen-driven interaction with intestinal epithelial cells independent of local dendritic cells. Gut. 2009;58:211–9.
213. Rothberg RM, Farr RS. Anti-bovine serum albumin and anti-alpha lactalbumin in the serum of children and adults. Pediatrics. 1965;35:571–88.
214. Scott H, Rognum TO, Midtvedt T, Brandtzaeg P. Age-related changes of human serum antibodies to dietary and colonic bacterial antigens measured by an enzyme-linked immunosorbent assay. Acta Pathol Microbiol Immunol Scand A. 1985;93: 65–70.
215. Korenblat PE, Rothberg RM, Minden P, Farr RS. Immune responses of human adults after oral and parenteral exposure to bovine serum albumin. J Allergy. 1968;41:226–35.
216. Husby S, Mestecky J, Moldoveanu Z, Holland S, Elson CO. Oral tolerance in humans. T cell but not B cell tolerance after antigen feeding. J Immunol. 1994;152:4663–70.
217. Waldo FB, van den Wall Bake AW, Mestecky J, Husby S. Suppression of the immune response by nasal immunization. Clin Immunol Immunopathol. 1994;72:30–4.
218. Kraus TA, Toy L, Chan L, Childs J, Mayer L. Failure to induce oral tolerance to a soluble protein in patients with inflammatory bowel disease. Gastroenterology. 2004;126:1771–8.
219. Kraus TA, Cheifetz A, Toy L, Meddings JB, Mayer L. Evidence for a genetic defect in oral tolerance induction in inflammatory bowel disease. Inflamm Bowel Dis. 2006;12:82–8.
220. Qiao L, Braunstein J, Golling M, Schürmann G, Autschbach F, Möller P, et al. Differential regulation of human T cell responsiveness by mucosal versus blood monocytes. Eur J Immunol. 1996;26:922–7.
221. Hausmann M, Kiessling S, Mestermann S, Webb G, Spöttl T, Andus T, et al. Toll-like receptors 2 and 4 are up-regulated during intestinal inflammation. Gastroenterology. 2002;122:1987–2000.
222. Rugtveit J, Nilsen EM, Bakka A, Carlsen H, Brandtzaeg P, Scott H. Cytokine profiles differ in newly recruited and resident subsets of mucosal macrophages from inflammatory bowel disease. Gastroenterology. 1997;112:1493–505.
223. Smythies LE, Sellers M, Clements RH, Mosteller-Barnum M, Meng G, Benjamin WH, et al. Human intestinal macrophages display profound inflammatory anergy despite avid phagocytic and bacteriocidal activity. J Clin Invest. 2005;115:66–75.
224. Smith PD, Smythies LE, Shen R, Greenwell-Wild T, Gliozzi M, Wahl SM. Intestinal macrophages and response to microbial encroachment. Mucosal Immunol. 2011;4:31–42.
225. Weber B, Saurer L, Mueller C. Intestinal macrophages: differentiation and involvement in intestinal immunopathologies. Semin Immunopathol. 2009;31:171–84.
226. Geissmann F, Manz MG, Jung S, Sieweke MH, Merad M, Ley K. Development of monocytes, macrophages, and dendritic cells. Science. 2010;327:656–61.
227. Denning TL, Wang YC, Patel SR, Williams IR, Pulendran B. Lamina propria macrophages and dendritic cells differentially induce regulatory and interleukin 17-producing T cell responses. Nat Immunol. 2007;8:1086–94.
228. Rescigno M. Before they were gut dendritic cells. Immunity. 2009;31:454–6.
229. Cheong C, Matos I, Choi JH, Dandamudi DB, Shrestha E, Longhi MP, et al. Microbial stimulation fully differentiates monocytes to DC-SIGN/$CD209^+$ dendritic cells for immune T cell areas. Cell. 2010;143:416–29.

230. Schulz O, Jaensson E, Persson EK, Liu X, Worbs T, Agace WW, et al. Intestinal CD103⁺, but not CX3CR1⁺, antigen sampling cells migrate in lymph and serve classical dendritic cell functions. J Exp Med. 2009;206:3101–14.
231. Mazzini E, Massimiliano L, Penna G, Rescigno M. Oral tolerance can be established via gap junction transfer of fed antigens from CX3CR1⁺ macrophages to CD103⁺ dendritic cells. Immunity. 2014;40:248–61. doi:10.1016/j.immuni.2013.12.012.
232. Shakhar G, Kolesnikov M. Intestinal macrophages and DCs close the gap on tolerance. Immunity. 2014;40:171–3. doi:10.1016/j.immuni.2014.01.008.
233. Matteoli G, Mazzini E, Iliev ID, Mileti E, Fallarino F, Puccetti P, et al. Gut CD103⁺ dendritic cells express indoleamine 2,3-dioxygenase which influences T regulatory/T effector cell balance and oral tolerance induction. Gut. 2010;59:595–604.
234. Rescigno M. Intestinal dendritic cells. Adv Immunol. 2010;107:109–38.
235. Grindebacke H, Stenstad H, Quiding-Järbrink M, Waldenström J, Adlerberth I, Wold AE, et al. Dynamic development of homing receptor expression and memory cell differentiation of infant $CD4^+CD25^{high}$ regulatory T cells. J Immunol. 2009;183:4360–70.
236. Hadis U, Wahl B, Schulz O, Hardtke-Wolenski M, Schippers A, Wagner N, et al. Intestinal tolerance requires gut homing and expansion of FoxP3+ regulatory T cells in the lamina propria. Immunity. 2011;34:237–46. doi:10.1016/j.immuni.2011.01.016.
237. Hammerschmidt SI, Ahrendt M, Bode U, Wahl B, Kremmer E, Förster R, et al. Stromal mesenteric lymph node cells are essential for the generation of gut-homing T cells in vivo. J Exp Med. 2008;205:2483–90.
238. Jaensson-Gyllenbäck E, Kotarsky K, Zapata F, Persson EK, Gundersen TE, Blomhoff R, et al. Bile retinoids imprint intestinal CD103+ dendritic cells with the ability to generate gut-tropic T cells. Mucosal Immunol. 2011;4:438–47. doi:10.1038/mi.2010.91.
239. Pantazi E, Marks E, Stolarczyk E, Lycke N, Noelle RJ, Elgueta R. Cutting edge: retinoic acid signaling in B cells is essential for oral immunization and microflora composition. J Immunol. 2015;195:1368–71. doi:10.4049/jimmunol.1500989.
240. Belkaid Y, Oldenhove G. Tuning microenvironments: induction of regulatory T cells by dendritic cells. Immunity. 2008;29:362–71.
241. Horwitz DA, Zheng SG, Gray JD. Natural and TGF-β-induced $Foxp3^+CD4^+$ $CD25^+$ regulatory T cells are not mirror images of each other. Trends Immunol. 2008;29:429–35.
242. Barnes MJ, Powrie F. Regulatory T cells reinforce intestinal homeostasis. Immunity. 2009;31:401–11.
243. Sakaguchi S, Wing K, Yamaguchi T. Dynamics of peripheral tolerance and immune regulation mediated by Treg. Eur J Immunol. 2009;39:2331–6.
244. Akbar AN, Vukmanovic-Stejic M, Taams LS, Macallan DC. The dynamic co-evolution of memory and regulatory $CD4^+$ T cells in the periphery. Nat Rev Immunol. 2007;7:231–7.
245. Booth NJ, McQuaid AJ, Sobande T, Kissane S, Agius E, Jackson SE, et al. Different proliferative potential and migratory characteristics of human $CD4^+$ regulatory T cells that express either CD45RA or CD45RO. J Immunol. 2010;184:4317–26.
246. Miyara M, Yoshioka Y, Kitoh A, Shima T, Wing K, Niwa A, et al. Functional delineation and differentiation dynamics of human $CD4^+$ T cells expressing the FoxP3 transcription factor. Immunity. 2009;30:899–911.
247. Sakaguchi S, Miyara M, Costantino CM, Hafler DA. $FOXP3^+$ regulatory T cells in the human immune system. Nat Rev Immunol. 2010;10:490–500.
248. Sakaguchi S. Immunology: Conditional stability of T cells. Nature. 2010;468:41–2.
249. Verhasselt V. Oral tolerance in neonates: from basics to potential prevention of allergic disease. Mucosal Immunol. 2010;3:326–33.
250. Honda K, Takeda K. Regulatory mechanisms of immune responses to intestinal bacteria. Mucosal Immunol. 2009;2:187–96.
251. Schnoeller C, Rausch S, Pillai S, Avagyan A, Wittig BM, Loddenkemper C, et al. A helminth immunomodulator reduces allergic and inflammatory responses by induction of IL-10-producing macrophages. J Immunol. 2008;180:4265–72.
252. Weinstock JV, Elliott DE. Helminths and the IBD hygiene hypothesis. Inflamm Bowel Dis. 2009;15:128–33.
253. Grainger JR, Smith KA, Hewitson JP, McSorley HJ, Harcus Y, Filbey KJ, et al. Helminth secretions induce de novo T cell Foxp3 expression and regulatory function through the TGF-β pathway. J Exp Med. 2010;207:2331–41.
254. Harnett W, Harnett MM. Helminth-derived immunomodulators: can understanding the worm produce the pill? Nat Rev Immunol. 2010;10:278–84.
255. Blümer N, Herz U, Wegmann M, Renz H. Prenatal lipopolysaccharide-exposure prevents allergic sensitization and airway inflammation, but not airway responsiveness in a murine model of experimental asthma. Clin Exp Allergy. 2005;35:397–402.
256. Gerhold K, Avagyan A, Seib C, Frei R, Steinle J, Ahrens B, et al. Prenatal initiation of endotoxin airway exposure prevents subsequent allergen-induced sensitization and airway inflammation in mice. J Allergy Clin Immunol. 2006;118:666–73.
257. Eder W, von Mutius E. Genetics in asthma: the solution to a lasting conundrum? Allergy. 2005;60:1482–4.
258. Hong X, Tsai HJ, Wang X. Genetics of food allergy. Curr Opin Pediatr. 2009;21:770–6.
259. Mathew CG, Lewis CM. Genetics of inflammatory bowel disease: progress and prospects. Hum Mol Genet. 2004;13(Spec No 1):R161–8.
260. Marks DJ, Harbord MW, MacAllister R, Rahman FZ, Young J, Al-Lazikani B, et al. Defective acute inflammation in Crohn's disease: a clinical investigation. Lancet. 2006;367:668–78. Erratum in: Lancet. 2007;370:318.
261. Fallon PG, Mangan NE. Suppression of TH2-type allergic reactions by helminth infection. Nat Rev Immunol. 2007;7:220–30.
262. Tang ML. Probiotics and prebiotics: immunological and clinical effects in allergic disease. In: Brandtzaeg P, Isolauri E, Prescott SL, editors. Microbial–host interaction: tolerance versus allergy. Nestlé nutr. workshop ser pediatr progr., vol 64. Basel: Nestec Ltd., Vevey/S, Karger AG; 2009. p. 219–38.
263. Hedin CR, Mullard M, Sharratt E, Jansen C, Sanderson JD, Shirlaw P, et al. Probiotic and prebiotic use in patients with inflammatory bowel disease: a case-control study. Inflamm Bowel Dis. 2010;16:2099–108.
264. Salminen S, Collado MC, Isolauri E, Gueimonde M. Microbial-host interactions: selecting the right probiotics and prebiotics for infants. In: Brandtzaeg P, Isolauri E, Prescott SL, editors. Microbial–host interaction: tolerance versus allergy. Nestlé Nutr Workshop Ser Pediatr Progr, vol 64. Basel: Nestec Ltd., Vevey/S, Karger AG; 2009. p. 201–17.
265. Hörmannsperger G, Haller D. Molecular crosstalk of probiotic bacteria with the intestinal immune system: clinical relevance in the context of inflammatory bowel disease. Int J Med Microbiol. 2010;300:63–73.
266. Mileti E, Matteoli G, Iliev ID, Rescigno M. Comparison of the immunomodulatory properties of three probiotic strains of Lactobacilli using complex culture systems: prediction for in vivo efficacy. PLoS One. 2009;4:e7056.
267. Rancé F, Boguniewicz M, Lau S. New visions for atopic eczema: an iPAC summary and future trends. Pediatr Allergy Immunol. 2008;19 Suppl 19:17–25.
268. Vercelli D. Discovering susceptibility genes for asthma and allergy. Nat Rev Immunol. 2008;8:169–82.
269. Qin J, Li R, Raes J, et al. A human gut microbial gene catalogue established by metagenomic sequencing. Nature. 2010;464:59–65.
270. Reyes A, Haynes M, Hanson N, Angly FE, Heath AC, Rohwer F, et al. Viruses in the faecal microbiota of monozygotic twins and their mothers. Nature. 2010;466:334–8.

271. Guo PF, Du MR, Wu HX, Lin Y, Jin LP, Li DJ. Thymic stromal lymphopoietin from trophoblasts induces dendritic cell-mediated regulatory TH2 bias in the deciduas during early gestation in humans. Blood. 2010;116:2061–9.
272. Herz U, Lacy P, Renz H, Erb K. The influence of infections on the development and severity of allergic disorders. Curr Opin Immunol. 2000;12:632–40.
273. Isolauri E, Grönlund MM, Salminen S, Arvilommi H. Why don't we bud? J Pediatr Gastroenterol Nutr. 2000;30:214–6.
274. Prescott SL, Macaubas C, Holt BJ, Smallacombe TB, Loh R, Sly PD, et al. Transplacental priming of the human immune system to environmental allergens: universal skewing of initial T cell responses toward the Th2 cytokine profile. J Immunol. 1998;160:4730–7.
275. Michaëlsson J, Mold JE, McCune JM, Nixon DF. Regulation of T cell responses in the developing human fetus. J Immunol. 2006;176:5741–8.
276. Cupedo T, Nagasawa M, Weijer K, Blom B, Spits H. Development and activation of regulatory T cells in the human fetus. Eur J Immunol. 2005;35:383–90.
277. Darrasse-Jèze G, Marodon G, Salomon BL, Catala M, Klatzmann D. Ontogeny of $CD4^{+}CD25^{+}$ regulatory/suppressor T cells in human fetuses. Blood. 2005;105:4715–21.
278. Renz H, Pfefferle PI, Teich R, Garn H. Development and regulation of immune responses to food antigens in pre- and postnatal life. In: Brandtzaeg P, Isolauri E, Prescott SL, editors. Microbial–host interaction: tolerance versus allergy. Nestlé Nutr Workshop Ser Pediatr Progr, vol 64. Basel: Nestec Ltd., Vevey/S, Karger AG; 2009. p. 139–57.
279. Huehn J, Polansky JK, Hamann A. Epigenetic control of FOXP3 expression: the key to a stable regulatory T-cell lineage? Nat Rev Immunol. 2009;9:83–9.
280. Wilson CB, Rowell E, Sekimata M. Epigenetic control of T-helper-cell differentiation. Nat Rev Immunol. 2009;9:91–105.
281. Conrad ML, Ferstl R, Teich R, Brand S, Blümer N, Yildirim AO, et al. Maternal TLR signaling is required for prenatal asthma protection by the nonpathogenic microbe *Acinetobacter lwoffii* F78. J Exp Med. 2009;206:2869–77.
282. Takahashi K, Sugi Y, Hosono A, Kaminogawa S. Epigenetic regulation of TLR4 gene expression in intestinal epithelial cells for the maintenance of intestinal homeostasis. J Immunol. 2009;183: 6522–9.
283. Alford SH, Zoratti E, Peterson EL, Maliarik M, Ownby DR, Johnson CC. Parental history of atopic disease: disease pattern and risk of pediatric atopy in offspring. J Allergy Clin Immunol. 2004;114:1046–50.
284. Thompson AI, Lees CW. Genetics of ulcerative colitis. Inflamm Bowel Dis. 2011;17:831–48. doi:10.1002/ibd.21375.
285. Renz H, Blümer N, Virna S, Sel S, Garn H. The immunological basis of the hygiene hypothesis. In: Crameri R, editor. The environment. allergy and asthma in modern society: a scientific approach. Chem Immunol Allergy, vol 91. Basel: Karger; 2006. p. 30–48.
286. van der Kleij D, Latz E, Brouwers JF, Kruize YC, Schmitz M, Kurt-Jones EA, et al. A novel host-parasite lipid cross-talk. Schistosomal lyso-phosphatidylserine activates Toll-like receptor 2 and affects immune polarization. J Biol Chem. 2002;277: 48122–9.
287. Sepp E, Julge K, Vasar M, Naaber P, Björksten B, Mikelsaar M. Intestinal microflora of Estonian and Swedish infants. Acta Paediatr. 1997;86:956–61.
288. Björkstén B, Naaber P, Sepp E, Mikelsaar M. The intestinal microflora in allergic Estonian and Swedish 2-year-old children. Clin Exp Allergy. 1999;29:342–6.
289. Kalliomäki M, Kirjavainen P, Eerola E, Kero P, Salminen S, Isolauri E. Distinct patterns of neonatal gut microflora in infants in whom atopy was and was not developing. J Allergy Clin Immunol. 2001;107:129–34.
290. Kuitunen M, Kukkonen K, Juntunen-Backman K, Korpela R, Poussa T, Tuure T, et al. Probiotics prevent IgE-associated allergy until age 5 years in cesarean-delivered children but not in the total cohort. J Allergy Clin Immunol. 2009;123:335–41.
291. Zeiger RS. Dietary aspects of food allergy prevention in infants and children. J Pediatr Gastroenterol Nutr. 2000;30(Suppl):S77–86.
292. Prescott SL. Role of dietary immunomodulatory factors in the development of immune tolerance. In: Brandtzaeg P, Isolauri E, Prescott SL, editors. Microbial–host interaction: tolerance versus allergy. Nestlé Nutr Workshop Ser Pediatr Progr, vol 64. Basel: Nestec Ltd., Vevey/S, Karger AG; 2009. p. 185–200.
293. Rautava S, Luoto R, Salminen S, Isolauri E. Microbial contact during pregnancy, intestinal colonization and human disease. Nat Rev Gastroenterol Hepatol. 2012;9:565–76. doi:10.1038/nrgastro.2012.144.
294. Miettinen M, Matikainen S, Vuopio-Varkila J, Pirhonen J, Varkila K, Kurimoto M, et al. Lactobacilli and streptococci induce interleukin-12 (IL-12), IL-18, and gamma interferon production in human peripheral blood mononuclear cells. Infect Immun. 1998;66:6058–62.
295. Hessle C, Hanson LA, Wold AE. Lactobacilli from human gastrointestinal mucosa are strong stimulators of IL-12 production. Clin Exp Immunol. 1999;116:276–82.
296. Hessle C, Andersson B, Wold AE. Gram-positive bacteria are potent inducers of monocytic interleukin-12 (IL-12) while gram-negative bacteria preferentially stimulate IL-10 production. Infect Immun. 2000;68:3581–6.
297. Caramalho I, Lopes-Carvalho T, Ostler D, Zelenay S, Haury M, Demengeot J. Regulatory T cells selectively express Toll-like receptors and are activated by lipopolysaccharide. J Exp Med. 2003;197:403–11.
298. Murai M, Turovskaya O, Kim G, Madan R, Karp CL, Cheroutre H, et al. Interleukin 10 acts on regulatory T cells to maintain expression of the transcription factor Foxp3 and suppressive function in mice with colitis. Nat Immunol. 2009;10:1178–84.
299. Steidler L, Hans W, Schotte L, Neirynck S, Obermeier F, Falk W, et al. Treatment of murine colitis by *Lactococcus lactis* secreting interleukin-10. Science. 2000;289:1352–5.
300. Lathrop SK, Bloom SM, Rao SM, Nutsch K, Lio CW, Santacruz N, et al. Peripheral education of the immune system by colonic commensal microbiota. Nature. 2011;478:250–4.
301. Josefowicz SZ, Niec RE, Kim HY, Treuting P, Chinen T, Zheng Y, et al. Extrathymically generated regulatory T cells control mucosal TH2 inflammation. Nature. 2012;482:395–9.
302. Geijtenbeek TB, den Dunnen J, Gringhuis SI. Pathogen recognition by DC-SIGN shapes adaptive immunity. Future Microbiol. 2009;4:879–90.
303. Zhou Y, Kawasaki H, Hsu SC, Lee RT, Yao X, Plunkett B, et al. Oral tolerance to food-induced systemic anaphylaxis mediated by the C-type lectin SIGNR1. Nat Med. 2010;16:1128–33.
304. O'Mahony C, Scully P, O'Mahony D, Murphy S, O'Brien F, Lyons A, et al. Commensal-induced regulatory T cells mediate protection against pathogen-stimulated NF-kB activation. PLoS Pathog. 2008;4:e1000112.
305. Lee JH, Ulrich B, Cho J, Park J, Kim CH. Progesterone promotes differentiation of human cord blood fetal T cells into T regulatory cells but suppresses their differentiation into Th17 cells. J Immunol. 2011;187:1778–87.
306. Atarashi K, Tanoue T, Shima T, Imaoka A, Kuwahara T, Momose Y, et al. Induction of colonic regulatory T cells by indigenous Clostridium species. Science. 2011;331:337–41.
307. Reading NC, Kasper DL. The starting lineup: key microbial players in intestinal immunity and homeostasis. Front Microbiol. 2011;2:148.
308. Baklien K, Brandtzaeg P. Comparative mapping of the local distribution of immunoglobulin-containing cells in ulcerative colitis and Crohn's disease of the colon. Clin Exp Immunol. 1975;22: 197–209.

309. Brandtzaeg P. The changing immunological paradigm in coeliac disease. Immunol Lett. 2006;105:127–39.
310. Brandtzaeg P. Update on mucosal immunoglobulin A in gastrointestinal disease. Curr Opin Gastroenterol. 2010;26:554–63.
311. Kleessen B, Kroesen AJ, Buhr HJ, et al. Mucosal and invading bacteria in patients with inflammatory bowel disease compared with controls. Scand J Gastroenterol. 2002;37:1034–41.
312. Kett K, Rognum TO, Brandtzaeg P. Mucosal subclass distribution of immunoglobulin G-producing cells is different in ulcerative colitis and Crohn's disease of the colon. Gastroenterology. 1987; 93:919–24.
313. Helgeland L, Tysk C, Järnerot G, et al. The IgG subclass distribution in serum and rectal mucosa of monozygotic twins with or without inflammatory bowel disease. Gut. 1992;33: 1358–64.
314. Brandtzaeg P, Korsrud FR. Significance of different J-chain profiles in human tissues: generation of IgA and IgM with binding site for secretory component is related to the J-chain expressing capacity of the total local immunocyte population, including IgG- and IgD-producing cells, and depends on the clinical state of the tissue. Clin Exp Immunol. 1984;58:709–18.
315. Kett K, Brandtzaeg P. Local IgA subclass alterations in ulcerative colitis and Crohn's disease of the colon. Gut. 1987;28: 1013–21.
316. Kett K, Brandtzaeg P, Fausa O. J-chain expression is more prominent in immunoglobulin A2 than in immunoglobulin A1 colonic immunocytes and is decreased in both subclasses associated with inflammatory bowel disease. Gastroenterology. 1988;94: 1419–25.
317. Van Den Bogaerde J, Cahill J, Emmanuel AV, et al. Gut mucosal response to food antigens in Crohn's disease. Aliment Pharmacol Ther. 2002;16:1903–15.
318. Montaldo E, Vitale C, Cottalasso F, Conte R, Glatzer T, Ambrosini P, et al. Human NK cells at early stages of differentiation produce CXCL8 and express CD161 molecule that functions as an activating receptor. Blood. 2012;119:3987–96. doi:10.1182/blood-2011-09-379693.
319. Cella M, Fuchs A, Vermi W, Facchetti F, Otero K, Lennerz JK, et al. A human natural killer cell subset provides an innate source of IL-22 for mucosal immunity. Nature. 2009;457:722–5. doi:10.1038/nature07537.
320. Cupedo T, Crellin NK, Papazian N, Rombouts EJ, Weijer K, Grogan JL, et al. Human fetal lymphoid tissue-inducer cells are interleukin 17-producing precursors to RORC^{+} CD127^{+} natural killer-like cells. Nat Immunol. 2009;10:66–74. doi:10.1038/ni.1668.
321. Kurashima Y, Goto Y, Kiyono H. Mucosal innate immune cells regulate both gut homeostasis and intestinal inflammation. Eur J Immunol. 2013;43:3108–15. doi:10.1002/eji.201343782.
322. Diefenbach A, Colonna M, Koyasu S. Development, differentiation, and diversity of innate lymphoid cells. Immunity. 2014;41:354–65. doi:10.1016/j.immuni.2014.09.005.
323. Fuchs A, Vermi W, Lee JS, Lonardi S, Gilfillan S, Newberry RD, et al. Intraepithelial type 1 innate lymphoid cells are a unique subset of IL-12- and IL-15-responsive IFN-γ-producing cells. Immunity. 2013;38:769–81. doi:10.1016/j.immuni.2013.02.010.
324. Van Kaer L, Algood HM, Singh K, Parekh VV, Greer MJ, Piazuelo MB, et al. CD8$\alpha\alpha^{+}$ innate-type lymphocytes in the intestinal epithelium mediate mucosal immunity. Immunity. 2014;41:451–64. doi:10.1016/j.immuni.2014.08.010. Erratum in: Immunity. 2014;41:1064.
325. Napier RJ, Adams EJ, Gold MC, Lewinsohn DM. The role of mucosal associated invariant T cells in antimicrobial immunity. Front Immunol. 2015;6:344. doi:10.3389/fimmu.2015.00344.
326. Macpherson A, Khoo UY, Forgacs I, et al. Mucosal antibodies in inflammatory bowel disease are directed against intestinal bacteria. Gut. 1996;38:365–75.
327. Foo MC, Lee A. Immunological response of mice to members of the autochthonous intestinal microflora. Infect Immun. 1972;6:525–32.
328. Berg RD, Savage DC. Immune responses of specific pathogen-free and gnotobiotic mice to antigens of indigenous and nonindigenous microorganisms. Infect Immun. 1975;11:320–9.
329. Slack E, Hapfelmeier S, Stecher B, et al. Innate and adaptive immunity cooperate flexibly to maintain host-microbiota mutualism. Science. 2009;325:617–20.
330. Landers CJ, Cohavy O, Misra R, et al. Selected loss of tolerance evidenced by Crohn's disease-associated immune responses to auto- and microbial antigens. Gastroenterology. 2002;123:689–99.
331. Garrett WS, Gallini CA, Yatsunenko T, Michaud M, DuBois A, Delaney ML, et al. Enterobacteriaceae act in concert with the gut microbiota to induce spontaneous and maternally transmitted colitis. Cell Host Microbe. 2010;8:292–300.
332. Garrett WS, Gordon JI, Glimcher LH. Homeostasis and inflammation in the intestine. Cell. 2010;140:859–70.
333. Boirivant M, Amendola A, Butera A, Sanchez M, Xu L, Marinaro M, et al. A transient breach in the epithelial barrier leads to regulatory T-cell generation and resistance to experimental colitis. Gastroenterology. 2008;135:1612–23.e5.
334. Karlsson MR, Rugtveit J, Brandtzaeg P. Allergen-responsive CD^{+}CD25^{+} regulatory T cells in children who have outgrown cow's milk allergy. J Exp Med. 2004;199:1679–88.

3 Understanding the Epithelial Barrier in IBD

Matthew A. Odenwald and Jerrold R. Turner

Mucosal surfaces are lined by epithelial cells, which form a barrier between the internal and external environment. The integrity of this barrier is critical, particularly within the intestine, where the luminal environment includes potentially pathogenic antigens and microorganisms. Although the term "barrier" may imply that the mucosa simply acts as a static impediment, preventing all transepithelial flux, this is not the case, as the epithelium must absorb and secrete the water, ions, and macromolecules that are necessary to maintain intestinal homeostasis and overall nutrition. Thus, the mucosa must integrate active, vectorial, and passive transport with a selectively permeable barrier that prevents entry of noxious luminal materials.

"Intestinal barrier function" is often used indiscriminately but is commonly thought of as either (1) the epithelial cells and materials they secrete, which provide a physical impediment to ion, water, and macromolecular flux, or (2) the defense provided by the mucosal immune system, which protects the host from potentially pathogenic luminal contents that have crossed the physical barrier. While both types of barriers are essential to epithelial homeostasis, the primary focus of this chapter is the former, i.e. the barrier formed by epithelial cells and the materials they secrete. The latter include mucins, secreted by intestinal goblet cells, which form a hydrated gel over the epithelial surface. As discussed elsewhere defects in mucin synthesis and the extracellular mucin layer have been associated with inflammatory bowel disease (IBD) in humans and spontaneous colitis in mice.

M.A. Odenwald, Ph.D.
Department of Pathology, The University of Chicago, 5841 South Maryland, MC 1089, Chicago, IL 60637, USA

J.R. Turner, M.D., Ph.D. (✉)
Department of Pathology, The University of Chicago, 5841 South Maryland, MC 1089, Chicago, IL 60637, USA

Departments of Pathology and Medicine (GI), Brigham and Women's Hospital and Harvard Medical School, 20 Shattuck St., TH1428, Boston, MA 02116, USA
e-mail: jturner@bsd.uchicago.edu

While mucin contributes to the development of the unstirred layer by limiting passage of large materials and trapping some bacteria, it is the epithelial cells that form the principal barrier to water and solute flux. The lipid bilayer of epithelial cells serves as a barrier to most hydrophilic solutes, and therefore, the majority of passive flux across epithelia occurs via the paracellular route. Changes in epithelial state can affect three distinct flux routes: the paracellular pore and leak pathways and the unrestricted pathway. The pore pathway is a high-capacity, size- and charge-selective route that mediates flux of small ions and water. In contrast, the leak pathway is a low-capacity, relatively size- and charge-non-selective pathway that facilitates passive transport of larger macromolecules. In the presence of erosions or ulcerations the epithelium is lost and, therefore, does not contribute to barrier function. In this case, flux of water, ions, macromolecules, and bacteria is unrestricted in terms of both capacity and selectivity. Molecules that permeate denuded epithelia are therefore said to cross the "unrestricted pathway." It is important to note that these pathways are not absolute, and as discussed below, there is cross-talk between elements of each pathway. When the unrestricted pathway is sealed, i.e. in the presence of an intact epithelial layer, the intercellular tight junctions define the selective permeability of the mucosal barrier.

The Epithelial Barrier Is Regulated in Response to Physiologic Stimuli

The intestinal epithelium is charged with the complex task of serving as a barrier that separates internal body cavities from potentially noxious luminal contents while simultaneously facilitating nutrient, ion, and water absorption and secretion. Physiologic regulation of epithelial barrier function has been studied extensively in the context of Na^+-glucose cotransport [1–4]. Upon activation of Na^+-glucose cotransport, a transepithelial osmotic gradient is developed and epithelial myosin light chain kinase (MLCK) is activated. Together, these

D.C. Baumgart (ed.), *Crohn's Disease and Ulcerative Colitis*, DOI 10.1007/978-3-319-33703-6_3

changes result in increased pore pathway flux, passive water absorption, and solvent-drag-mediated absorption of nutrient-sized molecules, such as glucose [1].

The Intestinal Barrier Is Compromised in IBD

Epithelial barrier function is compromised in many intestinal disorders. The association between decreased barrier function and intestinal disease was first reported in the early 1980s [5–7]. These studies, which made use of both ex vivo and in vivo approaches, demonstrated increased permeability in Crohn's disease (CD) and ulcerative colitis (UC) in the absence, as well as the presence, of ulcerations. Barrier defects are also present in conditions not typically associated with erosion and ulceration, e.g. celiac disease [8, 9], and in some healthy first-degree relatives of CD patients [10].

In patients, measurement of intestinal permeability typically involves measuring fractional urinary excretion of orally administered small molecules, such as ^{51}Cr-EDTA, polyethylene glycols, mannitol, lactulose, sucralose, or creatinine [11–14]. Intestinal absorption of these molecules occurs freely across erosions. When the epithelium is intact absorption is more restricted and defined by the tight junctions. These tracers are not metabolized in the circulation and are freely filtered at the glomerulus. Thus, fractional urinary recovery can be used as a noninvasive measure of intestinal permeability, assuming normal vascular perfusion, renal function, and intestinal motility. Lactulose and mannitol are used most commonly. With a small radius, mannitol is capable of crossing via the paracellular pore pathway, while lactulose is larger and can cross at sites of epithelial damage or through the paracellular leak pathway. Fractional excretion of lactulose can therefore be thought of as a measure of leak pathway permeability and intestinal damage while mannitol excretion can be used as a measure of intestinal surface area. Assessing the lactulose to mannitol ratio (LAMA) therefore corrects for confounding factors such as epithelial surface area, intestinal transit time, and renal function [12]. However, lactulose and mannitol are partially degraded by luminal bacteria within the colon, making these probes unsuitable analysis of colonic permeability [15, 16]. As a result, permeability has been studied to a far greater extent in patients with small intestinal Crohn's disease than in patients with Crohn's colitis or ulcerative colitis.

The contribution of the intestinal barrier to IBD was first suggested following the observation that increased permeability is present in a subset of healthy, asymptomatic first-degree relatives of CD patients [10, 17, 18]. The exact nature of these barrier defects is not known, and increased intestinal permeability may stem from increased susceptibility to epithelial ulceration, tight junction barrier defects, or subclinical immune activation. However, analysis of some of these healthy subjects failed to identify erosions or ulcers. Nevertheless, one clinical trial found hypersensitivity to NSAID-mediated increases in intestinal permeability in subjects with genetic susceptibility to CD, i.e. first-degree relatives [19]. Additional studies have linked barrier defects in healthy first-degree relatives to specific CD-associated mutations in NOD2, an immunoregulatory gene [20]. Finally, barrier loss in IBD has been correlated with altered tight junction organization, protein composition, cytoskeletal regulation, and epithelial damage [21–28]. It is important to note that these findings are not mutually exclusive as heightened immune activation may lead to increased tight junction permeability and ultimately epithelial damage.

Although the contribution of barrier defects in disease pathogenesis is unclear, it is interesting to note a case report describing the development of CD in a previously healthy relative with increased intestinal permeability [29]. While this single patient could be interpreted as support for a link between abnormal intestinal permeability and subsequent disease development, it is important to keep in mind that risk of disease was increased in this individual on a genetic basis. Indeed, first-degree relatives of patients affected by CD have an elevated risk of developing IBD [30]. Unfortunately, no studies have compared the long-term risk of developing CD in healthy relatives with or without increased permeability. However, increased small intestinal permeability is a known marker of impending relapse in CD patients with inactive disease [31].

The Epithelial Monolayer

In a reductionist view, the intestinal barrier is formed by a single layer of epithelial cells linked together by intercellular junctions. In the absence of specific transporters, the epithelial plasma membrane serves as a barrier to most hydrophilic molecules; thus, intercellular junctions are the limiting factor in transepithelial permeability. The most critical intercellular junctions are the tight junctions, adherens junctions, and desmosomes, which form the apical junctional complex [32]. The tight junction and adherens junctions are associated with a dense perijunctional ring of actin and myosin II that encircles the apical aspect of each epithelial cell. These form a network that connects neighboring cells and forms the selectively permeable paracellular barrier (Fig. 3.1a).

Molecular Anatomy of the Tight Junction

The adherens junction is formed by homotypic interactions between the epithelial cadherin isoform E-cadherin (Fig. 3.1B). The cytoplasmic domains of the cadherins interact with the catenins, which in turn bind to the actin

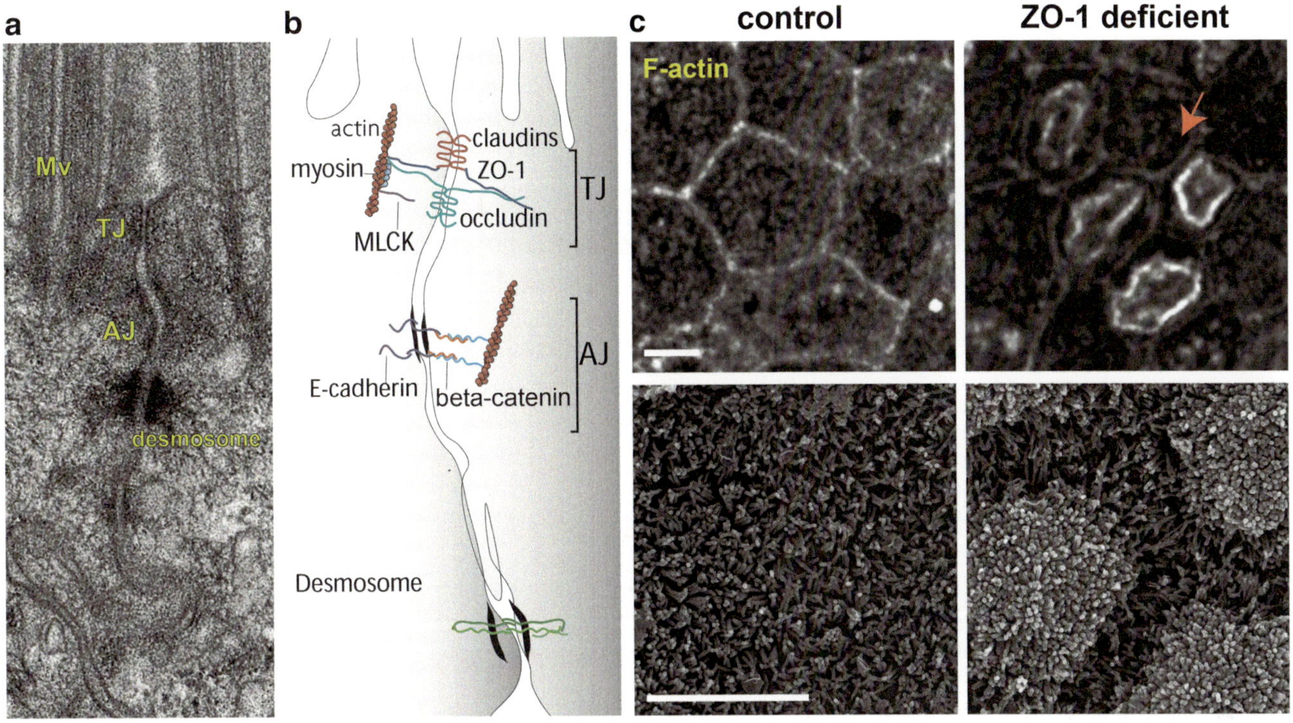

Fig. 3.1 Structure of the epithelial barrier. (**a**) Transmission electron micrograph depicting the apical junctional complex between two mouse enterocytes. From apical to basal, the apical junctional complex consists of the zonula occludens, also referred to as the tight junction (TJ); the zonula adherens, also referred to as the adherens junction (AJ); and macula adherens, also referred to as the desmosome. Microvilli (Mv) line the luminal surface of intestinal epithelia and are labeled for orientation. (**b**) The tight junction is spanned by occludin and claudin family members, which dynamically regulate permeability between cells. The plaque protein zonula ocludens-1 (ZO-1) interacts with transmembrane tight junction proteins and with the actomyosin cytoskeleton to regulate tight junction function. Myosin light chain kinase (MLCK) controls junction-associated myosin phosphorylation and myosin ATPase activity to regulate barrier function. (**c**) The cytosolic tight junction scaffolding protein ZO-1 is essential for cortical actin organization. Fluorescence microscopy (*top two panels*) and scanning electron microscopy (*bottom two panels*) of confluent epithelial monolayers show that ZO-1 deletion results in marked abnormalities of apical structure. *Top panels* are maximum intensity projections of confocal z-series through the entire epithelial monolayer. Scale bars = 5 μm

cytoskeleton to regulate cell structure and function [33–35]. The tight junction consists of many transmembrane proteins, including occludin and claudins [36–39] (Fig. 3.1b). Transmembrane tight junction proteins are linked to one another and to the actomyosin cytoskeleton by the cytosolic scaffolding protein zonula occludens (ZO)-1, thereby forming an elaborate protein network at the apical junctional complex [40–43]. The extracellular loops of claudins mediate homotypic interactions to form high-capacity size- and charge-selective paracellular pores [44, 45]. In contrast, occludin, ZO-1, and the actomyosin cytoskeleton are known to regulate leak pathway permeability [46–49]. These molecular components interact and can regulate both pathways, as occludin and ZO-1, which primarily regulate the leak pathway, can also affect claudin pore function [50]. ZO-1 may affect paracellular permeability through regulation of cortical actomyosin organization and contractile activity [43, 51]. Moreover, by integrating cortical actomyosin function, ZO-1 directs a diverse array of cellular processes; ZO-1 depletion has marked effects on epithelial morphology (Fig. 3.1c).

In vitro and in vivo studies have revealed that tight junction assembly is closely linked to adherens junction integrity, as confluent epithelial monolayers lacking E-cadherin or alpha-catenin are unable to efficiently recruit tight junction proteins or form effective barriers to ions and macromolecular flux [52–55].

Intercellular Junctions and IBD

The critical role of the adherens junction in intestinal physiology was demonstrated using chimeric mice in which some, but not all, villous enterocytes expressed a dominant-negative cytoplasmic tail of N-cadherin [52]. Expression of the dominant-negative N-cadherin tail disrupted E-cadherin function and resulted in the loss of intercellular junctions, aberrant epithelial differentiation, Crohn's-like disease, and epithelial dysplasia [52]. E-cadherin may also be relevant to human disease as data from recent genome-wide association studies (GWAS) suggest that polymorphisms within *CDH1*, the gene encoding E-cadherin, may be associated with ulcerative colitis [56].

Despite this critical role of the adherens junction, the tight junction is the primary determinant of paracellular permeability. It is, therefore, not surprising that alterations in tight junction structure and function are associated with increased permeability in IBD. For example, the normally complex anastomosing network of tight junction strands seen by freeze-fracture electron microscopy is simplified in IBD [26]. Moreover, the expression and distribution of individual tight junction proteins is altered in IBD [21, 22, 25]. Finally, increased expression and enzymatic activity of myosin light chain kinase, a key regulator of the perijunctional actomyosin ring and tight junction permeability, have been associated with active IBD [24]. As discussed below, this appears to be the primary intracellular signaling pathway by which TNF and related cytokines disrupt tight junction barrier function [48, 49, 57, 58].

Discovery of the claudins, a large family of proteins now recognized to define tight junction ion selectivity and to be essential for the development of the paracellular barrier, was a major breakthrough in tight junction biology [38]. The availability of reagents suitable for analyzing individual claudin proteins in human specimens revealed that expression of claudin-2 was upregulated in IBD [21, 23]. In parallel, in vitro studies demonstrated that claudin-2 expression increased the paracellular flux of cations, e.g. Na^+, and small uncharged molecules [59–61]. Furthermore, in vitro and in vivo studies have shown that claudin-2 upregulation alone is responsible for the increased pore pathway flux induced by IL-13 [61]. Thus, increased flux through claudin-2 is a potential mechanism for the elevated pore pathway paracellular permeability observed in IBD. IL-13 may not be the only mediator of claudin-2 induction in IBD [62, 63], but it is interesting to note that claudin-2 expression is greater in UC than CD, and that there is a greater elevation of IL-13 production by lamina propria mononuclear cells from UC, relative to CD [22, 23]. However, as discussed below, increased claudin-2 expression cannot fully explain the barrier defects present in IBD, and it remains uncertain whether this represents a beneficial adaptive, or detrimental maladaptive, process.

While elevated levels of IL-13 are highly relevant to IBD, the impact of IL-13 neutralization on intestinal permeability and disease activity in human IBD is untested. In contrast, TNF neutralization reduces disease severity and also restores intestinal barrier function in IBD patients [64]. While this does, in part, reflect healing of mucosal ulcers and global immune downregulation, TNF also plays a critical role in tight junction regulation. For example, studies in mice have shown that acute T cell activation causes a TNF-dependent increase in intestinal permeability. This is associated with endocytosis of the tight junction protein occludin and redistribution of the cytoplasmic plaque protein ZO-1 [47, 49]. Occludin internalization is directly related to TNF-induced barrier loss, as occludin overexpression in transgenic mice limits increases in permeability and prevents diarrhea following acute TNF exposure [47]. More recent in vitro studies have shown that occludin knockdown also protects from such barrier loss as occludin deficient monolayers are insensitive to TNF exposure. This barrier regulation relies on direct interactions between occludin and ZO-1 [46, 65]. This failure of occludin-deficient epithelia to regulate tight junction permeability following TNF exposure is likely explained by the fact that these monolayers have increased tight junction leak pathway permeability at baseline [46]. Notably, occludin expression is reduced in chronic experimental colitis as well as human IBD [22, 66].

TNF-induced barrier loss has also been shown, in vitro and in vivo, to require myosin light chain kinase- (MLCK-) dependent myosin II regulatory light chain (MLC) phosphorylation [48, 49]. TNF-induced MLCK activation precedes occludin internalization, as genetic or pharmacological MLCK inhibition prevents occludin redistribution, barrier loss, and diarrhea [49]. In contrast, inhibition of occludin endocytosis prevents barrier loss but does not block MLC phosphorylation. Beyond enzymatic activation, TNF increases MLCK transcription and protein synthesis in vitro and in vivo [67, 68]. Moreover, MLCK expression and enzymatic activity are both increased in human IBD, particularly in association with active disease [24]. MLCK activation is also required for barrier dysregulation by other cytokines relevant to IBD, including lymphotoxin-like inducible protein that competes with glycoprotein D for herpes virus entry on T cells (LIGHT), and interleukin-1β (IL-1β) [58, 69, 70]. As discussed below, these and other data [28] indicate that MLCK inhibition may have therapeutic efficacy in IBD, particularly as a maintenance therapy.

The ability of pro-inflammatory cytokines to regulate tight junction barrier function may explain the presence of increased permeability in human IBD. For example, the permeability increases that precede CD reactivation may be secondary to limited immune activation. This model is also consistent with the observation that barrier defects in first-degree relatives of CD patients are associated with mutations in NOD2, a known immunoregulatory gene [20]. However, the fact that these relatives, as well as other individuals with reduced barrier function, do not have disease as well as the absence of spontaneous disease in animal models of impaired intestinal tight junction barrier function demonstrate that increased intestinal permeability alone is insufficient to cause IBD [10, 71, 72]. How is it possible to integrate these data and understand the relationship between intestinal barrier function and disease? One animal model that clarifies the relationship between immune signaling and barrier function in disease is the interleukin-10 knockout (IL-10 KO) mouse.

This model is relevant to human disease, as polymorphisms of both the IL-10 promoter and the IL-10 receptor have been linked to ulcerative colitis and very eraly onset IBD [73, 74].

IL-10 knockout mice develop spontaneous colitis when housed under 'normal' specific pathogen-free conditions. However, like human IBD, development of disease in IL-10 KO mice is clearly multifactorial. Disease penetrance and presentation vary with genetic background and among different animal facilities, and disease does not develop at all in germ-free mice. Moreover, when disease does occur in IL-10 KO mice, clinical symptoms are not present at birth, but develop only after weeks or months [75]. Intestinal barrier defects are detectable in a large proportion of IL-10 KO mice within 4 weeks of birth, but are absent in antibiotic-treated or germ-free mice [76]. Thus, given that the primary defect in these mice is loss of the immunoregulatory cytokine IL-10, one can conclude that intestinal permeability defects arise secondary to an interaction between the immune system and luminal microbiota. This suggests that the barrier defects in IL-10 KO mice are a sensitive indicator of mucosal immune activation. Another study suggests that enhancing mucosal barrier function by undefined mechanisms may limit disease in IL-10 KO mice [77]. Thus, early permeability defects may contribute to disease progression in IL-10 KO mice.

Another observation that suggests a contribution of barrier defects to disease evolution in IL-10 KO mice is the synchronization of disease onset by treatment with the nonsteroidal anti-inflammatory drug (NSAID) piroxicam [78]. While the mechanisms by which piroxicam exerts these effects are unclear, NSAIDs are known to cause epithelial injury, including erosions that can enhance mucosal bacterial invasion in IL-10 KO mice. Thus, one might hypothesize that piroxicam triggers disease in IL-10 KO mice by enhancing intestinal permeability, although not by increasing tight junction permeability. This suggests that a transient elevation of intestinal permeability in a genetically susceptible host, e.g. IL-10 KO mice, is sufficient to initiate chronic disease. This model could also explain the observation, made in humans, that an acute episode of bacterial gastroenteritis is associated with increased risk of developing IBD [79]. Thus, the IL-10 KO mouse model emphasizes the interaction between genetic susceptibility, immune activation, intestinal microbiota, and epithelial barrier function in development of human IBD.

Barrier Defects and Mucosal Immune Regulation

The data discussed above suggest that barrier function can be a sensitive indicator of mucosal immune activation and that increased permeability may be able to amplify the effects of such immune activation. However, while the role of primary epithelial barrier dysfunction in IBD pathogenesis remains controversial, the associations are striking. For example, barrier defects precede clinical manifestations of disease in IL-10 KO mice, in which the primary defect is immunological [76]. Increased intestinal permeability has also been reported prior to clinical disease onset in the outbred SAMP1/YitFc mouse model of IBD [80]. Bone marrow chimera studies suggest that the primary defect in these mice is present within a radioresistant, non-bone marrow-derived cell population [80]. However, the precise abnormality that causes disease in SAMP1/YitFc mice has not been identified.

Studies of mice with targeted barrier defects provide further evidence that tight junction permeability may contribute to disease progression. One informative example comes from mice lacking junctional adhesion molecule A (JAM-A), an immunoglobulin superfamily member that facilitates tight junction assembly and leukocyte transmigration across endothelia and epithelia [72, 81]. Loss of JAM-A expression within intestinal epithelia led to increased colonic epithelial apoptosis in colitis, providing one potential mechanism by which JAM-A deficiency augments disease. Consistent with this, colonic neutrophil accumulation was increased in JAM-A KO mice, and these mice were also hypersensitive to dextran sulfate sodium- (DSS-) induced epithelial injury and colitis [72]. Because JAM-A is normally expressed ubiquitously, defects in these mice could not be linked directly to loss of intestinal epithelial JAM-A. However, endothelial specific JAM-A KO mice did not demonstrate increased DSS susceptibility, demonstrating that endothelial JAM-A loss was not responsible for the observed phenotype. In addition, the observation that intestinal epithelial, but not endothelial, JAM-A expression is reduced in human and experimental IBD supports the hypothesis that loss of intestinal epithelial JAM-A is responsible for the phenotype of JAM-A KO mice [72]. Although the phenotype of the JAM-A KO mice is informative and implicates tight junction proteins in epithelial repair processes, the cause of JAM-A loss in human and experimental IBD remains unclear. Moreover, despite the experimental simplicity of the model, the DSS model of colitis primarily reflects responses to acute epithelial damage and does not reflect the pathogenesis of human IBD. Some workers have attempted to correct this using a chronic DSS model, but that model suffers from the same problem in that it is caused by ongoing direct epithelial injury, which is unlikely to be the cause of human IBD.

Increased transcription and enzymatic activity of intestinal epithelial MLCK are well-documented in human and experimental IBD, and are regulated by proinflammatory cytokines such as TNF. Moreover, MLCK is required for in vitro and in vivo TNF-induced barrier loss [48, 49]. To model this form of barrier loss, transgenic mice that express constitutively active MLCK (CA-MLCK) from an intestinal epithelial-specific promoter were created [71]. These mice have

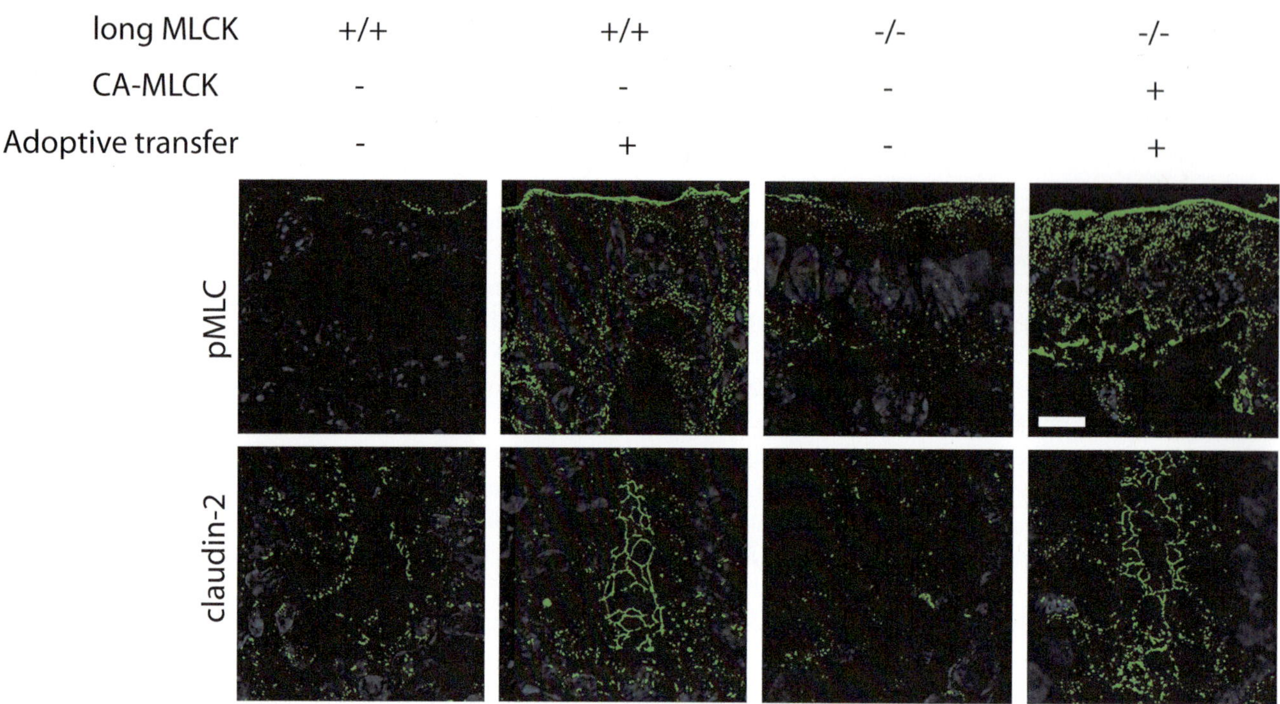

Fig. 3.2 Both leak and pore paracellular pathways are altered in immune-mediated colitis. All mice are RAG1$^{-/-}$ to allow for adoptive transfer colitis. Myosin light chain is phosphorylated in immune-mediated colitis in an MLCK-dependent manner (*top panels*). Transgenic, intestinal epithelial-restricted expression of constitutively active-MLCK restores disease-associated MLC phosphorylation to long MLCK$^{-/-}$ mice. Claudin-2 expression parallels MLC phosphorylation in CD4^{+}CD45RB^{hi} colitis (*bottom panels*). Increases in MLC phosphorylation and claudin-2 expression correspond with worsened clinical outcomes in early stages of colitis. Scale bar = 10 μm. From Su et al., 2013

increased small intestinal and colonic paracellular permeability and exhibit mucosal immune activation, as evidenced by elevated mucosal IFNγ (gamma), TNF, IL-10, and IL-13 transcription and increased numbers of colonic lamina propria T cells. However, despite mucosal immune activation, the mice thrive and do not develop spontaneous disease. While this absence of disease may reflect the activity of immunoregulatory cells, such as those responsible for the increase in IL-10 transcription, expression of CA-MLCK in RAG1-deficient (RAG1$^{-/-}$) mice, which lack regulatory T cells, also fails to induce disease [71]. However, when effector T lymphocytes are introduced into CA-MLCK/RAG1$^{-/-}$ mice, using the CD4+CD45Rbhi T lymphocyte adoptive transfer model of colitis, the onset of disease is accelerated and severity is increased relative to RAG1$^{-/-}$ littermates that lack CA-MLCK [71]. Therefore, these CA-MLCK transgenic mice recapitulate the observation in humans that primary barrier dysfunction is insufficient to cause disease, e.g. in healthy relatives of CD patients, and also provide evidence that barrier dysfunction can accelerate the onset and enhance the severity of immune-mediated colitis.

This interplay between TNF exposure, immune activation, MLCK, and intestinal barrier function has been further studied using immune-mediated adoptive transfer colitis in RAG1 knockout mice lacking either TNF receptor 1 (TNFR1) or TNFR2 [28]. CD4+CD45Rbhi T lymphocyte adoptive transfer into RAG1 deficient mice results in increased MLCK protein expression along with increased transcription of TNFR2 but not TNFR1 [28]. Adoptive transfer into RAG1 knockout mice lacking TNFR2 failed to induce MLCK expression, and mice lacking either TNFR2 or MLCK were at least partially protected from immune-mediated colitis [28]. These data, along with in vitro observations showing that TNF-induced, MLCK-dependent barrier loss requires TNFR2 function indicate that it is epithelial TNFR2, and not TNFR1, that drives MLCK transcription [28]. Remarkably, colitis-associated claudin-2 upregulation was also limited in MLCK-deficient mice (Fig. 3.2), demonstrating the in vivo interplay between paracellular leak and pore pathways [28]. Nevertheless, mice lacking either epithelial MLCK or TNFR2 did eventually develop colitis and unrestricted pathway barrier loss [28]. This occurred as a consequence of immune-mediated epithelial damage. Consistent with this, epithelial MLCK knockout mice were not protected from acute, TNF-induced epithelial apoptosis or DSS colitis [28]. These data reinforce the notion that MLCK inhibition may be beneficial in preventing relapse or progression to advanced IBD but may not be useful in treatment of active disease with ulcerations.

Isolated Barrier Defects Are Insufficient to Cause Disease

While data above link increased intestinal permeability to disease severity and relapse, mild barrier defects may actually trigger regulatory processes that prevent inappropriate immune responses in immunocompetent hosts. The clearest example of this may be data indicating that, despite the presence of increased permeability in patients with infectious gastroenteritis, most of these individuals recover fully and do not develop IBD [79]. Recent studies in mice have provided some insight into the immunoregulatory mechanisms that prevent development of chronic disease in this situation. In wild-type mice, when mucosal damage was induced by intrarectal ethanol administration, the resulting transient increase in permeability induced a population of regulatory T cells characterized by the surface expression of the TGFβ pro-peptide latency-associated peptide (LAP) and also increased IL-10 production by lamina propria mononuclear cells [82]. Moreover, this mild mucosal damage protected mice from colitis induced by subsequent intrarectal TNBS administration. While the detailed mechanisms by which transient increases in permeability invoke immunoregulatory responses are incompletely characterized, it is notable that mucosal IL-10 production was also increased in CA-MLCK transgenic mice [71]. Thus, chronic barrier defects may also induce immunoregulatory responses that prevent disease. On this basis, it can be inferred that, in an immunocompetent host, limited barrier defects induce a robust immunoregulatory response that prevents disease. If correct, this hypothesis suggests that the difference between CD patients and their healthy relatives with increased permeability may be the quality of this regulatory response and the ability to manage inflammation induced by barrier loss. Overall, these studies emphasize the need for further clarification of the complex interactions between the intestinal epithelial barrier and mucosal immune system.

A Multifactorial Model of IBD

The data discussed above suggest a model of IBD in which paracellular defects, mucosal immune activation, and the luminal microbiota are interrelated and act cooperatively in the prevention, induction, and progression of disease (Fig. 3.3). The epithelial barrier balances the interaction between immunostimulatory luminal materials and the

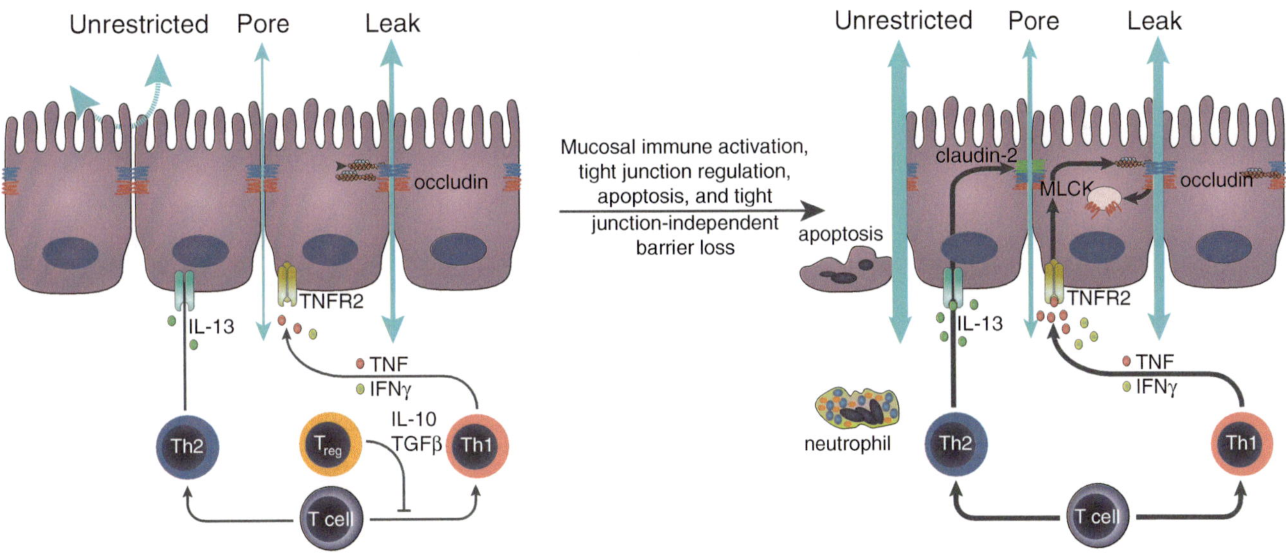

Fig. 3.3 The epithelial barrier regulates the balance between the luminal environment and mucosal immunity. Breaches in the epithelial barrier allow luminal material to cross the epithelium, where it may then activate mucosal immune responses. Under conditions of appropriate immune regulation, regulatory T cells (Tregs) produce anti-inflammatory signals to counter the pro-inflammatory immune response. A subset of these Tregs, those expressing latency-associated peptide (LAP), secrete IL-10 and TGF-β to attenuate disease. In contrast, under disease conditions, luminal material may activate Th1 or Th2 T cells. Th1 cells secrete TNF and IFNγ, which increase paracellular leak pathway permeability via MLCK-dependent mechanisms. Alternatively, Th2 cells secrete IL-13, which increases pore pathway permeability by upregulating claudin-2 expression. These increases in paracellular permeability may allow the passage of additional luminal material across the barrier. Amplification of this cycle of inflammation eventually leads to apoptosis of epithelial cells. Under these conditions, intestinal permeability is largely tight-junction independent and unrestricted. Due to the tight junction-independent nature of this unrestricted pathway in more advanced disease, therapeutics designed to restore tight junction barrier function will likely be most useful in early disease or in maintaining remission. Adapted from Su et al. 2013

mucosal immune system. In immunocompetent subjects, mild barrier defects activate regulatory immune responses that compensate for and prevent excessive immune activation. In contrast, barrier defects may trigger inappropriate immune activation and cytokine release in subjects who are unable to elicit effective immunoregulatory responses. These cytokines may then signal to epithelial cells to cause further increases in paracellular permeability, which, in turn, allows further transmucosal passage of immunostimulatory materials and an even greater degree of immune activation. Thus defects in either barrier function or immune activation may initiate the cycle of barrier-immune dysregulation, but defects in both are necessary for perpetuation of this cycle and disease pathogenesis. This model also suggests that, in addition to the immunosuppressive and immunomodulatory agents that have been central to IBD therapy, it may be possible to break the cycle by restoring barrier function prior to onset of clinical disease.

Barrier Restoration as a Future Therapeutic Intervention

Current immunosuppressive and immunomodulatory approaches are often effective in IBD management, but they treat the inflammation responsible for tissue damage rather than the underlying cause of inflammation. It has been recognized for some time that the epithelial barrier can be dysregulated by proinflammatory stimuli. The model described, which explains available data from in vitro and in vivo models as well as human studies, suggests that the barrier also regulates the immune response. Although increased paracellular permeability is a normal physiological response that is often beneficial and, in an immunocompetent host, triggers an immunoregulatory response, reduced barrier function may also be critical to disease pathogenesis. This is particularly true in individuals with immunoregulatory defects. For example, barrier loss precedes colitis in IL-10-deficient mice. Conversely, barrier restoration may blunt disease development. Similarly, genetic deletion of intestinal epithelial long MLCK, which is necessary for TNF-induced barrier loss, partially protects immunodeficient mice from colitis induced by CD4+CD45Rbhi adoptive transfer. These data suggest that barrier restoration may be therapeutically useful, particularly in patients with IL-10 receptor mutations or single nucleotide polymorphisms (SNPs) within the IL10 promoter.

Development of barrier restorative agents will require targeting the pore, leak, and unrestricted paracellular pathways, all of which are disrupted at different stages of colitis. While claudin-2 must be responsible for some of the increases in pore pathway permeability in colitis, no modulators of claudin-2 pore function are currently available.

Epithelial MLCK is clearly an attractive druggable target to restore leak pathway permeability early during disease development and promote maintenance of remission. However, the different MLCK isoforms expressed in smooth muscle and nonmuscle cells are encoded by a single gene and, therefore, have common catalytic and calmodulin-dependent regulatory domains [83, 84]. Knockout mouse studies clearly show that inhibition of smooth muscle MLCK has disastrous consequences [84]. Thus, alternatives to currently available MLCK inhibitors, all of which target the catalytic domain, will be necessary if MLCK is to be a viable therapeutic target.

Tight junctions play a lesser role in intestinal barrier loss in more advanced disease when increased permeability is primarily driven by epithelial damage and increased flux across the unrestricted pathway. Some of the epithelial wounds present are repaired by an actomyosin purse string-dependent mechanism that also requires epithelial MLCK activity [85]. Therefore, in order restore tight junction barrier function without disrupting other tissues or epithelial wound repair, it will be critical to develop a more targeted approach to inhibiting tight junction regulatory activities of epithelial MLCK in response to pathophysiologic stimuli, such as TNF, without impairing wound healing. If this can be achieved, barrier restoration may have a promising future in IBD therapy.

References

1. Turner JR, Rill BK, Carlson SL, Carnes D, Kerner R, Mrsny RJ, et al. Physiological regulation of epithelial tight junctions is associated with myosin light-chain phosphorylation. Am J Physiol. 1997;273:C1378–85.
2. Shiue H, Musch MW, Wang Y, Chang EB, Turner JR. Akt2 phosphorylates ezrin to trigger NHE3 translocation and activation. J Biol Chem. 2005;280:1688–95.
3. Turner JR, Black ED, Ward J, Tse CM, Uchwat FA, Alli HA, et al. Transepithelial resistance can be regulated by the intestinal brush border Na^+-H^+ exchanger NHE3. Am J Physiol Cell Physiol. 2000;279:C1918–24.
4. Turner JR, Cohen DE, Mrsny RJ, Madara JL. Noninvasive in vivo analysis of human small intestinal paracellular absorption: regulation by Na+-glucose cotransport. Dig Dis Sci. 2000;45:2122–6.
5. Ukabam SO, Clamp JR, Cooper BT. Abnormal small intestinal permeability to sugars in patients with Crohn's disease of the terminal ileum and colon. Digestion. 1983;27:70–4.
6. Hollander D. Crohn's disease—a permeability disorder of the tight junction? Gut. 1988;29:1621–4.
7. Pearson AD, Eastham EJ, Laker MF, Craft AW, Nelson R. Intestinal permeability in children with Crohn's disease and coeliac disease. Br Med J (Clin Res Ed). 1982;285:20–1.
8. Schulzke JD, Bentzel CJ, Schulzke I, Riecken EO, Fromm M. Epithelial tight junction structure in the jejunum of children with acute and treated celiac sprue. Pediatr Res. 1998;43:435–41.
9. Madara JL, Trier JS. Structural abnormalities of jejunal epithelial cell membranes in celiac sprue. Lab Invest. 1980;43:254–61.
10. Hollander D, Vadheim CM, Brettholz E, Petersen GM, Delahunty T, Rotter JI. Increased intestinal permeability in patients with Crohn's disease and their relatives. A possible etiologic factor. Ann Intern Med. 1986;105:883–5.
11. Jenkins RT, Ramage JK, Jones DB, Collins SM, Goodacre RL, Hunt RH. Small bowel and colonic permeability to 51Cr-EDTA in

patients with active inflammatory bowel disease. Clin Invest Med. 1988;11:151–5.
12. Bijlsma PB, Peeters RA, Groot JA, Dekker PR, Taminiau JA, Van Der Meer R. Differential in vivo and in vitro intestinal permeability to lactulose and mannitol in animals and humans: a hypothesis. Gastroenterology. 1995;108:687–96.
13. Arslan G, Atasever T, Cindoruk M, Yildirim IS. (51)CrEDTA colonic permeability and therapy response in patients with ulcerative colitis. Nucl Med Commun. 2001;22:997–1001.
14. Bjarnason I. Intestinal permeability. Gut. 1994;35:S18–22.
15. Keighley MR, Taylor EW, Hares MM, Arabi Y, Youngs D, Bentley S, et al. Influence of oral mannitol bowel preparation on colonic microflora and the risk of explosion during endoscopic diathermy. Br J Surg. 1981;68:554–6.
16. Vince A, Killingley M, Wrong OM. Effect of lactulose on ammonia production in a fecal incubation system. Gastroenterology. 1978;74:544–9.
17. Katz KD, Hollander D, Vadheim CM, McElree C, Delahunty T, Dadufalza VD, et al. Intestinal permeability in patients with Crohn's disease and their healthy relatives. Gastroenterology. 1989;97:927–31.
18. May GR, Sutherland LR, Meddings JB. Is small intestinal permeability really increased in relatives of patients with Crohn's disease? Gastroenterology. 1993;104:1627–32.
19. Hilsden RJ, Meddings JB, Sutherland LR. Intestinal permeability changes in response to acetylsalicylic acid in relatives of patients with Crohn's disease. Gastroenterology. 1996;110:1395–403.
20. Buhner S, Buning C, Genschel J, Kling K, Herrmann D, Dignass A, et al. Genetic basis for increased intestinal permeability in families with Crohn's disease: role of CARD15 3020insC mutation? Gut. 2006;55:342–7.
21. Prasad S, Mingrino R, Kaukinen K, Hayes KL, Powell RM, MacDonald TT, et al. Inflammatory processes have differential effects on claudins 2, 3 and 4 in colonic epithelial cells. Lab Invest. 2005;85:1139–62.
22. Heller F, Florian P, Bojarski C, Richter J, Christ M, Hillenbrand B, et al. Interleukin-13 is the key effector Th2 cytokine in ulcerative colitis that affects epithelial tight junctions, apoptosis, and cell restitution. Gastroenterology. 2005;129:550–64.
23. Zeissig S, Burgel N, Gunzel D, Richter J, Mankertz J, Wahnschaffe U, et al. Changes in expression and distribution of claudin 2, 5 and 8 lead to discontinuous tight junctions and barrier dysfunction in active Crohn's disease. Gut. 2007;56:61–72.
24. Blair SA, Kane SV, Clayburgh DR, Turner JR. Epithelial myosin light chain kinase expression and activity are upregulated in inflammatory bowel disease. Lab Invest. 2006;86:191–201.
25. Weber CR, Nalle SC, Tretiakova M, Rubin DT, Turner JR. Claudin-1 and claudin-2 expression is elevated in inflammatory bowel disease and may contribute to early neoplastic transformation. Lab Invest. 2008;88:1110–20.
26. Schmitz H, Barmeyer C, Fromm M, Runkel N, Foss HD, Bentzel CJ, et al. Altered tight junction structure contributes to the impaired epithelial barrier function in ulcerative colitis. Gastroenterology. 1999;116:301–9.
27. Zeissig S, Bojarski C, Buergel N, Mankertz J, Zeitz M, Fromm M, et al. Downregulation of epithelial apoptosis and barrier repair in active Crohn's disease by tumour necrosis factor alpha antibody treatment. Gut. 2004;53:1295–302.
28. Su L, Nalle SC, Shen L, Turner ES, Singh G, Breskin LA, et al. TNFR2 activates MLCK-dependent tight junction dysregulation to cause apoptosis-mediated barrier loss and experimental colitis. Gastroenterology. 2013;145:407–15.
29. Irvine EJ, Marshall JK. Increased intestinal permeability precedes the onset of Crohn's disease in a subject with familial risk. Gastroenterology. 2000;119:1740–4.
30. Sands BE. Inflammatory bowel disease: past, present, and future. J Gastroenterol. 2007;42:16–25.
31. Wyatt J, Vogelsang H, Hubl W, Waldhoer T, Lochs H. Intestinal permeability and the prediction of relapse in Crohn's disease. Lancet. 1993;341:1437–9.
32. Farquhar M, Palade G. Junctional complexes in various epithelia. J Cell Biol. 1963;17:375–412.
33. Ojakian GK, Nelson WJ, Beck KA. Mechanisms for de novo biogenesis of an apical membrane compartment in groups of simple epithelial cells surrounded by extracellular matrix. J Cell Sci. 1997;110:2781–94.
34. Nejsum LN, Nelson WJ. A molecular mechanism directly linking E-cadherin adhesion to initiation of epithelial cell surface polarity. J Cell Biol. 2007;178:323–35.
35. Buckley CD, Tan J, Anderson KL, Hanein D, Volkmann N, Weis WI, et al. Cell adhesion. The minimal cadherin-catenin complex binds to actin filaments under force. Science. 2014;346:1254211.
36. Furuse M, Hirase T, Itoh M, Nagafuchi A, Yonemura S, Tsukita S, et al. Occludin: a novel integral membrane protein localizing at tight junctions. J Cell Biol. 1993;123:1777–88.
37. McCarthy KM, Skare IB, Stankewich MC, Furuse M, Tsukita S, Rogers RA, et al. Occludin is a functional component of the tight junction. J Cell Sci. 1996;109(Pt 9):2287–98.
38. Furuse M, Fujita K, Hiiragi T, Fujimoto K, Tsukita S. Claudin-1 and -2: novel integral membrane proteins localizing at tight junctions with no sequence similarity to occludin. J Cell Biol. 1998;141:1539–50.
39. Furuse M, Sasaki H, Fujimoto K, Tsukita S. A single gene product, claudin-1 or -2, reconstitutes tight junction strands and recruits occludin in fibroblasts. J Cell Biol. 1998;143:391–401.
40. Fanning AS, Anderson JM. Zonula occludens-1 and -2 are cytosolic scaffolds that regulate the assembly of cellular junctions. Ann N Y Acad Sci. 2009;1165:113–20.
41. Furuse M, Hata M, Furuse K, Yoshida Y, Haratake A, Sugitani Y, et al. Claudin-based tight junctions are crucial for the mammalian epidermal barrier: a lesson from claudin-1-deficient mice. J Cell Biol. 2002;156:1099–111.
42. Umeda K, Ikenouchi J, Katahira-Tayama S, Furuse K, Sasaki H, Nakayama M, et al. ZO-1 and ZO-2 independently determine where claudins are polymerized in tight-junction strand formation. Cell. 2006;126:741–54.
43. Ikenouchi J, Umeda K, Tsukita S, Furuse M. Requirement of ZO-1 for the formation of belt-like adherens junctions during epithelial cell polarization. J Cell Biol. 2007;176:779–86.
44. Van Itallie CM, Anderson JM. Claudins and epithelial paracellular transport. Annu Rev Physiol. 2006;68:403–29.
45. Suzuki H, Nishizawa T, Tani K, Yamazaki Y, Tamura A, Ishitani R, et al. Crystal structure of a claudin provides insight into the architecture of tight junctions. Science. 2014;344:304–7.
46. Buschmann MM, Shen L, Rajapakse H, Raleigh DR, Wang Y, Wang Y, et al. Occludin OCEL-domain interactions are required for maintenance and regulation of the tight junction barrier to macromolecular flux. Mol Biol Cell. 2013;24:3056–68.
47. Marchiando AM, Shen L, Graham WV, Weber CR, Schwarz BT, Austin 2nd JR, et al. Caveolin-1-dependent occludin endocytosis is required for TNF-induced tight junction regulation in vivo. J Cell Biol. 2010;189:111–26.
48. Zolotarevsky Y, Hecht G, Koutsouris A, Gonzalez DE, Quan C, Tom J, et al. A membrane-permeant peptide that inhibits MLC kinase restores barrier function in in vitro models of intestinal disease. Gastroenterology. 2002;123:163–72.
49. Clayburgh DR, Barrett TA, Tang Y, Meddings JB, Van Eldik LJ, Watterson DM, et al. Epithelial myosin light chain kinase-dependent barrier dysfunction mediates T cell activation-induced diarrhea in vivo. J Clin Invest. 2005;115:2702–15.
50. Raleigh DR, Boe DM, Yu D, Weber CR, Marchiando AM, Bradford EM, et al. Occludin S408 phosphorylation regulates tight junction

protein interactions and barrier function. J Cell Biol. 2011;193:565–82.

51. Van Itallie CM, Fanning AS, Bridges A, Anderson JM. ZO-1 stabilizes the tight junction solute barrier through coupling to the perijunctional cytoskeleton. Mol Biol Cell. 2009;20:3930–40.
52. Hermiston ML, Gordon JI. Inflammatory bowel disease and adenomas in mice expressing a dominant negative N-cadherin. Science. 1995;270:1203–7.
53. Hermiston ML, Gordon JI. In vivo analysis of cadherin function in the mouse intestinal epithelium: essential roles in adhesion, maintenance of differentiation, and regulation of programmed cell death. J Cell Biol. 1995;129:489–506.
54. Capaldo CT, Macara IG. Depletion of E-cadherin disrupts establishment but not maintenance of cell junctions in Madin-Darby canine kidney epithelial cells. Mol Biol Cell. 2007;18:189–200.
55. Maiers JL, Peng X, Fanning AS, DeMali KA. ZO-1 recruitment to alpha-catenin—a novel mechanism for coupling the assembly of tight junctions to adherens junctions. J Cell Sci. 2013;126:3904–15.
56. Barrett JC, Hansoul S, Nicolae DL, Cho JH, Duerr RH, Rioux JD, et al. Genome-wide association defines more than 30 distinct susceptibility loci for Crohn's disease. Nat Genet. 2008;40:955–62.
57. Al-Sadi R, Guo S, Ye D, Dokladny K, Alhmoud T, Ereifej L, et al. Mechanism of IL-1beta modulation of intestinal epithelial barrier involves p38 kinase and activating transcription factor-2 activation. J Immunol. 2013;190:6596–606.
58. Schwarz BT, Wang F, Shen L, Clayburgh DR, Su L, Wang Y, et al. LIGHT signals directly to intestinal epithelia to cause barrier dysfunction via cytoskeletal and endocytic mechanisms. Gastroenterology. 2007;132:2383–94.
59. Furuse M, Furuse K, Sasaki H, Tsukita S. Conversion of zonulae occludentes from tight to leaky strand type by introducing claudin-2 into Madin-Darby canine kidney I cells. J Cell Biol. 2001;153: 263–72.
60. Amasheh S, Meiri N, Gitter AH, Schoneberg T, Mankertz J, Schulzke JD, et al. Claudin-2 expression induces cation-selective channels in tight junctions of epithelial cells. J Cell Sci. 2002;115:4969–76.
61. Weber CR, Raleigh DR, Su L, Shen L, Sullivan EA, Wang Y, et al. Epithelial myosin light chain kinase activation induces mucosal interleukin-13 expression to alter tight junction ion selectivity. J Biol Chem. 2010;285:12037–46.
62. Suzuki T, Yoshinaga N, Tanabe S. Interleukin-6 (IL-6) regulates claudin-2 expression and tight junction permeability in intestinal epithelium. J Biol Chem. 2011;286:31263–71.
63. Mankertz J, Amasheh M, Krug SM, Fromm A, Amasheh S, Hillenbrand B, et al. TNFalpha up-regulates claudin-2 expression in epithelial HT-29/B6 cells via phosphatidylinositol-3-kinase signaling. Cell Tissue Res. 2009;336:67–77.
64. Suenaert P, Bulteel V, Lemmens L, Noman M, Geypens B, Van Assche G, et al. Anti-tumor necrosis factor treatment restores the gut barrier in Crohn's disease. Am J Gastroenterol. 2002;97: 2000–4.
65. Van Itallie CM, Fanning AS, Holmes J, Anderson JM. Occludin is required for cytokine-induced regulation of tight junction barriers. J Cell Sci. 2010;123:2844–52.
66. Wang F, Schwarz BT, Graham WV, Wang Y, Su L, Clayburgh DR, et al. IFN-gamma-induced TNFR2 expression is required for TNF-dependent intestinal epithelial barrier dysfunction. Gastroenterology. 2006;131:1153–63.
67. Wang F, Graham WV, Wang Y, Witkowski ED, Schwarz BT, Turner JR. Interferon-gamma and tumor necrosis factor-alpha synergize to induce intestinal epithelial barrier dysfunction by up-regulating myosin light chain kinase expression. Am J Pathol. 2005;166:409–19.
68. Graham WV, Wang F, Clayburgh DR, Cheng JX, Yoon B, Wang Y, et al. Tumor necrosis factor-induced long myosin light chain kinase transcription is regulated by differentiation-dependent signaling events. Characterization of the human long myosin light chain kinase promoter. J Biol Chem. 2006;281:26205–15.
69. Al-Sadi R, Ye D, Dokladny K, Ma TY. Mechanism of IL-1beta-induced increase in intestinal epithelial tight junction permeability. J Immunol. 2008;180:5653–61.
70. Al-Sadi R, Ye D, Said HM, Ma TY. IL-1beta-induced increase in intestinal epithelial tight junction permeability is mediated by MEKK-1 activation of canonical NF-kappaB pathway. Am J Pathol. 2010;177:2310–22.
71. Su L, Shen L, Clayburgh DR, Nalle SC, Sullivan EA, Meddings JB, et al. Targeted epithelial tight junction dysfunction causes immune activation and contributes to development of experimental colitis. Gastroenterology. 2009;136:551–63.
72. Vetrano S, Rescigno M, Rosaria Cera M, Correale C, Rumio C, Doni A, et al. Unique role of junctional adhesion molecule-a in maintaining mucosal homeostasis in inflammatory bowel disease. Gastroenterology. 2008;135:173–84.
73. Tedde A, Laura Putignano A, Bagnoli S, Congregati C, Milla M, Sorbi S, et al. Interleukin-10 promoter polymorphisms influence susceptibility to ulcerative colitis in a gender-specific manner. Scand J Gastroenterol. 2008;43:712–8.
74. Glocker EO, Kotlarz D, Boztug K, Gertz EM, Schaffer AA, Noyan F, et al. Inflammatory bowel disease and mutations affecting the interleukin-10 receptor. N Engl J Med. 2009;361:2033–45.
75. Kuhn R, Lohler J, Rennick D, Rajewsky K, Muller W. Interleukin-10-deficient mice develop chronic enterocolitis. Cell. 1993;75: 263–74.
76. Madsen KL, Malfair D, Gray D, Doyle JS, Jewell LD, Fedorak RN. Interleukin-10 gene-deficient mice develop a primary intestinal permeability defect in response to enteric microflora. Inflamm Bowel Dis. 1999;5:262–70.
77. Arrieta MC, Madsen K, Doyle J, Meddings J. Reducing small intestinal permeability attenuates colitis in the IL10 gene-deficient mouse. Gut. 2009;58:41–8.
78. Narushima S, Spitz DR, Oberley LW, Toyokuni S, Miyata T, Gunnett CA, et al. Evidence for oxidative stress in NSAID-induced colitis in IL10−/− mice. Free Radic Biol Med. 2003;34:1153–66.
79. Gradel KO, Nielsen HL, Schonheyder HC, Ejlertsen T, Kristensen B, Nielsen H. Increased short- and long-term risk of inflammatory bowel disease after salmonella or campylobacter gastroenteritis. Gastroenterology. 2009;137:495–501.
80. Olson TS, Reuter BK, Scott KG, Morris MA, Wang XM, Hancock LN, et al. The primary defect in experimental ileitis originates from a nonhematopoietic source. J Exp Med. 2006;203:541–52.
81. Woodfin A, Reichel CA, Khandoga A, Corada M, Voisin MB, Scheiermann C, et al. JAM-A mediates neutrophil transmigration in a stimulus-specific manner in vivo: evidence for sequential roles for JAM-A and PECAM-1 in neutrophil transmigration. Blood. 2007;110:1848–56.
82. Boirivant M, Amendola A, Butera A, Sanchez M, Xu L, Marinaro M, et al. A transient breach in the epithelial barrier leads to regulatory T-cell generation and resistance to experimental colitis. Gastroenterology. 2008;135:1612–23.
83. Clayburgh DR, Rosen S, Witkowski ED, Wang F, Blair S, Dudek S, et al. A differentiation-dependent splice variant of myosin light chain kinase, MLCK1, regulates epithelial tight junction permeability. J Biol Chem. 2004;279:55506–13.
84. He WQ, Peng YJ, Zhang WC, Lv N, Tang J, Chen C, et al. Myosin light chain kinase is central to smooth muscle contraction and required for gastrointestinal motility in mice. Gastroenterology. 2008;135:610–20.
85. Russo JM, Florian P, Shen L, Graham WV, Tretiakova MS, Gitter AH, et al. Distinct temporal-spatial roles for rho kinase and myosin light chain kinase in epithelial purse-string wound closure. Gastroenterology. 2005;128:987–1001.

Intestinal Microbiology and Ecology in Crohn's Disease and Ulcerative Colitis

4

Ludovica F. Buttó and Dirk Haller

Inflammatory bowel diseases (IBD) include the two main phenotypes Crohn's disease (CD) and ulcerative colitis (UC) both characterized by intermittent conditions of chronic and relapsing inflammation in the entire gastrointestinal tract or colon, respectively. Disease initiation and perturbation is triggered by environmental factors in genetically susceptible individuals [1, 2]. Genome-wide association studies (GWAS) and animal data provide evidence for an interrelated role of the intestinal microbiota, epithelial interface, and immune system in the pathogenesis of IBD [3–6]. This chapter provides an overview of the current state of research on the role of the intestinal microbiota in CD and UC. In addition, approaches to the treatment of IBD by the modulation of the intestinal microbiota are discussed.

Structure and Functionality of the Intestinal Microbiota

The human intestinal microbiota encompasses a variety of microorganisms, including bacteria, archaea, viruses, yeasts, and protozoa. The totality of these microbes and their genes is referred to as "intestinal microbiome" [7]. The microbial colonization of the intestine of newborn depends on the type of delivery (natural birth versus caesarean section) and the type of food intake (breastfeeding versus bottle milk) [8]. The first 2 years of life intestinal communities undergo substantial compositional fluctuations reacting to the new environmental cues, such as changes in dietary patterns, and thus it represents a crucial phase for the maturation of the intestinal microbial ecosystem [9–11]. After this critical phase, a relatively stable adult microbiota is established and interference factors (i.e., antibiotics, drugs, infections, excessive hygiene, nutrition, lifestyle) may affect its composition leading to serious long-term consequences [12–16]. For instance, long-term dietary patterns have a significant influence on the selection of specific microbial networks, the so-called enterotypes. A diet rich in animal fat and protein is associated with the Bacteroides enterotype, while a high-carbohydrate diet corresponds to the Prevotella enterotype [13, 17]. The mammalian gut microbiota comprises several hundred different bacterial species, many of which have a beneficial effect on the host and correspond to up to 10^{12}–10^{14} organisms/g of colon content, exceeding greatly the number of eukaryotic cells. The totality of all microbial gene of the microbiota is called the metagenome and latest estimations suggest a reference catalogue of 9.9 million genes [18, 19]. The adult intestinal microbiota is dominated by the two phyla Bacteroidetes and Firmicutes accompanied at much lower abundance by Actinobacteria and Proteobacteria [7, 20–22]. At the species level, high-throughput 16S rRNA gene sequencing and metagenomic analysis allow the detection of approximately 100–200 operational taxonomic units (OTU) per individual [19, 23]. It should be pointed out that each human being has an individual gut microbiota composition, therefore the relative amounts of different phyla varies considerably between individuals. Overall, more than 1000 different species of bacteria were detected in human fecal samples and biopsies [7]. The high interindividual variability of the intestinal microbiota in healthy people hampers the identification of a reference microbiota. Nevertheless, metagenomic analysis revealed a core functional gut microbiome consisting in approximately 60 bacterial gene families shared by individual subjects with differences in bacterial phylotypes. Thus, different combinations of bacterial species, belonging to a common ecological niche, are able to carry out functions necessary for survival in the gut resulting in a stable microbiota [7, 21, 24, 25]. Hence, an extensive understanding of the functions of the microorganisms is

L.F. Buttó, Ph.D. • D. Haller, Ph.D. (✉)
Chair of Nutrition and Immunology, Technische Universität München, Gregor-Mendel-Str. 2, Freising-Weihenstephan 85354, Germany
e-mail: ludovica.butto@tum.de

D.C. Baumgart (ed.), *Crohn's Disease and Ulcerative Colitis*, DOI 10.1007/978-3-319-33703-6_4

crucial in order to explain the complex intestinal ecosystem and its interaction with the host. Integration of data from metagenomic, metatranscriptomic, metaproteomic, and metabolomics studies may aid to gain insights into the host–microbiota interactome [26]. Elucidating the functions of the microbiota is of enormous physiological relevance for humans, considering the central role the intestinal ecosystem exerts on host immune and metabolic functions [27]. The evidence that many chronic diseases, such as allergies, metabolic conditions, and autoimmune diseases, including IBD, are associated with compositional shifts of the gut microbiota in clinical and/or animal studies underlies the therapeutic importance of this field of research [28–31].

Factors Influencing the Intestinal Microbiota Composition

Under physiological conditions the microbiota is highly resilient to perturbations, such as moderate fluctuations in change in dietary-patterns, smoking, drugs or antibiotics. These factors, the so-called exposomal components, might temporarily or permanently modify the microbiota composition leading the bacterial ecosystem to stabilize within a new "alternative state" [32]. The ability of the microbiota to adapt to alterations in the intestinal milieu maintains intestinal homeostasis. In addition, a variety of host factors, including gender, genotype, age, psychological stress, and health status have been reported to shape the intestinal microbiota [8, 33].

The increased incidence of IBD in more developed country is speculated to be partially due to westernized dietary habits and overuse of antibiotics that disrupt mechanisms involved in development of immune tolerance altering dramatically the microbiota composition [15, 34, 35].

Smoking (e.g., nicotine) is an example of a disease specific modifier that seems to exacerbate CD [36] increasing the risk of surgical and clinical recurrence [37], while being protective against UC [38]. One explanation for the dichotomous effect of smoking in patients with UC and CD is based on the evidence that smoking (e.g., nicotine) impairs autophagy [39]. In contrast, recent findings in animal models of IBD suggested that the cytokine milieu characteristic of UC or CD may differentially regulate the expression of nicotinic receptors harbored by colonic CD4 T cells and therefore inhibiting or promoting their pro-inflammatory function [40].

Drug therapy administered to CD patients, such as anti-TNF-α antibody treatment, has been investigated for its ability to alter the microbiota composition, showing an increase in *Faecalibacterium prausnitzii* [41, 42]. This evidence indicates that this species is affected by inflammation and reducing it leads to a repopulation. This suggests that the inflammatory milieu may impact the microbiota composition selecting a specific combination of bacterial species.

The Role of the Intestinal Microbiota in IBD

Several lines of evidence implicate the microbiota in the pathogenesis of IBD. For instance, animal models for chronic ileitis and colitis require the presence of gut microbiota to trigger the disease [43–47]. Additionally, inflammation occurs at sites with higher bacterial concentration and the administration of antibiotics usually leads to a reduction of inflammation in IBD patients and animal models [44, 48, 49]. The central role of the intestinal microbiota in the development of IBD was confirmed by GWAS and animal studies. Currently, 163 variant loci are associated with an increased risk of IBD. Their functions are attributed to microbial recognition or defense, epithelial cell function or the activation and regulation of innate as well as adaptive immune functions [50]. In line with this, IBD patients harbor exacerbated immune responses directed against the normal intestinal microbiota due to aberrant immunoregulatory mechanisms and/or mucosal barrier defects. In fact, IBD patients exhibit spatial and compositional modifications within the gut compared to healthy individuals. Clinical data report that the rigorous spatial separation between the epithelial surface and the intestinal microbiota is ablated in biopsies from CD patients [51–53]. The number of mucosa-associated microorganisms increase and the distance between the intestinal microbiota and the intestinal epithelium is reduced by a thinner or more permeable mucous layer [1, 54]. A large number of studies have reported that IBD patients display compositional changes in the microbiota, so-called dysbiosis, compared to healthy individuals [1, 55–59]. Dysbiosis can be defined an alteration in the bacterial ecosystem associated to pathology [55, 60–62]. Intestinal dysbiosis has been associated with a variety of human disease, other than IBD, such as irritable bowel syndrome [63], chronic diarrhea [64], obesity [65], diabetes [31], autism [66], colorectal cancer [67], cardiovascular [68], and liver disease [69]. It is still unclear to what extent the observed changes of the intestinal microbiota are a cause or consequence of the disease, or to what extent they contribute to the further course of the disease.

Intestinal Microbiota Composition in IBD

Several studies compared the gut microbiota of IBD patients and healthy individuals in order to determine microbial signatures associated with disease or healthy status. Changes in the microbiota composition in IBD encompass decrease in α-diversity [61, 70, 71], in Firmicutes, including Erysipelotrichales and Ruminococcaceae [72], especially *F. prausnitzii* [41, 58, 59], in Bacteroidales, specifically *Bacteroides fragilis* and *vulgatus* [73], with concomitant overrepresentation of Fusobacteria [72, 74], of Firmicutes, such as Veillonellaceae [72], and of Gammaproteobacteria, i.e., Pasteurellaceae [75] and Enterobacteriaceae, such as *Escherichia coli* (*E. coli*) and specifically adherent-invasive *E. coli* (AIEC) [60, 74, 76, 77]. It has been observed that infectious bacteria, such as AIEC and mycobacterium avium subsp. paratuberculosis, are frequently associated with the pathogenesis of inflammation in CD patients [77–81]. This observation leads to the tempting speculation that transient infection with pathogens could act as environmental trigger to initiate inflammatory responses. These responses may become chronic and persistent under the stimulation offered by commensal bacteria once the pathogen has been cleared by the host. It is still debated whether bacterial infection is causal or secondary to underlying immune dysregulation in CD patients, such as macrophages unable to clear pathogens in the lamina propria of CD patients [82]. Furthermore, it is suggested that inflammation may lead to modifications in the composition of gut bacterial communities. Animal studies show that the induction of acute inflammation, for example, by chemical substances, such as DSS [83–85], or to a less extend by infectious bacteria such as *Citrobacter rodentium* [83], can cause changes of the intestinal microbiota.

In a twin cohort study, the authors showed that patients with ileal CD had significantly lower levels of Faecalibacterium and Roseburia and higher levels of Enterobacteriaceae and Ruminococcus compared to their discordant healthy twins [56, 62]. Another study carried out in UC patients and their discordant twins revealed the presence of a dysbiotic microbiota in UC subjects characterized by a reduced bacterial diversity and more Actinobacteria (mostly Rhodococcus genus) and Proteobacteria (mainly Enterobacteriaceae, i.e., *Shigella/Escherichia*) than that of their healthy siblings [61]. This evidence is of particular importance because it indicates that the gut microbiota composition is affected much more by the disease state rather than the genetic component in the context of ileitis and colitis.

IBD patients displayed an unusually higher amount of mucosa-associated aerobic and facultative-anaerobic bacteria [61, 86, 87], supporting the oxygen hypothesis [88]. This theory proposes that an increase in oxygen tension in the gut leads to a bloom of facultative anaerobes and to the ablation of obligate anaerobes. A well-recognized example of bacterial species highly reduced in IBD patients and dramatically affected by oxygen levels is *Faecalibacterium prausnitzii* [58, 59]. Similarly, the pullulation of facultative-anaerobic members of Enterobacteriaceae, especially *E. coli*, has been reported in IBD patients [60, 74, 76, 77]. It has been proposed that alteration in oxygen composition may be due to the inflammation status which is characterized by an oxidative burst in the intestinal tissue with release of reactive oxygen species (ROS) [89]. An attractive and innovative strategy will be to balance dysbiosis by modulating the level of oxygen in distal segments of the gut, for instance via drugs or probiotics selected for their ability to consume oxygen. In line with this, it is possible to speculate that small bowel resection, frequently performed in CD to eliminate the inflamed gastrointestinal portion, causes per se the exposition of gut segments to atmospheric oxygen. Thus, bacteria that are able to cope with oxidative stress would be favored to proliferate and this dysbiosis would lead to disease reoccurrence.

Concomitant with changes in microbiota composition, IBD patients display alterations in function and metabolic capacity of the intestinal microbiota. The decreased production of short chain fatty acids (SCFAs) or the ability of host tissues to use SCFAs might be altered under conditions of chronic inflammation [90]. For instance, butyrate is a major nutrient for enterocytes and lack of this energy source leads to energy deprivation, to impaired barrier function, and to increased bacterial translocation [91]. Several butyrate-producing bacterial species, such as *Roseburia hominis* and *Faecalibacterium prausnitzii*, were found to be decreased in UC patients compared to their healthy siblings [61], or to healthy controls [92]. By harboring anti-inflammatory properties [93–95], these bacteria may represent an attractive strategy for therapeutic intervention. Another possibility is to establish these indicator species as diagnostic markers for IBD. Examples are provided by studies on the butyrate-producing bacterium *Butyricicoccus pullicaecorum* which is underrepresented in fecal samples from IBD patients and it is able to reduce trinitrobenzenesulfonic acid-induced colitis in rats [96].

Genetic Background Contribution in IBD

The contribution of genetic factors to the etiology of IBD has been estimated in monozygotic twins to be lower than 50 %, indicating a more predominant role for environmental factors in the development of the disease [56, 97]. Nevertheless, host genomic loci (i.e., NOD2, ATG16L1, and XBP1) have an impact on the composition and functionality of the bacterial community [14, 98, 99]. This concept has been supported by in vivo data generated in Nod2- and Xbp1-deficient mice, which harbor dysbiotic microbiota compared to the WT counterparts [45, 100]. However, these genetically driven changes are not sufficient to trigger the development of IBD, as confirmed by studies in germ-free mice deficient in specific IBD susceptibility loci [45]. Further evidence has been provided by clinical data, which report a reduced diversity of mucosa-associated bacteria in UC patients and in their discordant monozygotic twins compared to healthy subjects [3, 61, 101]. This observation emphasizes that familial aggregation, and thus genetic background and environment, may promote low microbial diversity. How these factors favor the development of IBD in some individuals and not in their siblings is still a forum of speculations. Another piece of evidence supporting the influence of IBD susceptibility loci on the microbiota composition is that subtle immunodeficiency, such as

ATG16L1 and NOD2 deficiency, licenses AIEC bacteria to proliferate as a consequence of decreased capacity to kill intracellular organisms due to defective autophagy [102, 103].

Intestinal Microbiota–Immune System Interaction in IBD

Many studies investigated and reviewed the role of the intestinal microbiota in driving the development and maintenance of the gut immune system [104–106]. Members of the microbiota or their metabolites can activate anti-inflammatory immune response by the induction of regulatory T-cells [107]. On the other hand, T cell subpopulations may also cause shifts in bacterial composition of the microbiota, and thereby contribute to dysbiosis and inflammation. Pathogenic NKG2D expressing $CD4^+$ T-cells are preferentially recruited to the ileum in CD and their presence in non-inflamed gut segments correlates with post-resection relapse [108–110]. These cells induce Th17-like responses secreting high level of interleukin (IL)-17 and IL-22 and their clonal expansion is bacterial antigen-specific [109].

It is possible to speculate that the depletion of bacterial species or the selection of more aggressive ones may enhance bacterial recognition by the immune system promoting pro-inflammatory responses, fueling the question whether dysbiosis may lead to immune system dysregulation. An example is provided by a recent study which reports an increased number of cells expressing CD11c and TLR4 in mesenteric lymph nodes of DSS-treated mice. The high number of these enriched immune cells correlates with the increasing amount of mucin-degrading Enterobacteriaceae and Akkermansia in the colonic mucosa [84]. This evidence is in agreement with clinical data indicating an increase in TLR4 expressing dendritic cells in inflamed tissue of UC patients [111].

Manipulation of the Intestinal Microbiota in IBD

Despite the strong correlative evidence of changes in the gut microbial ecosystem and disease activity, functional prove for the causative nature of microbe–host interactions especially the role of complex changes in community structure (dysbiosis) and related clinical adaptation is still lacking in IBD.

At present, microbial therapies are intensively studied with the aim to influence the disease activity by modulating the intestinal milieu. Four therapeutic intention strategies are applied to modulate the intestinal microbiota including the administration of antibiotics, prebiotics (i.e., dietary components that promote the growth and metabolic activity of beneficial bacteria), probiotics (i.e., beneficial bacteria), or fecal transplantation (bacteriotherapy).

Antibiotic treatment is well-known to affect microbiota composition leading to the reduction or elimination of specific taxa within microbial communities [112]. This is an efficient way to eradicate infectious organisms but on the other hand the chronic use of antibiotics may promote dysbiosis [113]. Especially the repeated consumption of antibiotics at an early age lead to persistent disturbances of the microbial ecosystem and associates with an increased risk for the later occurrence of IBD [113, 114].

Several clinical studies have reported the efficacy of probiotics, such as *Escherichia coli Nissle* 1917, *Lactobacillus* GG, *Bifidobacterium longum*, *Lactobacillus reuteri*, and VSL#3, in maintaining remission in UC [115–120]. In contrast, clinical trials of probiotics in CD have generated heterogeneous results and up to date probiotics have shown to be ineffective in inducing or in maintaining remission in CD patients [121, 122]. Clinical improvement has been achieved with a combination strategy, the so-called symbiotics, of probiotic bacteria, e.g., *B. longum*, and prebiotics [123]. These data suggest that combination strategies including bacteriotherapy and milieu modifiers offer an additional approach to treat CD.

While the intake of probiotics has only a minor influence on the intestinal ecosystem, relevant changes in the microbiota of the recipient may be induced by the introduction of complex bacterial communities through bacteriotherapy, the so-called fecal microbiota transplantation (FMT). In patients with refractory *Clostridium difficile*-associated diarrhea, therapeutic success can be achieved by FMT, which corresponds to the transfer of a "normal" microbiota [124, 125]. The potential of bacteriotherapy is intriguing and applicable to diseases associated with intestinal dysbiosis. Nevertheless, the therapeutic efficacy of FMT in IBD patients is not yet clear. Borody and colleagues exploited FMT to successfully treat six patients with refractory UC [126]. A patient with severe CD complicated by refractory *Clostridium difficile* infection has been successfully treated by FMT [127]. A pilot study with 30 refractory CD patients showed clinical improvement and clinical remission (>76 %) after FMT up to 15 months follow up [128]. However, a systematic review in 2014 of FMT for IBD revealed that only half of the patients experienced symptoms improvement, disease remission and cessation of medication after FMT treatment [129]. Another systematic review in the same year described studies which report a success rate for the treatment of CD via FMT in the range of 80–100 %, indicating that the outcome of FMT is patient-specific [130], and in some cases no clinical benefit of FMT has been observed [131]. Two recent double-blind randomized control trials investigated the efficacy of FMT in UC patients. While the study from Moayyed et al. reported efficacy of FMT in active UC [132], the trial carried out by Ponsioen group showed that FMT may be beneficial only for some patients [133]. The contrasting results may be explained by the different approach adopted by the two research teams, including mode of administration and the composition and the dose of the donor microbiota used.

Conclusion

A growing body of evidence indicates that the intestinal microbiota play an essential role in IBD pathogenesis, potentially by exacerbation of host immune responses in genetically susceptible host. Consequently, the modulation of microbial communities is an attractive therapeutic option. Despite the residual risk of transmission of pathogens, the unresolved long-term effects, as well as the use of functionally uncharacterized bacterial consortia, bacteriotherapy represents a more promising therapeutic approach to restore eubiosis.

References

1. Baumgart DC, Sandborn WJ. Crohn's disease. Lancet. 2012; 380(9853):1590–605.
2. Danese S, Fiocchi C. Ulcerative colitis. N Engl J Med. 2011;365(18):1713–25.
3. Buhner S, Buning C, Genschel J, Kling K, Herrmann D, Dignass A, et al. Genetic basis for increased intestinal permeability in families with Crohn's disease: role of CARD15 3020insC mutation? Gut. 2006;55(3):342–7.
4. Wehkamp J, Salzman NH, Porter E, Nuding S, Weichenthal M, Petras RE, et al. Reduced Paneth cell alpha-defensins in ileal Crohn's disease. Proc Natl Acad Sci U S A. 2005;102(50): 18129–34.
5. Xavier RJ, Podolsky DK. Unravelling the pathogenesis of inflammatory bowel disease. Nature. 2007;448(7152):427–34.
6. Cobrin GM, Abreu MT. Defects in mucosal immunity leading to Crohn's disease. Immunol Rev. 2005;206:277–95.
7. Human Microbiome Project C. Structure, function and diversity of the healthy human microbiome. Nature. 2012;486(7402):207–14.
8. Dominguez-Bello MG, Costello EK, Contreras M, Magris M, Hidalgo G, Fierer N, et al. Delivery mode shapes the acquisition and structure of the initial microbiota across multiple body habitats in newborns. Proc Natl Acad Sci U S A. 2010;107(26): 11971–5.
9. Koenig JE, Spor A, Scalfone N, Fricker AD, Stombaugh J, Knight R, et al. Succession of microbial consortia in the developing infant gut microbiome. Proc Natl Acad Sci U S A. 2011;108 Suppl 1:4578–85.
10. Turnbaugh PJ, Ridaura VK, Faith JJ, Rey FE, Knight R, Gordon JI. The effect of diet on the human gut microbiome: a metagenomic analysis in humanized gnotobiotic mice. Sci Transl Med. 2009;1(6):6ra14.
11. Cotillard A, Kennedy SP, Kong LC, Prifti E, Pons N, Le Chatelier E, et al. Dietary intervention impact on gut microbial gene richness. Nature. 2013;500(7464):585–8.
12. Leone VA, Cham CM, Chang EB. Diet, gut microbes, and genetics in immune function: can we leverage our current knowledge to achieve better outcomes in inflammatory bowel diseases? Curr Opin Immunol. 2014;31:16–23.
13. Wu GD, Chen J, Hoffmann C, Bittinger K, Chen YY, Keilbaugh SA, et al. Linking long-term dietary patterns with gut microbial enterotypes. Science. 2011;334(6052):105–8.
14. Benson AK, Kelly SA, Legge R, Ma F, Low SJ, Kim J, et al. Individuality in gut microbiota composition is a complex polygenic trait shaped by multiple environmental and host genetic factors. Proc Natl Acad Sci U S A. 2010;107(44):18933–8.
15. David LA, Maurice CF, Carmody RN, Gootenberg DB, Button JE, Wolfe BE, et al. Diet rapidly and reproducibly alters the human gut microbiome. Nature. 2014;505(7484):559–63.
16. Cox LM, Yamanishi S, Sohn J, Alekseyenko AV, Leung JM, Cho I, et al. Altering the intestinal microbiota during a critical developmental window has lasting metabolic consequences. Cell. 2014;158(4):705–21.
17. Arumugam M, Raes J, Pelletier E, Le Paslier D, Yamada T, Mende DR, et al. Enterotypes of the human gut microbiome. Nature. 2011;473(7346):174–80.
18. Sommer F, Backhed F. The gut microbiota—masters of host development and physiology. Nat Rev Microbiol. 2013;11(4):227–38.
19. Li J, Jia H, Cai X, Zhong H, Feng Q, Sunagawa S, et al. An integrated catalog of reference genes in the human gut microbiome. Nat Biotechnol. 2014;32(8):834–41.
20. Lozupone CA, Stombaugh J, Gonzalez A, Ackermann G, Wendel D, Vazquez-Baeza Y, et al. Meta-analyses of studies of the human microbiota. Genome Res. 2013;23(10):1704–14.
21. Lozupone CA, Stombaugh JI, Gordon JI, Jansson JK, Knight R. Diversity, stability and resilience of the human gut microbiota. Nature. 2012;489(7415):220–30.
22. Eckburg PB, Bik EM, Bernstein CN, Purdom E, Dethlefsen L, Sargent M, et al. Diversity of the human intestinal microbial flora. Science. 2005;308(5728):1635–8.
23. Greenblum S, Carr R, Borenstein E. Extensive strain-level copy-number variation across human gut microbiome species. Cell. 2015;160(4):583–94.
24. Turnbaugh PJ, Hamady M, Yatsunenko T, Cantarel BL, Duncan A, Ley RE, et al. A core gut microbiome in obese and lean twins. Nature. 2009;457(7228):480–4.
25. Qin J, Li R, Raes J, Arumugam M, Burgdorf KS, Manichanh C, et al. A human gut microbial gene catalogue established by metagenomic sequencing. Nature. 2010;464(7285):59–65.
26. Fiocchi C. Integrating omics: the future of IBD? Dig Dis. 2014;32 Suppl 1:96–102.
27. O'Hara AM, Shanahan F. The gut flora as a forgotten organ. EMBO Rep. 2006;7(7):688–93.
28. Hormannsperger G, Clavel T, Haller D. Gut matters: microbe-host interactions in allergic diseases. J Allergy Clin Immunol. 2012;129(6):1452–9.
29. Renz H, von Mutius E, Brandtzaeg P, Cookson WO, Autenrieth IB, Haller D. Gene-environment interactions in chronic inflammatory disease. Nat Immunol. 2011;12(4):273–7.
30. Karlsson FH, Tremaroli V, Nookaew I, Bergstrom G, Behre CJ, Fagerberg B, et al. Gut metagenome in European women with normal, impaired and diabetic glucose control. Nature. 2013;498(7452):99–103.
31. Qin J, Li Y, Cai Z, Li S, Zhu J, Zhang F, et al. A metagenome-wide association study of gut microbiota in type 2 diabetes. Nature. 2012;490(7418):55–60.
32. Faust K, Lahti L, Gonze D, de Vos WM, Raes J. Metagenomics meets time series analysis: unraveling microbial community dynamics. Curr Opin Microbiol. 2015;25:56–66.
33. Claesson MJ, Jeffery IB, Conde S, Power SE, O'Connor EM, Cusack S, et al. Gut microbiota composition correlates with diet and health in the elderly. Nature. 2012;488(7410):178–84.
34. Dethlefsen L, Relman DA. Incomplete recovery and individualized responses of the human distal gut microbiota to repeated antibiotic perturbation. Proc Natl Acad Sci U S A. 2011;108 Suppl 1:4554–61.
35. Willing BP, Russell SL, Finlay BB. Shifting the balance: antibiotic effects on host-microbiota mutualism. Nat Rev Microbiol. 2011;9(4):233–43.

36. Lindberg E, Tysk C, Andersson K, Jarnerot G. Smoking and inflammatory bowel disease. A case control study. Gut. 1988;29(3):352–7.
37. Reese GE, Nanidis T, Borysiewicz C, Yamamoto T, Orchard T, Tekkis PP. The effect of smoking after surgery for Crohn's disease: a meta-analysis of observational studies. Int J Colorectal Dis. 2008;23(12):1213–21.
38. Thomas GA, Rhodes J, Green JT, Richardson C. Role of smoking in inflammatory bowel disease: implications for therapy. Postgrad Med J. 2000;76(895):273–9.
39. Monick MM, Powers LS, Walters K, Lovan N, Zhang M, Gerke A, et al. Identification of an autophagy defect in smokers' alveolar macrophages. J Immunol. 2010;185(9):5425–35.
40. Galitovskiy V, Qian J, Chernyavsky AI, Marchenko S, Gindi V, Edwards RA, et al. Cytokine-induced alterations of alpha7 nicotinic receptor in colonic CD4 T cells mediate dichotomous response to nicotine in murine models of Th1/Th17- versus Th2-mediated colitis. J Immunol. 2011;187(5):2677–87.
41. Lopez-Siles M, Martinez-Medina M, Abella C, Busquets D, Sabat-Mir M, Duncan SH, et al. Mucosa-associated Faecalibacterium prausnitzii phylotype richness is reduced in inflammatory bowel disease patients. Appl Environ Microbiol. 2015;81(21):7582–92.
42. Busquets D, Mas-de-Xaxars T, Lopez-Siles M, Martinez-Medina M, Bahi A, Sabat M, et al. Anti-tumour Necrosis Factor Treatment with Adalimumab Induces Changes in the Microbiota of Crohn's Disease. J Crohns Colitis. 2015;9(10):899–906.
43. Adolph TE, Tomczak MF, Niederreiter L, Ko HJ, Bock J, Martinez-Naves E, et al. Paneth cells as a site of origin for intestinal inflammation. Nature. 2013;503(7475):272–6.
44. Schaubeck M, Clavel T, Calasan J, Lagkouvardos I, Haange SB, Jehmlich N, et al. Dysbiotic gut microbiota causes transmissible Crohn's disease-like ileitis independent of failure in antimicrobial defence. Gut. 2015;65(2):225–37.
45. Couturier-Maillard A, Secher T, Rehman A, Normand S, De Arcangelis A, Haesler R, et al. NOD2-mediated dysbiosis predisposes mice to transmissible colitis and colorectal cancer. J Clin Invest. 2013;123(2):700–11.
46. Ocvirk S, Sava IG, Lengfelder I, Lagkouvardos I, Steck N, Roh JH, et al. Surface-associated lipoproteins link Enterococcus faecalis virulence to colitogenic activity in IL-10-deficient mice independent of their expression levels. PLoS Pathog. 2015;11(6):e1004911.
47. Patwa LG, Fan TJ, Tchaptchet S, Liu Y, Lussier YA, Sartor RB, et al. Chronic intestinal inflammation induces stress-response genes in commensal Escherichia coli. Gastroenterology. 2011;141(5):1842–51.e1–10.
48. Khan KJ, Ullman TA, Ford AC, Abreu MT, Abadir A, Marshall JK, et al. Antibiotic therapy in inflammatory bowel disease: a systematic review and meta-analysis. Am J Gastroenterol. 2011;106(4):661–73.
49. Prantera C, Lochs H, Grimaldi M, Danese S, Scribano ML, Gionchetti P, et al. Rifaximin-extended intestinal release induces remission in patients with moderately active Crohn's disease. Gastroenterology. 2012;142(3):473–81.e4.
50. Jostins L, Ripke S, Weersma RK, Duerr RH, McGovern DP, Hui KY, et al. Host-microbe interactions have shaped the genetic architecture of inflammatory bowel disease. Nature. 2012; 491(7422):119–24.
51. Swidsinski A, Weber J, Loening-Baucke V, Hale LP, Lochs H. Spatial organization and composition of the mucosal flora in patients with inflammatory bowel disease. J Clin Microbiol. 2005;43(7):3380–9.
52. Fu J, Wei B, Wen T, Johansson ME, Liu X, Bradford E, et al. Loss of intestinal core 1-derived O-glycans causes spontaneous colitis in mice. J Clin Invest. 2011;121(4):1657–66.
53. Buisine MP, Desreumaux P, Debailleul V, Gambiez L, Geboes K, Ectors N, et al. Abnormalities in mucin gene expression in Crohn's disease. Inflamm Bowel Dis. 1999;5(1):24–32.
54. Johansson ME, Gustafsson JK, Holmen-Larsson J, Jabbar KS, Xia L, Xu H, et al. Bacteria penetrate the normally impenetrable inner colon mucus layer in both murine colitis models and patients with ulcerative colitis. Gut. 2014;63(2):281–91.
55. Manichanh C, Rigottier-Gois L, Bonnaud E, Gloux K, Pelletier E, Frangeul L, et al. Reduced diversity of faecal microbiota in Crohn's disease revealed by a metagenomic approach. Gut. 2006;55(2):205–11.
56. Willing B, Halfvarson J, Dicksved J, Rosenquist M, Jarnerot G, Engstrand L, et al. Twin studies reveal specific imbalances in the mucosa-associated microbiota of patients with ileal Crohn's disease. Inflamm Bowel Dis. 2009;15(5):653–60.
57. Michail S, Durbin M, Turner D, Griffiths AM, Mack DR, Hyams J, et al. Alterations in the gut microbiome of children with severe ulcerative colitis. Inflamm Bowel Dis. 2012;18(10):1799–808.
58. Sokol H, Pigneur B, Watterlot L, Lakhdari O, Bermudez-Humaran LG, Gratadoux JJ, et al. Faecalibacterium prausnitzii is an anti-inflammatory commensal bacterium identified by gut microbiota analysis of Crohn disease patients. Proc Natl Acad Sci U S A. 2008;105(43):16731–6.
59. Sokol H, Seksik P, Furet JP, Firmesse O, Nion-Larmurier I, Beaugerie L, et al. Low counts of Faecalibacterium prausnitzii in colitis microbiota. Inflamm Bowel Dis. 2009;15(8):1183–9.
60. Frank DN, St Amand AL, Feldman RA, Boedeker EC, Harpaz N, Pace NR. Molecular-phylogenetic characterization of microbial community imbalances in human inflammatory bowel diseases. Proc Natl Acad Sci U S A. 2007;104(34):13780–5.
61. Lepage P, Hasler R, Spehlmann ME, Rehman A, Zvirbliene A, Begun A, et al. Twin study indicates loss of interaction between microbiota and mucosa of patients with ulcerative colitis. Gastroenterology. 2011;141(1):227–36.
62. Willing BP, Dicksved J, Halfvarson J, Andersson AF, Lucio M, Zheng Z, et al. A pyrosequencing study in twins shows that gastrointestinal microbial profiles vary with inflammatory bowel disease phenotypes. Gastroenterology. 2010;139(6):1844–54.e1.
63. Collins SM. A role for the gut microbiota in IBS. Nat Rev Gastroenterol Hepatol. 2014;11(8):497–505.
64. Swidsinski A, Loening-Baucke V, Verstraelen H, Osowska S, Doerffel Y. Biostructure of fecal microbiota in healthy subjects and patients with chronic idiopathic diarrhea. Gastroenterology. 2008;135(2):568–79.
65. Le Chatelier E, Nielsen T, Qin J, Prifti E, Hildebrand F, Falony G, et al. Richness of human gut microbiome correlates with metabolic markers. Nature. 2013;500(7464):541–6.
66. Adams JB, Johansen LJ, Powell LD, Quig D, Rubin RA. Gastrointestinal flora and gastrointestinal status in children with autism—comparisons to typical children and correlation with autism severity. BMC Gastroenterol. 2011;11:22.
67. Schwabe RF, Jobin C. The microbiome and cancer. Nat Rev Cancer. 2013;13(11):800–12.
68. Serino M, Blasco-Baque V, Nicolas S, Burcelin R. Far from the eyes, close to the heart: dysbiosis of gut microbiota and cardiovascular consequences. Curr Cardiol Rep. 2014;16(11):540.
69. Abu-Shanab A, Quigley EM. The role of the gut microbiota in nonalcoholic fatty liver disease. Nat Rev Gastroenterol Hepatol. 2010;7(12):691–701.
70. Ott SJ, Musfeldt M, Wenderoth DF, Hampe J, Brant O, Folsch UR, et al. Reduction in diversity of the colonic mucosa associated bacterial microflora in patients with active inflammatory bowel disease. Gut. 2004;53(5):685–93.
71. Scanlan PD, Shanahan F, O'Mahony C, Marchesi JR. Culture-independent analyses of temporal variation of the dominant fecal microbiota and targeted bacterial subgroups in Crohn's disease. J Clin Microbiol. 2006;44(11):3980–8.
72. Gevers D, Kugathasan S, Denson LA, Vazquez-Baeza Y, Van Treuren W, Ren B, et al. The treatment-naive microbiome in new-onset Crohn's disease. Cell Host Microbe. 2014;15(3):382–92.

73. Takaishi H, Matsuki T, Nakazawa A, Takada T, Kado S, Asahara T, et al. Imbalance in intestinal microflora constitution could be involved in the pathogenesis of inflammatory bowel disease. Int J Med Microbiol. 2008;298(5–6):463–72.
74. Strauss J, Kaplan GG, Beck PL, Rioux K, Panaccione R, Devinney R, et al. Invasive potential of gut mucosa-derived Fusobacterium nucleatum positively correlates with IBD status of the host. Inflamm Bowel Dis. 2011;17(9):1971–8.
75. Minamoto Y, Otoni CC, Steelman SM, Buyukleblebici O, Steiner JM, Jergens AE, et al. Alteration of the fecal microbiota and serum metabolite profiles in dogs with idiopathic inflammatory bowel disease. Gut Microbes. 2015;6(1):33–47.
76. Rehman A, Lepage P, Nolte A, Hellmig S, Schreiber S, Ott SJ. Transcriptional activity of the dominant gut mucosal microbiota in chronic inflammatory bowel disease patients. J Med Microbiol. 2010;59(Pt 9):1114–22.
77. Barnich N, Denizot J, Darfeuille-Michaud A. E. coli-mediated gut inflammation in genetically predisposed Crohn's disease patients. Pathol Biol (Paris). 2013;61(5):e65–9.
78. Rhodes JM. The role of Escherichia coli in inflammatory bowel disease. Gut. 2007;56(5):610–2.
79. Chassaing B, Garenaux E, Carriere J, Rolhion N, Guerardel Y, Barnich N, et al. Analysis of the sigmaE regulon in Crohn's disease-associated Escherichia coli revealed involvement of the waaWVL operon in biofilm formation. J Bacteriol. 2015;197(8): 1451–65.
80. Chassaing B, Koren O, Carvalho FA, Ley RE, Gewirtz AT. AIEC pathobiont instigates chronic colitis in susceptible hosts by altering microbiota composition. Gut. 2014;63(7):1069–80.
81. Behr MA, Kapur V. The evidence for Mycobacterium paratuberculosis in Crohn's disease. Curr Opin Gastroenterol. 2008;24(1): 17–21.
82. Glasser AL, Boudeau J, Barnich N, Perruchot MH, Colombel JF, Darfeuille-Michaud A. Adherent invasive Escherichia coli strains from patients with Crohn's disease survive and replicate within macrophages without inducing host cell death. Infect Immun. 2001;69(9):5529–37.
83. Rautava J, Pinnell LJ, Vong L, Akseer N, Assa A, Sherman PM. Oral microbiome composition changes in mouse models of colitis. J Gastroenterol Hepatol. 2015;30(3):521–7.
84. Hakansson A, Tormo-Badia N, Baridi A, Xu J, Molin G, Hagslatt ML, et al. Immunological alteration and changes of gut microbiota after dextran sulfate sodium (DSS) administration in mice. Clin Exp Med. 2015;15(1):107–20.
85. Schwab C, Berry D, Rauch I, Rennisch I, Ramesmayer J, Hainzl E, et al. Longitudinal study of murine microbiota activity and interactions with the host during acute inflammation and recovery. ISME J. 2014;8(5):1101–14.
86. Walujkar SA, Dhotre DP, Marathe NP, Lawate PS, Bharadwaj RS, Shouche YS. Characterization of bacterial community shift in human Ulcerative Colitis patients revealed by Illumina based 16S rRNA gene amplicon sequencing. Gut Pathog. 2014;6:22.
87. Conte MP, Schippa S, Zamboni I, Penta M, Chiarini F, Seganti L, et al. Gut-associated bacterial microbiota in paediatric patients with inflammatory bowel disease. Gut. 2006;55(12):1760–7.
88. Rigottier-Gois L. Dysbiosis in inflammatory bowel diseases: the oxygen hypothesis. ISME J. 2013;7(7):1256–61.
89. Zhu H, Jia Z, Misra H, Li YR. Oxidative stress and redox signaling mechanisms of alcoholic liver disease: updated experimental and clinical evidence. J Dig Dis. 2012;13(3):133–42.
90. Huda-Faujan N, Abdulamir AS, Fatimah AB, Anas OM, Shuhaimi M, Yazid AM, et al. The impact of the level of the intestinal short chain Fatty acids in inflammatory bowel disease patients versus healthy subjects. Open Biochem J. 2010;4:53–8.
91. Morgan XC, Tickle TL, Sokol H, Gevers D, Devaney KL, Ward DV, et al. Dysfunction of the intestinal microbiome in inflammatory bowel disease and treatment. Genome Biol. 2012;13(9):R79.
92. Machiels K, Joossens M, Sabino J, De Preter V, Arijs I, Eeckhaut V, et al. A decrease of the butyrate-producing species Roseburia hominis and Faecalibacterium prausnitzii defines dysbiosis in patients with ulcerative colitis. Gut. 2014;63(8):1275–83.
93. Segain JP, Raingeard de la Bletiere D, Bourreille A, Leray V, Gervois N, Rosales C, et al. Butyrate inhibits inflammatory responses through NFkappaB inhibition: implications for Crohn's disease. Gut. 2000;47(3):397–403.
94. Ploger S, Stumpff F, Penner GB, Schulzke JD, Gabel G, Martens H, et al. Microbial butyrate and its role for barrier function in the gastrointestinal tract. Ann N Y Acad Sci. 2012;1258: 52–9.
95. Wong JM, de Souza R, Kendall CW, Emam A, Jenkins DJ. Colonic health: fermentation and short chain fatty acids. J Clin Gastroenterol. 2006;40(3):235–43.
96. Eeckhaut V, Machiels K, Perrier C, Romero C, Maes S, Flahou B, et al. Butyricicoccus pullicaecorum in inflammatory bowel disease. Gut. 2013;62(12):1745–52.
97. Halfvarson J. Genetics in twins with Crohn's disease: less pronounced than previously believed? Inflamm Bowel Dis. 2011; 17(1):6–12.
98. Spor A, Koren O, Ley R. Unravelling the effects of the environment and host genotype on the gut microbiome. Nat Rev Microbiol. 2011;9(4):279–90.
99. Zhang Q, Pan Y, Yan R, Zeng B, Wang H, Zhang X, et al. Commensal bacteria direct selective cargo sorting to promote symbiosis. Nat Immunol. 2015;16(9):918–26.
100. Adolph TE, Niederreiter L, Blumberg RS, Kaser A. Endoplasmic reticulum stress and inflammation. Dig Dis. 2012;30(4):341–6.
101. Orholm M, Munkholm P, Langholz E, Nielsen OH, Sorensen TI, Binder V. Familial occurrence of inflammatory bowel disease. N Engl J Med. 1991;324(2):84–8.
102. Lapaquette P, Glasser AL, Huett A, Xavier RJ, Darfeuille-Michaud A. Crohn's disease-associated adherent-invasive E. coli are selectively favoured by impaired autophagy to replicate intracellularly. Cell Microbiol. 2010;12(1):99–113.
103. Cooney R, Baker J, Brain O, Danis B, Pichulik T, Allan P, et al. NOD2 stimulation induces autophagy in dendritic cells influencing bacterial handling and antigen presentation. Nat Med. 2010;16(1):90–7.
104. Mazmanian SK, Liu CH, Tzianabos AO, Kasper DL. An immunomodulatory molecule of symbiotic bacteria directs maturation of the host immune system. Cell. 2005;122(1):107–18.
105. Wu HJ, Wu E. The role of gut microbiota in immune homeostasis and autoimmunity. Gut Microbes. 2012;3(1):4–14.
106. Round JL, Mazmanian SK. The gut microbiota shapes intestinal immune responses during health and disease. Nat Rev Immunol. 2009;9(5):313–23.
107. Atarashi K, Tanoue T, Shima T, Imaoka A, Kuwahara T, Momose Y, et al. Induction of colonic regulatory T cells by indigenous Clostridium species. Science. 2011;331(6015):337–41.
108. Connor SJ, Paraskevopoulos N, Newman R, Cuan N, Hampartzoumian T, Lloyd AR, et al. CCR2 expressing CD4+ T lymphocytes are preferentially recruited to the ileum in Crohn's disease. Gut. 2004;53(9):1287–94.
109. Camus M, Esses S, Pariente B, Le Bourhis L, Douay C, Chardiny V, et al. Oligoclonal expansions of mucosal T cells in Crohn's disease predominate in NKG2D-expressing CD4 T cells. Mucosal Immunol. 2014;7(2):325–34.
110. Allez M, Tieng V, Nakazawa A, Treton X, Pacault V, Dulphy N, et al. CD4+NKG2D+ T cells in Crohn's disease mediate inflammatory and cytotoxic responses through MICA interactions. Gastroenterology. 2007;132(7):2346–58.
111. Hart AL, Al-Hassi HO, Rigby RJ, Bell SJ, Emmanuel AV, Knight SC, et al. Characteristics of intestinal dendritic cells in inflammatory bowel diseases. Gastroenterology. 2005;129(1): 50–65.

112. Bartosch S, Fite A, Macfarlane GT, McMurdo ME. Characterization of bacterial communities in feces from healthy elderly volunteers and hospitalized elderly patients by using real-time PCR and effects of antibiotic treatment on the fecal microbiota. Appl Environ Microbiol. 2004;70(6):3575–81.
113. Vangay P, Ward T, Gerber JS, Knights D. Antibiotics, pediatric dysbiosis, and disease. Cell Host Microbe. 2015;17(5):553–64.
114. Kronman MP, Zaoutis TE, Haynes K, Feng R, Coffin SE. Antibiotic exposure and IBD development among children: a population-based cohort study. Pediatrics. 2012;130(4):e794–803.
115. Kruis W, Fric P, Pokrotnieks J, Lukas M, Fixa B, Kascak M, et al. Maintaining remission of ulcerative colitis with the probiotic Escherichia coli Nissle 1917 is as effective as with standard mesalazine. Gut. 2004;53(11):1617–23.
116. Bibiloni R, Fedorak RN, Tannock GW, Madsen KL, Gionchetti P, Campieri M, et al. VSL#3 probiotic-mixture induces remission in patients with active ulcerative colitis. Am J Gastroenterol. 2005;100(7):1539–46.
117. Tursi A, Brandimarte G, Papa A, Giglio A, Elisei W, Giorgetti GM, et al. Treatment of relapsing mild-to-moderate ulcerative colitis with the probiotic VSL#3 as adjunctive to a standard pharmaceutical treatment: a double-blind, randomized, placebo-controlled study. Am J Gastroenterol. 2010;105(10):2218–27.
118. Zocco MA, Dalverme LZ, Cremonini F, Piscaglia AC, Nista EC, Candelli M, et al. Efficacy of Lactobacillus GG in maintaining remission of ulcerative colitis. Aliment Pharmacol Ther. 2006;23(11):1567–74.
119. Furrie E, Macfarlane S, Kennedy A, Cummings JH, Walsh SV, O'Neil DA, et al. Synbiotic therapy (Bifidobacterium longum/Synergy 1) initiates resolution of inflammation in patients with active ulcerative colitis: a randomised controlled pilot trial. Gut. 2005;54(2):242–9.
120. Oliva S, Di Nardo G, Ferrari F, Mallardo S, Rossi P, Patrizi G, et al. Randomised clinical trial: the effectiveness of Lactobacillus reuteri ATCC 55730 rectal enema in children with active distal ulcerative colitis. Aliment Pharmacol Ther. 2012;35(3):327–34.
121. Doherty GA, Bennett GC, Cheifetz AS, Moss AC. Meta-analysis: targeting the intestinal microbiota in prophylaxis for post-operative Crohn's disease. Aliment Pharmacol Ther. 2010;31(8):802–9.
122. Whelan K, Quigley EM. Probiotics in the management of irritable bowel syndrome and inflammatory bowel disease. Curr Opin Gastroenterol. 2013;29(2):184–9.
123. Steed H, Macfarlane GT, Blackett KL, Bahrami B, Reynolds N, Walsh SV, et al. Clinical trial: the microbiological and immunological effects of synbiotic consumption—a randomized double-blind placebo-controlled study in active Crohn's disease. Aliment Pharmacol Ther. 2010;32(7):872–83.
124. van Nood E, Vrieze A, Nieuwdorp M, Fuentes S, Zoetendal EG, de Vos WM, et al. Duodenal infusion of donor feces for recurrent Clostridium difficile. N Engl J Med. 2013;368(5):407–15.
125. Cammarota G, Masucci L, Ianiro G, Bibbo S, Dinoi G, Costamagna G, et al. Randomised clinical trial: faecal microbiota transplantation by colonoscopy vs. vancomycin for the treatment of recurrent Clostridium difficile infection. Aliment Pharmacol Ther. 2015; 41(9):835–43.
126. Borody TJ, Campbell J. Fecal microbiota transplantation: techniques, applications, and issues. Gastroenterol Clin North Am. 2012;41(4):781–803.
127. Duplessis CA, You D, Johnson M, Speziale A. Efficacious outcome employing fecal bacteriotherapy in severe Crohn's colitis complicated by refractory Clostridium difficile infection. Infection. 2012;40(4):469–72.
128. Cui B, Feng Q, Wang H, Wang M, Peng Z, Li P, et al. Fecal microbiota transplantation through mid-gut for refractory Crohn's disease: safety, feasibility, and efficacy trial results. J Gastroenterol Hepatol. 2015;30(1):51–8.
129. Colman RJ, Rubin DT. Fecal microbiota transplantation as therapy for inflammatory bowel disease: a systematic review and meta-analysis. J Crohns Colitis. 2014;8(12):1569–81.
130. Sha S, Liang J, Chen M, Xu B, Liang C, Wei N, et al. Systematic review: faecal microbiota transplantation therapy for digestive and nondigestive disorders in adults and children. Aliment Pharmacol Ther. 2014;39(10):1003–32.
131. Wei Y, Zhu W, Gong J, Guo D, Gu L, Li N, et al. Fecal microbiota transplantation improves the quality of life in patients with inflammatory bowel disease. Gastroenterol Res Pract. 2015;2015:517597.
132. Moayyedi P, Surette MG, Kim PT, Libertucci J, Wolfe M, Onischi C, et al. Fecal microbiota transplantation induces remission in patients with active ulcerative colitis in a randomized, controlled trial. Gastroenterology. 2015;149(1):102–9.e6.
133. Rossen NG, Fuentes S, van der Spek MJ, Tijssen JG, Hartman JH, Duflou A, et al. Findings from a randomized controlled trial of fecal transplantation for patients with ulcerative colitis. Gastroenterology. 2015;149(1):110–8.e4.

The Immune System in IBD: Antimicrobial Peptides

5

Charles L. Bevins

Introduction

The causes of Crohn's disease (CD) and ulcerative colitis (UC), the two major idiopathic inflammatory bowel diseases, are incompletely understood, despite having been defined many decades ago on the basis of their clinical manifestations [1–4]. For both UC and CD, most theories on pathogenesis include intestinal microbes in either initiating and/or perpetuating mucosal inflammation in genetically susceptible hosts [5–9]. Abnormalities of intestinal microbes found in IBD include alterations in the composition (dysbiosis), the presence (or absence) of particular bacterial species, and the adherence of bacteria to the mucosal surface [7, 10, 11]. Evidence supports that host factors have a major role in regulating intestinal microbes [12]. Antimicrobial peptides are a class of innate immune system mediators that serve as endogenous antibiotics [13] and likely constitute a major type of host factor to regulate these microbes [12]. This chapter provides an overview on the proposed biological role of intestinal antimicrobial peptides relevant to IBD pathogenesis and develops a hypothesis to link altered expression of antimicrobial peptides in the pathogenesis of CD.

Intestinal Microbiota in IBD

The intestine harbors an astonishingly numerous and diverse collection of microbes. Most studies have focused on bacteria, because of their high abundance, but archaea, fungi, and viruses also contribute to the intestinal microbiome [14, 15]. Humans typically harbor more bacteria in their intestines than the total number of human cells in the body [15]. The intestinal bacteria are quite diverse, with a thousand or more different bacterial species represented [16]. Most of these bacteria are resident organisms (microbiota), but also include food- and water-borne organisms in transit through the intestine. Opportunistic and potentially virulent pathogens may be found in both resident and transiting groups.

The gut microbiota occupies anatomical and physiological niches that are vital to many physiological and homeostatic functions [17, 18]. For example, the commensal microbiota have important roles in nutrition by fermenting indigestible components in the diet and synthesizing vitamins, amino acids and short-chain fatty acids, in host defense through colonization resistance, and in the development and regulation of the mucosal immune system [17–22]. Despite these host-beneficial effects, the microbiota poses a perpetual threat of microbial disease owing to the shear numbers of bacteria and the close contact with the mucosal surface. As a countermeasure, the host relies on barriers and multifaceted defenses that involve both the innate and adaptive immune systems. The intestinal epithelium serves as a critical component of the innate immune system [23, 24], both by providing a physical barrier (cells, tight junctions, and mucus), and by secreting various antimicrobial factors, including antimicrobial peptides [21, 25, 26].

Clinical observations support that intestinal bacteria are critical in IBD pathogenesis [11, 27]. In IBD, the microbiota loses diversity and has altered composition [10, 11, 27]. The presence of granulomas associated with CD has suggested one or more specific pathogens as potential causative agents. Although some data support that specific pathogens could cause CD [28], this is not a widely held hypothesis [10]. More favored are hypotheses invoking detrimental influences of altered composition, termed dysbiosis [5, 11, 27]. The dysbiosis in CD includes increases in *Enterobacteriaceae* [29], a change that may be linked intimately to mucosal inflammation [30]. In addition, the dysbiosis is accompanied by a striking increase in mucosal-adherent bacteria [31–33]. There is also a decrease in some populations that are considered protective, such *Faecalibacterium prausnitzii* [34]. Finally, the ability of intestinal bacteria to incite and perpetuate intestinal

C.L. Bevins, M.D., Ph.D. (✉)
Department of Microbiology and Immunology, University of California Davis School of Medicine, Davis, CA 95616, USA
e-mail: clbevins@ucdavis.edu

D.C. Baumgart (ed.), *Crohn's Disease and Ulcerative Colitis*, DOI 10.1007/978-3-319-33703-6_5

inflammation has been demonstrated in a variety of rodent models [35–41]. Together, accumulating evidence points to a central pathogenic role for intestinal microbes in IBD, although multiple mechanisms are likely and many details remain unresolved [7, 10, 11, 27].

The Host Shapes the Microbiota

The intestinal microbiota is a complex ecosystem whose composition depends on both endogenous and exogenous factors. The microbes themselves influence their own environment (pH, nutrients, etc.), which in turn affects microbe composition. The exogenous factors come from the environment and from the host. Environmental factors include: ingested microbes from food- and water-borne sources, maternal sources of microbes [42, 43], dietary nutrients [44–46], and antibiotic exposure [47]. These factors can have longstanding significant influence on composition of intestinal microbiota. In addition to these determinants, host factors likely have an overarching influence on the make-up of the microbiota [12, 24, 48, 49].

Experimental evidence supports the idea that all metazoans shape the composition of their colonizing microbiota. For example, studies involving transplantation of intestinal microbiota from mice and zebrafish into their reciprocal germ-free host (i.e., zebrafish microbiota into germ-free mice and visa versa) resulted in dramatic shifts in composition, whereby the recipient host selected microbes that much more closely approximated their own native microbiota than composition observed in the transplanted microbiota [50]. In studies of nonhuman primates, the phylogeny of the host superseded both diet and environmental influences in determining fecal microbial community structure [51]. No doubt, there are many host factors that influence the make-up of the colonizing microbes, and we are only beginning to unravel an understanding of these factors.

The host immune system is likely to be a key driving force in shaping the composition of the colonizing microbiota under baseline, as well as inflammatory conditions. This idea is supported in studies of basal metazoans, such as Hydra [52], in insects [53], as well as in mammals. In humans and other mammals, immunoglobulin-A (IgA) and defensins are two implicated effector molecules in this function. IgA can influence the composition of the intestinal microbiota [54], and an absence of IgA results in notable changes in microbial colonization [55]. Moreover, there is a dynamic interaction between intestinal IgA and microbial colonization [56–63]. Defensins are the second identified host factor that shapes the structure of the microbial community. Experimentally, Paneth cell α(alpha)-defensins have significant impact on the composition of intestinal microbiota [64]. This concept will be detailed below.

Complementary evidence for the role of host factors in altering the composition of the microbiota stems from analysis of the acute response to enteric pathogens. Interestingly, an important aspect of virulence for some enteric pathogens involves eliciting a mucosal inflammatory response, which then creates an environment favoring the pathogen as it strives to out-compete the residing microbiota. For example, *Salmonella enterica* serovar Typhimurium (*S.* typhimurium) induces intestinal inflammation that can impede the commensal microbiota via various mechanisms. Concurrently, this pathogen uses multiple virulence factors to evade (and even profit from) the host-generated lethal antimicrobial inflammatory milieu [30, 65, 66]. One factor released from epithelial cells during the mucosal inflammatory response is lipocalin-2 (also known as siderocalin, neutrophil gelatinase-associated lipocalin, or 24p3), a 23-kDa antimicrobial "peptide." As discussed below lipocalin-2 sequesters bacterial siderophores, the bacterial proteins used for iron acquisition, thereby suppressing bacterial growth. However, *S. typhimurium* expresses a variant siderophore (called salmochelin) that is not recognized or inhibited by lipocalin-2 [67]. Thus, during *S.* typhimurium infection, the elicited lipocalin-2 selectively suppresses growth of the indigenous microbiota dependent on siderophor-acquisition of iron, providing an advantage to *S.* typhimurium [68]. An analogous virulence strategy involving defensin peptides has been proposed for *Helicobacter pylori* [69]. Together, these data support that host factors, including antimicrobial peptides, mold the composition of the microbiota, both in baseline and in inflammatory conditions.

Antimicrobial Peptides

Antimicrobial peptides are among the most ancient elements of the immune system, and arguably are the most widely utilized host-defense effector molecules found in nature [13]. Antimicrobial peptides are ribosome-synthesized antibiotics, differentiated from other antibiotics in nature, such as penicillin, which are typically products of secondary metabolism of microorganisms. Studies of lower organisms have established that antimicrobial peptides are key to both host defense [53] and mucosal colonization by beneficial bacteria [70]. Most often, a size of about 100 amino acids differentiates "peptide" from "protein," but this size limit is rather arbitrary. Rather than size, the characteristic of being a gene-encoded, ribosome-synthesized antibiotic is most germane to the antimicrobial peptide designation [13]. Therefore, several small proteins fall under the umbrella of antimicrobial peptide in this discussion. So defined, intestinal antimicrobial "peptides" (Table 5.1) function by mechanisms that include membrane disruption, inhibition of cell wall biosynthesis, cell wall degradation and vital nutrient scavenging.

Table 5.1 Major antimicrobial peptides of the human small intestine and colon

Antimicrobial	Size (kDa)	Antibacterial activity	Cellular source
α-Defensin 1–4	3.4	Gm+ and Gm–	Neutrophils
α-Defensin 5	3.6	Gm+ and Gm–	Paneth cells
α-Defensin 6	3.7	Self-assembles Forms protective nets	Paneth cells
β-Defensin 1–3	4	Gm+ and Gm–	Colonocytes
Lysozyme	14	Gm+>Gm–	Paneth cells, mØ
sPLA2	16	Gm+>Gm–	Paneth cells, colonocytes, mØ
Reg3A/HIP/PAP	16	Lectin, Gm+	Paneth cells, enterocytes
Lipocalin 2	24	Selectively bacteriostatic (Sequesters chelated iron)	Colonocytes

Defensins are a major family of antimicrobial peptide of mammals [71–75], and in vivo models have provided compelling support for their innate immune functions in the intestinal tract [64, 76–78]. Characteristically, defensins are 18–40 amino acids in length and contain three intramolecular disulfide bonds [71, 72]. In the course of evolution, the genes encoding defensins have undergone duplication and diversity, accompanied by relatively rapid changes in primary sequence attributed to host's interactions with microbes in the internal and external environment [79]. Together these sequence changes have resulted in much diversity in the defensin family between species. However, a conserved sequence feature is the alignment of the six cysteines that participate in the three-disulfide bonds, which helps define the two subfamilies of defensins expressed in humans. One of these subfamilies, α(alpha)-defensins, is expressed most highly in neutrophils and in Paneth cells. In both of these cell types, α(alpha)-defensin expression is constitutive and part of the cellular differentiation of these cells as they mature. While this expression pattern is observed in marsupials, glires (including rats) and some other mammals, mice are a striking exception, where defensins are expressed in Paneth cells (where they are called "cryptdins," to emphasize *crypt* de*fensins*), but not neutrophils [71, 73]. Paneth cells granules contain proteolytic enzymes that mediate processing of α(alpha)-defensin precursors [76, 80]. In humans, Paneth cell trypsin is the processing enzyme of pro-α(alpha)-defensins, while in mice matrix metalloproteinase (MMP)-7, also called matrilysin, serves this function [76, 80]. The β(beta)-defensin sub-family is expressed in many epithelial cells, including colonocytes. In the intestine, epithelial expression of β(beta)-defensin is inducible, except for the apparent constitutive expression of HBD-1. In summary, in the human intestine, α(alpha)-defensins are highly expressed in Paneth cells of the small intestine, and β(beta)-defensins are expressed in the colon. At both locations, infiltrating neutrophils also carry an abundant stockpile of α(alpha)-defensins.

Both α(alpha)- and β(beta)-defensins typically have bactericidal activity against both Gm– and Gm+ bacteria. Some defensins also have activity against fungi, viruses, and protozoa [72, 81]. Many defensins kill their target microbes by disrupting membrane integrity, but recent studies find that some defensin peptides interfere specifically with lipid II function and thereby block bacterial wall biosynthesis [82–84]. Curiously, while Paneth cell HD5 has potent bactericidal activity, the second Paneth cell α(alpha)-defensin, HD6, does not have cidal activity against bacteria [78, 85] (at least while its tri-disulfide bonds are intact [86]). Nevertheless, HD6 has significant mucosal protective function via a novel mechanism. HD6 can block the ability of enteric bacterial pathogens to invade cultured epithelial cells in vitro [78, 87], and HD6 expressed in Paneth cells at physiological levels can protect mice from oral challenge by *S.* typhimurium in vivo [78]. The protection was attributable to unique binding and self-association properties of HD6, resulting in formation of nanofibrils and nanonets, which can surround and entangle the targeted microbes. This unique mechanism helps explain the sequence conservation of HD6 throughout primate evolution and suggests a key role for HD6 in protecting the human small intestine against invasion by diverse enteric pathogens [78].

Besides their antimicrobial activities, some defensins have additional activities that suggest their capacity to help coordinate host defense responses in the intestine [72, 73]. For example, human β(beta)-defensin-1 and -2 have chemoattractant activity for cells expressing the chemokine receptor CCR-6, including dendritic cells [88, 89]. Human α(alpha)-defensin 5 is a potent lectin [90] and can neutralize bacterial exotoxins [90]. Certain other α(alpha)-defensins promote ion fluxes in epithelial cells [91, 92]. These and other activities of intestinal defensins suggest a broad role where these peptides likely contribute in several ways to innate immunity.

Lysozyme is an enzyme that specifically hydrolyzes peptidoglycan. This enzyme is very abundant in the surface-lining fluid of many organs, including the intestine where it is chiefly made by Paneth cells. In addition, lysozyme is abundant in macrophages and neutrophils. Its high concentration in these cells and at mucosal surfaces supports that lysozyme has a substantial role as an antimicrobial agent in vivo, even though specific activity in vitro is modest.

In addition to its role as an antimicrobial agent, analysis of knockout mice points to another key in vivo role for lysozyme—an ability to impede peptidoglycan accumulation in tissue. By enzymatic degradation of peptidoglycan, lysozyme activity appears to help avoid prolonged inflammatory responses that otherwise would result from persistence of bacterial cell wall antigens [93]. Thus, whether eliminating peptidoglycan from crypts and intestinal tissue, and/or antibacterial activity against lumenal microbes is the chief role for intestinal lysozyme remains an open question.

Phosholipase A2 enzymes are a large family of catalytic molecules that hydrolyze the fatty acid ester bond at position sn-2 of membrane phosphotriglycerides. Paneth cells granules contain abundant quantities of one specific member of this family that has selective activity on bacterial membranes [94, 95]. Colonic epithelial cells also express this enzyme, which is named group IIA secretory phospholipase A2 (PLA2G2A, or simply sPLA2) [96]. Like lysozyme, sPLA2 is not only expressed in epithelial cells, but also in macrophages [95]. Bacterial membranes, rich in phosphatidylglycerol and phosphatidylethanolamine, are the key targets of sPLA2, but the enzyme can cleave other phosphotriglyceride substrates [95, 97]. The enzyme is bactericidal, with preferential activity against Gm+ bacteria [97, 98]. Interestingly, genetic evidence found that the gene encoding sPLA2 is a key modifier gene in mouse lines that spontaneously form intestinal adenomas and tumors [99, 100], but the mechanism leading to increased neoplastic growth is unknown [101].

An interesting C-type lectin with a single carbohydrate recognition domain is expressed in the human intestine, named REG3A (also called hepatocarcinoma-intestine-pancreas (HIP) or pancreatitis-associated protein (PAP)). Like its mouse ortholog, Reg3γ(gamma), this lectin binds peptidoglycan and is bactericidal against Gm+ bacteria [102–105]. This lectin is abundantly expressed in Paneth cells and enterocytes [102, 106, 107]. Another lectin abundantly expressed in Paneth cells (although without direct antimicrobial activity) is intelectin-1 [108, 109], which is encoded by *INTL1*, a gene that was identified in genetic screens for IBD-susceptibility loci [110].

Lipocalin-2 binds bacterial siderophores, which are the catechol-related iron chelators secreted by bacteria to acquire iron from their environment. Sequestering these iron chelators prevents this mode of bacterial iron acquisition and inhibits bacterial growth [111]. Many cells express lipocalin-2 inducibly, including liver, macrophages and epithelial cells of the lung and intestine [68, 112, 113]. In the intestine, lipocalin-2 may selectively inhibit growth of siderocalin-dependent bacteria at the mucosal surface.

Mouse Paneth cells express certain antimicrobial peptides that have not been identified in humans, including a group of peptides called cryptdin-related sequences (CRS) [114, 115]. The genes encoding CRS peptides are homologs of α(alpha)-defensins [116]. The CRS peptides are highly expressed, cationic and cysteine-rich, like α(alpha)-defensins, and they have similar antimicrobial activity, but differ in many structural features [73]. Angiogenin-4 is another antimicrobial peptide that does not have a clear human ortholog. Originally identified as a Paneth cell product induced when germ-free mice were colonized [117], angiogenin-4 belongs to a subfamily of ribonuclease enzymes that have antibacterial and antiviral activities [118].

Before leaving the topic of intestinal antimicrobial peptides, it must be mentioned that the host is not the sole source of antimicrobial peptides in the intestinal lumen. While antimicrobial peptides in the intestinal tract are chiefly derived from the host epithelium, some Gm+ and Gm– bacteria also secrete ribosome-synthesized antimicrobial peptides called bacteriocins [119–123]. Bacteria seem to use these peptides to establish or protect an environmental niche. The bacterial strains producing bacteriocins will affect, like their host-derived counterparts, the composition of complex bacterial communities, adding considerable complexity to the dynamics of the intestinal microbiota [119, 121–123].

Paneth Cells, An Antimicrobial Peptide Factory

Paneth cells are epithelial cells with intensive secretory activity. Their large secretory granules contain massive concentrations of antimicrobial peptides [26, 124–126]. The cells reside in small clusters at the base of the small intestinal crypts. Although difficult to maintain in tissue culture with conventional approaches, new "organoid" models hold promise for facilitating in vitro studies of Paneth cell function [127, 128]. In the crypt, Paneth cells discharge their granules into the crypt lumen, and their contents diffuse from the crypt to target microbes at the intestinal surface and in the lumen, including both resident and newly acquired microbes. In so doing, Paneth cells antimicrobials can maintain host sovereignty at its surface interface with the intestinal lumen, provide protection from food and water-borne pathogens and help shape the composition of the endogenous microbiota (Fig. 5.1) [26, 126]. In vivo studies in mouse models have provided strong support for these proposed antimicrobial functions [64, 76–78, 104, 129, 130]. The biological activities of Paneth cell antimicrobial peptides may be evident not only in the small intestine, but also in the colon, as lumenal contents transit via peristalsis [131].

A direct role of Paneth cell antimicrobials in regulating the small intestinal microbiome was investigated using complementary mouse models [64]. In α(alpha)-defensin-deficient mice (via MMP7 gene knockout, encoding the processing enzyme for α(alpha)-defensins), there was decreased abundance of Bacteroidetes and increased

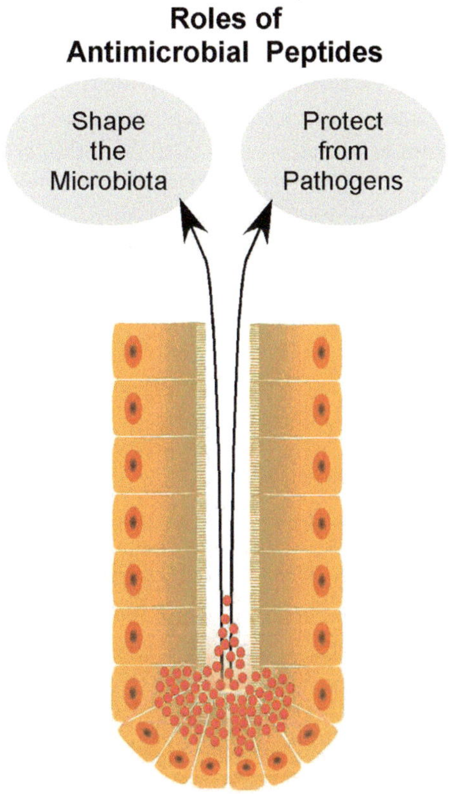

Roles of Antimicrobial Peptides

Shape the Microbiota

Protect from Pathogens

Fig. 5.1 Proposed roles for enteric antimicrobial peptides. The two principal roles for antimicrobial peptides in the intestine, such as Paneth cell α-defensins, are to protect the host from ingested pathogens and to help shape the composition of the colonizing microbiota. Depicted here in cartoon form is the release of secretory granules, chock-full of antimicrobial peptides, from Paneth cells in the crypts of the small intestine

Firmicutes, as compared to wild-type littermate controls. In HD5 transgenic mice, the abundance of Bacteroides species increased and the Firmicutes dropped inversely. Thus, Paneth cell α(alpha)-defensin expression had significant impact on the colonizing microbiota under baseline conditions. In addition to these shifts in the dominant phyla of the small intestinal microbiota, transgenic expression of HD5 also eliminated colonization by *Candidatus* Arthromitus, also referred to as segmented filamentous bacteria (SFB) [64]. SFB is a bacterium that directly contacts the surface of the small intestinal epithelium. The loss of SFB in the HD5 transgenic mice resulted in a significant decrease of Th17 cells in the small intestinal lamina propria, highlighting that Paneth cell antimicrobials can indirectly affect lymphocyte populations in intestinal tissues [64]. Interestingly, a converse SFB increase was reported in a mouse model that had marked Paneth cell dysfunction [132]. Together these data support that Paneth cell antimicrobials have an important homeostatic role in regulating the small intestinal microbiome. Furthermore, in their capacity to regulate the composition of the microbiome, Paneth cell antimicrobials can indirectly alter the abundance of subsets of lymphocytes in the lamina propria. Taken together, it seems clear that genetic or acquired abnormalities in Paneth cell function may have significant impact on host–microbe homeostasis.

While antimicrobial peptides are the most abundant component of the secretory granules, other secretory peptides and proteins impart additional biological roles for Paneth cells [124, 126]. Many molecules that have likely roles in innate immunity, or bridge between innate and adaptive immunity, are expressed in Paneth cells [124, 125, 133–136]. For example, Paneth cells express *NOD2*, the gene encoding nuclear oligomerization domain 2 protein, an intracellular receptor for muramyl dipeptide of bacterial cell walls [133]. New data reveals that Paneth cells also express several molecules that serves as ligands for the adjacent intestinal stem cells, providing them with vital trophic factors [137]. It is likely that these cells have a much more fundamental and sophisticated role in intestinal homeostasis than currently acknowledged [126], although caveats have been highlighted in experimental approaches to study these intriguing cells [138].

Paneth Cells and Crohn's Disease

CD is often involves the distal portions of the small intestine where Paneth cells are abundant [1, 139, 140]. CD is associated with dysbiosis and abnormal bacterial adherence to the intestinal mucosal surface [5], consistent with impaired innate antimicrobial defenses. The identification of several CD susceptibility genes has placed a focus of CD pathogenesis squarely on Paneth cells and their antimicrobial products [140]. Indeed, Paneth cell structural abnormalities detected by routine histology are associated with inherited CD-susceptibility alleles [141–143]. Although the risk-alleles in these susceptibility genes are found in only a subset of patients with CD, and all of these genes are expressed in other cells in the body, a compelling thread connects them to suggest that Paneth cell dysfunction [144] leads to an antimicrobial peptide deficiency [107], which underlies disease pathogenesis in predisposed hosts (Fig. 5.2). The name "Paneth Disease" has been suggested to describe CD of the ileum [140].

Wehkamp and colleagues found reduced Paneth cell α(alpha)-defensin expression in ileal CD compared to controls [107, 153]. Similar reduced expression of defensins was not observed in either UC or CD limited to the colon (L2) [107]. The decrease in Paneth cell α(alpha)-defensin was independent of intestinal inflammation [107]. This suggests that reduced α(alpha)-defensin expression is not the result of inflammation, but rather an intrinsic and early event in the pathophysiology of CD. Individuals with L1007fs (SNP13) *NOD2* mutations, have especially low α(alpha)-defensin levels, which are significantly lower than others

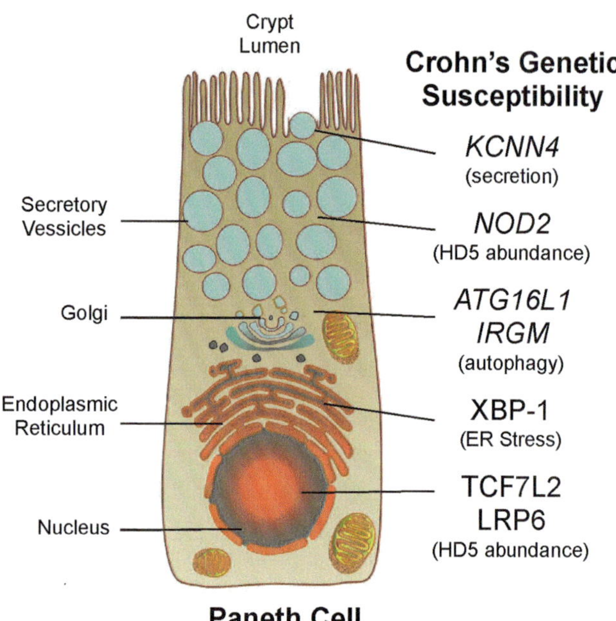

Fig. 5.2 Genetic associations implicating Paneth cells in Crohn's disease pathogenesis. Paneth cells are quintessential secretory cells of the small intestinal epithelium. Their functions contribute to intestinal homeostasis. Several genetic susceptibility factors for IBD may have their phenotypic underpinnings in Paneth cell dysfunction. These include *KCNN4* (encoding KCa3.1) [145], *NOD2* [146, 147], *ATG16L1* [148], *XBP1* [149], *IRGM* [150], *TCF7L2* (encoding TCF7L2, formerly TCF4) [151], and *LRP6* [152]

with ileal CD but without this specific genetic variant [107]. This specific genetic polymorphism in *NOD2* is also linked to increased disease severity and more significant ileal involvement [2, 154, 155]. Additional studies show that deficiency of TCF7L2 (formerly TCF4) is associated with ileal CD [156]. TCF7L2 is an integral transcription factor that drives both Paneth cell differentiation and α(alpha)-defensin expression [157]. The decrease in TCF7L2 expression was not dependent on an abnormal *NOD2* genotype, and was independent of the degree of tissue inflammation, again suggesting that α(alpha)-defensin-deficiency may be a common inciting event in CD pathogenesis. A genetic association of *TCF7L2* with ileal CD provides evidence that a decrease in Paneth cell α(alpha)-defensins is a primary factor in disease pathogenesis for some individuals [151]. Despite the aggregate of supportive data, the role of reduced α(alpha)-defensin expression is a subject of some residual controversy [158, 159].

NOD2 was the first susceptibility gene identified for IBD and is especially linked to CD [146, 147]. Epithelial expression of *NOD2* in the small intestine is restricted to Paneth cells [160]. *Nod2*$^{-/-}$ mice have reduced Paneth cell α(alpha)-defensin expression [133] and are deficient in immune response to enteric pathogens, including *Listeria monocytogenes* [133] and *Helicobacter hepaticus* [38]. Other investigations of *Nod2*$^{-/-}$ mice have found conflicting results [161]. Interestingly, *Nod2*$^{-/-}$ mice develop granulomatous lesions in the ileal mucosa when challenged with *H. hepaticus*, a phenotype that is rescued by transgenic expression of HD5 in the mouse Paneth cells [38]. In addition, *Nod2*$^{-/-}$ mice have alterations in their small intestinal microbial microbiota [162].

Other CD susceptibility genes are associated with dysfunction of Paneth cell secretory pathways, rather than antimicrobial expression. One such susceptibility gene is *ATG16L1*, which is homologous to the yeast autophagy gene *ATG16* [148]. Autophagy is an essential cellular process for renewal and homeostasis, whereby organelles and other components (including secretory granules) are recycled following targeting to lysosomes for degradation [163, 164]. Mouse strains with reduced expression of the gene encoding Atg16l1 resulted in abnormalities in Paneth cell granule form and function [144, 165–167]. CD patients with the *ATG16L1* (T300A) mutation have similar abnormalities of their Paneth cell granules [143, 165, 168], and have both alterations in their microbiota [169] and increases in mucosal-adherent *E. coli* [168]. The mouse phenotype in *Atg16l1* hypomorphic mice is triggered by viral infection [170]. Interestingly, viral triggers have been implicated in human IBD [171].

Studies have linked CD to polymorphisms in another gene encoding a protein involved in autophagy, the immune-related GTPase M (IRGM) [150, 172, 173]. *Irgm1* k/o mice are susceptible to ileal inflammation upon ingestion of dextran sodium sulfate [174]. Abnormalities in Paneth cells of *Irgm1* k/o mice, including abnormalities in Paneth cell granule size and histology, support the purported perturbations in autophagy processes [174]. In patients with CD, there was also evidence of autophagy in Paneth cells with or without disease-associated variants of *IRGM* and *ATG16L1*, where a significant decrease in number and morphology of secretory granules was noted [141]. Finally, like with ATG16L1, there is a tantalizing connection of IRGM with viral infection [175] that potentially could have relevance in CD [141].

Variants of the transcription factor X-box binding protein 1 (XBP1) have been associated with increased risk for CD [149]. XBP1 is involved in maintaining endoplasmic reticulum (ER) function, especially important in intensive secretory cells, such as Paneth cells [176]. Selectively deletion of *Xbp1* in intestinal epithelial cells leads to Paneth cell (and goblet cell) dysfunction and results in intestinal inflammation in mice [149]. Genetic variations in the gene encoding XBP1 are associated with IBD susceptibility, and some uncommon variants may also predispose to CD [149]. A recently reported striking link between Xbp1 and Atg16L1 function further advances a mechanistic model for Paneth cell dysfunction in CD pathogenesis [144]. Mice with lineage-specific *Xbp1* gene knockout in Paneth cells showed induced autophagy in these epithelial cells and had aberrant secretory granules. A majority of these mice developed spontaneous enteritis. Conversely, lineage-specific *Atg16l1* gene knockout in intestinal epithelial cells increases susceptibility to ER stress. Mice with the genetic deficits in both pathways developed severe spontaneous transmural ileitis [144], supporting the notion that small intestinal CD is a specific disorder of Paneth cell function [140].

Another gene implicated in CD susceptibility may have pathogenic roots in Paneth cell secretion. *KCNN4*, which encodes for the calcium-activated potassium channel KCa3.1, was identified in a CD susceptibility genome-wide association study [145]. KCa3.1 is expressed in Paneth cells where it is involved in granule secretion [177]. One might speculate that disruption of the KCa3.1 channel would disrupt Paneth cell granule secretion, and result in deficiency of α(alpha)-defensins and other Paneth cell antimicrobials.

Finally, two genes in the WNT signaling pathway, *TCF7L2* and *LRP6*, are implicated in CD pathogenesis [151, 152, 156]. Wnt signaling is a key regulatory circuit for Paneth cell differentiation and α-defensin expression [126]. Levels of TCF7L2 mRNA showed a high degree of correlation with both HD5 and HD6 mRNA [156]. The levels of TCF7L2 mRNA and TCF7L2 α(alpha)-defensin gene-promoter binding activity were decreased in CD patients with ileal disease, but were not decreased in colonic CD (L2) or UC [156]. Reduced expression of Tcf7l2 in heterozygous (+/−) mice caused a significant decrease of both Paneth cell α(alpha)-defensin levels and bacterial killing activity [156]. Furthermore, genetic study identified an association of sequence variants in the *TCF7L2* promoter region with ileal CD [151]. The co-receptor named low-density lipoprotein receptor related protein 6 (LRP6) is a crucial WNT signaling pathway factor [178]. A rare sequence variant of LRP6 (I1062V) was linked with early onset ileal CD and with penetrating ileal CD behavior, but not to adult onset ileal CD, colonic CD, or UC [152]. This variant was also linked to particularly low defensin levels in ileal CD patients who were carrying this genetic alteration [152].

Taken together, these puzzle pieces merge to implicate Paneth cells, and their arsenal of antimicrobial peptides in the pathogenesis of CD (Fig. 5.3) [140]. It seems likely that the aforementioned susceptibility genes may manifest part of their phenotypic effects through compromise of Paneth cell function. The aberrant function may lead to chronic alterations in microbiota, establishing dysbiosis [179], or limitations in the ability of these cells to successfully cope with acute microbial challenges.

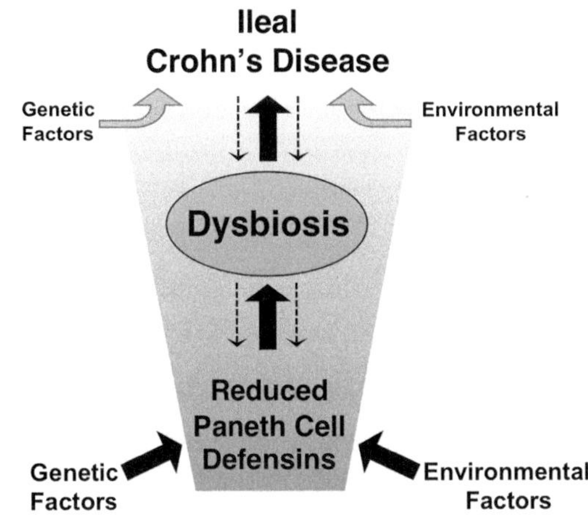

Fig. 5.3 Hypothesis on the possible link of Paneth cell α(alpha)-defensins and ileal Crohn's disease (CD). Reduced expression of Paneth cell α(alpha)-defensins is characteristic of CD of the ileum (*bottom*), but not ulcerative colitis or CD of the colon [107]. Genetic and environmental factors reduce expression of Paneth cell α(alpha)-defensins (*solid arrows*). The resulting α(alpha)-defensin deficit is thought to contribute to dysbiosis (*solid arrow*). In turn, the dysbiosis (*solid arrow*), when combined with perhaps additional independent genetic susceptibility factors and environmental triggers (*gray arrows*), leads to CD. Mucosal pathology may further promote dysbiosis and further impairment of Paneth cell function (*dashed arrows*)

Conclusions

The human intestine is colonized by a diverse, abundant, and dynamic microbial ecosystem. These microbes are key to physiological homeostasis and proper balance of the immune system. The interactions between antimicrobial peptides and this intestinal microbiota may have a significant impact on both health and disease, and many aspects of this dynamic interplay are areas of current investigation. Paneth cell antimicrobial peptides, including α-defensins, are likely fundamental host factors that determine the composition of the colonizing microbiota. Perturbations of Paneth cell function, and α-defensin expression in particular, may be a fundamental factor in the pathogenesis of ileal CD. A vital link could be aberrant interactions with the intestinal microbiota that initiate and/or propagate ileal inflammation. Future studies to further define the function(s) and regulation of enteric antimicrobial peptides will enhance our understanding of normal intestinal physiology and homeostasis. This knowledge may provide new therapeutic targets for treating inflammatory diseases in the intestine.

References

1. Podolsky DK. Inflammatory bowel disease. N Engl J Med. 2002;347:417–29.
2. Cho JH. The genetics and immunopathogenesis of inflammatory bowel disease. Nat Rev Immunol. 2008;8(6):458–66.
3. Khor B, Gardet A, Xavier RJ. Genetics and pathogenesis of inflammatory bowel disease. Nature. 2011;474(7351):307–17.
4. Baumgart DC, Sandborn WJ. Crohn's disease. Lancet. 2012;380(9853):1590–605.
5. Sartor RB. Microbial influences in inflammatory bowel diseases. Gastroenterology. 2008;134(2):577–94.
6. Nell S, Suerbaum S, Josenhans C. The impact of the microbiota on the pathogenesis of IBD: lessons from mouse infection models. Nat Rev Microbiol. 2010;8(8):564–77.
7. Sokol H, Seksik P. The intestinal microbiota in inflammatory bowel diseases: time to connect with the host. Curr Opin Gastroenterol. 2010;26(4):327–31.
8. Kaser A, Zeissig S, Blumberg RS. Inflammatory bowel disease. Annu Rev Immunol. 2010;28:573–621.
9. Jostins L, Ripke S, Weersma RK, Duerr RH, McGovern DP, Hui KY, et al. Host-microbe interactions have shaped the genetic architecture of inflammatory bowel disease. Nature. 2012; 491(7422):119–24.
10. Packey CD, Sartor RB. Commensal bacteria, traditional and opportunistic pathogens, dysbiosis and bacterial killing in inflammatory bowel diseases. Curr Opin Infect Dis. 2009;22(3):292–301.
11. Manichanh C, Borruel N, Casellas F, Guarner F. The gut microbiota in IBD. Nat Rev Gastroenterol Hepatol. 2012;9(10):599–608.
12. Bevins CL, Salzman NH. The potter's wheel: the host's role in sculpting its microbiota. Cell Mol Life Sci. 2011;68(22): 3675–85.
13. Zasloff M. Antimicrobial peptides of multicellular organisms. Nature. 2002;415:389–95.
14. Reyes A, Haynes M, Hanson N, et al. Viruses in the faecal microbiota of monozygotic twins and their mothers. Nature. 2010;466(7304):334–8.
15. Lozupone CA, Stombaugh JI, Gordon JI, Jansson JK, Knight R. Diversity, stability and resilience of the human gut microbiota. Nature. 2012;489(7415):220–30.
16. Consortium THMP. Structure, function and diversity of the healthy human microbiome. Nature. 2012;486(7402):207–14.
17. O'Hara AM, Shanahan F. The gut flora as a forgotten organ. EMBO Rep. 2006;7(7):688–93.
18. Tremaroli V, Backhed F. Functional interactions between the gut microbiota and host metabolism. Nature. 2012;489(7415):242–9.
19. Sekirov I, Finlay BB. The role of the intestinal microbiota in enteric infection. J Physiol. 2009;587(Pt 17):4159–67.
20. Round JL, Mazmanian SK. The gut microbiota shapes intestinal immune responses during health and disease. Nat Rev Immunol. 2009;9(5):313–23.
21. Hooper LV, Macpherson AJ. Immune adaptations that maintain homeostasis with the intestinal microbiota. Nat Rev Immunol. 2010;10(3):159–69.
22. Sommer F, Backhed F. The gut microbiota—masters of host development and physiology. Nat Rev Microbiol. 2013;11(4): 227–38.
23. Mowat AM, Agace WW. Regional specialization within the intestinal immune system. Nat Rev Immunol. 2014;14(10):667–85.
24. Mukherjee S, Hooper LV. Antimicrobial defense of the intestine. Immunity. 2015;42(1):28–39.
25. Wehkamp J, Fellermann K, Herrlinger K, Bevins CL, Stange EF. Defensins in gastrointestinal diseases. Nat Clin Pract (Gastroenterol Hepatol). 2005;2:406–15.
26. Bevins CL, Salzman NH. Paneth cells, antimicrobial peptides and maintenance of intestinal homeostasis. Nat Rev Microbiol. 2011;9(5):356–68.
27. Kostic AD, Xavier RJ, Gevers D. The microbiome in inflammatory bowel disease: current status and the future ahead. Gastroenterology. 2014;146(6):1489–99.
28. Chacon O, Bermudez LE, Barletta RG. Johne's disease, inflammatory bowel disease, and Mycobacterium paratuberculosis. Annu Rev Microbiol. 2004;58:329–63.
29. Frank DN, St Amand AL, Feldman RA, Boedeker EC, Harpaz N, Pace NR. Molecular-phylogenetic characterization of microbial community imbalances in human inflammatory bowel diseases. Proc Natl Acad Sci U S A. 2007;104(34):13780–5.
30. Winter SE, Baumler AJ. Dysbiosis in the inflamed intestine: chance favors the prepared microbe. Gut Microbes. 2014;5(1):71–3.
31. Darfeuille-Michaud A, Boudeau J, Bulois P, et al. High prevalence of adherent-invasive Escherichia coli associated with ileal mucosa in Crohn's disease. Gastroenterology. 2004;127(2):412–21.
32. Swidsinski A, Weber J, Loening-Baucke V, Hale LP, Lochs H. Spatial organization and composition of the mucosal flora in patients with inflammatory bowel disease. J Clin Microbiol. 2005;43(7):3380–9.
33. Baumgart M, Dogan B, Rishniw M, et al. Culture independent analysis of ileal mucosa reveals a selective increase in invasive Escherichia coli of novel phylogeny relative to depletion of Clostridiales in Crohn's disease involving the ileum. ISME J. 2007;1(5):403–18.
34. Sokol H, Pigneur B, Watterlot L, et al. Faecalibacterium prausnitzii is an anti-inflammatory commensal bacterium identified by gut microbiota analysis of Crohn disease patients. Proc Natl Acad Sci U S A. 2008;105(43):16731–6.
35. Kim SC, Tonkonogy SL, Albright CA, et al. Variable phenotypes of enterocolitis in interleukin 10-deficient mice monoassociated with two different commensal bacteria. Gastroenterology. 2005;128(4):891–906.
36. Elson CO, Cong Y, McCracken VJ, Dimmitt RA, Lorenz RG, Weaver CT. Experimental models of inflammatory bowel disease reveal innate, adaptive, and regulatory mechanisms of host dialogue with the microbiota. Immunol Rev. 2005;206:260–76.
37. Lupp C, Robertson ML, Wickham ME, et al. Host-mediated inflammation disrupts the intestinal microbiota and promotes the overgrowth of Enterobacteriaceae. Cell Host Microbe. 2007;2(2): 119–29.
38. Biswas A, Liu YJ, Hao L, et al. Induction and rescue of Nod2-dependent Th1-driven granulomatous inflammation of the ileum. Proc Natl Acad Sci U S A. 2010;107(33):14739–44.
39. Garrett WS, Gallini CA, Yatsunenko T, et al. Enterobacteriaceae act in concert with the gut microbiota to induce spontaneous and maternally transmitted colitis. Cell Host Microbe. 2010;8(3):292–300.
40. Schaubeck M, Clavel T, Calasan J, et al. Dysbiotic gut microbiota causes transmissible Crohn's disease-like ileitis independent of failure in antimicrobial defence. Gut. 2016;65(2):225–37.
41. Hoffmann TW, Pham HP, Bridonneau C, et al. Microorganisms linked to inflammatory bowel disease-associated dysbiosis differentially impact host physiology in gnotobiotic mice. ISME J. 2016;10(2):460–77.
42. Dominguez-Bello MG, Costello EK, Contreras M, et al. Delivery mode shapes the acquisition and structure of the initial microbiota across multiple body habitats in newborns. Proc Natl Acad Sci U S A. 2010;107(26):11971–5.
43. Funkhouser LJ, Bordenstein SR. Mom knows best: the universality of maternal microbial transmission. PLoS Biol. 2013;11(8): e1001631.
44. Ley RE, Backhed F, Turnbaugh P, Lozupone CA, Knight RD, Gordon JI. Obesity alters gut microbial ecology. Proc Natl Acad Sci U S A. 2005;102:11070–5.
45. Turnbaugh PJ, Backhed F, Fulton L, Gordon JI. Diet-induced obesity is linked to marked but reversible alterations in the mouse distal gut microbiome. Cell Host Microbe. 2008;3(4):213–23.

46. David LA, Maurice CF, Carmody RN, et al. Diet rapidly and reproducibly alters the human gut microbiome. Nature. 2014;505(7484):559–63.
47. Willing BP, Russell SL, Finlay BB. Shifting the balance: antibiotic effects on host-microbiota mutualism. Nat Rev Microbiol. 2011;9(4):233–43.
48. Spor A, Koren O, Ley R. Unravelling the effects of the environment and host genotype on the gut microbiome. Nat Rev Microbiol. 2011;9(4):279–90.
49. Jacobs JP, Braun J. Immune and genetic gardening of the intestinal microbiome. FEBS Lett. 2014;588(22):4102–11.
50. Rawls JF, Mahowald MA, Ley RE, Gordon JI. Reciprocal gut microbiota transplants from zebrafish and mice to germ-free recipients reveal host habitat selection. Cell. 2006;127(2):423–33.
51. Ochman H, Worobey M, Kuo CH, et al. Evolutionary relationships of wild hominids recapitulated by gut microbial communities. PLoS Biol. 2010;8(11):e1000546.
52. Bosch TC. Cnidarian-microbe interactions and the origin of innate immunity in metazoans. Annu Rev Microbiol. 2013;67:499–518.
53. Charroux B, Royet J. Drosophila immune response From systemic antimicrobial peptide production in fat body cells to local defense in the intestinal tract. Fly. 2010;4(1):40–7.
54. Cerutti A, Rescigno M. The biology of intestinal immunoglobulin A responses. Immunity. 2008;28(6):740–50.
55. Suzuki K, Meek B, Doi Y, et al. Aberrant expansion of segmented filamentous bacteria in IgA-deficient gut. Proc Natl Acad Sci U S A. 2004;101:1981–6.
56. Peterson DA, McNulty NP, Guruge JL, Gordon JI. IgA response to symbiotic bacteria as a mediator of gut homeostasis. Cell Host Microbe. 2007;2(5):328–39.
57. Hapfelmeier S, Lawson MAE, Slack E, et al. Reversible microbial colonization of germ-free mice reveals the dynamics of IgA immune responses. Science. 2010;328(5986):1705–9.
58. Wei M, Shinkura R, Doi Y, Maruya M, Fagarasan S, Honjo T. Mice carrying a knock-in mutation of Aicda resulting in a defect in somatic hypermutation have impaired gut homeostasis and compromised mucosal defense. Nat Immunol. 2011;12(3):264-U102.
59. Kawamoto S, Tran TH, Maruya M, et al. The inhibitory receptor PD-1 regulates IgA selection and bacterial composition in the gut. Science. 2012;336(6080):485–9.
60. Mirpuri J, Raetz M, Sturge CR, et al. Proteobacteria-specific IgA regulates maturation of the intestinal microbiota. Gut Microbes. 2014;5(1):28–39.
61. Kawamoto S, Maruya M, Kato LM, et al. Foxp3(+) T cells regulate immunoglobulin a selection and facilitate diversification of bacterial species responsible for immune homeostasis. Immunity. 2014;41(1):152–65.
62. Kau AL, Planer JD, Liu J, et al. Functional characterization of IgA-targeted bacterial taxa from undernourished Malawian children that produce diet-dependent enteropathy. Sci Transl Med. 2015;7(276):276ra224.
63. Moon C, Baldridge MT, Wallace MA, Burnham CA, Virgin HW, Stappenbeck TS. Vertically transmitted faecal IgA levels determine extra-chromosomal phenotypic variation. Nature. 2015;521(7550):90–3.
64. Salzman NH, Hung K, Haribhai D, et al. Enteric defensins are essential regulators of intestinal microbial ecology. Nat Immunol. 2010;11(1):76–83.
65. Stecher B, Robbiani R, Walker AW, et al. Salmonella enterica serovar typhimurium exploits inflammation to compete with the intestinal microbiota. PLoS Biol. 2007;5(10):2177–89.
66. Winter SE, Thiennimitr P, Winter MG, et al. Gut inflammation provides a respiratory electron acceptor for Salmonella. Nature. 2010;467(7314):426–9.
67. Fischbach MA, Lin HN, Zhou L, et al. The pathogen-associated iroA gene cluster mediates bacterial evasion of lipocalin 2. Proc Natl Acad Sci U S A. 2006;103(44):16502–7.
68. Raffatellu M, George MD, Akiyama Y, et al. Lipocalin-2 resistance confers an advantage to Salmonella enterica serotype Typhimurium for growth and survival in the inflamed intestine. Cell Host Microbe. 2009;5(5):476–86.
69. Hornsby MJ, Huff JL, Kays RJ, Canfield DR, Bevins CL, Solnick JV. Helicobacter pylori induces an antimicrobial response in rhesus macaques in a cag pathogenicity island-dependent manner. Gastroenterology. 2008;134(4):1049–57.
70. Franzenburg S, Walter J, Kunzel S, et al. Distinct antimicrobial peptide expression determines host species-specific bacterial associations. Proc Natl Acad Sci U S A. 2013;110(39):E3730–8.
71. Ganz T. Defensins: antimicrobial peptides of innate immunity. Nat Rev Immunol. 2003;3(9):710–20.
72. Lehrer RI. Primate defensins. Nat Rev Microbiol. 2004;2:727–38.
73. Selsted ME, Ouellette AJ. Mammalian defensins in the antimicrobial immune response. Nat Immunol. 2005;6:551–7.
74. Lehrer RI, Lu W. Alpha-defensins in human innate immunity. Immunol Rev. 2012;245(1):84–112.
75. Bevins CL. Innate immune functions of alpha-defensins in the small intestine. Dig Dis. 2013;31(3–4):299–304.
76. Wilson CL, Ouellette AJ, Satchell DP, et al. Regulation of intestinal alpha-defensin activation by the metalloproteinase matrilysin in innate host defense. Science. 1999;286(5437):113–7.
77. Salzman NH, Ghosh D, Huttner KM, Paterson Y, Bevins CL. Protection against enteric salmonellosis in transgenic mice expressing a human intestinal defensin. Nature. 2003;422(6931):522–6.
78. Chu H, Pazgier M, Jung G, et al. Human alpha-defensin 6 promotes mucosal innate immunity through self-assembled peptide nanonets. Science. 2012;337(6093):477–81.
79. Lynn DJ, Lloyd AT, Fares MA, O'Farrelly C. Evidence of positively selected sites in mammalian alpha-defensins. Mol Biol Evol. 2004;21:819–27.
80. Ghosh D, Porter E, Shen B, et al. Paneth cell trypsin is the processing enzyme for human defensin-5. Nat Immunol. 2002;3(6):583–90.
81. Lehrer RI, Lichtenstein AK, Ganz T. Defensins: antimicrobial and cytotoxic peptides of mammalian cells. Annu Rev Immunol. 1993;11:105–28.
82. de Leeuw E, Li C, Zeng P, et al. Functional interaction of human neutrophil peptide-1 with the cell wall precursor lipid II. FEBS Lett. 2010;584(8):1543–8.
83. Sass V, Schneider T, Wilmes M, et al. Human beta-defensin 3 inhibits cell wall biosynthesis in Staphylococci. Infect Immun. 2010;78(6):2793–800.
84. Schneider T, Kruse T, Wimmer R, et al. Plectasin, a fungal defensin, targets the bacterial cell wall precursor Lipid II. Science. 2010;328(5982):1168–72.
85. Ericksen B, Wu Z, Lu W, Lehrer RI. Antibacterial activity and specificity of the six human {alpha}-defensins. Antimicrob Agents Chemother. 2005;49(1):269–75.
86. Schroeder BO, Ehmann D, Precht JC, et al. Paneth cell alpha-defensin 6 (HD-6) is an antimicrobial peptide. Mucosal Immunol. 2015;8(3):661–71.
87. Chairatana P, Nolan EM. Molecular basis for self-assembly of a human host-defense peptide that entraps bacterial pathogens. J Am Chem Soc. 2014;136:13267–76.
88. Yang D, Chertov O, Bykovskaia SN, et al. Beta-defensins: linking innate and adaptive immunity through dendritic and T cell CCR6. Science. 1999;286:525–8.
89. Yang D, Biragyn A, Kwak LW, Oppenheim JJ. Mammalian defensins in immunity: more than just microbicidal. Trends Immunol. 2002;23:291–6.

90. Lehrer RI, Jung G, Ruchala P, Andre S, Gabius HJ, Lu W. Multivalent binding of carbohydrates by the human {alpha}-defensin, HD5. J Immunol. 2009;183(1):480–90.
91. Lencer WI, Cheung G, Strohmeier GR, et al. Induction of epithelial chloride secretion by channel-forming cryptins 2 and 3. Proc Natl Acad Sci U S A. 1997;94:8585–9.
92. Yue G, Merlin D, Selsted ME, Lencer WI, Madara JL, Eaton DC. Cryptdin 3 forms anion selective channels in cytoplasmic membranes of human embryonic kidney cells. Am J Physiol Gastrointest Liver Physiol. 2002;282:G757–65.
93. Ganz T, Gabayan V, Liao HI, et al. Increased inflammation in lysozyme M-deficient mice in response to Micrococcus luteus and its peptidoglycan. Blood. 2003;101:2388–92.
94. Lambeau G, Gelb MH. Biochemistry and physiology of mammalian secreted phospholipases A(2). Annu Rev Biochem. 2008;77:495–520.
95. Murakami M, Taketomi Y, Girard C, Yamamoto K, Lambeau G. Emerging roles of secreted phospholipase A(2) enzymes: lessons from transgenic and knockout mice. Biochimie. 2010;92(6):561–82.
96. Qu XD, Lloyd KC, Walsh JH, Lehrer RI. Secretion of type II phospholipase A2 and cryptdin by rat small intestinal Paneth cells. Infect Immun. 1996;64:5161–5.
97. Nevalainen TJ, Graham GG, Scott KF. Antibacterial actions of secreted phospholipases A(2). Review. Biochim Biophys Acta. 2008;1781(1–2):1–9.
98. Harwig SSL, Tan L, Qu X-D, Cho Y, Eisenhauer PB, Lehrer RI. Bactericidal properties of murine intestinal phospholipase A2. J Clin Invest. 1995;95:603–10.
99. MacPhee M, Chepenik KP, Liddell RA, Nelson KK, Siracusa LD, Buchberg AM. The secretory phospholipase A2 gene is a candidate for the Mom1 locus, a major modifier of ApcMin-induced intestinal neoplasia. Cell. 1995;81:957–66.
100. Cormier RT, Hong KH, Halberg RB, et al. Secretory phospholipase Pla2g2a confers resistance to intestinal tumorigenesis. Nat Genet. 1997;17(1):88–91.
101. Fijneman RJA, Cormier RT. The roles of sPLA2-IIA (Pla2g2a) in cancer of the small and large intestine. Front Biosci. 2008;13:4144–74.
102. Cash HL, Whitham CV, Behrendt CL, Hooper LV. Symbiotic bacteria direct expression of an intestinal bactericidal lectin. Science. 2006;313:1126–30.
103. Mukherjee S, Partch CL, Lehotzky RE, et al. Regulation of C-type lectin antimicrobial activity by a flexible N-terminal prosegment. J Biol Chem. 2009;284(8):4881–8.
104. Brandl K, Plitas G, Schnabl B, DeMatteo RP, Pamer EG. MyD88-mediated signals induce the bactericidal lectin RegIII gamma and protect mice against intestinal Listeria monocytogenes infection. J Exp Med. 2007;204(8):1891–900.
105. Mukherjee S, Zheng H, Derebe MG, et al. Antibacterial membrane attack by a pore-forming intestinal C-type lectin. Nature. 2014;505(7481):103–7.
106. Christa L, Carnot F, Simon MT, et al. HIP/PAP is an adhesive protein expressed in hepatocarcinoma, normal Paneth, and pancreatic cells. Am J Physiol. 1996;271(6 Pt 1):993–1002.
107. Wehkamp J, Salzman NH, Porter E, et al. Reduced Paneth cell alpha-defensins in ileal Crohn's disease. Proc Natl Acad Sci U S A. 2005;102(50):18129–34.
108. Komiya T, Tanigawa Y, Hirohashi S. Cloning of the novel gene intelectin, which is expressed in intestinal paneth cells in mice. Biochem Biophys Res Commun. 1998;251:759–62.
109. Wesener DA, Wangkanont K, McBride R, et al. Recognition of microbial glycans by human intelectin-1. Nat Struct Mol Biol. 2015;22(8):603–10.
110. Barrett JC, Hansoul S, Nicolae DL, et al. Genome-wide association defines more than 30 distinct susceptibility loci for Crohn's disease. Nat Genet. 2008;40(8):955–62.
111. Ganz T. Iron in innate immunity: starve the invaders. Curr Opin Immunol. 2009;21(1):63–7.
112. Flo TH, Smith KD, Sato S, et al. Lipocalin 2 mediates an innate immune response to bacterial infection by sequestrating iron. Nature. 2004;432:917–21.
113. Sunil VR, Patel KJ, Nilsen-Hamilton M, Heck DE, Laskin JD, Laskin DL. Acute endotoxemia is associated with upregulation of lipocalin 24p3/Lcn2 in lung and liver. Exp Mol Pathol. 2007;83(2):177–87.
114. Huttner KM, Ouellette AJ. A family of defensin-like genes codes for diverse cysteine-rich peptides in mouse Paneth cells. Genomics. 1994;24:99–109.
115. Hornef MF, Pütsep K, Karlsson J, Refai E, Andersson M. Increased variability of intestinal antimicrobial peptides by covalent dimer formation. Nat Immunol. 2004;5:836–43.
116. Shanahan MT, Vidrich A, Shirafuji Y, et al. Elevated expression of Paneth cell CRS4C in ileitis-prone SAMP1/YitFc mice: regional distribution, subcellular localization, and mechanism of action. J Biol Chem. 2010;285(10):7493–504.
117. Hooper LV, Stappenbeck TS, Hong CV, Gordon JI. Angiogenins: a new class of microbicidal proteins involved in innate immunity. Nat Immunol. 2003;4:269–73.
118. Harder J, Schroder J-M. RNase 7, a novel innate immune defense antimicrobial protein of healthy human skin. J Biol Chem. 2002;277(48):46779–84.
119. Czaran TL, Hoekstra RF, Pagie L. Chemical warfare between microbes promotes biodiversity. Proc Natl Acad Sci U S A. 2002;99(2):786–90.
120. Duquesne S, Destoumieux-Garzon D, Peduzzi J, Rebuffat S. Microcins, gene-encoded antibacterial peptides from enterobacteria. Nat Prod Rep. 2007;24(4):708–34.
121. Gillor O, Etzion A, Riley MA. The dual role of bacteriocins as anti- and probiotics. Appl Microbiol Biotechnol. 2008;81(4):591–606.
122. Dobson A, Cotter PD, Ross RP, Hill C. Bacteriocin production: a probiotic trait? Appl Environ Microbiol. 2012;78(1):1–6.
123. Nishie M, Nagao J, Sonomoto K. Antibacterial peptides "bacteriocins": an overview of their diverse characteristics and applications. Biocontrol Sci. 2012;17(1):1–16.
124. Porter EM, Bevins CL, Ghosh D, Ganz T. The multifaceted Paneth cell. Cell Mol Life Sci. 2002;59(1):156–70.
125. Ouellette AJ. Paneth cells and innate mucosal immunity. Curr Opin Gastroenterol. 2010;26(6):547–53.
126. Clevers HC, Bevins CL. Paneth cells: maestros of the small intestinal crypts. Annu Rev Physiol. 2013;75:289–311.
127. Watson CL, Mahe MM, Munera J, et al. An in vivo model of human small intestine using pluripotent stem cells. Nat Med. 2014;20(11):1310–4.
128. Wilson SS, Tocchi A, Holly MK, Parks WC, Smith JG. A small intestinal organoid model of non-invasive enteric pathogen-epithelial cell interactions. Mucosal Immunol. 2015;8(2):352–61.
129. Vaishnava S, Behrendt CL, Ismail AS, Eckmann L, Hooper LV. Paneth cells directly sense gut commensals and maintain homeostasis at the intestinal host-microbial interface. Proc Natl Acad Sci U S A. 2008;105(52):20858–63.
130. Zhang Q, Pan Y, Yan R, et al. Commensal bacteria direct selective cargo sorting to promote symbiosis. Nat Immunol. 2015;16:918–26.
131. Mastroianni JR, Ouellette AJ. Alpha-defensins in enteric innate immunity: functional Paneth cell alpha-defensins in mouse colonic lumen. J Biol Chem. 2009;284(41):27848–56.
132. Nieuwenhuis EE, Matsumoto T, Lindenbergh D, et al. Cd1d-dependent regulation of bacterial colonization in the intestine of mice. J Clin Invest. 2009;119(5):1241–50.
133. Kobayashi KS, Chamaillard M, Ogura Y, et al. Nod2-dependent regulation of innate and adaptive immunity in the intestinal tract. Science. 2005;307(5710):731–4.

134. George MD, Wehkamp J, Kays RJ, et al. In vivo gene expression profiling of human intestinal epithelial cells: analysis by laser microdissection of formalin fixed tissues. BMC Genomics. 2008;9:209.
135. Wolfs TG, Derikx JP, Hodin CM, et al. Localization of the lipopolysaccharide recognition complex in the human healthy and inflamed premature and adult gut. Inflamm Bowel Dis. 2010;16(1):68–75.
136. Untersmayr E, Bises G, Starkl P, et al. The high affinity IgE receptor Fc epsilonRI is expressed by human intestinal epithelial cells. PLoS One. 2010;5(2):e9023.
137. Sato T, van Es JH, Snippert HJ, et al. Paneth cells constitute the niche for Lgr5 stem cells in intestinal crypts. Nature. 2011;469(7330):415–8.
138. Shanahan MT, Carroll IM, Gulati AS. Critical design aspects involved in the study of Paneth cells and the intestinal microbiota. Gut Microbes. 2014;5(2):208–14.
139. Abraham C, Cho JH. Inflammatory bowel disease. N Engl J Med. 2009;361(21):2066–78.
140. Wehkamp J, Stange EF. Paneth's disease. J Crohns Colitis. 2010;4(5):523–31.
141. Thachil E, Hugot JP, Arbeille B, et al. Abnormal activation of autophagy-induced crinophagy in Paneth cells from patients with Crohn's disease. Gastroenterology. 2012;142(5):1097–9. e1094.
142. Liu TC, Gao F, McGovern DP, Stappenbeck TS. Spatial and temporal stability of paneth cell phenotypes in Crohn's disease: implications for prognostic cellular biomarker development. Inflamm Bowel Dis. 2014;20(4):646–51.
143. VanDussen KL, Liu TC, Li D, et al. Genetic variants synthesize to produce paneth cell phenotypes that define subtypes of Crohn's disease. Gastroenterology. 2014;146(1):200–9.
144. Adolph TE, Tomczak MF, Niederreiter L, et al. Paneth cells as a site of origin for intestinal inflammation. Nature. 2013;503(7475): 272–6.
145. Simms LA, Doecke JD, Roberts RL, et al. KCNN4 gene variant is associated with ileal Crohn's Disease in the Australian and New Zealand population. Am J Gastroenterol. 2010;105(10):2209–17.
146. Hugot JP, Chamaillard M, Zouali H, et al. Association of NOD2 leucine-rich repeat variants with susceptibility to Crohn's disease. Nature. 2001;411:599–603.
147. Ogura Y, Bonen DK, Inohara N, et al. A frameshift mutation in NOD2 associated with susceptibility to Crohn's disease. Nature. 2001;411:603–6.
148. Rioux JD, Xavier RJ, Taylor KD, et al. Genome-wide association study identifies new susceptibility loci for Crohn disease and implicates autophagy in disease pathogenesis. Nat Genet. 2007;39(5):596–604.
149. Kaser A, Lee AH, Franke A, et al. XBP1 links ER stress to intestinal inflammation and confers genetic risk for human inflammatory bowel disease. Cell. 2008;134(5):743–56.
150. Brest P, Lapaquette P, Souidi M, et al. A synonymous variant in IRGM alters a binding site for miR-196 and causes deregulation of IRGM-dependent xenophagy in Crohn's disease. Nat Genet. 2011;43(3):242–5.
151. Koslowski MJ, Kubler I, Chamaillard M, et al. Genetic variants of Wnt transcription factor TCF-4 (TCF7L2) putative promoter region are associated with small intestinal Crohn's disease. PLoS One. 2009;4(2):e4496.
152. Koslowski MJ, Teltschik Z, Beisner J, et al. Association of a functional variant in the Wnt co-receptor LRP6 with early onset ileal Crohn's disease. PLoS Genet. 2012;8(2):e1002523.
153. Wehkamp J, Harder J, Weichenthal M, et al. NOD2 (CARD15) mutations in Crohn's disease are associated with diminished mucosal alpha-defensin expression. Gut. 2004;53(11):1658–64.
154. Russell RK, Drummond HE, Nimmo EE, et al. Genotype-phenotype analysis in childhood-onset Crohn's disease: NOD2/CARDI 5 variants consistently predict phenotypic characteristics of severe disease. Inflamm Bowel Dis. 2005;11(11):955–64.
155. Seiderer J, Schnitzler F, Brand S, et al. Homozygosity for the CARD15 frameshift mutation 1007fs is predictive of early onset of Crohn's disease with ileal stenosis, entero-enteral fistulas, and frequent need for surgical intervention with high risk of re-stenosis. Scand J Gastroenterol. 2006;41(12): 1421–32.
156. Wehkamp J, Wang G, Kubler I, et al. The Paneth cell {alpha}-defensin deficiency of ileal Crohn's disease is linked to Wnt/Tcf-4. J Immunol. 2007;179(5):3109–18.
157. van Es JH, Jay P, Gregorieff A, et al. Wnt signalling induces maturation of Paneth cells in intestinal crypts. Nat Cell Biol. 2005;7(4):381–6.
158. Simms LA, Doecke JD, Walsh MD, Huang N, Fowler EV, Radford-Smith GL. Reduced alpha-defensin expression is associated with inflammation and not NOD2 mutation status in ileal Crohn's disease. Gut. 2008;57:903–10.
159. Bevins CL, Stange EF, Wehkamp J. Decreased Paneth cell defensin expression in ileal Crohn's disease is independent of inflammation, but linked to the NOD2 1007fs genotype. Gut. 2009;58(6):882–3. discussion 883–4.
160. Ogura Y, Lala S, Xin W, et al. Expression of NOD2 in Paneth cells: a possible link to Crohn's ileitis. Gut. 2003;52: 1591–7.
161. Shanahan MT, Carroll IM, Grossniklaus E, et al. Mouse Paneth cell antimicrobial function is independent of Nod2. Gut. 2014;63(6):903–10.
162. Petnicki-Ocwieja T, Hrncir T, Liu YJ, et al. Nod2 is required for the regulation of commensal microbiota in the intestine. Proc Natl Acad Sci U S A. 2009;106(37):15813–8.
163. Levine B, Kroemer G. Autophagy in the pathogenesis of disease. Cell. 2008;132(1):27–42.
164. Ravikumar B, Sarkar S, Davies JE, et al. Regulation of mammalian autophagy in physiology and pathophysiology. Physiol Rev. 2010;90(4):1383–435.
165. Cadwell K, Liu JY, Brown SL, et al. A key role for autophagy and the autophagy gene Atg16l1 in mouse and human intestinal Paneth cells. Nature. 2008;456(7219):259–63.
166. Conway KL, Kuballa P, Song JH, et al. Atg16l1 is required for autophagy in intestinal epithelial cells and protection of mice from Salmonella infection. Gastroenterology. 2013;145(6): 1347–57.
167. Lassen KG, Kuballa P, Conway KL, et al. Atg16L1 T300A variant decreases selective autophagy resulting in altered cytokine signaling and decreased antibacterial defense. Proc Natl Acad Sci U S A. 2014;111(21):7741–6.
168. Deuring JJ, Fuhler GM, Konstantinov SR, et al. Genomic ATG16L1 risk allele-restricted Paneth cell ER stress in quiescent Crohn's disease. Gut. 2014;63(7):1081–91.
169. Frank DN, Robertson CE, Hamm CM, et al. Disease phenotype and genotype are associated with shifts in intestinal-associated microbiota in inflammatory bowel diseases. Inflamm Bowel Dis. 2010;17(1):179–84.
170. Cadwell K, Patel KK, Maloney NS, et al. Virus-plus-susceptibility gene interaction determines Crohn's disease gene Atg16L1 phenotypes in intestine. Cell. 2010;141(7):1135–45.
171. Kangro HO, Chong SKF, Hardiman A, Heath RB, Walkersmith JA. A prospective-study of viral and mycoplasma-infections in chronic inflammatory bowel-disease. Gastroenterology. 1990; 98(3):549–53.
172. Parkes M, Barrett JC, Prescott NJ, et al. Sequence variants in the autophagy gene IRGM and multiple other replicating loci contribute to Crohn's disease susceptibility. Nat Genet. 2007;39(7): 830–2.
173. McCarroll SA, Huett A, Kuballa P, et al. Deletion polymorphism upstream of IRGM associated with altered IRGM expression and Crohn's disease. Nat Genet. 2008;40(9):1107–12.

174. Liu B, Gulati AS, Cantillana V, et al. Irgm1-deficient mice exhibit Paneth cell abnormalities and increased susceptibility to acute intestinal inflammation. Am J Physiol Gastrointest Liver Physiol. 2013;305(8):G573–84.
175. Gregoire IP, Richetta C, Meyniel-Schicklin L, et al. IRGM is a common target of RNA viruses that subvert the autophagy network. PLoS Pathog. 2011;7(12):e1002422.
176. Hosomi S, Kaser A, Blumberg RS. Role of endoplasmic reticulum stress and autophagy as interlinking pathways in the pathogenesis of inflammatory bowel disease. Curr Opin Gastroenterol. 2015;31(1):81–8.
177. Ayabe T, Wulff H, Darmoul D, Cahalan MD, Chandy KG, Ouellette AJ. Modulation of mouse Paneth cell alpha-defensin secretion by mIKCa1, a Ca2+-activated, intermediate conductance potassium channel. J Biol Chem. 2002;277:3793–800.
178. He X, Semenov M, Tamai K, Zeng X. LDL receptor-related proteins 5 and 6 in Wnt/beta-catenin signaling: arrows point the way. Development. 2004;131(8):1663–77.
179. Salzman NH, Bevins CL. Dysbiosis—a consequence of Paneth cell dysfunction. Semin Immunol. 2013;25(5):334–41.

Vascular Responses to Intestinal Inflammation

6

D. Neil Granger and Norman R. Harris

Introduction

It is now well recognized that the blood and lymph vascular systems play an important role in the genesis and perpetuation of an inflammatory response. Evidence accumulated from decades of clinical and basic research has revealed that the vasculature of the inflamed intestine undergoes a variety of functional and structural changes that influences the quality and intensity of the inflammatory and tissue injury responses, and sets the stage for tissue repair and regeneration. All segments of the vascular tree (arterial, capillary, venous) exhibit characteristic changes in response to inflammation. These include an altered reactivity of arterioles to vasodilators and vasoconstrictors, impaired capillary perfusion, the adhesion of leukocytes and platelets to venular endothelium, enhanced coagulation and thrombus formation, increased vascular permeability with accelerated fluid and protein filtration, and the proliferation of blood and lymphatic vessels. Since virtually every cell that either resides within or courses through the inflamed gut is activated, it is generally believed that multiple cell types and mediators activate the signaling mechanisms that account for the altered vascular function that accompanies inflammation. This chapter provides a brief summary of the vascular responses to gut inflammation and addresses the potential mechanisms that underlie these diverse vascular changes (Fig. 6.1) that contribute to the pathogenesis of inflammatory bowel diseases (IBD) [1–4].

D. Neil Granger and Norman R. Harris are supported by a grant from the National Institutes of Diabetes and Digestive and Kidney Diseases (P01 DK43785-19).

D.N. Granger, Ph.D. (✉) • N.R. Harris, Ph.D.
Department of Molecular & Cellular Physiology, Louisiana State University Health Sciences Center—Shreveport,
1501 Kings Highway, Shreveport, LA 71130-3932, USA
e-mail: dgrang@lsuhsc.edu

Vasomotor Dysfunction

Intestinal blood flow can be altered profoundly by chronic gut inflammation. However, the nature and magnitude of the change in intestinal blood flow appear to be dependent on the stage of progression of the inflammatory response. During the early "exudative" phase of colonic inflammation in patients with either ulcerative colitis (UC) or Crohn's disease (CD), colonic blood flow (particularly in the mucosal and submucosal layers) is increased significantly (two- to sixfold) [5]. However, in the late "fibrosing" stage of the disease, colonic blood flow is reduced below normal. A reduction in blood flow also has been reported in colonic arterioles of mice with experimental colitis induced by either dextran sodium sulfate (DSS) or T-cell transfer into immunodeficient mice [6, 7]. However, despite the arteriolar constriction and lower blood flow rates in the individual vessels, overall blood flow rates to the ileum and colon in both models were only marginally reduced as a result of an approximate twofold increase in vascular density [6–10]. A subset of mice in the T-cell transfer model does exhibit a significantly reduced overall blood flow, and this is accompanied by mucosal hypoxia and only mild signs of inflammation [11]. There is also evidence that leukocytes recruited into the inflamed bowel may also influence vasoactivity [12]. In a T-cell transfer model of chronic colitis, vasodilation of first-order colonic arterioles and venules was found to correlate with the number of circulating leukocytes [13]. However, it should be noted that the dilation was not accompanied by an increase in blood flow, possibly due to the constriction of smaller arterioles mentioned earlier [6].

Studies on colonic arterioles derived from patients with IBD and from animal models of experimental colitis have revealed an impaired ability of the resistance vessels to respond to endothelium-dependent vasodilators [2, 7, 14]. The arteriolar dysfunction detected in vessels derived from IBD patients is severe, with acetylcholine-induced dilation reduced to only about 10 % of the response detected in

D.C. Baumgart (ed.), *Crohn's Disease and Ulcerative Colitis*, DOI 10.1007/978-3-319-33703-6_6

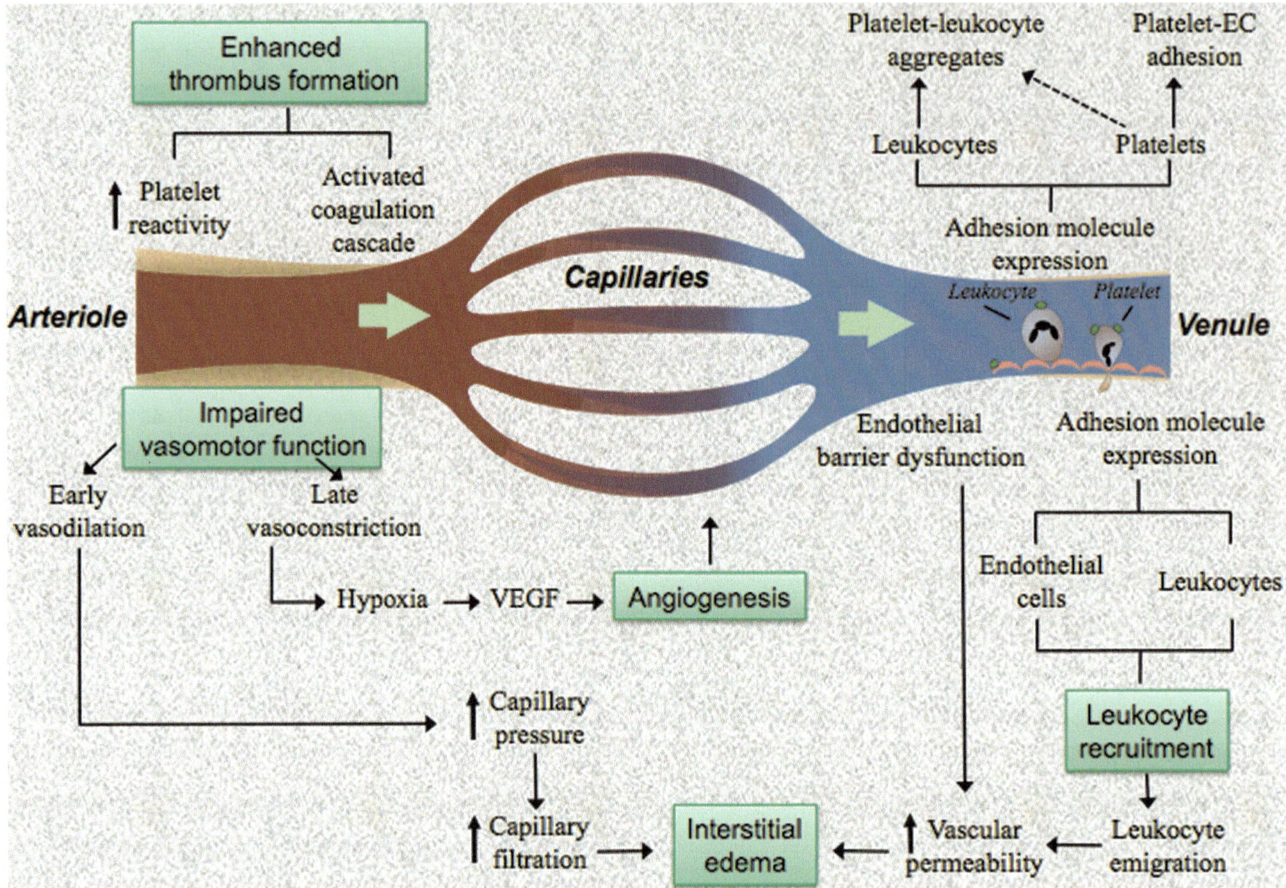

Fig. 6.1 Microvascular responses to intestinal inflammation. Arterioles exhibit impaired vasomotor function that is manifested as an early hyperemia and a later phase of vasoconstriction. The hyperemic response may contribute to the edema associated with inflammation by virtue of the effect of arteriolar dilation on capillary pressure. The late phase vasoconstriction may result in tissue hypoxia, a stimulus for VEGF production and angiogenesis. Arterioles are also the primary site of microvascular thrombosis in experimental IBD. Increased platelet reactivity and an activated coagulation system render the arterioles vulnerable to thrombus formation during inflammation. Increased endothelial cell adhesion molecule expression occurs in inflamed venules, which promotes the recruitment of both leukocytes and platelets. Leukocytes and platelet can bind directly to the vessel wall or adhere to each other. The enhanced leukocyte emigration across inflamed venules can, along with the direct actions of many inflammatory mediators, cause endothelial barrier dysfunction and an increased vascular permeability, leading to plasma protein extravasation and interstitial edema

normal arterioles. The impaired vasodilatory response appears to result from a diminished capacity of arteriolar endothelial cells (EC) to produce nitric oxide (NO), rather than prostacyclin. The NO deficiency results from an excessive production of superoxide, which rapidly reacts with and inactivates NO, thereby inhibiting smooth muscle relaxation [2, 7, 14]. The deficient dilation appears to be a consequence of endothelial dysfunction, inasmuch as vascular smooth muscle function appears to remain unchanged [15]. Recent work has also implicated circulating microparticles, which are elevated in plasma of CD patients, in the impaired flow (and NO)-dependent dilation that accompanies IBD [16].

The changes in colonic blood flow during IBD may also reflect an altered production of endogenous vasoconstrictors [10, 17]. Several reports describe increased levels of thromboxane synthase and/or thromboxane B_2 in the colon of IBD patients, with a correlation noted between thromboxane synthase and disease activity. It remains unclear whether thromboxane-induced vasoconstriction contributes to disease progression because thromboxane synthase inhibitors showed little effectiveness in promoting remission of IBD. Angiotensin II and endothelin-1, other endogenous vasoconstrictors generated by the gut, are also elevated in the colonic mucosa of CD patients [17]. Endothelin-1 has been implicated in the tissue hypoxia that accompanies the ischemic phase of IBD progression [18].

Leukocyte- and Platelet-Endothelial Cell Adhesion

The adhesion of leukocytes to vascular endothelium is a hallmark of the inflammatory response. This adhesive interaction between blood cells and the vessel wall largely occurs

Table 6.1 Endothelial cell adhesion molecules: ligands and functions

Adhesion molecule	Leukocyte receptors	Adhesion response
P-selectin	L-selectin, PSGL-1	Rolling
E-selectin	L-selectin	Rolling
ICAM-1	CD11/CD18	Adherence, emigration
VCAM-1	VLA_4	Adherence, emigration
MAdCAM-1	alpha4beta7	Adherence, emigration
PECAM-1	PECAM-1	Emigration

ICAM-1 intercellular cell adhesion molecule-1, *PSGL-1* P-selectin glycoprotein ligand, *VCAM-1* vascular cell adhesion molecule-1, *VLA4* very late antigen-4, *MAdCAM-1* mucosal addressin cell adhesion molecule-1, *PECAM-1* platelet endothelial cell adhesion molecule-1

in postcapillary venules and is critical for the recruitment of inflammatory cells to sites of infection and/or tissue injury. An important determinant of whether leukocytes adhere to vascular endothelium is the pro-adhesive force that is generated by adhesion molecules expressed on the surface of activated leukocytes and endothelial cells (EC). Table 6.1 summarizes some of the EC adhesion glycoproteins that have been implicated in the recruitment of leukocytes in inflamed colonic venules, their ligands (counter-receptors) on leukocytes, and the type of adhesive interaction mediated by the glycoprotein pairs. Studies in animal models of IBD have demonstrated a time-dependent increase in the expression of P- and E-selectins, ICAM-1, VCAM-1, and MAdCAM-1 in the vasculature of the inflamed colon [1, 19, 20]. Similar findings have been reported for mucosal biopsy samples derived patients with active (but not quiescent) ulcerative or Crohn's colitis. This upregulation of EC adhesion molecules is accompanied by the recruitment of large numbers of rolling, firmly adherent and emigrated (extravasated) leukocytes within (and surrounding) inflamed colonic venules. The critical importance of adhesion molecules in the genesis of experimental IBD is evidenced by a number of studies demonstrating attenuated inflammatory and tissue injury responses in mice that are genetically deficient in specific leukocyte or endothelial cell adhesion molecules, and in animals treated with blocking antibodies directed against these adhesion glycoproteins [1, 19, 20].

A variety of factors contribute to the modulation of leukocyte–endothelial cell adhesion during gut inflammation either by affecting the intensity of adhesion molecule expression and/or the ability of these glycoproteins to sustain strong adhesive interactions between the blood cell and vascular endothelium. Nitric oxide, adenosine, and prostacyclin produced by EC tend to prevent leukocyte–EC adhesion while reactive oxygen species (superoxide, hydrogen peroxide) produced by activated leukocytes and EC appear to promote leukocyte adhesion [14, 15]. These endogenous regulators of leukocyte adhesion exert either a direct (transcription-dependent) or indirect (i.e., altering the production of inflammatory cytokines) effect on the production/expression of EC adhesion molecules. Vasoactive agents (e.g., nitric oxide) can also influence the quality of the adhesive interaction between glycoproteins expressed on leukocytes and EC by altering shear forces generated by the movement of blood through the microvasculature. The number of leukocytes recruited in inflamed venules is inversely related to wall shear rate, suggesting that it is easier for leukocytes to create strong adhesive bonds with ECs at low shear rates and that high shear rates are likely to prevent the creation of such bonds. This dependency of leukocyte adhesion on shear rate suggests that the changes in blood flow associated with the early and late stages (discussed above) of inflammation may significantly influence the intensity of leukocyte recruitment during IBD [19–21].

Platelets also accumulate in the microvasculature of the inflamed colon. The adhesion of platelets to the walls of colonic venules appears to reflect platelet binding to activated ECs rather than adhesion to the collagen-rich subendothelial surface of damaged blood vessels [22, 23]. Intravital microscopic evaluation of platelet binding in inflamed colonic venules has revealed that a relatively small proportion (<10 %) of the platelets bind directly to ECs, while most attach to leukocytes that are already bound to the vessel wall. P-selectin blockade effectively inhibits both the leukocyte-dependent and -independent components of platelet adhesion in colonic venules of colitic mice, suggesting that P-selectin (whether expressed on the platelet or EC) contributes to both recruitment processes [23]. While platelet binding to EC is not altered by ICAM-1 or CD18 immunoblockade, the accumulation of leukocyte-bound platelets is dramatically reduced. The findings are consistent with a model wherein leukocytes require P-selectin to roll on venular endothelium and subsequently establish firm adhesion via CD18-ICAM-1 interactions. The adherent leukocytes, which constitutively express PSGL-1, then create a platform onto which platelets can bind using P-selectin. Similar P-selectin (platelet-associated)-PSGL-1 (leukocyte-associated) interactions also likely account for the platelet-leukocyte aggregates that are detected in blood of IBD patients. Platelet recruitment into inflamed microvessels may be important because, upon activation, platelets produce/release a variety of pro-inflammatory mediators. Furthermore, platelets attachment to neutrophils enhances superoxide production by the latter cells [24].

Coagulation and Thrombosis

Additional consequences of the altered platelet function that occurs during IBD include hyper-reactivity, hyper-aggregability, and an increased propensity for thrombus formation in large and microscopic blood vessels [3, 20–23]. Intravascular platelet aggregates are detected in mucosal biopsies from patients with ulcerative colitis, and the number of platelet aggregates in mesenteric venous blood is increased in IBD. The enhanced reactivity and aggregability of platelets in IBD are accompanied by evidence of significant systemic activation of the coagulation system. The anticoagulant role of ECs is diminished during inflammation, which is reflected in an increased expression of tissue factor, downregulation of anticoagulant protein C pathway, and the inactivation of nitric oxide by superoxide. Collectively, the hemostatic alterations that accompany inflammation tip the balance between procoagulant and anticoagulant mechanisms in favor of thrombus formation. This combination of a hypercoagulable state and platelet hyper-reactivity/aggregability in IBD likely accounts for the fact that vascular beds distant from the inflamed bowel are vulnerable to thrombosis [3, 25–29].

Systemic thromboembolic events (TE) are a significant cause of morbidity and mortality in IBD patients. Clinical studies have revealed that the incidence of TE events in IBD patients is ~6.2 %, with a 3.6-fold increase in risk for TE complications compared to the general population [3, 30, 31]. A much higher incidence of systemic TE (41 %) is predicted from postmortem studies. Both the arterial and venous circulations appear to be involved in IBD-associated TE, although venous complications occur more frequently. TE is most commonly manifested as deep vein thrombosis (DVT) or pulmonary embolism (PE), although thromboses have been detected in other regional circulations, including brain, retina, and liver [3].

Many of the hemostatic alterations reported in patients with IBD have been recapitulated in animal models [3]. These include increases in blood levels of fibrinogen and TAT complexes, thrombocytosis, and a reduced capacity for protein C activation [32, 33]. Mice with experimental colitis also exhibit an increased vulnerability to microvascular thrombus formation in extra-intestinal tissues, a response that is largely confined to arterioles [3, 32]. Tissue factor activation, an impaired protein C pathway, and thrombin have all been implicated in the enhanced extra-intestinal thrombosis in experimental IBD models. While the chemical and/or cellular signals produced by the inflamed gut that initiates this distant organ thrombogenic response remain undefined, there is evidence implicating the cytokines, interleukin-1beta, tumor necrosis factor-alpha, and interleukin-6 (IL-6) [3, 34]. Immunoblockade of these cytokines, particularly IL-6, appears to largely prevent the enhanced extra-intestinal thrombosis associated with DSS-induced murine colitis [34]. The DSS model has also been useful in demonstrating a role for procoagulants (tissue factor) and anticoagulants (activated protein C) in modulating the initiation and perpetuation of gut inflammation, findings consistent with the view that inflammation and coagulation are interdependent processes that can initiate a vicious cycle wherein each process propagates and intensifies the other [35].

Angiogenesis and Vascular Permeability

There is a growing body of evidence that IBD is associated with the development of new blood (angiogenesis) and lymph (lymphangiogenesis) vessels from the existing vascular network and that the angiogenic response tends to prolong and intensify the inflammatory response [4, 8, 36, 37]. Mucosal biopsies from inflamed bowel in IBD patients have revealed a significant increase in the density of microscopic blood vessels, compared to normal bowel samples. Similar evidence for increased vascularity has been reported in different models of experimental colitis. A dependency of the inflammatory response on angiogenesis is supported by animal studies that demonstrate significant positive correlations between angiogenic and inflammatory disease activity [36, 37]. Further support is provided by reports that describe diminished disease activity, tissue injury, and colonic inflammation in mice treated with (or that genetically overexpress) antiangiogenic agents (e.g., soluble VEGF-1 receptor), while a worsening of disease activity, injury, and inflammation is noted in colitic animals treated with (or that genetically overexpress) pro-angiogenic agents such as VEGF-A (vascular endothelial growth factor-A). The dependency of the inflammatory response on angiogenesis has been explained by the fact that newly formed blood vessels are immature and dysfunctional (e.g., leaky) which tends to promote the recruitment and emigration of inflammatory cells [36, 37].

Angiogenesis is a complex process that begins with an initiating event, such as inflammation, which involves the activation of different cell populations that release angiogenic factors, such as VEGF, PDGF (platelet derived growth factor), FGF (fibroblast growth factor), tumor necrosis factor-alpha (TNF-alpha), and adenosine [20, 36, 37]. This is followed by a proliferation/invasion phase that involves changes in the vessel wall (e.g., increased vascular permeability, dissolution of the basement membrane) that allow for the migration and proliferation of ECs. The final stage (maturation/differentiation) includes tube formation and restoration of a normal vessel wall. The rate of angiogenesis is governed by the balance between angiogenic and angiostatic factors produced by the tissue. During inflammation, this balance favors angiogenesis. Because sites of inflammation are often hypoxic, the low tissue oxygen tension also contributes to angiogenesis by virtue of its induction of hypoxia-inducible factor (HIF), which elicits the transcription-dependent production of VEGF and FGF. [18] The leukocytes, platelets, and macrophages that are recruited and activated in inflamed tissue are also capable of producing large quantities of pro-angiogenic factors, including VEGF and cytokines.

In contrast to the deleterious effects of angiogenesis in colonic inflammation, the lymphatic proliferation that also accompanies this condition appears to facilitate disease resolution [38, 39]. Lymphatic stasis, a potent stimulant for lymphatic proliferation, has been described in human and experimental IBD. Interference with lymphatic proliferation in experimental IBD is associated with enhanced inflammation and edema, while treatments that promote lymphangiogenesis (e.g., adenoviral induction of VEGF-C) tend to afford protection against the development of colonic inflammation [38, 39].

Inflammation is generally associated with impaired endothelial barrier function and an increased vascular permeability [40, 41]. While this response is a critical component of the angiogenic response, it is not confined to those regions of the vascular bed that sprout new blood vessels. Inflamed postcapillary venules exhibit an increased permeability to plasma proteins which leads to increased tissue oncotic pressure, withdrawal of fluid from the intravascular compartment (capillaries and venules), increased interstitial fluid volume, and ultimately interstitial edema (Fig. 6.1). Studies in animal models of IBD support the view that substances released by recruited inflammatory cells, and resident mast cells and macrophages mediate the endothelial cell contraction and diminished barrier function noted in the inflamed gut [42]. Potential candidate mediators include histamine, VEGF, cytokines (interleukin-8), lipid mediators (e.g., platelet activating factor), leukocyte-derived proteases (e.g., elastase), and reactive oxygen and nitrogen species.

References

1. Laroux FS, Grisham MB. Immunological basis of inflammatory bowel disease: role of the microcirculation. Microcirculation. 2001;8(5):283–301.
2. Hatoum OA, Binion DG. The vasculature and inflammatory bowel disease: contribution to pathogenesis and clinical pathology. Inflamm Bowel Dis. 2005;11(3):304–13.
3. Yoshida H, Granger DN. Inflammatory bowel disease: a paradigm for the link between coagulation and inflammation. Inflamm Bowel Dis. 2009;15(8):1245–55.
4. Alexander JS, Chaitanya GV, Grisham MB, Boktor M. Emerging roles of lymphatics in inflammatory bowel disease. Ann N Y Acad Sci. 2010;1207 Suppl 1:E75–85.
5. Hulten L, Lindhagen J, Lundgren O, Fasth S, Ahren C. Regional intestinal blood flow in ulcerative colitis and Crohn's disease. Gastroenterology. 1977;72:388–96.
6. Harris NR, Carter PR, Lee S, Watts MN, Zhang S, Grisham MB. Association between blood flow and inflammatory state in a T-cell transfer model of inflammatory bowel disease in mice. Inflamm Bowel Dis. 2010;16:776–82.
7. Mori M, Stokes KY, Vowinkel T, Watanabe N, Elrod JW, Harris NR. Colonic blood flow responses in experimental colitis: time course and underlying mechanisms. Am J Physiol Gastrointest Liver Physiol. 2005;289:G1024–9.
8. Chidlow Jr JH, Langston W, Greer JJ, Ostanin D, Abdelbaqi M, Houghton J. Differential angiogenic regulation of experimental colitis. Am J Pathol. 2006;169:2014–30.
9. Harris NR, Whatley JR, Carter PR, Morgan GA, Grisham MB. Altered microvascular hemodynamics during the induction and perpetuation of chronic gut inflammation. Am J Physiol Gastrointest Liver Physiol. 2009;296:G750–4.
10. Lee S, Carter PR, Watts MN, Bao JR, Harris NR. Effects of the endothelin-converting enzyme inhibitor SM-19712 in a mouse model of dextran sodium sulfate-induced colitis. Inflamm Bowel Dis. 2009;15:1007–13.
11. Harris NR, Carter PR, Yadav AS, Watts MN, Zhang S, Kosloski-Davidson M, et al. Relationship between inflammation and tissue hypoxia in a mouse model of chronic colitis. Inflamm Bowel Dis. 2011;17:742–6.
12. Sasaki T, Kunisaki R, Kinoshita H, Kimura H, Kodera T, Nozawa A, et al. Doppler ultrasound findings correlate with tissue vascularity and inflammation in surgical pathology specimens from patients with small intestinal Crohn's disease. BMC Res Notes. 2014;7:363.
13. Harris NR, Carter PR, Watts MN, Zhang S, Kosloski-Davidson M, Grisham MB, et al. Relationship among circulating leukocytes, platelets, and microvascular responses during induction of chronic colitis. Pathophysiology. 2011;18:305–11.
14. Hatoum OA, Binion DG, Otterson MF, Gutterman DD. Acquired microvascular dysfunction in inflammatory bowel disease: loss of nitric oxide-mediated vasodilation. Gastroenterology. 2003; 125:58–69.
15. Neill LA, Saundry CM, Hyman NH, Wellman GC. Evidence against a systemic arterial defect in patients with inflammatory bowel disease. J Surg Res. 2014;191:318–22.
16. Leonetti D, Reimund JM, Tesse A, Viennot S, Martinez MC, Bretagne AL, et al. Circulating microparticles from Crohn's disease patients cause endothelial and vascular dysfunctions. PLoS One. 2013;8:e73088.
17. Grisham MB, Kevil CG, Harris NR, Granger DN. Role of the microcirculation in chronic gut inflammation. In: Targan SR, Shanahan F, Karp LC, editors. Inflammatory bowel disease: translating basic science into clinical practice. Oxford: Blackwell Publishing; 2010. p. 157–69.
18. Colgan SP, Taylor CT. Hypoxia: an alarm signal during intestinal inflammation. Nat Rev Gastroenterol Hepatol. 2010;7:281–7.
19. Panés J, Granger DN. Leukocyte-endothelial cell interactions: molecular mechanisms and implications in gastrointestinal disease. Gastroenterology. 1998;114(5):1066–90.
20. Granger DN, Senchenkova E. Inflammation and the microcirculation. In: Granger DN, Granger JP, editors. Integrated systems physiology: from cell to function. Morgan & Claypool; 2010. ISBN: 9781615041657
21. Granger DN, Kubes P. The microcirculation and inflammation: modulation of leukocyte-endothelial cell adhesion. J Leukoc Biol. 1994;55(5):662–75.
22. Tailor A, Cooper D, Granger DN. Platelet-vessel wall interactions in the microcirculation. Microcirculation. 2005;12(3):275–85.
23. Vowinkel T, Wood KC, Stokes KY, Russell J, Tailor A, Anthoni C, et al. Mechanisms of platelet and leukocyte recruitment in experimental colitis. Am J Physiol Gastrointest Liver Physiol. 2007;293(5):G1054–60.
24. Suzuki K, Sugimura K, Hasegawa K, Yoshida K, Suzuki A, Ishizuka K, et al. Activated platelets in ulcerative colitis enhance the production of reactive oxygen species by polymorphonuclear leukocytes. Scand J Gastroenterol. 2001;36(12):1301–6.
25. Larsen TB, Nielsen JN, Fredholm L, Lund ED, Brandslund I, Munkholm P, et al. Platelets and anticoagulant capacity in patients with inflammatory bowel disease. Pathophysiol Haemost Thromb. 2002;32:92–6.
26. Collins CE, Rampton DS. Platelets dysfunction: a new dimension in inflammatory bowel disease. Gut. 1995;36:5–8.

27. Collins CE, Rampton DS. Review article: platelets in inflammatory bowel disease—pathogenetic role and therapeutic implications. Aliment Pharmacol Ther. 1997;11:237–47.
28. Webberley MJ, Hart MT, Melikian V. Thromboembolism in inflammatory bowel disease: role of platelets. Gut. 1993;34:247–51.
29. Twig G, Zandman-Goddard G, Szyper-Kravitz M, Shoenfeld Y. Systemic thromboembolism in inflammatory bowel disease: mechanisms and clinical applications. Ann N Y Acad Sci. 2005;1051:166–73.
30. Solem CA, Loftus EV, Tremaine WJ, Sandborn WJ. Venous thromboembolism in inflammatory bowel disease. Am J Gastroenterol. 2004;99:97–101.
31. Irving PM, Pasi KJ, Rampton DS. Thrombosis and inflammatory bowel disease. Clin Gastroenterol Hepatol. 2005;3:617–28.
32. Anthoni C, Russell J, Wood KC, Stokes KY, Vowinkel T, Kirchofer D, et al. Tissue factor: a mediator of inflammatory cell recruitment, tissue injury, and thrombus formation in experimental colitis. J Exp Med. 2007;204:1595–601.
33. Scaldaferri F, Sans M, Vetrano S, Graziani C, De Cristofaro R, Gerlitz B et al. Crucial role of the protein C pathway in governing microvascular inflammation in inflammatory bowel disease. J Clin Invest. 2007;117:1951–60.
34. Senchenkova EY, Komoto S, Russell J,Almeida-Paula LD, Yan LS, Zhang S et al. Interleukin-6 mediates the platelet abnormalities and thrombogenesis associated with experimental colitis. Am J Pathol. 2013;183:173–81.
35. Esmon CT. Inflammation and thrombosis. J Thromb Haemost. 2003;1:1343–8.
36. Chidlow Jr JH, Shukla D, Grisham MB, Kevil CG. Pathogenic angiogenesis in IBD and experimental colitis: new ideas and therapeutic avenues. Am J Physiol Gastrointest Liver Physiol. 2007; 293(1):G5–18.
37. D'Alessio S, Tacconi C, Fiocchi C, Danese S. Advances in therapeutic interventions targeting the vascular and lymphatic endothelium in inflammatory bowel disease. Curr Opin Gastroenterol. 2013;29:608–13.
38. Becker F, Yi P, Al-Kofahi M, Ganta VC, Morris J, Alexander JS. Lymphatic dysregulation in intestinal inflammation: new insights into inflammatory bowel disease pathomechanisms. Lymphology. 2014;47:3–27.
39. Kim H, Kataru RP, Koh GY. Inflammation-associated lymphangiogenesis: a double-edged sword? J Clin Invest. 2014;124:936–42.
40. Kumar P, Shen Q, Pivetti CD, Lee ES, Wu MH, Yuan SY. Molecular mechanisms of endothelial hyperpermeability: implications in inflammation. Expert Rev Mol Med. 2009;11:e19.
41. Weber C, Fraemohs L,. Dejana E. The role of junctional adhesion molecules in vascular inflammation. Nat Rev Immunol. 2007;7(6): 467–77.
42. Mori M, Salter JW, Vowinkel T, Krieglstein CF, Stokes KY, Granger DN. Molecular determinants of the prothrombogenic phenotype assumed by inflamed colonic venules. Am J Physiol Gastrointest Liver Physiol. 2005;288(5):G920–6.

Immunobiology of Human Dendritic Cells in Inflammatory Bowel Disease

7

Daniel C. Baumgart

Introduction

Breakdown of immunological tolerance towards the commensal microflora in genetically susceptible individuals is believed to be the key event in the pathogenesis of inflammatory bowel disease [1, 2].

Dendritic cells control the critical balance between anergy and immunity due to their functional dichotomy of being either the most potent antigen presenters or effective inducers of (peripheral) tolerance. Due to their expression of the entire spectrum of pattern recognition receptors (PRRs), such as TLR and NOD they can sense virtually all microbial associated molecular patterns (MAMPs). This puts them in a pivotal position for understanding the distinct innate and adaptive immune responses intestinal microbiota induce in inflammatory bowel disease. Following microbial recognition and interpretation, dendritic cells direct the innate and adaptive immune response of effector cells towards regulation vs. inflammation [3, 4].

Thus, dendritic cells are considered key for the initiation, perpetuation and control of inflammation in inflammatory bowel disease. Animal and in vitro studies suggest that DC falsely recognize commensal bacteria and may induce a T_H1 or T_H17, pro-inflammatory immune response normally directed at pathogens. Activated DC have been demonstrated in IBD animal models which may prolong the survival of activated T-cells, thereby maintaining inflammation [5–8].

Human dendritic cell populations in Crohn's disease and ulcerative are insufficiently characterized. This is due to their generally low frequency in accessible tissues and further complicated by our still incomplete understanding of human dendritic cell origins and ontogeny and the resulting problem to unequivocally identify the human counterparts of the various murine dendritic cell subsets [9–11].

D.C. Baumgart, M.D., Ph.D., M.B.A., F.A.C.P. (✉)
Inflammatory Bowel Disease Center, Department of Gastroenterology and Hepatology, Charité Medical School—Humboldt-University of Berlin, 13344 Berlin, Germany
e-mail: daniel.baumgart@charite.de

This chapter focuses exclusively on human dendritic cells in human inflammatory bowel disease, while the data on inflammatory bowel disease animal model derived dendritic cell data has been extensively reviewed elsewhere [12].

Distribution, Phenotype, and Function of Human Dendritic Cells in Inflammatory Bowel Disease

Peripheral (Circulating) Blood Dendritic Cells

A number of studies have looked at peripheral blood dendritic cells from patients with inflammatory bowel disease. We and others found an activated (mature) phenotype indicated by higher expression of CD40, CD83, or CD86 and on freshly isolated myeloid dendritic cells from Crohn's patients and ulcerative colitis compared with healthy controls [13, 14]. Myeloid dendritic cells from Crohn's and ulcerative colitis patients show an exaggerated response to lipopolysaccharide, stimulate T-cells significantly more in mixed lymphocyte reactions and are important producers and secretors of key inflammatory cytokines such as IL-1 [15], IL-6 [13], IL-8 [13, 15], TNF-α [13], and nitric oxide [16]. The anti-inflammatory capacity of TGF-β and IL10 to inhibit proinflammatory cytokine production by monocyte-derived dendritic cells (MoDC) was not disturbed in one pediatric IBD study [17]. However, the IL-17A response in allogeneic T helper memory cells in the presence of LPS stimulated moDCs of Crohn's disease was attenuated compared with controls [18].

The frequency of peripheral blood dendritic cells is already low compared with primary lymphatic organs such as the spleen or mesenteric lymph nodes [19]. Data from our group demonstrated a decreased frequency of both plasmacytoid and myeloid dendritic cells in IBD patients that strikingly correlates with disease activity [20]. This also applies to circulating 6-sulfo LacNAc DC (slanDC). The frequency of CD14dullSlan DCs was reduced in patients in Crohn's

D.C. Baumgart (ed.), *Crohn's Disease and Ulcerative Colitis*, DOI 10.1007/978-3-319-33703-6_7

disease refractory to immunosuppressive drugs or TNF-alpha blockers relative to untreated CD, UC, and healthy subjects. In blood of CD patients, SlanDCs expressed CD172a, as detected by CD47 fusion protein binding, when compared with its lack of expression in control subjects [21]. slanDC establish a network with human neutrophils and KK cells which ultimately serves to upregulate NK-derived IFN-γ. LPS and IL-2 or IL-15/IL-18 stimulation of neutrophils potentiates the activity of both slanDCs and NK cells. Neutrophils augment the release of IL-12p70 by slanDCs via a CD18 via ICAM-1. Colocalization of neutrophils, NK cells, and slanDCs, as well as of IL-12p70 and IFNgamma, in inflamed tissues of Crohn disease provides strong evidence for a novel cellular and cytokine cooperation within the innate immune system [22].

This peripheral depletion and their accumulation at the sites of inflammation (see below) suggest recruitment of dendritic cells to the gut in active inflammatory bowel disease. In fact their expression of transmigration, gut homing and chemokine/chemoattractant receptors such as intercellular adhesion molecule-1 (ICAM-1), the integrin $\alpha 4\beta 7$ (CD49d) [20], CCR6 [23], and CCR7 (CD197) [24, 25] and CCR8 [26] has been shown and supports this hypothesis [13, 20, 27]. It is conceivable that dendritic cells are attracted to the mucosa and mesenteric lymph nodes by the stromal expression of chemokines or chemoattractants such as lymphotactin [28], CXCL-8 [29], CXCL9 [29], CXCL10 (IFN-γ induced protein 10 kDa [IP-10]) [29] and CXCL13 (also called B cell-attracting chemokine 1 [BCA-1] or B-lymphocyte chemoattractant [BLC]) [30, 31] as well as CCL19 [25, 32], CCL20 [25, 33], and CCL21 [21, 25, 32, 34].

To investigate the role of microRNA (miR)-10a, a small, noncoding RNA, in the regulation of innate and adaptive responses to microbiota in IBD human MoDC and IBD CD4+ T cells were transfected with miR-10a precursor to define their effect on the function of DC and CD4+ T cells. The expression of miR-10a was markedly decreased, while NOD2 and interleukin (IL)-12/IL-23p40 were significantly increased, in the inflamed mucosa of IBD patients compared with those in healthy controls. Anti-TNF mAb treatment significantly promoted miR-10a expression, whereas it markedly inhibited NOD2 and IL-12/IL-23p40 in the inflamed mucosa. The authors further identified NOD2, in addition to IL-12/IL-23p40, as a target of miR-10a. The ectopic expression of the miR-10a precursor inhibited IL-12/IL-23p40 and NOD2 in DC. Moreover, miR-10a was found to markedly suppress IBD T helper (Th)1 and Th17 cell responses [35].

A functional defect in myeloid dendritic cells potentially explain the suspected defect in innate immunity was suggested by this study, where the authors reported that pattern-recognition receptor (PRR)-induced cytokine secretion was diminished in human monocyte-derived dendritic cells (MDDC) from rs7282490 ICOSLG GG risk carriers [36].

More recent research aimed potentially therapeutically exploitable modulation of human peripheral blood dendritic cells. Retinaldehyde dehydrogenase (RALDH) RALDH activity is known to upregulated in CD103(+) and CD103(−) DCs from Crohn's disease patients [37]. One approach, based on the evolving concept that retinoic acid an enhances the transforming growth factor TGFβ dependent conversion of naive T-cells into regulatory T (Treg) cells, used peripheral blood monocyte derived DC (MoDC) with or without synthetic retinoid acid (Am80). The authors found that (Am80-MoDC) compared with conventional MoDC showed macrophage like adherent phenotype and lacked the expression of the typical DC marker CD1a. Am80-MoDC produced less IL-12p70 and revealed less polarizing ability toward Th1 by allogeneic mixed lymphocyte reaction with naive T-cells [38]. Another group reported that MoDC and circulating $CD1c^{+}$ myeloid DC conditioned with supernatants from intestinal epithelial cells from healthy donors promoted the differentiation of tolerogenic DC able to drive the development of adaptive $Foxp3^{+}$ Treg cells [39].

Vitamin-D supplementation changed the phenotype of LPS stimulated MoDC with educed expression of CD80 and production of the cytokines IL-10, IL-1beta, and IL-6 following 26 weeks of oral vitamin D3 oral supplementation, while MoDC remained unaffected [40].

Cigarette smoking extracts also affects MoDC phenotypes including increased MHC-II, CXCL10, and CCL3 expression in ulcerative colitis vs. Crohn's disease patients. CSE exposed MoDC also drive T-cell proliferation and Th1 polarization in Crohn's as doing the opposite in ulcerative colitis [41].

Mucosal Dendritic Cells

Initially a subpopulation of gut mononuclear phagocytes were suspected to be dendritic cells based on their long dendritic cytoplasmic projections [42]. The studies employing a marker that identifies interdigitating cells antigen presenting (RFD1) hypothesized distinct phenotypic change in macrophages away from an interdigitating phenotype towards mature tissue macrophages (RFD7) in actively inflamed intestinal segments and pouches [43–45]. A later study showed that aphthoid lesions in the colonic mucosa of Crohn's disease patients contained densely aggregated CD68+ macrophages surrounded by numerous ICAM-1, HLA-DR, ID-1 positive dendritic cells [27].

With the availability of a novel dendritic cell marker DC-specific ICAM-3 grabbing non-integrin (DC-SIGN), two recent histochemical studies identified additional distinct populations of DC present in Crohn's disease patients: a DC-SIGN positive population that was present scattered throughout the mucosa, and a CD83 positive population that was present in aggregated lymphoid nodules and as single cells in the lamina propria [46, 47]. Another immunohistochemical study reported M-DC8$^+$ myeloid dendritic cells localized in the T cell area in the subepithelial dome region of Peyer's patches the inflamed ileal mucosa of patients with active Crohn's disease [48]. Interleukin-27, a newly described member of the IL-12 family, is a heterodimeric cytokine composed of two subunits, p28 and Epstein-Barr virus-induced gene 3 (EBI3) and mainly produced by activated dendritic cells and monocytes. EBI3 expressing dendritic cells were described in the in the lamina propria of Crohn's patients with a pattern of reactivity was similar to control mucosa [49]. Bone loss is a major clinical problem in Crohn's disease. Receptor activator of NF-kB ligand (RANKL) and its receptor RANK are potentially associated with non-steroid attributable bone loss and controlled by pro-inflammatory cytokines. RANK, CD68, S100$^+$ (myeloid dendritic) cells were increased in inflamed areas of colonic mucosa from Crohn's disease patients [50]. CD14+ myeloid DC from Crohn's disease patients control promote the polarization from innate lymphoid cells (ILC) ILC3 to CD127(+) ILC1. In contrast, CD14(−) DCs promoted differentiation from CD127(+) ILC1 toward ILC3. These observations suggest that environmental cues determine the composition, function, and phenotype of CD127(+) ILC1 and ILC3 in the gut [51].

The accumulation of mucosal dendritic cells is not restricted to Crohn's disease. Immunohistochemical studies in ulcerative colitis patients revealed an increased number of follicular dendritic cells and myeloid cells dendritic cells basal lymphocyte aggregates of colonic lamina propria and inflamed crypts of ulcerative colitis patients [21, 23, 25, 52, 53].

These early immunohistochemical data have been corroborated by a number of functional flow cytometry studies with different marker panels focused on myeloid dendritic cells. Several studies reported an increased frequency of activated, i.e., CD40, CD83, and/or CD86 expressing myeloid, dendritic cells in the inflamed mucosa of both Crohn's and ulcerative colitis [13–15, 54–56].

Knowing their mature state it's perhaps not surprising that mucosal myeloid dendritic cells are also an important source of inflammatory cytokines such as TNF-α, IL-1b, IL-6, IL-8(CXCL8), IL-12, IL-17, IL-23, and IL-27 mostly in patients with Crohn's disease [29, 48, 49, 56–58]. However, the production of IL-12 and more recently also IL-23 in Crohn's disease has been called into questions by a study of mucosal monocyte derived dendritic cells in children with Crohn's disease [59]. Colonic myeloid dendritic cells are also strong drivers of Th17 differentiation of naïve T-cells in Crohn's disease [58].

Mesenteric Lymph Node Dendritic Cells

Dendritic cells have been linked to a hallmark feature of Crohn's disease—granuloma formation [60–62]. Early immunohistochemical studies in granulomatous lymphadenitis in Crohn's patients investigated the cellular composition of the granulomas in mesenteric lymph nodes and found an increased number of interdigitating reticulum cells with characteristics of antigen-presenting cells, that we would now classify as dendritic cell subsets [63].

More recent studies using more refined markers identified mature myeloid CD83$^+$ dendritic cells, DC-SIGN positive dendritic cells and CD141$^+$ dendritic cells in mesenteric lymph nodes clustered around T-cells of Crohn's disease patients [46]. Another study that looked at IL-27 expressing myeloid dendritic cells demonstrated, that granulomas, present in the intestinal wall or in mesenteric draining lymph nodes of Crohn's disease patients stained positive with both anti-EBI3 and anti-p28 antibodies localized to the cytoplasm of epithelia and multinucleate giant cells [49].

The expression of chemokines that regulate homing of T-cells and promote recirculating T-cell and dendritic cell interactions, CCL19 and CCL21, was studied in surgically resected mesenteric lymph nodes from controls and patients with Crohn's disease and ulcerative colitis. Mesenteric lymph nodes from Crohn's disease patients displayed an increased expression of CCL21 and CCL19, mainly in high endothelial venules (HEV), mature DC and lymphatic vessels. CCR7 mRNA was increased in T cell areas. This data indirectly supports the hypothesis of homing T-cells and mature myeloid dendritic cells to mesenteric lymph nodes in Crohn's disease [32].

More recently CD103$^+$ DCs described in the mesenteric lymph nodes draining the normal small intestine, although the percentage of showed considerable variation. Human CD103$^+$ mesenteric lymph node DC displayed a more mature phenotype compared with their CD103$^-$ counterparts, as judged by expression of CD40 and CD83. In mixed lymphocyte reactions with allogeneic peripheral blood lymphocytes human CD103$^+$ mesenteric lymph node DC induced significantly higher levels of CCR9 on responding CD8$^+$ T cells than their CD103$^-$ counterparts. Both, CD103$^+$ and CD103$^-$ populations induced similar expression of α4β7. No difference was seen with their counterparts isolated from mesenteric lymph nodes from patients with Crohn's disease. The induction of CCR9$^+$ and α4β7$^+$ by human CD103+ mesenteric lymph node DC was dependent on RAR signaling as gut-homing receptor expression was inhibited by addition of LE540 to the cultures [64]. Human CD103$^+$ DC also express leucine rich repeat kinase 2 (LRRK2), an IFN-γ target gene and its expression increased in intestinal tissues upon Crohn's disease inflammation. LRRK2 expression enhances NF-kB-dependent transcription [65].

When stimulated with exogenous bacterial derivative, mesenteric lymph node myeloid DC from Crohn's disease produce a higher amounts of IL-23 and a lower amount of IL-10 compared with controls and induce stronger Th1 immune responses in mixed lymphocyte reactions compared with those from ulcerative colitis and normal controls [57].

Dendritic Cells in Extraintestinal Tissues in Inflammatory Bowel Disease

The distribution of DC in Crohn's disease patients is not restricted to classical lymphatic spaces and compartments. Adipose tissue is reported to contain monocyte-like preadipocytes, which may mature into macrophages, contributing to local inflammation. Myeloid dendritic cells originate from monocytes [10]. Accumulating dendritic cells enriched from "creeping fat" were potent stimulators of primary proliferation of allogeneic T-cells in mixed leukocyte reactions in one study [66]. Another study investigating corneal changes of patients with Crohn's disease using confocal microscopy found that patients with Crohn's disease had a lower corneal density of dendritic cells [67].

Interaction of Human Dendritic Cells with Microbial Antigens in Ulcerative Colitis and Crohn's Disease

Interaction My Microbial Antigens

Both peripheral blood [13] and mucosal [47, 56, 68, 69] dendritic cells from patients with Crohn's disease and ulcerative colitis express the microbial pattern recognition receptors TLR2 and/or TLR4. TLR4 expression may correlate with positively with disease activity and inversely with *F. prausnitzii* in Crohn's disease [70]. Myeloid DC from patients with inflammatory bowel disease have been shown to respond with an exaggerated immune response to lipopolysaccharide—the principal ligand of TLR4 [13]. Single nucleotide polymorphisms (SNPs) in the TLR4 receptor have been reported to be associated with Crohn's disease in some cohorts and were indeed shown to modulate dendritic cell response towards TLR4 agonists to the generation of strongly polarized Th1 responses against common commensal microorganisms [71].

Myeloid dendritic cells also express the intracellular pattern recognition receptor NOD2. A study comparing NOD2 dependent genome wide expression profiles of muramyldipeptide (MDP) MDP—a derivative of bacterial peptidoglycan—stimulated MoDC from Crohn's disease NOD2 SNP carriers and controls showed that the transcription of pathogen response genes was absent [72].

There is evidence that these expression profile differences translate into actual functional defects. One group was able to link the development of Th17 through the NOD2 ligand. The role of NOD2 in this IL-23-IL-1-IL-17 axis could be confirmed in NOD2 deficient DCs from selected Crohn's disease patients [73]. These data were corroborated by the work of several other groups that NOD2 mutant MoDC from Crohn's disease patients were unable to react appropriately to MDP and promoted the development of Th1 cells [71, 74, 75].

NOD2 triggering by MDP normally induces autophagy in myeloid DC and requires receptor-interacting serine–threonine kinase-2 (RIPK-2), autophagy-related protein-5 (ATG5), ATG7, and ATG16L1 but not NLR family, pyrin domain containing-3 (NALP3) [76]. Two studies showed that that NOD2 mediated autophagy is required for both bacterial handling and generation of major histocompatibility complex (MHC) class II antigen-specific CD4^{+} T-cell responses in DC and that DC from individuals with Crohn's disease expressing Crohn's disease associated NOD2 or ATG16L1 risk variants are defective in autophagy induction, bacterial trafficking, and antigen presentation [76, 77]. Moreover, the T300A variant of autophagy ATG16L1 gene is associated with decreased antigen sampling and processing by DC in pediatric Crohn's disease [78].

The production of cytokines by DC is also dependent on the microbiota composition. In one study IL-12p40 and IL-6 production correlated with the ratio of *Bacteroides* and *Bifidobacteria*, IL-10 production with *Bifidobacteria*, and IL-6 inversely with *F. prausnitzii* [70].

Therapeutic Modulation of the Microbial Response

Based on diversity of the commensal flora in the human gut, the importance of microbial antigen recognition and preliminary evidence that that intestinal dendritic cell function may be influenced by the composition of the commensal microbiota encouraged pilot studies with different probiotic microbial species to exploit this important aspect of the immune response therapeutically [79].

In one study human MoDC were cultured in vitro with different *Lactobacilli* species. *Lactobacillus reuteri* and *Lactobacillus casei*, but not *Lactobacillus plantarum* primed MoDC to drive the development of IL-10 producing Treg through binding of the C-type lectin DC-specific intercellular adhesion molecule 3-grabbing non-integrin (DC-SIGN) [80]. However, these findings are partial contradicted by a study where *Lactobacillus rhamnosus* treated MoDC decreased T cell proliferation and cytokine production of IL-2, IL-4, and IL-10 [81]. The bacterial serine–threonine peptide conditioning of colonic DC in vitro reduced TLR expression, increased CD40 and CD80 expression, and restored their stimulatory capacity [82].

Not only bacteria have therapeutic potential with IBD DC. Culture of primary human myeloid CD1c⁺CD11c⁺CD123⁻ myeloid DC in the presence of *Saccharomyces boulardii* culture supernatant (active component molecular weight <3 kDa, as evaluated by membrane partition chromatography) reduced significantly the expression of CD40, CD80, and CCR7 (CD197) induced by the prototypical microbial antigen and TLR4 ligand lipopolysaccharide. Moreover,

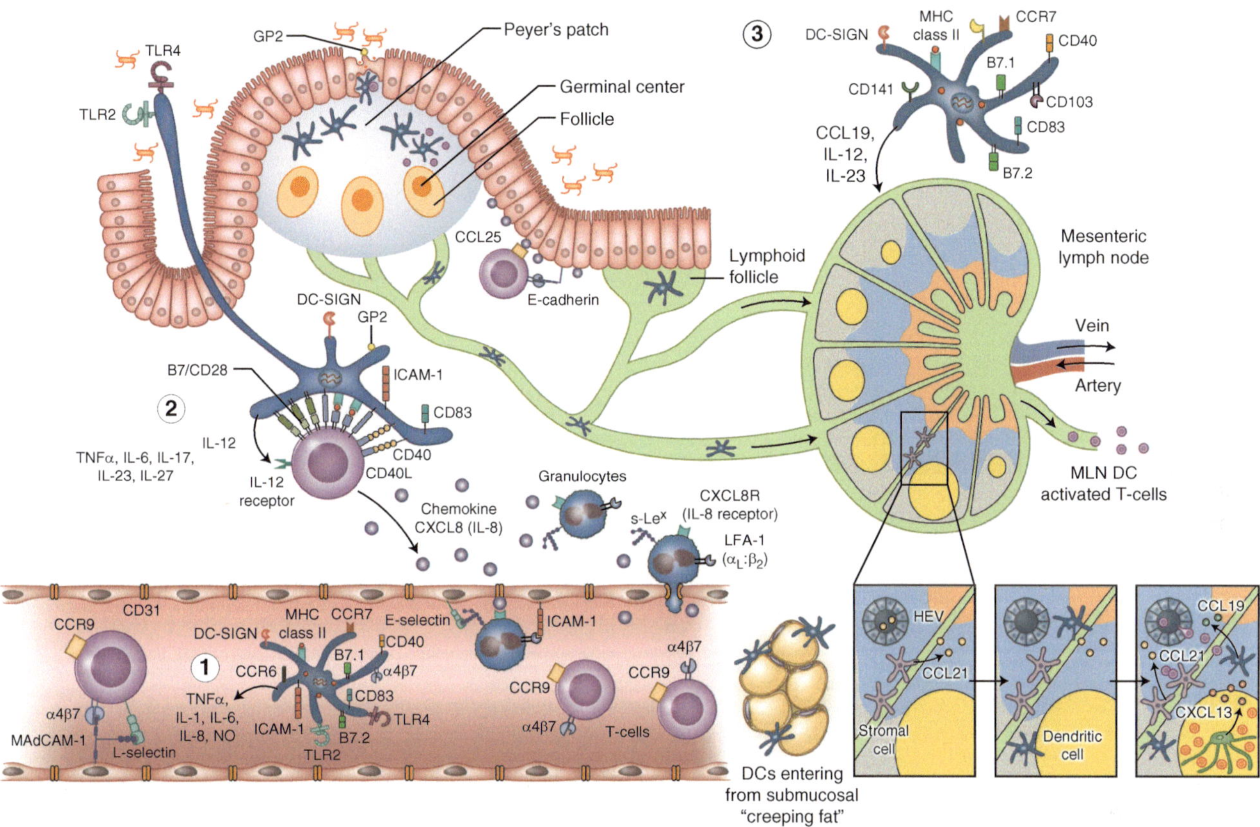

Fig. 7.1 Model of the three major myeloid dendritic cell populations and their hypothesized (dys)function in human inflammatory bowel disease (The majority of pathways were identified for Crohn's disease and to a lesser degree for ulcerative colitis. See text and references for details. For clarity no distinction between Crohn's disease and ulcerative colitis was made and to bring out cellular details this cartoon is not to scale.). (*1*) Peripheral blood myeloid dendritic cells: In IBD patients these cells display an activated phenotype and have been demonstrated to express HLA-DR, CCR6, CCR7(CD197), CCR8, CD80, CD83, CD86, CD40, ICAM-1 (CD49d), TLR2, and TLR4. In acute flares circulating dendritic cells evade the peripheral blood pool and probably migrate to the mucosal sites of the inflammation. Their secretion of chemokines like CXCL8 (IL-8) attracts innate immune cells such as granulocytes expressing its cognate receptor CXCR8 and homing CCR9⁺ α4β7⁺ T-lymphocytes that transmigrate into the tissue mediate, amplify and perpetuate the inflammation. (*2*) Mucosal myeloid dendritic cells: In IBD they show an activated phenotype as well. These cells inspect molecular microbial associated patterns (MAMP) of the intestinal microbiota with their own TLR2 and TLR4 receptors directly through their epithelial layer penetrating dendrites or are fed microbial antigens via M-cells in Peyer's patches that transport them into the lamina propria. Moreover, antigens are recognized by intracellular NOD. In the small intestine this happens in the subepithelial dome area of Peyer's patches or isolated lymph follicles in other parts of the small and large intestine. DC-SIGN and CD83 expressing myeloid dendritic cells have been described in isolated lymph follicles as well. Misinterpretation of MAMPs perhaps due to single nucleotide polymorphisms of TLR4 and NOD2 reported in IBD and absent tolerogenic effects of TGFβ and retinoid acid on mucosal dendritic cells normally secreted intestinal epithelia triggers immunity against the normally tolerated flora. The distinct pro-inflammatory cytokine profile (TNFα, IL-6, IL-17, IL-23, and IL-27) of myeloid mucosal dendritic cells in IBD promotes the development of inflammatory Th1 and Th17 T-lymphocytes and attracts other leukocytes to transmigrate through the endothelial layer into the lamina propria. (*3*) Mesenteric lymph node myeloid dendritic cells: Stromal cells and high endothelial venules (HEV) secrete the chemokine CCL21 and attract circulating dendritic cells that recognize it through their expression of its native receptor CCR7. Mucosal dendritic cells migrate along the chemokine gradient via efferent lymphatic vessels from the lamina propria into the afferent lymphatic of the mesenteric lymph node (MLN). In the paracortex mesenteric myeloid lymph node dendritic cell function depends on their expression of CD103. Once arrived in the T-cell zone CD103⁺ dendritic cells secrete CCL19 that increases via feedback loop the expression of CCR7—the CCL19 receptor on dendritic cells—and also attract CCR9⁺ α4β7⁺ T-lymphocytes to arrive through high endothelial venules from the blood. These T-cells start to proliferate once they recognize their cognate antigens presented by the mesenteric lymph node dendritic cells and leave the lymph node activated through the efferent lymphatic further aggravating inflammation. The expression of CCL19 and CCL21 suggests that B-cells are also attracted to mesenteric lymph nodes which may induce follicular dendritic cells that secrete CXCL13 (BCA-1 or BLC) that drives more B-cell migration. While the chemokine expression has been described in IBD, the interaction is speculative

secretion of TNFα and IL-6 were notably reduced, while the secretion of IL-10 increased. Finally, Sb supernatant inhibited the proliferation of naive T cells in a mixed lymphocyte reaction with myeloid DC [24].

A different approach was taken by another group of investigators based on the fact that some *Bifidobacteria* species are immunoregulatory, induce increased dendritic cell interleukin IL-10 release in vitro and that administration of fructooligosaccharides increases fecal and mucosal bifidobacteria. The found the percentage of IL-10 and TLR2 and TLR4 positive dendritic cells in fructooligosaccharide treated Crohn's disease patients [68]. Unfortunately, these data could not be validated in a randomized trial [83] (see Fig. 7.1).

References

1. Baumgart DC, Sandborn WJ. Crohn's disease. Lancet. 2012;380:1590–605.
2. Ordas I, Eckmann L, Talamini M, Baumgart DC, Sandborn WJ. Ulcerative colitis. Lancet. 2012;380:1606–19.
3. Iwasaki A, Medzhitov R. Toll-like receptor control of the adaptive immune responses. Nat Immunol. 2004;5:987–95.
4. Iwasaki A. Mucosal dendritic cells. Annu Rev Immunol. 2007;25:381–418.
5. Malmstrom V, Shipton D, Singh B, Al-Shamkhani A, Puklavec MJ, Barclay AN, et al. CD134L expression on dendritic cells in the mesenteric lymph nodes drives colitis in T cell-restored SCID mice. J Immunol. 2001;166:6972–81.
6. Leithauser F, Trobonjaca Z, Moller P, Reimann J. Clustering of colonic lamina propria CD4(+) T cells to subepithelial dendritic cell aggregates precedes the development of colitis in a murine adoptive transfer model. Lab Invest. 2001;81:1339–49.
7. Krajina T, Leithauser F, Moller P, Trobonjaca Z, Reimann J. Colonic lamina propria dendritic cells in mice with CD4+ T cell-induced colitis. Eur J Immunol. 2003;33:1073–83.
8. Cruickshank SM, English NR, Felsburg PJ, Carding SR. Characterization of colonic dendritic cells in normal and colitic mice. World J Gastroenterol. 2005;11:6338–47.
9. Reizis B. Regulation of plasmacytoid dendritic cell development. Curr Opin Immunol. 2010;22:206–11.
10. Geissmann F, Manz MG, Jung S, Sieweke MH, Merad M, Ley K. Development of monocytes, macrophages, and dendritic cells. Science. 2010;327:656–61.
11. Liu K, Victora GD, Schwickert TA, Guermonprez P, Meredith MM, Yao K, et al. In vivo analysis of dendritic cell development and homeostasis. Science. 2009;324:392–7.
12. Kelsall BL, Leon F. Involvement of intestinal dendritic cells in oral tolerance, immunity to pathogens, and inflammatory bowel disease. Immunol Rev. 2005;206:132–48.
13. Baumgart DC, Thomas S, Przesdzing I, Metzke D, Bielecki C, Lehmann SM, et al. Exaggerated inflammatory response of primary human myeloid dendritic cells to lipopolysaccharide in patients with inflammatory bowel disease. Clin Exp Immunol. 2009;157:423–36.
14. Vuckovic S, Florin TH, Khalil D, Zhang MF, Patel K, Hamilton I, et al. CD40 and CD86 upregulation with divergent CMRF44 expression on blood dendritic cells in inflammatory bowel diseases. Am J Gastroenterol. 2001;96:2946–56.
15. Murakami H, Akbar SM, Matsui H, Horiike N, Onji M. Macrophage migration inhibitory factor activates antigen-presenting dendritic cells and induces inflammatory cytokines in ulcerative colitis. Clin Exp Immunol. 2002;128:504–10.
16. Ikeda Y, Akbar F, Matsui H, Onji M. Characterization of antigen-presenting dendritic cells in the peripheral blood and colonic mucosa of patients with ulcerative colitis. Eur J Gastroenterol Hepatol. 2001;13:841–50.
17. Begue B, Verdier J, Rieux-Laucat F, Goulet O, Morali A, Canioni D, et al. Defective IL10 signaling defining a subgroup of patients with inflammatory bowel disease. Am J Gastroenterol. 2011;106:1544–55.
18. Nieminen JK, Sipponen T, Farkkila M, Vaarala O. Monocyte-derived dendritic cells from Crohn's disease patients exhibit decreased ability to activate T helper type 17 responses in memory cells. Clin Exp Immunol. 2014;177:190–202.
19. MacDonald KP, Munster DJ, Clark GJ, Dzionek A, Schmitz J, Hart DN. Characterization of human blood dendritic cell subsets. Blood. 2002;100:4512–20.
20. Baumgart DC, Metzke D, Schmitz J, Scheffold A, Sturm A, Wiedenmann B, et al. Patients with active inflammatory bowel disease lack immature peripheral blood plasmacytoid and myeloid dendritic cells. Gut. 2005;54:228–36.
21. Bsat M, Chapuy L, Baba N, Rubio M, Panzini B, Wassef R, et al. Differential accumulation and function of proinflammatory 6-sulfo LacNAc dendritic cells in lymph node and colon of Crohn's versus ulcerative colitis patients. J Leukoc Biol. 2015;98:671–81.
22. Costantini C, Calzetti F, Perbellini O, Micheletti A, Scarponi C, Lonardi S, et al. Human neutrophils interact with both 6-sulfo LacNAc+DC and NK cells to amplify NK-derived IFN{gamma}: role of CD18, ICAM-1, and ICAM-3. Blood. 2011;117:1677–86.
23. Watanabe S, Yamakawa M, Hiroaki T, Kawata S, Kimura O. Correlation of dendritic cell infiltration with active crypt inflammation in ulcerative colitis. Clin Immunol. 2007;122:288–97.
24. Thomas S, Przesdzing I, Metzke D, Schmitz J, Radbruch A, Baumgart DC. Saccharomyces boulardii inhibits lipopolysaccharide-induced activation of human dendritic cells and T cell proliferation. Clin Exp Immunol. 2009;156:78–87.
25. Middel P, Raddatz D, Gunawan B, Haller F, Radzun HJ. Increased number of mature dendritic cells in Crohn's disease: evidence for a chemokine mediated retention mechanism. Gut. 2006;55:220–7.
26. Bernardo D, Vallejo-Diez S, Mann ER, Al-Hassi HO, Martinez-Abad B, Montalvillo E, et al. IL-6 promotes immune responses in human ulcerative colitis and induces a skin-homing phenotype in the dendritic cells and Tcells they stimulate. Eur J Immunol. 2012;42:1337–53.
27. Morise K, Yamaguchi T, Kuroiwa A, Kanayama K, Matsuura T, Shinoda M, et al. Expression of adhesion molecules and HLA-DR by macrophages and dendritic cells in aphthoid lesions of Crohn's disease: an immunocytochemical study. J Gastroenterol. 1994;29:257–64.
28. Middel P, Thelen P, Blaschke S, Polzien F, Reich K, Blaschke V, et al. Expression of the T-cell chemoattractant chemokine lymphotactin in Crohn's disease. Am J Pathol. 2001;159:1751–61.
29. Damen GM, Hol J, de Ruiter L, Bouquet J, Sinaasappel M, van der Woude J, et al. Chemokine production by buccal epithelium as a distinctive feature of pediatric Crohn disease. J Pediatr Gastroenterol Nutr. 2006;42:142–9.
30. Carlsen HS, Baekkevold ES, Johansen FE, Haraldsen G, Brandtzaeg P. B cell attracting chemokine 1 (CXCL13) and its receptor CXCR5 are expressed in normal and aberrant gut associated lymphoid tissue. Gut. 2002;51:364–71.
31. Carlsen HS, Baekkevold ES, Morton HC, Haraldsen G, Brandtzaeg P. Monocyte-like and mature macrophages produce CXCL13 (B cell-attracting chemokine 1) in inflammatory lesions with lymphoid neogenesis. Blood. 2004;104:3021–7.
32. Kawashima D, Oshitani N, Jinno Y, Watanabe K, Nakamura S, Higuchi K, et al. Augmented expression of secondary lymphoid tissue chemokine and EBI1 ligand chemokine in Crohn's disease. J Clin Pathol. 2005;58:1057–63.
33. Kaser A, Ludwiczek O, Holzmann S, Moschen AR, Weiss G, Enrich B, et al. Increased expression of CCL20 in human inflammatory bowel disease. J Clin Immunol. 2004;24:74–85.

34. Manzo A, Bugatti S, Caporali R, Prevo R, Jackson DG, Uguccioni M, et al. CCL21 expression pattern of human secondary lymphoid organ stroma is conserved in inflammatory lesions with lymphoid neogenesis. Am J Pathol. 2007;171:1549–62.
35. Wu W, He C, Liu C, Cao AT, Xue X, Evans-Marin HL, et al. miR-10a inhibits dendritic cell activation and Th1/Th17 cell immune responses in IBD. Gut. 2014;64(11):1755–64.
36. Hedl M, Lahiri A, Ning K, Cho JH, Abraham C. Pattern recognition receptor signaling in human dendritic cells is enhanced by ICOS ligand and modulated by the Crohn's disease ICOSLG risk allele. Immunity. 2014;40:734–46.
37. Sanders TJ, McCarthy NE, Giles EM, Davidson KL, Haltalli ML, Hazell S, et al. Increased production of retinoic acid by intestinal macrophages contributes to their inflammatory phenotype in patients with Crohn's disease. Gastroenterology. 2014;146:1278–88.e1–2.
38. Wada Y, Hisamatsu T, Kamada N, Okamoto S, Hibi T. Retinoic acid contributes to the induction of IL-12-hypoproducing dendritic cells. Inflamm Bowel Dis. 2009;15:1548–56.
39. Iliev ID, Spadoni I, Mileti E, Matteoli G, Sonzogni A, Sampietro GM, et al. Human intestinal epithelial cells promote the differentiation of tolerogenic dendritic cells. Gut. 2009;58:1481–9.
40. Bartels LE, Bendix M, Hvas CL, Jorgensen SP, Agnholt J, Agger R, et al. Oral vitamin D3 supplementation reduces monocyte-derived dendritic cell maturation and cytokine production in Crohn's disease patients. Inflammopharmacology. 2014;22:95–103.
41. Ueno A, Jijon H, Traves S, Chan R, Ford K, Beck PL, et al. Opposing effects of smoking in ulcerative colitis and Crohn's disease may be explained by differential effects on dendritic cells. Inflamm Bowel Dis. 2014;20:800–10.
42. Seldenrijk CA, Drexhage HA, Meuwissen SG, Pals ST, Meijer CJ. Dendritic cells and scavenger macrophages in chronic inflammatory bowel disease. Gut. 1989;30:484–91.
43. Allison MC, Poulter LW. Changes in phenotypically distinct mucosal macrophage populations may be a prerequisite for the development of inflammatory bowel disease. Clin Exp Immunol. 1991;85:504–9.
44. Allison MC, Cornwall S, Poulter LW, Dhillon AP, Pounder RE. Macrophage heterogeneity in normal colonic mucosa and in inflammatory bowel disease. Gut. 1988;29:1531–8.
45. de Silva HJ, Jones M, Prince C, Kettlewell M, Mortensen NJ, Jewell DP. Lymphocyte and macrophage subpopulations in pelvic ileal pouches. Gut. 1991;32:1160–5.
46. te Velde AA, van Kooyk Y, Braat H, Hommes DW, Dellemijn TA, Slors JF, et al. Increased expression of DC-SIGN+IL-12+IL-18+ and CD83+IL-12-IL-18− dendritic cell populations in the colonic mucosa of patients with Crohn's disease. Eur J Immunol. 2003;33:143–51.
47. Salim SY, Silva MA, Keita AV, Larsson M, Andersson P, Magnusson KE, et al. CD83+CCR7− dendritic cells accumulate in the subepithelial dome and internalize translocated Escherichia coli HB101 in the Peyer's patches of ileal Crohn's disease. Am J Pathol. 2009;174:82–90.
48. de Baey A, Mende I, Baretton G, Greiner A, Hartl WH, Baeuerle PA, et al. A subset of human dendritic cells in the T cell area of mucosa-associated lymphoid tissue with a high potential to produce TNF-alpha. J Immunol. 2003;170:5089–94.
49. Larousserie F, Pflanz S, Coulomb-L'Hermine A, Brousse N, Kastelein R, Devergne O. Expression of IL-27 in human Th1-associated granulomatous diseases. J Pathol. 2004;202:164–71.
50. Franchimont D, Vermeire S, El Housni H, Pierik M, Van Steen K, Gustot T, et al. Deficient host-bacteria interactions in inflammatory bowel disease? The toll-like receptor (TLR)-4 Asp299gly polymorphism is associated with Crohn's disease and ulcerative colitis. Gut. 2004;53:987–92.
51. Bernink JH, Krabbendam L, Germar K, de Jong E, Gronke K, Kofoed-Nielsen M, et al. Interleukin-12 and -23 control plasticity of CD127(+) group 1 and group 3 innate lymphoid cells in the intestinal lamina propria. Immunity. 2015;43:146–60.
52. Yeung MM, Melgar S, Baranov V, Oberg A, Danielsson A, Hammarstrom S, et al. Characterisation of mucosal lymphoid aggregates in ulcerative colitis: immune cell phenotype and TcR-gammadelta expression. Gut. 2000;47:215–27.
53. Silva MA, Lopez CB, Riverin F, Oligny L, Menezes J, Seidman EG. Characterization and distribution of colonic dendritic cells in Crohn's disease. Inflamm Bowel Dis. 2004;10:504–12.
54. Bell SJ, Rigby R, English N, Mann SD, Knight SC, Kamm MA, et al. Migration and maturation of human colonic dendritic cells. J Immunol. 2001;166:4958–67.
55. Ikeda Y, Akbar SM, Matsui H, Onji M. Antigen-presenting dendritic cells in ulcerative colitis. J Gastroenterol. 2002;37 Suppl 14:53–5.
56. Hart AL, Al-Hassi HO, Rigby RJ, Bell SJ, Emmanuel AV, Knight SC, et al. Characteristics of intestinal dendritic cells in inflammatory bowel diseases. Gastroenterology. 2005;129:50–65.
57. Sakuraba A, Sato T, Kamada N, Kitazume M, Sugita A, Hibi T. Th1/Th17 immune response is induced by mesenteric lymph node dendritic cells in Crohn's disease. Gastroenterology. 2009;137:1736–45.
58. Ogino T, Nishimura J, Barman S, Kayama H, Uematsu S, Okuzaki D, et al. Increased Th17-inducing activity of CD14+ CD163 low myeloid cells in intestinal lamina propria of patients with Crohn's disease. Gastroenterology. 2013;145:1380–91.e1.
59. Damen GM, van Lierop P, de Ruiter L, Escher JC, Donders R, Samsom JN, et al. Production of IL12p70 and IL23 by monocyte-derived dendritic cells in children with inflammatory bowel disease. Gut. 2008;57:1480.
60. Crohn BB, Ginzburg L, Oppenheimer GD. Landmark article Oct 15, 1932. Regional ileitis. A pathological and clinical entity. By Burril B. Crohn, Leon Ginzburg, and Gordon D. Oppenheimer. JAMA. 1984;251:73–9.
61. Crohn BB. Granulomatous diseases of the small and large bowel. A historical survey. Gastroenterology. 1967;52:767–72.
62. Patel P, Barone F, Nunes C, Boursier L, Odell E, Escudier M, et al. Subepithelial dendritic B cells in orofacial granulomatosis. Inflamm Bowel Dis. 2010;16:1051–60.
63. Geboes K, van den Oord J, De Wolf-Peeters C, Desmet V, Rutgeerts P, Janssens J, et al. The cellular composition of granulomas in mesenteric lymph nodes from patients with Crohn's disease. Virchows Arch A Pathol Anat Histopathol. 1986;409:679–92.
64. Jaensson E, Uronen-Hansson H, Pabst O, Eksteen B, Tian J, Coombes JL, et al. Small intestinal CD103+ dendritic cells display unique functional properties that are conserved between mice and humans. J Exp Med. 2008;205:2139–49.
65. Gardet A, Benita Y, Li C, Sands BE, Ballester I, Stevens C, et al. LRRK2 is involved in the IFN-gamma response and host response to pathogens. J Immunol. 2010;185:5577–85.
66. Bedford PA, Todorovic V, Westcott ED, Windsor AC, English NR, Al-Hassi HO, et al. Adipose tissue of human omentum is a major source of dendritic cells, which lose MHC Class II and stimulatory function in Crohn's disease. J Leukoc Biol. 2006;80:546–54.
67. Ceresara G, Fogagnolo P, De Cilla S, Panizzo V, Danelli PG, Orzalesi N, et al. Corneal involvement in Crohn's disease: an in vivo confocal microscopy study. Cornea. 2011;30:136–42.
68. Lindsay JO, Whelan K, Stagg AJ, Gobin P, Al-Hassi HO, Rayment N, et al. Clinical, microbiological, and immunological effects of fructo-oligosaccharide in patients with Crohn's disease. Gut. 2006;55:348–55.
69. Silva MA, Quera R, Valenzuela J, Salim SY, Soderholm JD, Perdue MH. Dendritic cells and toll-like receptors 2 and 4 in the ileum of Crohn's disease patients. Dig Dis Sci. 2008;53:1917–28.
70. Ng SC, Benjamin JL, McCarthy NE, Hedin CR, Koutsoumpas A, Plamondon S, et al. Relationship between human intestinal dendritic cells, gut microbiota, and disease activity in Crohn's disease. Inflamm Bowel Dis. 2011;17:2027–37.

71. Butler M, Chaudhary R, van Heel DA, Playford RJ, Ghosh S. NOD2 activity modulates the phenotype of LPS-stimulated dendritic cells to promote the development of T-helper type 2-like lymphocytes—possible implications for NOD2-associated Crohn's disease. J Crohns Colitis. 2007;1:106–15.
72. Zelinkova Z, van Beelen AJ, de Kort F, Moerland PD, Ver Loren van Themaat E, te Velde AA, et al. Muramyl dipeptide-induced differential gene expression in NOD2 mutant and wild-type Crohn's disease patient-derived dendritic cells. Inflamm Bowel Dis. 2008;14:186–94.
73. van Beelen AJ, Zelinkova Z, Taanman-Kueter EW, Muller FJ, Hommes DW, Zaat SA, et al. Stimulation of the intracellular bacterial sensor NOD2 programs dendritic cells to promote interleukin-17 production in human memory T cells. Immunity. 2007;27:660–9.
74. Granzotto M, Fabbro E, Maschio M, Martelossi S, Quaglia S, Tommasini A, et al. Heterozygous nucleotide-binding oligomerization domain-2 mutations affect monocyte maturation in Crohn's disease. World J Gastroenterol. 2007;13:6191–6.
75. Salucci V, Rimoldi M, Penati C, Sampietro GM, van Duist MM, Matteoli G, et al. Monocyte-derived dendritic cells from Crohn patients show differential NOD2/CARD15-dependent immune responses to bacteria. Inflamm Bowel Dis. 2008;14:812–8.
76. Cooney R, Baker J, Brain O, Danis B, Pichulik T, Allan P, et al. NOD2 stimulation induces autophagy in dendritic cells influencing bacterial handling and antigen presentation. Nat Med. 2010;16:90–7.
77. Homer CR, Richmond AL, Rebert NA, Achkar JP, McDonald C. ATG16L1 and NOD2 interact in an autophagy-dependent anti-bacterial pathway implicated in Crohn's disease pathogenesis. Gastroenterology. 2010;139:1630–41, 41.e1–2.
78. Strisciuglio C, Miele E, Wildenberg ME, Giugliano FP, Andreozzi M, Vitale A, et al. T300A variant of autophagy ATG16L1 gene is associated with decreased antigen sampling and processing by dendritic cells in pediatric Crohn's disease. Inflamm Bowel Dis. 2013;19:2339–48.
79. Bengtson MB, Solberg C, Aamodt G, Sauar J, Jahnsen J, Moum B, et al. Familial aggregation in Crohn's disease and ulcerative colitis in a Norwegian population-based cohort followed for ten years. J Crohns Colitis. 2009;3:92–9.
80. Smits HH, Engering A, van der Kleij D, de Jong EC, Schipper K, van Capel TM, et al. Selective probiotic bacteria induce IL-10-producing regulatory T cells in vitro by modulating dendritic cell function through dendritic cell-specific intercellular adhesion molecule 3-grabbing nonintegrin. J Allergy Clin Immunol. 2005;115:1260–7.
81. Braat H, van den Brande J, van Tol E, Hommes D, Peppelenbosch M, van Deventer S. Lactobacillus rhamnosus induces peripheral hyporesponsiveness in stimulated CD4+ T cells via modulation of dendritic cell function. Am J Clin Nutr. 2004;80:1618–25.
82. Al-Hassi HO, Mann ER, Sanchez B, English NR, Peake ST, Landy J, et al. Altered human gut dendritic cell properties in ulcerative colitis are reversed by Lactobacillus plantarum extracellular encrypted peptide STp. Mol Nutr Food Res. 2014;58:1132–43.
83. Benjamin JL, Hedin CR, Koutsoumpas A, Ng SC, McCarthy NE, Hart AL, et al. Randomised, double-blind, placebo-controlled trial of fructo-oligosaccharides in active Crohn's disease. Gut. 2011;60:923–9.

Immunobiology of T-Cells in Inflammatory Bowel Disease

8

S. Snapper, D. Nguyen, and A. Biswas

Introduction

The adaptive immune system plays a central role in the pathogenesis of inflammatory bowel disease (IBD). In a healthy state, both CD8^{+} and CD4^{+} subsets of T cells are present in the intestines in small numbers; the former are found mostly in the epithelial layer while the latter are located deeper in the lamina propria. In an inflammatory state, however, the number of CD4^{+} T cells is often vastly magnified. Early research efforts were largely centered on T lymphocytes given evidence that CD4^{+} T cells from colitic animals and human IBD patients expressed activation markers and produced pro-inflammatory cytokines [1–5] and adoptive transfer of CD4^{+} T cells from several animal models of colitis into immunodeficient mice could transfer disease [6–8]. While still controversial, it seems likely in most IBD patients that altered T cells are not the critical initiating signal driving inflammation, but rather are an essential mediator and propagator of disease resulting from aberrant innate immune function [1].

T lymphocytes are broadly classified as regulatory or effector T cells. The latter is crucial in the protective immune response against infections. In contrast, the function of regulatory T cells is to maintain mucosal homeostasis by limiting the immune response to pathogens and by disarming any self-reactive effector T cells that escape negative selection in the thymus. Both T cell subsets are present in the gut-associated lymphoid tissue. Thus, inflammation can result from an imbalance of the number and/or function of these two T cell arms of the homeostatic T cell equation. Most studies on the role of T lymphocytes in IBD pathogenesis have centered on the CD4^{+} T cell subset, which is the main focus of this chapter; however, other T cell subsets are briefly covered at the end of the chapter.

Effector T Cells

In the human gut, immune homeostasis requires exquisitely regulated responses to rare pathogens among a preponderance of seemingly harmless commensal microorganisms. Effector T cells are critical for protecting against intestinal pathogens and are broadly classified into Th1, Th2, or Th17 cells based on their cytokine secretion profile. Interferon-(γ) gamma and TNF-(α)alpha are the predominant cytokines produced by Th1 cells whereas Th2 cells produce interleukin (IL)-4, IL-5, and/or IL-13. Th17 cells secrete IL-17, a phenotype that is perpetuated by IL-23. In a physiologic state, Th1 and Th2 cytokines are necessary to restrain pathogens: Th2 cytokines are secreted in response to parasitic infections, whereas Th1 cytokines are secreted in response to the presence of intracellular bacteria and viruses. Th17 cell produced IL-17, on the other hand, plays a role in protection against pathogenic bacteria, viruses, and fungi, namely by recruitment of other immune subsets to mucosal sites [9, 10].

Inappropriately activated effector T cells can lead to pathology. Crohn's disease was classically considered a Th1-associated disease [3, 5], but more recently, Crohn's disease has been reclassified as a mixed Th1/17 disease as mucosal tissue from Crohn's patients have been found to produce IL-17 in addition to TNF-(α)alpha and interferon-(γ) gamma [11]. Ulcerative colitis, on the other hand, has been described by some but not all studies to be a Th2-associated disease with elevated levels of IL-5 and IL-13 (but not the classic Th2 cytokine IL-4) detected in diseased mucosa [4, 11]. More recent studies, however, have reported detection of IL-17 in ulcerative colitis tissues [11]. A relatively new subset of T-helper cells, Th9 cells, defined by their secretion

S. Snapper (✉)
Division of Gastroenterology, Hepatology and Nutrition, Boston Children's Hospital, Boston, MA 02115, USA

Division of Gastroenterology, Brigham and Women's Hospital, Boston, MA 02115, USA
e-mail: ssnapper@hms.harvard.edu

D. Nguyen • A. Biswas
Division of Gastroenterology, Hepatology and Nutrition, Boston Children's Hospital, Boston, MA 02115, USA

D.C. Baumgart (ed.), *Crohn's Disease and Ulcerative Colitis*, DOI 10.1007/978-3-319-33703-6_8

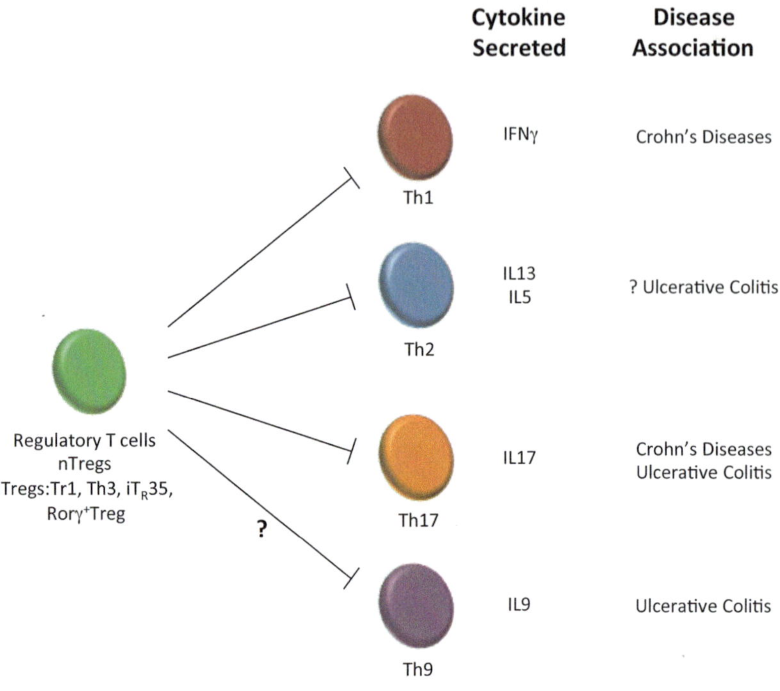

Fig. 8.1 Regulatory and Effector T cell populations controlling IBD. Various effector T cells (Th1, Th2, Th17, and Th9) are depicted and their cytokine secretion patterns as well as potential IBD disease associations. Regulatory T cells (nTregs and iTregs) can suppress effector T cell function employing diverse mechanisms including anti-inflammatory cytokine secretion (e.g., IL-10, TGF-β, and IL-35)

of interleukin-9, has been implicated in the pathogenesis of IBD [12–14]. Patients with active Crohn's disease or ulcerative colitis have elevated numbers of CD4$^+$PU.1$^+$ and CD4$^+$IRF4$^+$ T cells in the intestinal mucosa compared to control patients [12, 13]. Interestingly, only ulcerative colitis patients showed elevated expression of IL-9 by these cells, and there was an association of IL-9 expression and IL-9$^+$ T cells with the severity of the disease [12, 13]. Ulcerative colitis patients also showed elevated expression of IL-9R in intestinal epithelial cells [12, 13] and it has been proposed that Th9 cell-derived IL9 alters tight junction protein composition in the intestinal epithelium and thereby increases intestinal permeability leading to disease [12, 14]. The association of Crohn's disease and ulcerative colitis with particular T helper cell subsets is summarized in Fig. 8.1. Please refer to Chaps. 15 and 16 on Th1/2/17 cells and animal models of IBD, respectively, for further details.

Regulatory T Cells

The proinflammatory capacity of effector cells is kept in balance by regulatory T cells. These cells are classically hypoproliferative, hyporesponsive, and potent in their suppressive capacity to inhibit proliferation and activation of non-regulatory T cell counterparts. Regulatory T cells are classically divided into at least two distinct populations (summarized in Fig. 8.1): naturally occurring regulatory T cells (nTregs) that are generated in the thymus and "induced" regulatory T cells (iTregs) that are generated in peripheral tissues or are generated in vitro in the presence of certain anti-inflammatory cytokines. Both populations are likely essential, with distinct and nonredundant functions in maintaining mucosal homeostasis [14–16].

Naturally Occurring Tregs

Easily detected in the peripheral blood and peripheral immune compartments, such as the spleen, lymph nodes, and the intestines, nTregs express Foxp3, a member of the forkhead family of transcription factors that is crucial for their development and function. Scurfy mice, that have mutant *FOXP3*, are devoid of nTregs, die soon after birth from autoimmunity, a phenotype that can be rescued by transfer of regulatory T cells within a few days after birth [15]. Similarly, humans without functional Foxp3 develop immune dysregulation, polyendocrinopathy, enteropathy, X-linked (IPEX) syndrome and also suffer from multiple autoimmune manifestations, including enteropathy [17–19]. In addition to IPEX, other genetic deficiencies including mutations in WASP, CD25, and IL-10 all lead to abnormal Treg cell numbers and/or function, and are associated with increased risk of IBD [20, 21]. In the mouse, Foxp3 is a reliable marker of Tregs. However, in human cells, CD4$^+$ T cells can transiently express low levels of Foxp3 when activated, thus, making Foxp3 an ambiguous marker of nTregs [22]. Some cell surface markers have been described, albeit inconsistently, to be expressed by nTregs, such as GITR, GARP, CD49d, ICOS, CD25, and CTLA-4 [23, 24]. Unfortunately, these cell surface markers are not specific to nTregs and, therefore, leave room for better markers for identification of nTregs. Liu et al. proposed a strategy to identify "pure" FOXP3$^+$ Treg cells, devoid of activated T cells, by inclusion of the IL-7 receptor alpha chain (CD127) in their flow cytometry-based purification protocols. More specifically, low expression of CD127, in conjunction with CD25 expression, provides a useful strategy for the identification of a highly enriched FOXP3$^+$ cells in humans [15, 25, 26].

Despite the fact that they make up only 5–10 % of the total CD4$^+$ cell population, nTregs are critical in maintaining immunologic homeostasis. In the mouse, co-transfer of nTregs with CD45RB^{hi} T cells into immunodeficient mice not only protect against colitis but can also reverse ongoing colitis [27, 28]. Transfer of nTregs into susceptible animals can also ameliorate other autoimmune diseases, such as experimental autoimmune encephalopathy (a model of multiple sclerosis), or nonobese diabetic (NOD) mice (a model of type I diabetes), or systemic lupus erythematosus [29–31]. Along the same line, mice depleted of CD25$^+$ T cells, which consist mainly of nTregs, develop significant autoimmune diseases [32]. In the in vitro setting, nTregs can potently suppress proliferation of cocultured naïve T cells [23, 33].

Naturally occurring Tregs function partly through secretion of a multitude of anti-inflammatory cytokines, including IL-10, TGFβ, and IL-35 [34]. Tregs deficient in TGFβ or WT Tregs transferred with neutralizing antibodies to TGFβ were not able to suppress disease in an adoptive cell transfer model of colitis [35, 36]. The data regarding IL-10 are not as clear; Tregs deficient in IL-10 or WT Tregs transferred with neutralizing antibodies to IL-10R are defective in colitis protection in some, but not all, settings [6, 37]. Moreover, deletion of IL-10 from Foxp3$^+$ Treg leads to less severe intestinal inflammation compared to deletion in total CD4$^+$ T cells, implicating CD4$^+$ Foxp3$^-$ cells as a functional source of IL-10 that contributes to intestinal homeostasis [16, 38]. On the other hand, IL-35, which is a heterodimer of Epstein-Barr-virus-induced gene 3 (EBI3) and IL-12α, appears crucial to the regulatory function of Tregs, since EBI3-deficient and IL-12α deficient Tregs lose their suppressive properties both in vitro and in vivo in a model of colitis [34, 39]. In addition to cytokine-mediated regulation, Tregs can also modulate antigen presenting cell and effector T cell function by alteration of cellular metabolism by surface expression of enzymes CD39 and CD73 that convert proinflammatory extracellular ATP into the immunosuppressive nucleoside adenosine [40, 41]. Whether or not all these regulatory mechanism are necessary for mucosal homeostasis in a normal mouse is not clear, but collectively they play important roles in the suppressive function of Tregs in different settings [16, 42].

Inducible Tregs

In addition to nTregs that are generated in the thymus, regulatory T cells can be “induced” in vivo outside of the thymus in peripheral lymphoid tissue under tolerogenic conditions. The majority of peripheral Foxp3$^+$ cells in the spleen and lymph nodes are thymically established nTreg cells. In contrast, the inducible Tregs (iTregs) make up a large fraction of T cells in the lamina propria (LP) and gut-associated lymphoid tissue (GALT) of the intestine [15, 16, 43]. Observed by transferring Foxp3$^-$ cells from reporter animals into lymphopenic mice and identified by the induced expression of FoxP3, these iTregs were demonstrated to be as suppressive as nTregs in an in vitro suppression assay [44]. In addition, antigen administration at low dose can lead to oral tolerance, a condition of systemic and/or local immunological tolerance, through the generation of iTregs that secrete both TGF-β and IL-10 [45].

Similarly, iTregs can also be induced ex vivo in the cell culture system when naïve T cells are stimulated through the TCR in the presence of different anti-inflammatory cytokines. For example, Th3 cells can be generated in vivo by exposure to oral antigen at low dose or in vitro by stimulating naïve T cells in the presence of TGF-β, along with other cytokines. Tr1 cells result when naïve T cells are stimulated in the presence of IL-10 either in vitro or in vivo. Th3 cells secrete abundant amounts of TGF-β and have been described to express Foxp3. Th3 cells can protect against colitis alone but also synergize with nTregs in an adoptive cell transfer model of colitis [46]. Tr1 cells, which secrete large amounts of IL-10 and some TGF-β but do not express Foxp3, also have been shown to prevent a similar model of colitis by adoptive cell transfer [47, 48]. Although Tr1 cells certainly can be generated in vitro from both human and murine naïve T cells [47], they can also be found in the GALT of normal mice [49] and have been detected in humans in the setting of transplantation, autoimmune diseases, and exposure to allergens (reviewed in ref. [50]). Recently Gagliani and colleagues identified the surface markers CD49b and lymphocyte activation gene 3 (LAG-3) as being co-expressed on mouse and human Tr1 cells [51]. The use of these markers makes it possible to track and purify Tr1 cells to explore there immune regulatory potential in cell based therapy.

Another Treg population, iTr35 cells, was identified that are generated in the setting of IL-35 stimulation [52]. Culture of either mouse or human CD4$^+$ T cells with IL-35 leads to iTR35 cells, which are potent secretors of IL-35. These cells are highly effective suppressors of T cell proliferation in vitro and autoimmune diseases in vivo [52], as shown in both experimental models of multiple sclerosis and colitis [52]. Unlike other regulatory T cells, iTR35 cells appear stable and retain suppressive properties in vivo after transfer into recipient mice [52].

A new population of iTreg co-expressing FoxP3 and Rorγ was recently described by several groups in both mice and human [53, 54]. They comprise 40–60 % of colonic Tregs in inbreed mouse strains raised in specific pathogen free conditions; the frequency are much lower in germ-free settings. Microbial colonization of intestinal mucosa induces generation of these CD4⁺Helios⁻FoxP3⁺Rorγ⁺ Tregs. They also found that these cells protect from colonic inflammation in TNBS-induced colitis model [53].

Plasticity of T Cells

T cell differentiation was once considered linear and irreversible, but recent findings indicate that this process is flexible and committed cells can acquire features of different effector cells upon adequate stimuli [55]. Tregs co-expressing Foxp3 and IL-17 have been described at mucosal sites and Tregs can be induced to express IFN-γ potentially leading to tissue damage by certain microbial infections (reviewed in refs. [56, 57]). In fact, cells that were previously Tregs have been demonstrated to lose their Foxp3 expression, gain a memory T cell phenotype, produce inflammatory cytokines, and lead to diabetes in an adaptive cell transfer model [58]. Moreover, IL17 producing Treg cells were also identified in inflamed intestinal mucosa of patients with Crohn's disease [59]. Similarly, trans-differentiation of Th17 cells into a regulatory Tr1 cells can occur during an immune response. Conversion of Th17 cells into Tr1 cells are promoted by activation of Ahr signaling in presence of TGF-β1 and contribute to the resolution of inflammation [60]. Previously it has been shown by the same group that anti-CD3 treatment leads to the generation of regulatory Th17 (rTh17) cell in the small intestine. rTh17 cells express high level of anti-inflammatory cytokine IL10 and suppressive capacity of these cells was dependent of the expression of IL10, TGF-β, and CTLA-4 [61]. Collectively, it can be concluded that both Treg and Th17 lymphocytes possess an intrinsic functional plasticity, which must be considered in attempts to target these cells therapeutically.

Less Conventional T Cell Subsets

In addition to $CD4^+$ T cells, other T lymphocyte subsets have potential effector or regulatory properties. In the lamina propria, $CD8^+$ cells possess regulatory function and have been noted to be decreased in IBD tissues compared to controls [62, 63]. Likewise, in the intraepithelial compartment, $TCR\alpha\alpha^+$ $CD8^+$ T cells have been shown to be protective in animal models of colitis using adoptive cell transfer [64, 65] whereas $TCR\gamma\delta^+$ cells appear to limit the extent of injury and promote tissue healing in a chemically induced model of colitis [66]. However, others have demonstrated a potential pathogenic role of $TCR\gamma\delta^+$ cells given absence of these cells in a transgenic colitis model leads to attenuated disease [67]. These findings may have implications for the pathogenesis of ulcerative colitis given higher frequency of these $TCR\gamma\delta^+$ cells has been noted in colonic tissue from UC patients [67]. Another less common subset of T cell is NK-T cells, which express surface markers and possess certain functional properties typical of both NK cells and T cells. In addition to expressing components of the T cell receptor complex, CD3, they express semi-invariant CD1d-restricted αβ TCRs recognizing glycolipid antigens. Some regard these cells as potentially pathogenic in inflammatory bowel disease. In fact, Fuss et al. demonstrated circumstantial evidence for NK-T cells being the source of high IL-13 levels noted in samples from patients with active UC, suggestive of a pathogenic role of these cells [4]. Likewise, in the oxazolone-induced murine model of ulcerative colitis, depletion of NK-T cells led to protection against disease [68]. However, in a chemically induced model of colitis (with dextran sodium sulfate), NK-T cells have been demonstrated to possess a regulatory function [69]. A recent murine study showed that microbial exposure during early life leads to the generation of mucosal invariant (i)-NKT cell tolerance. In absence of such tolerogenic commensal exposure in germ-free mice leads to CXCL16-mediated iNKT cell driven intestinal inflammation in oxazolone-induced colitis model [70]. Although these less conventional T cell subsets typically have reduced frequencies when compared with the more conventional $CD4^+$ T cells, their pathogenic/regulatory properties may contribute, at least in part, to overall mucosal homeostasis [70].

The Role of T Cells in Colitis

T cells have been long recognized to be central to the mucosal inflammatory process and thought early on to even be the instigator of disease given the marked expansion of activated $CD4^+$ T cells in the lamina propria of both inflamed mouse and human intestinal tissues [1, 2, 10]. $CD4^+$ T cells from intestinal samples isolated from Crohn's disease and ulcerative colitis patients were found to be resistant to apoptosis [71], which may be one mechanism for such seemingly inadequately controlled expansion of T cells. The ability to transfer colitis by adoptively transferring $CD4^+$ T cells from a colitic mouse to an immunodeficient host in many animal models also implicated the colitogenic potential of $CD4^+$ T cells [6–8]. Even transfer of $CD4^+$ T cells depleted of $CD25^+$ regulatory T cells from normal animals could lead to disease in a lymphocyte-deficient host [27], demonstrating the pro-inflammatory nature of effector T cells and its usual tight regulation by regulatory T cells during homeostasis.

Similar to that seen in a variety of murine models of IBD, $CD4^+$ T cells isolated from patients with Crohn's disease or ulcerative colitis express large quantities of pro-inflammatory cytokines [3, 5, 11, 72]. Interferon-(γ)gamma, tumor necrosis factor-(α)alpha and IL-2 have been demonstrated repeatedly to be elevated in Crohn's disease mucosa, whereas IL-5 and IL-13 have been associated with ulcerative colitis. Early studies demonstrating an abundance of Th1 type cytokines in Crohn's disease suggested IFN-γ^+ Th1 cells to be a major mediator of disease, while ulcerative colitis was suggested in some studies to be mediated primarily by excessive Th2 responses. Interestingly, despite an elevated level of IL-5 and IL-13 associated with ulcerative colitis, there is evidence of surprisingly reduced expression of IL4$^+$ Th2 cells [3, 4, 10]. More recent reports demonstrating increased population of IL-5 and IL-13 expressing atypical natural killer T (NKT) cells in ulcerative colitis provided one explanation for this apparent anomaly [4, 10]. More recent studies have shown that tissues from both Crohn's disease and ulcerative colitis patients have a massive infiltration of Th17 cells and Th17-related cytokines [10, 73, 74]. Apart from activating cellular targets like epithelium, endothelium, monocytes/macrophages, and neutrophils, IL-17 is known to induce proinflammatory cytokines (TNF-α, IL-1B, GM-CSF, G-CSF, IL-6), chemokines (CXCL8, CXCL9, CXCL10), and metalloproteases [74–76]. Interestingly, several signature cytokines involved in Th17 differentiation and expansion, including IL-23R, IL-12B, JAK2, STAT3, CCR6, and TNFSF15, have been identified as susceptibility genes of Crohn's disease and ulcerative colitis in genome-wide association studies [77–79].

On the basis of the observations that IFNγ, IL-17, IL-3 may play a key role in the pathogenesis of Crohn's disease and ulcerative colitis, both in mouse models and in humans, these cytokines have been considered as potential targets for the treatment of IBD. However the outcome in several studies has not been met with much success. Several groups have studied the effect of humanized antibody against IFN-γ, fontolizumab, in patients with Crohn's disease; however, the efficacy of anti-IFN-γ treatment remains unclear [80–82]. Blockade of IL-17 pathway was also not effective in Crohn's disease: secukinumab, a fully humanized anti-IL-17A monoclonal antibody, failed to control symptoms and was associated with severe adverse effects [83]. Finally, two anti-IL-13 monoclonal antibodies, tralokinumab [84] and anrunkinzumab [85], recently failed in phase II clinical trials in ulcerative colitis patients [86]. The failure of these agents, which target adaptive immune responses, has led to some rethinking of the central role of these cytokines in the pathogenesis of both Crohn's disease and ulcerative colitis.

Recent data has suggested that the initial aberrant signal may derive from defects in the innate immune system (such as an epithelial cell, macrophages, dendritic cells, NK cells, etc.). Polymorphisms in genes (e.g., NOD2, *ATG16L1*, and *IRGM*) that code for proteins important in recognizing and handling intracellular microbes, processes that occur in innate immune cells, have been recognized to be associated with Crohn's disease risk in genome-wide association studies [87]. Data from animal studies have also implicated professional antigen presenting cells or epithelial cells in playing a more direct role in colitis induction [37, 88, 89]. Nonetheless, T cells are still thought to be an important mediator of disease, contributing to either the initiation or perpetuation of disease [1]. In this latter context, once activated by soluble factors and/or by cell–cell contact, T cells are able to expand and secrete chemokines and cytokines that recruit and activate, respectively, other immune cell subsets to perpetuate an inflammatory signal.

In order to damage the gut, effector T cells need to adhere and migrate into intestinal mucosa, a process which depends on the recognition between adhesion receptors (CCR9 and α4β7) expressed on the T cell surface and their ligands (MAdCAM-1) on the gut vascular endothelial surface [90]. CCR9 and α4β7 are the two most well characterized gut-homing receptors on T cells, and blocking the interaction between these receptors and their ligands on endothelial cells prevents T cells from entering the gut. This serves as the basis for the development of biologic therapies for Crohn's disease such as natalizumab, which is a monoclonal antibody against the integrin α4, and vedolizumab, a monoclonal antibody against α4β7. Both agents interfere with T cell homing to the gut and consequently decrease inflammatory activities leading to clinical efficacy in both Crohn's disease and ulcerative colitis [91–94]. Additional anti-adhesion molecule strategies including the anti-β7 antibody etrolizumab [95] and anti-MAdCAM-1 antibody targeting the α4β7 ligand [96] are currently being tested in IBD [97]. Moreover, a CCR9 chemokine receptor small-molecule antagonist targeting the CCR9-CCL25 interaction has recently failed in a large [96–98]. Other agents blocking such signals crucial to T cell gut homing are also under development.

One may also hypothesize that T cell suppression is diminished in IBD either from a qualitative or quantitative defect in Treg function. However, a defect in Treg numbers appears not to be a principal cause of IBD, since their proportions are noted to be increased in inflamed IBD tissue when compared to non-inflamed samples from IBD patients or samples from healthy control patients [99]. In fact, during periods of active disease, fewer Tregs are seen in the peripheral blood and more are found in the mucosa, suggesting an increase (through homing) or retention of Treg to sites of inflammation. Moreover, peripheral blood, mesenteric lymph node, and mucosal Tregs when removed from IBD patients retain in vitro suppressive function [99–101]. Thus, Tregs from IBD patients have the capacity for functional activity. However, the increase in Treg proportions in inflamed mucosa from IBD patients appear to be quantitatively less than that seen in non-IBD inflammatory control samples (those with diverticulitis), suggesting the increase in Treg numbers seen in IBD is not as robust as seen in other inflammatory disorders. Nonetheless, despite the presence of regulatory T cells in IBD associated mucosa these cells are not sufficient in situ to control inflammation.

Regulatory T Cells as Potential Therapy for IBD

Given the potent suppressive properties of regulatory T cells, one potential therapeutic option for IBD is quantitative enhancement of Treg numbers and/or functional capacity [21]. One theoretical approach is to isolate Tregs from a patient's peripheral blood, followed by augmentation of cell function/numbers in vitro, and subsequent infusion of these cells into the patient. However, this idea has been hindered by difficulty in Treg expansion given their tendency for hypoproliferation, poorly defined surface markers, and uncertain stability and longevity in vivo. One potential way of overcoming these difficulties is to generate and expand inducible Tregs in vitro from naïve T cells, such as iTr35 cells, Tr1 cells, or regulatory $CD8^+$ cells [47, 52, 63]. Even then, it is difficult to purify some of these populations due to the lack of specific cell surface markers. In addition, this technique will still require peripheral blood cell isolation; immediate processing or cryopreservation; in vitro culture and stimulation; vigorous testing for function, purity, and viability; and reinfusion of newly induced Tregs, posing technical challenges to avoid infection and maintain quality control. Recently Canavan and colleague have shown that Tregs can be expanded from the blood of patients with Crohn's disease. They demonstrated that the expanded cells were epigenetically stable and home to human small bowel in a C.B-17 severe combined immune deficiency (SCID) xenotransplant model [102]. In a phase 1/2a study 40 % of the patients showed a clinical response after a single injection of ovalbumin-specific Treg cells in 20 Crohn's disease patients [97, 103]. In this study autologous Treg cells were expanded in vitro, cloned by limiting dilution, and selected for IL-10 production in response to ovalbumin before transfer [15, 103]. An alternative option is to pharmacologically expand the already existing pool of Tregs or induction of an iTreg population. The latter could be done with an agent such as oral anti-CD3 antibody, which has been shown to expand a particular type of Tregs and has been shown to suppress EAE, SLE, and diabetes in mice [104, 105]. In another study Koreth et al. showed that daily administration of low-dose interleukin-2 in patients with active chronic GVHD that was refractory to glucocorticoid therapy was associated with preferential sustained Treg cell expansion in vivo and amelioration of the manifestations of chronic GVHD in a substantial proportion of patients [106]. Phase 1 studies investigating the role of oral OKT3 (anti-CD3) and low-dose IL2 have been initiated for ulcerative colitis (ClinicalTrials.gov: NCT02200445; ClinicalTrials.gov: NCT01287195). Taken together therapies targeting the immunomodulatory potential of Treg cells seem to be a promising approach for treatments of IBD.

Summary

T cells have been clearly implicated as a mediator and propagator of disease in many animal models of IBD. In patient samples, T cells secrete an abundance of pro-inflammatory cytokines suggesting a central role of T cells in the pathogenesis of disease. Despite the large body of knowledge regarding the role of T cells in mucosal homeostasis, much still remains to be understood with regard to how these T cell subsets interact with each other and with other immune cell subsets to lead to IBD and how these interactions can be repaired to restore intestinal homeostasis.

References

1. Maynard CL, Weaver CT. Intestinal effector T cells in health and disease. Immunity. 2009;31:389–400.
2. Elson CO, Cong Y, McCracken VJ, Dimmitt RA, Lorenz RG, Weaver CT. Experimental models of inflammatory bowel disease reveal innate, adaptive, and regulatory mechanisms of host dialogue with the microbiota. Immunol Rev. 2005;206:260–76.
3. Fuss IJ et al. Disparate CD4+ lamina propria (LP) lymphokine secretion profiles in inflammatory bowel disease. Crohn's disease LP cells manifest increased secretion of IFN-gamma, whereas ulcerative colitis LP cells manifest increased secretion of IL-5. J Immunol. 1996;157:1261–70.
4. Fuss IJ et al. Nonclassical CD1d-restricted NK T cells that produce IL-13 characterize an atypical Th2 response in ulcerative colitis. J Clin Invest. 2004;113:1490–7. doi:10.1172/JCI19836.
5. MacDonald TT, Hutchings P, Choy MY, Murch S, Cooke A. Tumour necrosis factor-alpha and interferon-gamma production measured at the single cell level in normal and inflamed human intestine. Clin Exp Immunol. 1990;81:301–5.
6. Asseman C, Read S, Powrie F. Colitogenic Th1 cells are present in the antigen-experienced T cell pool in normal mice: control by CD4+ regulatory T cells and IL-10. J Immunol. 2003;171: 971–8.
7. Wirtz S et al. Cutting edge: chronic intestinal inflammation in STAT-4 transgenic mice: characterization of disease and adoptive transfer by TNF- plus IFN-gamma-producing CD4+ T cells that respond to bacterial antigens. J Immunol. 1999;162:1884–8.
8. Nguyen DD et al. Lymphocyte-dependent and Th2 cytokine-associated colitis in mice deficient in Wiskott-Aldrich syndrome protein. Gastroenterology. 2007;133:1188–97. doi:S0016-5085(07)01311-X [pii].
9. Khader SA, Gaffen SL, Kolls JK. Th17 cells at the crossroads of innate and adaptive immunity against infectious diseases at the mucosa. Mucosal Immunol. 2009;2:403–11.
10. Shale M, Schiering C, Powrie F. CD4(+) T-cell subsets in intestinal inflammation. Immunol Rev. 2013;252:164–82. doi:10.1111/imr.12039.
11. Fujino S et al. Increased expression of interleukin 17 in inflammatory bowel disease. Gut. 2003;52:65–70.
12. Gerlach K et al. TH9 cells that express the transcription factor PU.1 drive T cell-mediated colitis via IL-9 receptor signaling in intestinal epithelial cells. Nat Immunol. 2014;15:676–86. doi:10.1038/ni.2920.
13. Nalleweg N et al. IL-9 and its receptor are predominantly involved in the pathogenesis of UC. Gut. 2015;64:743–55. doi:10.1136/gutjnl-2013-305947.

14. Kaplan MH, Hufford MM, Olson MR. The development and in vivo function of T helper 9 cells. Nat Rev Immunol. 2015;15:295–307. doi:10.1038/nri3824.
15. Mayne CG, Williams CB. Induced and natural regulatory T cells in the development of inflammatory bowel disease. Inflamm Bowel Dis. 2013;19:1772–88. doi:10.1097/MIB.0b013e318281f5a3.
16. Harrison OJ, Powrie FM. Regulatory T cells and immune tolerance in the intestine. Cold Spring Harb Perspect Biol. 2013;5. doi:10.1101/cshperspect.a018341.
17. Bennett CL et al. The immune dysregulation, polyendocrinopathy, enteropathy, X-linked syndrome (IPEX) is caused by mutations of FOXP3. Nat Genet. 2001;27:20–1. doi:10.1038/83713.
18. Wildin RS et al. X-linked neonatal diabetes mellitus, enteropathy and endocrinopathy syndrome is the human equivalent of mouse scurfy. Nat Genet. 2001;27:18–20. doi:10.1038/83707.
19. Wildin RS, Smyk-Pearson S, Filipovich AH. Clinical and molecular features of the immunodysregulation, polyendocrinopathy, enteropathy, X linked (IPEX) syndrome. J Med Genet. 2002;39:537–45.
20. Maillard MH et al. The Wiskott-Aldrich syndrome protein is required for the function of CD4(+)CD25(+)Foxp3(+) regulatory T cells. J Exp Med. 2007;204:381–91. doi:10.1084/jem.20061338.
21. Boden EK, Snapper SB. Regulatory T cells in inflammatory bowel disease. Curr Opin Gastroenterol. 2008;24:733–41.
22. Gavin MA et al. Single-cell analysis of normal and FOXP3-mutant human T cells: FOXP3 expression without regulatory T cell development. Proc Natl Acad Sci U S A. 2006;103:6659–64.
23. Takahashi T et al. Immunologic self-tolerance maintained by CD25(+)CD4(+) regulatory T cells constitutively expressing cytotoxic T lymphocyte-associated antigen 4. J Exp Med. 2000;192:303–10.
24. Shimizu J, Yamazaki S, Takahashi T, Ishida Y, Sakaguchi S. Stimulation of CD25(+)CD4(+) regulatory T cells through GITR breaks immunological self-tolerance. Nat Immunol. 2002;3:135–42.
25. Liu W et al. CD127 expression inversely correlates with FoxP3 and suppressive function of human CD4+ T reg cells. J Exp Med. 2006;203:1701–11. doi:10.1084/jem.20060772.
26. Seddiki N et al. Expression of interleukin (IL)-2 and IL-7 receptors discriminates between human regulatory and activated T cells. J Exp Med. 2006;203:1693–700. doi:10.1084/jem.20060468.
27. Powrie F, Leach MW, Mauze S, Caddle LB, Coffman RL. Phenotypically distinct subsets of CD4+ T cells induce or protect from chronic intestinal inflammation in C. B-17 scid mice. Int Immunol. 1993;5:1461–71.
28. Mottet C, Uhlig HH, Powrie F. Cutting edge: cure of colitis by CD4+CD25+ regulatory T cells. J Immunol. 2003;170:3939–43.
29. Tang Q et al. In vitro-expanded antigen-specific regulatory T cells suppress autoimmune diabetes. J Exp Med. 2004;199:1455–65.
30. Kohm AP, Carpentier PA, Anger HA, Miller SD. Cutting edge: CD4+CD25+ regulatory T cells suppress antigen-specific autoreactive immune responses and central nervous system inflammation during active experimental autoimmune encephalomyelitis. J Immunol. 2002;169:4712–6.
31. Scalapino KJ, Tang Q, Bluestone JA, Bonyhadi ML, Daikh DI. Suppression of disease in New Zealand Black/New Zealand White lupus-prone mice by adoptive transfer of ex vivo expanded regulatory T cells. J Immunol. 2006;177:1451–9.
32. Asano M, Toda M, Sakaguchi N, Sakaguchi S. Autoimmune disease as a consequence of developmental abnormality of a T cell subpopulation. J Exp Med. 1996;184:387–96.
33. Thornton AM, Shevach EM. Suppressor effector function of CD4+CD25+ immunoregulatory T cells is antigen nonspecific. J Immunol. 2000;164:183–90.
34. Collison LW et al. The inhibitory cytokine IL-35 contributes to regulatory T-cell function. Nature. 2007;450:566–9.
35. Li MO, Wan YY, Flavell RA. T cell-produced transforming growth factor-beta1 controls T cell tolerance and regulates Th1- and Th17-cell differentiation. Immunity. 2007;26:579–91.
36. Asseman C, Mauze S, Leach MW, Coffman RL, Powrie F. An essential role for interleukin 10 in the function of regulatory T cells that inhibit intestinal inflammation. J Exp Med. 1999;190:995–1004.
37. Murai M et al. Interleukin 10 acts on regulatory T cells to maintain expression of the transcription factor Foxp3 and suppressive function in mice with colitis. Nat Immunol. 2009;10:1178–84.
38. Rubtsov YP et al. Regulatory T cell-derived interleukin-10 limits inflammation at environmental interfaces. Immunity. 2008;28:546–58. doi:10.1016/j.immuni.2008.02.017.
39. Liu JQ et al. Increased Th17 and regulatory T cell responses in EBV-induced gene 3-deficient mice lead to marginally enhanced development of autoimmune encephalomyelitis. J Immunol. 2012;188:3099–106. doi:10.4049/jimmunol.1100106.
40. Borsellino G et al. Expression of ectonucleotidase CD39 by Foxp3+ Treg cells: hydrolysis of extracellular ATP and immune suppression. Blood. 2007;110:1225–32. doi:10.1182/blood-2006-12-064527.
41. Deaglio S et al. Adenosine generation catalyzed by CD39 and CD73 expressed on regulatory T cells mediates immune suppression. J Exp Med. 2007;204:1257–65. doi:10.1084/jem.20062512.
42. Bettini M, Vignali DA. Regulatory T cells and inhibitory cytokines in autoimmunity. Curr Opin Immunol. 2009;21:612–8.
43. Bilate AB, Lafaille JJ. It takes two to tango. Immunity. 2011;35:6–8. doi:10.1016/j.immuni.2011.07.003.
44. Haribhai D et al. A central role for induced regulatory T cells in tolerance induction in experimental colitis. J Immunol. 2009;182:3461–8.
45. Chen Y et al. Oral tolerance in myelin basic protein T-cell receptor transgenic mice: suppression of autoimmune encephalomyelitis and dose-dependent induction of regulatory cells. Proc Natl Acad Sci U S A. 1996;93:388–91.
46. Fantini MC et al. Transforming growth factor beta induced FoxP3+ regulatory T cells suppress Th1 mediated experimental colitis. Gut. 2006;55:671–80.
47. Groux H et al. A CD4+ T-cell subset inhibits antigen-specific T-cell responses and prevents colitis. Nature. 1997;389:737–42.
48. Faria AM, Weiner HL. Oral tolerance. Immunol Rev. 2005;206:232–59.
49. Kamanaka M et al. Expression of interleukin-10 in intestinal lymphocytes detected by an interleukin-10 reporter knockin tiger mouse. Immunity. 2006;25:941–52. doi:10.1016/j.immuni.2006.09.013.
50. Battaglia M, Gregori S, Bacchetta R, Roncarolo MG. Tr1 cells: from discovery to their clinical application. Semin Immunol. 2006;18:120–7.
51. Gagliani N et al. Coexpression of CD49b and LAG-3 identifies human and mouse T regulatory type 1 cells. Nat Med. 2013;19:739–46. doi:10.1038/nm.3179.
52. Collison LW et al. IL-35-mediated induction of a potent regulatory T cell population. Nat Immunol. 2010;11:1093–101.
53. Sefik E et al. Individual intestinal symbionts induce a distinct population of RORgamma+regulatory T cells. Science. 2015;349:993–7. doi:10.1126/science.aaa9420.
54. Ohnmacht C et al. The microbiota regulates type 2 immunity through RORgammat+T cells. Science. 2015;349:989–93. doi:10.1126/science.aac4263.
55. Cosmi L, Maggi L, Santarlasci V, Liotta F, Annunziato F. T helper cells plasticity in inflammation. Cytometry A. 2014;85:36–42. doi:10.1002/cyto.a.22348.

56. Wohlfert E, Belkaid Y. Plasticity of Treg at infected sites. Mucosal Immunol. 2010;3:213–5.
57. Lee YK, Mukasa R, Hatton RD, Weaver CT. Developmental plasticity of Th17 and Treg cells. Curr Opin Immunol. 2009;21:274–80.
58. Zhou X et al. Instability of the transcription factor Foxp3 leads to the generation of pathogenic memory T cells in vivo. Nat Immunol. 2009;10:1000–7. doi:10.1038/ni.1774.
59. Hovhannisyan Z, Treatman J, Littman DR, Mayer L. Characterization of interleukin-17-producing regulatory T cells in inflamed intestinal mucosa from patients with inflammatory bowel diseases. Gastroenterology. 2011;140:957–65. doi:10.1053/j.gastro.2010.12.002.
60. Gagliani N et al. Th17 cells transdifferentiate into regulatory T cells during resolution of inflammation. Nature. 2015;523:221–5. doi:10.1038/nature14452.
61. Esplugues E et al. Control of TH17 cells occurs in the small intestine. Nature. 2011;475:514–8. doi:10.1038/nature10228.
62. Brimnes J et al. Defects in CD8+ regulatory T cells in the lamina propria of patients with inflammatory bowel disease. J Immunol. 2005;174:5814–22.
63. Allez M, Brimnes J, Dotan I, Mayer L. Expansion of CD8+ T cells with regulatory function after interaction with intestinal epithelial cells. Gastroenterology. 2002;123:1516–26.
64. Poussier P, Ning T, Banerjee D, Julius M. A unique subset of self-specific intraintestinal T cells maintains gut integrity. J Exp Med. 2002;195:1491–7.
65. Das G et al. An important regulatory role for CD4+CD8 alpha alpha T cells in the intestinal epithelial layer in the prevention of inflammatory bowel disease. Proc Natl Acad Sci U S A. 2003;100:5324–9.
66. Chen Y, Chou K, Fuchs E, Havran WL, Boismenu R. Protection of the intestinal mucosa by intraepithelial gamma delta T cells. Proc Natl Acad Sci U S A. 2002;99:14338–43.
67. Nanno M et al. Exacerbating role of gammadelta T cells in chronic colitis of T-cell receptor alpha mutant mice. Gastroenterology. 2008;134:481–90.
68. Heller F, Fuss IJ, Nieuwenhuis EE, Blumberg RS, Strober W. Oxazolone colitis, a Th2 colitis model resembling ulcerative colitis, is mediated by IL-13-producing NK-T cells. Immunity. 2002;17:629–38.
69. Saubermann LJ et al. Activation of natural killer T cells by alpha-galactosylceramide in the presence of CD1d provides protection against colitis in mice. Gastroenterology. 2000;119:119–28.
70. Olszak T et al. Microbial exposure during early life has persistent effects on natural killer T cell function. Science (New York, NY). 2012;336(6080):489–93. doi:10.1126/science.1219328.
71. Matsuura T, West GA, Youngman KR, Klein JS, Fiocchi C. Immune activation genes in inflammatory bowel disease. Gastroenterology. 1993;104:448–58.
72. Boirivant M et al. Lamina propria T cells in Crohn's disease and other gastrointestinal inflammation show defective CD2 pathway-induced apoptosis. Gastroenterology. 1999;116:557–65.
73. Galvez J. Role of Th17 cells in the pathogenesis of human IBD. ISRN Inflamm. 2014;2014:928461. doi:10.1155/2014/928461.
74. Wallace KL, Zheng LB, Kanazawa Y, Shih DQ. Immunopathology of inflammatory bowel disease. World J Gastroenterol. 2014;20:6–21. doi:10.3748/wjg.v20.i1.6.
75. Awane M, Andres PG, Li DJ, Reinecker HC. NF-kappa B-inducing kinase is a common mediator of IL-17-, TNF-alpha-, and IL-1 beta-induced chemokine promoter activation in intestinal epithelial cells. J Immunol. 1999;162:5337–44.
76. Witowski J et al. IL-17 stimulates intraperitoneal neutrophil infiltration through the release of GRO alpha chemokine from mesothelial cells. J Immunol. 2000;165:5814–21.
77. Franke A et al. Genome-wide meta-analysis increases to 71 the number of confirmed Crohn's disease susceptibility loci. Nat Genet. 2010;42:1118–25. doi:10.1038/ng.717.
78. Franke A et al. Genome-wide association study for ulcerative colitis identifies risk loci at 7q22 and 22q13 (IL17REL). Nat Genet. 2010;42:292–4. doi:10.1038/ng.553.
79. McGovern DP et al. Genome-wide association identifies multiple ulcerative colitis susceptibility loci. Nat Genet. 2010;42:332–7. doi:10.1038/ng.549.
80. Cui D, Huang G, Yang D, Huang B, An B. Efficacy and safety of interferon-gamma-targeted therapy in Crohn's disease: a systematic review and meta-analysis of randomized controlled trials. Clin Res Hepatol Gastroenterol. 2013;37:507–13. doi:10.1016/j.clinre.2012.12.004.
81. Reinisch W et al. Fontolizumab in moderate to severe Crohn's disease: a phase 2, randomized, double-blind, placebo-controlled, multiple-dose study. Inflamm Bowel Dis. 2010;16:233–42. doi:10.1002/ibd.21038.
82. Reinisch W et al. A dose escalating, placebo controlled, double blind, single dose and multidose, safety and tolerability study of fontolizumab, a humanised anti-interferon gamma antibody, in patients with moderate to severe Crohn's disease. Gut. 2006;55:1138–44. doi:10.1136/gut.2005.079434.
83. Hueber W et al. Secukinumab, a human anti-IL-17A monoclonal antibody, for moderate to severe Crohn's disease: unexpected results of a randomised, double-blind placebo-controlled trial. Gut. 2012;61:1693–700. doi:10.1136/gutjnl-2011-301668.
84. Danese S et al. Tralokinumab for moderate-to-severe UC: a randomised, double-blind, placebo-controlled, phase IIa study. Gut. 2015;64:243–9. doi:10.1136/gutjnl-2014-308004.
85. Reinisch W et al. Anrukinzumab, an anti-interleukin 13 monoclonal antibody, in active UC: efficacy and safety from a phase IIa randomised multicentre study. Gut. 2015;64:894–900. doi:10.1136/gutjnl-2014-308337.
86. Amiot A, Peyrin-Biroulet L. Current, new and future biological agents on the horizon for the treatment of inflammatory bowel diseases. Therap Adv Gastroenterol. 2015;8:66–82. doi:10.1177/1756283X14558193.
87. Abraham C, Cho JH. Inflammatory bowel disease. N Engl J Med. 2009;361:2066–78.
88. Abe K et al. Conventional dendritic cells regulate the outcome of colonic inflammation independently of T cells. Proc Natl Acad Sci U S A. 2007;104:17022–7. doi:0708469104 [pii].
89. Shouval DS et al. Interleukin-10 receptor signaling in innate immune cells regulates mucosal immune tolerance and anti-inflammatory macrophage function. Immunity. 2014;40:706–19. doi:10.1016/j.immuni.2014.03.011.
90. Podolsky DK. Selective adhesion-molecule therapy and inflammatory bowel disease—a tale of Janus? N Engl J Med. 2005;353:1965–8. doi:10.1056/NEJMe058212.
91. Feagan BG et al. Treatment of active Crohn's disease with MLN0002, a humanized antibody to the alpha4beta7 integrin. Clin Gastroenterol Hepatol. 2008;6:1370–7.
92. Sandborn WJ et al. Natalizumab induction and maintenance therapy for Crohn's disease. N Engl J Med. 2005;353:1912–25. doi:10.1056/NEJMoa043335.
93. Feagan BG et al. Treatment of ulcerative colitis with a humanized antibody to the alpha4beta7 integrin. N Engl J Med. 2005;352:2499–507.
94. Sandborn WJ et al. Vedolizumab as induction and maintenance therapy for Crohn's disease. N Engl J Med. 2013;369:711–21. doi:10.1056/NEJMoa1215739.
95. Rutgeerts PJ et al. A randomised phase I study of etrolizumab (rhuMAb beta7) in moderate to severe ulcerative colitis. Gut. 2013;62:1122–30. doi:10.1136/gutjnl-2011-301769.

96. Thomas S, Baumgart DC. Targeting leukocyte migration and adhesion in Crohn's disease and ulcerative colitis. Inflammopharmacology. 2012;20:1–18. doi:10.1007/s10787-011-0104-6.
97. Neurath MF. New targets for mucosal healing and therapy in inflammatory bowel diseases. Mucosal Immunol. 2014;7:6–19. doi:10.1038/mi.2013.73.
98. Papadakis KA et al. CC chemokine receptor 9 expression defines a subset of peripheral blood lymphocytes with mucosal T cell phenotype and Th1 or T-regulatory 1 cytokine profile. J Immunol. 2003;171:159–65.
99. Maul J et al. Peripheral and intestinal regulatory CD4+ CD25(high) T cells in inflammatory bowel disease. Gastroenterology. 2005;128:1868–78.
100. Yu QT et al. Expression and functional characterization of FOXP3+ CD4+ regulatory T cells in ulcerative colitis. Inflamm Bowel Dis. 2007;13:191–9.
101. Kelsen J et al. FoxP3(+)CD4(+)CD25(+) T cells with regulatory properties can be cultured from colonic mucosa of patients with Crohn's disease. Clin Exp Immunol. 2005;141:549–57.
102. Canavan JB et al. Developing in vitro expanded CD45RA+ regulatory T cells as an adoptive cell therapy for Crohn's disease. Gut. 2015;65:584–94. doi:10.1136/gutjnl-2014-306919.
103. Desreumaux P et al. Safety and efficacy of antigen-specific regulatory T-cell therapy for patients with refractory Crohn's disease. Gastroenterology. 2012;143:1207–17. doi:10.1053/j.gastro.2012.07.116. e1201–2.
104. Ochi H et al. Oral CD3-specific antibody suppresses autoimmune encephalomyelitis by inducing CD4+ CD25− LAP+ T cells. Nat Med. 2006;12:627–35.
105. Ishikawa H et al. Inhibition of autoimmune diabetes by oral administration of anti-CD3 monoclonal antibody. Diabetes. 2007;56:2103–9.
106. Koreth J et al. Interleukin-2 and regulatory T cells in graft-versus-host disease. N Engl J Med. 2011;365:2055–66. doi:10.1056/NEJMoa1108188.

Immunobiology of B Cells in Inflammatory Bowel Disease

9

Atsushi Mizoguchi and Atul K. Bhan

As B cells predominate at inflamed mucosal sites and possess multiple functions including the ability to recognize microbial TLR ligands, they are likely to play a role in the pathogenesis of inflammatory bowel disease (IBD) [1–3]. In this chapter, the impact of B cells on IBD pathogenesis is discussed in relation to the recently accumulating knowledge of B cell functions: antibody production, antigen presentation and interaction with T cells, and cytokine production (Fig. 9.1). Since most of the information regarding the immunopathogenesis of IBD in the last two decades has been obtained by the use of experimental models, the emphasis is on IBD models [4–6] rather than on human studies.

Antibody Production

B cells in the intestine are primarily located in the lymphoid follicles and as plasma cells in the lamina propria [7]. The activation of mucosal B cells occurs in the lymphoid follicles and mesenteric lymph nodes (MLN) with subsequent migration and differentiation to predominantly IgA secreting plasma cells in the lamina propria. The circulating B cells with activated phenotype (TLR2$^+$) that are capable of migrating to mucosal sites may either represent activated mucosal B cells or B cells activated in circulation, perhaps by translocated enteric bacteria/bacterial antigens [8]. The histological evidence of prominent lymphoid follicles and lymphoplasmacytic infiltrate in the inflamed intestine suggests involvement of B cells in IBD, in particular ulcerative colitis (UC). Recent studies suggest that plasma may play a pathogenic role in addition to their known function of producing antibodies. Plasma cells characterized by CD19$^+$ CD20$^-$CD27^{low} CXCR4^{high} unique immature phenotype are increased in the inflamed mucosa of UC patients, and they are capable of activating pathogenic CD14$^+$ macrophages via IgG-IC-FcγR signaling [9]. Furthermore, CD27$^+$ CD38^{high} CD20$^-$ IgA$^+$ plasma cells, which expand in the inflamed mucosa of both UC and CD patients, could provide cytotoxicity to epithelial cells by producing granzyme B in response to IL-21 [10]. IgM$^+$ CD19$^+$ CD138$^+$ plasma cells are capable of producing IL-10 [11].

The frequent presence of several types of circulating antibodies reactive with both microbial antigens and self-antigens in IBD supports the notion that dysregulated immune response to normal enteric microorganisms represents the primary pathogenic event in IBD. The antibodies include anti-Saccharomyces cerevisiae antibodies (ASCA), anti-neutrophilic cytoplasmic antibodies (ANCA), and antibodies to outer membrane porin (OMP), Pseudomonas fluorescence-related sequence I2, and Cbir (see below), and anti-carbohydrate antibodies (ALCA, ACCA, AMCA) [12, 13]. However, most of the studies performed with circulating antibodies have focused on their diagnostic or prognostic utility rather than their role in IBD pathogenesis [12–15]. ASCA are detected frequently in CD, whereas seropositivity for ANCA predominates in UC.

The normal IgA dominant immune response at the mucosal sites is skewed towards IgG in chronically inflamed mucosa of IBD [16]. The isolated cells from the inflamed mucosa have been shown to secrete antibodies to bacteria to *Escherichia coli* strains [16, 17] as well as antibodies against colonic epithelial antigens [18]. Antibodies to *Escherichia coli* are more often detected in CD, whereas anti-colonic epithelial antibodies are particularly seen in UC. The colonic epithelial antigens that are reactive with antibodies include tropomyosin (40 kDa) isoforms (TM1 and TM5) and 200 kDa colon epithelial protein [19]. Studies performed in Per Brandtzaeg's laboratory have provided evidence for a pathogenic role of antibodies in UC by showing complement

A. Mizoguchi, M.D., Ph.D.
Department of Immunology, Kurume University School of Medicine, Fukuoka, Japan

A.K. Bhan, M.B.B.S., M.D. (✉)
Department of Pathology, Massachusetts General Hospital, Harvard Medical School, 55 Fruit Street, Warren 501A, Boston, MA 02114-2698, USA
e-mail: abhan@mgh.harvard.edu

D.C. Baumgart (ed.), *Crohn's Disease and Ulcerative Colitis*, DOI 10.1007/978-3-319-33703-6_9

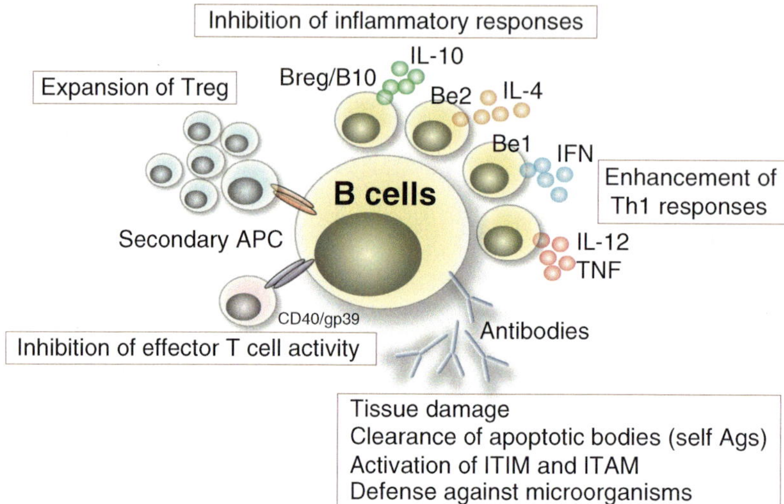

Fig. 9.1 Functional diversity of B cells in IBD: Immunoglobulins (Igs) produced by B cells may have both deleterious and protective roles in IBD. Binding of autoantibodies to colonic tissues or IgG Fc fragment-mediated ITAM-dependent activation of immune responses could result in tissue damage. Antibodies could provide protection by altering the diversity of enteric microorganisms that are required for the development of IBD and by helping the clearance of apoptotic bodies that may serve as a source of self-antigens for eliciting autoimmune responses. Furthermore, IgG may suppress immune response through the ITIM by binding to inhibitory FcγRIIb receptors expressed on immune cells. B-cell subsets could modulate inflammatory responses depending on their distinct cytokine production profiles. IL-10-producing B cells ("Breg") inhibit chronic colitis progression. B-cell subsets producing IL-12p70 or IFN-γ may have a pathogenic effect in CD, but a beneficial role in UC. B cells may also regulate immune responses by serving as a second line of APCs, by enhancing expansion of $CD4^+$ $Foxp3^+$ Tregs, and by inhibiting proliferation of effector $CD4^+$ T cells in a contact-dependent manner

activation in relation to IgG1 deposited at the apical aspect of the colonic epithelium [16, 20]. It is not clear whether above findings represent primary pathogenic events or a secondary phenomenon due to local immune response in the setting of chronic inflammation and tissue injury. In any case, the locally produced antibodies help maintain epithelial barrier, and may play a role in regulating enteric flora repertoire and excluding invading microorganisms. Decreased J-chain production with resultant reduced secretion of dimeric IgA has been reported in IBD [16, 21]. However, IgG antibodies, because of their phagocytotic enhancing properties, are likely to be more efficient than IgA in removing invading microorganisms and antigens, and could compensate for abnormality of the IgA response in IBD [16]. They could be also involved in the pathogenesis of IBD (see discussion of IgG Fcγ receptors below) [22].

Circulating autoantibodies and antimicrobial antibodies have also been reported in experimental models of IBD [5, 23–25]. The IL-4-mediated spontaneous çolitis in T-cell receptor α knockout (TCRαKO) mice resembles ulcerative colitis, and is associated with expansion of MLN B cells, increased production of antibodies (ANCA, anti-nuclear, and anti-tropomyosin), and alteration of polyclonal to an oligoclonal immune response to cecal bacterial antigens [23, 24]. This raised the possibility that B cells or antibodies may be pathogenic in this model. However, B cell-deficient mice TCRαKO mice developed more severe colitis (see below) [26]. Transfer of autoantibodies or purified immunoglobulin from TCRαKO mice to B- cell-deficient TCRαKO led to attenuation of colitis and decrease in the apoptotic cells, supporting the notion that autoantibodies may have a role in clearance of self-antigens released from apoptotic cells [26]. In addition, B-1 B cells, which represent a major source of natural IgM antibodies that provide first line of defense against microorganisms, are fully activated in conventional facility as compared to specific pathogen-free facility, resulting in the inhibition of colitis in TCRαKO mice [27]. These results support a role of B cells in the "hygiene hypothesis", which is based on the observation that repeated childhood infections lead to decreased incidence of allergic diseases in adulthood [27].

The spontaneous colitis in C3H/HeJBir mice is associated with both B and T cells responses to selective enteric bacterial antigens; the colitis can be transferred with T cells. Unlike TCRαKO mice, the oligoclonal response to enteric bacteria is detected even in young C3H/HeJBir mice [25]. Serologic expression cloning of cecal bacterial antigens in C3H/HeJBir mice led to the identification of previously unknown microbial flagellins [28]. The flagellin, CBir1, was found to be the dominant antigen capable of inducing T-cell-mediated colitis. Interestingly, sera from about 50 % of patients with Crohn's disease are reactive with CBir1; the CBir1 sera reactivity identified a subset of patients with complicated CD [29].

It is well established that humoral immunity can be regulated by Fc fragments of IgG [22]. Although most receptors of IgG, FcγRs are activating receptors due to the presence of the immunoreceptor tyrosine-based activation motif (ITAM), FcγRIIB is the only FcγR that has been shown to have inhibitory functions through immunoreceptor tyrosine-based inhibitory motif (ITIM), which includes suppression of B cells, macrophages, dendritic cells, mast cells and basophils [22]. FcγRIIB is involved in the pathogenesis of autoimmune disease, in particular lupus erythematosus. Recent studies indicate that intravenous immunoglobulin (IVIG) in autoimmune diseases and infliximab [anti-TNFα antibodies] in rheumatoid arthritis may partly act through FcγRIIB [30, 31]. Since FcγRIIB also effects antimicrobial immune responses [22], it is likely that this receptor may play an important role in the pathogenesis of IBD. FcγRIIB KO mice exhibit less distal colon inflammation during *Citrobacter rodentium* infection, probably due to increased phagocytic function of macrophages as compared to wild type mice [32]. Granulomatous inflammation developing in B cell and IL-4 deficient TCRα triple knockout mice can be suppressed by the administration of Fc fragments of IgG [33]. The importance on Fc-mediated pathway in IBD is highlighted by recent genome-wide association studies identifying FcγRIIA an UC-associated gene [34].

Antigen Presentation and Interaction with T Cells

It has become increasingly clear that B cells have functional capabilities that are not directly related to secreted immunoglobulins. B cells have been shown to serve as *a* "second line" of antigen presenting cells (secondary APCs) by conditioning the activity of effector memory T cells that have already been primed by professional antigen presenting cells such as dendritic cells [35, 36]. Indeed, B cells can suppress proliferation of effector CD4$^+$ T cells in a contact dependent manner through the interaction of CD40 on B cells and gp39 on effector T cells [37, 38]; this interaction contributes to the suppression of colitis in TCRαKO mice [37]. This observation is supported by a study showing that forced ectopic overexpression of gp39 on B cells, leading to the impairment of interaction of CD40 (B cells) and gp39 (T cells), induces the development of colitis [39]. In Gαi2 knockout mice, B cells facilitate expansion of CD4$^+$CD8α$^+$ intraepithelial T cells and CD3$^+$ CD4$^-$ NKT cells with consequent suppression of colitis [40]. MHC class I-mediated antigen presentation is required for this B-cell-mediated induction of regulatory CD8$^+$ T cell subset capable of controlling colitis through the production of perforin [41].

Since autophagy is a cellular degradation system, which is used not only for the elimination of intracellular bacteria but is also involved in adaptive immune responses as well as MHC-dependent antigen presentation [42], it is likely that autophagy plays an important role in secondary APC function of B cells. Autophagy is also required for B cell development [43], and for B cells to induce tolerance of CD4$^+$ T cells [44]. Genome-wide association studies have identified autophagy-related gene (Atg) 16L1 as a CD susceptibility gene [1] and a deletion polymorphism upstream of IRGM, a gene essential for autophagy, is also associated with the development of CD [45].

A number of studies suggest that regulatory B cells function through interaction with regulatory CD4$^+$ Foxp3$^+$ (Treg) cells that are known to suppress a wide range of murine and human inflammatory responses [46]. B cells may enhance the expansion of Tregs either in a contact-dependent manner or a contact-independent manner through the production of IL-10 [38, 47, 48] or maximize their regulatory activity. Spontaneous colitis in mice expressing T-cell-specific dominant negative TGFβ receptor II is exacerbated when they are crossed with B-cell-deficient mice, and the B-cell deficiency is associated with a significant reduction of Tregs [49]. In addition, an acute colitis induced by dextran sulfate sodium (DSS) was exacerbated in the absence of B cells, and adoptive transfer of B cells improved it in an IL-10-independent manner [50]. These regulatory interactions of regulatory B-cells and Tregs support the findings of recent genetic studies in IBD patients, which highlight the significance of immune regulatory network to prevent the development of IBD [1].

Cytokine Production

The recent recognition of B cells as cytokine-producing cells represents a major advancement in understanding the function of B cells in inflammatory disorders. Both human and murine B cells can produce a spectrum of cytokines, especially under inflammatory conditions. The cytokines include IL-4, IFN-γ [51], IL-2, TNF-α [52], GM-CSF [53], TGF-β [54], and IL-12p70 [55]. Therefore, like CD4$^+$ T cells, B cells may be classified into functionally different subsets: IFN-γ-producing B effector 1 (Be1) and IL-4-producing B effector 2 (Be2) cells [51, 52].

Our studies in TCRαKO mice have identified a B-cell subset that regulates inflammation by the production of a regulatory cytokine IL-10; we have called these regulatory *B* cells ("Breg") [56]. As stated above, TCRαKO mice spontaneously develop a Th2-mediated chronic colitis, and B-cell-deficient TCRα double knockout mice develop much more exacerbated form of colitis as compared to TCRαKO mice indicating a protective role of B cells in this colitis model [26]. IL-10-producing B cells, which are characterized by high expression levels of CD1d, appear in the MLN of this model after, but not before, the development of colitis. Cell transfer studies conclusively showed that the inducible IL-10-producing B cells attenuate ongoing colitis [57]. A recent study using a reporter mouse system that expresses green fluorescent protein (GFP) when IL-10 expressions are induced confirms that a major source of IL-10 in the MLN under inflammatory condition is B cells [58]. Importantly, B-cell-specific deletion of IL-10 cannot cause spontaneous colitis [58], consistent with previous reports that IL-10-producing Breg is involved in controlling the progression, but not induction, of colitis [56].

Several other studies have also identified IL-10 producing B cells to suppress diverse inflammatory diseases including IBD, graft versus host diseases (GVHD), experimental allergic encephalomyelitis and collagen-induced rheumatoid arthritis [56, 59–62]. IL-10-producing B10 cells are involved in suppressing different types of colitis, including DSS-induced acute colitis and Th1-mediated chronic colitis seen in IL-10 KO mice and CD45RB model in which colitis is induced in immunodeficient recipients by transfer of splenic CD45RB^{high} CD4^{+} T cells [63–65]. As stated above, IL-10-producing regulatory B cells exist at a very low number in normal conditions and expand under inflammatory conditions [56, 59]; these cells function primarily to suppress ongoing inflammation rather than inhibit the initiation of inflammatory process. The regulatory B cells exhibit unique phenotypic characteristics. This includes expression of both immature transitional type 2 B cells and fully matured marginal zone B cells [57, 61]. Although IL-10-producing regulatory B cells originate from B2 B cell lineage, some of these cells express a CD5, a marker associated with B1 B cells [66, 67]. Like dendritic cells, high levels of MHC class II may be expressed by some regulatory B cells [47, 48]. The development of Breg under intestinal inflammatory conditions may be induced by apoptotic cells [68].

IL-10-producing regulatory B-cell subsets may originate from either immature/naïve or activated memory B cells. Like regulatory T-cell subsets (Treg, Tr1, and Th3), it is likely that regulatory B cells also originate in the gut-associated lymphoid tissues (GALT) containing about 80 % of activated B cells [6, 7]. Our studies in TCRαKO mice indicate that “Bregs” appear in the mesenteric lymph nodes (MLNs) only under intestinal inflammatory conditions [56, 57] and are capable of expanding throughout the body [40]. Bregs, which are phenotypically characterized by high expression levels of CD1d, represents immature/naïve B cells that are polyclonally activated, presumably by stimulation with enteric microorganisms. Functionally, Bregs attenuate ongoing colitis by inhibiting proinflammatory responses such as the production of IL-1β [56, 57]. Recent studies have identified a spleen-specific IL-10-producing regulatory B cells termed “B10”, which are characterized by a CD1d^{high} CD5^{+} surface phenotype [66]. The B10 cells originate from memory follicular B cell pool and develop in an antigen-dependent manner [59, 66]. B10 cells, unlike Bregs, regulate the initiation, but not progression, of inflammatory conditions such as murine lupus and experimental autoimmune encephalomyelitis by down-regulating the ability of dendritic cells to act as APCs for priming effector CD4^{+} T cells [66, 67, 69]. Another difference between B10 cells and Breg is that B10 cells are detected in the systemic circulation, but not in lymph nodes, where Bregs develop [66].

In addition to IL-10-producing Bregs, another unique B cell population, capable of producing IL-12p70 but not IL-10, is also generated in the MLN of TCRαKO mice during colitis development and participates in the attenuation of this Th2-mediated colitis [55]. Interestingly, a unique B-cell subset, which is characterized by high expression levels of MHC class II and its ability to produce IL-12p70 in response to a bacterial product CpG (toll-like receptor 9 ligand), has been identified in the colon of these mice [70]. These unique colonic B cells are recruited from immature/transitional and recirculating naïve B2 B-cell pools. Like Bregs, they are inducible; they exist in normal colon at a very low number and expand during the recovery phase of intestinal inflammation [70]. IL-10 producing Bregs may have a wider role in inhibiting a large spectrum of inflammatory conditions, whereas IL-12p70 producing B cells may have a more limited role in suppressing Th-2-mediated colitis. Recent studies indicate that CD40L-expressing B cells suppress a CD8^{+} T cell-induced colitis by inducing IL-10 expression in the pathogenic CD8^{+} T cells [71]. B cells stimulated with *Hymenolepis diminuta* infection improved oxazolone colitis by producing TGF-β and cooperating with regulatory macrophages [72], and B cells expressing an ectoenzyme CD73 suppress DSS-induced colitis by producing adenosine [73].

A protective role of IL-10-producing B cells has also been demonstrated in IBD experimental models with features of human CD. These models include Gαi2 knockout mice in which the ability of regulatory B cells to produce IL-10 is impaired [74], CD45RB transfer model [75], and mice expressing T cell-specific dominant negative TGFβ receptor II in which B cells regulate colitis in an IL-10-independent manner [49]. Polyclonally activated B cells have been shown to suppress an innate immune-mediated spontaneous colitis in nuclear factor of activated T cells (NFAT) C2-deficient RAG2 double knockout mice; this suppression is not dependent on IL-10 [76]. In contrast to above studies, a pathogenic role of B cells has been reported in ileitis developing in the SAMP1/Yit congenic mouse model and in the TCRβ×TCRδ double knockout mouse model with the reconstitution of WT mouse-derived naïve CD4^{+} T cells [77, 78]. It is possible that the function of B cells differs depending on the site of inflammation: a pathogenic role in small intestine (ileitis), but a regulatory role in large intestine (colitis). Since a recent study indicates that the development of IL-10-producing regulatory B cells is impaired in SAMP1/Yit mice [79], a pathogenic role of B may be exhibited in the absence of regulatory B cells.

Human Mucosal and Regulatory B cells

There have been a limited number of studies regarding the functional characterization of mucosal B cells in human IBD. In a recent study [8], circulating and mucosal tissue B cells (isolated from surgical resection specimens) from CD patients showed elevated levels of basal activation as indicated by TLR2 expression, spontaneous IL-8 secretion, and increased levels of phosphorylated signaling proteins. Correlation between increased expression of TLR2 and IL-8 and clinical activity was observed in CD but not in UC. Whether the hyperactivated B cells reflect a pathogenic role or merely reflect a secondary response to microbes in diseased mucosa is not clarified in the study. A more recent study [80] suggests that in IBD patients B cells could be modulated by TLR ligands towards proinflammatory or autoinflammatory activity depending on the predominance of systemic TLR ligands (LPS/endotoxin and high mobility group box 1). B cells from IBD patients also produce chemokine eotaxin in response to TLR ligands and may regulate directly or indirectly eosinophil tissue migration patterns [81].

A unique phenotype of $CD19^{+}$ $CD24^{high}$ $CD38^{high}$ $CD1d^{high}$ $CD5^{+}$ $CD27^{-}$ of human IL-10 producing regulatory B cells in peripheral blood lymphocytes (PBL) has been reported [38]. These regulatory B cells require in vitro CD40 stimulation to exhibit IL-10 production and inhibit differentiation of Th1 cells in vitro. This regulatory capacity is lacking in patients with systemic lupus erythematosus [38]. A recent study reports an increase of IL-35-producing $CD20^{+}$ regulatory B cells in the inflamed colon of CD patients as compared to UC and healthy controls [82].

A possible role of B cells in IBD has been suggested by B-cell depletion studies. In one study, UC was induced in a patient with Graves' disease after depletion of B cells through treatment with rituximab, a mouse–human chimeric anti-CD20 mAb [83, 84]. In another study, administration of this antibody in a UC patient led to the exacerbation of colitis [85]. Interestingly, the exacerbation of colitis was associated with a reduction of IL-10 production in the colon, supporting the possible protective role of IL-10-producing Bregs in UC. Recently, a clinical trial of B cell depletion by rituximab showed no significant effect of B cell depletion on inducing remission in moderately active UC [86]. However, there appeared to be increased in remission at week 4 but was not sustained.

Concluding Remarks

It is now well established that dysregulation of mucosal immune response to enteric bacteria is the underlying factor in the development of IBD. B cells form an important component of mucosal immune system for maintaining an epithelial barrier, regulation of the enteric microflora diversity, and development of adequate immune response to both enteric floral and food antigens. A compelling case for regulatory B cells has been made in IBD experimental models; however, a pathogenic role of B cells has not been excluded. The presence of circulating antibodies to self-antigens and enteric bacteria in many patients indicates B cell involvement in human IBD. Whether or not B cells play an important role in UC and CD pathogenesis has yet to be defined. Further understanding of the role of B cells in IBD would require functional characterization of human mucosal B cells in normal and diseased states. Genome-wide association studies of IBD may lead to the identification of B-cell-associated genes that may be candidate genes involved in the pathogenesis of chronic intestinal inflammation.

References

1. Abraham C, Cho JH. Inflammatory bowel disease. N Engl J Med. 2009;361(21):2066–78.
2. Xavier RJ, Podolsky DK. Unravelling the pathogenesis of inflammatory bowel disease. Nature. 2007;448(7152):427–34.
3. Strober W, Fuss I, Mannon P. The fundamental basis of inflammatory bowel disease. J Clin Invest. 2007;117(3):514–21.
4. Bhan AK, Mizoguchi E, Smith RN, Mizoguchi A. Colitis in transgenic and knockout animals as models of human inflammatory bowel disease. Immunol Rev. 1999;169:195–207.
5. Mizoguchi A, Mizoguchi E, Bhan AK. Immune networks in animal models of inflammatory bowel disease. Inflamm Bowel Dis. 2003;9(4):246–59.
6. Mizoguchi A, Mizoguchi E. Inflammatory bowel disease, past, present and future: lessons from animal models. J Gastroenterol. 2008;43(1):1–17.
7. Brandtzaeg P, Johansen FE. Mucosal B cells: phenotypic characteristics, transcriptional regulation, and homing properties. Immunol Rev. 2005;206:32–63.
8. Noronha AM, Liang Y, Hetzel JT, Hasturk H, Kantarci A, Stucchi A, et al. Hyperactivated B cells in human inflammatory bowel disease. J Leukoc Biol. 2009;86(4):1007–16.
9. Uo M, Hisamatsu T, Miyoshi J, Kaito D, Yoneno K, Kitazume MT, et al. Mucosal CXCR4+ IgG plasma cells contribute to the pathogenesis of human ulcerative colitis through FcgammaR-mediated CD14 macrophage activation. Gut. 2013;62(12):1734–44.
10. Cupi ML, Sarra M, Marafini I, Monteleone I, Franze E, Ortenzi A, et al. Plasma cells in the mucosa of patients with inflammatory bowel disease produce granzyme B and possess cytotoxic activities. J Immunol. 2014;192(12):6083–91.
11. Fillatreau S. Regulatory plasma cells. Curr Opin Pharmacol. 2015;23:1–5.
12. Peyrin-Biroulet L, Standaert-Vitse A, Branche J, Chamaillard M. IBD serological panels: facts and perspectives. Inflamm Bowel Dis. 2007;13(12):1561–6.
13. Ferrante M, Henckaerts L, Joossens M, Pierik M, Joossens S, Dotan N, et al. New serological markers in inflammatory bowel disease are associated with complicated disease behaviour. Gut. 2007;56(10):1394–403.
14. Sellin JH, Shah RR. The promise and pitfalls of serologic testing in inflammatory bowel disease. Gastroenterol Clin North Am. 2012;41(2):463–82.
15. Kuna AT. Serological markers of inflammatory bowel disease. Biochem Med. 2013;23(1):28–42.

16. Brandtzaeg P, Carlsen HS, Halstensen TS. The B-cell system in inflammatory bowel disease. Adv Exp Med Biol. 2006;579: 149–67.
17. Heddle RJ, La Brooy JT, Shearman DJ. Escherichia coli antibody-secreting cells in the human intestine. Clin Exp Immunol. 1982;48(2):469–76.
18. Hibi T, Ohara M, Toda K, Hara A, Ogata H, Iwao Y, et al. In vitro anticolon antibody production by mucosal or peripheral blood lymphocytes from patients with ulcerative colitis. Gut. 1990;31(12):1371–6.
19. Das KM. Relationship of extraintestinal involvements in inflammatory bowel disease: new insights into autoimmune pathogenesis. Dig Dis Sci. 1999;44(1):1–13.
20. Halstensen TS, Das KM, Brandtzaeg P. Epithelial deposits of immunoglobulin G1 and activated complement colocalise with the M(r) 40 kD putative autoantigen in ulcerative colitis. Gut. 1993;34(5):650–7.
21. Brandtzaeg P, Korsrud FR. Significance of different J chain profiles in human tissues: generation of IgA and IgM with binding site for secretory component is related to the J chain expressing capacity of the total local immunocyte population, including IgG and IgD producing cells, and depends on the clinical state of the tissue. Clin Exp Immunol. 1984;58(3):709–18.
22. Smith KG, Clatworthy MR. FcgammaRIIB in autoimmunity and infection: evolutionary and therapeutic implications. Nat Rev Immunol. 2010;10(5):328–43.
23. Mizoguchi A, Mizoguchi E, Chiba C, Spiekermann GM, Tonegawa S, Nagler-Anderson C, et al. Cytokine imbalance and autoantibody production in T cell receptor-alpha mutant mice with inflammatory bowel disease. J Exp Med. 1996;183(3):847–56.
24. Mizoguchi A, Mizoguchi E, Tonegawa S, Bhan AK. Alteration of a polyclonal to an oligoclonal immune response to cecal aerobic bacterial antigens in TCR alpha mutant mice with inflammatory bowel disease. Int Immunol. 1996;8(9):1387–94.
25. Brandwein SL, McCabe RP, Cong Y, Waites KB, Ridwan BU, Dean PA, et al. Spontaneously colitic C3H/HeJBir mice demonstrate selective antibody reactivity to antigens of the enteric bacterial flora. J Immunol. 1997;159(1):44–52.
26. Mizoguchi A, Mizoguchi E, Smith RN, Preffer FI, Bhan AK. Suppressive role of B cells in chronic colitis of T cell receptor alpha mutant mice. J Exp Med. 1997;186(10):1749–56.
27. Shimomura Y, Mizoguchi E, Sugimoto K, Kibe R, Benno Y, Mizoguchi A, et al. Regulatory role of B-1 B cells in chronic colitis. Int Immunol. 2008;20(6):729–37.
28. Elson CO, Cong Y, Qi F, Hershberg RM, Targan SR. Molecular approaches to the role of the microbiota in inflammatory bowel disease. Ann N Y Acad Sci. 2006;1072:39–51.
29. Targan SR, Landers CJ, Yang H, Lodes MJ, Cong Y, Papadakis KA, et al. Antibodies to CBir1 flagellin define a unique response that is associated independently with complicated Crohn's disease. Gastroenterology. 2005;128(7):2020–8.
30. Tackenberg B, Jelcic I, Baerenwaldt A, Oertel WH, Sommer N, Nimmerjahn F, et al. Impaired inhibitory Fcgamma receptor IIB expression on B cells in chronic inflammatory demyelinating polyneuropathy. Proc Natl Acad Sci U S A. 2009;106(12): 4788–92.
31. Belostocki K, Pricop L, Redecha PB, Aydin A, Leff L, Harrison MJ, et al. Infliximab treatment shifts the balance between stimulatory and inhibitory Fcgamma receptor type II isoforms on neutrophils in patients with rheumatoid arthritis. Arthritis Rheum. 2008;58(2): 384–8.
32. Masuda A, Yoshida M, Shiomi H, Ikezawa S, Takagawa T, Tanaka H, et al. Fcgamma receptor regulation of Citrobacter rodentium infection. Infect Immun. 2008;76(4):1728–37.
33. Mizoguchi A, Ogawa A, Takedatsu H, Sugimoto K, Shimomura Y, Shirane K, et al. Dependence of intestinal granuloma formation on unique myeloid DC-like cells. J Clin Invest. 2007;117(3):605–15.
34. McGovern DP, Gardet A, Torkvist L, Goyette P, Essers J, Taylor KD, et al. Genome-wide association identifies multiple ulcerative colitis susceptibility loci. Nat Genet. 2010;42(4):332–7.
35. Wolf SD, Dittel BN, Hardardottir F, Janeway Jr CA. Experimental autoimmune encephalomyelitis induction in genetically B cell-deficient mice. J Exp Med. 1996;184(6):2271–8.
36. Knoechel B, Lohr J, Kahn E, Abbas AK. The link between lymphocyte deficiency and autoimmunity: roles of endogenous T and B lymphocytes in tolerance. J Immunol. 2005;175(1):21–6.
37. Mizoguchi E, Mizoguchi A, Preffer FI, Bhan AK. Regulatory role of mature B cells in a murine model of inflammatory bowel disease. Int Immunol. 2000;12(5):597–605.
38. Blair PA, Norena LY, Flores-Borja F, Rawlings DJ, Isenberg DA, Ehrenstein MR, et al. CD19(+)CD24(hi)CD38(hi) B cells exhibit regulatory capacity in healthy individuals but are functionally impaired in systemic Lupus Erythematosus patients. Immunity. 2010;32(1):129–40.
39. Kawamura T, Kanai T, Dohi T, Uraushihara K, Totsuka T, Iiyama R, et al. Ectopic CD40 ligand expression on B cells triggers intestinal inflammation. J Immunol. 2004;172(10):6388–97.
40. Wei B, Velazquez P, Turovskaya O, Spricher K, Aranda R, Kronenberg M, et al. Mesenteric B cells centrally inhibit CD4+ T cell colitis through interaction with regulatory T cell subsets. Proc Natl Acad Sci U S A. 2005;102(6):2010–5.
41. McPherson M, Wei B, Turovskaya O, Fujiwara D, Brewer S, Braun J. Colitis immunoregulation by CD8+ T cell requires T cell cytotoxicity and B cell peptide antigen presentation. Am J Physiol Gastrointest Liver Physiol. 2008;295(3):G485–92.
42. Munz C. Enhancing immunity through autophagy. Annu Rev Immunol. 2009;27:423–49.
43. Miller BC, Zhao Z, Stephenson LM, Cadwell K, Pua HH, Lee HK, et al. The autophagy gene ATG5 plays an essential role in B lymphocyte development. Autophagy. 2008;4(3):309–14.
44. Su Y, Carey G, Maric M, Scott DW. B cells induce tolerance by presenting endogenous peptide-IgG on MHC class II molecules via an IFN-gamma-inducible lysosomal thiol reductase-dependent pathway. J Immunol. 2008;181(2):1153–60.
45. McCarroll SA, Huett A, Kuballa P, Chilewski SD, Landry A, Goyette P, et al. Deletion polymorphism upstream of IRGM associated with altered IRGM expression and Crohn's disease. Nat Genet. 2008;40(9):1107–12.
46. Izcue A, Coombes JL, Powrie F. Regulatory lymphocytes and intestinal inflammation. Annu Rev Immunol. 2009;27:313–38.
47. Singh A, Carson WF, Secor Jr ER, Guernsey LA, Flavell RA, Clark RB, et al. Regulatory role of B cells in a murine model of allergic airway disease. J Immunol. 2008;180(11):7318–26.
48. Rafei M, Hsieh J, Zehntner S, Li M, Forner K, Birman E, et al. A granulocyte-macrophage colony-stimulating factor and interleukin-15 fusokine induces a regulatory B cell population with immune suppressive properties. Nat Med. 2009;15(9):1038–45.
49. Moritoki Y, Lian ZX, Lindor K, Tuscano J, Tsuneyama K, Zhang W, et al. B-cell depletion with anti-CD20 ameliorates autoimmune cholangitis but exacerbates colitis in transforming growth factor-beta receptor II dominant negative mice. Hepatology. 2009;50(6):1893–903.
50. Wang L, Ray A, Jiang X, Wang JY, Basu S, Liu X, et al. T regulatory cells and B cells cooperate to form a regulatory loop that maintains gut homeostasis and suppresses dextran sulfate sodium-induced colitis. Mucosal Immunol. 2015;8(6):1297–312.
51. Harris DP, Haynes L, Sayles PC, Duso DK, Eaton SM, Lepak NM, et al. Reciprocal regulation of polarized cytokine production by effector B and T cells. Nat Immunol. 2000;1(6):475–82.
52. Wojciechowski W, Harris DP, Sprague F, Mousseau B, Makris M, Kusser K, et al. Cytokine-producing effector B cells regulate type 2 immunity to H. polygyrus. Immunity. 2009;30(3):421–33.
53. Rauch PJ, Chudnovskiy A, Robbins CS, Weber GF, Etzrodt M, Hilgendorf I, et al. Innate response activator B cells protect against microbial sepsis. Science. 2012;335(6068):597–601.

54. Olkhanud PB, Damdinsuren B, Bodogai M, Gress RE, Sen R, Wejksza K, et al. Tumor-evoked regulatory B cells promote breast cancer metastasis by converting resting CD4(+) T cells to T-regulatory cells. Cancer Res. 2011;71(10):3505–15.
55. Sugimoto K, Ogawa A, Shimomura Y, Nagahama K, Mizoguchi A, Bhan AK. Inducible IL-12-producing B cells regulate Th2-mediated intestinal inflammation. Gastroenterology. 2007;133(1): 124–36.
56. Mizoguchi A, Bhan AK. A case for regulatory B cells. J Immunol. 2006;176(2):705–10.
57. Mizoguchi A, Mizoguchi E, Takedatsu H, Blumberg RS, Bhan AK. Chronic intestinal inflammatory condition generates IL-10-producing regulatory B cell subset characterized by CD1d upregulation. Immunity. 2002;16(2):219–30.
58. Madan R, Demircik F, Surianarayanan S, Allen JL, Divanovic S, Trompette A, et al. Nonredundant roles for B cell-derived IL-10 in immune counter-regulation. J Immunol. 2009;183(4):2312–20.
59. Bouaziz JD, Yanaba K, Tedder TF. Regulatory B cells as inhibitors of immune responses and inflammation. Immunol Rev. 2008;224: 201–14.
60. Jamin C, Morva A, Lemoine S, Daridon C, de Mendoza AR, Youinou P. Regulatory B lymphocytes in humans: a potential role in autoimmunity. Arthritis Rheum. 2008;58(7):1900–6.
61. Lund FE, Randall TD. Effector and regulatory B cells: modulators of CD4+ T cell immunity. Nat Rev Immunol. 2010;10(4):236–47.
62. Thaunat O, Morelon E, Defrance T. Am"B"valent: anti-CD20 antibodies unravel the dual role of B cells in immunopathogenesis. Blood. 2010;116(4):515–21.
63. Yanaba K, Yoshizaki A, Asano Y, Kadono T, Tedder TF, Sato S. IL-10-producing regulatory B10 cells inhibit intestinal injury in a mouse model. Am J Pathol. 2011;178(2):735–43.
64. Schmidt EG, Larsen HL, Kristensen NN, Poulsen SS, Claesson MH, Pedersen AE. B cells exposed to enterobacterial components suppress development of experimental colitis. Inflamm Bowel Dis. 2012;18(2):284–93.
65. Maseda D, Candando KM, Smith SH, Kalampokis I, Weaver CT, Plevy SE, et al. Peritoneal cavity regulatory B cells (B10 cells) modulate IFN-gamma+CD4+ T cell numbers during colitis development in mice. J Immunol. 2013;191(5):2780–95.
66. Yanaba K, Bouaziz JD, Haas KM, Poe JC, Fujimoto M, Tedder TF. A regulatory B cell subset with a unique CD1dhiCD5+ phenotype controls T cell-dependent inflammatory responses. Immunity. 2008;28(5):639–50.
67. Matsushita T, Yanaba K, Bouaziz JD, Fujimoto M, Tedder TF. Regulatory B cells inhibit EAE initiation in mice while other B cells promote disease progression. J Clin Invest. 2008;118(10):3420–30.
68. Ansary MM, Ishihara S, Oka A, Kusunoki R, Oshima N, Yuki T, et al. Apoptotic cells ameliorate chronic intestinal inflammation by enhancing regulatory B-cell function. Inflamm Bowel Dis. 2014;20(12):2308–20.
69. Matsushita T, Horikawa M, Iwata Y, Tedder TF. Regulatory B cells (B10 cells) and regulatory T cells have independent roles in controlling experimental autoimmune encephalomyelitis initiation and late-phase immunopathogenesis. J Immunol. 2010;185(4):2240–52.
70. Shimomura Y, Ogawa A, Kawada M, Sugimoto K, Mizoguchi E, Shi HN, et al. A unique B2 B cell subset in the intestine. J Exp Med. 2008;205(6):1343–55.
71. Koni PA, Bolduc A, Takezaki M, Ametani Y, Huang L, Lee JR, et al. Constitutively CD40-activated B cells regulate CD8 T cell inflammatory response by IL-10 induction. J Immunol. 2013; 190(7):3189–96.
72. Reyes JL, Wang A, Fernando MR, Graepel R, Leung G, van Rooijen N, et al. Splenic B cells from Hymenolepis diminuta-infected mice ameliorate colitis independent of T cells and via cooperation with macrophages. J Immunol. 2015;194(1):364–78.
73. Kaku H, Cheng KF, Al-Abed Y, Rothstein TL. A novel mechanism of B cell-mediated immune suppression through CD73 expression and adenosine production. J Immunol. 2014;193(12):5904–13.
74. Dalwadi H, Wei B, Schrage M, Spicher K, Su TT, Birnbaumer L, et al. B cell developmental requirement for the G alpha i2 gene. J Immunol. 2003;170(4):1707–15.
75. Ostanin DV, Pavlick KP, Bharwani S, D'Souza D, Furr KL, Brown CM, et al. T cell-induced inflammation of the small and large intestine in immunodeficient mice. Am J Physiol Gastrointest Liver Physiol. 2006;290(1):G109–19.
76. Gerth AJ, Lin L, Neurath MF, Glimcher LH, Peng SL. An innate cell-mediated, murine ulcerative colitis-like syndrome in the absence of nuclear factor of activated T cells. Gastroenterology. 2004;126(4):1115–21.
77. Olson TS, Bamias G, Naganuma M, Rivera-Nieves J, Burcin TL, Ross W, et al. Expanded B cell population blocks regulatory T cells and exacerbates ileitis in a murine model of Crohn disease. J Clin Invest. 2004;114(3):389–98.
78. Dohi T, Fujihashi K, Koga T, Shirai Y, Kawamura YI, Ejima C, et al. T helper type-2 cells induce ileal villus atrophy, goblet cell metaplasia, and wasting disease in T cell-deficient mice. Gastroenterology. 2003;124(3):672–82.
79. Mishima Y, Ishihara S, Aziz MM, Oka A, Kusunoki R, Otani A, et al. Decreased production of interleukin-10 and transforming growth factor-beta in Toll-like receptor-activated intestinal B cells in SAMP1/Yit mice. Immunology. 2010;131(4):473–87.
80. McDonnell M, Liang Y, Noronha A, Coukos J, Kasper DL, Farraye FA, et al. Systemic Toll-like receptor ligands modify B-cell responses in human inflammatory bowel disease. Inflamm Bowel Dis. 2011;17(1):298–307.
81. Rehman MQ, Beal D, Liang Y, Noronha A, Winter H, Farraye FA, et al. B cells secrete eotaxin-1 in human inflammatory bowel disease. Inflamm Bowel Dis. 2013;19(5):922–33.
82. Fonseca-Camarillo G, Furuzawa-Carballeda J, Yamamoto-Furusho JK. Interleukin 35 (IL-35) and IL-37: Intestinal and peripheral expression by T and B regulatory cells in patients with Inflammatory Bowel Disease. Cytokine. 2015;75:389–402.
83. El Fassi D, Nielsen CH, Kjeldsen J, Clemmensen O, Hegedus L. Ulcerative colitis following B lymphocyte depletion with rituximab in a patient with Graves' disease. Gut. 2008;57(5):714–5.
84. El Fassi D, Nielsen CH, Junker P, Hasselbalch HC, Hegedus L. Systemic adverse events following rituximab therapy in patients with Graves' disease. J Endocrinol Invest. 2011;34(7):e163–7.
85. Goetz M, Atreya R, Ghalibafian M, Galle PR, Neurath MF. Exacerbation of ulcerative colitis after rituximab salvage therapy. Inflamm Bowel Dis. 2007;13(11):1365–8.
86. Leiper K, Martin K, Ellis A, Subramanian S, Watson AJ, Christmas SE, et al. Randomised placebo-controlled trial of rituximab (anti-CD20) in active ulcerative colitis. Gut. 2011;60(11):1520–6.

Immune Cells: Monocytes and Macrophages

10

Gerhard Rogler

Introduction

Monocytes and macrophages are important components of the innate immune system [1]. The innate immune system provides the first defense line against external or internal pathogens and danger signals (e.g., danger associated molecular pattern molecules, DAMPs), by triggering a protective inflammatory response that normally is self-limiting after clearance of the initial trigger [2]. In addition, an adaptive and longer lasting adaptive and specific immune response may be initiated by the same cells. The innate immune response provided by monocytes and macrophages (but also by other cellular components of the innate immune system) aims to directly destroy pathogens. This is followed by a phase in which the destroyed pathogens such as bacteria as well as cell detritus and damaged extracellular matrix material are taken up ("phagocytosed") by the cells, degraded and such removed by the same cells to allow tissue repair and recovery of the healthy situation [3].

Besides monocytes and macrophages the mononuclear phagocyte system (MPS) is composed of lineage-committed bone marrow precursors, circulating monocytes, resident tissue macrophages, and dendritic cells (DC) [1].

Monocytes and macrophages have been shown to play an important role during the initiation and chronification of inflammatory bowel disease (IBD) [4–6]. They contain many functionally important proteins that carry potential variants known to be associated with the risk for developing IBD. Macrophage differentiation from monocytes occurs in the intestine associated with the acquisition of a typical functional phenotype that is tissue specific depending on microenvironmental signals, such as signal from the gut lumen (e.g., products of the intestinal microbiota) [5, 6]. Obviously a differentiation of monocytes into macrophages in the intestine normally occurs under "non-inflammatory" or "minor inflammatory" conditions. With respect to this a "normal" non-activated monocyte will differentiate into a "normal" intestinal macrophage after entering the mucosa form the blood stream [7, 8]. Under inflammatory conditions such as IBD the differentiation is altered but not completely blocked [9–15]. A different phenotype with most likely different functions will occur [9–15].

The mechanisms how the various risk genes for IBD—and especially the ones that are associated with functions of the innate immune response—influence this process of tissue specific and inflammation-modified macrophage differentiation so far is largely unclear.

Monocytes

Monocytes represent 5–10 % of peripheral blood leukocytes in humans but only 2–4 % of the total leukocytes in mice [1]. Therefore differences in monocyte function are likely and results obtained from mouse experiments may be not easily transferable to the human "monocyte situation." Circulating monocytes together with lymphocytes morphologically belong to the group of "mononuclear cells" with mainly round but frequently also somewhat irregular cell shape, oval- or kidney-shaped nuclei, and cytoplasmic vesicles. In contrast to lymphocytes monocytes have a high cytoplasm-to-nucleus ratio. Monocytes usually remain in the blood stream and circulate through the blood vessels for 24–48 h and then migrate into tissues or are removed. Before entering the blood stream monocytes originate and differentiate in the bone marrow from hematopoietic stem cells (HSCs) through several sequential differentiation stages such as the common myeloid progenitor (CMP), the granulocyte-macrophage progenitor (GMP) as well as the common macrophage and DC precursor (MDP) [1].

Macrophage colony-stimulating factor (M-CSF) (also known as colony stimulating factor-1, CSF-1) is the most important

G. Rogler (✉)
Division of Gastroenterology and Hepatology, University Hospital of Zürich, Rämistrasse 100, 8091 Zürich, Switzerland
e-mail: gerhard.rogler@usz.ch

D.C. Baumgart (ed.), *Crohn's Disease and Ulcerative Colitis*, DOI 10.1007/978-3-319-33703-6_10

growth factor and essential component for the differentiation of monocytes/macrophages [1, 16, 17]. Granulocyte-macrophage colony-stimulating factor (GM-CSF) also is involved in the development of monocytes/macrophages especially under inflammatory conditions [1, 16, 17].

Monocytes as important component of the innate immune system initiate inflammatory responses to invading pathogens by killing, neutralizing and removing them via phagocytosis, production of reactive oxygen species (ROS), production of nitric oxide (NO), of myeloperoxidase, and secretion of cytokines and/or chemokines. As mentioned above monocytes can trigger T-cell responses and direct T-cell differentiation (e.g., by secretion of interferon gamma (IFNγ) or IL-12) [4, 18, 19].

Monocyte Heterogeneity

Circulating human peripheral blood monocytes are a heterogeneous cell population that can be discriminated by their surface antigen expression [20]. Mainly three functional subsets of human monocytes have been identified. The discrimination of the three subsets is mainly based on two surface antigens: CD14 (part of the LPS receptor) or CD16 (Fcγ RIII) [20]. Up to 90 % of human monocytes display high CD14 but no CD16 surface expression in flow cytometry (FACS) analyses (usually they are annotated as CD14++CD16− or CD14+CD16−). They may be seen as the "classical monocytes" as this population has been described first and also represents the majority of the circulating monocytes. The remaining 10 % of circulating monocytes can be split into two subtypes: A population with high CD14 and low (but not absent in contrast to the "classical" monocytes) CD16 expression (usually annotated as: CD14++CD16+ or CD14+CD16+), and a so called "non-classical subset" with low CD14 but high CD16 expression (CD14+CD16++ or CD14dimCD16+) [20].

Whether there are significant functional differences between those subpopulations is not completely clear and still a matter of discussion [1, 20]. Differences between these monocyte subpopulations with respect to their capacity to be activated by bacterial products and secrete pro-inflammatory cytokines have been described [1, 20]. This may be obvious as CD14 is part of the LPS receptor complex and subsequently a lower expression may limit the ability to react to LPS exposure. Further differences with respect to antigen presentation, phagocytosis, and oxidative burst have been reported [1, 20]. In a recent review article functional differences between the subsets have been described and discussed in detail [21]. In general, "classical" human monocytes have the ability to induce a pro-inflammatory reaction similar to the murine Ly6C+ monocytes (also termed "inflammatory" monocytes) [1]. In contrast, the "non-classical", high CD16 expressing monocytes may have properties similar to those of murine Ly6C− monocytes (also termed "alternative" or "patrolling" monocytes) [1]. Whereas classical inflammatory monocytes respond to the chemokine CCL2 as they express the respective receptor triggering recruitment to inflammatory sites the CD16++ monocytes respond to CX3C-chemokine ligand 1 [CX3CL1, the human fractalkine and mouse neurotactin] as chemokine [1].

Tissue Macrophages

Resident macrophages are found in virtually all tissues of adult mammals, where they usually represent up to 10–15 % of the total cell number [22–24]. In the intestinal mucosa they are mainly localized in the lamina propria [25]. The specific tissue environment is thought to influence the differentiation of monocytes into the organ or tissue specific macrophage phenotype explaining a significant heterogeneity between macrophages isolated from different organs or tissues [1].

The tissue macrophages found in the gut wall represent one of the largest—if not the largest—compartments of the mononuclear phagocyte system in the body. They are localized preferentially at the sites of antigen entry, e.g., in the periepithelial region of the small intestine and in the subepithelial domes of Peyer's patches. Macrophages constitute 10–20 % of the mononuclear cells in the lamina propria, as determined by immunohistochemistry and tissue disaggregation experiments [25].

Intestinal macrophages are involved in the pathogenesis of IBD. With respect to their transcriptional profile they differ from macrophages in other tissues such as Kupffer cell in the liver, alveolar macrophages or osteoclasts [26–29]. Intestinal macrophages show a specific phenotype with low expression of typical monocyte antigens such as CD14 or CD16 [13]. The differentiation of intestinal macrophages is partly regulated by epithelial cells as it can be in vitro induced in spheroid cultures of intestinal epithelial cells [7, 8]. They display a more "anergic," "regulatory," "tolerogenic," or M2 phenotype with also low expression of costimulatory molecules such as CD80 or CD86 and low expression of pattern recognition receptors such as TLR4 or TLR2 [12, 30].

The phenotype and the functional characteristics of intestinal macrophages are altered during chronic inflammation in IBD [10–12, 14, 15, 31]. Whether this is only due to a disturbed differentiation of invading monocytes remains to be elucidated and is not clear so far.

During acute flares of IBD the heterogeneity of the intestinal macrophage population is strongly increased. In mouse models of colitis such as the acute DSS colitis model an early influx of monocytes/macrophages into the mucosa is observed [32–34]. There usually is a concomitant "loss" of resident macrophages, due to tissue adherence, emigration, or death. This is also called "macrophages disappearance reaction" and has mainly been described for peritoneal and alveolar macrophages (as it is easier to describe and analyze in those tissues) [35].

Inflammatory macrophages most likely derive from recruited blood monocytes that do not undergo the normal process of differentiation into intestinal macrophages in the mucosa [15, 36].

There are two main chemokines and related receptors found to be responsible for the recruitment of monocytes into the inflamed intestinal mucosa: CCL2/CCR2 and CX3CL1/CX3CR1, respectively [37–39]. CCL2 is produced by mucosal fibroblasts, intestinal epithelial cells as well as endothelial cells in response to the inflammatory environment and in response to invading microbes.

Intestinal Macrophage Differentiation and Function

The intestinal mucosa is challenged by a permanent contact to an indeterminable multiplicity of bacterial and food antigens from the intestinal lumen. Mechanisms must exist, which facilitate an immediate immune reaction against pathogens penetrating into the mucosa. On the other hand, ongoing immune reactions against commensal bacteria or food antigens must be effectively prevented—otherwise the consequence is a chronic mucosal inflammation—as we find it in patients with IBD.

In general two major types of macrophages have been described in recent years: M2 macrophages are tolerogenic, promote tissue healing and growth whereas M1 macrophages have easily activated defense functions and kill bacteria as well as initiate inflammation [1]. This is associated with a shift in cell metabolism: In M1 macrophages the arginine metabolism is shifted to NO and citrulline [1]. In contrast in M2 macrophages it is shifted to ornithine and polyamines [1].

However, the M1 and M2 polarization may not represent a final differentiation status but more a reversible form of functional specialization [40, 41].

As mentioned above intestinal macrophages in normal, non-inflamed mucosa have lost a whole number of "typical" macrophage abilities as a consequence of their specific differentiation. In contrast to blood monocytes or in vitro differentiated macrophages intestinal macrophages are rather irresponsive to LPS as LPS receptors (TLR4 and CD14) are not expressed [30, 42]. Besides that, normal intestinal macrophages cannot induce clonal T-cell reactions, because they do not express T-cell co-stimulatory molecules such as CD80 (B7-1) and CD86 (B7-2), necessary for a clonal T-cell expansion [12]. These data point to an anergic, tolerance-inducing intestinal macrophages-type in the normal intestinal mucosa. Normal intestinal macrophages have the task to prevent a perpetuation of inflammatory reactions against bacteria of the commensal intestinal flora. However, the tolerogenic intestinal macrophages' function so far is only partially understood. Better knowledge of the specific immunomodulatory functions of normal intestinal macrophages would allow specific interventions during intestinal inflammation targeted to reinduce the normal intestinal macrophages-phenotype—in the sense of a "reestablishment of physiological conditions."

Conclusion

Polymorphisms in molecules of the innate immune system have been shown to be risk factors for IBD. Very important components of the innate immune system are monocytes/macrophages. Intestinal macrophages usually show a tolerogenic phenotype (M2 like) and are important for the mediation of tolerance (prevention of inflammation) to commensal bacteria. In IBD monocytes invade the mucosa and do not completely differentiate into the M2 phenotype but rather stay in a M1 state. Understanding the reasons for this lack of proper intestinal macrophage differentiation will provide new insights into IBD pathophysiology and will open up new therapeutic possibilities and approaches.

References

1. Italiani P, Boraschi D. From monocytes to M1/M2 macrophages: phenotypical vs. functional differentiation. Front Immunol. 2014;5:514.
2. Moretta A, Marcenaro E, Sivori S, Della Chiesa M, Vitale M, Moretta L. Early liaisons between cells of the innate immune system in inflamed peripheral tissues. Trends Immunol. 2005;26:668–75.
3. Liddiard K, Taylor PR. Understanding local macrophage phenotypes in disease: shape-shifting macrophages. Nat Med. 2015;21:119–20.
4. Mann ER, Li X. Intestinal antigen-presenting cells in mucosal immune homeostasis: crosstalk between dendritic cells, macrophages and B-cells. World J Gastroenterol. 2014;20:9653–64.
5. Bain CC, Mowat AM. Macrophages in intestinal homeostasis and inflammation. Immunol Rev. 2014;260:102–17.
6. Steinbach EC, Plevy SE. The role of macrophages and dendritic cells in the initiation of inflammation in IBD. Inflamm Bowel Dis. 2014;20:166–75.
7. Spoettl T, Hausmann M, Menzel K, Piberger H, Herfarth H, Schoelmerich J, et al. Role of soluble factors and three-dimensional culture in in vitro differentiation of intestinal macrophages. World J Gastroenterol. 2007;13:1032–41.
8. Spottl T, Hausmann M, Kreutz M, Peuker A, Vogl D, Scholmerich J, et al. Monocyte differentiation in intestine-like macrophage phenotype induced by epithelial cells. J Leukoc Biol. 2001;70:241–51.
9. Hausmann M, Bataille F, Spoettl T, Schreiter K, Falk W, Schoelmerich J, et al. Physiological role of macrophage inflammatory protein-3 alpha induction during maturation of intestinal macrophages. J Immunol. 2005;175:1389–98.

10. Hausmann M, Obermeier F, Schreiter K, Spottl T, Falk W, Scholmerich J, et al. Cathepsin D is up-regulated in inflammatory bowel disease macrophages. Clin Exp Immunol. 2004;136:157–67.
11. Hausmann M, Spottl T, Andus T, Rothe G, Falk W, Scholmerich J, et al. Subtractive screening reveals up-regulation of NADPH oxidase expression in Crohn's disease intestinal macrophages. Clin Exp Immunol. 2001;125:48–55.
12. Rogler G, Hausmann M, Spottl T, Vogl D, Aschenbrenner E, Andus T, et al. T-cell co-stimulatory molecules are upregulated on intestinal macrophages from inflammatory bowel disease mucosa. Eur J Gastroenterol Hepatol. 1999;11:1105–11.
13. Rogler G, Hausmann M, Vogl D, Aschenbrenner E, Andus T, Falk W, et al. Isolation and phenotypic characterization of colonic macrophages. Clin Exp Immunol. 1998;112:205–15.
14. Rogler G, Brand K, Vogl D, Page S, Hofmeister R, Andus T, et al. Nuclear factor kappaB is activated in macrophages and epithelial cells of inflamed intestinal mucosa. Gastroenterology. 1998;115:357–69.
15. Rogler G, Andus T, Aschenbrenner E, Vogl D, Falk W, Scholmerich J, et al. Alterations of the phenotype of colonic macrophages in inflammatory bowel disease. Eur J Gastroenterol Hepatol. 1997;9:893–9.
16. Ziegler-Heitbrock L. The CD14+ CD16+ blood monocytes: their role in infection and inflammation. J Leukoc Biol. 2007;81:584–92.
17. Kumar S, Jack R. Origin of monocytes and their differentiation to macrophages and dendritic cells. J Endotoxin Res. 2006;12:278–84.
18. Chakarov S, Fazilleau N. Monocyte-derived dendritic cells promote T follicular helper cell differentiation. EMBO Mol Med. 2014;6:590–603.
19. Slingluff Jr CL, Petroni GR, Olson WC, Smolkin ME, Ross MI, Haas NB, et al. Effect of granulocyte/macrophage colony-stimulating factor on circulating CD8+ and CD4+ T-cell responses to a multipeptide melanoma vaccine: outcome of a multicenter randomized trial. Clin Cancer Res. 2009;15:7036–44.
20. Ziegler-Heitbrock L. Monocyte subsets in man and other species. Cell Immunol. 2014;289:135–9.
21. Wong KL, Yeap WH, Tai JJ, Ong SM, Dang TM, Wong SC. The three human monocyte subsets: implications for health and disease. Immunol Res. 2012;53:41–57.
22. Weiss G, Schaible UE. Macrophage defense mechanisms against intracellular bacteria. Immunol Rev. 2015;264:182–203.
23. Sica A, Erreni M, Allavena P, Porta C. Macrophage polarization in pathology. Cell Mol Life Sci. 2015;72(21):4111–26.
24. Motwani MP, Gilroy DW. Macrophage development and polarization in chronic inflammation. Semin Immunol. 2015;27:257–66.
25. Brandtzaeg P. Nature and function of gastrointestinal antigen-presenting cells. Allergy. 2001;56 Suppl 67:16–20.
26. Schultze JL, Freeman T, Hume DA, Latz E. A transcriptional perspective on human macrophage biology. Semin Immunol. 2015;27:44–50.
27. Lawrence T, Natoli G. Transcriptional regulation of macrophage polarization: enabling diversity with identity. Nat Rev Immunol. 2011;11:750–61.
28. Hume DA, Wells CA, Ravasi T. Transcriptional regulatory networks in macrophages. Novartis Found Symp. 2007;281:2–18. discussion –24, 50–3, 208–9.
29. Hawiger J. Innate immunity and inflammation: a transcriptional paradigm. Immunol Res. 2001;23:99–109.
30. Hausmann M, Kiessling S, Mestermann S, Webb G, Spottl T, Andus T, et al. Toll-like receptors 2 and 4 are up-regulated during intestinal inflammation. Gastroenterology. 2002;122: 1987–2000.
31. Hetzenecker AM, Seidl MC, Kosovac K, Herfarth H, Kellermeier S, Obermeier F, et al. Downregulation of the ubiquitin-proteasome system in normal colonic macrophages and reinduction in inflammatory bowel disease. Digestion. 2012;86:34–47.
32. Abdelouhab K, Rafa H, Toumi R, Bouaziz S, Medjeber O, Touil-Boukoffa C. Mucosal intestinal alteration in experimental colitis correlates with nitric oxide production by peritoneal macrophages: effect of probiotics and prebiotics. Immunopharmacol Immunotoxicol. 2012;34:590–7.
33. Crielaard BJ, Lammers T, Morgan ME, Chaabane L, Carboni S, Greco B, et al. Macrophages and liposomes in inflammatory disease: friends or foes? Int J Pharm. 2011;416:499–506.
34. Ghia JE, Galeazzi F, Ford DC, Hogaboam CM, Vallance BA, Collins S. Role of M-CSF-dependent macrophages in colitis is driven by the nature of the inflammatory stimulus. Am J Physiol Gastrointest Liver Physiol. 2008;294:G770–7.
35. Barth MW, Hendrzak JA, Melnicoff MJ, Morahan PS. Review of the macrophage disappearance reaction. J Leukoc Biol. 1995;57: 361–7.
36. Spoettl T, Hausmann M, Herlyn M, Gunckel M, Dirmeier A, Falk W, et al. Monocyte chemoattractant protein-1 (MCP-1) inhibits the intestinal-like differentiation of monocytes. Clin Exp Immunol. 2006;145:190–9.
37. Schmall A, Al-Tamari HM, Herold S, Kampschulte M, Weigert A, Wietelmann A, et al. Macrophage and cancer cell cross-talk via CCR2 and CX3CR1 is a fundamental mechanism driving lung cancer. Am J Respir Crit Care Med. 2015;191:437–47.
38. Lionakis MS, Swamydas M, Fischer BG, Plantinga TS, Johnson MD, Jaeger M, et al. CX3CR1-dependent renal macrophage survival promotes Candida control and host survival. J Clin Invest. 2013;123:5035–51.
39. Medina-Contreras O, Geem D, Laur O, Williams IR, Lira SA, Nusrat A, et al. CX3CR1 regulates intestinal macrophage homeostasis, bacterial translocation, and colitogenic Th17 responses in mice. J Clin Invest. 2011;121:4787–95.
40. Lissner D, Schumann M, Batra A, Kredel LI, Kuhl AA, Erben U, et al. Monocyte and M1 macrophage-induced barrier defect contributes to chronic intestinal inflammation in IBD. Inflamm Bowel Dis. 2015;21:1297–305.
41. Kredel LI, Batra A, Stroh T, Kuhl AA, Zeitz M, Erben U, et al. Adipokines from local fat cells shape the macrophage compartment of the creeping fat in Crohn's disease. Gut. 2013;62:852–62.
42. Salem M, Seidelin JB, Eickhardt S, Alhede M, Rogler G, Nielsen OH. Species-specific engagement of human nucleotide oligomerization domain 2 (NOD)2 and Toll-like receptor (TLR) signalling upon intracellular bacterial infection: role of Crohn's associated NOD2 gene variants. Clin Exp Immunol. 2015;179:426–34.

Immune Functions of Epithelial Cells in Inflammatory Bowel Disease

11

Eric L. Campbell and Sean P. Colgan

Introduction

Epithelial cells, which line organs such as the intestine, are uniquely positioned to serve as a direct conduit of communication between the immune system and the external environment. While carrying out nutrient absorption functions, mucosal surfaces of the alimentary tract are constantly exposed on the luminal surface to microbes and foreign antigens. For years, the sole role ascribed to the epithelium was acting as a highly selective barrier. Dynamic cross talk between the epithelium and the immune system, via the intimately associated subepithelial lymphoid tissue, has more recently been appreciated [1]. For these reasons, intestinal epithelial cells (IEC) lie at the heart of innate immunity. IEC rely on a diverse set of pathogen recognition receptors (PRR) to recognize and respond to this diverse set of microbial antigens. A common feature of patients with active ulcerative colitis and Crohn's disease (collectively termed inflammatory bowel disease, IBD) is disruption of the intestinal epithelial lining [2, 3]. Ongoing studies have identified multiple genetic mutations associated with the innate immune response that could contribute to abnormal epithelial responses to microbial antigens. Here, we discuss the contribution of IEC to immune responses in health and during ongoing mucosal inflammation.

Dynamic Nature of Intestinal Epithelial Cells

Historically, IEC were considered passive players to the immune response. For decades, epithelial cells were thought to provide a selective barrier to allow nutrient absorption and provide for electrolyte transport. This view has changed considerably in the past two decades. Epithelial cells are now considered an active participant of a successful immune response, to the extent that primary defects within the epithelium likely determine the limit of many autoimmune diseases, including IBD [2, 3].

Studies in the 1980s and 1990s revealed that epithelial cells have the capacity to "phenotype switch" from a cell primarily expressing machinery for barrier function and electrolyte transport to one well adapted to interacting and directing the innate and adaptive immune system. These studies were founded on original observations that epithelial cells express and respond to cytokines such as IFNγ through a loss of barrier function and an induction of immune accessory features that promote immune cell interactions [4, 5]. This focus on IFNγ at the time was important, as it was demonstrated that in the basal state, IFNγ production is readily detectable in the mucosa [6]. During active immune responses, the number of lymphocytes increase, and upon antigenic challenge of mucosal T-lymphocytes, the IFNγ signal is markedly enhanced in the mucosa [6]. It was subsequently shown that IFNγ was capable of eliciting the surface expression of MHC class II on intestinal epithelial cells [7] and that human intestinal epithelia could function as antigen presenting cells to lymphocytes in classic mixed lymphocyte reactions [8]. These studies revealed the dynamic nature of IEC phenotype and demonstrated that IFNγ induces a global shift in phenotype from one expressing classic epithelial features (barrier function, ion transport, electrolyte movement) to one harboring considerable immune accessory functions (induction of MHC class I/II, upregulation of ICAM-1, regulated leukocyte recruitment, see Fig. 11.1) [5]. Extensions of these studies have revealed, and continue to reveal, that IEC are a source and/or a first responder to multiple cytokines and chemokines found within the inflammatory milieu, including IL-4, IL-6, IL-7, IL-8, IL-13, IL-15, IL-18, GM-CSF, and TGFβ [9].

NFkB is a quintessential inflammatory transcription factor that functions as a signaling hub to direct the immune

E.L. Campbell, Ph.D. • S.P. Colgan, Ph.D. (✉)
Department of Medicine and the Mucosal Inflammation Program, University of Colorado School of Medicine,
12700 East 19th Ave., MS B-146, Aurora, CO 80045, USA
e-mail: Sean.Colgan@UCDenver.edu

D.C. Baumgart (ed.), *Crohn's Disease and Ulcerative Colitis*, DOI 10.1007/978-3-319-33703-6_11

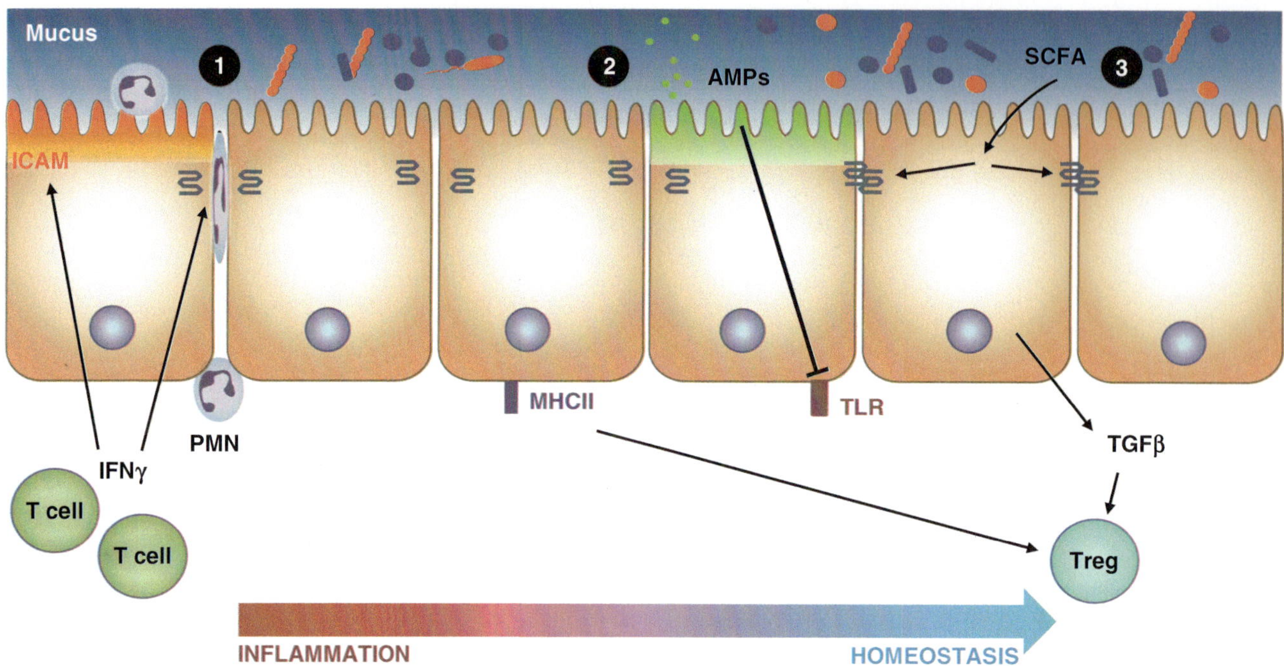

Fig. 11.1 Epithelial cells and the coordination of immune homeostasis: (*1*) IFN-gamma released by T-cells can increase tight junction permeability and induce apical expression of ICAM-1. Together this allows migration and apical localization of neutrophils (PMN). (*2*) IECs can kill bacteria to maintain the sterility of the mucus layer and neutralize gram-negative LPS through the activity of AMPs (antimicrobial peptides), both secreted (e.g., defensins, BPI) and apically expressed (e.g., ALPI), preventing TLR4 stimulation. (*3*) Commensal bacterial-derived SCFA (short chain fatty acids) provide an energy source to the IECs and in combination with antigen presentation can stimulate IEC TGF-beta production to promote tolerance through regulatory T cell (Treg) homing

response and has been linked to autoimmunity, cancer, and chronic inflammation [10]. One particularly interesting observation has been the function of NFkB within the intestinal epithelium. Indeed, NF-kB activation has been associated with disease activity in IBD. For example, lamina propria macrophages and colonic biopsies from IBD patients show enhanced NF-kB activity. Likewise, a polymorphism in the promoter region of the *Nfkb1* gene, which encodes the p105 precursor of the NF-kB p50 subunit, has been associated with an increased risk of developing IBD [11]. Thus, it was somewhat surprising that multiple genetic studies in mice have revealed that conditional loss of function deletions of components of the NF-kB pathway within the epithelium significantly increased susceptibility to colitis [12]. These studies indicated a protective role for epithelial NF-kB in inflammation through a mechanism involving the expression of anti-apoptotic genes in the IEC resulting in enhanced epithelial barrier function and mucosal homeostasis [12].

Expression of Co-stimulatory Molecules, Classical/Non-Classical MHC, TLRs

IEC represent a first line of defense to invasion by pathogens [13]. Intestinal epithelial cells are equipped with a diverse array of PRR that, upon ligand binding results in the induction of a diverse set of chemokines that recruit circulating leukocytes to initiate innate immune responses [9]. Colonic epithelial cells, for example, express surface TLRs, including TLR2, 3, 4, and 5, that are selectively polarized to the basolateral surface [14], ensuring that only invasive bacteria that have breached the barrier trigger TLR's in the epithelium (see Fig. 11.1).

While specialized gut-associated lymphoid tissues (GALT), including Peyer's patches, exist throughout the GI tract and are dedicated to sampling luminal contents at steady state, in fact any IEC can adopt such functions under inflammatory conditions. In addition to relaying luminal signals to the lamina propria, Mayer et al. have provided significant evidence that IEC can recognize, process and even present antigens to antigen-specific lymphocytes [1]. IEC constitutively express MHC class I along the length of the small and large intestine as well as MHC class II in the small intestine, the latter of which can be significantly induced by cytokines such as IFNγ [15]. Polarized antigen sorting and processing in late endosomes is similarly regulated by IFNγ, where antigens are subsequently processed into appropriate immunogenic peptides for presentation to CD4+ T-cells [1]. While IEC do not express classical co-stimulatory molecules such as CD80 or CD86, IEC from IBD patients express novel members of the B7 family (B7h and B7H1) that when paired CD28 or CD152 can produce a co-stimulatory signals [16].

In addition to expression of MHC class I and II, IEC have been shown to express functional non-classical MHC molecules, particularly CD1d [17]. The CD1 family of molecules present self and microbial glycolipids to CD1-restricted T cells (NKT cells in the case of CD1d). Ligation of IEC CD1d has been shown to result in the production of the immunoregulatory cytokine IL-10 [18], for which IEC have been demonstrated to express IL-10 receptors on the luminal surface [19]. Olszak et al., recently demonstrated that IEC-specific deletion of CD1d resulted in a severe NKT cell-mediated intestinal inflammation in a mouse model [20]. Moreover, the decreased expression of CD1d on IEC of patients with IBD may contribute to perpetuation of intestinal inflammation [21].

Coordination of Inflammatory and Resolution Responses

The successful inflammatory response is initiated by recruitment of leukocytes to sites of infection/injury. Leukocyte migration into and across the epithelium is orchestrated through a highly coordinated series of steps, mediated by cell adhesion molecules and integrins. The molecular details of this cascade have been extensively summarized elsewhere [22, 23]. These seminal studies have revealed that IEC surface molecules and IEC secreted factors play a central role in recruiting and coordinating leukocyte migration to the mucosa (Fig. 11.1).

Crypt abscesses, the accumulation of large numbers of leukocytes to the luminal surface, represent one of the pathological hallmarks of active IBD [22]. There is significant recent interest in understanding how such crypt abscesses might impact mucosal tissue function, particularly related to inflammatory resolution or progression toward chronicity. A recent study examined the influence of neutrophil (polymorphonuclear leukocyte, PMN) transepithelial migration on epithelial gene programming and the resolution response [24]. In this study, gene expression changes within the epithelium were attributable to the consumption of large amounts of O_2 by PMN through the activation of the NADPH oxidase. These studies revealed that O_2 consumption by activated PMN resulted in the stabilization of the transcription factor hypoxia-inducible factor (HIF) within the epithelium. Utilizing murine models of colitis, the authors demonstrated that both the presence of PMNs as well as PMN-elicited hypoxia were necessary for mucosal progressive resolution of inflammation. Depletion of PMNs led to exacerbated tissue destruction during colitis. These observations have also been validated in human patients. For example, human IBD specimens containing crypt abscesses were examined for the localized expression of the HIF gene target gene Glut1. Areas adjacent to the human crypt abscess revealed marked upregulation of Glut-1 relative to healthy controls. Also notable is the observation that patients lacking a functional NADPH oxidase (i.e., chronic granulomatous disease, CGD) often present with an IBD-like syndrome [25]. This NADPH oxidase complex is responsible for the generation of reactive oxygen species (ROS) and used by innate immune cells (esp. PMN) to kill invading pathogens. CGD patients exhibit congenital defects in genes coding the subunits of the neutrophil NADPH oxidase complex (e.g., mutations in CYBA, CYBB, NCF, RAC1, and RAC2). Approximately 40 % of CGD patients develop IBD-like symptoms [26]. Such clinical observations suggest that CGD-associated IBD could represent a failure to resolve acute mucosal insults. These findings have given rise to significant interest in developing therapies around the concept of hypoxia-associated metabolism and HIF expression in the mucosa [27].

Epithelial Antimicrobial Defense and Innate Immunity

The mammalian gastrointestinal tract is home to trillions of bacteria. A finely regulated commensal relationship exists within the intestinal mucosa, where microbes, essential for host health, can also initiate and perpetuate mucosal disease [28]. As part of their contribution to overall innate immunity, IEC actively defend the mucosa through the production of antimicrobial peptides. As an example, actively produce defensins, a prominent class of antimicrobial peptides which are cationic, cysteine-rich, and possess broad antimicrobial activity [29, 30]. Defensins are classified as α- or β-defensins based on structural differences in cysteine bond pairing [31]. Crohn's disease patients have been shown to express defects in α-defensin 5 and α-defensin 6 from Paneth cells of the small intestine [31]. The nature of this defect is not completely understood but is thought to relate to defects in the Nod2 and Atg16l1 genes. Up to 35 % of Crohn's disease patients carry a mutation in NOD2 and correlates with defective secretion of defensins [31], which may contribute to the dysbiosis observed in some IBD patients.

Human β defensin-1 (hBD1) is notable within the IEC that it is constitutively secreted, whereas others are induced by inflammatory mediators [32, 33]. Constitutive expression of hBD1 was recently shown to depend on the tissue microenvironment (e.g., low oxygen levels found in the colon) [34]. Another distinguishing feature of hBD1 is that the full spectrum of its antimicrobial activity is only revealed when its disulfide bonds are reduced [35]. Reduction of the hBD1 disulfide bonds is accomplished by thioredoxin that localizes with hBD1 in the colonic mucus; oxidation of hBD1 is prevented by the low pO_2 environment of the lumen [36].

Among the other innate antimicrobial defense molecules expressed by IEC is bactericidal permeability-increasing protein (BPI), originally found in neutrophil and eosinophil granules [37]. Subsequently, BPI was found to be expressed in IEC [38]. Based on an original transcriptional profiling approach to identify lipid-mediator regulation of mucosal inflammation, BPI was found to be expressed in both human and murine epithelial cells of wide origin (oral, pulmonary, and gastrointestinal mucosa). Additional studies in human and murine tissue ex vivo revealed that BPI is diffusely expressed along the crypt-villous axis [38, 39], and that epithelial BPI protein levels decrease along the length of the intestine [40]. As its name infers, BPI selectively exerts multiple antimicrobial actions against gram-negative bacteria, including cytotoxicity through damage to bacterial inner/outer membranes, neutralization of bacterial lipopolysaccharide (endotoxin), as well as functioning as an opsonin for phagocytosis of gram-negative bacteria by neutrophils [41, 42]. The high affinity of BPI for the lipid A region of LPS [43] targets its cytotoxic activity to gram-negative bacteria. Binding of BPI to the gram-negative bacterial outer membrane is followed by a time-dependent penetration of the molecule to the bacterial inner membrane where damage results in loss of membrane integrity, dissipation of electrochemical gradients, and bacterial death [44]. BPI binds the lipid A region of LPS with high affinity [45, 46] and thereby prevents its interaction with other (pro-inflammatory) LPS-binding molecules, including LBP and CD14 [47]. Since BPI binds the lipid A region common to all LPS, it is able to neutralize endotoxin from a broad array of gram-negative pathogens [42].

Intestinal alkaline phosphatase (ALPI) represents another recently appreciated antimicrobial molecule expressed on apical (luminal) aspect of IEC [48]. In the past, this molecule was viewed as one of the better epithelial differentiation markers, with little understanding of the true function of this molecule in the mucosa. More recent studies have identified this molecule as a central player in microbial homeostasis [49–51]. Surface expressed ALPI was shown to retard gram-negative bacterial growth and to potently neutralize LPS through a mechanism involving dephosphorylation of 1,4′-bisphosphorylated glucosamine disaccharide of LPS lipid A [50, 51]. This observation was translated to a murine colitis model and revealed that the expression of ALPI strongly correlated with the resolution phase of inflammation. Moreover, inhibition of ALPI activity was shown to increase the severity of colitic disease [52]. Like those defining epithelial expression of BPI [38], these studies provide an example of the critical interface between inflammatory resolution and the importance of epithelial antimicrobial defense mechanisms (see Fig. 11.1).

Intestinal Epithelia and Dysbiosis in IBD

The intestinal microbiota, in addition to aiding in digestion, produce a number of vitamins and benefit the host through the local synthesis of short-chain fatty acids (SCFAs), including butyrate, propionate, and acetate. Butyrate can reach luminal concentrations of 30 mM in the colon and serves as a preferred metabolic substrate for colonic epithelial cells [53]. Butyrate is efficiently absorbed and metabolized by epithelia, and in contrast to other SCFAs, very little butyrate is released into portal circulation [53]. One factor contributing to the preference of the colonic epithelium for butyrate is that butyrate stimulates expression of pyruvate dehydrogenase kinases, which inhibit the pyruvate dehydrogenase complex [54]. This inhibition prevents conversion of glucose-derived pyruvate to acetyl-CoA. Yet, because formation of acetyl-CoA from butyrate is not dependent on pyruvate dehydrogenase, butyrate-derived acetyl-CoA is available for oxidative phosphorylation. Significant literature supports an immunological homeostatic role for SCFA in the distal gut [53, 55]. For example, the protection elicited by fiber and resistant starch in experimental colitis are thought to depend on SCFA production [56–58], and administration of exogenous butyrate promotes resistance to experimental colitis [59, 60]. Recent studies investigating dysbiosis in inflammatory bowel disease identified lower concentrations of luminal butyrate and reduced abundance of butyrate-producing organisms (e.g., certain *Roseburia* and *Faecalibacterium* species) with disease [61–63]. The importance of butyrate as the preferred epithelial substrate has been highlighted by demonstration that pharmacologic inhibition of β-oxidation induces colitis [64] and that mice with mitochondrial polymorphisms that maintain increased oxidative phosphorylation activity are resistant to colitis [65]. Several trials have evaluated the efficacy of butyrate in the treatment of human disease, primarily ulcerative colitis, with mixed results [53].

The intestinal microbiota shifts in fundamental ways during inflammation. It remains unclear exactly what these shifts in the microbiota might mean to tissue and immune function [66]. Microbial signals, such as those delivered by a mix of *Clostridia* species, induce mucosal tolerance by promoting the formation of regulatory T cells [67]. Moreover, studies have implicated SCFAs as critical products of tolerogenic *Clostridia* species [68]. In addition to functioning as a direct energy source, SCFAs can signal through a series of G-protein coupled receptors (GPR) to mediate their biological functions [69, 70]. In mice, deletion of *Gpr41* and *Gpr43* mediate protective immunity in inflammatory models [69, 70]. Also notable is the observation that treatment of mice with the SCFA propionate promotes colonic protection during inflammation [70] and that the major butyrate receptor (GPR109a) functions to suppress colonic carcinogenesis and inflammation [71]. Such studies clearly implicate that targeting SCFA and SCFA receptors/transporters as promising strategies for the development of new lines of treatment for IBD.

Conclusions

Multiple lines of evidence now support the concept that epithelial cells function as an integral part of the innate immune system (see Fig. 11.1). The intimate interactions between epithelial cells and the various components of the immune system contribute fundamentally to maintenance of health in the gut but also to the development of both acute and chronic inflammatory diseases, most particularly IBD. A further understanding of the genetic links to the luminal triggers associated with IBD will go far in developing effective therapies that enhance epithelial innate immune responses.

Acknowledgments This work was supported by NIH grants DK50189/DK104713/DK095491/DK103639, VA Merit Award 1I01BX002182 and by the Crohn's and Colitis Foundation of America.

The authors declare no financial interests in any of the work submitted here.

References

1. Hershberg RM, Mayer LF. Antigen processing and presentation by intestinal epithelial cells—polarity and complexity. Immunol Today. 2000;21:123–8.
2. Turner JR. Intestinal mucosal barrier function in health and disease. Nat Rev Immunol. 2009;9(11):799–809.
3. Koch S, Nusrat A. The life and death of epithelia during inflammation: lessons learned from the gut. Annu Rev Pathol. 2012;7:35–60.
4. Madara JL, Stafford J. Interferon-gamma directly affects barrier function of cultured intestinal epithelial monolayers. J Clin Invest. 1989;83:724–7.
5. Colgan SP, Parkos CA, Matthews JB, D'Andrea L, Awtrey CS, Lichtman A, et al. Interferon-γ induces a surface phenotype switch in intestinal epithelia: downregulation of ion transport and upregulation of immune accessory ligands. Am J Physiol. 1994;267:C402–10.
6. Quiding M, Nordstrom I, Kilander A, Andersson G, Hanson LA, Holmgren J, et al. Intestinal immune responses in humans: oral cholera vaccination induces strong intestinal antibody responses and interferon-gamma production and evokes local immunological memory. J Clin Invest. 1991;88:143–8.
7. Mayer L, Eisenhardt D, Salomon P, Bauer W, Plous R, Piccinini L. Expression of class II molecules on intestinal epithelial cells in humans: differences between normal and inflammatory bowel disease. Gastroenterology. 1991;100:3–12.
8. Mayer L, Panja A, Li Y, Siden E, Pizzimenti A, Gerardi F, et al. Unique features of antigen presentation in the intestine. Ann N Y Acad Sci. 1992;664:39–46.
9. Kagnoff MF. The intestinal epithelium is an integral component of a communications network. J Clin Invest. 2014;124(7):2841–3.
10. Pasparakis M. Role of NF-kappaB in epithelial biology. Immunol Rev. 2012;246(1):346–58. doi:10.1111/j.600-065X.2012.01109.x.
11. Borm ME, van Bodegraven AA, Mulder CJ, Kraal G, Bouma G. A NFKB1 promoter polymorphism is involved in susceptibility to ulcerative colitis. Int J Immunogenet. 2005;32(6):401–5.
12. Pasparakis M. IKK/NF-kappaB signaling in intestinal epithelial cells controls immune homeostasis in the gut. Mucosal Immunol. 2008;1 Suppl 1:S54–7. doi:10.1038/mi.2008.53.
13. Iwasaki A, Medzhitov R. Control of adaptive immunity by the innate immune system. Nat Immunol. 2015;16(4):343–53.
14. Abreu MT. Toll-like receptor signalling in the intestinal epithelium: how bacterial recognition shapes intestinal function. Nat Rev Immunol. 2010;10(2):131–44.
15. Salomon P, Pizzimenti A, Panja A, Reisman A, Mayer L. The expression and regulation of class II antigens in normal and inflammatory bowel disease peripheral blood monocytes and intestinal epithelium. Autoimmunity. 1991;9(2):141–9.
16. Nakazawa A, Dotan I, Brimnes J, Allez M, Shao L, Tsushima F, et al. The expression and function of costimulatory molecules B7H and B7-H1 on colonic epithelial cells. Gastroenterology. 2004;126(5):1347–57.
17. Bleicher PA, Balk SP, Hagen SJ, Blumberg RS, Flotte TJ, Terhorst C. Expression of murine CD1 on gastrointestinal epithelium. Science. 1990;250:679–82.
18. Colgan SP, Hershberg RM, Furuta GT, Blumberg RS. Ligation of intestinal epithelial CD1d induces bioactive IL-10: critical role of the cytoplasmic tail in autocrine signaling. Proc Natl Acad Sci U S A. 1999;96:13938–43.
19. Kominsky DJ, Campbell EL, Ehrentraut SF, Wilson KE, Kelly CJ, Glover LE, et al. IFN-gamma-mediated induction of an apical IL-10 receptor on polarized intestinal epithelia. J Immunol. 2014;192(3):1267–76.
20. Olszak T, Neves JF, Dowds CM, Baker K, Glickman J, Davidson NO, et al. Protective mucosal immunity mediated by epithelial CD1d and IL-10. Nature. 2014;509(7501):497–502. doi:10.1038/nature13150. Epub 2014 Apr 6.
21. Perera L, Shao L, Patel A, Evans K, Meresse B, Blumberg R, et al. Expression of nonclassical class I molecules by intestinal epithelial cells. Inflamm Bowel Dis. 2007;13(3):298–307.
22. Chin AC, Parkos CA. Pathobiology of neutrophil transepithelial migration: implications in mediating epithelial injury. Annu Rev Pathol. 2007;2:111–43.
23. Voisin MB, Nourshargh S. Neutrophil transmigration: emergence of an adhesive cascade within venular walls. J Innate Immun. 2013;5(4):336–47. doi:10.1159/000346659. Epub 2013 Mar 2.
24. Campbell EL, Bruyninckx WJ, Kelly CJ, Glover LE, McNamee EN, Bowers BE, et al. Transmigrating neutrophils shape the mucosal microenvironment through localized oxygen depletion to influence resolution of inflammation. Immunity. 2014;40(1):66–77.
25. Huang JS, Noack D, Rae J, Ellis BA, Newbury R, Pong AL, et al. Chronic granulomatous disease caused by a deficiency in p47(phox) mimicking Crohn's disease. Clin Gastroenterol Hepatol. 2004;2(8):690–5.
26. Werlin SL, Chusid MJ, Caya J, Oechler HW. Colitis in chronic granulomatous disease. Gastroenterology. 1982;82(2):328–31.
27. Eltzschig HK, Bratton DL, Colgan SP. Targeting hypoxia signalling for the treatment of ischaemic and inflammatory diseases. Nat Rev Drug Discov. 2014;13(11):852–69.
28. Lozupone CA, Stombaugh JI, Gordon JI, Jansson JK, Knight R. Diversity, stability and resilience of the human gut microbiota. Nature. 2012;489(7415):220–30.
29. Ganz T. Defensins: antimicrobial peptides of innate immunity. Nat Rev Immunol. 2003;3(9):710–20.
30. Pazgier M, Hoover DM, Yang D, Lu W, Lubkowski J. Human beta-defensins. Cell Mol Life Sci. 2006;63(11):1294–313.

31. Ramasundara M, Leach ST, Lemberg DA, Day AS. Defensins and inflammation: the role of defensins in inflammatory bowel disease. J Gastroenterol Hepatol. 2009;24(2):202–8. doi:10.1111/j.440-746.2008.05772.x.
32. O'Neil DA, Porter EM, Elewaut D, Anderson GM, Eckmann L, Ganz T, et al. Expression and regulation of the human beta-defensins hBD-1 and hBD-2 in intestinal epithelium. J Immunol. 1999;163(12):6718–24.
33. Harder J, Bartels J, Christophers E, Schroder JM. Isolation and characterization of human beta -defensin-3, a novel human inducible peptide antibiotic. J Biol Chem. 2001;276(8):5707–13.
34. Kelly CJ, Glover LE, Campbell EL, Kominsky DJ, Ehrentraut SF, Bowers BE, et al. Fundamental role for HIF-1alpha in constitutive expression of human beta defensin-1. Mucosal Immunol. 2013;6(10):1110–8.
35. Schroeder BO, Wu Z, Nuding S, Groscurth S, Marcinowski M, Beisner J, et al. Reduction of disulphide bonds unmasks potent antimicrobial activity of human beta-defensin 1. Nature. 2011;469(7330):419–23.
36. Jaeger SU, Schroeder BO, Meyer-Hoffert U, Courth L, Fehr SN, Gersemann M, et al. Cell-mediated reduction of human beta-defensin 1: a major role for mucosal thioredoxin. Mucosal Immunol. 2013;6(6):1179–90.
37. Canny G, Levy O. Bactericidal/permeability-increasing protein (BPI) and BPI homologs at mucosal sites. Trends Immunol. 2008;29:541–7.
38. Canny G, Levy O, Furuta GT, Narravula-Alipati S, Sisson RB, Serhan CN, et al. Lipid mediator-induced expression of bactericidal/ permeability- increasing protein (BPI) in human mucosal epithelia. Proc Natl Acad Sci U S A. 2002;99:3902–7.
39. Canny G, Cario E, Lennartsson A, Gullberg U, Brennan C, Levy O, et al. Functional and biochemical characterization of epithelial bactericidal/permeability-increasing protein. Am J Physiol Gastrointest Liver Physiol. 2006;290(3):G557–67.
40. Canny GO, Trifonova RT, Kindelberger DW, Colgan SP, Fichorova RN. Expression and function of bactericidal/permeability-increasing protein in human genital tract epithelial cells. J Infect Dis. 2006;194(4):498–502.
41. Elsbach P, Weiss J. Role of the bactericidal/permeability-increasing protein in host defence. Curr Opin Immunol. 1998;10:45–9.
42. Levy O. A neutrophil-derived anti-infective molecule: bactericidal/ permeability- increasing protein. Antimicrob Agents Chemother. 2000;44:2925–31.
43. Gazzano-Santoro H, Parent JB, Grinna L, Horwitz A, Parsons T, Theofan G, et al. High-affinity binding of the bactericidal/ permeability-increasing protein and a recombinant amino-terminal fragment to the lipid A region of lipopolysaccharide. Infect Immun. 1992;60(11):4754–61.
44. Mannion BA, Weiss J, Elsbach P. Separation of sublethal and lethal effects of the bactericidal/permeability increasing protein on Escherichia coli. J Clin Invest. 1990;85(3):853–60.
45. Levy O, Ooi CE, Elsbach P, Doerfler ME, Lehrer RI, Weiss J. Antibacterial proteins of granulocytes differ in interaction with endotoxin. Comparison of bactericidal/permeability-increasing protein, p15s, and defensins. J Immunol. 1995;154(10):5403–10.
46. Ulevitch RJ, Tobias PS. Recognition of gram-negative bacteria and endotoxin by the innate immune system. Curr Opin Immunol. 1999;11(1):19–22.
47. Gazzano-Santoro H, Meszaros K, Birr C, Carroll SF, Theofan G, Horwitz AH, et al. Competition between rBPI23, a recombinant fragment of bactericidal/permeability-increasing protein, and lipopolysaccharide (LPS)-binding protein for binding to LPS and gram-negative bacteria. Infect Immun. 1994;62(4):1185–91.
48. Vaishnava S, Hooper LV. Alkaline phosphatase: keeping the peace at the gut epithelial surface. Cell Host Microbe. 2007;2(6):365–7.
49. Goldberg RF, Austen Jr WG, Zhang X, Munene G, Mostafa G, Biswas S, et al. Intestinal alkaline phosphatase is a gut mucosal defense factor maintained by enteral nutrition. Proc Natl Acad Sci U S A. 2008;105(9):3551–6.
50. Mata-Haro V, Cekic C, Martin M, Chilton PM, Casella CR, Mitchell TC. The vaccine adjuvant monophosphoryl lipid A as a TRIF-biased agonist of TLR4. Science. 2007;316(5831):1628–32.
51. Moyle PM, Toth I. Self-adjuvanting lipopeptide vaccines. Curr Med Chem. 2008;15(5):506–16.
52. Campbell EL, MacManus CF, Kominsky DJ, Keely S, Glover LE, Bowers BE, et al. Resolvin E1-induced intestinal alkaline phosphatase promotes resolution of inflammation through LPS detoxification. Proc Natl Acad Sci U S A. 2010;107(32):14298–303.
53. Hamer HM, Jonkers D, Venema K, Vanhoutvin S, Troost FJ, Brummer RJ. Review article: the role of butyrate on colonic function. Aliment Pharmacol Ther. 2008;27(2):104–19. Epub 2007 Oct 25.
54. Blouin JM, Penot G, Collinet M, Nacfer M, Forest C, Laurent-Puig P, et al. Butyrate elicits a metabolic switch in human colon cancer cells by targeting the pyruvate dehydrogenase complex. Int J Cancer. 2011;128(11):2591–601.
55. Ploger S, Stumpff F, Penner GB, Schulzke JD, Gabel G, Martens H, et al. Microbial butyrate and its role for barrier function in the gastrointestinal tract. Ann N Y Acad Sci. 2012;1258:52–9.
56. Ito H, Tanabe H, Kawagishi H, Tadashi W, Yasuhiko T, Sugiyama K, et al. Short-chain inulin-like fructans reduce endotoxin and bacterial translocations and attenuate development of TNBS-induced colitis in rats. Dig Dis Sci. 2009;54(10):2100–8.
57. Morita T, Tanabe H, Sugiyama K, Kasaoka S, Kiriyama S. Dietary resistant starch alters the characteristics of colonic mucosa and exerts a protective effect on trinitrobenzene sulfonic acid-induced colitis in rats. Biosci Biotechnol Biochem. 2004;68(10):2155–64.
58. Videla S, Vilaseca J, Antolin M, Garcia-Lafuente A, Guarner F, Crespo E, et al. Dietary inulin improves distal colitis induced by dextran sodium sulfate in the rat. Am J Gastroenterol. 2001;96(5):1486–93.
59. Cresci G, Nagy LE, Ganapathy V. Lactobacillus GG and tributyrin supplementation reduce antibiotic-induced intestinal injury. JPEN J Parenter Enteral Nutr. 2013;37(6):763–74.
60. Leonel AJ, Teixeira LG, Oliveira RP, Santiago AF, Batista NV, Ferreira TR, et al. Antioxidative and immunomodulatory effects of tributyrin supplementation on experimental colitis. Br J Nutr. 2013;109(8):1396–407.
61. Machiels K, Joossens M, Sabino J, De Preter V, Arijs I, Eeckhaut V, et al. A decrease of the butyrate-producing species Roseburia hominis and Faecalibacterium prausnitzii defines dysbiosis in patients with ulcerative colitis. Gut. 2014;63(8):1275–83.
62. Eeckhaut V, Machiels K, Perrier C, Romero C, Maes S, Flahou B, et al. Butyricicoccus pullicaecorum in inflammatory bowel disease. Gut. 2013;62(12):1745–52. doi:10.1136/gutjnl-2012-303611. Epub 2012 Dec 22.
63. Sokol H, Seksik P, Furet JP, Firmesse O, Nion-Larmurier I, Beaugerie L, et al. Low counts of Faecalibacterium prausnitzii in colitis microbiota. Inflamm Bowel Dis. 2009;15(8):1183–9. doi:10.1002/ibd.20903.
64. Roediger WEW, Lawson MJ, Nance SH, Radcliffe BC. Detectable colonic nitrite levels in inflammatory bowel disease—mucosal or bacterial malfunction? Digestion. 1986;35:199–204.
65. Bar F, Bochmann W, Widok A, von Medem K, Pagel R, Hirose M, et al. Mitochondrial gene polymorphisms that protect mice from colitis. Gastroenterology. 2013;145(5):1055–63. e3.
66. Jostins L, Ripke S, Weersma RK, Duerr RH, McGovern DP, Hui KY, et al. Host-microbe interactions have shaped the genetic architecture of inflammatory bowel disease. Nature. 2012; 491(7422):119–24.

67. Atarashi K, Tanoue T, Oshima K, Suda W, Nagano Y, Nishikawa H, et al. Treg induction by a rationally selected mixture of Clostridia strains from the human microbiota. Nature. 2013;500(7461):232–6.
68. Smith PM, Howitt MR, Panikov N, Michaud M, Gallini CA, Bohlooly YM, et al. The microbial metabolites, short-chain fatty acids, regulate colonic Treg cell homeostasis. Science. 2013; 341(6145):569–73.
69. Kim MH, Kang SG, Park JH, Yanagisawa M, Kim CH. Short-chain fatty acids activate GPR41 and GPR43 on intestinal epithelial cells to promote inflammatory responses in mice. Gastroenterology. 2013;145(2):396–406.
70. Maslowski KM, Vieira AT, Ng A, Kranich J, Sierro F, Yu D, et al. Regulation of inflammatory responses by gut microbiota and chemoattractant receptor GPR43. Nature. 2009;461(7268):1282–6.
71. Singh N, Gurav A, Sivaprakasam S, Brady E, Padia R, Shi H, et al. Activation of Gpr109a, receptor for niacin and the commensal metabolite butyrate, suppresses colonic inflammation and carcinogenesis. Immunity. 2014;40(1):128–39.

Autophagy and Endoplasmic Reticulum Stress

12

Arthur Kaser

The two main types of inflammatory bowel disease (IBD), Crohn's disease (CD) and ulcerative colitis (UC), are characterized by pathologic immune activation directed toward the microbial flora, which arises from a complex gene–environment interaction [1]. While major inroads have been made into the genetic underpinning of disease [2], the environmental factors that trigger disease that could explain the dramatic rise in incidence and prevalence of CD and UC, initially in Europe and North America and more recently globally [3], remain entirely unknown.

Numerous innate and adaptive cell types have been demonstrated to have a role in the pathogenesis of IBD [1]. The intestinal epithelium with its specialized cell types has only more recently emerged as an important orchestrator of the mucosal immune response contributing an important homeostatic function, and importantly also providing a pathophysiologic function in the context of IBD. In particular, stress in the endoplasmic reticulum (ER) is commonly observed in the IBD epithelium, irrespective on the presence or absence of local inflammation [4–6]. ER stress arises when misfolded and hence potentially dysfunctional or toxic proteins accumulate in the rough ER [7]. Highly secretory cells are naturally particularly sensitive to ER stress due to stochastically occurring misfolding and the requirement that the cell's folding capacity closely follows its translational output. In response to this type of stress, the Unfolded Protein Response (UPR) is elicited, which is aimed at resolving stress by adapting the translational and protein folding capacity in the ER to increased demands, and by degrading misfolded proteins via ER associated degradation (ERAD) [7].

The UPR is organized along three main branches, each of which is characterized by a pair of an ER transmembrane sensor of misfolded proteins and its downstream transcription factor (IRE1–XBP1, PERK–ATF4, ATF6–ATF6f). In addition to transactivation of their specific target genes, the PERK branch of the UPR also triggers a transient halt in translation via phosphorylation of the elongation initiation factor 2α (eIF2α) [7]. The IRE1–XBP1 branch is the evolutionary most conserved branch. Remarkably, in addition to ubiquitously expressed IRE1α, the intestinal and bronchial epithelium expresses a second isoform of IRE1, IRE1β, possibly hinting toward a particularly important role of this UPR branch at inner body surfaces [8].

It has been demonstrated that genetic deletion of *Xbp1* in intestinal epithelial cells results in ER stress due to a consequent impairment in the cells' capacity to elicit the aforementioned adaptive program [6]. Remarkably, this cell-type specific induction of ER stress causes mild, superficial inflammation that is confined to the small intestine [6]. This is associated with a secretory defect and condensation of the ER in Paneth cells, specialized highly secretory cells at the base of intestinal crypts that are most well known for secreting large amounts of antimicrobial peptides [9]. This type of ER stress-induced small intestinal inflammation has been shown to be dependent on microbial signals as it does not develop in mice re-derived germ-free, and involves IRE1α overactivation and tumor necrosis receptor type 1 (TNFR1) signaling [10].

Importantly, manipulation of further UPR components also affects mucosal homeostasis. Deletion of *Atf6α* or *P58*^{IPK}, the latter an important ER chaperone, results in increased sensitivity to dextran sodium sulfate (DSS)-induced colitis [11], while deletion of *Agr2* (anterior gradient 2), a ER protein disulphide isomerase gene family member, results in spontaneous ileocolitis and aberrant Paneth cell secretory apparatus [12, 13]. Furthermore, deletion of Chop, which is downstream of PERK-eIF2α and involved in mediating a terminal UPR with induction of apoptosis, is protective in DSS colitis [14]. Finally, a forward genetic screen has identified two independent mutations in *Muc2*, the gene encoding the major mucin component, which result in spontaneous colitis development [15]. Misfolding of the large MUC2

A. Kaser (✉)
Division of Gastroenterology and Hepatology, Department of Medicine, Addenbrooke's Hospital, University of Cambridge, Cambridge, UK
e-mail: ak729@cam.ac.uk

D.C. Baumgart (ed.), *Crohn's Disease and Ulcerative Colitis*, DOI 10.1007/978-3-319-33703-6_12

protein has been demonstrated to cause ER stress, and unresolved ER stress is thought to drive the colitis in this model [15]. Altogether, these data demonstrate the close mechanistic relationship between unresolved ER stress and the induction and propagation of intestinal inflammation.

The identification of a coding polymorphism in the autophagy gene *ATG16L1*, which leads to an alanine for threonine substitution at amino acid position 300 (*ATG16L1T300A*), exposed autophagy as a genetically affected mechanism involved in the pathogenesis of CD [16]. Despite its high prevalence in the general population (risk allele frequency in the Caucasian population is 52%), *ATG16L1T300A* is indeed one of the strongest genetic risk factors of CD [2]. Macro-autophagy (herein further referred to as "autophagy") is a fundamental biological process that describes the engulfment of intracellular content in double-layered membranes that form autophagosomes [17]. Autophagosomes fuse with lysosomes prompting the subsequent degradation of their content. Cargo that can be engulfed by autophagosomes includes any type of cytoplasmic content, organelles such as mitochondria ("mitophagy"), infectious agents that have gained cytoplasmic access ("xenophagy"), and macromolecular complexes (e.g., inflammasomes) [17]. Lysosomal degradation of this cargo releases amino acids and other basic building blocks of life, and hence autophagy is a central catabolic process of the cell. Consistent with this, evolutionarily it is thought to have evolved as a response to starvation. The T300A variant is juxtaposed to a caspase-3 cleavage site, rendering the risk variant susceptible to caspase-3-mediated cleavage of ATG16L1. Hence, under conditions of caspase-3 activation, such as during metabolic stress, death receptor signaling, or intracellular infection, ATG16L1 protein is degraded via this mechanism, resulting in hypomorphic autophagy induction in risk variant carriers [18]. *ATG16l1T300A* is amongst the genetic risk factors with the largest effect size in Crohn's disease, and it is indeed notable that the intracellular pattern recognition receptor NOD2, variants of which account for the largest fraction of heritability amongst all genetic loci associated with risk for inflammatory bowel disease (IBD) [2, 19, 20], can physically interact with ATG16L1, and this interaction is reciprocally impaired with *ATG16L1* and *NOD2* risk variants [21, 22]. Indeed it has been demonstrated that NOD2 is involved in induction of xenophagy upon intracellular bacterial infection with for example *Shigella* and *Salmonella* species [21, 22]. Altogether, this implicates two of the strongest genetic risk factors of Crohn's disease involved in autophagy and suggests that their function may be directly related to each other under certain conditions. In addition to *ATG16L1* and *NOD2*, variants of additional genes which encode for proteins involved in autophagy confer risk for IBD. This includes *IRGM* [23], an immunity related GTPase which binds to cardiolipin and induces autophagy via a mechanism that involves mitochondrial fission [24, 25]; *NDP52* [26], a receptor involved in specific autophagy [27]; and *LRRK2*, encoding a protein that acts as a signaling hub, and which also mediates an important regulatory function on autophagy [28]. Altogether, these genetic observations hint toward alterations in autophagy as a major theme in IBD, in particular CD.

Remarkably, hypomorphic function of ATG16L1 [29, 30], NOD2 [31, 32], and LRRK2 [33] is associated with abnormalities in the secretory compartment of Paneth cells, both in murine genetic models and individuals and patients carrying risk alleles. As alluded to above, Paneth cells are specialized intestinal epithelial cells which reside at the base of small intestinal crypts, interspersed with crypt stem cells from which they differentiate and for which they provide the physiological niche [9]. Paneth cells are highly secretory cells with a characteristic elaborate granule network at their apical side that faces the crypt lumen. This granule network contains lysozyme and α-defensins (also known as cryptdins), with granules secreted into the crypt lumen, thereby thought to protect the crypt by keeping this locale sterile [9]. Secretion of antimicrobial peptides by Paneth cells exerts a protective function towards pathogens and profoundly affects the composition of the intestinal microbiota [34, 35]. It has been speculated that alterations in microbial ecology ("dysbiosis") imposed by host genetic alterations affecting Paneth cell function might play an important role in the pathogenesis of Crohn's disease [36]. Indeed, alterations in the microbiota can indeed aggravate models of colitis exogenously induced via DSS [37], and specific constituents of the microbiota have an important role in the maturation and responsiveness of the mucosal (and indeed systemic) immune system [38]. However, since mice rendered genetically deficient or hypomorphic for NOD2 [31], ATG16L1 [29, 30] or LRRK2 [33] function do not develop any form of spontaneous intestinal inflammation, the cause-effect relationship of such microbial alterations for the initiation or propagation of intestinal inflammation remains a critically important, unresolved question. The lack of spontaneous inflammation in these murine models is also an important reminder on the critical importance of—entirely unknown—environmental factors that trigger disease in genetically susceptible individuals. Consistent with this, only 1 in 20 individuals homozygous for the *NOD23020insC* variant does actually develop Crohn's disease [1].

Strikingly, hypomorphic function of ATG16L1 in healthy individuals and patients with CD carrying the *ATG16L1T300A* risk allele [39], or in mice with genetic deletion of *Atg16l1* in the intestinal epithelium [10] is associated with evidence of ER stress at the base of their intestinal crypts in Paneth cells. Conversely, ER stress induced via genetic deletion of *Xbp1* in the intestinal epithelium causes autophagosome formation, again localized to Paneth cells [10]. The mechanism underlying autophagosome formation involves the PERK–eIF2α–ATF4–Chop branch of the UPR [10]. Pharmacological augmentation of autophagosome formation alleviates the superficial type of ileitis emanating from *Xbp1* deletion in the intestinal epithelium, and this protective function is indeed only observable when autophagy function was intact in the intestinal epithelium [10]. Importantly, mice carrying deletions in both *Xbp1* and *Atg16l1* (‘*Atg16l1;Xbp1ΔIEC*’) in their intestinal epithelium spontaneously develop discontinuous, transmural fissuring ulceration in their terminal ileum, which closely resembles the histological presentation of ileal CD [10]. Notably, no inflammation is observed in the colon. Altogether, these data suggest that autophagy serves an important function in relieving ER stress, and in its absence unresolved ER stress can trigger a disease phenotype originating from the epithelium that phenocopies ileal CD. In this context it is also notable that amongst clinical phenotypes, *ATG16L1T300A* is most strongly associated with ileal CD.

The intestinal epithelium and Paneth cells in particular appear particularly sensitive to the perturbations in their capacity to resolve ER stress. Protein folding is an energy-dependent process, profoundly influenced by perturbations in oxygen and nutrient (e.g., glucose) availability, which in itself might make the locale of the intestinal epithelium particularly susceptible. Furthermore, the cell's protein folding capacity needs to strike a fine balance with the translational burden it experiences. A classic example is the transition of an activated B cells to a plasma cells with its associated vast expansion in ER and overall secretory apparatus, which is critically dependent on the UPR, in particular the IRE1-XBP1 branch [40, 41]. Consistent with this notion are also data that demonstrate that infection and immune activation with the associated inherent increase in protein production burden due to activation of transcription factors requires a fully operative UPR [42, 43]. Finally, microbial metabolites have also been shown to directly affect UPR function. It is therefore intriguing to speculate whether environmental factors may play a role as triggers for ER stress in the intestinal epithelium [44]. Remarkably, UPR-associated genes have indeed been identified as associated with genetic risk for developing IBD. Specifically, rare variants of *XBP1* have been associated with both forms of IBD [6], and several other genes (e.g., *ORMDL3*, *LRRK2*) have been prioritized as highly likely causative genes located at established IBD risk loci [2].

While the *Atg16l1;Xbp1ΔIEC* model system alluded to above demonstrates the critical role that autophagy has in restraining ER stress within the intestinal epithelium and hence the close interrelatedness of these fundamental biological mechanisms, it is critical to note that ATG16L1-dependent autophagy fulfills numerous other biological functions within the intestinal epithelium, and importantly also in a variety of other cell types. As an example, ATG16L1 has been demonstrated to have an important role in the xenophagic response [45, 46], and also in the handling of intestinal infections. This function extends to adherent-invasive *Escherichia coli* (AIEC) [47], whose presence has been linked with ileal CD [48]. Impaired ATG16L1 function in myeloid cells leads to increased NLRP3 inflammasome activation with consecutive increased release of IL-1β and IL-18 [49]. Hypomorphic autophagy function has also been associated with perturbed thymic selection [50, 51], and with alterations in T cell receptor synapse formation of dendritic cells [52]. Undoubtedly, germ line variation in *ATG16L1T300A* might very likely involve multiple biological functions beyond restraining ER stress as described above, which contribute to the pathogenesis of CD and the complex immune alterations associated with it.

In conclusion, autophagy and ER stress mechanisms have emerged as important and closely intertwined mechanisms, which can trigger small intestinal inflammation originating from the intestinal epithelium, and in particular Paneth cells, if perturbed. Insight into these mechanisms might open new therapeutic avenues that may be targetable in the context of precision medicine.

References

1. Kaser A, Zeissig S, Blumberg RS. Inflammatory bowel disease. Annu Rev Immunol. 2010;28:573–621.
2. Jostins L, Ripke S, Weersma RK, Duerr RH, McGovern DP, Hui KY. Host-microbe interactions have shaped the genetic architecture of inflammatory bowel disease. Nature. 2012;491:119–24.
3. Molodecky NA et al. Increasing incidence and prevalence of the inflammatory bowel diseases with time, based on systematic review. Gastroenterology. 2012;142:46–54 e42; quiz e30.
4. Treton X et al. Altered endoplasmic reticulum stress affects translation in inactive colon tissue from patients with ulcerative colitis. Gastroenterology. 2011;141:1024–35.
5. Shkoda A et al. Interleukin-10 blocked endoplasmic reticulum stress in intestinal epithelial cells: impact on chronic inflammation. Gastroenterology. 2007;132:190–207.
6. Kaser A et al. XBP1 links ER stress to intestinal inflammation and confers genetic risk for human inflammatory bowel disease. Cell. 2008;134:743–56.
7. Walter P, Ron D. The unfolded protein response: from stress pathway to homeostatic regulation. Science. 2011;334:1081–6.
8. Bertolotti A et al. Increased sensitivity to dextran sodium sulfate colitis in IRE1beta-deficient mice. J Clin Invest. 2001;107:585–93.
9. Clevers HC, Bevins CL. Paneth cells: maestros of the small intestinal crypts. Annu Rev Physiol. 2013;75:289–311.
10. Adolph TE et al. Paneth cells as a site of origin for intestinal inflammation. Nature. 2013;503:272–6.
11. Cao SS et al. The unfolded protein response and chemical chaperones reduce protein misfolding and colitis in mice. Gastroenterology. 2013;144(5):989–1000.e6.
12. Park SW et al. The protein disulfide isomerase AGR2 is essential for production of intestinal mucus. Proc Natl Acad Sci U S A. 2009;106:6950–5.
13. Zhao F et al. Disruption of Paneth and goblet cell homeostasis and increased endoplasmic reticulum stress in Agr2−/− mice. Dev Biol. 2010;338:270–9.

14. Namba T et al. Positive role of CCAAT/enhancer-binding protein homologous protein, a transcription factor involved in the endoplasmic reticulum stress response in the development of colitis. Am J Pathol. 2009;174:1786–98.
15. Heazlewood CK et al. Aberrant mucin assembly in mice causes endoplasmic reticulum stress and spontaneous inflammation resembling ulcerative colitis. PLoS Med. 2008;5:e54.
16. Hampe J et al. A genome-wide association scan of nonsynonymous SNPs identifies a susceptibility variant for Crohn disease in ATG16L1. Nat Genet. 2007;39:207–11.
17. Levine B, Kroemer G. Autophagy in the pathogenesis of disease. Cell. 2008;132:27–42.
18. Murthy A et al. A Crohn's disease variant in Atg16l1 enhances its degradation by caspase 3. Nature. 2014;506:456–62.
19. Hugot JP et al. Association of NOD2 leucine-rich repeat variants with susceptibility to Crohn's disease. Nature. 2001;411:599–603.
20. Ogura Y et al. A frameshift mutation in NOD2 associated with susceptibility to Crohn's disease. Nature. 2001;411:603–6.
21. Travassos LH et al. Nod1 and Nod2 direct autophagy by recruiting ATG16L1 to the plasma membrane at the site of bacterial entry. Nat Immunol. 2010;11:55–62.
22. Homer CR, Richmond AL, Rebert NA, Achkar JP, McDonald C. ATG16L1 and NOD2 interact in an autophagy-dependent antibacterial pathway implicated in Crohn's disease pathogenesis. Gastroenterology. 2010;139:1630–41, 1641 e1631–2.
23. Parkes M et al. Sequence variants in the autophagy gene IRGM and multiple other replicating loci contribute to Crohn's disease susceptibility. Nat Genet. 2007;39:830–2.
24. Singh SB, Davis AS, Taylor GA, Deretic V. Human IRGM induces autophagy to eliminate intracellular mycobacteria. Science. 2006;313:1438–41.
25. Singh SB et al. Human IRGM regulates autophagy and cell-autonomous immunity functions through mitochondria. Nat Cell Biol. 2010;12:1154–65.
26. Ellinghaus D et al. Association between variants of PRDM1 and NDP52 and Crohn's disease, based on exome sequencing and functional studies. Gastroenterology. 2013;145:339–47.
27. Till A et al. Autophagy receptor CALCOCO2/NDP52 takes center stage in Crohn disease. Autophagy. 2013;9:1256–7.
28. Lewis PA, Manzoni C. LRRK2 and human disease: a complicated question or a question of complexes? Sci Signal. 2012;5:pe2.
29. Cadwell K et al. A key role for autophagy and the autophagy gene Atg16l1 in mouse and human intestinal Paneth cells. Nature. 2008;456:259–63.
30. Cadwell K et al. Virus-plus-susceptibility gene interaction determines Crohn's disease gene Atg16L1 phenotypes in intestine. Cell. 2010;141:1135–45.
31. Kobayashi KS et al. Nod2-dependent regulation of innate and adaptive immunity in the intestinal tract. Science. 2005;307:731–4.
32. Wehkamp J et al. Reduced Paneth cell alpha-defensins in ileal Crohn's disease. Proc Natl Acad Sci U S A. 2005;102:18129–34.
33. Zhang Q et al. Commensal bacteria direct selective cargo sorting to promote symbiosis. Nat Immunol. 2015;16:918–26.
34. Bevins CL, Salzman NH. Paneth cells, antimicrobial peptides and maintenance of intestinal homeostasis. Nat Rev Microbiol. 2011;9:356–68.
35. Salzman NH et al. Enteric defensins are essential regulators of intestinal microbial ecology. Nat Immunol. 2010;11:76–83.
36. Hansen J, Gulati A, Sartor RB. The role of mucosal immunity and host genetics in defining intestinal commensal bacteria. Curr Opin Gastroenterol. 2010;26:564–71.
37. Elinav E et al. NLRP6 inflammasome regulates colonic microbial ecology and risk for colitis. Cell. 2011;145:745–57.
38. Ivanov II et al. Induction of intestinal Th17 cells by segmented filamentous bacteria. Cell. 2009;139:485–98.
39. Deuring JJ et al. Genomic ATG16L1 risk allele-restricted Paneth cell ER stress in quiescent Crohn's disease. Gut. 2013;63:1081–91.
40. Reimold AM et al. Plasma cell differentiation requires the transcription factor XBP-1. Nature. 2001;412:300–7.
41. Iwakoshi NN et al. Plasma cell differentiation and the unfolded protein response intersect at the transcription factor XBP-1. Nat Immunol. 2003;4:321–9.
42. Martinon F, Chen X, Lee AH, Glimcher LH. TLR activation of the transcription factor XBP1 regulates innate immune responses in macrophages. Nat Immunol. 2010;11:411–8.
43. Richardson CE, Kooistra T, Kim DH. An essential role for XBP-1 in host protection against immune activation in C. elegans. Nature. 2010;463:1092–5.
44. Kaser A, Adolph TE, Blumberg RS. The unfolded protein response and gastrointestinal disease. Semin Immunopathol. 2013;35:307–19.
45. Marchiando AM et al. A deficiency in the autophagy gene Atg16L1 enhances resistance to enteric bacterial infection. Cell Host Microbe. 2013;14:216–24.
46. Kuballa P, Huett A, Rioux JD, Daly MJ, Xavier RJ. Impaired autophagy of an intracellular pathogen induced by a Crohn's disease associated ATG16L1 variant. PLoS One. 2008;3:e3391.
47. Lapaquette P, Glasser AL, Huett A, Xavier RJ, Darfeuille-Michaud A. Crohn's disease-associated adherent-invasive E. coli are selectively favoured by impaired autophagy to replicate intracellularly. Cell Microbiol. 2010;12:99–113.
48. Darfeuille-Michaud A et al. High prevalence of adherent-invasive Escherichia coli associated with ileal mucosa in Crohn's disease. Gastroenterology. 2004;127:412–21.
49. Saitoh T et al. Loss of the autophagy protein Atg16L1 enhances endotoxin-induced IL-1beta production. Nature. 2008;456:264–8.
50. Schuster C et al. The autoimmunity-associated gene CLEC16A modulates thymic epithelial cell autophagy and alters T cell selection. Immunity. 2015;42:942–52.
51. Nedjic J, Aichinger M, Emmerich J, Mizushima N, Klein L. Autophagy in thymic epithelium shapes the T-cell repertoire and is essential for tolerance. Nature. 2008;455:396–400.
52. Wildenberg ME et al. Autophagy attenuates the adaptive immune response by destabilizing the immunologic synapse. Gastroenterology. 2012;142:1493–503 e1496.

Matrix Metalloproteinases

13

Paolo Biancheri and Thomas T. MacDonald

Abbreviations

ADAM	A Disintegrin and A Metalloproteinase-containing protease
CD	Crohn's disease
DSS	dextran sodium sulfate
ECM	extracellular matrix
IBD	inflammatory bowel disease
Ig	immunoglobulin
IL	interleukin
JAM-A	junctional adhesion molecule-A
MMP	matrix metalloproteinase
MT	membrane-bound
PGP	proline–glycine–proline
TIMP	tissue inhibitor of metalloproteinases
TNBS	trinitrobenzene sulfonic acid
TNF	tumor necrosis factor
UC	ulcerative colitis

Introduction

Matrix metalloproteinases (MMPs) belong to the protease superfamily of metzincins, which also includes snake venom MMPs and the adamalysins, also known as A Disintegrin and A Metalloproteinase-containing proteases (ADAMs) [1]. MMPs are structurally related, as they contain a catalytic domain with a highly conserved zinc-binding sequence essential for their action, and a pro-domain, which maintains the enzyme in inactive form and is cleaved by trypsin, plasmin, plasminogen or active MMPs during the activation process [2]. MMPs can collectively degrade all extracellular matrix (ECM) components [3] and, according to their main substrates, have been traditionally classified as collagenases, such as MMP-1 (collagenase 1), MMP-8 (collagenase 2) and MMP-13 (collagenase 3); gelatinases, including MMP-2 (gelatinase A) and MMP-9 (gelatinase B); stromelysins, such as MMP-3 (stromelysin 1), MMP-10 (stromelysin 2) and MMP-11; matrilysins, including MMP-7 and MMP-26; macrophage metalloelastase (MMP-12) [4]. The majority of MMPs are released into the ECM, whereas membrane-bound (MT)-MMPs are activated intracellularly by furin and subsequently anchored to the cell surface by a transmembrane domain [5]. MMPs can be produced by most immune and non immune cells, including macrophages, neutrophils, T cells, mast cells, epithelial cells, and mesenchymal cells [6]. Similar to MT-MMPs, ADAMs are transmembrane metalloproteinases, and are centrally implicated in ectodomain shedding of molecules such as cytokines, cytokine receptors and growth factors [7]. In inflammatoryss bowel disease (IBD) there is a marked upregulation of mucosal MMPs and other proteolytic enzymes [6]. MMPs contribute to mucosal lesions in IBD not only by their broad tissue-degrading actions on ECM substrates, but also by their recently investigated specific effects on non-matrix substrates, such as intercellular junctions, cytokines/chemokines and therapeutic antibodies (Table 13.1).

The Diverse Range of MMP Substrates and Targets

ECM Components

In physiological conditions, controlled expression of MMPs plays a central role in ECM turnover and wound healing after injury. In this setting, MMPs exert their actions on different constituents of the ECM, thereby regulating key pathways of tissue repair, such as re-epithelization and

P. Biancheri, M.D., Ph.D.
T.T. MacDonald, Ph.D., F.R.C.Path., F.Med.Sci. (✉)
Centre for Immunobiology, Barts and The London School of Medicine and Dentistry, Queen Mary University of London, London E1 2AT, UK
e-mail: t.t.macdonald@qmul.ac.uk

D.C. Baumgart (ed.), *Crohn's Disease and Ulcerative Colitis*, DOI 10.1007/978-3-319-33703-6_13

Table 13.1 Substrates and targets of MMP action

Type of substrate/target	Molecule/species	MMPs	Effect
ECM components	Collagen I–IV	MMP-1, MMP-3, MMP-7, MMP-8, MMP-10, MMP-12, MMP-13, MT1-MMP	Degradation
	Collagen V	MMP-1, MMP-3, MMP-8, MMP-13	Degradation
	Collagen IX	MMP-1, MMP-3, MMP-8, MMP-13	Degradation
	Collagen X	MMP-3	Degradation
	Elastin	MMP-2, MMP-7, MMP-12	Degradation
	Laminin	MMP-2, MMP-3, MMP-7, MMP-9, MMP-10, MMP-12	Degradation
	Fibronectin	MMP-2, MMP-3, MMP-7, MMP-10, MMP-12, MT-MMP-1	Degradation
	Gelatin	MMP-2, MMP-9, MMP-10, MMP-13, MT1-MMP	Degradation
	Proteoglycan	MMP-3, MMP-7, MMP-10	Degradation
	Chondroitin sulfate	MMP-12	Degradation
	Aggrecan	MMP-2, MT1-MMP	Degradation
Intercellular junction proteins	E-cadherin	MMP-7, enterotoxin, gelatinase E	Degradation
Cytokines/chemokines	Pro-IL-1β	MMP-2, MMP-3, MMP-9	Activation (by cleavage)
	IL-1β	MMP-3	Inactivation (by cleavage)
	mTNF-α	MMP-7, MMP-12, MMP-13	Conversion into soluble TNF-α
	CXCL5/CXCL6	MMP-8	Activation (by cleavage)
	CXCL8 (IL-8)	MMP-9	Activation (by cleavage)
	CCCL7	MMP-2	Inactivation (by cleavage)
	CXCL1	MMP-7	Generation of a chemotactic gradient by cleavage of CXCL1 ligand syndecan-1
Antibodies	IgG_1	MMP-3, MMP-7, MMP-12	Cleavage
Bacteria	*Staphylococcus aureus*	MMP-12	Inhibition
	Escherichia coli	MMP-12	Inhibition
	Citrobacter rodentium	MMP-3	Increased clearance via regulation of T cell migration

CCCL7 CC-chemokine ligand, *CXCL* CXC-chemokine ligand, *ECM* extracellular matrix, *Ig* immunoglobulin, *IL* interleukin, *MMP* matrix metalloproteinase, *MT* membrane-bound, *m* transmembrane, *TNF* tumor necrosis factor

angiogenesis. In particular, MMP-1, MMP-7, and MMP-10 modulate enterocyte migration and re-epithelialization through their action on collagens I–V, elastin, laminin, and fibronectin. MMP-3, produced by subepithelial myofibroblasts, degrades laminin and collagens IV, V, IX, and X, and is centrally involved in scar formation and consequent tissue remodeling [8]. On the other hand, increased levels of MMPs—such as MMP-1, MMP-2, MMP-3, MMP-8, MMP-9, MMP-10, MMP-12, and MT1-MMP—can degrade ECM components such as the collagen subtypes, fibronectin, gelatin, proteoglycans, laminin, elastin, chondroitin sulfate, and aggrecan and plays a central role in tissue injury during inflammation [9].

Intercellular Junction Proteins

MMPs and other extracellular or transmembrane proteases play a central role in the regulation of mucosal barrier functions by exerting specific effects on intercellular junction proteins. MMP-7, *Bacteroides fragilis* enterotoxin and *Enterococcus faecalis* gelatinase E can degrade the epithelial adherens junction protein E-cadherin [10–12]. Interestingly, the transmembrane proteases matriptase and ADAM19 co-localize respectively with E-cadherin in the apical junctional complex and with zonula occludens-1, a tight junction-associated protein, on epithelial cell membrane; knockdown of matriptase results in claudin-2 overexpression and an increase in epithelial permeability [13–15]. Addition of mast cell tryptase (a serine protease) to gut epithelial cell lines results in a marked decrease in expression of junctional adhesional molecule-A (JAM-A), claudin-1, and zonula occludens-1 and a substantial reduction in epithelial permeability [16].

Cytokines/Chemokines

It is becoming increasingly clear that MMPs exert an important influence on the mucosal immune response by specifically cleaving cytokines and chemokines. MMP-7, MMP-12, and MMP-13 can cleave and convert transmembrane tumor necrosis factor (TNF)-α into soluble TNF-α [17]. MMP-2,

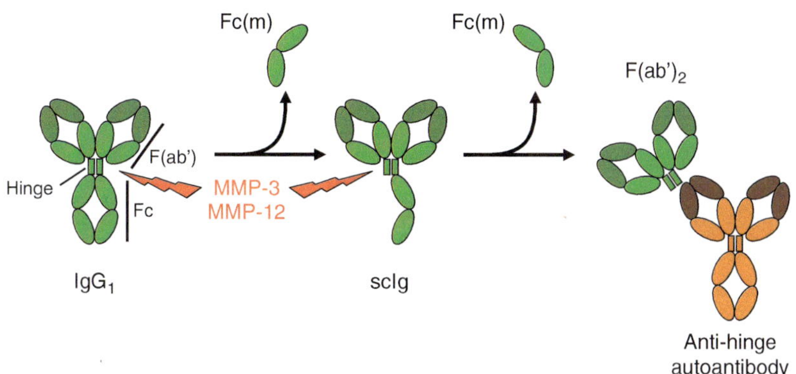

Fig. 13.1 Sequential proteolytic cleavage of IgG_1 by MMP-3 and MMP-12 promotes the development of anti-hinge autoantibodies. Several MMPs can cleave human IgG_1 near the hinge region, thereby exposing immunogenic amino acid sequences. In particular, human IgG_1 have a Pro-Glu scissile bond in the lower hinge susceptible to cleavage by MMP-3 and MMP-12, which act in a sequential manner by removing first a single chain 32 kDa Fc monomer (Fc(m)), with the formation of a single-cleaved intermediate (sc)Ig. Subsequently, MMP-3 and MMP-12 cleave the second single chain Fc(m), with the formation of a $F(ab')_2$. The exposure of the resulting neo-epitope on the hinge region promotes the formation of anti-hinge autoantibodies, which may be relevant in the mucosal immune response in the context of upregulated MMP expression such as in IBD

MMP-3, and MMP-9 activate pro-interleukin (IL)-1β; however, MMP-3 can also inactivate the mature form of IL-1β [18, 19]. MMP-8 and MMP-9 activate by cleavage the chemokines CXCL5/CXCL6 and CXCL8 (IL-8) respectively, thereby promoting leukocyte recruitment at the site of damage, whereas MMP-2 degrades and inactivates CC-chemokine ligands [20]. Finally, MMP-7 can generate a chemotactic gradient by cleaving from the epithelial cell surface the proteoglycan syndecan-1, the ligand for the neutrophil chemoattractant CXCL1 [21].

Antibodies

Several MMPs can clip human immunoglobulin $(Ig)G_1$ in the hinge region, releasing single-chain Fc monomers. As a result of MMP action, IgG_1 can therefore become a single-cleaved intermediate with a single heavy chain or a $F(ab')_2$ when both the chains forming the Fc are cleaved (Fig. 13.1) [22]. In particular, MMP-3 and MMP-12 clip IgG_1 at the same point on the lower hinge, next to the MMP-7 cleavage site, and there is a Thr-His neutrophil elastase cleavage site in the upper hinge of IgG_1 [23]. We have recently shown that MMP-3 and MMP-12 can differentially cleave TNF-α neutralizing agents, and this mechanism may contribute to lack of response to biologic treatment [24]. In particular when etanercept, a TNF-α receptor-IgG Fc fusion protein is cleaved with MMPs, it loses its ability to neutralize TNF-α [24].

Bacteria

Specific intestinal MMPs can exert direct or indirect bactericidal properties. In particular, MMP-12 has a direct inhibitory effect on *Staphylococcus aureus* and *Escherichia coli* [25], whereas MMP-7 promotes bacterial killing by activating α-defensins within Paneth cells [26]. Clearance of *Citrobacter rodentium* is delayed in MMP-$3^{-/-}$ mice due to impaired migration of $CD4^+$ cells in the lamina propria [27]. Interestingly, the acidic protease cathepsin K has potent antimicrobial activity, and it has been shown that cathepsin K null mice are more prone to developing dextran sodium sulfate (DSS) colitis, whereas intrarectal cathepsin K administration improves DSS colitis [28].

Role of MMPs in IBD

In the normal intestinal mucosa, various pathways, including inhibition of MMP activity by the four tissue inhibitors of metalloproteinases (TIMP1-4) and differential transcription, activation, and substrate availability, maintain MMP activity in a tightly regulated balance, necessary for physiological tissue renewal [4]. The balance between tissue levels of MMPs and their inhibitors is a major determinant in the formation of ulcers in the gut. Excessive immune activity and increased cytokine concentrations drive epithelial injury and mucosal lesions in ulcerative colitis (UC) and the transmural lesions in Crohn's disease (CD) [29, 30]. Dysregulation of MMP expression and activity in IBD mucosa has been repeatedly and consistently reported in several studies [8]. MMP-1, MMP-2, MMP-3, MMP-7, MMP-8, MMP-9, MMP-10, MMP-12, MMP-13, and MT1-MMP are all upregulated in IBD inflamed mucosa [8, 9]. Overexpressed epithelial-derived MMP-7 can disrupt the gut mucosal barrier, and a similar effect is exerted by MMP-9. The latter is normally produced at very low levels by macrophages and neutrophils, whereas in intestinal inflammation epithelial cells produce high amounts of MMP-9 levels, which correlate with disease activity in IBD [9, 31]. MMP-1, MMP-3,

MMP-12, and MMP-13, produced by stromal and immune cells in the lamina propria, are highly expressed in the proximity of intestinal ulcers in IBD [32–34]. Interestingly, in IBD high levels of MMP-3 are also produced by long-lived lamina propria IgG plasma cells [35]. Elastinolytic activity is higher in biopsies from patients with IBD compared to control subjects, suggesting that the serine protease neutrophil elastase may play an important role in tissue degradation particularly in inflamed UC mucosa, where there is abundant infiltration by neutrophils [36]. Unexpectedly, MMP-28 (epilysin) is reduced in the inflamed mucosa of UC patients, possibly as epithelial cells are the main cellular source of MMP-28 [37], however the substrates of MMP-28 are still not clear. The trypsin-like transmembrane serine protease matriptase, that is expressed in the apical junctional complex of epithelial cells and plays a central role in maintaining the integrity of the gut barrier, is also reduced in IBD mucosa [38]. There is however considerable heterogeneity in the MMP mucosal expression profile in different IBD patients, which requires further investigation.

The contribution of MMP upregulation to the induction of gut lesions in IBD has been studied in various experimental models. Culture of human fetal gut explants with nanomolar concentrations of recombinant human MMP-3 causes tissue destruction in 24 h, and can be prevented by the addition of an MMP-3 inhibitor to the culture [39]. Most pro-inflammatory cytokines centrally involved in IBD pathogenesis have an important influence on MMP and TIMP expression. For instance, IL-1β, IL-17A, and TNF-α induce an increase in MMP-3 and MMP-12 expression, but also TIMP-1 expression by intestinal myofibroblasts cultured in vitro [40, 41]. The study of MMP knockout mice has provided useful insights into the in vivo effect of MMPs in intestinal inflammation. While deletion of MMP-9 protects mice from DSS- and trinitrobenzene sulfonic acid (TNBS)-induced colitis, MMP-2 and MMP-10 knockout mice are more susceptible to DSS colitis [42–44]. This suggests that different MMPs may have opposite effects on the gut barrier and on tissue disruption in intestinal inflammation. Recently, it has been shown that the combined action of MMP-8, MMP-9 and prolyl-endopeptidase generates collagen cleavage products, such as the tripeptide proline–glycine–proline (PGP) and its acetylated form N-acetyl-PGP, with chemoattractive effects on neutrophils, and that PGP is increased in IBD mucosa [45]. Of note, TIMP-3, the endogenous inhibitor of ADAM17, also known as TNF-α converting enzyme due to its ability to cleave transmembrane TNF-α into soluble TNF-α, is downregulated in CD mucosa, resulting in increased ADAM17 activity and increased TNF-α shedding from the cell membrane [46].

While intestinal lesions are limited to the mucosa in UC, repeated cycles of tissue damage and abnormal repair in CD may be accompanied by the development of transmural complications such as fistulae and/or fibrotic strictures. Both these lesions are characterized by aberrant ECM turnover and dysregulated MMP expression. In particular, MMP-2, MMP-3, and MMP-9 are highly overexpressed in CD fistulae [47], whereas MMP-3 and MMP-12 are downregulated in the mucosa overlying intestinal strictures in CD [48]. Additionally, blocking the pro-fibrotic cytokine transforming growth factor (TGF)-β increases MMP-12 production by intestinal myofibroblasts [48].

The central involvement of MMPs in IBD points to this class of proteolytic enzymes as a potentially attractive therapeutic target. Indeed, broad-spectrum MMP inhibitors, such as marimastat and batimastat, ameliorate DSS colitis [8], however lack of selective compounds, together with probable toxicity due to the ubiquitous expression and the important physiological functions of MMPs, limit targeting MMPs to treat intestinal inflammation. More interestingly, selective neutralization of MMP-9 using a monoclonal antibody has been shown to effectively reduce the severity of DSS colitis [49], and recently a humanized anti-MMP-9 monoclonal antibody has entered a phase I clinical trial in UC [50]. Finally, the adamalysin ADAM17 has traditionally been considered as an inappropriate target because of its wide range of substrates and the fact that most mutant null mice die before or soon after birth. However, humans are more resilient than mice, and the identification of an adult individual who is a functional ADAM17 knockout suggests that this protease should be reexamined as a therapeutic target in chronic inflammatory conditions [51].

Use of MMPs as Biomarkers in IBD

Since MMPs are consistently upregulated in IBD inflamed mucosa, measurement of fecal and serum levels of MMPs has been recently explored as a noninvasive diagnostic tool for IBD. Fecal MMP-9 is upregulated and correlates with fecal calprotectin in UC, and has shown promising potential to separate IBD from non-IBD patients in a pediatric population [52, 53]. More recently, a prospective study in adult IBD showed that fecal MMP-9 correlates with fecal calprotectin and endoscopic activity in UC and pouchitis, but not in CD [54]. The EMBARK study [55], which analyzed various different biomarkers in IBD, showed that active intestinal inflammation is associated most strongly with increased serum MMP-9 and fecal calprotectin for UC, and with raised serum MMP-9, serum IL-22, and fecal calprotectin for CD. Also serum levels of MMP degradation products may be promising biomarkers in IBD. In particular, fragments of MMP-degraded vimentin and type III collagen are elevated in IBD and have shown potential to discriminate UC patients from CD patients and control subjects [56]. In addition to degrading ECM components and therapeutic antibodies,

MMPs can also cleave endogenous IgG_1. The consequent exposure of the hinge region on cleaved IgG is immunogenic and leads to the formation of anti-hinge autoantibodies [57]. In our pilot study on a small cohort of patients, we observed that patients with active IBD and IBD patients who do not respond to biologic therapy have higher serum levels of MMP-3/MMP-12-cleaved IgG and anti-hinge autoantibodies compared to control subjects and responders [24].

Conclusions

There is no doubt that MMPs and their inhibitors are critically important as the end-stage effectors of immune-mediated injury in IBD. At the same time, epithelial expression of MMPs such as MMP-7 is important in epithelial restitution and healing after injury. Inhibitors of MMP-1, MMP-3, MMP-10, and MMP-12 would undoubtedly be therapeutic in IBD, but unfortunately the lack of selectivity and the disruptive effects on homeostatic remodeling preclude their use. Some consideration however is being made to generating neutralizing and highly specific monoclonal antibodies to selectively target the various MMPs. Although it has been appreciated for many years that MMPs have non-matrix substrates, the authors' own recent work has identified that some biologic agents lose function when cleaved by MMPs, suggesting that engineering antibodies or Fc-receptor fusion proteins in order to eliminate cleavage sites may lead to a new generation of therapeutics [24]. In addition, the neo-epitope exposed upon MMP cleavage onto the hinge region of both biologic agents and IgG stimulates IgG autoantibody formation [56], so there is the possibility in vivo that biologic agents cleaved by MMPs are restored to intact antibodies and indeed perhaps to dimers by these autoantibodies.

References

1. Huxley-Jones J, Clarke TK, Beck C, Toubaris G, Robertson DL, Boot-Handford RP. The evolution of the vertebrate metzincins; insights from Ciona intestinalis and Danio rerio. BMC Evol Biol. 2007;7:63.
2. Nagase H, Visse R, Murphy G. Structure and function of matrix metalloproteinases and TIMPs. Cardiovasc Res. 2006;69:562–73.
3. Sorokin L. The impact of the extracellular matrix on inflammation. Nat Rev Immunol. 2010;10:712–23.
4. Biancheri P, Di Sabatino A, Corazza GR, MacDonald TT. Proteases and the gut barrier. Cell Tissue Res. 2013;351:269–80.
5. Parks WC, Wilson CL, López-Boado YS. Matrix metalloproteinases as modulators of inflammation and innate immunity. Nat Rev Immunol. 2004;4:617–29.
6. Giuffrida P, Biancheri P, MacDonald TT. Proteases and small intestinal barrier function in health and disease. Curr Opin Gastroenterol. 2014;30:147–53.
7. Edwards DR, Handsley MM, Pennington CJ. The ADAM metalloproteinases. Mol Aspects Med. 2008;29:258–89.
8. O'Shea NR, Smith AM. Matrix metalloproteases role in bowel inflammation and inflammatory bowel disease: an up to date review. Inflamm Bowel Dis. 2014;20:2379–93.
9. Ravi A, Garg P, Sitaraman SV. Matrix metalloproteinases in inflammatory bowel disease: boon or a bane? Inflamm Bowel Dis. 2007;13:97–107.
10. Noë V, Fingleton B, Jacobs K, Crawford HC, Vermeulen S, Steelant W, et al. Release of an invasion promoter E-cadherin fragment by matrilysin and stromelysin-1. J Cell Sci. 2001;114:111–8.
11. Wu S, Lim KC, Huang J, Saidi RF, Sears CL. *Bacteroides fragilis* enterotoxin cleaves the zonula adherens protein, E-cadherin. Proc Natl Acad Sci U S A. 1998;95:14979–84.
12. Steck N, Hoffmann M, Sava IG, Kim SC, Hahne H, Tonkonogy SL, et al. *Enterococcus faecalis* metalloprotease compromises epithelial barrier and contributes to intestinal inflammation. Gastroenterology. 2011;141:959–71.
13. Buzza MS, Martin EW, Driesbaugh KH, Désilets A, Leduc R, Antalis TM. Prostasin is required for matriptase activation in intestinal epithelial cells to regulate closure of the paracellular pathway. J Biol Chem. 2013;288:10328–37.
14. Franzè E, Caruso R, Stolfi C, Sarra M, Cupi ML, Ascolani M, et al. High expression of the "A Disintegrin And Metalloprotease" 19 (ADAM19), a sheddase for TNF-α in the mucosa of patients with inflammatory bowel diseases. Inflamm Bowel Dis. 2013;19:501–11.
15. Buzza MS, Netzel-Arnett S, Shea-Donohue T, Zhao A, Lin CY, List K, et al. Membrane-anchored serine protease matriptase regulates epithelial barrier formation and permeability in the intestine. Proc Natl Acad Sci U S A. 2010;107:4200–5.
16. Wilcz-Villega EM, McClean S, O'Sullivan MA. Mast cell tryptase reduces junctional adhesion molecule-A (JAM-A) expression in intestinal epithelial cells: implications for the mechanisms of barrier dysfunction in irritable bowel syndrome. Am J Gastroenterol. 2013;108:1140–51.
17. Vandenbroucke RE, Dejonckheere E, Van Hauwermeiren F, Lodens S, De Rycke R, Van Wonterghem E, et al. Matrix metalloproteinase 13 modulates intestinal epithelial barrier integrity in inflammatory diseases by activating TNF. EMBO Mol Med. 2013;5:932–48.
18. Schönbeck U, Mach F, Libby P. Generation of biologically active IL-1 beta by matrix metalloproteinases: a novel caspase-1-independent pathway of IL-1 beta processing. J Immunol. 1998;161:3340–6.
19. Ito A, Mukaiyama A, Itoh Y, Nagase H, Thogersen IB, Enghild JJ, et al. Degradation of interleukin 1beta by matrix metalloproteinases. J Biol Chem. 1997;271:14657–60.
20. Van Den Steen PE, Wuyts A, Husson SJ, Proost P, Van Damme J, Opdenakker G. Gelatinase B/MMP-9 and neutrophil collagenase/MMP-8 process the chemokines human GCP-2/CXCL6, ENA-78/CXCL5 and mouse GCP-2/LIX and modulate their physiological activities. Eur J Biochem. 2003;270:3739–49.
21. Li Q, Park PW, Wilson CL, Parks WC. Matrilysin shedding of syndecan-1 regulates chemokine mobilization and transepithelial efflux of neutrophils in acute lung injury. Cell. 2002;111:635–46.
22. Brezski RJ, Vafa O, Petrone D, Tam SH, Powers G, Ryan MH, et al. Tumor-associated and microbial proteases compromise host IgG effector functions by a single cleavage proximal to the hinge. Proc Natl Acad Sci U S A. 2009;106:17864–9.
23. Brezski RJ, Jordan RE. Cleavage of IgGs by proteases associated with invasive diseases: an evasion tactic against host immunity? MAbs. 2010;2:212–20.
24. Biancheri P, Brezski RJ, Di Sabatino A, Greenplate AR, Soring KL, Corazza GR, et al. Proteolytic cleavage and loss of function of biologic agents that neutralize tumor necrosis factor in the mucosa of patients with inflammatory bowel disease. Gastroenterology. 2015;149(6):1564–74.e3.
25. Houghton AM, Hartzell WO, Robbins CS, Gomis-Rüth FX, Shapiro SD. Macrophage elastase kills bacteria within murine macrophages. Nature. 2009;460:637–41.

26. Wilson CL, Ouellette AJ, Satchell DP, Ayabe T, López-Boado YS, Stratman JL, et al. Regulation of intestinal alpha-defensin activation by the metalloproteinase matrilysin in innate host defense. Science. 1999;286:113–7.
27. Li CK, Pender SL, Pickard KM, Chance V, Holloway JA, Huett A, et al. Impaired immunity to intestinal bacterial infection in stromelysin-1 (matrix metalloproteinase-3)-deficient mice. J Immunol. 2004;173:5171–9.
28. Sina C, Lipinski S, Gavrilova O, Aden K, Rehman A, Till A, et al. Extracellular cathepsin K exerts antimicrobial activity and is protective against chronic intestinal inflammation in mice. Gut. 2013;62:520–30.
29. Baumgart DC, Sandborn WJ. Crohn's disease. Lancet. 2012;380: 1590–605.
30. Ordás I, Eckmann L, Talamini M, Baumgart DC, Sandborn WJ. Ulcerative colitis. Lancet. 2012;380:1606–19.
31. Baugh MD, Perry MJ, Hollander AP, Davies DR, Cross SS, Lobo AJ, et al. Matrix metalloproteinase levels are elevated in inflammatory bowel disease. Gastroenterology. 1999;117:814–22.
32. Di Sabatino A, Saarialho-Kere U, Buckley MG, Gordon JN, Biancheri P, Rovedatti L, et al. Stromelysin-1 and macrophage metalloelastase expression in the intestinal mucosa of Crohn's disease patients treated with infliximab. Eur J Gastroenterol Hepatol. 2009;21:1049–55.
33. Saarialho-Kere UK, Vaalamo M, Puolakkainen P, Airola K, Parks WC, Karjalainen-Lindsberg ML. Enhanced expression of matrilysin, collagenase, and stromelysin-1 in gastrointestinal ulcers. Am J Pathol. 1996;148:519–26.
34. Vaalamo M, Karjalainen-Lindsberg ML, Puolakkainen P, Kere J, Saarialho-Kere U. Distinct expression profiles of stromelysin-2 (MMP-10), collagenase-3 (MMP-13), macrophage metalloelastase (MMP-12), and tissue inhibitor of metalloproteinases-3 (TIMP-3) in intestinal ulcerations. Am J Pathol. 1998;152: 1005–14.
35. Gordon JN, Pickard KM, Di Sabatino A, Prothero JD, Pender SL, Goggin PM, et al. Matrix metalloproteinase-3 production by gut IgG plasma cells in chronic inflammatory bowel disease. Inflamm Bowel Dis. 2008;14:195–203.
36. Motta JP, Bermúdez-Humarán LG, Deraison C, Martin L, Rolland C, Rousset P, et al. Food-grade bacteria expressing elafin protect against inflammation and restore colon homeostasis. Sci Transl Med. 2012;4:158ra144.
37. Rath T, Roderfeld M, Halwe JM, Tschuschner A, Roeb E, Graf J, et al. Cellular sources of MMP-7, MMP-13 and MMP-28 in ulcerative colitis. Scand J Gastroenterol. 2010;45:1186–96.
38. Netzel-Arnett S, Buzza MS, Shea-Donohue T, Désilets A, Leduc R, Fasano A, et al. Matriptase protects against experimental colitis and promotes intestinal barrier recovery. Inflamm Bowel Dis. 2012;18:1303–14.
39. Pender SL, Tickle SP, Docherty AJ, Howie D, Wathen NC, MacDonald TT. A major role for matrix metalloproteinases in T cell injury in the gut. J Immunol. 1997;158:1582–90.
40. Biancheri P, Pender SL, Ammoscato F, Giuffrida P, Sampietro G, Ardizzone S, et al. The role of interleukin 17 in Crohn's disease-associated intestinal fibrosis. Fibrogenesis Tissue Repair. 2013;6:13.
41. Andoh A, Bamba S, Fujiyama Y, Brittan M, Wright NA. Colonic subepithelial myofibroblasts in mucosal inflammation and repair: contribution of bone marrow-derived stem cells to the gut regenerative response. J Gastroenterol. 2005;40:1089–99.
42. Castaneda FE, Walia B, Vijay-Kumar M, Patel NR, Roser S, Kolachala VL, et al. Targeted deletion of metalloproteinase 9 attenuates experimental colitis in mice: central role of epithelial-derived MMP. Gastroenterology. 2005;129:1991–2008.
43. Garg P, Rojas M, Ravi A, Bockbrader K, Epstein S, Vijay-Kumar M, et al. Selective ablation of matrix metalloproteinase-2 exacerbates experimental colitis: contrasting role of gelatinases in the pathogenesis of colitis. J Immunol. 2006;177:4103–12.
44. Koller FL, Dozier EA, Nam KT, Swee M, Birkland TP, Parks WC, et al. Lack of MMP10 exacerbates experimental colitis and promotes development of inflammation associated colonic dysplasia. Lab Invest. 2012;92:1749–59.
45. Koelink PJ, Overbeek SA, Braber S, Morgan ME, Henricks PA, Abdul Roda M, et al. Collagen degradation and neutrophilic infiltration: a vicious circle in inflammatory bowel disease. Gut. 2014;63:578–87.
46. Monteleone I, Federici M, Sarra M, Franzè E, Casagrande V, Zorzi F, et al. Tissue inhibitor of metalloproteinase-3 regulates inflammation in human and mouse intestine. Gastroenterology. 2012;143:1277–87.
47. Kirkegaard T, Hansen A, Bruun E, Brynskov J. Expression and localisation of matrix metalloproteinases and their natural inhibitors in fistulae of patients with Crohn's disease. Gut. 2004;53:701–9.
48. Di Sabatino A, Jackson CL, Pickard KM, Buckley M, Rovedatti L, Leakey NAB, et al. Transforming growth factor β signalling and matrix metalloproteinases in the mucosa overlying Crohn's disease strictures. Gut. 2009;58:777–89.
49. Sela-Passwell N, Kikkeri R, Dym O, Rozenberg H, Margalit R, Arad-Yellin R, et al. Antibodies targeting the catalytic zinc complex of activated matrix metalloproteinases show therapeutic potential. Nat Med. 2012;18:143–7.
50. Shimshoni E, Yablecovitch D, Baram L, Dotan I, Sagi I. ECM remodelling in IBD: innocent bystander or partner in crime? The emerging role of extracellular molecular events in sustaining intestinal inflammation. Gut. 2015;64:367–72.
51. Blaydon DC, Biancheri P, Di WL, Plagnol V, Cabral RM, Brooke MA, et al. Inflammatory skin and bowel disease linked to ADAM17 deletion. N Engl J Med. 2011;365:1502–8.
52. Annahazi A, Molnar T, Farkas K, Rosztoczy A, Izbeki F, Gecse K, et al. Fecal MMP-9: a new noninvasive differential diagnostic and activity marker in ulcerative colitis. Inflamm Bowel Dis. 2013;19:316–20.
53. Kolho KL, Sipponen T, Valtonen E, Savilahti E. Fecal calprotectin, MMP-9, and human beta-defensin-2 levels in pediatric inflammatory bowel disease. Int J Colorectal Dis. 2014;29:43–50.
54. Farkas K, Saródi Z, Bálint A, Földesi I, Tiszlavicz L, Szűcs M, et al. The diagnostic value of a new fecal marker, matrix metalloprotease-9, in different types of inflammatory bowel diseases. J Crohns Colitis. 2015;9:231–7.
55. Faubion WA, Fletcher JG, O'Byrne S, Feagan BG, de Villiers WJ, Salzberg B, et al. EMerging BiomARKers in Inflammatory Bowel Disease (EMBARK) study identifies fecal calprotectin, serum MMP9, and serum IL-22 as a novel combination of biomarkers for Crohn's disease activity: role of cross-sectional imaging. Am J Gastroenterol. 2013;108:1891–900.
56. Mortensen JH, Godskesen LE, Jensen MD, Van Haaften WT, Klinge LG, Olinga P, et al. Fragments of citrullinated and MMP degraded vimentin and MMP-degraded type III collagen are novel serological biomarkers to differentiate Crohn's disease from ulcerative colitis. J Crohns Colitis. 2015;9(10):863–72.
57. Brezski RJ, Luongo JL, Petrone D, Ryan MH, Zhong D, Tam SH, et al. Human anti-IgG1 hinge autoantibodies reconstitute the effector functions of proteolytically inactivated IgGs. J Immunol. 2008;181:3183–92.

Paradigm of T Cell Differentiation in IBD

14

Takashi Nagaishi and Mamoru Watanabe

Introduction

Inflammatory bowel disease (IBD) may occur only once in a patient's lifetime, but often it recurs and becomes refractory [1]. This feature suggests "pathogenic memory" that hints the importance of acquired immunity in the pathogenesis of IBD. Therefore, helper T (Th) cells differentiated from CD4$^+$ naïve T cells play central roles in the acquired immune system. Thus, each Th cell subset secretes various cytokines, which activate other immune cells. Original Th cell subsets only included type 1 (Th1) or type 2 (Th2). Subsequent recognition of regulatory T cells (Treg), which regulates effector T cell functions negatively, and Th17 cells added to the complexity of the system [2].

The effectiveness of monoclonal antibody against TNF-α, which is one of the proinflammatory cytokines secreted by several Th subsets as well as macrophages, for the treatment for both Crohn's disease (CD) and ulcerative colitis (UC) has changed natural history of IBD pathogenesis [3]. This has encouraged many scientists to develop more effective therapies targeting other T cell activation pathways. Furthermore, Th17 has also been highlighted in the pathogenesis of IBD due to significant association between the genetic polymorphisms in the Th17/IL-23 pathway. In this section, the role of each Th subset in the pathogenesis of IBD is discussed since this will be the fundamental basis for the future development of IBD treatment.

T. Nagaishi, M.D., Ph.D. (✉) • M. Watanabe, M.D., Ph.D.
Department of Gastroenterology, Tokyo Medical and Dental University, Tokyo, Japan
e-mail: tnagaishi.gast@tmd.ac.jp

Differentiation of Helper T Cells

When CD4$^+$ T cells are developed in thymus and migrated to the peripheral tissues, they are called naïve T cells, which secret minimal cytokines and no efficient effector function. However, they are activated when specific antigens are presented to their T cell receptors (TCR) via antigen presenting cells (APC) through MHC class-II with co-stimulatory signaling. Moreover, cytokines in the environment where the antigen presentation occurs determine the polarization of these Th cells. Thus, expression of the specific transcription factors such as T-bet, GATA-3, and retinoic acid receptor-related orphan receptor (ROR-γτ) is induced in these cells. Such an event allows naïve T cells to differentiate into various Th cells that secrete characteristic type of cytokines [4] (Fig. 14.1).

Th1 Differentiation

Classically, helper CD4$^+$ T cells were classified as Th1 or Th2. Th1 cells differentiate in the presence of IL-12 and secrete IFN-γ, TNF-α, and IL-2. Th1 cells play an important role in the cellular immunity against tumors and intracellular viral and/or bacterial infections. IL-12 is secreted by APC such as macrophages and dendritic cells (DC). IL-12 activates STAT4 pathway through IL-12 receptor (IL-12R) signaling and T-bet, a transcription factor which promotes specific gene expression profile including IFN-γ. This expression of IFN-γ is also one of the important factors for Th1 differentiation, because such differentiation can be inhibited by IFN-γ neutralization according to in vitro experiments. However, T-bet, a member of the T-box family, is thought to be the master regulator of the Th1 differentiation. While artificial transduction of T-bet in polarized Th2 cells converts them into Th1 cells, its absence causes disorder of Th1 differentiation in vitro and in vivo. T-bet prompts IL-12R expression and activates IFN-γ gene, which results in a positive feedback of Th1 polarization [4, 5].

D.C. Baumgart (ed.), *Crohn's Disease and Ulcerative Colitis*, DOI 10.1007/978-3-319-33703-6_14

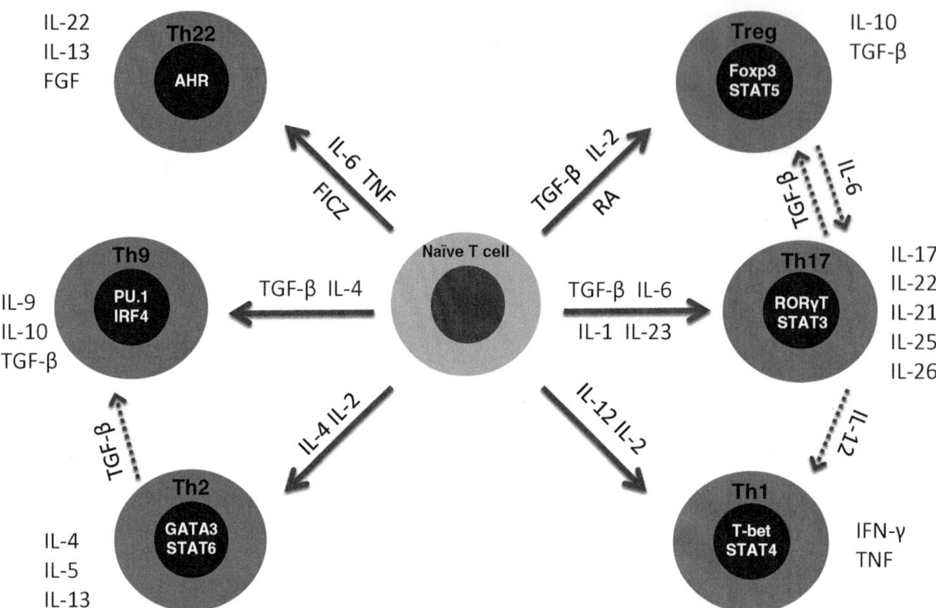

Fig. 14.1 Differentiation of helper CD4⁺ T cells. When antigens specific for their own TCR are presented to naïve T cells by APC through MHC class-II/TCR signal with co-stimulatory signals, naïve T cells differentiate to helper T cells, which secrete characteristic types of cytokines and express specific transcription factors. Cytokines in the environment where the antigen presentation occurs determine the polarization of these helper T cells. Th1 cells differentiate in the presence of IL-12, and secrete IFN-γ, TNF-α, and IL-2. IL-12 activates STAT4 pathway through IL-12R and promotes T-bet, which is a master regulator for the Th1 differentiation. Th2 cells differentiate in the presence of IL-4, and secrete IL-4, IL-5, and IL-13. IL-4 activates STAT6 pathway through IL-4R and promotes GATA-3, which is a master regulator of the Th2 differentiation. Th17 cells produce L-17A, IL-17F, IL-21, IL-22, and TNF-α. Th17 cells differentiate in the presence of IL-6 and TGF-β, through the expression of ROR-γt, which is a master regulator of Th17. While TGF-β drives Smad signaling, IL-6 activates STAT3 pathway, which promotes the expression of RORγt. IL-21 is an important cytokine for the amplification of Th17, while IL-23 is important for their stabilization. Th9 cells differentiate in the presence of TGF-β and IL-4, and secrete IL-9. IL-9 expression in these cells is regulated by transcription factors such as PU.1, STAT6, Batf, GATA3, and IRF4. Particularly, PU.1, which is induced by TGFβ, is thought to be a master regulator for Th9, and inhibits the development of Th2. Th22 cells differentiate in the presence of IL-6, TNF, and FICZ, and secrete IL-22, but not IL-17. FICZ activates AHR, which is thought to be a master regulator for the Th22 differentiation. Th22 cells are also known to produce IL-13 and FGF. On the other hand, TGF-β is known to suppress Th22. iTreg is derived from naïve T cells in the presence of TGF-β and the absence of IL-6 through the expression of Foxp3. RA and IL-2 promote iTreg differentiation. In addition, IL-2 is an important survival factor for Treg. On the other hand, IL-6 prevents iTreg differentiation and promotes Th17 differentiation

Th2 Differentiation

Th2 cells are differentiated in the presence of IL-4 when specific antigens are presented to their TCR by APC, and these cells then start to secrete IL-4, IL-5, and IL-13. Th2 cells play an important role mainly in humoral immunity against parasites and some allergens. IL-4 activates STAT6 pathway through IL-4 receptor (IL-4R) signaling and promotes expression of GATA-3, which is a master regulator of the Th2 differentiation. In the absence of GATA-3, Th2 development is inhibited in vitro and in vivo, while transduction of GATA-3 in the polarized Th1 cells results in IL-4 secretion. GATA-3 induces IL-4 gene expression, which forms a positive feedback of Th2 polarization. IL-12 inhibits Th2 polarization, while IL-4 inhibits Th1 differentiation, which makes these subsets reciprocal [4, 5].

Th17 Differentiation

Th17 cells have been reported to produce L-17A, IL-17F, IL-21, IL-22, and TNF-α, and these cells play an important role in the protective immunity against the extracellular pathogens such as bacteria [6]. Th17 cells are differentiated in the presence of IL-6 and TGF-β at the antigen presentation through the expression of RORγt. While TGF-β drives Smad signaling, IL-6 activates STAT3 pathway, which promotes the expression of RORγt [2]. RORγt, a transcription factor expressed on double positive (DP) T cells in the thymus and type 3 innate lymphoid cells (ILC3), is thought to be the master regulator of Th17 differentiation. Transduction of RORγt to CD4⁺ T cells results in significant IL-17A secretion, while depletion in Th17 cells results in decreased IL-17A production. In addition to RORγt, Th17 cells may also express RORα, which is upregulated by STAT3 pathway. RORα deficient mice are still able to produce normal level of IL-17A, while RORγt deficient mice have impaired production of IL-17A. However, IL-17A production in RORγt deficient mice is dependent on the expression of RORα, and thus RORα and RORγt double deficient mice cannot produce any IL-17A [7]. In addition, IL-21 is also important cytokine for the differentiation of Th17. IL-6 promotes the production of IL-21 from Th17 cells independent of RORγt, and subsequently IL-21 upregulates the expression of RORγt through the activation of STAT3 pathway. This process forms a positive feedback in the Th17 differentiation and is thus called "amplification". Therefore, it is necessary for the amplification of Th17 cells although IL-21 is not essential for h17 polarization. In fact, IL-21 deficient mice show a reduction in the number of Th17 cells [8]. IL-23 is also important for the Th17 pathway. However, IL-23 receptor (IL-23R) is not originally expressed on naïve T cells. TGF-β signal mediates IL-23R expression on Th17 cells, which makes them responsive to IL-23. IL-23 is essential to the maintenance of the Th17 phenotype in long-term cultures. Therefore, the effect of IL-23 on Th17 is defined as "stabilization" [8]. IL-23 is highly expressed in mucosa of human ileum, and there are many Th17 cells in the human GALT. These Th17 cells play an important role for protective immunity against intestinal pathogens. Intestinal microbiota is essential for the development of Th17, since mice in germ-free condition show decreased number of Th17 cells [9].

Treg Differentiation

Regulatory T cells (Treg) play a crucial role in peripheral tolerance to prevent autoimmune disease development and chronic inflammation. Thus, Treg is one of the $CD4^+$ T cell subsets that inhibit other Th cells, and this subset consists of two distinct subpopulations, naturally occurring Treg (nTreg) and induced Treg (iTreg) [10]. While nTreg is generated during T cell development in the thymus, iTreg is differentiated from naïve T cells in the peripheral tissues during an immune response.

In the thymus, nTreg is identified as $CD4^+CD25^+$ autoreactive T cells expressing TCR specific for auto-antigens. Although CD25 (also known as IL-2Rα chain) was previously thought to be an activation marker of effector T cells, it is notably expressed on nTreg in response to auto-antigens. nTreg may also express GITR and CTLA-4, as well as Foxp3 which is thought to be the master regulator of nTreg. Genetic depletion of Foxp3 leads to various autoimmune disease and chronic intestinal inflammation similar to that of IBD. Furthermore, induction of Foxp3 to $CD4^+$ T cells causes inhibition of effector T cells [10].

The other Treg subset, iTreg, may be derived from peripheral naïve T cells in the presence of TGF-β and the absence of IL-6 through the expression of Foxp3. It is believed that retinoic acid (RA) and IL-2 promote iTreg differentiation. IL-2 is especially important for the survival factor of Treg. On the other hand, IL-6 prevents iTreg differentiation and promotes Th17 differentiation instead [4–6, 10]. In this manner, IL-6 may be an important cytokine that regulates the balance between Treg and Th17. However, these findings are according to in vitro assays, and whether they can be applied in vivo is still largely unknown.

Role of Each Th Subset in IBD Models

In the past, CD was originally thought to be a Th1-mediated disease, while UC was Th2-mediated. Accordingly, the pathogenesis of animal models of IBD was understood to be either Th1- or Th2-mediated intestinal inflammation. However, many studies have already demonstrated that both Th1 and Th2 conditions can exist in most of animal models (Table 14.1) as well as IBD patients (Table 14.2). Moreover, recent studies also showed plasticity of Th cells differentiating into other subsets. Also, newly defined Th subsets, such as Th9 and Th22, have been added to the mix (Fig. 14.1).

Th1 in Animal Models

It is known that naïve T cells derived from wild type mice can be differentiated into colitogenic effector T cells after transferring to the recipients such as RAG-deficient and SCID mice. Chronic colitis in this animal model was originally thought to be induced by Th1 inflammation. Thus, it has been reported that naïve T cells from T-bet deficient mice are unable to induce colitis in the recipient RAG-deficient mice, and the overexpression of T-bet in naive T cells results in exacerbation of colitis [11]. In addition, naïve T cells from STAT4 deficient mice cause less severe colitis in the recipients [12]. On the other hand, it is known that the lack of *IL10* gene results in spontaneous chronic colitis which was also thought to be Th1-mediated. In fact, administration of antagonistic antibody against IFN-γ abrogates colitis in IL-10 deficient mice as well as T cell-reconstituted RAG-deficient mice [13, 14]. However, naïve T cells from IFN-γ deficient mice may induce colitis [12]. Furthermore, IL-10 and IFN-γ double-deficient mice develop colitis equally as IL-10 deficient mice when they are infected with *H. hepaticus* [15]. These findings suggest that IFN-γ may not be essential for the development of colitis in these models.

Table 14.1 Effector T cells involved in the pathogenesis of murine models of IBD

Animal models	Type of Th	Mechanisms
Dysfunction of intestinal epithelial barrier		
DSS colitis	Th1, Th2, Th17	Direct damage to epithelial barrier
Gαi2−/−	Th1	Defect of intestinal epithelial barrier Defect of regulatory B cells
Dysregulation of innate immune system		
C3H/HeJBir	Th1,Th17	Dysfunction of sensitivity of TLR
Dysregulation of acquired immune system		
TNFαΔARE	Th1	Overexpression of TNF-α Activation of effector T cells
IL-7-Tg	Th1	Overexpression of IL-7 Activation of effector T cells
T bet Tg	Th1	Activation of effector T cells
STAT4 Tg	Th1	Activation of effector T cells
Bone marrow-reconstituted Tgε26	Th1	Activation of effector T cells
TCRα−/−	Th2	Activation of effector T cells
Dysfunction or decrease of Treg		
T cell-reconstituted RAG$^{-/-}$	Th1, Th17	Decrease of Treg Activation of effector T cells
IL-10−/−	Th1, Th17	Dysfunction of Treg
TGFβ1−/−, TGFβR2−/−	Th1	Decrease of Treg
IL2−/−, IL2R−/−	Th1	Decrease of Treg
Smad3−/−	Th1	Decrease of Treg
WASP−/−	Th2	Dysfunction of Treg
Other mechanisms		
TNBS colitis	Th1, Th2, Th17	Increase of activated effector T cells SJL/J mice: Th1, Th17 Balb/c mice: Th2
Oxazolone colitis	Th2, NKT, Th9	Increase of activated effector T cells
SAMP1/Yit mutant mice	Th1, Th2	Dysfunction of intestinal epithelial cells Increase of activated effector T cells Increase of activated B cells

Th2 in Animal Models

While Th1 plays important role in the pathogenesis of most animal models of IBD, there are few IBD models that are thought to be Th2 related [16]. Oxazolone-induced colitis, one of the models induced by haptens, reveals acute inflammation limited to colonic mucosa lasting for 4–5 days [17]. CD4^{+} T cells in the intestinal mucosa in oxazolone-treated mice produce large amounts of Th2 cytokines such as IL-4 and IL-5. Therefore it is believed that Th2 cells plays an important role in this model [17], while CD4^{+} T cells in TNBS-induced colitis model, which is also hapten-induced, produce Th1 cytokines such as IL-2 and IFN-γ [18]. Neutralization of IL-4 can attenuate the severity of oxazolone-induced colitis [17]. When mice are exposed to oxazolone prior to the rectal administration, chronic inflammation is induced and production of IL-4 is increased in the early phase followed by IL-13 elevation in the chronic phase [18]. In this chronic model, it is reported that the main sources of IL-13 are not only Th2 cells but also CD1d-restricted invariant NKT cells. In fact, either depletion of NKT cells or inhibition of CD1-restricted antigen presentation suppresses the development of colitis in this model [19, 20].

Th17 in Animal Models

IL-23 forms a heterodimer made of p19 subunit and p40 subunit, which is also a subunit of IL-12. Therefore it was previously difficult to determine whether IL-12/Th1 or IL-23/Th17 pathway was more critical in the pathogenesis in many animal models since the antibody used in these experiments targeted IL-12p40. In fact, it has been reported the increase of Th17 cells in several colitis models are IL-12 dependent [5]. For example, in both IL-10 deficient mice and T cell-reconstituted RAG deficient mice, both of which have been thought as Th1 models previously, CD4^{+} T cells producing a

Table 14.2 Th subsets involved in the pathogenesis of UC and CD patients

	CD		UC	
Th1				
T-bet	LP CD4+ T cells (mRNA)	↑	LP CD4+ T cells (mRNA)	→
IL-12	LPMC LP macrophages	↑ ↑	LPMC	→
IL-12R	LPL	↑	not clear	
TNF-α	Inflamed mucosa (mRNA) LP CD3+ T cells LP macrophages	↑ ↑ ↑	Inflamed mucosa (mRNA) LP CD3+ T cells LP macrophages	↑ ↑ ↑
IFN-γ	Inflamed mucosa LP CD4+ T cells PB CD4+ T cells	↑ ↑ ↑	Inflamed mucosa PB CD4+ T cells	→ →
IL-2	LP CD4+ T cells PB CD4+ T cells	↓ ↓	LP CD4+ T cells	→
IL-18	Intestinal mucosa LPMC	↑↑ ↑↑	Intestinal mucosa LPMC	↑ ↑
Th2				
IL-4	LP CD4+ T cells	↓	LP CD4+ T cells	↓
IL-5	LP CD4+ T cells PB CD4+ T cells	↓ →	LP CD4+ T cells PB CD4+ T cells	↑ →
IL-13	LPL PB CD4+ T cells	↑ →	LPL PB CD4+ T cells	↑↑ →
Th17				
RORγt	LP CD4+ T cells (mRNA)	↑	LP CD4+ T cells (mRNA)	↑
IL-6	Inflamed mucosa (mRNA)	↑	Inflamed mucosa (mRNA)	↑
IL-17A	Sera LP CD3+ T cells LP macrophages PB CD4+ T cells	↑ ↑ ↑ ↑	Sera LP CD3+ T cells LP macrophages PB CD4+ T cells	↑ ↑ ↑ ↑
IL-17F	Inflamed mucosa (mRNA)	↑	Intestinal mucosa (mRNA)	↑
IL-21	Inflamed mucosa	↑↑	Inflamed mucosa	↑
IL-23	Inflamed mucosa (mRNA) LP MC	↑↑ ↑	Inflamed mucosa (mRNA) LP MC	↑ ↑
IL-23R	LP CD4+ T cells (mRNA)	↑	LP CD4+ T cells (mRNA)	↑
Th9				
IL-9	LP CD4+ T cells	↑	LP CD4+ T cells	↑↑
Th22				
IL-22	LP CD4+ T cells	↑	LP CD4+ T cells	↓
Treg				
FOXP3	Intestinal mucosa (mRNA) LP CD4+ PB CD4+	↑ ↓[a] ↓	Intestinal mucosa (mRNA) LP CD4+ PB CD4+	↑ ↓[a] ↓
IL-10	LP CD3+ T cells (mRNA)	→	LP CD3+ T cells (mRNA)	↑
TGF-β	LP CD3+ T cells (mRNA)	→	LP CD3+ T cells (mRNA)	↑

LP intestinal lamina propria, *LPL* intestinal lamina propria lymphocytes
LPMC intestinal lamina propria mononuclear cells
PB peripheral blood, *PBMC* peripheral blood mononuclear cells
[a]Compared with other inflammatory disease such as diverticulitis

large amount of IL-17 are increased as well as IFN-γ producing cells [21, 22]. IL-23p19 transgenic mice develop colitis and systemic autoimmune disease [23]. Administration of recombinant IL-23 exacerbates colitis in RAG deficient mice that has with naïve T cells from IL-10 deficient mice [22]. Genetic depletion or neutralization of IL-23p19 ameliorates colitis in both IL-10 deficient and T cell-transferred RAG deficient mice [22, 24]. IL-21 is important for the amplification of Th17 cell, and IL-21 depletion can ameliorates DSS colitis and TNBS colitis [25]. These observations suggest that Th17/IL-23 is more important than IL-12/Th1 in the pathogenesis in this model.

IL-17, including various subtypes such as IL-17A and IL-17F, is a main effector cytokine of Th17. However, the role of IL-17 in the pathogenesis of IBD is controversial, and there are different arguments that it exacerbates, ameliorates, or does not influence colitis. IL-17A deficient mice developed more severe colitis than wild type mice in the TNBS colitis model, and administration of antibody against IL-17A exacerbates colitis induced by DSS [26]. In addition, although IL-23 is not dispensable for the development of colitis in T cell-reconstituted RAG deficient mice, IL-17 is not essential [21]. IL-17A suppresses DSS colitis, while IL-17F accelerates colitis in this model [27]. Similarly, IL-17A suppresses colitis in T cell-transferred RAG deficient mice, inhibiting the polarization of Th1 [28]. In summary, effects of IL-17 in colitis differ among the various colitis models or experimental methods such as genetic depletion or neutralization antibodies.

In the oxazolone colitis model, depletion of IRF-4, an important factor for the Th2 differentiation, can suppress colitis [29]. However, IRF-4 is also associated with the Th17 differentiation, and therefore the importance of Th17 rather than Th2 cannot be excluded. In addition, it is known that depletion of IL-6, important factor for the differentiation of Th17, leads to suppression of oxazolone colitis, suggesting that Th17 may be critical in the pathogenesis of this model. Furthermore, recent studies reported that Th17 cells may trans-differentiate into Th1 or Treg [30, 31], and Treg cells may trans-differentiate into Th17 cells [32–34]. Taken together, further investigations are needed on Th17 functions in IBD.

Th9 in Animal Models

The expression of a cytokine IL-9 was originally associated with Th2 phenotype such as the one during infection with *Leishmania major*. However, Th9, a specialized IL-9-producing T cell subset induced by IL-4 and TGFβ, has been recently reported [35–37]. In this subset, IL-9 expression has been reported to be regulated by transcription factors such as PU.1, STAT6, Batf, GATA3, and IRF4. Particularly, IL-9 transcription is controlled by PU.1, which is induced by TGFβ. Therefore, PU.1 is thought to be a master regulator for Th9 (Fig. 14.1). PU.1, which is encoded by *Spi1* gene, is known to inhibit the development of Th2.

The exacerbation of colitis in the T cell-reconstituted RAG deficient mice by co-transfer of IL-10 and IL-9 double positive T cells with naïve T cells has been reported [35]. And recently, it has been reported that Th9 subset is also induced in the oxazolone-induced colitis model. Neutralization of IL-9 with antibodies or deficiency in PU.1 results in amelioration of colitis [38]. IL-9 was found to have epithelial cells with impaired intestinal barrier function and poor mucosal healing.

Th22 in Animal Models

IL-22 is known to be produced by Th17 cells. It is an inhibitory cytokine unlike other Th17 cytokines. IL-22 is also produced by ILC3 including lymphoid inducer cells (LTi) and one of the NK cell subset. Recently it is reported that IL-22 producing RORγt$^+$NKp46$^+$ cells play a critical role in the homeostasis of intestinal mucosal immune system. In addition, a newly defined Th subset called Th22 producing IL-22, but not IL-17, has been recently reported [39, 40]. Th22 cells are differentiated in the presence of IL-6, TNF and the tryptophan metabolite 6-formylindolo [3,2-b] carbazole (FICZ), and secrete IL-22, but not IL-17. FICZ is known to be a natural ligand for aryl hydrocarbon receptor (AHR). AHR is a ligand-dependent transcription factor, and thought to be a master regulator for the Th22 differentiation (Fig. 14.1). Th22 cells are also known to produce IL-13 and fibroblast growth factor (FGF). On the other hand, TGF-β is known to suppress Th22 differentiation.

Either genetic depletion or neutralization of IL-22 exacerbates colitis in T cell-reconstituted RAG deficient and DSS-treated mice [41]. IL-22 not only prevents excess activation of immune system but also induces anti-apoptotic molecules in the intestinal epithelial cells to ameliorate epithelial dysfunction in colitis [42].

Each Th Subset in IBD Patients

Th1 had been originally thought to play important roles in the pathogenesis of CD and Th2 in UC. However, it has also been reported that Th17 may be involved in the pathogenesis of CD and UC. In addition, significant associations between genomic regions of Th17/IL-23 pathway and IBD have been reported from genome wide association studies (GWAS) [43]. On the other hand, the roles of the newly defined Th9 and Th22 subsets in the pathogenesis of UC have been accumulating (Table 14.2).

CD Patients

A large number of CD4$^+$ T cells that highly express T-bet and STAT-4 have been found in the intestinal mucosa of CD patients [11, 44]. In fact, CD4$^+$ T cells in the intestinal lamina propria of CD patients produce a large amount of IFN-γ and lower amount of IL-4 when compared to that of healthy control [44]. Macrophages in the intestinal lamina propria of CD patients produce a large amount of IL-12 [45]. Lymphocytes in the intestinal lamina propria of CD patients express high levels of IL-12R, and produce a large amount of IFN-γ in response to IL-12 [46]. Although treatment with blocking antibody against IFN-γ has not been effective in CD patient, treatment of monoclonal antibody against IL-12p40 may be effective [47]. These data show that Th1 is also strongly associated with the pathogenesis of CD.

On the other hand, it is reported that IL-17A, IL-17F, IL-21, IL-22, IL-23, RORγt, and IL-23R are highly expressed in the intestinal mucosa of CD patients [4, 48]. Furthermore, a unique macrophage producing IL-23, TNF and IL-6 are found to be increased in the intestinal mucosa of CD patients [49]. IL-17 and IL-23 in CD patients decrease after treatment with steroids or neutralizing antibody against IL-12p40 [50]. As mentioned above, several GWAS proved significant associations between the genomic regions of Th17/IL-23 pathway and IBD [43]. Although Th17 is believed to be an important factor in IBD development, human data are weak, and further studies are still needed.

UC Patients

UC has traditionally been thought of as Th2-mediated, because IFN-γ in the colon of UC patients has always found to be very low. In UC patients, CD4$^+$ T cells in the intestinal lamina propria secretes higher amount of IL-5 and IL-13 compared to that of CD patients or healthy control [44, 51]. On the other hand, IL-4, the predominant Th2 cytokine, level in the intestine of UC is lower than that of CD patients or healthy control [44], and this suggests that UC cannot be defined as merely a Th2-mediated disease. Similarly to the oxazolone-induced colitis model, the main sources of IL-13 in the colonic mucosa of UC patients are CD1d-restricted invariant NKT cells. In fact, there are many NKT cells in the inflamed mucosa of UC patients [51]. However, the role of IL-13 and NKT cells in the pathogenesis of UC is not clear, and further investigations are still needed.

Th17 cytokines, such as IL-17A, IL-17F, IL-21, IL-22, IL-23, RORγt, and IL-23R, are highly expressed in the intestinal mucosa of UC patients [4, 48]. Moreover, Th9 subset expressing the transcription factor PU.1 and IL-9, as well as the epithelial cells expressing IL-9R, has been recently reported in the patients with UC [38]. PU.1 expression is known to be induced by TGF-β signaling. In addition, there is a reduced number of IL-22⁺ cells in actively inflamed tissue in UC patients despite increase of mono-IL-17-producing cells [40]. It is suggested that such decrease of Th22 cells is associated with increased TGF-β expression. This is consistent with the finding that Th22 population was decreased in lamina propria mononuclear cell culture in vitro by stimulation with recombinant TGF-β, whereas anti-TGF-β antibody increased IL-22 production. Loss of Th22 by increased TGF-β may be associated with alterations of mucosal microbiota in the inflamed colonic tissues of UC.

Treg in Animal Models and IBD Patients

There are several animal models that relates to the importance of regulatory T cells for the homeostasis of intestinal mucosal immune system. Both CTLA4 deficient mice and Foxp3 deficient mice develop colitis, and transferring of Treg suppresses colitis in multiple IBD models [10]. These findings suggest that dysfunction or decrease in Treg may cause IBD.

The number of $CD4^+CD25^+FOXP3^+$ T cells in the peripheral blood of both CD and UC patients is decreased when compared to that of the healthy control [52, 53]. On the other hand, the number of $CD4^+CD25^+FOXP3^+$ T cells in intestinal mucosa of both CD and UC patients is increased [53, 54]. Furthermore, these Treg from IBD patients can suppress effector T cells in vitro [54]. These findings of either decrease in the effector site or dysfunction of Treg are not observed in IBD patients, and thus they raise doubts regarding the importance of Tregs in the pathogenesis of IBD. However, as compared with other intestinal inflammatory diseases such as diverticulitis, intestinal Treg in IBD patients is decreased [52, 53], and it is thought that there exists an imbalance between Treg and effector T cells in IBD patients.

IL-10 is one of the regulatory cytokines produced by Treg. It is known that IL-10 deficient mice develop colitis. Administration of recombinant IL-10 or transgenic overexpression of IL-10 suppresses colitis in T cell-reconstituted RAG deficient mice. In human, there is a strong association between polymorphism at *IL10* locus and UC [55]. Rare alleles of *IL10R* locus associated with familial enterocolitis [56] have also been reported.

Conclusion

Previously, anti-inflammatory and/or nonspecific immunosuppression drugs have been used to treat IBD. Recently, anti-TNF therapies including chimeric or humanized monoclonal antibody have advanced and revolutionized the disease management. The traditional Th1/Th2 paradigm is augmented by the discovery of other equally important cells and cytokines such as Treg, Th17, Th9, and Th22. Also, follicular helper T cell subset supporting the differentiation and immunoglobulin secretion of B cells has been recently identified [57]. Definitions of such Th subsets have become more complex. However, understanding the role of each Th subset will accelerate the development of new IBD therapies.

References

1. Abraham C, Cho JH. Inflammatory bowel disease. N Engl J Med. 2009;361(21):2066–78. Review.
2. Manel N, Unutmaz D, Littman DR. The differentiation of human T(H)-17 cells requires transforming growth factor-beta and induction of the nuclear receptor RORgammat. Nat Immunol. 2008;9(6):641–9.
3. Hanauer SB, Feagan BG, Lichtenstein GR, Mayer LF, Schreiber S, Colombel JF, et al. Maintenance infliximab for Crohn's disease: the ACCENT I randomised trial. Lancet. 2002;359(9317):1541–9.
4. Zenewicz LA, Antov A, Flavell RA. CD4 T-cell differentiation and inflammatory bowel disease. Trends Mol Med. 2009;15(5):199–207. Review.
5. Maynard CL, Weaver CT. Intestinal effector T cells in health and disease. Immunity. 2009;31(3):389–400. Review.
6. Weaver CT, Hatton RD, Mangan PR, Harrington LE. IL-17 family cytokines and the expanding diversity of effector T cell lineages. Annu Rev Immunol. 2007;25:821–52. Review.
7. Yang XO, Pappu BP, Nurieva R, et al. T helper 17 lineage differentiation is programmed by orphan nuclear receptors ROR alpha and ROR gamma. Immunity. 2008;28(1):29–39.
8. Abraham C, Cho JH. IL-23 and autoimmunity: new insights into the pathogenesis of inflammatory bowel disease. Annu Rev Med. 2009;60:97–110. Review.
9. Atarashi K, Nishimura J, Shima T, et al. ATP drives lamina propria T(H)17 cell differentiation. Nature. 2008;455(7214):808–12.
10. Sakaguchi S, Yamaguchi T, Nomura T, Ono M. Regulatory T cells and immune tolerance. Cell. 2008;133(5):775–87. Review.
11. Neurath MF, Weigmann B, Finotto S, et al. The transcription factor T-bet regulates mucosal T cell activation in experimental colitis and Crohn's disease. J Exp Med. 2002;195(9):1129–43.
12. Simpson SJ, Shah S, Comiskey M, et al. T cell-mediated pathology in two models of experimental colitis depends predominantly on the interleukin 12/Signal transducer and activator of transcription (Stat)-4 pathway, but is not conditional on interferon gamma expression by T cells. J Exp Med. 1998;187(8):1225–34.
13. Berg DJ, Davidson N, Kühn R, et al. Enterocolitis and colon cancer in interleukin-10-deficient mice are associated with aberrant cytokine production and CD4(+) TH1-like responses. J Clin Invest. 1996;98(4):1010–20.
14. Powrie F, Leach MW, Mauze S, et al. Inhibition of Th1 responses prevents inflammatory bowel disease in scid mice reconstituted with CD45RBhi CD4+ T cells. Immunity. 1994;1(7):553–62.
15. Kullberg MC, Rothfuchs AG, Jankovic D, et al. Helicobacter hepaticus-induced colitis in interleukin-10-deficient mice: cytokine requirements for the induction and maintenance of intestinal inflammation. Infect Immun. 2001;69(7):4232–41.
16. Strober W, Fuss IJ, Blumberg RS. The immunology of mucosal models of inflammation. Annu Rev Immunol. 2002;20:495–549. Review.
17. Boirivant M, Fuss IJ, Chu A, Strober W. Oxazolone colitis: a murine model of T helper cell type 2 colitis treatable with antibodies to interleukin 4. J Exp Med. 1998;188(10):1929–39.

18. Neurath MF, Fuss I, Kelsall BL, et al. Antibodies to interleukin 12 abrogate established experimental colitis in mice. J Exp Med. 1995;182(5):1281–90.
19. Heller F, Fuss IJ, Nieuwenhuis EE, et al. Oxazolone colitis, a Th2 colitis model resembling ulcerative colitis, is mediated by IL-13-producing NK-T cells. Immunity. 2002;17(5):629–38.
20. Brozovic S, Nagaishi T, Yoshida M, et al. CD1d function is regulated by microsomal triglyceride transfer protein. Nat Med. 2004;10(5):535–9.
21. Izcue A, Hue S, Buonocore S, et al. Interleukin-23 restrains regulatory T cell activity to drive T cell-dependent colitis. Immunity. 2008;28(4):559–70.
22. Yen D, Cheung J, Scheerens H, et al. IL-23 is essential for T cell-mediated colitis and promotes inflammation via IL-17 and IL-6. J Clin Invest. 2006;116(5):1310–6.
23. Wiekowski MT, Leach MW, Evans EW, et al. Ubiquitous transgenic expression of the IL-23 subunit p19 induces multiorgan inflammation, runting, infertility, and premature death. J Immunol. 2001;166(12):7563–70.
24. Elson CO, Cong Y, Weaver CT, et al. Monoclonal anti-interleukin 23 reverses active colitis in a T cell-mediated model in mice. Gastroenterology. 2007;132(7):2359–70.
25. Fina D, Sarra M, Fantini MC, et al. Regulation of gut inflammation and th17 cell response by interleukin-21. Gastroenterology. 2008;134(4):1038–48.
26. Ogawa A, Andoh A, Araki Y, et al. Neutralization of interleukin-17 aggravates dextran sulfate sodium-induced colitis in mice. Clin Immunol. 2004;110(1):55–62.
27. Yang XO, Chang SH, Park H, et al. Regulation of inflammatory responses by IL-17F. J Exp Med. 2008;205(5):1063–75.
28. Awasthi A, Kuchroo VK. IL-17A directly inhibits TH1 cells and thereby suppresses development of intestinal inflammation. Nat Immunol. 2009;10(6):568–70.
29. Mudter J, Amoussina L, Schenk M, et al. The transcription factor IFN regulatory factor-4 controls experimental colitis in mice via T cell-derived IL-6. J Clin Invest. 2008;118(7):2415–26.
30. Lee YK, Turner H, Maynard CL, et al. Late developmental plasticity in the T helper 17 lineage. Immunity. 2009;30(1):92–107.
31. Gagliani N, Amezcua-Vesely MC, Iseppon A, et al. Th17 cells transdifferentiate into regulatory T cells during resolution of inflammation. Nature. 2015;253(7559):221–5.
32. Xu L, Kitani A, Fuss I, Strober W. Regulatory T cells induce CD4+CD25−Foxp3− T cells or are self-induced to become Th17 cells in the absence of exogeneous TGF-beta. J Immunol. 2007;178(11):6725–9.
33. Zhou L, Lopes JE, Chong MM, et al. TGF-beta-induced Foxp3 inhibits T(H)17 cell differentiation by antagonizing RORgamma function. Nature. 2008;453(7192):236–40.
34. Hoechst B, Gamrekelashvili J, Manns MP, et al. Plasticity of human Th17 cells and iTregs is orchestrated by different subsets of myeloid cells. Blood. 2011;117(24):6532–41.
35. Darvalhon V, Awasthi A, Kwon H, et al. IL-4 inhibits TGF-beta-induced Foxp3+ T cells, and together with TGF-beta, generates IL-9+ IL-10+ Foxp3− effector T cells. Nat Immunol. 2008; 9(12):1347–55.
36. Veldhoen M, Uyttenhove C, van Snick J, et al. Transforming growth factor-beta 'reprograms' the differentiation of T helper 2 cells and promotes an interleukin 9-producing subset. Nat Immunol. 2008;9(12):1341–6.
37. Licona-Limon P, Henao-Mejia J, Temann AU, et al. Th9 cells drive host immunity against gastrointestinal worm infection. Immunity. 2013;39(4):744–57.
38. Gerlach K, Hwang Y, Nikolaev A, et al. Th9 cells that express the transcription factor PU.1 drive T cell-mediated colitis via IL-9 receptor signaling in intestinal epithelial cells. Nat Immunol. 2014;15(7):676–86.
39. Trifari S, Spits H. IL-22producing CD4+ T cells: middle-men between the immune system and its environment. Eur J Immunol. 2010;40(9):2369–71.
40. Leuing JM, Davenport M, Wolff MJ, et al. IL-22-producing CD4+ T cells are depleted in actively inflamed colitis tissue. Mucosal Immunol. 2014;7(1):124–33.
41. Zenewicz LA, Yancopoulos GD, Valenzuela DM, et al. Innate and adaptive interleukin-22 protects mice from inflammatory bowel disease. Immunity. 2008;29(6):947–57.
42. Luci C, Reynders A, Ivanov II, et al. Influence of the transcription factor RORgammat on the development of NKp46+ cell populations in gut and skin. Nat Immunol. 2009;10(1):75–82.
43. Duerr RH, Taylor KD, Brant SR, et al. A genome-wide association study identifies IL23R as an inflammatory bowel disease gene. Science. 2006;314:1461–3.
44. Fuss IJ, Neurath M, Boirivant M, et al. Disparate CD4+ lamina propria (LP) lymphokine secretion profiles in inflammatory bowel disease. Crohn's disease LP cells manifest increased secretion of IFN-gamma, whereas ulcerative colitis LP cells manifest increased secretion of IL-5. J Immunol. 1996;157(3):1261–70.
45. Monteleone G, Biancone L, Marasco R, et al. Interleukin 12 is expressed and actively released by Crohn's disease intestinal lamina propria mononuclear cells. Gastroenterology. 1997;112(4):1169–78.
46. Okazawa A, Kanai T, Watanabe M, et al. Th1-mediated intestinal inflammation in Crohn's disease may be induced by activation of lamina propria lymphocytes through synergistic stimulation of interleukin-12 and interleukin-18 without T cell receptor engagement. Am J Gastroenterol. 2002;97(12):3108–17.
47. Mannon PJ, Fuss IJ, Mayer L, et al. Anti-interleukin-12 antibody for active Crohn's disease. N Engl J Med. 2004;351(20):2069–79.
48. Abraham C, Cho J. Interleukin-23/Th17 pathways and inflammatory bowel disease. Inflamm Bowel Dis. 2009;15(7):1090–100. Review.
49. Kamada N, Hisamatsu T, Okamoto S, et al. Unique CD14 intestinal macrophages contribute to the pathogenesis of Crohn disease via IL-23/IFN-gamma axis. J Clin Invest. 2008;118(6):2269–80.
50. Fuss IJ, Becker C, Yang Z, et al. Both IL-12p70 and IL-23 are synthesized during active Crohn's disease and are down-regulated by treatment with anti-IL-12 p40 monoclonal antibody. Inflamm Bowel Dis. 2006;12(1):9–15.
51. Fuss IJ, Heller F, Boirivant M, et al. Nonclassical CD1d-restricted NK T cells that produce IL-13 characterize an atypical Th2 response in ulcerative colitis. J Clin Invest. 2004;113(10):1490–7.
52. Maul J, Loddenkemper C, Mundt P, et al. Peripheral and intestinal regulatory CD4+ CD25(high) T cells in inflammatory bowel disease. Gastroenterology. 2005;128(7):1868–78.
53. Himmel ME, Hardenberg G, Piccirillo CA, et al. The role of T-regulatory cells and Toll-like receptors in the pathogenesis of human inflammatory bowel disease. Immunology. 2008;125(2):145–53. Review.
54. Makita S, Kanai T, Oshima S, et al. CD4+CD25bright T cells in human intestinal lamina propria as regulatory cells. J Immunol. 2004;173(5):3119–30.
55. Franke A, Balschun T, Karlsen TH, et al. Sequence variants in IL10, ARPC2 and multiple other loci contribute to ulcerative colitis susceptibility. Nat Genet. 2008;40(11):1319–23.
56. Glocker EO, Kotlarz D, Boztug K, et al. Inflammatory bowel disease and mutations affecting the interleukin-10 receptor. N Engl J Med. 2009;361(21):2033–45.
57. Tsuji M, Komatsu N, Kawamoto S, et al. Preferential generation of follicular B helper T cells from Foxp3+ T cells in gut Peyer's patches. Science. 2009;323(5920):1488–92.

Mouse Models of Chronic Intestinal Inflammation: Characterization and Use in Pharmacological Intervention Studies

15

Cynthia Reinoso Webb and Matthew B. Grisham

Introduction

A number of different animal models have been used over the past 50 years to better understand the immunopathogenesis of autoimmune and chronic inflammatory diseases as well as to assess the therapeutic efficacy of new and potentially more potent therapeutic agents. Retrospective meta-analyses of these preclinical studies report that very few of the promising, therapeutic studies were replicated in clinical trials [1–7]. A recent, non-exhaustive search of PubMed using *mouse and colitis* as search terms revealed ~6200 published studies. The vast majority of these studies have focused on the use of mouse models of the inflammatory bowel diseases (IBD; Crohn's disease, ulcerative colitis). This search also identified several hundred studies that have reported major anti-inflammatory properties of novel small molecules, biologics, genetic alterations or immune manipulations using these mouse models of IBD. However, only a very small fraction of these promising results have been replicated by other investigators and evaluated in clinical studies. Indeed, Valatas et al. have recently summarized the bench-to-bedside success rates of >50 novel small molecules, biologics and cell-based therapies that have been reported to attenuate intestinal inflammation in different mouse models of IBD *and* have been or are currently being evaluated in large numbers of phase I–III clinical studies [8]. They report that of the numerous new targets and therapeutic strategies identified in preclinical studies, only two classes of novel therapeutics are currently approved for treatment of IBD (Reviewed in ref. [8]; http://wwwclinicaltrials.gov). Indeed, the newest of these therapies are new generation preparations of biologics that have been used for the past several years including monoclonal antibodies directed against TNF (e.g., infliximab, adalimumab, certolizumab, golimumab) or the integrins α_4 or α_4 β_7 (e.g., natalizumab, vedolizumab). The reasons for the lack of translation of promising preclinical results to the clinics are not known with certainty; however, several possible factors may contribute to this lack of *bench-to-bedside* transition.

One obvious reason for the lack of translation is the use of mouse models that do not recapitulate the *chronic* immunopathology that is observed in human IBD. Currently, there are several dozen mouse models of intestinal inflammation with the large majority of these mice expressing acute or chronic colitis (Table 15.1) [1, 9–16]. A cursory survey of PubMed reveals that >2000 studies have been published using the two most popular, chemically-induced models of experimental colitis, i.e., dextran sulfate sodium (DSS) and trinitrobenzene sulfonic acid (TNBS) models. A large number of these studies have reported significant protective or anti-inflammatory activity of novel small molecules, biologics, immune manipulations or genetic alterations. Yet, few of these potential "targets" or therapeutic agents have been evaluated in animal models of chronic intestinal inflammation. When assessed in mouse models of chronic gut inflammation, investigators have been unable to reproduce many of the promising anti-inflammatory results reported using the DSS or TNBS models of erosive, self-limiting colitis [1, 17–21]. Examples of the disparity between preclinical studies using chemically induced models and clinical efficacy can be found in studies describing the development of the different leukotriene B_4 receptor antagonists and 5-lipoxygenase inhibitors for the treatment of IBD [1]. Although these novel anti-inflammatory agents appeared to be quite effective in preclinical experiments using erosive models of self-limiting colitis in rodents, investigators failed to demonstrate significant anti-inflammatory effects in patients with Crohn's disease (CD) or ulcerative colitis (UC) when evaluated in blinded, multicenter, placebo-controlled clinical studies [22, 23].

C.R. Webb, B.S., M(ASCP) • M.B. Grisham, Ph.D. (✉)
Department of Immunology and Molecular Microbiology, Texas Tech University Health Sciences Center,
3601 4th Street STOP 6591, Lubbock, TX 79430-6591, USA
e-mail: matthew.grisham@ttuhsc.edu

D.C. Baumgart (ed.), *Crohn's Disease and Ulcerative Colitis*, DOI 10.1007/978-3-319-33703-6_15

Table 15.1 Representative mouse models of chronic small and large bowel inflammation

T cell transfer	Genetic	Spontaneous	Bacterial
CD45RB^{high} → RAG$^{-/-}$ (*SB* + *C*)	IL-2$^{-/-}$	SAMP1/Yit (*SB*)	*H. hepaticus*
	IL-2Rα$^{-/-}$		
	IL-10$^{-/-}$		
WT → CD3εtg	TCR$^{-/-}$	C3H/HeJBr	
	Gαi2$^{-/-}$		
	Mdr1a$^{-/-}$		
	TNF$^{\Delta ARE}$ (*SB*)		
	STAT3$^{-/-}$		
	STAT4 tg		
	CD40L tg		
	A20$^{-/-}$		
	TGFβ1$^{-/-}$		
	TGFβR2$^{-/-}$		
	N-Cadherin DN		
	GPx 1 + 2$^{-/-}$		
	EP4$^{-/-}$		
	R59D-JAB tg (SOCs-1 tg)		
	WASP$^{-/-}$		
	MUC2$^{-/-}$		
	IL10R2 × TGFβR DN		
	IEC/IKK$^{-/-}$		
	Tbet$^{-/-}$ × RAG$^{-/-}$(TRUC)		
	CD4^{+}/TGFβRII DN		
	IL-7 tg		

Compiled from references cited in Refs. 1, 8. *SB* small bowel inflammation, *SB* + *C* small bowel and colonic inflammation, *tg* transgenic, *DN* dominant negative

In retrospect, these results are not surprising given the differences in the immunopathogenetic mechanisms that promote intestinal inflammation in the DSS and TNBS models. For example, it is well known that the adaptive immune system is *not* required for development of DSS- or TNBS-induced colitis as distal bowel inflammation occurs in the absence of T and B cells [24, 25]. Indeed, recent studies have demonstrated that lymphocyte homing plays virtually not role in the pathogenesis of DSS- or TNBS-induced colitis [26–28]. There is also convincing evidence that the acute/self-limiting inflammation is a secondary response following the erosive and nonspecific injury of the colonic epithelium. Although these models are excellent in vivo systems for investigating wound responses in the gut, very few preclinical studies using these mouse models actually demonstrate how various pharmacologic agents or genetic manipulations affect epithelial cell restitution, proliferation, and/or mucosal barrier repair [1]. It is very likely that the vast majority of reports demonstrating anti-inflammatory properties of different therapeutics or experimental maneuvers may in fact be the result of more effective repair of the mucosal epithelium. When viewed in context of our current understanding of the immunopathogenesis of human IBD, these data indicate that erosive, self-limiting models of colitis may be of limited value for preclinical studies.

Other factors that have been suggested to limit the translation of preclinical data is the use of inbred strains of mice as surrogates for heterogeneous human populations as well as differences in intestinal microbiota [1, 16]. Flawed experimental design and/or data analyses as well as publication bias have also received a great deal of attention as factors that limit effective translation of preclinical studies to disease treatment [1–7, 29]. Furthermore, the inability of investigators within the academic and pharmaceutical/biotechnology communities to reproduce published studies demonstrating therapeutic efficacy of novel, small molecules or biologics in mouse models of disease has received a great deal of discussion in recent months. This is a particularly troubling situation that has garnered a great deal of attention by funding agencies and the publishing community [1, 2, 30–35]. In a recent review of the quality of methods reported in 58 studies using four of the most popular mouse models of IBD, Bramhall et al. reported that <2 % of these articles described all of the criteria that are considered to be essential for promoting reproducibility of mouse models of IBD [36]. They noted that while many of the studies described some of the criteria in reasonable detail, animal age, gender, housing conditions, and mortality/morbidity were poorly reported. When taken together, it appears clear that in order to more efficiently utilize the limited resources available for preclinical studies and accelerate the bench-to-bedside transition for promising therapeutics, investigators should utilize well-characterized, models of *chronic* intestinal inflammation that more closely mimics the immunopathology of human IBD [1, 16, 35, 37].

Mouse Models of Chronic Intestinal Inflammation

No single mouse model of chronic intestinal inflammation completely recapitulates the clinical and histopathological characteristics of human IBD; however, a number of different mouse models of *chronic* small and/or large bowel inflammation have been developed over the past two decades that have greatly advanced our understanding of disease pathogenesis (Table 15.1). Data obtained from numerous studies using a variety of chronic models have revealed several recurring themes. First, *chronic* gut inflammation requires the presence of a functioning adaptive immune system. Second, intestinal microbiota are required for the induction and/or perpetuation of chronic gut inflammation. Third, defective immuno-regulation of mucosal immune responses induces chronic intestinal inflammation and finally, the onset and severity of inflammation may be greatly dependent upon the genetic background of the animal. Taken together, these studies suggest that chronic intestinal inflammation develops as a result of a dysregulated immune response to components of the intestinal microbiota [38–40]. In addition, these data strongly suggest that mouse models of *chronic gut inflammation* are in general, much more relevant to human IBD than are acute/self-limiting models. Of the many mouse models of chronic gut inflammation that have been developed, a few of these have been used by sufficient numbers of investigators to yield detailed information on the penetrance, severity and pathogenesis of the inflammation. Below, we discuss a few of these models focusing on the immunopathology and their use in preclinical studies.

Mouse Models of Chronic Colitis

One of the best-characterized mouse models of chronic colitis is the CD45RB^{high} T cell transfer model (Table 15.1) [41, 42]. Adoptive transfer of antigen inexperienced (i.e., naïve) CD4^{+}CD45RB^{high} T cells from healthy wild type mice into syngeneic, lymphopenic recipients results in the generation and expansion of large numbers of Th1 and Th17 effector cells but few, if any, regulatory T cells (Tregs; CD4^{+}Foxp3^{+}) [42]. This unregulated immune response requires the presence of *intestinal microbiota* and ultimately induces chronic and unrelenting pancolitis at 6–8 weeks following T cell transfer [41–43]. This model illustrates the concept that in the absence of effective immunoregulation (due to the paucity of Tregs), naïve T cells undergo microbial antigen-driven priming, polarization, and expansion to yield large numbers of colitogenic effector cells within the gut-draining mesenteric lymph nodes (MLNs) and colon [39, 41–43]. Because naïve T cells will, by default, convert to disease-producing effector cells in the absence of Tregs, virtually any T cell deficient recipient (e.g., SCID, RAG-1$^{-/-}$, RAG-2$^{-/-}$, nude, CD3$^{-/-}$, TCRβ$^{-/-}$ × TCRδ$^{-/-}$) can be used as recipients [39, 42, 44]. We have also observed that the presence of B cells delays modestly the onset but not severity of colitis supporting the concept that B cells may act to suppress colonic inflammation in mice [43, 45, 46]. Histopathological analysis of colons obtained from mice with active disease reveals transmural inflammation, epithelial cell hyperplasia, PMN and mononuclear leukocyte infiltration, occasional crypt abscesses and epithelial cell erosions. Depending upon the strain of the donor and recipient, reconstituted mice may exhibit varying degrees of weight loss, diarrhea/loose stools, and severity of disease. Historically, the T-cell transfer model has been described as a Th1 model of colitis because of the large increase in IFN-γ production within the inflamed tissue [43]. However, we and others have found that the inflammation induced in this model represents a mixed Th1/Th17 inflammation because CD4^{+} T cells isolated from the spleen, mesenteric lymph nodes, and colonic lamina propria of colitic mice produce IFN-γ, IL-17 or both cytokines.

The original reports describing this model suggested that the inflammation was largely confined to the colon; however, more recent data demonstrates that the transfer of naïve T cells into RAG-1$^{-/-}$ (or TCRβ$^{-/-}$ × δ$^{-/-}$) mice induces both colitis and small bowel inflammation [43, 47, 48]. We and others have found that the small intestine of these reconstituted RAG-1$^{-/-}$ mice exhibited loss of goblet and Paneth cells along the entire length of small intestine, which was most noticeable in the distal portion [43]. This model may prove useful for investigators who wish to ascertain whether the immunological mechanisms responsible for colitis are similar to those that induce inflammation of the small intestine. The reasons for the relative paucity of reports by other laboratories describing small intestine inflammation in this model are not known; however, most of the original studies used SCID recipients whereas we have used RAG-1$^{-/-}$ mice. It is well known that SCID mice are "leaky" in that they can begin to develop T and B cells with age which may influence the development of intestinal inflammation. In addition to the small intestine, reconstitution of RAG-1$^{-/-}$ mice with naïve T cells induces chronic liver and lung inflammation. We have observed extensive periportal and lobular lymphocytic inflammation, hepatocellular necrosis but no bile duct damage [42]. In addition, we and others have found that the majority of colitic mice develop chronic bronchitis/pulmonary inflammation [1, 49]. In the majority of mice, we observed confluent inflammation merged together between small and medium sized bronchi. Varying degrees of perivascular lymphocytic cuffing were also observed in virtually all of the mice; however, few PMNs were observed and vasculitis was absent.

The major advantages of this model are that one may examine the earliest immunological events associated with the induction of gut inflammation as well as the time-dependent development of disease. In addition, chronic colitis can be attenuated by treatment with a variety of different pharmacologic, immunologic, and biologic treatment protocols (Table 15.2) [8, 10, 50–57]. Furthermore, this model has been proven to be very useful to study the role that Tregs play in suppressing or limiting the onset and/or severity of colonic inflammation [58–61]. Te Velde and coworkers have found, using genome-wide gene expression profiling of inflamed colons, that the pattern of gene expression in the CD45RB^{high} T cell transfer model most closely reflects the altered expression profile observed in human IBD when compared to the erosive, self-limiting models of colitis [20, 62, 63]. Disadvantages of this model include the expense and the requirement for cell sorting. In our experience, differences in animal housing, food and water may influence greatly the onset and severity of disease. It has also been suggested that homeostatic proliferation of disease-producing T cells in lymphopenic recipients may not accurately represent the immunopathological mechanisms responsible for human disease [58]. However, a number of features of this model strongly suggest that the development of chronic colitis is not simply the result of homeostatic proliferation of T cells in a lymphopenic environment. For example, colitis does not develop following transfer of naïve T cells into antibiotic-treated or germ-free recipients [58]. These observations together with those demonstrating reduced accumulation of naïve T cells suggest that pathology is driven by intestinal bacterial antigens and not by "space" [58]. In addition, there is a great deal of evidence demonstrating a strong correlation between genes involved in the immunopathogenesis of chronic colitis in the T cell transfer model and those linked to human susceptibility alleles from genome wide association studies performed on patients with CD suggesting that this model may in fact represent a very good model for pre-clinical studies [58].

A second, widely used model of chronic colitis is the interleukin-10 deficient (IL-10$^{-/-}$) model (Table 15.1). Mice

Table 15.2 Pharmacological studies using mouse models of chronic gut inflammation

Model	Therapeutic	Efficacy
IL-10$^{-/-}$	TNF/TNFR antisense	Yes
	IL-6/IL-6R mAb	Yes
	IFNγ/IFNγR mAb	Depends on timing
	IL-12/IL-23 mAb	Yes
CD45RB^{high} → SCID/RAG	TNF mAb	Yes
	OX40L mAb	Yes
	B7-H1 mAb	Yes
	CD70 mAb	Yes
	Antiangiogenic peptide	Yes
	FTY720	Yes
	FASL mAb	No
	Dexamethasone/prednisolone	Yes
	Azathioprine	No
	Sulfasalazine/5-ASA	No
	Cyclosporine	No
	Tacrolimus	No
	TNF/TNFR mAb	Yes
	Integrins mAb (β7, MAC-1, LFA-1, α4)	Yes
	IL-6/IL-6R mAb	Yes
	IFNγ/IFNγR mAb	Yes
	IL-12/IL-23 mAb	Yes
	IL-17 mAb	No
TNF^{ΔARE}	CCR6 mAb	No
	Integrins mAb (β7)	Yes
	TNF/TNFR mAb	Yes
	IL-12/IL-23 mAb	Yes
	IFNγ mAb	Yes
SAMP1/Yitc	Dexamethasone	Yes
	TNF/TNFR mAb	Yes
	Integrins mAb (β7, MAC-1, LFA-1, α4)	Yes
	IL-6/IL-6R mAb	Yes
	IFNγ/IFNγR mAb	Yes
	IL-12/IL-23 mAb	Yes
	CCR9 mAb	Yes

Compiled from references cited in Refs. 1, 8; mAb signifies monoclonal antibody with targeted disruption (i.e., deletion) of the *IL10* gene develop spontaneous pancolitis and cecal inflammation by 2–4 months of age. Again, this model of chronic colitis illustrates the recurrent paradigm that *defective immunoregulation*, via the loss of IL-10 production, leads to a dysregulated immune response to intestinal microbiota resulting in the development of chronic inflammation [64, 65]. Histopathological analysis of colons obtained from mice with active disease show many of the same characteristics as those observed in human CD including transmural infiltration of mononuclear leukocytes, T cells, and plasma cells. The genetic background of the mouse is a major modifier of disease with disease penetrance and severity occurring to a much greater extent in 129SvEv IL-$10^{-/-}$ and Balb/c IL-$10^{-/-}$ mice when compared to the C57Bl/6 IL-$10^{-/-}$ strain. The advantage of using the IL-$10^{-/-}$ model is that it is a well-established Th1 model of transmural colitis and cecal inflammation that can be attenuated by administration of various pharmacologic, immunologic, and biologic agents (Table 15.2) [8, 10]. A disadvantage of this model is the onset and severity of disease may be quite variable and in some cases requires several months to develop.

The variability in penetrance and severity as well as the delayed onset of disease in genetically engineered models of chronic colitis involving single mutations of specific genes (e.g., IL-$10^{-/-}$ model) limit an investigator's ability to more fully characterize the time course and immunopathogenesis of disease, as well as evaluate new therapeutic strategies for treatment of chronic colitis. Indeed, investigators have demonstrated that genetic manipulations in two (or more) loci appear to enhance the penetrance of robust colitis as well as accelerate the onset of disease [8, 66, 67]. Recent data derived from genome-wide association studies have identified ~163 different susceptibility loci for CD and/or UC [68]. Of these, alterations in genes involved in IL-10 and TGFβ signaling have been described with polymorphisms in each increasing modestly the risk of developing disease [69]. Furthermore, recent clinical studies have determined that mutations in the IL-10 receptor (IL-10R) results in very early onset IBD in young children [70]. Capitalizing on these observations, Kang et al. generated a novel, "2 hit" mouse model of fulminant and unrelenting colitis [67]. To do this, investigators bred dominant negative TGFβRII (dnTGFβRII) mice with IL-10R$2^{-/-}$ mice to generate dnTGFβRII × IL-10R$2^{-/-}$ offspring referred to as dnKO mice. These offspring have defective IL-10R2 signaling in all tissues and TGFβ signaling only in T cells [67]. Compared to their littermate controls (i.e., IL-10R$2^{-/-}$ or dnTGFβRII), dnKO mice fail to gain weight following birth and develop an accelerated and severe colitis with a 100 % penetrance by 4 weeks of age. Kang et al. show that broad spectrum antibiotics rescued the dnKO offspring, thereby preventing the development of colitis [67]. Additional studies by this same group show that an isolate of *Bacteroides* but not *Enterobacteriaceae* induces robust disease in dnKO but not controls [66, 69]. Taken together, these studies clearly demonstrate the need to assess colitogenic potential rather than relying solely on 16S rRNA quantification. Although this model represents a major advancement in mouse models of IBD using IBD-relevant deficiencies in IL-10 and TGFβ signaling, the time commitment and resources necessary to generate sufficient dnKO offspring for studying immunopathogenesis or performing pharmacologic intervention studies are substantially higher than for other mouse models.

Another, well-characterized mouse model of chronic colitis that has been used by different groups of investigators is the multidrug resistance pump 1a-deficient (Mdr1$a^{-/-}$) mouse (Table 15.1) [71]. Mdr1a is a P-glycoprotein expressed on the surface of several different cell populations including intestinal epithelial cells, T cells, monocytes, macrophages, natural killer cells, dendritic cells, and brain microvascular endothelial cells. This transport protein pumps small amphiphilic and hydrophobic molecules across the cell membrane in an ATP-dependent manner. Of note is that the *mdr1a* gene is located on chromosome 7q21.1 which is a susceptibility locus for human IBD [71]. Approximately 25 % of the Mdr1$a^{-/-}$ mice develop colitis beginning at 8–12 weeks of age when housed under specific pathogen-free conditions [71, 72]. The colonic inflammation can be delayed for up to 16 weeks of age by the administration of antibiotics [72] or eliminated when raised under germ-free housing conditions demonstrating yet another model of IBD where inflammation is dependent upon the presence of commensal bacteria. Histopathological analysis of colons obtained from these mice reveals an inflammation that is similar to human UC. There is substantial thickening of the mucosa, extensive infiltration of inflammatory cells into the lamina propria and occasional crypt abscesses and ulcerations. The mechanisms by which ablation of the *mdr1a* gene induces chronic gut inflammation are not known at the present time; however, it is known that the induction of colitis in these mice is dependent upon defective *Mdr1a* activity on the intestinal epithelial cells and not the lymphocytes [72]. It may be that the lack of intestinal epithelial cell Mdr1 results in increased accumulation of enteric antigens within these cells. Antigen-loaded cells could then process and present these microbial antigens to T cells immediately underlying the epithelium, thereby priming the T cells to become "hyper-reactive" to the enteric microbiota thereby driving colonic inflammation [71, 72]. More recent studies have demonstrated a significant dysregulation of expression of cytokines and chemokines prior to onset of colitis in young Mdr1$a^{-/-}$ mice. These data suggest that the intestinal immune system in these mice may be in a continuous state of immune activation and thus are particularly susceptible to induction of chronic gut inflammation [71].

Collett et al. [73] have shown that older FVB.mdr1a$^{-/-}$ mice (12–16 weeks) have increased colonic mucosal permeability that is associated with tissue inflammation. Tissue from these mice reveal an upregulation in genes involved in bacterial recognition, a downregulation in anti-inflammatory pancreatitis-associated protein (PAP) and RegIIIγ genes and appear to be more responsive to lipopolysaccharide (LPS). Interestingly, although younger Mdr1a$^{-/-}$ mice (4–5 weeks) lack histological evidence of inflammation or increased permeability, they have increased cytokine and chemokine secretion (IFNγ, MIP2, TNFα, and IL1β) that is similar to that of older mice with active colitis [73]. These data could suggest an inappropriate immune response to luminal antigens prior to the induction of chronic inflammation. It has also been shown that FVB.mdr1a$^{-/-}$ mice have decreased amounts of inducible Tregs (iTregs; CD4$^+$Foxp3$^+$) in the intestinal lamina propria and Peyer's patches prior to and following the onset of colonic inflammation [74]. P-glycoprotein (P-gp) was found to be expressed in these cells and it appears to be restricting the development of iTregs from naïve FVB. mdr1a T cells, as demonstrated both, in vivo and in vitro [74]. P-gp deficiency phenotype conferred by knocking out of the Mdr1a$^{-/-}$ gene has been shown to be modified by the genetic background strain [75]. When the FVB.mdr1a strain is crossed with a C57BL/6 mouse (C57BL/6.*mdrla* deficient), it no longer develops spontaneous colitis nor is it sensitive to the induction of colitis by piroxicam or *Helicobacter bilis*. However, this strain shows an increased susceptibility to DSS-induced colitis, which has been attributed to the possible impaired cell cycling associated with P-gp deficiency that then affects wound repair [75, 76].

In order to further investigate the effect of other genes associated with human IBD, Ey et al. produced the Mdr1a$^{-/-}$TLR2$^{-/-}$ double knockout on the FVB strain. TLR2 is another susceptibility gene identified by GWAS in UC patients and it has been associated with a more severe disease phenotype [37, 77]. The inflammation in this model is spontaneous in nature and is characterized by an excessive release of IL-1β that requires MD2- and MyD88-mediated signaling. Colonic inflammation is characterized by mucosal thickening and inflammatory cell infiltration beginning at 5 weeks of age, which represents an acceleration in disease onset and severity when compared to Mdr1a$^{-/-}$ animals. Deletion of the *MyD88* gene in these mice to create triple knockout mice lacking all three genes (Mdr1a$^{-/-}$TLR2$^{-/-}$MyD88$^{-/-}$) prevents induction of colonic inflammation suggesting that MyD88-dependent signaling is required for induction of disease in Mdr1a$^{-/-}$TLR2$^{-/-}$ mice [37].

The large majority of mouse models displaying chronic colitis require the participation of the adaptive immune system for expression of disease. However, recent evidence suggests that innate immune cell activation alone is capable of inducing and perpetuating protracted colonic inflammation. For example, Maloy et al. have developed a mouse model of innate immune cell-mediated chronic colitis that is induced by associating lymphopenic RAG-1 or -2$^{-/-}$ animals with the *Helicobacter hepaticus* (Hp; Table 15.1) [13, 78, 79]. Although Hp does not normally induce chronic gut inflammation in healthy/immunocompetent mice, introduction of this Gram negative, spiral bacterium into RAG-2$^{-/-}$ animals establishes a lifelong colonization that ultimately induces chronic cecal and colonic inflammation (typhlocolitis) [78, 79]. This IL-23-driven inflammation is characterized by epithelial cell hyperplasia and extensive infiltration of PMNs and monocytes which is more severe in the cecum than in the colon [78, 80]. A recent variation of this model has been described in which chronic colitis can be induced in immunocompetent mice by combining the introduction of Hp with systemic administration of a mAb to IL10R [81–83].

Another interesting model of chronic colitis driven by innate immune cells has been described by Garrett and coworkers [84]. These investigators demonstrated that the ablation of *T-bet* (a T-box transcription factor family member) in RAG-2$^{-/-}$ mice results in the development of spontaneous and *communicable* colitis that is similar to human UC (Table 15.1). The colonic inflammation in these ***T***-bet$^{-/-}$ × ***R***AG-2$^{-/-}$ ***u***lcerative ***c***olitis (TRUC) mice is characterized by remarkable PMN and monocyte inflammation, crypt abscesses, bowel wall thickening, erosions, and ulcerations. These investigators also demonstrated colonic epithelial barrier disruption prior to the onset of active colitis. The fact that colitis is communicable and will develop in wild type mice when housed with TRUC mice suggest the selection of a pathogenic microbiota that develops in response to immune defects and/or inflammation [84]. Indeed, these investigators characterized the intestinal microbiota in TRUC mice and found that the overabundance of *Klebsiella pneumoniae* and *Proteus mirabilis* correlated with the onset of disease. Furthermore, TRUC-associated bacterial strains in association with maternally transmitted microbiota have the ability to induce disease in WT and RAG$^{-/-}$ mice [85]. Not surprisingly, these two organisms, as well as other members of *the Enterobacteriaceae family*, have been shown to be increased in human IBD [85–87]. Certain species within *Enterobacteriaceae* are thought to thrive in the inflamed gut due to the ability of these facultative anaerobes to proliferate in the presence of small, but significant amounts of oxygen adjacent to the inflamed tissue [85, 88]. In addition, the relative overabundance of some members of the *Enterobacteriaceae* family may be due to their ability to utilize certain electron acceptors (e.g., tetrathionate and nitrate) that are present in the inflamed lumen for anaerobic respiration, thereby outcompeting obligate anaerobes [88–90]. Not only does the microbial structure differ during active colitis and treatment-induced remission, but so do the major metabolic functions of the microbiota [88]. Some of the major differences that are seen in microbial function during active colitis are their decreased ability to harvest energy (i.e., lipid metabolism, xenobiotics biodegradation, and metabolism) and dysregulated pathways of microbial signaling and processing [88].

In addition to chronic colitis, TRUC mice develop colitis-associated colorectal cancer (caCRC) that resembles human disease. Virtually all TRUC mice develop colonic dysplasia and adenocarcinoma (ADA) by 6 weeks of age [91]. Selective depletion of dendritic cells (DCs) prevents inflammation and cancer progression in these mice, demonstrating the critical interplay between the innate immune system and intestinal microbiota in the induction of inflammation and associated malignant disease. As with other models of chronic colitis, disease incidence and severity in the TRUC model depends upon background strain. Ermann et al. showed that the severity of colitis in TRUC mice bred onto the C57BL/6 background (B6.TRUC) was less severe when compared to mice bred onto the BALB/c background (BALB/c.TRUC) [92]. These investigators found that when the suspected susceptibility locus *Cdcs1* (cytokine deficiency-induced colitis susceptibility-1) was introduced into the B6.TRUC mice, severity of colitis was found to be similar to that observed in BALB/c.TRUC animals. The *Cdcs1* locus, among others, has been described in the IL-$10^{-/-}$ and Gαi$2^{-/-}$ mouse models of chronic colitis and it is thought to control disease severity via its effects on innate immune cell function and maintenance of mucosal homeostasis [92, 93]. Although this model represents an important addition to the toolbox for IBD investigators who wish to examine the relationship among the innate immune system and chronic gut inflammation, it should be noted that currently, little or no evidence exists suggesting that human CD or UC can be transferred to healthy children or adults.

Models of Chronic Small Bowel Inflammation

In addition to the well-characterized models of chronic colitis described above, two models of spontaneous, small bowel inflammation are gaining increasing interest for studying the immunopathology of Crohn's ileitis as well as for evaluating new drug therapies. One model is the homozygous TNF-overexpressing TNF$^{\Delta ARE/\Delta ARE}$ mouse (Table 15.1). These mice were developed by targeted deletion of a 69 base-pair region of the AU-rich elements in the 3′ UTR region of the *TNF-α* gene [94]. The deletion results in increased TNF-α mRNA stability and enhanced TNF-α protein production. Mice possessing the deletion in the homozygous state display severe and rapid wasting disease and die within 1–3 months of age. These mice are runted in appearance, exhibit alopecia-like lesions, develop chronic and degenerative inflammatory arthritis and express severe inflammatory changes in the distal small bowel similar to CD by 4 weeks of age [94]. Interestingly, there appears to be a gene dosage effect as heterozygote littermates (HET; TNF$^{\Delta ARE/+}$) have a gradual development of inflammation and live at least 7–8 months, showing severe intestinal inflammation at 8 weeks of age [94]. HET mice models are useful because as in human disease, they show a malabsorption phenotype characterized by weight loss, increase fecal energy loss, fecal fat excretion and bone alterations possibly due to calcium malabsorption [95, 96]. Lesions consist of villous blunting (and broadening) associated with the transmural infiltration of acute and chronic inflammatory cells, including mononuclear leukocytes, plasma cells, and PMNs. This transmural inflammation extends deep into the muscular layers of the bowel wall, displaying characteristics of Crohn's ileitis. The severity and location of the inflammation (ileum) in this model seems to be dependent on the dysbiotic microbiota, according to Schaubeck et al.[97]. When transferred into germ–free TNF$^{\Delta ARE/\Delta ARE}$ mice, this dysbiotic microbiota induced Crohn's-like ileitis and decreased antimicrobial lysozymes and defensins. This is yet another mouse model of IBD that demonstrates the role of intestinal microbiota in disease as antibiotic treatment or raising mice under germ-free conditions eliminates intestinal inflammation [97]. In addition, different environmental and dietary factors may alter the microbiota thereby altering the onset and/or severity of disease. For example, Wernet et al. have shown depletion of luminal iron alters the gut microbiota and prevents Crohn's disease-like ileitis suggesting that luminal (oral) supplementation with iron for patients with IBD may be problematic [98]. The inflammation observed in this model can be treated with several biologics and immune-modifying drugs used in human medicine (Table 15.2). This model also offers the unique opportunity to examine the immunopathological mechanisms underlying TNF-induced ileitis *and* arthritis with the possibility of identifying new therapeutic strategies to treat patients with CD.

The *SAMP1/Yit* model of chronic ileitis is another model that is gaining increased attention and is readily available to interested investigators (Table 15.1). As with TNF$^{\Delta ARE/\Delta ARE}$ mice, these animals are useful for studying the underlying mechanisms involved in the pathogenesis of Crohn's ileitis and preclinical evaluation of new drug therapies. This model of spontaneous ileitis was originally generated by >20 generations of brother–sister mating of a senescence-accelerated mouse line [99]. SAMP1/Yit mice are unique in that 100 % of these animals develop spontaneous ileitis at ~30 weeks of age without any genetic, immunological or environmental manipulation. Histopathological analysis of these mice reveals robust and chronic ileitis as well as extraintestinal manifestations similar to human CD. The segmental inflammation is localized to the terminal ileum and displays transmural involvement and occasional granulomas. Chronic ileitis can be adoptively transferred by CD4⁺ T cells to SCID or RAG$^{-/-}$ recipients suggesting that activated CD4⁺ T cells home specifically to and recognize antigens within the terminal ileum [100]. Over the past few years, it has been found that with further brother–sister matings for an additional 20 generations, a new phenotype emerged in which chronic ileitis developed by 10 weeks of age with the occurrence of perianal disease, ulceration and fistula in a small subset of these mice as well as periodontal disease [101]. This substrain has been renamed SAMP1/YitFc and has been propagated through continued brother–sister mating [102]. Given its well-defined progression of disease in the SAMP1/YitFc model, it has shown to be very useful in studying the immunological changes before and during inflammation [103]. Pizzarro et al. demonstrated two clear phases of disease [103]: The inductive phase occurs between 4–7 weeks of age that is characterized by intense upregulation of Th1 and proinflammatory cytokines that precede histological evidence of overt inflammation. The chronic phase occurs at 9–10 weeks of age and is characterized by a Th1/Th2 response that correlates with robust intestinal inflammation [103]. It should be noted that the Tregs in this mouse model have been shown to be dysfunctional in vivo, whereas, these cells seem to have normal suppressive activity in vitro [104]. This paradoxical observation has also been made in human IBD in which investigators have noted an expansion of Tregs in the lamina propria of inflamed intestinal tissue obtained from CD patients [105]. Although these data imply Treg dysfunction, Ishikawa et al. and Fantini et al. have demonstrated normal suppressive activity of Tregs obtained from inflamed tissue in vitro [104] [106]. Fantini et al. further showed that the apparent lack of effect of Tregs in chronic gut inflammation is most likely due to resistance of colitogenic effector T cells to Treg-mediated suppression [106].

This model of chronic ileitis has also been helpful in defining the role of the innate immune system in chronic inflammation. As described above, it is widely believed the adaptive immune system plays a major role in induction and perpetuation of chronic intestinal inflammation. However, Corridoni et al. hypothesize that: "CD may occur as a deficit in innate immunity as opposed to an overly aggressive immune response" [107, 108]. It is also important to point out that although the microbiota seem to play a role in the SAMP/Yit model, it is not required for induction of disease as in other models given that some germ-free animals still develop small bowel inflammation [103]. Studies using the SAMP1/YitFc model have shown that immune-blockade of Th1- polarizing cytokines or certain T-cell adhesion molecules attenuate the severity of ileitis (Table 15.2). Thus, both the TNF$^{\Delta ARE/\Delta ARE}$ and the SAMP1/YitFc mice provide the investigator with the unique ability to study the underlying immunopathological mechanisms responsible for the development of ileal inflammation.

Humanized Mouse Models of Autoimmune and Chronic Inflammatory Diseases

There is no question that mouse models have provided investigators with valuable information on the immunopathogenesis of chronic intestinal inflammation as well as other autoimmune and chronic inflammatory diseases [109–112]. Despite revealing a number of different targets and therapeutic strategies from preclinical studies, few new therapies have been demonstrated to be effective in well-controlled clinical trials. This is not entirely surprising given the fact that the structure and function of the mouse immune system differs substantially from humans [113, 114]. It has been estimated that >80 major differences exist between the mouse and human immune systems. [35, 114]. Thus, even with the use of standardized and reproducible mouse models of chronic gut inflammation, it may be difficult to accurately model human disease. In response to these concerns, investigators have been actively working to develop mice with a functional human immune system [35]. By utilizing long-term engraftment of the human hemato-lymphoid cells (e.g., hematopoietic stem cells or lymphocytes) in severely immunodeficient recipients, investigators have been successful in producing humanized mouse models of some acute and chronic inflammatory diseases. Furthermore, some of these models have been used to evaluate certain human-specific therapies in vivo. This approach has been particularly successful using humanized mouse models of infectious diseases (e.g., HIV) [29, 110, 112, 115]. In addition, great strides have been made in using humanized mice to study the pathogenesis and human-specific therapies in different chronic diseases such as diabetes, arthritis, graft-vs.-host disease, transplant rejection and cancer [109–112, 116–118].

A major breakthrough came in the humanization of the murine immune system with the discovery that targeted mutation of the IL-2 receptor common gamma chain (IL-2γ) in NOD/scid mice (termed NOD/scid-IL2rγ$^{-/-}$ or NSG mice) greatly enhanced the long-term engraftment of human hemato-lymphoid cells in these severely immunodeficient mice [35, 119–122]. It was well known that IL-2rγ was a required component for receptor complexes specific for IL-2, IL-4, IL-7, IL-9, IL-15, and IL-21 (Fig. 15.1) [123, 124]. In addition, studies had demonstrated that these cytokines are critical for generation of T, B and NK cells. Thus, deletion or inactivation of IL-2rγ created mice devoid of T, B and NK cells [125–127]. Several laboratories have developed different stocks of immunodeficient mice devoid of IL-2rγ that differ with respect to strain background and the type of IL-2rγ mutation (reviewed in 35). These novel platforms have been used to engraft different populations of human hemato-lymphoid cells, thereby producing three major models of humanized mice (Table 15.3). The reader is referred to recent reviews for more detailed discussions of these models

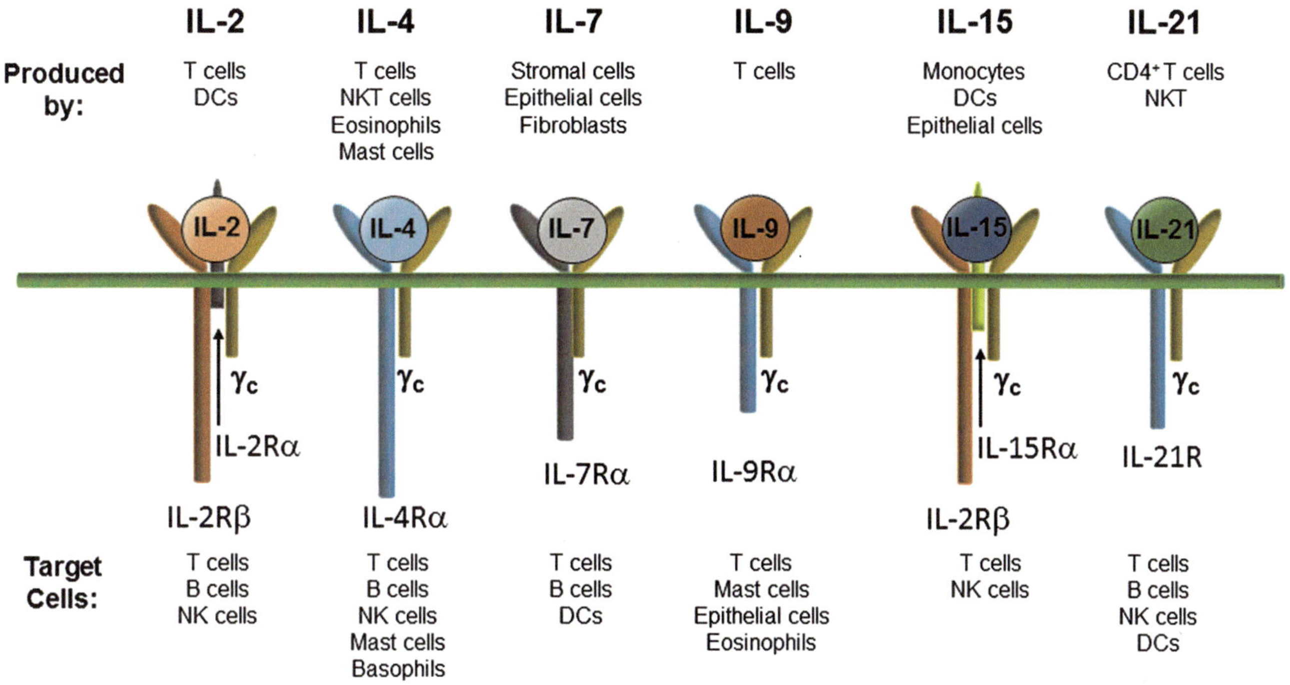

Fig. 15.1 The IL-2 receptor common γ chain plays a critical role in the development of immune cells. The common γ chain is associated with the high affinity receptors for IL-2, IL-4, IL-7, IL-9, IL-15, and IL-21. These cytokines are produced by different immune cells, stromal cells, and epithelial cells. Cytokine-receptor signaling is critically important for the generation of different populations of immune cells (Modified from Ref. 127 with permission)

[35, 128, 129]. It is theoretically possible to model most, if not all of the human autoimmune and chronic inflammatory diseases using one or more of the immunodeficient IL-2rγ$^{-/-}$ strains. Below is a brief overview of the generation, uses and limitations of the 3 major humanized mouse models.

Engraftment of Human Peripheral Blood Mononuclear Cells into Immunodeficient Mice Devoid of IL-2rγ

There is a long history of attempts to engraft (via adoptive transfer) human peripheral mononuclear cells (PBMCs) into immunodeficient mice such as SCID or RAG-1$^{-/-}$ or -2$^{-/-}$ mice [35, 130]. However, very small numbers of T cells and few if any B cells engraft in this model due to the presence of a fully functional innate immune system that destroys xenogeneic (human) cells [131–133]. As pointed out above, the development and use of immunodeficient mice that lack IL-2rγ greatly enhanced the engraftment of T cells in these novel lymphopenic recipients devoid of T, B, and NK cells [112, 134–136]. This model, which we have termed the *Hu-PBMC-IL-2rγ$^{-/-}$* model, has been used to investigate immunological mechanisms involved in allograft rejection, cancer, autoimmunity, regenerative medicine, and infectious diseases [29, 112, 116, 134, 137] (Table 15.3). This model has also been used to evaluate novel, human-specific therapies including cell-based therapies [138]. It should be noted that this model is particularly useful for investigating T cell-mediated immune responses following engraftment of PBMCs obtained from patients with autoimmune or chronic inflammation diseases; however, the usefulness of this model is limited by the development of lethal, xenogeneic graft versus host disease (GVHD) within 3–4 weeks post T cell engraftment [139]. King and coworkers discovered that GVHD developed as a result of aggressive immune responses of human T cells towards murine MHC class I and II [139]. A delay in GVHD in NSG mice devoid of murine MHC class I and II may prove useful in extending the observation period in the *Hu-PBMC-IL-2rγ$^{-/-}$* model in future studies [139].

Engraftment of Human Hematopoietic Stem Cells into Immunodeficient Mice Devoid of IL-2rγ

While enhanced engraftment of PBMCs into lymphopenic IL-2rγ$^{-/-}$ mice was a major step forward in creating a humanized immune system in these animals, the usefulness of this model was limited by the absence of significant numbers of B cells and myeloid cells as well as the development of GVHD within the first 3–4 weeks post transfer. In an attempt to circumvent these limitations, investigators undertook a series of studies to determine whether human hematopoietic stem

Table 15.3 Models of human hemato-lymphoid cell engraftment into immunodeficient IL-2rγ$^{-/-}$ mice

Model name	Description	Advantages	Applications	Limitations
Hu-PBMC-IL-2rγ$^{-/-}$ (*Hu*man *P*eripheral *B*lood *M*ononuclear *C*ells engrafted into lymphopenic IL-2rγ$^{-/-}$ mice)	Lymphopenic IL-2rγ$^{-/-}$ mice are injected with human peripheral mononuclear cells	• Technically simple model • Good engraftment of effector and memory T cells	• Induced models of inflammation (e.g., sepsis, arthritis, colitis) • Model of *xenogeneic* GVHD • Assess effector functions of T cells obtained from patients with RA, lupus, MS, diabetes or IBD • Human-specific infectious diseases (HIV) • Allograft tissue rejection	• Only activated/memory T cells are present • Lack of mature human B cells, myeloid cells, DCs, platelets and erythrocytes • Xenogeneic GVHD develops after 4–5 weeks due to human T cell reactivity against mouse MHC molecules • Limited primary immune responses
Hu-HSC-IL-2rγ$^{-/-}$ (*Hu*man *H*ematopoietic *S*tem *C*ells engrafted into lymphopenic IL-2rγ$^{-/-}$ mice)	Lymphopenic IL-2rγ$^{-/-}$ mice are injected with CD34^{+} HSCs derived from fetal liver, cord blood, bone marrow, or from peripheral blood following G-CSF-mediated mobilization	• Generates a naïve human immune system • Development of T and B cells, APCs, myeloid cells, and NK cells	• Human hematopoiesis • Induced models of inflammation (e.g., sepsis, arthritis, colitis) • Engraft human HSCs from patients with autoimmune or chronic inflammatory diseases • Human-specific infectious diseases • Transplantation biology	• Low rate of T cell engraftment • Impaired T and B functions • No mucosal immune system • Lack of expression of human HLA within the thymus prevents education and development of HLA-restricted CD4^{+} and CD8^{+} T cells (DTH response is suboptimal) • Only small numbers of PMNs, RBCs, and megakaryocytes are present in the blood
BLT-IL-2rγ$^{-/-}$ (*B*one marrow, *L*iver, *T*hymus engrafted into lymphopenic IL-2rγ$^{-/-}$ mice)	Lymphopenic IL-2rγ$^{-/-}$ mice are implanted with small pieces of human fetal liver and autologous thymus under the renal capsule; the mice are then injected with human CD34^{+} HSCs purified from the same fetal liver sample	• Human immune system engraftment is much more robust than in the Hu-SRC-NSG model • Sustained high level of T cell development; T cells are educated by the human thymus and are HLA restricted • Produces human mucosal immune system	• Human hematopoiesis • Engraft human HSCs from patients with autoimmune or chronic inflammatory diseases • Human-specific infectious diseases • Transplantation biology	• Surgical expertise and fetal tissue are required • Responses to vaccination protocols are limited to IgM antibody production • A delayed xenogeneic GVHD (>4 months) occurs in these mice that results from the lack of negative selection against murine antigens in human thymus and/or to lack of peripheral regulation

Table derived from Ref. 35 (with permission)

cells (HSCs; CD34+ cells) could engraft and differentiate into the different immune cell lineages in lymphopenic IL-2rγ$^{-/-}$ recipients (Table 15.3) (reviewed in 35). Investigators found that HSCs derived from granulocyte-colony stimulating factor (G-CSF)-mobilized peripheral blood, bone marrow, fetal liver, or umbilical cord blood (UC) were capable of engrafting in different strains of lymphopenic IL-2rγ$^{-/-}$ mice [128, 140, 141]. The investigators determined that depending upon the strain and route of administration of the human HSCs, greater numbers of HSCs engrafted and differentiated into immune cell subsets than had been observed in previous studies using more traditional lymphopenic recipients (i.e. scid or RAG$^{-/-}$ mice) [142, 143]. Adoptive transfer of human HSCs into lymphopenic IL-2rγ$^{-/-}$ mice resulted in the generation of T and B cells and small but significant numbers of myeloid cells and dendritic cells (DCs) [35, 119–121, 135, 144, 145]. This model, which we have termed the Hu-HSC-IL-2rγ$^{-/-}$ model to avoid confusion with previous HSC models, represented a major leap forward in the humanization of the mouse immune system [35]. Additionally, because human T cells were selected (positively and negatively) within the mouse thymus, circulating human T cells were incapable of reacting with murine MHC I and II and thus xenogeneic GVHD did not develop [146]. Unfortunately, this also meant that human T cells (or B cells) failed to react to antigens presented by human DCs or other human antigen presenting cells that develop within the different lymphoid and nonlymphoid tissue [147]. In addition, it became clear that despite the presence of human T cells within these novel immunodeficient recipients, their development was suboptimal due to defective thymopoiesis within the mouse thymus [144]. It was also noted that only very small numbers of human platelets, erythrocytes, and granulocytes were observed in these mice [112, 137, 147]. Nevertheless, the Hu-HSC-IL-2r$\gamma^{-/-}$ model has provided invaluable information of human immuno-biology.

Engraftment of Human Hematopoietic Stem Cells into Immunodeficient IL-2r$\gamma^{-/-}$ Mice Containing Human Fetal Thymic and Liver Tissues

The problems associated with human T cell development and differentiation described above for the Hu-HSC-IL-2r$\gamma^{-/-}$ model prompted investigators to develop the *Bone marrow–Liver–Thymus* (BLT) mouse model (Table 15.3). The BLT model was originally developed in NOD/*scid* mice in which small fragments of human fetal liver and thymus were surgically implanted under the kidney capsules [29, 112, 148, 149]. These mice were then injected (I.V.) with varying numbers of autologous human HSCs obtained from a portion of the same fetal human liver implanted into the recipients [150]. Using this approach, investigators observed long-term engraftment and differentiation of multiple human immune cell subsets including T and B cells, DCs, monocytes, macrophages, erythrocytes, and platelets [29, 135, 148, 149, 151]. An advantage of this model is that human T cells are selected within the human thymus implanted under the kidney capsule, thereby making the mouse capable of mounting adaptive immune responses in vivo [29, 135, 148, 149, 151]. Furthermore, BLT mice developed a humanized mucosal immune system as well as lymph nodes, thereby making this the model of choice for HIV investigations [29, 135, 148, 149, 151]. While engraftment of human HSCs was similar to or even greater in NSG-BLT recipients when compared to NOD/scid-BLT mice [119, 120, 129, 152–155], Denton and coworkers discovered that NSG-BLT mice contain significantly fewer T cells within the lamina propria and intraepithelial cell compartments when compared to their NOD/scid BLT counterparts [153]. Furthermore, Nochi et al. observed little or no evidence of cryptopatches and gut associated lymphoid tissue (GALT) in NSG-BLT mice whereas both were readily apparent in NOD/scid-BLT mice [156]. Taken together, these studies revealed the crucial role of the IL-2rγ chain in GALT development [156].

Despite their differences, both the NOD/*scid*-BLT and NSG-BLT models are regarded as the most immunologically relevant mouse models for studying human hematopoiesis, infectious diseases, acute and chronic diseases and therapeutic/vaccine development. Indeed, these animals possess a well-integrated immune system that is reasonably adept at mounting both direct and indirect delayed type hypersensitivity (DTH) responses [157]. As with the other humanized mouse models, the BLT model possess several shortcomings such as the requirement for small animal surgery, procurement and utilization of human fetal tissue, generation of small numbers of certain immune cell subsets (e.g., granulocytes, myeloid cells, B cells) and delayed xenogeneic GVHD [150, 158–161]. The mechanisms responsible for the GVHD have not been clearly identified; however, it does appears that a loss of tolerance of human T and/or B cells toward murine MHC class I and II antigens may not be responsible [150]. Recent studies by Lavender and coworkers demonstrate that the presence of CD47 in RAG-2$^{-/-}$IL-2r$\gamma^{-/-}$-BLT recipients may play an important role in the pathogenesis of xenogeneic GVHD because genetic ablation of CD47 renders the triple knockout (CD47$^{-/-}$RAG-2$^{-/-}$IL-2r$\gamma^{-/-}$) animals resistant to GVHD in the BLT model [162, 163].

Humanized Mouse Models of the Inflammatory Bowel Diseases

The three major humanized mouse models described above have been used extensively for studies involved in infectious diseases, autoimmunity and cancer; however only a handful of studies have reported their use in studying the immunopathogenesis and/or treatment of IBD. Recent studies by Nolte and coworkers reported the use of Hu-PBMC-NSG mice in a chemically induced model of self-limiting colitis [164]. NSG mice were engrafted with human PBMCs obtained from healthy donors (HD) or from individuals suffering from UC or atopic dermatitis (AD). Mice were then sensitized, via dermal application, to the vehicle (ethanol) or the hapten oxazalone (OXA) and challenged 24 h later via intrarectal administration of either 50 % ethanol or OXA in 50 % ethanol [164, 165]. Although these investigators observed significant colonic inflammation in all groups of mice, they did not observe significant differences between or among the different groups [164]. These results are not entirely surprising given the way in which inflammation is induced in this model. As discussed in more detail in this and our previous review [1], intrarectal administration of erosive chemicals (i.e., organic acids, ethanol) injures the colonic epithelium, thereby initiating an intense inflammatory response that may conceal more subtle immune responses induce by the "hapten" OXA.

In a preliminary report (abstract only), using a method similar to that described by Nolte et al., Goettel and coworkers utilized transgenic NSG mice that expressed human HLADR1 but lacked murine MHC class II (called NSGAb0DR1 mice) [166]. These mice were then engrafted with HLA-matched $CD4^+$ T cells and sensitized (via skin painting) with the hapten, trinitrobenzene sulfonic acid (TNBS). Seven days following sensitization, mice were challenged with a single intrarectal infusion of TNBS in ethanol. These investigators observed colonic inflammation in mice that received TNBS in ethanol; however, colitis was not evident in those mice that received TNBS in ethanol but no human T cells [166]. As noted above, the use of erosive chemicals to induce self-limiting colitis is problematic if one desires to recapitulate the immunopathology of human disease. A second, more interesting study reported by this same group, demonstrated that adoptive transfer of HLA-matched $CD34^+$ HSCs obtained from patients with immunodysregulation polyendocrinopathy enteropathy X-linked (IPEX) syndrome into NSGAb0DR1 mice induces a systemic and lethal autoimmunity similar to that observed in humans with IPEX [167]. Conceptually, this study is quite exciting as it provides proof of principle for modeling human autoimmune diseases via engraftment of patient HSCs.

Improving Humanized Mouse Models of IBD: Remaining Issues and Questions

The generation of humanized mouse models of IBD would greatly advance our understanding of the immunopathogenesis of UC and CD as well as provide preclinical platforms to evaluate human-specific therapeutic agents; however, progress in developing these types of mouse models has been disappointingly slow compared to other autoimmune disease models. The reasons for this are not clear at the present time but most likely represent the complex relationship between genetics and environmental factors required for full expression of these diseases. Because of the low concordance rates in identical twins for UC and CD, we know that the environment plays an important role in disease pathogenesis [168–173]. Thus, several issues and fundamental questions must be considered when attempting to model human IBD in humanized mice. For example, it may not be possible to generate chronic intestinal inflammation in immunodeficient IL-2r$\gamma^{-/-}$ mice by simple transfer of PBMCs or HSCs from patients with CD or UC. We know that the intestinal microbiome plays an important role in both experimental and human IBD. Even though the general composition of human and mouse microbiota are quite similar, significant differences do exist that may greatly affect our ability to induce chronic gut inflammation [29]. Chung and coworkers have clearly demonstrated species-specific effects on immune system development in germ free mice. These investigators found that colonization of germ free mice with human microbiota essentially prevents the development of the murine immune system whereas colonization of these gnotobiotic mice with murine microbiota induces a fully functional innate and adaptive immune system [174]. These data suggest that humanized mice may require colonization with healthy or disease-specific microbiota obtained from human donors in order to induce intestinal inflammation.

Alternatively, development of disease may require transplant of fecal microbiota obtained from the same patient(s) that donated their PBMCs or HSCs. Theoretically, this could be accomplished by initial antibiotic treatment of the immunodeficient mice followed by donor specific human fecal colonization [175]. Another variation that could be evaluated is transfer of autologous PBMCs into immunodeficient mice previously engrafted with HSCs from IBD patients in order to provide memory T cells. One issue that has received little attention is whether murine endothelial cells are replaced with human cells following engraftment of $CD34^+$ HSCs [29]. This is an important consideration because of the possible problems associated with human leukocyte trafficking to lymphoid and nonlymphoid tissue. Despite this concern, studies have demonstrated human leukocyte infiltration into the inflamed gut in the xenogeneic GVHD that develops in the Hu-PBMC- IL-2r$\gamma^{-/-}$ and BLT-IL-2r$\gamma^{-/-}$ mouse models [160, 176]. In conclusion, the prospects for developing humanized mouse models of IBD are quite good but will require systematic studies that address the issues discussed above.

Acknowledgements Some of the work reported in this manuscript was supported by a grant from DOD (W81XWH-11-1-0666; MBG) and the NIH (R01-DK091269; MBG).

Some of this chapter was reproduced from a review entitled "Pharmacological Intervention Studies Using Mouse Models of the Inflammatory Bowel Diseases:

Translating Preclinical Data into New Drug Therapies" published in Inflammatory Bowel Diseases, 2011. This material is reproduced with permission of John Wiley and Sons, Inc.

References

1. Koboziev I, Karlsson F, Zhang S, Grisham MB. Pharmacological intervention studies using mouse models of the inflammatory bowel diseases: translating preclinical data into new drug therapies. Inflamm Bowel Dis. 2011;17(5):1229–45.
2. DeVoss J, Diehl L. Murine models of inflammatory bowel disease (IBD): challenges of modeling human disease. Toxicol Pathol. 2014;42(1):99–110.
3. Hackam DG, Redelmeier DA. Translation of research evidence from animals to humans. JAMA. 2006;296(14):1731–2.
4. Hackam DG. Translating animal research into clinical benefit. BMJ. 2007;334(7586):163–4.

5. Sena ES, van der Worp HB, Bath PM, Howells DW, Macleod MR. Publication bias in reports of animal stroke studies leads to major overstatement of efficacy. PLoS Biol. 2010;8(3), e1000344.
6. Sena ES, Currie GL, McCann SK, Macleod MR, Howells DW. Systematic reviews and meta-analysis of preclinical studies: why perform them and how to appraise them critically. J Cereb Blood Flow Metab. 2014;34(5):737–42.
7. van der Worp HB, Howells DW, Sena ES, Porritt MJ, Rewell S, O'Collins V, et al. Can animal models of disease reliably inform human studies? PLoS Med. 2010;7(3), e1000245.
8. Valatas V, Vakas M, Kolios G. The value of experimental models of colitis in predicting efficacy of biological therapies for inflammatory bowel diseases. Am J Physiol Gastrointest Liver Physiol. 2013;305(11):G763–85.
9. Elson CO, Cong Y, McCracken VJ, Dimmitt RA, Lorenz RG, Weaver CT. Experimental models of inflammatory bowel disease reveal innate, adaptive, and regulatory mechanisms of host dialogue with the microbiota. Immunol Rev. 2005;206:260–76.
10. Maxwell JR, Viney JL. Overview of mouse models of inflammatory bowel disease and their use in drug discovery. Curr Protoc Pharmacol. 2009;47:5.57.1–19.
11. Strober W, Fuss IJ, Blumberg RS. The immunology of mucosal models of inflammation. Annu Rev Immunol. 2002;20:495–549.
12. Strober W, Fuss I, Mannon P. The fundamental basis of inflammatory bowel disease. J Clin Invest. 2007;117(3):514–21.
13. Uhlig HH, Powrie F. Mouse models of intestinal inflammation as tools to understand the pathogenesis of inflammatory bowel disease. Eur J Immunol. 2009;39(8):2021–6.
14. Cho JH, Weaver CT. The genetics of inflammatory bowel disease. Gastroenterology. 2007;133(4):1327–39.
15. Xavier RJ, Podolsky DK. Unravelling the pathogenesis of inflammatory bowel disease. Nature. 2007;448(7152):427–34.
16. Jones-Hall YL, Grisham MB. Immunopathological characterization of selected mouse models of inflammatory bowel disease: comparison to human disease. Pathophysiology. 2014;21(4):267–88.
17. Chidlow Jr JH, Langston W, Greer JJ, Ostanin D, Abdelbaqi M, Houghton J, et al. Differential angiogenic regulation of experimental colitis. Am J Pathol. 2006;169(6):2014–30.
18. Siegmund B, Lehr HA, Fantuzzi G. Leptin: a pivotal mediator of intestinal inflammation in mice. Gastroenterology. 2002;122(7):2011–25.
19. Siegmund B, Sennello JA, Lehr HA, Batra A, Fedke I, Zeitz M, et al. Development of intestinal inflammation in double IL-10- and leptin-deficient mice. J Leukoc Biol. 2004;76(4):782–6.
20. Te Velde AA, de KF, Sterrenburg E, Pronk I, ten Kate FJ, Hommes DW, et al. Comparative analysis of colonic gene expression of three experimental colitis models mimicking inflammatory bowel disease. Inflamm Bowel Dis. 2007;13(3):325–30.
21. Vowinkel T, Anthoni C, Wood KC, Stokes KY, Russell J, Gray L, et al. CD40-CD40 ligand mediates the recruitment of leukocytes and platelets in the inflamed murine colon. Gastroenterology. 2007;132(3):955–65.
22. Hawkey CJ, Dube LM, Rountree LV, Linnen PJ, Lancaster JF. A trial of zileuton versus mesalazine or placebo in the maintenance of remission of ulcerative colitis. The European Zileuton Study Group For Ulcerative Colitis. Gastroenterology. 1997;112(3):718–24.
23. Roberts WG, Simon TJ, Berlin RG, Haggitt RC, Snyder ES, Stenson WF, et al. Leukotrienes in ulcerative colitis: results of a multicenter trial of a leukotriene biosynthesis inhibitor, MK-591. Gastroenterology. 1997;112(3):725–32.
24. Dieleman LA, Ridwan BU, Tennyson GS, Beagley KW, Bucy RP, Elson CO. Dextran sulfate sodium-induced colitis occurs in severe combined immunodeficient mice. Gastroenterology. 1994;107(6):1643–52.
25. Fiorucci S, Mencarelli A, Palazzetti B, Sprague AG, Distrutti E, Morelli A, et al. Importance of innate immunity and collagen binding integrin alpha1beta1 in TNBS-induced colitis. Immunity. 2002;17(6):769–80.
26. Nguyen LP, Pan J, Dinh TT, Hadeiba H, O'Hara III E, Ebtikar A, et al. Role and species-specific expression of colon T cell homing receptor GPR15 in colitis. Nat Immunol. 2015;16(2):207–13.
27. Soriano A, Salas A, Salas A, Sans M, Gironella M, Elena M, et al. VCAM-1, but not ICAM-1 or MAdCAM-1, immunoblockade ameliorates DSS-induced colitis in mice. Lab Invest. 2000;80(10):1541–51.
28. Wang C, Hanly EK, Wheeler LW, Kaur M, McDonald KG, Newberry RD. Effect of alpha4beta7 blockade on intestinal lymphocyte subsets and lymphoid tissue development. Inflamm Bowel Dis. 2010;16(10):1751–62.
29. Rongvaux A, Takizawa H, Strowig T, Willinger T, Eynon EE, Flavell RA, et al. Human hemato-lymphoid system mice: current use and future potential for medicine. Annu Rev Immunol. 2013;31:635–74.
30. Receptive to replication. Nat Biotechnol 2013;31(11):943.
31. Arrowsmith J. Trial watch: phase II failures: 2008–2010. Nat Rev Drug Discov. 2011;10(5):328–9.
32. Begley CG, Ellis LM. Drug development: raise standards for preclinical cancer research. Nature. 2012;483(7391):531–3.
33. Couzin-Frankel J. When mice mislead. Science. 2013;342(6161):922–3. 925.
34. Prinz F, Schlange T, Asadullah K. Believe it or not: how much can we rely on published data on potential drug targets? Nat Rev Drug Discov. 2011;10(9):712.
35. Koboziev I, Jones-Hall Y, Valentine JF, Reinoso WC, Furr KL, Grisham MB. Use of humanized mice to study the pathogenesis of autoimmune and inflammatory diseases. Inflamm Bowel Dis. 2015;21(7):1652–73.
36. Bramhall M, Florez-Vargas O, Stevens R, Brass A, Cruickshank S. Quality of methods reporting in animal models of colitis. Inflamm Bowel Dis. 2015;21(6):1248–59.
37. Ey B, Eyking A, Klepak M, Salzman NH, Gothert JR, Runzi M, et al. Loss of TLR2 worsens spontaneous colitis in MDR1A deficiency through commensally induced pyroptosis. J Immunol. 2013;190(11):5676–88.
38. Feng T, Wang L, Schoeb TR, Elson CO, Cong Y. Microbiota innate stimulation is a prerequisite for T cell spontaneous proliferation and induction of experimental colitis. J Exp Med. 2010;207(6):1321–32.
39. Powrie F. T cells in inflammatory bowel disease: protective and pathogenic roles. Immunity. 1995;3(2):171–4.
40. Powrie F, Read S, Mottet C, Uhlig H, Maloy K. Control of immune pathology by regulatory T cells. Novartis Found Symp. 2003;252:92–8.
41. Powrie F, Leach MW, Mauze S, Caddle LB, Coffman RL. Phenotypically distinct subsets of CD4+ T cells induce or protect from chronic intestinal inflammation in C. B-17 scid mice. Int Immunol. 1993;5(11):1461–71.
42. Ostanin DV, Bao J, Koboziev I, Gray L, Robinson-Jackson SA, Kosloski-Davidson M, et al. T cell transfer model of chronic colitis: concepts, considerations, and tricks of the trade. Am J Physiol Gastrointest Liver Physiol. 2009;296(2):G135–46.
43. Ostanin DV, Pavlick KP, Bharwani S, D'Souza D, Furr KL, Brown CM, et al. T cell-induced inflammation of the small and large intestine in immunodeficient mice. Am J Physiol Gastrointest Liver Physiol. 2006;290(1):G109–19.
44. Kanai T, Kawamura T, Dohi T, Makita S, Nemoto Y, Totsuka T, et al. TH1/TH2-mediated colitis induced by adoptive transfer of CD4+CD45RBhigh T lymphocytes into nude mice. Inflamm Bowel Dis. 2006;12(2):89–99.

45. Mizoguchi A, Mizoguchi E, Takedatsu H, Blumberg RS, Bhan AK. Chronic intestinal inflammatory condition generates IL-10-producing regulatory B cell subset characterized by CD1d upregulation. Immunity. 2002;16(2):219–30.
46. Mizoguchi E, Mizoguchi A, Preffer FI, Bhan AK. Regulatory role of mature B cells in a murine model of inflammatory bowel disease. Int Immunol. 2000;12(5):597–605.
47. Dohi T, Fujihashi K, Koga T, Shirai Y, Kawamura YI, Ejima C, et al. T helper type-2 cells induce ileal villus atrophy, goblet cell metaplasia, and wasting disease in T cell-deficient mice. Gastroenterology. 2003;124(3):672–82.
48. Dohi T, Fujihashi K, Koga T, Etani Y, Yoshino N, Kawamura YI, et al. CD4+CD45RBHi interleukin-4 defective T cells elicit antral gastritis and duodenitis. Am J Pathol. 2004;165(4):1257–68.
49. Nemoto Y, Kanai T, Takahara M, Oshima S, Okamoto R, Tsuchiya K, et al. Th1/Th17-mediated interstitial pneumonia in chronic colitis mice independent of intestinal microbiota. J Immunol. 2013;190(12):6616–25.
50. Hirano D, Kudo S. Usefulness of CD4+CD45RBhigh. J Pharmacol Sci. 2009;110(2):169–81.
51. Dan N, Kanai T, Totsuka T, Iiyama R, Yamazaki M, Sawada T, et al. Ameliorating effect of anti-Fas ligand MAb on wasting disease in murine model of chronic colitis. Am J Physiol Gastrointest Liver Physiol. 2003;285(4):G754–60.
52. Fujii R, Kanai T, Nemoto Y, Makita S, Oshima S, Okamoto R, et al. FTY720 suppresses CD4+CD44highC. Am J Physiol Gastrointest Liver Physiol. 2006;291(2):G267–74.
53. Kanai T, Totsuka T, Uraushihara K, Makita S, Nakamura T, Koganei K, et al. Blockade of B7-H1 suppresses the development of chronic intestinal inflammation. J Immunol. 2003;171(8):4156–63.
54. Leon F, Contractor N, Fuss I, Marth T, Lahey E, Iwaki S, et al. Antibodies to complement receptor 3 treat established inflammation in murine models of colitis and a novel model of psoriasiform dermatitis. J Immunol. 2006;177(10):6974–82.
55. Liu Z, Geboes K, Colpaert S, Overbergh L, Mathieu C, Heremans H, et al. Prevention of experimental colitis in SCID mice reconstituted with CD45RBhigh CD4+ T cells by blocking the CD40 – CD154 interactions. J Immunol. 2000;164(11):6005–14.
56. Manocha M, Rietdijk S, Laouar A, Liao G, Bhan A, Borst J, et al. Blocking CD27 – CD70 costimulatory pathway suppresses experimental colitis. J Immunol. 2009;183(1):270–6.
57. Totsuka T, Kanai T, Uraushihara K, Iiyama R, Yamazaki M, Akiba H, et al. Therapeutic effect of anti-OX40L and anti-TNF-alpha MAbs in a murine model of chronic colitis. Am J Physiol Gastrointest Liver Physiol. 2003;284(4):G595–603.
58. Barnes MJ, Powrie F. Regulatory T cells reinforce intestinal homeostasis. Immunity. 2009;31(3):401–11.
59. Izcue A, Coombes JL, Powrie F. Regulatory lymphocytes and intestinal inflammation. Annu Rev Immunol. 2009;27:313–38.
60. Karlsson F, Robinson-Jackson SA, Gray L, Zhang S, Grisham MB. Ex vivo generation of regulatory T cells: characterization and therapeutic evaluation in a model of chronic colitis. Methods Mol Biol. 2011;677:47–61.
61. Karlsson F, Martinez NE, Gray L, Zhang S, Tsunoda I, Grisham MB. Therapeutic evaluation of ex vivo-generated versus natural regulatory T-cells in a mouse model of chronic gut inflammation. Inflamm Bowel Dis. 2013;19(11):2282–94.
62. Fang K, Zhang S, Glawe J, Grisham MB, Kevil CG. Temporal genome expression profile analysis during t-cell-mediated colitis: identification of novel targets and pathways. Inflamm Bowel Dis. 2012;18(8):1411–23.
63. Fang K, Grisham MB, Kevil CG. Application of comparative transcriptional genomics to identify molecular targets for pediatric IBD. Front Immunol. 2015;6:165.
64. Berg DJ, Davidson N, Kuhn R, Muller W, Menon S, Holland G, et al. Enterocolitis and colon cancer in interleukin-10-deficient mice are associated with aberrant cytokine production and CD4(+) TH1-like responses. J Clin Invest. 1996;98(4):1010–20.
65. Kuhn R, Lohler J, Rennick D, Rajewsky K, Muller W. Interleukin-10-deficient mice develop chronic enterocolitis. Cell. 1993;75(2):263–74.
66. Hickey CA, Kuhn KA, Donermeyer DL, Porter NT, Jin C, Cameron EA, et al. Colitogenic Bacteroides thetaiotaomicron antigens access host immune cells in a sulfatase-dependent manner via outer membrane vesicles. Cell Host Microbe. 2015;17(5):672–80.
67. Kang SS, Bloom SM, Norian LA, Geske MJ, Flavell RA, Stappenbeck TS, et al. An antibiotic-responsive mouse model of fulminant ulcerative colitis. PLoS Med. 2008;5(3), e41.
68. Jostins L, Ripke S, Weersma RK, Duerr RH, McGovern DP, Hui KY, et al. Host-microbe interactions have shaped the genetic architecture of inflammatory bowel disease. Nature. 2012;491(7422):119–24.
69. Bloom SM, Bijanki VN, Nava GM, Sun L, Malvin NP, Donermeyer DL, et al. Commensal Bacteroides species induce colitis in host-genotype-specific fashion in a mouse model of inflammatory bowel disease. Cell Host Microbe. 2011;9(5):390–403.
70. Glocker EO, Kotlarz D, Boztug K, Gertz EM, Schaffer AA, Noyan F, et al. Inflammatory bowel disease and mutations affecting the interleukin-10 receptor. N Engl J Med. 2009;361(21):2033–45.
71. Wilk JN, Bilsborough J, Viney JL. The mdr1a–/– mouse model of spontaneous colitis: a relevant and appropriate animal model to study inflammatory bowel disease. Immunol Res. 2005;31(2):151–9.
72. Panwala CM, Jones JC, Viney JL. A novel model of inflammatory bowel disease: mice deficient for the multiple drug resistance gene, mdr1a, spontaneously develop colitis. J Immunol. 1998;161(10):5733–44.
73. Collett A, Higgs NB, Gironella M, Zeef LA, Hayes A, Salmo E, et al. Early molecular and functional changes in colonic epithelium that precede increased gut permeability during colitis development in mdr1a(–/–) mice. Inflamm Bowel Dis. 2008;14(5):620–31.
74. Tanner SM, Staley EM, Lorenz RG. Altered generation of induced regulatory T cells in the FVB.mdr1a–/– mouse model of colitis. Mucosal Immunol. 2013;6(2):309–23.
75. Staley EM, Schoeb TR, Lorenz RG. Differential susceptibility of P-glycoprotein deficient mice to colitis induction by environmental insults. Inflamm Bowel Dis. 2009;15(5):684–96.
76. Pallis M, Turzanski J, Higashi Y, Russell N. P-glycoprotein in acute myeloid leukaemia: therapeutic implications of its association with both a multidrug-resistant and an apoptosis-resistant phenotype. Leuk Lymphoma. 2002;43(6):1221–8.
77. Pierik M, Joossens S, Van SK, Van SN, Vlietinck R, Rutgeerts P, et al. Toll-like receptor-1, -2, and -6 polymorphisms influence disease extension in inflammatory bowel diseases. Inflamm Bowel Dis. 2006;12(1):1–8.
78. Maloy KJ, Salaun L, Cahill R, Dougan G, Saunders NJ, Powrie F. CD4+CD25+ T(R) cells suppress innate immune pathology through cytokine-dependent mechanisms. J Exp Med. 2003;197(1):111–9.
79. Uhlig HH, McKenzie BS, Hue S, Thompson C, Joyce-Shaikh B, Stepankova R, et al. Differential activity of IL-12 and IL-23 in mucosal and systemic innate immune pathology. Immunity. 2006;25(2):309–18.
80. Hue S, Ahern P, Buonocore S, Kullberg MC, Cua DJ, McKenzie BS, et al. Interleukin-23 drives innate and T cell-mediated intestinal inflammation. J Exp Med. 2006;203(11):2473–83.
81. Asquith DL, Miller AM, McInnes IB, Liew FY. Animal models of rheumatoid arthritis. 2009;2009/08/13(8):2040–4.

82. Boulard O, Asquith MJ, Powrie F, Maloy KJ. TLR2-independent induction and regulation of chronic intestinal inflammation. Eur J Immunol. 2010;40(2):516–24.
83. Kullberg MC, Jankovic D, Feng CG, Hue S, Gorelick PL, McKenzie BS, et al. IL-23 plays a key role in Helicobacter hepaticus-induced T cell-dependent colitis. J Exp Med. 2006;203(11):2485–94.
84. Garrett WS, Lord GM, Punit S, Lugo-Villarino G, Mazmanian SK, Ito S, et al. Communicable ulcerative colitis induced by T-bet deficiency in the innate immune system. Cell. 2007;131(1):33–45.
85. Garrett WS, Gallini CA, Yatsunenko T, Michaud M, DuBois A, Delaney ML, et al. Enterobacteriaceae act in concert with the gut microbiota to induce spontaneous and maternally transmitted colitis. Cell Host Microbe. 2010;8(3):292–300.
86. Cooper R, Fraser SM, Sturrock RD, Gemmell CG. Raised titres of anti-klebsiella IgA in ankylosing spondylitis, rheumatoid arthritis, and inflammatory bowel disease. Br Med J (Clin Res Ed). 1988;296(6634):1432–4.
87. Kanareykina SK, Misautova AA, Zlatkina AR, Levina EN. Proteus dysbioses in patients with ulcerative colitis. Nahrung. 1987; 31(5–6):557–61.
88. Rooks MG, Veiga P, Wardwell-Scott LH, Tickle T, Segata N, Michaud M, et al. Gut microbiome composition and function in experimental colitis during active disease and treatment-induced remission. ISME J. 2014;8(7):1403–17.
89. Winter SE, Thiennimitr P, Winter MG, Butler BP, Huseby DL, Crawford RW, et al. Gut inflammation provides a respiratory electron acceptor for Salmonella. Nature. 2010;467(7314):426–9.
90. Winter SE, Winter MG, Xavier MN, Thiennimitr P, Poon V, Keestra AM, et al. Host-derived nitrate boosts growth of E. coli in the inflamed gut. Science. 2013;339(6120):708–11.
91. Garrett WS, Punit S, Gallini CA, Michaud M, Zhang D, Sigrist KS, et al. Colitis-associated colorectal cancer driven by T-bet deficiency in dendritic cells. Cancer Cell. 2009;16(3):208–19.
92. Ermann J, Garrett WS, Kuchroo J, Rourida K, Glickman JN, Bleich A, et al. Severity of innate immune-mediated colitis is controlled by the cytokine deficiency-induced colitis susceptibility-1 (Cdcs1) locus. Proc Natl Acad Sci U S A. 2011;108(17):7137–41.
93. Borm ME, He J, Kelsall B, Pena AS, Strober W, Bouma G. A major quantitative trait locus on mouse chromosome 3 is involved in disease susceptibility in different colitis models. Gastroenterology. 2005;128(1):74–85.
94. Kontoyiannis D, Pasparakis M, Pizarro TT, Cominelli F, Kollias G. Impaired on/off regulation of TNF biosynthesis in mice lacking TNF AU-rich elements: implications for joint and gut-associated immunopathologies. Immunity. 1999;10(3):387–98.
95. Baur P, Martin FP, Gruber L, Bosco N, Brahmbhatt V, Collino S, et al. Metabolic phenotyping of the Crohn's disease-like IBD etiopathology in the TNF(DeltaARE/WT) mouse model. J Proteome Res. 2011;10(12):5523–35.
96. Huybers S, Apostolaki M, van der Eerden BC, Kollias G, Naber TH, Bindels RJ, et al. Murine TNF(DeltaARE) Crohn's disease model displays diminished expression of intestinal Ca2+ transporters. Inflamm Bowel Dis. 2008;14(6):803–11.
97. Schaubeck M, Clavel T, Calasan J, Lagkouvardos I, Haange SB, Jehmlich N, et al. Dysbiotic gut microbiota causes transmissible Crohn's disease-like ileitis independent of failure in antimicrobial defence. Gut. 2015 Apr 17.
98. Werner T, Wagner SJ, Martinez I, Walter J, Chang JS, Clavel T, et al. Depletion of luminal iron alters the gut microbiota and prevents Crohn's disease-like ileitis. Gut. 2011;60(3):325–33.
99. Matsumoto S, Okabe Y, Setoyama H, Takayama K, Ohtsuka J, Funahashi H, et al. Inflammatory bowel disease-like enteritis and caecitis in a senescence accelerated mouse P1/Yit strain. Gut. 1998;43(1):71–8.
100. Kosiewicz MM, Nast CC, Krishnan A, Rivera-Nieves J, Moskaluk CA, Matsumoto S, et al. Th1-type responses mediate spontaneous ileitis in a novel murine model of Crohn's disease. J Clin Invest. 2001;107(6):695–702.
101. Pietropaoli D, Del PR, Corridoni D, Rodriguez-Palacios A, Di SG, Monaco A, et al. Occurrence of spontaneous periodontal disease in the SAMP1/YitFc murine model of Crohn disease. J Periodontol. 2014;85(12):1799–805.
102. Rivera-Nieves J, Bamias G, Vidrich A, Marini M, Pizarro TT, McDuffie MJ, et al. Emergence of perianal fistulizing disease in the SAMP1/YitFc mouse, a spontaneous model of chronic ileitis. Gastroenterology. 2003;124(4):972–82.
103. Pizarro TT, Pastorelli L, Bamias G, Garg RR, Reuter BK, Mercado JR, et al. SAMP1/YitFc mouse strain: a spontaneous model of Crohn's disease-like ileitis. Inflamm Bowel Dis. 2011;17(12): 2566–84.
104. Ishikawa D, Okazawa A, Corridoni D, Jia LG, Wang XM, Guanzon M, et al. Tregs are dysfunctional in vivo in a spontaneous murine model of Crohn's disease. Mucosal Immunol. 2013;6(2): 267–75.
105. Saruta M, Yu QT, Fleshner PR, Mantel PY, Schmidt-Weber CB, Banham AH, et al. Characterization of FOXP3+CD4+ regulatory T cells in Crohn's disease. Clin Immunol. 2007;125(3):281–90.
106. Fantini MC, Rizzo A, Fina D, Caruso R, Sarra M, Stolfi C, et al. Smad7 controls resistance of colitogenic T cells to regulatory T cell-mediated suppression. Gastroenterology. 2009;136(4): 1308–16.
107. Corridoni D, Kodani T, Rodriguez-Palacios A, Pizarro TT, Xin W, Nickerson KP, et al. Dysregulated NOD2 predisposes SAMP1/YitFc mice to chronic intestinal inflammation. Proc Natl Acad Sci U S A. 2013;110(42):16999–7004.
108. Corridoni D, Arseneau KO, Cominelli F. Functional defects in NOD2 signaling in experimental and human Crohn disease. Gut Microbes. 2014;5(3):340–4.
109. Brehm MA, Shultz LD, Greiner DL. Humanized mouse models to study human diseases. Curr Opin Endocrinol Diabetes Obes. 2010;17(2):120–5.
110. Shultz LD, Ishikawa F, Greiner DL. Humanized mice in translational biomedical research. Nat Rev Immunol. 2007;7(2):118–30.
111. Shultz LD, Brehm MA, Bavari S, Greiner DL. Humanized mice as a preclinical tool for infectious disease and biomedical research. Ann N Y Acad Sci. 2011;1245:50–4.
112. Shultz LD, Brehm MA, Garcia-Martinez JV, Greiner DL. Humanized mice for immune system investigation: progress, promise and challenges. Nat Rev Immunol. 2012;12(11):786–98.
113. Haley PJ. Species differences in the structure and function of the immune system. Toxicology. 2003;188(1):49–71.
114. Mestas J, Hughes CC. Of mice and not men: differences between mouse and human immunology. J Immunol. 2004;172(5): 2731–8.
115. Brehm MA, Jouvet N, Greiner DL, Shultz LD. Humanized mice for the study of infectious diseases. Curr Opin Immunol. 2013 Jun 7.
116. Brehm MA, Wiles MV, Greiner DL, Shultz LD. Generation of improved humanized mouse models for human infectious diseases. J Immunol Methods. 2014 Mar 4.
117. Pearson T, Greiner DL, Shultz LD. Creation of "humanized" mice to study human immunity. Curr Protoc Immunol. 2008;Chapter 15:Unit.
118. Zhou Q, Facciponte J, Jin M, Shen Q, Lin Q. Humanized NOD-SCID IL2rg–/– mice as a preclinical model for cancer research and its potential use for individualized cancer therapies. Cancer Lett. 2014;344(1):13–9.
119. Ishikawa F, Yasukawa M, Lyons B, Yoshida S, Miyamoto T, Yoshimoto G, et al. Development of functional human blood and

immune systems in NOD/SCID/IL2 receptor {gamma} chain(null) mice. Blood. 2005;106(5):1565–73.
120. Ito M, Hiramatsu H, Kobayashi K, Suzue K, Kawahata M, Hioki K, et al. NOD/SCID/gamma(c)(null) mouse: an excellent recipient mouse model for engraftment of human cells. Blood. 2002;100(9):3175–82.
121. Shultz LD, Lyons BL, Burzenski LM, Gott B, Chen X, Chaleff S, et al. Human lymphoid and myeloid cell development in NOD/LtSz-scid IL2R gamma null mice engrafted with mobilized human hemopoietic stem cells. J Immunol. 2005;174(10):6477–89.
122. Traggiai E, Chicha L, Mazzucchelli L, Bronz L, Piffaretti JC, Lanzavecchia A, et al. Development of a human adaptive immune system in cord blood cell-transplanted mice. Science. 2004; 304(5667):104–7.
123. DiSanto JP, Muller W, Guy-Grand D, Fischer A, Rajewsky K. Lymphoid development in mice with a targeted deletion of the interleukin 2 receptor gamma chain. Proc Natl Acad Sci U S A. 1995;92(2):377–81.
124. Sugamura K, Asao H, Kondo M, Tanaka N, Ishii N, Ohbo K, et al. The interleukin-2 receptor gamma chain: its role in the multiple cytokine receptor complexes and T cell development in XSCID. Annu Rev Immunol. 1996;14:179–205.
125. Kovanen PE, Leonard WJ. Cytokines and immunodeficiency diseases: critical roles of the gamma(c)-dependent cytokines interleukins 2, 4, 7, 9, 15, and 21, and their signaling pathways. Immunol Rev. 2004;202:67–83.
126. Leonard WJ. Cytokines and immunodeficiency diseases. Nat Rev Immunol. 2001;1(3):200–8.
127. Rochman Y, Spolski R, Leonard WJ. New insights into the regulation of T cells by gamma(c) family cytokines. Nat Rev Immunol. 2009;9(7):480–90.
128. Brehm MA, Cuthbert A, Yang C, Miller DM, Diiorio P, Laning J, et al. Parameters for establishing humanized mouse models to study human immunity: analysis of human hematopoietic stem cell engraftment in three immunodeficient strains of mice bearing the IL2rgamma(null) mutation. Clin Immunol. 2010;135(1): 84–98.
129. McDermott SP, Eppert K, Lechman ER, Doedens M, Dick JE. Comparison of human cord blood engraftment between immunocompromised mouse strains. Blood. 2010;116(2):193–200.
130. Mosier DE, Gulizia RJ, Baird SM, Wilson DB. Transfer of a functional human immune system to mice with severe combined immunodeficiency. Nature. 1988;335(6187):256–9.
131. Bock TA, Orlic D, Dunbar CE, Broxmeyer HE, Bodine DM. Improved engraftment of human hematopoietic cells in severe combined immunodeficient (SCID) mice carrying human cytokine transgenes. J Exp Med. 1995;182(6):2037–43.
132. Greiner DL, Hesselton RA, Shultz LD. SCID mouse models of human stem cell engraftment. Stem Cells. 1998;16(3):166–77.
133. Shultz LD, Schweitzer PA, Christianson SW, Gott B, Schweitzer IB, Tennent B, et al. Multiple defects in innate and adaptive immunologic function in NOD/LtSz-scid mice. J Immunol. 1995;154(1): 180–91.
134. Hogenes M, Huibers M, Kroone C, de WR. Humanized mouse models in transplantation research. Transplant Rev (Orlando). 2014;28(3):103–10.
135. Shultz LD, Pearson T, King M, Giassi L, Carney L, Gott B, et al. Humanized NOD/LtSz-scid IL2 receptor common gamma chain knockout mice in diabetes research. Ann N Y Acad Sci. 2007; 1103:77–89.
136. King M, Pearson T, Shultz LD, Leif J, Bottino R, Trucco M, et al. A new Hu-PBL model for the study of human islet alloreactivity based on NOD-scid mice bearing a targeted mutation in the IL-2 receptor gamma chain gene. Clin Immunol. 2008;126(3):303–14.
137. Brehm MA, Shultz LD, Luban J, Greiner DL. Overcoming current limitations in humanized mouse research. J Infect Dis. 2013;208 Suppl 2:S125–30.
138. Spranger S, Frankenberger B, Schendel DJ. NOD/scid IL-2Rg(null) mice: a preclinical model system to evaluate human dendritic cell-based vaccine strategies in vivo. J Transl Med. 2012;10:30.
139. King MA, Covassin L, Brehm MA, Racki W, Pearson T, Leif J, et al. Human peripheral blood leucocyte non-obese diabetic-severe combined immunodeficiency interleukin-2 receptor gamma chain gene mouse model of xenogeneic graft-versus-host-like disease and the role of host major histocompatibility complex. Clin Exp Immunol. 2009;157(1):104–18.
140. Lepus CM, Gibson TF, Gerber SA, Kawikova I, Szczepanik M, Hossain J, et al. Comparison of human fetal liver, umbilical cord blood, and adult blood hematopoietic stem cell engraftment in NOD-scid/gammac-/-, Balb/c-Rag1-/-gammac-/-, and C.B-17-scid/bg immunodeficient mice. 2009;2009/06/16(10):790–802.
141. Matsumura T, Kametani Y, Ando K, Hirano Y, Katano I, Ito R, et al. Functional CD5+ B cells develop predominantly in the spleen of NOD/SCID/gammac(null) (NOG) mice transplanted either with human umbilical cord blood, bone marrow, or mobilized peripheral blood CD34+ cells. Exp Hematol. 2003;31(9):789–97.
142. Choi B, Chun E, Kim M, Kim SY, Kim ST, Yoon K, et al. Human T cell development in the liver of humanized NOD/SCID/IL-2Rgamma(null)(NSG) mice generated by intrahepatic injection of CD34(+) human (h) cord blood (CB) cells. Clin Immunol. 2011;139(3):321–35.
143. Misharin AV, Haines III GK, Rose S, Gierut AK, Hotchkiss RS, Perlman H. Development of a new humanized mouse model to study acute inflammatory arthritis. J Transl Med. 2012;10:190.
144. Yahata T, Ando K, Nakamura Y, Ueyama Y, Shimamura K, Tamaoki N, et al. Functional human T lymphocyte development from cord blood CD34+ cells in nonobese diabetic/Shi-scid, IL-2 receptor gamma null mice. J Immunol. 2002;169(1):204–9.
145. Tanaka S, Saito Y, Kunisawa J, Kurashima Y, Wake T, Suzuki N, et al. Development of mature and functional human myeloid subsets in hematopoietic stem cell-engrafted NOD/SCID/IL2rgammaKO mice. J Immunol (Baltimore, MD: 1950). 2012;2012/05/23: 6145–55.
146. Lapidot T, Pflumio F, Doedens M, Murdoch B, Williams DE, Dick JE. Cytokine stimulation of multilineage hematopoiesis from immature human cells engrafted in SCID mice. Science. 1992; 255(5048):1137–41.
147. Watanabe Y, Takahashi T, Okajima A, Shiokawa M, Ishii N, Katano I, et al. The analysis of the functions of human B and T cells in humanized NOD/shi-scid/gammac(null) (NOG) mice (hu-HSC NOG mice). Int Immunol. 2009;21(7):843–58.
148. Lan P, Tonomura N, Shimizu A, Wang S, Yang YG. Reconstitution of a functional human immune system in immunodeficient mice through combined human fetal thymus/liver and CD34+ cell transplantation. Blood. 2006;108(2):487–92.
149. Melkus MW, Estes JD, Padgett-Thomas A, Gatlin J, Denton PW, Othieno FA, et al. Humanized mice mount specific adaptive and innate immune responses to EBV and TSST-1. Nat Med. 2006;12(11):1316–22.
150. Covassin L, Jangalwe S, Jouvet N, Laning J, Burzenski L, Shultz LD, et al. Human immune system development and survival of NOD-scid IL2rgamma (NSG) mice engrafted with human thymus and autologous hematopoietic stem cells. Clin Exp Immunol. 2013 Jul 19.
151. Tonomura N, Habiro K, Shimizu A, Sykes M, Yang YG. Antigen-specific human T-cell responses and T cell-dependent production of human antibodies in a humanized mouse model. Blood. 2008;111(8):4293–6.
152. Brainard DM, Seung E, Frahm N, Cariappa A, Bailey CC, Hart WK, et al. Induction of robust cellular and humoral virus-specific adaptive immune responses in human immunodeficiency virus-infected humanized BLT mice. J Virol. 2009;83(14):7305–21.

153. Denton PW, Nochi T, Lim A, Krisko JF, Martinez-Torres F, Choudhary SK, et al. IL-2 receptor gamma-chain molecule is critical for intestinal T-cell reconstitution in humanized mice. Mucosal Immunol. 2012;5(5):555–66.
154. Strowig T, Rongvaux A, Rathinam C, Takizawa H, Borsotti C, Philbrick W, et al. Transgenic expression of human signal regulatory protein alpha in Rag2-/-gamma(c)-/- mice improves engraftment of human hematopoietic cells in humanized mice. Proceedings National Academy of Sciences. 2011;108:13218–23.
155. Stoddart CA, Maidji E, Galkina SA, Kosikova G, Rivera JM, Moreno ME, et al. Superior human leukocyte reconstitution and susceptibility to vaginal HIV transmission in humanized NOD-scid IL-2Rgamma(-/-) (NSG) BLT mice. Virology. 2011;417(1): 154–60.
156. Nochi T, Denton PW, Wahl A, Garcia JV. Cryptopatches are essential for the development of human GALT. Cell Rep. 2013;3: 1874–84.
157. Rajesh D, Zhou Y, Jankowska-Gan E, Roenneburg DA, Dart ML, Torrealba J, et al. Th1 and Th17 immunocompetence in humanized NOD/SCID/IL2rgammanull mice. Hum Immunol. 2010;71(6): 551–9.
158. Villaudy J, Schotte R, Legrand N, Spits H. Critical assessment of human antibody generation in humanized mouse models. J Immunol Methods. 2014;410:18–27.
159. Ali N, Flutter B, Sanchez RR, Sharif-Paghaleh E, Barber LD, Lombardi G, et al. Xenogeneic graft-versus-host-disease in NOD-scid IL-2Rgammanull mice display a T-effector memory phenotype. PLoS One. 2012;7(8), e44219.
160. Greenblatt MB, Vrbanac V, Tivey T, Tsang K, Tager AM, Aliprantis AO. Graft versus host disease in the bone marrow, liver and thymus humanized mouse model. 2012;2012/09/08(9):e44664.
161. Lockridge JL, Zhou Y, Becker YA, Ma S, Kenney SC, Hematti P, et al. Mice engrafted with human fetal thymic tissue and hematopoietic stem cells develop pathology resembling chronic graft-versus-host disease. Biol Blood Marrow Transplant. 2013;19(9): 1310–22.
162. Lavender KJ, Pang WW, Messer RJ, Duley AK, Race B, Phillips K, et al. BLT-humanized C57BL/6 Rag2-/-gammac-/-CD47-/- mice are resistant to GVHD and develop B- and T-cell immunity to HIV infection. Blood. 2013;122(25):4013–20.
163. Lavender KJ, Messer RJ, Race B, Hasenkrug KJ. Production of bone marrow, liver, thymus (BLT) humanized mice on the C57BL/6 Rag2(-/-)gammac(-/-)CD47(-/-) background. J Immunol Methods. 2014;407:127–34.
164. Nolte T, Zadeh-Khorasani M, Safarov O, Rueff F, Gülberg V, Herbach N, et al. Oxazolone and ethanol induce colitis in non-obese diabetic-severe combined immunodeficiency interleukin-2Rγ(null) mice engrafted with human peripheral blood mononuclear cells. 2013;172:349–62.
165. Nolte T, Zadeh-Khorasani M, Safarov O, Rueff F, Varga R, Herbach N, et al. Induction of oxazolone-mediated features of atopic dermatitis in NOD-scid IL2Rgamma(null) mice engrafted with human peripheral blood mononuclear cells. Dis Model Mech. 2013;6(1):125–34.
166. Goettel JA, Biswas S, Lexmond WS, YUeste A, Passerinin L, Patel B, Yang S, Sun J, Ouahed J, et. al. Fatal autoimmunity inmice reconsitituted with human hematopoietic stem cells encouding defective FOXP3. Blood. 2015;125(25):3886–95.
167. Goettel JA, Biswas S, Lexmond WS, Sun J, Ouahed J, McCann K, et al. Human hematopoietic stem cells with a defined immunodeficiency and enteropathy transfer clinical phenotype to a novel humanized mouse strain. Inflamm Bowel Dis. 2014;146:S-81.
168. Jess T, Riis L, Jespersgaard C, Hougs L, Andersen PS, Orholm MK, et al. Disease concordance, zygosity, and NOD2/CARD15 status: follow-up of a population-based cohort of Danish twins with inflammatory bowel disease. Am J Gastroenterol. 2005;100: 2486–92.
169. Bernstein CN, Shanahan F. Disorders of a modern lifestyle: reconciling the epidemiology of inflammatory bowel diseases. Gut. 2008;57(9):1185–91.
170. Cosnes J, Gower-Rousseau C, Seksik P, Cortot A. Epidemiology and natural history of inflammatory bowel diseases. Gastroenterology. 2011;140(6):1785–94.
171. Khor B, Gardet A, Xavier RJ. Genetics and pathogenesis of inflammatory bowel disease. Nature. 2011;474(7351):307–17.
172. Molodecky NA, Soon IS, Rabi DM, Ghali WA, Ferris M, Chernoff G, et al. Increasing incidence and prevalence of the inflammatory bowel diseases with time, based on systematic review. Gastroenterology. 2012;142(1):46–54.
173. Ventham NT, Kennedy NA, Nimmo ER, Satsangi J. Beyond gene discovery in inflammatory bowel disease: the emerging role of epigenetics. Gastroenterology. 2013 Jun 8.
174. Chung H, Pamp SJ, Hill JA, Surana NK, Edelman SM, Troy EB, et al. Gut immune maturation depends on colonization with a host-specific microbiota. Cell. 2012;149(7):1578–93.
175. Hintze KJ, Cox JE, Rompato G, Benninghoff AD, Ward RE, Broadbent J, et al. Broad scope method for creating humanized animal models for animal health and disease research through antibiotic treatment and human fecal transfer. 2014;5:183–91.
176. Zheng J, Liu Y, Liu Y, Liu M, Xiang Z, Lam KT, et al. Human CD8+ regulatory T cells inhibit GVHD and preserve general immunity in humanized mice. Sci Transl Med. 2013;5:168ra9.

Stem Cells and Organoids to Study Epithelial Cell Biology in IBD

16

Jorge O. Múnera and James M. Wells

Introduction

Inflammatory bowel disease presents with chronic inflammation which damages normal intestinal mucosa. Because the disease is an inflammatory disease, much of the research on IBD has focused on the role of immune cells. However, it has become clear that the epithelial integrity as well as factors involved in healing of mucosa may also play a role in the pathogenesis of the disease. Genome-wide association studies of patients with Crohn's and colitis have identified genes involved in epithelial biology such as CDH1, HNF4, and SATB2 [1]. Thus, examining epithelial biology is critical for understanding how barrier function and dysfunction in IBD impacts epithelial health and regeneration. Regeneration is important because "mucosal healing" predicts long-term remission in patients treated for IBD.

In the past, models utilizing intestinal epithelial monolayers have been used to study epithelial mechanisms of IBD and in the development of therapies. Despite providing some insight into IBD mechanisms, these two-dimensional in vitro models have several disadvantages. (1) They typically require the use of transformed or cancer cell lines that lack normal physiological properties of intestinal epithelium. (2) They are largely enterocyte models and lack the other differentiated cell types and thus do not reflect intestinal physiology. (3) Mesenchymal cells are also absent in these models. The presence of multiple cell types is particularly important for accurate modeling of disease since IBD could have effects on multiple cell types. For example, depletion of goblet cells is often observed in biopsies from ulcerative colitis (UC) patients and Muc2 deficient mice develop spontaneous colitis, suggesting a role of goblet cells in pathogenesis. Glucagon like peptide-2, a product of enteroendocrine cells (EECs), has been shown to ameliorate experimental colitis in mice, suggesting that EECs may play a role in regeneration. In addition, Lgr5 positive stem cells are depleted in sites of injury in DSS treated mice [2]. Taken together these observations suggest that most differentiated cell types found in the intestine are involved in the pathology of IBD. Thus an organoid system containing multiple differentiated and stem cell types would more accurately mimic intestinal physiology.

In the past few years the identification of adult intestinal stem cell markers and the ability to isolate and culture these cells have led to significant advances in our understanding of intestinal stem cell function, differentiation, and gastrointestinal cancer [3–9]. Adult intestinal organoids (also called enteroids) can be grown in 3D culture from single Lgr5+ cells. These intestinal organoids display remarkable similarity to intestinal epithelium in vivo. Intestinal organoids contain a central lumen surrounded by a single cell layer of polarized epithelial cells. In addition, this single cell layer is organized into crypt-villus like domains containing the main differentiated cell types. Lgr5+ stem cells, Paneth cells, and proliferative progenitors localize in the crypt-like structures. Polarized enterocytes line the central lumen, while goblet cells and enteroendocrine cells are scattered throughout the organoid.

Since the discovery of Lgr5 as a marker of intestinal stem cells, several other markers of intestinal stem cells have been identified including Bmi1, Sox9, HopX, Lrig, and mTert [10–14]. Several of these markers are present in label retaining cells located at the +4 position in the crypt. These cells cycle slowly and are now believed to be a reserve stem cell population. Following damage of the intestine, these cells lose their quiescence and contribute to regeneration of the intestine while giving rise to new Lgr5+ stem cells which will maintain homeostasis [15–17]. It is likely that the quiescent stem cell contributes to regeneration in mouse models of colitis since Lgr5+ stem cells are lost during DSS induced colitis. Thus studies using organoid models could elucidate mechanisms by which the intestinal epithelium can

J.O. Múnera • J.M. Wells, Ph.D. (✉)
Division of Developmental Biology, Cincinnati Children's Hospital Research Foundation, 3333 Burnet Avenue, Cincinnati, OH 45229, USA
e-mail: james.wells@cchmc.org

D.C. Baumgart (ed.), *Crohn's Disease and Ulcerative Colitis*, DOI 10.1007/978-3-319-33703-6_16

regenerate following damage since these organoids contain reserve stem cells [18].

In this chapter we review the available intestinal organoid models and how they have been used in the study of epithelial biology and IBD (Fig. 16.1). For clarity we use three different terms to describe the different "organoid" types. Whole organoid units are derived from adult intestine and contain epithelial, mesenchymal, and neuronal cell types. Enteroids (as designated by the NIH Intestinal Stem Cell Consortium) are derived from adult intestinal stem cells or crypts and are purely epithelial organoids [19]. Induced human intestinal organoids (iHIOs) are derived from embryonic and induced pluripotent stem cells (collectively called PSCs) and contain both epithelial and mesenchymal cell types. In addition, we discuss the advantages and disadvantages of each model. Finally, we discuss emerging technologies and how they will contribute to understanding the molecular basis of IBD.

Organoid Models

Whole Organoid Units

One organoid model system was developed by Ootani et al. [20], whereby pieces of whole intestine or colon (including mesenchymal cells and enteric nerves) are grown in a liquid–air interface, which allows for long-term growth of organoid structures. These organoids contain the major differentiated intestinal cell types found in vivo. Furthermore, the presence of a mesenchyme within these organoids allows growth of the organoids without supplementation with niche factors such as Noggin and R-spondin. Thus, this system would be advantageous for examining the effects of epithelial–mesenchymal interactions in the context of inflammation or regeneration; however, to date it has not been used to study IBD. However, the system has been used to effectively investigate the effects of oncogene activation and inactivation of tumor

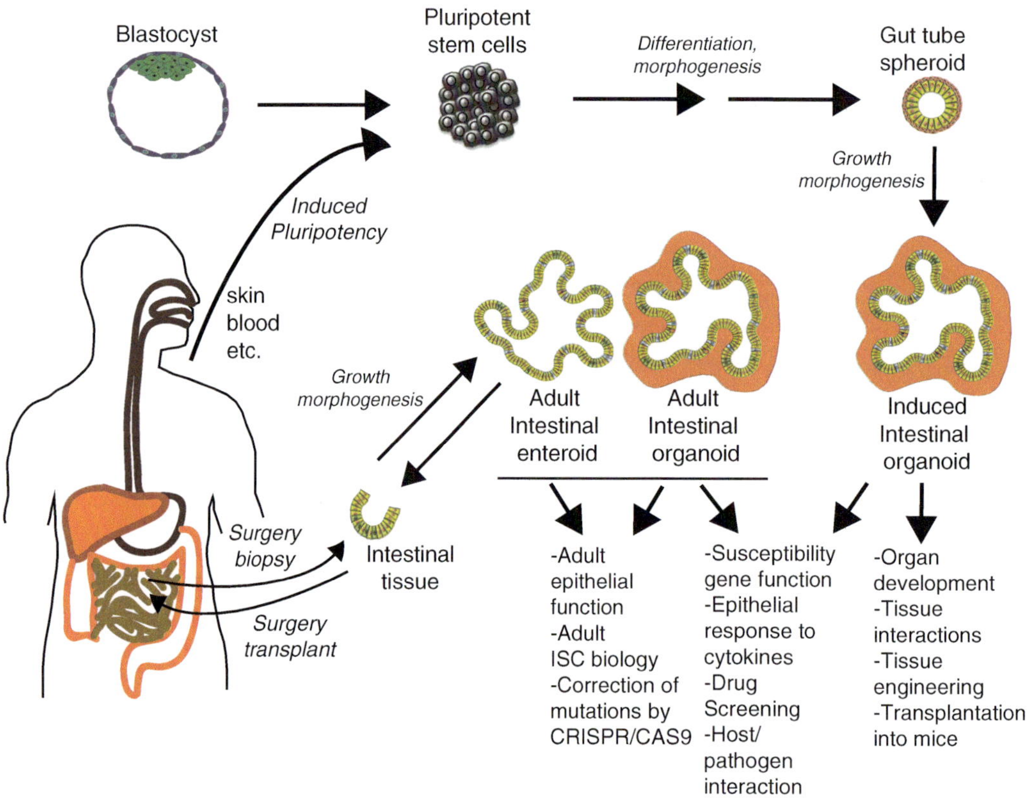

Fig. 16.1 Overview of Intestinal Organoid systems. Intestinal organoids can be derived by a variety of methods. Intestinal crypts and LGR5-expressing stem cells can be isolated from IBD patient biopsies and grown as human intestinal enteroids, which contain epithelium only. Thus these human intestinal enteroids can be used to study epithelial functions and mutations can be corrected using CRISPR\Cas9 gene editing technology. In addition, human intestinal organoids can be grown from whole intestinal tissue which will include stromal cells and enteric nerves. These human intestinal organoids can be used to study the interaction between epithelial, mesenchymal, and neuronal cell types. Induced human intestinal organoids (iHIOs) can be generated from human pluripotent stem cells (hPSCs) which are either from human embryonic stem cells or from induced pluripotent stem cells (iPSCs) generated from any somatic cell (blood and urine are easily obtained sources of somatic cells). Mutations in hPSCs can also be corrected using CRISPR/CAS9. iHIOs can be used to study organ development, tissue–tissue interactions, and to model intestinal disease. iHIOs resemble human fetal intestine when grown in vitro. However, iHIOs can be transplanted in vivo under the mouse kidney capsule to generate more mature, functional human intestine

suppressor genes in mouse models and could be used to study these changes in the context of IBD. For example, loss of the APC tumor suppressor gene allows for faster recovery in response to DSS-mediated epithelial injury [21].

Lgr5-Based Mouse Enteroids

The most commonly used intestinal organoid model was developed in the lab of Hans Clevers [9], and these will be referred to as enteroids because they are purely epithelial. Sato and colleagues demonstrated that single Lgr5+ stem cells could be grown into 3D enteroids in Matrigel culture in medium containing EGF, Noggin (BMP antagonist), and R-spondin (ENR). Interestingly enteroids were able to proliferate and differentiate spontaneously despite the lack of any mesenchymal cells, suggesting that ENR media was sufficient to replace the signals derived from supporting mesenchymal cell types. In addition, this system was used to demonstrate that the Paneth cells act as an ISC niche cell by supplying Wnt3a [5]. Although there are numerous studies that have used the mouse enteroid system to address questions about epithelial biology in an IBD context, we focus on several key examples.

One study by Günther and coworkers examined the role of caspase 8 in epithelial cell death and inflammation of the ileum [22]. This work was based on the observation that mice deficient in caspase 8 within the intestinal epithelium ($Casp8^{\Delta IEC}$) have depleted Paneth and goblets cells and develop spontaneous ileitis. Examination of enteroids derived from the intestines of Wild Type (WT) and $Casp8^{\Delta IEC}$ mice revealed no differences in the number of Paneth cells, suggesting that a factor present in vivo affected the differentiation or survival of this cell type. To further explore this possibility, the authors examined the effect of TNF-α stimulation on organoids from WT and $Casp8^{\Delta IEC}$ mice. Interestingly, 24 h after stimulation, WT enteroids appeared normal while $Casp8^{\Delta IEC}$ enteroids underwent nec-1-dependent necrosis. In addition, the authors presented evidence that RIP-mediated necroptosis of Paneth cells was also present in samples from patients with Crohn's disease and suggested that this may be the cause of the defective antimicrobial defense that is observed in these patients.

In another study, Farin and Karthaus et al. used enteroids to examine the effect of bacterial antigens on Paneth and goblet cells [23]. Interestingly these antigens had little effect on these cell types regardless of whether they were administered apically or basolaterally. However, when inflammatory cytokines were applied to these organoids, only IFN-γ caused degranulation of Paneth cells. In addition, IFN-γ stimulation led to loss of mucus containing goblet cells and mature enterocytes. As a consequence of the loss of Paneth cells, organoid growth was severely compromised likely due to the role of Paneth cells as a niche cell for intestinal stem cells. Taken together, these studies demonstrate how this organoid system can be used to interrogate the effect of inflammatory cytokines on various cell types.

Human Enteroids

Human enteroids (as designated by the NIH Intestinal Stem Cell Consortium [19]) can be grown from isolated intestinal crypts or $CD44^{+}CD166^{+}CD24^{lo}$ single cells in Matrigel based 3D culture [9, 24]. In the case of colon, single cells can be grown into colonoids by FACS sorting based on the expression of ephrin type-B receptor 2 (EPHB2) [7]. Enteroids have been generated from small and large intestine and require a unique set of growth factors. Cultured human intestinal enteroids (and colonoids) require Wnt3a, gastrin, nicotinamide, A-83-01 (Alk4/5/6 inhibitor) and SB202190 (p38 inhibitor) in addition to basic growth media containing EGF, Noggin, and R-spondin-1 [8]. These enteroids display remarkable similarity to intestinal tissue in vivo. Enteroids self-organize into structures containing a central lumen surrounded by a single cell layer of polarized epithelial cells. In addition, this single cell layer is organized into crypt-villus like structures which can differentiate into the main differentiated cell types following withdrawal of Wnt3a, nicotinamide, and SB202190. Interestingly, like their mouse counterparts, these organoids lack mesenchymal cells, suggesting that growth factors produced by mesenchymal cells (rather than physical interaction with these cells) are necessary for maintenance of the intestinal stem cell niche.

Directed Differentiation of Pluripotent Stem Cells into Induced Human Intestinal Organoids (iHIOs)

Another method for deriving intestinal organoids is through directed differentiation of human pluripotent stem cells in a manner that approximates embryonic development of the intestines [25–27]. First pluripotent stem cells are differentiated into definitive endoderm by treatment with Activin A. Subsequent activation of Wnt and FGF pathways promotes a posterior endoderm fate and induces morphogenesis into mid/hingut spheroids. Once formed, these midgut/hindgut spheroids can be grown into iHIOs in three-dimensional culture conditions that favor intestinal growth [9, 26]. Moreover, growth of these spheroids into iHIOs recapitulates developmental events that occur in vivo. Midgut/hindgut spheroids transition from a simple cuboidal epithelium into a pseudostratified epithelium, which then undergoes cytodifferentiation and transitions into a polarized epithelium which contains zones of differentiation and proliferation. When compared to developing mouse intestine, these intestinal organoid cultures undergo strikingly similar transitions [28]. In addition, iHIOs also contain a layer of mesenchymal cells which also mature along with the epithelium, giving rise to fibroblasts, smooth muscle cells, and subepithelial fibroblasts.

Transplantation of iHIOs in vivo allows for substantial growth maturation of the intestinal tissue [29]. Transplanted iHIOs form crypts and villi as well as circular and longitudinal muscle layers. Furthermore, these tissues are functional as demonstrated by brush border activity, mucus secretion and polypeptide uptake. Since iHIOs generated from IPSCs can also grow and mature in vivo, IBD patient specific organoids could be generated and transplanted and immune cells from the patients could be injected to study inflammatory responses of the intestinal tissue. This would allow for a humanized mouse model of IBD that could aid in personalized drug development.

One example of the use of the iHIO system for IBD research is work by Xue and colleagues [30]. In this work, iHIOs were used to model inflammatory hypoxia. When iHIOs were grown in 1 % oxygen, they increased their expression of TNF-α when compared to organoids grown in ambient oxygen. When the hypoxia inducible factor EPAS1 was inhibited by a chemical antagonist, the increase in TNF-α expression was inhibited. This work suggests that iHIOs are capable of expressing proinflammatory cytokines in the context of hypoxia. However, it was unclear if TNF-α expression was initiated by the epithelium or mesenchyme of the iHIOs.

Choosing an Organoid Model

Because of the variety of organoid models available, the advantages and disadvantages of each model should be taken into consideration. The use of the right model is dependent on the biological question to be addressed and cell type(s) to be examined. Here we discuss the advantages and disadvantages of the three main organoid models.

Enteroids from mouse intestine are a great model system for many reasons. First, these organoids are strictly epithelial and can be used to study epithelial biology directly. Second, genetic tools are available to examine lineage tracing, generating conditional knockouts and for visualizing epithelial architecture in live organoids. The availability of these tools is advantageous especially in the context of gene knockouts which may affect organoid viability. In this case, organoids can be grown and the gene of interested can be excised using an inducible Cre. Another advantage of this system is that organoids maintain zones of proliferation and differentiation. This is especially important when examination of multiple cell types is desired. There are several properties of this system that may limit its utility for human IBD studies, for example as a murine system it may not reflect human pathobiology. Second, enteroids being epithelial only, can not be used to study the role of mesenchymal/stromal cell types in IBD. Lastly, one limitation of all organoids is that there are no immune cells present; however, addition of exogenous immune cells is possible.

Human intestinal enteroids offer an alternative to mouse enteroids. The most obvious advantage is that human intestinal enteroids are derived from humans and thus may more accurately reflect human intestinal epithelial cell biology. Furthermore, human intestinal enteroids can be generated from normal and diseased patients in order to examine epithelial biology within a disease context. In addition, enteroids are amenable to CRISPR\Cas9 mediated gene editing, which can allow for correction of mutated genes [31] or to modify tumor suppressor and oncogenes for modeling colorectal cancer [32, 33]. This system does have some disadvantages. First, generation of these enteroids requires human patient samples which may be difficult to obtain. Second, the majority of surgical samples are from diseased patients so these organoids may not reflect normal intestinal physiology. Moreover, enteroids do not maintain proliferation and differentiation to the extent that mouse organoids do. Thus, this system may be impractical when interrogating questions which require the presence of the main intestinal call types. As with mouse enteroids, human enteroids are only epithelial and therefore mesenchymal interactions cannot be studied.

Induced Human intestinal organoids derived from human pluripotent stem cells also have unique advantages and disadvantages. First, these organoids are human and they can be generated from human pluripotent stem cells, which can be grown and expanded infinitely. Second, these organoids contain a mesenchymal layer that matures with the epithelium and thus can be used to study epithelial–mesenchymal interactions. This is especially important when examining a susceptibility gene like NKX2-3 which is expressed in the intestinal mesenchyme [1, 34]. Furthermore, human pluripotent stem cells are amenable to viral based transgene delivery as well as CRISPR\Cas9 mediated gene editing [26, 35]. Lastly, as describe above, human intestinal organoids can be grown in vivo, whereby they mature and form crypts from which enteroids can be derived [29]. This allows for patient-specific derivation of organoids and enteroids without the need for surgical acquisition of intestinal tissues. However, iHIOs have limitations. First, in vitro grown organoids are fetal in nature, which inhibits the examination of mature differentiated cell types. Second, these organoids lack regional specificity, which may be crucial for accurate modeling since IBD often presents in specific regions of the small and large intestine.

Translation of Organoid Models of IBD

Organoid model systems have revolutionized the field of gastrointestinal biology by fostering the interrogation of biological question in a complex ex vivo model which recapitulates many aspects of normal intestinal physiology. Importantly, human organoid systems can eliminate concerns about species differences where human pathology is not adequately modeled in murine systems. So how can these systems be translated into medical applications? In this section we discuss how emerging technologies advance the use of organoid systems in medicine.

Because IBD is a multifactorial disease, epithelium only organoid systems may not fully recapitulate aspects of disease. As mentioned previously, some IBD susceptibility genes are expressed specifically in the mesenchyme. To study mesenchymal factors, the iHIO system, which contains mesenchyme, would allow interrogation of the role of mesenchymal factors in IBD. The microbiota constitute another system that is perturbed in IBD but has not been studied in an organoid system. Although the microbiota exist in an anoxic environment, the ability of organoids to grow in low oxygen, and the relatively hypoxic nature of the organoid lumen open the possibility for incorporation of microbiota. Finally incorporation of immune cells into organoid cultures would be essential for elucidating mechanisms of communication between these cells and the intestinal epithelium. Given that immune cells are largely housed in the stroma, whole organoid units and iHIOs, both containing mesenchyme, might be good systems to start with for incorporation of immune cells. A comparison of enteroids and mesenchyme-containing systems would allow for systematic analysis of how different cell types interact with immune cells.

With the advent of CRISPR\Cas9 technology, an efficient method for gene editing, it is now possible to generate genetically modified organoid systems containing cell reporters for live cell imaging and monitoring organoid function. With regard to IBD research, CRISPR\Cas9 technology could be used to generate organoids that contain mutations associated with IBD susceptibility. Alternatively, enteroids or organoids could be generated from IBD patients to examine the effects of mutations on epithelial biology. CRISPR\Cas9 technology could then be used to correct the mutation to determine if phenotype can be reversed. Proof of concept for this approach has been demonstrated in enteroids from cystic fibrosis patients which could be corrected using CRISPR\Cas9 technology [31].

Regenerative medicine is another possible therapeutic use of organoid systems. Intestinal tissue generated ex vivo could be used to replace damaged intestinal tissue in IBD patients. Proof of concept for this approach has been shown in mice. Colonoids generated from single Lrg5+ colonic stem cells are able to engraft into the colon of mice with chemically induced mucosal lesions [36]. Generation of enteroids from IBD patient biopsies or generation of iHIOs from patient derived induced pluripotent stem cells could be used to generate tissue for transplantation. In addition, patient mutations could be corrected using gene editing technology. Despite the promise of regenerative medicine, vastly improved methods to efficiently and safely incorporate engineered intestinal tissue will need to be developed before tissues could be used therapeutically.

Lastly, intestinal organoids hold promise for the field of personalized medicine. Patient derived enteroids or organoids could be used to screen drugs that may be effective in treating IBD. This approach has been used, whereby a biobank of human colorectal cancers was used for drug screening [37]. Such studies could be aided further by new high-throughput microfluidic technologies that allow screening of thousands of organoids [18].

Conclusions and Future Directions

The development of organoid methodologies has led to an expanded knowledge of intestinal epithelial cell biology. Organoid systems are well suited for use in personalized medicine and regenerative medicine. Important improvements to organoid-based systems could include incorporation of additional cellular complexity, such as immune cells, which would allow for better modeling of IBD. Being able to manipulate cell types, genetically or via the culture conditions, should allow for a mechanistic dissection of the cellular and molecular mechanisms that participate in the pathogenesis of IBD. With the evolution of new technologies for gene editing and high-throughput analysis of organoids using microfluidic platforms, as well as the feasibility of whole-genome sequencing, the use of organoid systems for personalized medicine should be greatly expedited.

References

1. McGovern DP, Gardet A, Torkvist L, Goyette P, Essers J, Taylor KD, et al. Genome-wide association identifies multiple ulcerative colitis susceptibility loci. Nat Genet. 2010;42:332–7.
2. Davidson LA, Goldsby JS, Callaway ES, Shah MS, Barker N, Chapkin RS. Alteration of colonic stem cell gene signatures during the regenerative response to injury. Biochim Biophys Acta. 2012;1822:1600–7.
3. Barker N, Ridgway RA, van Es JH, van de Wetering M, Begthel H, van den Born M, et al. Crypt stem cells as the cells-of-origin of intestinal cancer. Nature. 2009;457:608–11.
4. Barker N, van Es JH, Kuipers J, Kujala P, van den Born M, Cozijnsen M, et al. Identification of stem cells in small intestine and colon by marker gene Lgr5. Nature. 2007;449:1003–7.

5. Sato T, van Es JH, Snippert HJ, Stange DE, Vries RG, van den Born M, et al. Paneth cells constitute the niche for Lgr5 stem cells in intestinal crypts. Nature. 2011;469:415–8.
6. Snippert HJ, van der Flier LG, Sato T, van Es JH, van den Born M, Kroon-Veenboer C, et al. Intestinal crypt homeostasis results from neutral competition between symmetrically dividing Lgr5 stem cells. Cell. 2010;143:134–44.
7. Jung P, Sato T, Merlos-Suarez A, Barriga FM, Iglesias M, Rossell D, et al. Isolation and in vitro expansion of human colonic stem cells. Nat Med. 2011;17:1225–7.
8. Sato T, Stange DE, Ferrante M, Vries RG, Van Es JH, Van den Brink S, et al. Long-term expansion of epithelial organoids from human colon, adenoma, adenocarcinoma, and Barrett's epithelium. Gastroenterology. 2011;141:1762–72.
9. Sato T, Vries RG, Snippert HJ, van de Wetering M, Barker N, Stange DE, et al. Single Lgr5 stem cells build crypt-villus structures in vitro without a mesenchymal niche. Nature. 2009;459:262–5.
10. Gracz AD, Ramalingam S, Magness ST. Sox9 expression marks a subset of CD24-expressing small intestine epithelial stem cells that form organoids in vitro. Am J Physiol Gastrointest Liver Physiol. 2010;298:G590–600.
11. Montgomery RK, Carlone DL, Richmond CA, Farilla L, Kranendonk ME, Henderson DE, et al. Mouse telomerase reverse transcriptase (mTert) expression marks slowly cycling intestinal stem cells. Proc Natl Acad Sci U S A. 2011;108:179–84.
12. Powell AE, Wang Y, Li Y, Poulin EJ, Means AL, Washington MK, et al. The pan-ErbB negative regulator Lrig1 is an intestinal stem cell marker that functions as a tumor suppressor. Cell. 2012;149:146–58.
13. Sangiorgi E, Capecchi MR. Bmi1 is expressed in vivo in intestinal stem cells. Nat Genet. 2008;40:915–20.
14. Takeda N, Jain R, LeBoeuf MR, Wang Q, Lu MM, Epstein JA. Interconversion between intestinal stem cell populations in distinct niches. Science. 2011;334:1420–4.
15. Metcalfe C, Kljavin NM, Ybarra R, de Sauvage FJ. Lgr5+ stem cells are indispensable for radiation-induced intestinal regeneration. Cell Stem Cell. 2014;14:149–59.
16. Tian H, Biehs B, Warming S, Leong KG, Rangell L, Klein OD, et al. A reserve stem cell population in small intestine renders Lgr5-positive cells dispensable. Nature. 2011;478:255–9.
17. Yan KS, Chia LA, Li X, Ootani A, Su J, Lee JY, et al. The intestinal stem cell markers Bmi1 and Lgr5 identify two functionally distinct populations. Proc Natl Acad Sci U S A. 2012;109: 466–71.
18. Gracz AD, Williamson IA, Roche KC, Johnston MJ, Wang F, Wang Y, et al. A high-throughput platform for stem cell niche co-cultures and downstream gene expression analysis. Nat Cell Biol. 2015;17:340–9.
19. Stelzner M, Helmrath M, Dunn JC, Henning SJ, Houchen CW, Kuo C, et al. A nomenclature for intestinal in vitro cultures. Am J Physiol Gastrointest Liver Physiol. 2012;302:G1359–63.
20. Ootani A, Li X, Sangiorgi E, Ho QT, Ueno H, Toda S, et al. Sustained in vitro intestinal epithelial culture within a Wnt-dependent stem cell niche. Nat Med. 2009;15:701–6.
21. Li X, Nadauld L, Ootani A, Corney DC, Pai RK, Gevaert O, et al. Oncogenic transformation of diverse gastrointestinal tissues in primary organoid culture. Nat Med. 2014;20:769–77.
22. Gunther C, Buchen B, He GW, Hornef M, Torow N, Neumann H, et al. Caspase-8 controls the gut response to microbial challenges by TNF-alpha-dependent and independent pathways. Gut. 2015;64:601–10.
23. Farin HF, Karthaus WR, Kujala P, Rakhshandehroo M, Schwank G, Vries RG, et al. Paneth cell extrusion and release of antimicrobial products is directly controlled by immune cell-derived IFN-gamma. J Exp Med. 2014;211:1393–405.
24. Wang F, Scoville D, He XC, Mahe MM, Box A, Perry JM, et al. Isolation and characterization of intestinal stem cells based on surface marker combinations and colony-formation assay. Gastroenterology. 2013;145:383–95. e1–21.
25. McCracken KW, Howell JC, Wells JM, Spence JR. Generating human intestinal tissue from pluripotent stem cells in vitro. Nat Protoc. 2011;6:1920–8.
26. Spence JR, Mayhew CN, Rankin SA, Kuhar MF, Vallance JE, Tolle K, et al. Directed differentiation of human pluripotent stem cells into intestinal tissue in vitro. Nature. 2011;470:105–9.
27. Wells JM, Spence JR. How to make an intestine. Development. 2014;141:752–60.
28. Spence JR, Lauf R, Shroyer NF. Vertebrate intestinal endoderm development. Dev Dyn. 2011;240:501–20.
29. Watson CL, Mahe MM, Munera J, Howell JC, Sundaram N, Poling HM, et al. An in vivo model of human small intestine using pluripotent stem cells. Nat Med. 2014;20:1310–4.
30. Xue X, Ramakrishnan S, Anderson E, Taylor M, Zimmermann EM, Spence JR, et al. Endothelial PAS domain protein 1 activates the inflammatory response in the intestinal epithelium to promote colitis in mice. Gastroenterology. 2013;145:831–41.
31. Schwank G, Koo BK, Sasselli V, Dekkers JF, Heo I, Demircan T, et al. Functional repair of CFTR by CRISPR/Cas9 in intestinal stem cell organoids of cystic fibrosis patients. Cell Stem Cell. 2013;13:653–8.
32. Drost J, van Jaarsveld RH, Ponsioen B, Zimberlin C, van Boxtel R, Buijs A, et al. Sequential cancer mutations in cultured human intestinal stem cells. Nature. 2015;521:43–7.
33. Matano M, Date S, Shimokawa M, Takano A, Fujii M, Ohta Y, et al. Modeling colorectal cancer using CRISPR-Cas9-mediated engineering of human intestinal organoids. Nat Med. 2015;21:256–62.
34. Pabst O, Schneider A, Brand T, Arnold HH. The mouse Nkx2-3 homeodomain gene is expressed in gut mesenchyme during pre- and postnatal mouse development. Dev Dyn. 1997;209:29–35.
35. McGrath PS, Watson CL, Ingram C, Helmrath MA, Wells JM. The basic helix-loop-helix transcription factor NEUROG3 is required for development of the human endocrine pancreas. Diabetes. 2015;64:2497–505.
36. Yui S, Nakamura T, Sato T, Nemoto Y, Mizutani T, Zheng X, et al. Functional engraftment of colon epithelium expanded in vitro from a single adult Lgr5(+) stem cell. Nat Med. 2012;18:618–23.
37. van de Wetering M, Francies HE, Francis JM, Bounova G, Iorio F, Pronk A, et al. Prospective derivation of a living organoid biobank of colorectal cancer patients. Cell. 2015;161:933–45.

Part III

Diagnostic Approach

17 Enhanced Endoscopy

R. Kiesslich

Introduction

Patients with long-standing extensive ulcerative colitis as well as patients with Crohn's associated colitis are at increased risk of developing colorectal cancer [1]. Colonoscopic surveillance is recommended in those patients to reduce associated mortality [2]. Surveillance relies on the detection of premalignant dysplastic tissue, and where multifocal dysplasia is detected, proctocolectomy remains the management of choice for colitis-associated neoplasia.

In general, the prognosis for patients with malignancies of the GI-tract is strictly dependent on early detection of premalignant and malignant lesions. However, small, flat or depressed neoplastic lesions [like colitis associated neoplasias] remain difficult to detect with conventional endoscopic technologies (e.g. standard resolution colonoscopy), thereby limiting their value for polyp detection and cancer screening.

Thus, what should an ideal enhance imaging method to be able to accomplish?

Three diagnostic steps are important: recognition; characterization and confirmation (see Fig. 17.1).

Recognition of lesions in the gut can be improved using better scopes, which have better imaging modalities like high resolution or high definition. Characterization of lesion type and surface architecture is important to predict histology, which can be eased with conventional chromoendoscopy or digital chromoendoscopy or magnifying or close focus endoscopy.

Here, a proposal for a consensus terminology for new imaging modalities is available and should be used [3].

R. Kiesslich (✉)
Klinik für Innere Medizin II (ZIM II), HELIOS Dr. Horst Schmidt Kliniken Wiesbaden, Ludwig-Erhard-Straße 100, 65199 Wiesbaden, Germany
e-mail: ralf.kiesslich@helios-kliniken.de

Finally, histological confirmation is needed to define whether cancer is present or not. This can be accomplished by conventional histology or with in vivo histology using endocytoscopy or confocal laser endomicroscopy. Confocal laser endomicroscopy with specific contrast agents will open a new door of tailored and individualised diagnosis.

High-Resolution, High-Definition and Magnifying Endoscopy

High-resolution and magnification endoscopes offer image quality that is significantly better than that of first-generation video endoscopes or the older fiber-optic systems. The *resolution* of an endoscopic image is a different quality from the *magnification*, and is defined as the ability to distinguish between two points that are close together. High-resolution imaging improves the ability to discriminate details while magnification enlarges the image. In digital video imaging, resolution is a function of pixel density. By incorporating high-pixel density charged-coupled devices (CCD), high-resolution endoscopes provide slightly magnified views of the gastrointestinal tract with greater mucosal detail. Magnification endoscopy utilises a movable lens controlled by the endoscopist to vary the degree of magnification, which ranges from ×1.5 to ×150. Newly designed magnification endoscopes provide high-resolution and magnification features [4].

Super magnifying endoscopes provide magnification up to 1100-fold. These endoscopes are called endocytoscopes. Endocytoscopy allows in conjunction with intravital staining identification of cellular structures [5].

High definition endoscopes are currently broadly available. Here, CCDs convert light information into an electronic signal. This signal is processed in the video-processor into an image. The standard analogue broadcasting systems (PAL or NTSC) generate approximately 480–576 scanning lines on a screen. The new high definition endoscopes can generate up to 1080 scanning lines on a screen, which further

D.C. Baumgart (ed.), *Crohn's Disease and Ulcerative Colitis*, DOI 10.1007/978-3-319-33703-6_17

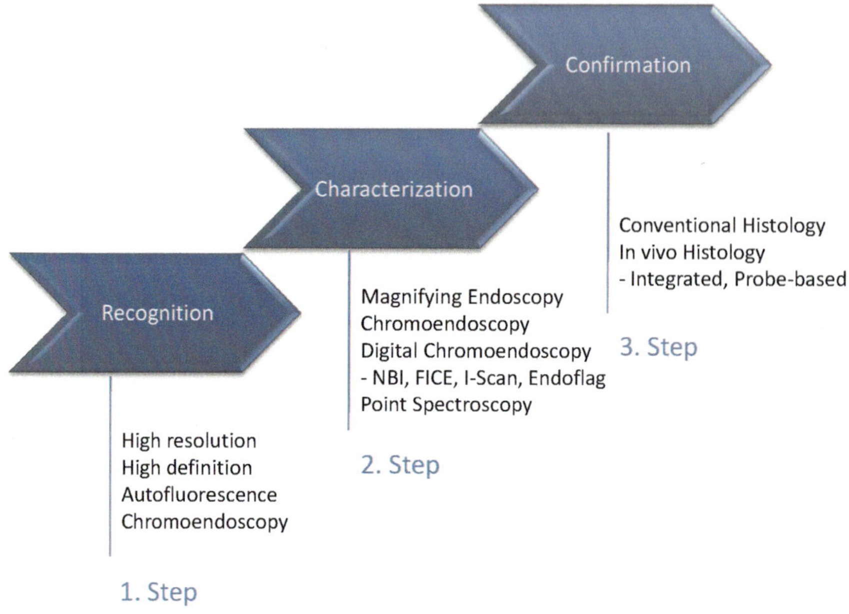

Fig. 17.1 Enhanced endoscopic technologies to improve the three essential steps to final diagnosis

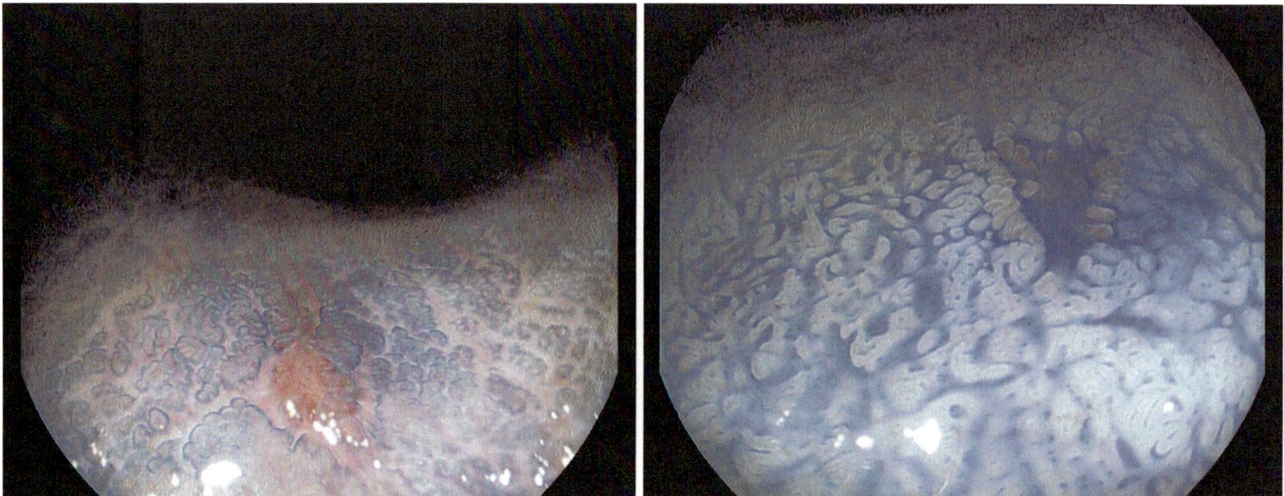

Fig. 17.2 Flat and depressed colitis-associated neoplasia diagnosed with chromoendoscopy [methylene blue]

increases the resolution. Surface analysis on distinct lesions can be done even before magnification (see Fig. 17.2). There are convincing data about screening colonoscopy emerging showing that high definition endoscopy lead to an increased detection of patients having at least one adenoma [6].

Wide View Colonoscopes and Balloon Assisted Colonoscopy

The so-called FUSE-colonoscope (Endoschoice, USA) has three optics at the distal tip of the colonoscope. Fuse colonoscopes feature cameras at the tip as well as on the sides of the scope providing a panoramic 330° view of the colon. The wide view facilitates navigation to the cecum as well as intubation of the terminal ileum. Studies have demonstrated that the adenoma detection rate can be significantly increased and the miss rate of adenomas can be significantly reduced [7].

Balloon assisted colonoscopy (G-EYE Colonoscopy) allows straightening colonic folds during withdrawal. Furthermore, endoscope slippage is reduced and the insufflated distal ballon of the colonoscope canters the endoscopic image and facilitates polyp removal by "anchoring" the endoscope in front of the polyp.

The silicone balloon is permanently mounted on any desirable colonoscope. The balloon is insufflated during withdrawal and pressure of the balloon is automatically controlled.

Studies have proven the benefit of the G-EYE system. Adenoma detection rates are significantly improved and adenoma miss rates are significantly reduced [8].

However, the benefit of wide viewing colonoscopy and balloon-assisted colonoscopy for IBD patients is not determined yet.

Chromoendoscopy

Chromoendoscopy or tissue staining is a relatively "old" endoscopic technique that has been used for decades. It involves the topical application of stains or pigments to improve localization, characterization, or diagnosis of lesions [9]. It is a useful adjunct to endoscopy; the contrast between normally stained and abnormally stained epithelium enables the endoscopist to make a diagnosis and/or to direct biopsies based on a specific reaction or enhancement of surface morphology (see Fig. 17.2).

The technique for staining is simple and easy to learn. Chromoendoscopy can be done in an untargeted fashion of the whole segment (Panchromoendoscopy) or directed towards a specific lesion (targeted staining). While spraying dyes in the colon in an untargeted fashion, the endoscopist needs to direct the endoscope and catheter tip towards the colorectal mucosa and use a combination of rotational clockwise-counter clockwise movements with simultaneous withdrawal of the endoscope tip.

Surface analysis of stained colorectal lesions was a new optical impression for the endoscopists in the nineties. First, Kudo et al. described that some of the regular staining patterns are often seen in hyperplastic polyps or normal mucosa, whereas unstructured surface architecture was associated with malignancy. Also the kind of adenoma (tubular vs. villous) can be seen by detailed inspection. This experience has lead to a categorization of the different staining patterns in the colon: The so-called pit-pattern classification [10] differentiated five types and several subtypes. Types 1 and 2 are staining patterns predicting non-neoplastic lesions, whereas types 3–5 are predicting neoplastic lesions. With the help of this classification the endoscopist may predict histology with good accuracy. Although the pit-pattern classification was developed by the help of magnifying endoscopes the question arises whether an endoscopic differentiation of different staining patterns can also be done with the help of the more common high-resolution endoscopes.

Chromoendoscopy has shown significant advantages in the detection of flat colorectal neoplasia and in colitis associated neoplasia [11].

Magnifying chromoendoscopy using either methylene blue or indigo carmine is a valid and proven tool for improving endoscopic detection of intraepithelial neoplasia in patients with long-standing ulcerative colitis. Chromoendoscopy increased the diagnostic yield of intraepithelial neoplasia as compared with conventional colonoscopy 3- to 4.5-fold. Differentiation of non-neoplastic from neoplastic lesions is possible with a high overall sensitivity and specificity. Chromoendoscopy is endorsed in multiple guidelines as a superior and recommended alternative to conventional colonoscopy with random biopsies [12].

An international guideline (SCENIC) was published 2015 underlining the importance of chromoendoscopy with guided biopsies as the standard for surveillance in patients with IBD [13].

Digital Chromoendoscopy

Conventional white light endoscopy uses the full visible wavelength range to produce a red-green-blue image. In contrast, narrow band imaging, in combination with magnification endoscopy, illuminates the tissue surface using special filters that narrow the respective red-green-blue bands. This enhances the tissue microvasculature mainly as a result of the differential optical absorption of light by haemoglobin in the mucosa associated with initiation and progression of dysplasia, particularly in the blue range. To some extent, the resulting images look like "chromoendoscopy without dyes" (see Figs. 17.3 and 17.4).

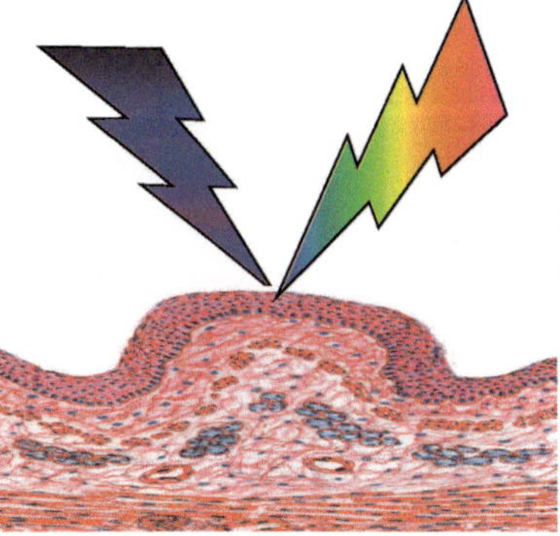

Fig. 17.3 Types and function of digital chromoendoscopy (filter aided endoscopy)

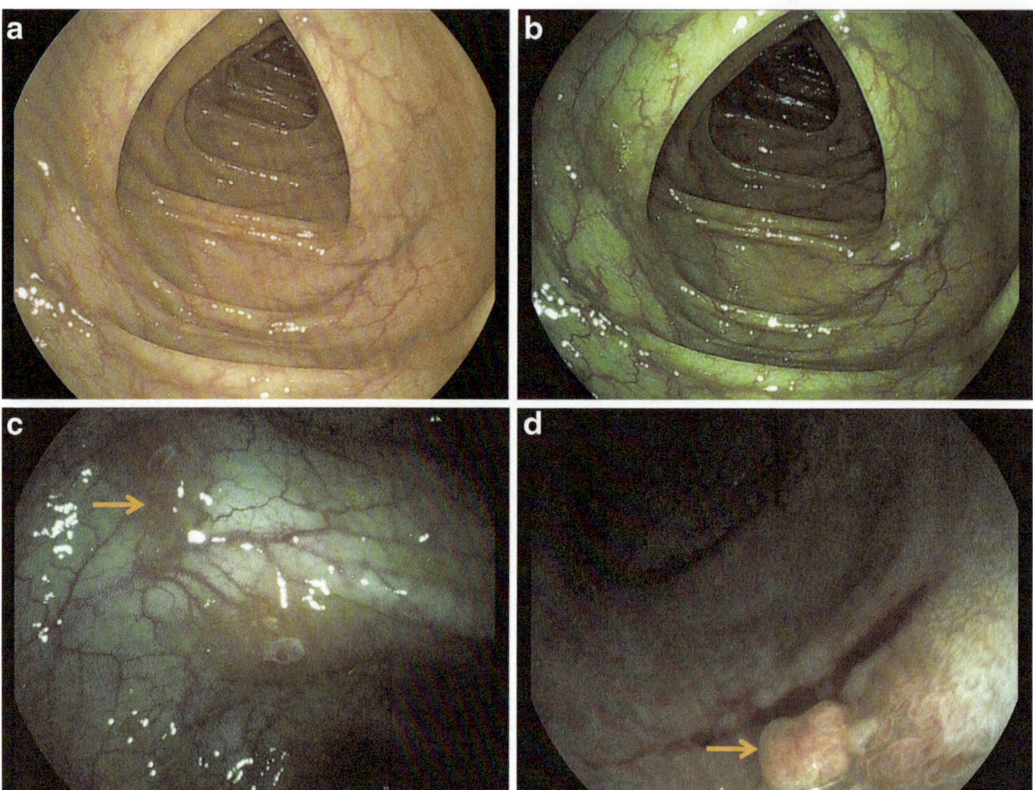

Fig. 17.4 Filter aided colonoscopy in IBD. (**A**, **B**): Normal colonic mucosa with (*a*) and without (*b*) i-scan imaging. (**C**, **D**) Inflamed mucosa (*see arrow*) (*c*) and neoplastic changes (*see arrow*) visualised with i-scan

Alternatively, the light which is reflected from the mucosal can be modified using post processing computer algorithms (FICE, i-Scan, SPIES). This can modulate different forms of enhancement, which leads to an accentuation of the vasculature, the surface architecture or the pattern visualisation (see Figs. 17.3 and 17.4). However, none of these filters has proven so far any benefit diagnosing colitis associated neoplasia [14, 15].

Autofluorescence Imaging

Autofluorescence imaging systems are available that use video endoscopes with two CCDs: one for high-resolution white light endoscopy and one for autofluorescence imaging (AFI). The autofluorescence image is a pseudo-colour image composed from three integrated images: (1) the total autofluorescence after blue light excitation (395–475 nm); (2) the green reflectance (540–560 nm); and (3) the red reflectance (600–620 nm).

A new system has become available that incorporates high-resolution endoscopy, AFI and NBI in one single system: endoscopic tri-modality imaging (ETMI). This system has a new autofluorescence algorithm in which the fluorescence image is composed of two integrated images instead of three images: total autofluorescence after blue light excitation (395–475 nm) and green reflectance. Autofluorescence in conjunction with NBI can help to unmask colitis-associated neoplasias [16].

Optical Coherence Tomography

Optical coherence tomography (OCT) is a high-resolution cross-sectional imaging technique. It is analogous to B-mode high-resolution endosonography but uses light waves instead of acoustic waves. As a result, OCT has a high resolution, up to ten times higher than high-frequency ultrasound, enabling microstructural features of tissue to be identified, but it has a limited sampling depth of 1–2 mm [17] OCT measures the intensity of back scattered light from tissue at various depths using low-coherence interferometry.

OCT is a probe-based technique in which the probe is passed through the accessory channel of an endoscope. Unlike endosonography, OCT can be performed without a coupling media (e.g. water). The OCT catheter has to be positioned adjacent to the mucosa within the system's focal distance (1-5 mm), which may be difficult due to the movement of the oesophagus by peristalsis and heart beat. In addition, compression artefacts may be seen when the probe comes in contact with the mucosa. OCT can easily differentiate normal epithelium from abnormal tissue with high accuracy. However, the detection and grading of high-grade dysplasia and early cancer remain still challenging [18].

Future developments in OCT, such as ultra-high resolution OCT, spectroscopic OCT, Doppler OCT and optical frequency-domain imaging, may enhance the accuracy of OCT for the detection of dysplasia and give rise to other applications.

Endocytoscopy

Endocytoscopy is based on the principle of light contact microscopy. The first studies using this system were performed in the field of otolaryngology. After application of methylene blue the tip of a rigid endoscope was placed in direct contact with the surface. With this method cytological details can be directly visualised, making direct observation of living cells feasible [5, 19]. The first endocytoscopy system was, however, a rigid instrument, which is not practical for use in the gastrointestinal tract. Therefore, a novel endocytoscope system has been developed, the Endocytoscope. This system consists of two flexible endoscopes with a diameter of 3.2 mm that can easily pass through an accessory channel with a diameter of 3.7 mm: one low-magnification endocytoscope with a maximal magnification of 450× and a high-magnification endocytoscope with a maximal magnification of 1100×. Recently, the integration of the endocytoscope within an otherwise conventional endoscope could be achieved.

Endocytoscopy is used to identify cellular and nuclei architecture of the surface layer of the epithelium. Residual mucin and moving artefacts can alter its accuracy. However, the combination of macroscopy (white light endoscopy) and microscopy (endocytoscopy) has lead to better understanding of the surface micro-architecture.

The current system, however, cannot visualise the deeper layers of the epithelium and is, therefore, not yet suited for evaluating early neoplasia with respect to depth of invasion. However, automated surface analysis has shown to be highly accurate diagnosing neoplastic and non-neoplastic tissue [20].

Confocal Laser Endomicroscopy

Confocal laser endomicroscopy is a new imaging modality for gastrointestinal endoscopy. It offers in vivo imaging of the mucosal layer at cellular and even subcellular resolution. Thus, in vivo histology becomes possible during ongoing endoscopy. This new imaging modality provides more than conventional histology, because cellular interaction can be observed over time (physiology) and distinct changes can be identified (pathophysiology) [21].

Principle of Confocal Microscopy and Types of Endoscopic Endomicroscopes

Confocal microscopy allows a better spatial resolution compared with conventional fluorescence microscopy, because images are not contaminated by light scattering from other focal planes. A low power laser is focused to a single point in a defined microscopic field of view and the same lens is used as both condenser and objective folding optical path. Thus, the point of illumination coincides with the point of detection within the specimen. Light emanating from that point is focused through a pinhole to a detector and light emanating from outside the illuminated spot is rejected from detection. Illumination and detection system are at the same focal plane and termed as "confocal". All detected signals from the illuminated spot are captured and measured. The created greyscale image is an optical section representing one focal plane within the examined specimen. The image of a scanned region can now be constructed and digitised by measuring light returning to the detector from successive points.

The first publication about an integrated confocal fluorescence microscope into the distal tip of a conventional colonoscope (Pentax EC 3830FK, Tokyo, Japan) was made 2004 [22] showing that in vivo microscopy at subcellular resolution (0.7 μm) simultaneously displayed to white light endoscopy became possible and achieved high accuracy. This approach, designated confocal laser endomicroscopy (CLE), permitted immediate diagnosis of colorectal intraepithelial neoplasias using fluorescein or acriflavin as contrast agents. The integrated endomicroscopic system is no longer commercially available. Probe based confocal endomicroscope has replaced it. Here, an endomicroscopic probe can be passed over the working channel of standard endoscopes [23] (see Fig. 17.5).

Contrast Agents

Fluorescence confocal imaging is only possible using exogenous fluorescence contrast agents. Potentially suitable agents are fluorescein, acriflavine or cresyl violet [24]. The most common and safe contrast agent is fluorescein sodium (5–10 ml of a 10 % solution; intravenous application) [5].

Fig. 17.5 Types of endomicroscopy

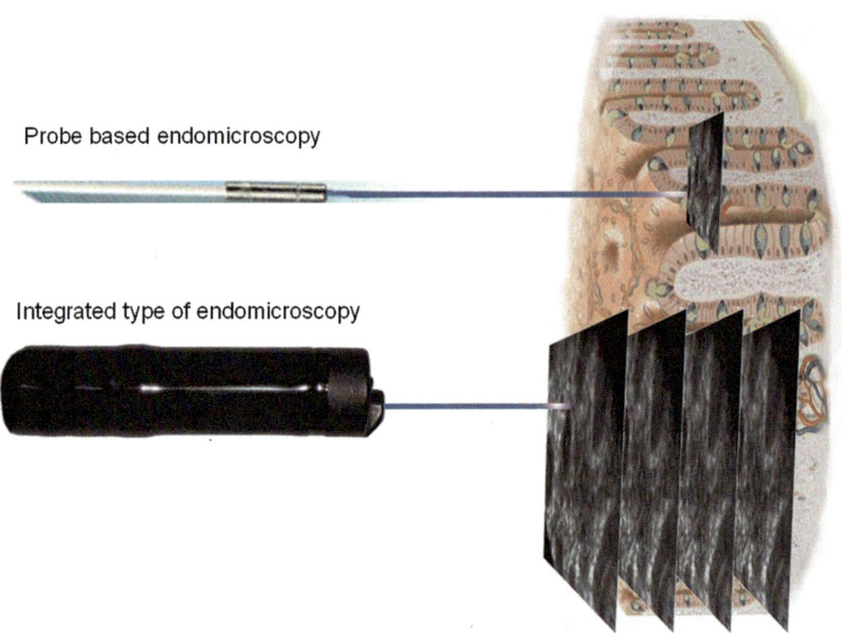

Clinical Data of Endomicroscopy

Endomicroscopy enables to predict and see histological changes with high accuracy based on simple classifications, which includes vessel and cellular changes [5]. Endomicroscopy is more accurate than high definition or filter aided endoscopy [25] (see Fig. 17.6).

Endomicroscopy further expands the diagnostic possibilities of chromoendoscopy in patients with inflammatory bowel diseases. Chromoendoscopy is able to reveal circumscribed lesions, and confocal laser microscopy can be used to confirm intraepithelial neoplasias with a high degree of accuracy [26]. Biopsies can therefore be limited to targeted sampling of relevant lesions. In vivo histology with endomicroscopy may lead to significant improvements in the clinical management of patients with ulcerative colitis, with reduced numbers of biopsies being needed for confirmation of the condition and time being gained for immediate therapeutic intervention.

Functional and Molecular Imaging

Endomicroscopy can not only be used to receive histology. The great potential of endomicroscopy is to display and observe physiologic and pathophysiologic changes during ongoing endoscopy. Furthermore molecular imaging becomes possible.

Cell shedding is a physiologic process. After cell shedding an epithelial gap occurs, this is sealed within seconds. Patients with inflammatory bowel disease show malfunction of gap closure, which can lead to invasion of bacteria into the lamina propria and represents the “leakiness” of the gut. These changes can be observed with endomicroscopy and predict the clinical course of the disease [27]. Endomicroscopy displays not only tissue also bacterial interaction with the mucosal layer can be seen [28] (see Fig. 17.7).

Molecular imaging is already achieved [29]. Dysplastic colonic crypts could be selectively stained with fluorescence heptapeptides. Also labelled adalimumab can be visualised within the mucosal layer [30]. This approach will open the door for new clinical algorithms, which will be dependent on the endomicroscopic findings (e.g. prediction of the efficiency of chemotherapy with biological). Also distinct receptors can be visualised [31, 32] (see Fig. 17.7).

Conclusion

New imaging modalities of gastrointestinal endoscopy are rapidly evolving, and they will greatly influence everyday work in the very near future. Patients with IBD will substantial profit of these new developments because they face an increased cancer risk even at young age.

The progress of endoscopic techniques follows substantial innovations in IT (information technology), biotechnology

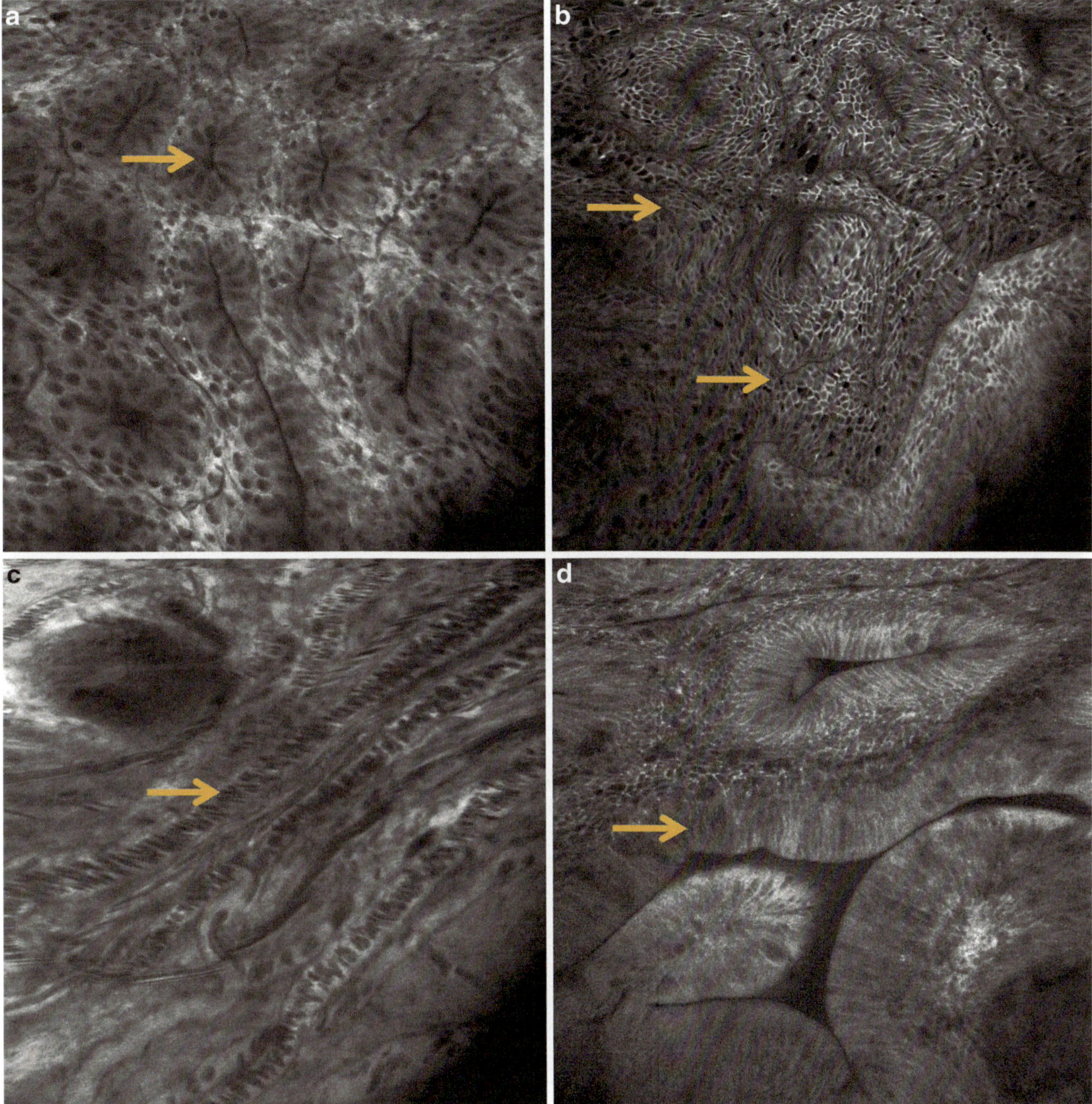

Fig. 17.6 Image examples of endomicroscopy. (**A**, **B**) Normal colonic crypts (*arrow*) with goblet cells (*a*) and hyperplastic changes (*b*; *arrow*). (**C**, **D**) Vessels (*c*) in inflamed mucosa with visible red blood cells (*arrow*). Tubular changes (*d*) with loss of goblet cells (low-grade intraepithelial neoplasia) (*d*)

and multimedia. We are currently facing only the beginning of a new era where computer assisted solutions and technical innovations will greatly influence our diagnostic strategies.

A main goal is the early detection of gastrointestinal cancer, because it is highly cost effective and convincing. Evolving technologies are helping to improve our diagnosis from recognition over characterization to confirmation.

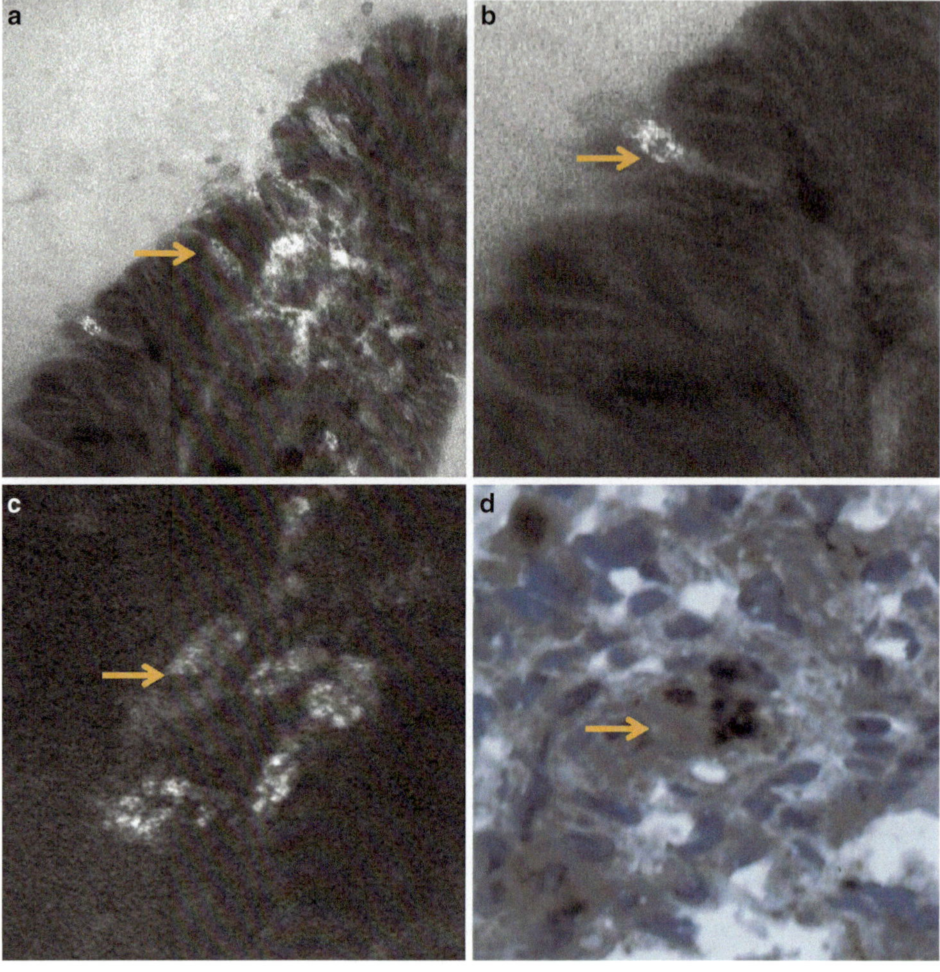

Fig. 17.7 Functional and molecular imaging using endomicroscopy. (**A**, **B**) Cell shedding with visible gap in the terminal ileum (epithelial cell layer) of a patient with Crohn's disease (*a*). Translocation of bacteria (bright spots) can be visualised. (**C**, **D**) Fluorescein labelled antibodies can visualise VEGF-receptors (*c*) in vivo which correlates with ex vivo immunohistochemistry (*d*)

References

1. Gilat T, Fireman Z, Grossman A, et al. Colorectal cancer in patients with ulcerative colitis. Gastroenterology. 1988;94:870–7.
2. Winawer S et al. Colorectal cancer screening and surveillance: clinical guidelines and rationale-Update based on new evidence. Gastroenterology. 2003;124(2):544–60.
3. Tajiri H, Niwa H. Proposal for a consensus terminology in endoscopy: how should different endoscopic imaging techniques be grouped and defined? Endoscopy. 2008;40(9):775–8.
4. Nelson DB, Block KP, Bosco JJ, et al. High resolution and high magnification endoscopy. Guidelines: Technology Status Evaluation Report. Gastrointest Endosc. 2000;52:864–6.
5. Goetz M, Malek NP, Kiesslich R. Microscopic imaging in endoscopy: endomicroscopy and endocytoscopy. Nat Rev Gastroenterol Hepatol. 2014;11(1):11–8.
6. Dik VK, Moons LM, Siersema PD. Endoscopic innovations to increase the adenoma detection rate during colonoscopy. World J Gastroenterol. 2014;20(9):2200–11.
7. Gralnek IM, Siersema PD, Halpern Z, et al. Standard forward-viewing colonoscopy versus full-spectrum endoscopy: an international, multicentre, randomised, tandem colonoscopy trial. Lancet Oncol. 2014;15(3):353–60.
8. Halpern Z, Gross SA, Gralnek IM, et al. Comparison of adenoma detection and miss rates between a novel balloon colonoscope and standard colonoscopy: a randomized tandem study. Endoscopy. 2015;47(3):238–44.
9. Canto MI. Staining in gastrointestinal endoscopy: the basics. Endoscopy. 1999;31:479–86.
10. Kudo S, Tamura S, Nakajima T, et al. Diagnosis of colorectal tumorous lesions by magnifying endoscopy. Gastrointest Endosc. 1996;44:8–14.
11. Kiesslich R, Fritsch J, Holtmann M, Koehler HH, Stolte M, Kanzler S, et al. Methylene blue-aided chromoendoscopy for the detection of intraepithelial neoplasia and colon cancer in ulcerative colitis. Gastroenterology. 2003;124(4):880–8.
12. Van Assche G, Dignass A, Reinisch W, et al. The second European evidence-based consensus on the diagnosis and management of Crohn's disease: special situations. J Crohns Colitis. 2010;4(1): 63–101.
13. Laine L, Kaltenbach T, Barkun A, et al. SCENIC international consensus statement on surveillance and management of dysplasia in inflammatory bowel disease. Gastroenterology. 2015;148(3):639–51.e28.
14. van den Broek FJ, Fockens P, van Eeden S, et al. Narrow-band imaging versus high-definition endoscopy for the diagnosis of neoplasia in ulcerative colitis. Endoscopy. 2010 Dec 16 [Epub ahead of print].
15. Dekker E, van den Broek FJ, Reitsma JB, et al. Narrow-band imaging compared with conventional colonoscopy for the detection of dysplasia in patients with longstanding ulcerative colitis. Endoscopy. 2007;39(3):216–21.
16. van den Broek FJ, Fockens P, van Eeden S, et al. Endoscopic tri-modal imaging for surveillance in ulcerative colitis: randomised comparison of high-resolution endoscopy and autofluorescence

imaging for neoplasia detection; and evaluation of narrow-band imaging for classification of lesions. Gut. 2008;57(8):1083–9. Epub 26 Mar 2008.
17. Wong Kee Song LM, Wilson BC. Endoscopic detection of early upper GI cancers. Best Pract Res Clin Gastroenterol. 2005;19: 833–56.
18. Shen B, Zuccaro Jr G, Gramlich TL, et al. In vivo colonoscopic optical coherence tomography for transmural inflammation in inflammatory bowel disease. Clin Gastroenterol Hepatol. 2004;2(12):1080–7.
19. Inoue H, Sasajima K, Kaga M, Sugaya S, Sato Y, Wada Y, et al. Endoscopic in vivo evaluation of tissue atypia in the esophagus using a newly designed integrated endocytoscope: a pilot trial. Endoscopy. 2006;38(9):891–5.
20. Tontini GE, Pastorelli L, Ishaq S, Neumann H. Advances in endoscopic imaging in ulcerative colitis. Expert Rev Gastroenterol Hepatol. 2015;12:1–13.
21. Kiesslich R, Galle PR, Neurath MF, editors. Atlas of endomicroscopy, 2008. Springer. ISBN 978-3-540-34757-6.
22. Kiesslich R, Burg J, Vieth M, Gnaendiger J, Enders M, Delaney P, et al. Confocal laser endoscopy for diagnosing intraepithelial neoplasias and colorectal cancer in vivo. Gastroenterology. 2004; 127(3):706–13.
23. Meining A, Saur D, Bajbouj M, Becker V, Peltier E, Höfler H, et al. In vivo histopathology for detection of gastrointestinal neoplasia with a portable, confocal miniprobe: an examiner blinded analysis. Clin Gastroenterol Hepatol. 2007;5(11):1261–7. Epub 6 Aug 2007.
24. Wallace MB, Meining A, Canto MI, et al. The safety of intravenous fluorescein for confocal laser endomicroscopy in the gastrointestinal tract. Aliment Pharmacol Ther. 2010;31(5):548–52.
25. Buchner AM, Shahid MW, Heckman MG, et al. Comparison of probe-based confocal laser endomicroscopy with virtual chromoendoscopy for classification of colon polyps. Gastroenterology. 2010;138(3):834–42.
26. Kiesslich R, Goetz M, Lammersdorf K, Schneider C, Burg J, Stolte M, et al. Chromoscopic-guided endomicroscopy increases the diagnostic yield of intraepithelial neoplasia in ulcerative colitis. Gastroenterology. 2007;132(3):874–82.
27. Kiesslich R, Goetz M, Angus EM, Hu Q, Guan Y, Potten C, et al. Identification of epithelial gaps in human small and large intestine by confocal endomicroscopy. Gastroenterology. 2007;133(6): 1769–78.
28. Moussata D, Goetz M, Gloeckner A, et al. Confocal laser endomicroscopy is a new imaging modality for recognition of intramucosal bacteria in inflammatory bowel disease in vivo. Gut. 2011; 60(1):26–33.
29. Hsiung PL, Hardy J, Friedland S, Soetikno R, et al. Detection of colonic dysplasia in vivo using a targeted heptapeptide and confocal microendoscopy. Nat Med. 2008;14(4):454–8. Epub 16 Mar 2008.
30. Atreya R, Neumann H, Neufert C, et al. In vivo imaging using fluorescent antibodies to tumor necrosis factor predicts therapeutic response in Crohn's disease. Nat Med. 2014;20(3):313–8.
31. Foersch S, Kiesslich R, Waldner MJ, et al. Molecular imaging of VEGF in gastrointestinal cancer in vivo using confocal laser endomicroscopy. Gut. 2010;59(8):1046–55.
32. Goetz M, Ziebart A, Foersch S, et al. In vivo molecular imaging of colorectal cancer with confocal endomicroscopy by targeting epidermal growth factor receptor. Gastroenterology. 2010;138(2): 435–46.

Magnetic Resonance Enterography

18

Patrik Rogalla and Luís Guimarães

The assessment of small bowel pathology has always been a difficult task for radiologists and gastroenterologists, mainly due to its remoteness from the mouth and anus and to the length of small bowel loops [1]. The wide range of methods currently available for the evaluation of the small bowel, including radiologic and endoscopic techniques, is a confirmation of this difficulty. The radiologic techniques include small bowel follow-through (SBFT), fluoroscopic enteroclysis, ultrasound (US), conventional computed tomography (CT), CT enteroclysis (CTe), CT enterography (CTE), magnetic resonance (MR) enteroclysis (MRe) and MR enterography (MRE). Endoscopic methods include ileoscopy, enteroscopy and wireless capsule endoscopy (CE).

Magnetic resonance enterography and enteroclysis consist in the high spatial resolution imaging of the small bowel with MR following the administration of large amounts of an enteric contrast agent, either orally (enterography) or using a nasojejunal tube (enteroclysis). The techniques would not be as accurate as we know them today without the last decade advances in MR technology. New scanners and new pulse sequences have been developed, allowing, for instance, for breath-hold isotropic or near-isotropic spatial resolution, robust cine-imaging and diffusion-weighted imaging. Moreover, the combined use of intravenous (IV) and specific enteric contrast agents optimizes luminal distension and permits the distinction of the layers of the bowel wall, the fluid-filled lumen and the adjacent mesenteric fat.

Compared with the traditional SBFT examination, CT and MR have several advantages: (1) they display the entire thickness of the bowel wall, (2) they permit the examination of the deep ileal loops in the pelvis without superimposition and (3) they allow the evaluation of the perienteric fat and mesentery. They also allow assessment of the remaining abdominopelvic organs. Because of the abovementioned reasons, CT and MR enterography have been promptly implemented by many institutions as the primary techniques used to image the small bowel, especially for Crohn's disease (CD), which is by far the most common indication.

Reasons of Success of CT and MR Enterography

The volume of CTE and MRE exams ordered to study diagnosed or suspected CD has progressively increased over the last decade in the vast majority of the institutions that have this exam available [2]. We believe there are three main reasons that motivate this growth: (1) the emergence of wireless capsule endoscopy, (2) the availability of new drugs, like infliximab, (3) the growing body of evidence about CTE/MRE performance and the proven clinical benefit of their use. We now discuss a little further these three aspects.

The Influence of the Emergence of Wireless Capsule Endoscopy

Wireless capsule endoscopy was introduced in 2000 and since then it has been demonstrated in repeated studies that the fluoroscopic radiological studies provide incomplete information about CD presence and extent [3].

In a prospective study comparing CE with SBFT and CT in 35 patients with suspected CD (using ileoscopy as the reference standard), the diagnostic yield of CE was 77 %, versus 23 % of fluoroscopic radiological techniques ($p<0.05$) [4]. The CE identified all true lesions found by SBFT, expanded the regions of involvement in some patients, established a diagnosis in one-fourth of the patients when the SBFT was interpreted as normal and excluded the diagnosis suspected by the radiological studies in 10/35 patients (29 %).

Just to give another example, in a prospective study comparing four small-bowel imaging techniques (SBFT, CTE, ileoscopy and CE) for depiction of abnormal findings in

P. Rogalla, BS, MD (✉) • L. Guimarães
Department of Medical Imaging, Princess Margaret Hospital, 610 University Ave, Toronto, ON M5G 2M, Canada
e-mail: Patrik.Rogalla@uhn.on.ca

D.C. Baumgart (ed.), *Crohn's Disease and Ulcerative Colitis*, DOI 10.1007/978-3-319-33703-6_18

patients known to have or suspected of having CD, small-bowel findings positive for CD were present in 12 of 17 (71 %) CE examinations, 11 of 17 (65 %) ileoscopic examinations and 9 of 17 (53 %) CTE examinations; however, fluoroscopic radiological examinations only found abnormalities in 4 of these 17 patients (24 %) [5].

These results are not surprising, as fluoroscopic small-bowel studies were known to have some important limitations: the changeable examination techniques of SBFT, the patient discomfort of enteroclysis, the low sensitivity for the detection of mild disease (such as aphthous ulcers), the lack of assessment of the entire bowel wall, the difficulty in the evaluation of some ileal loops due to superimposition [6], etc. However, these drawbacks became much more evident with the beginning of CE utilization. Simultaneously, CTE and MRE performance and clinical impact started to be proven (as discussed below). These factors profoundly contributed to the significant decrease in the number of fluoroscopic small-bowel examinations ordered by the clinicians and their replacement by CTE or MRE.

The Influence of the Development of New Medications for CD

Infliximab is a monoclonal antibody against tumour necrosis factor alpha (TNFα). TNFα has diverse pro-inflammatory effects within the intestinal mucosa and is a pivotal cytokine in the inflammatory cascade [7]. The first study demonstrating the efficacy of Infliximab in CD was published in the New England Journal of Medicine (NEJM) in 1997 [8]. This study was a randomized, double-blind, placebo-controlled trial. Eighty-one percent of patients treated with a single dose of Infliximab 5 mg/kg achieved clinical response at the fourth week, while only 16 % of patients treated with placebo accomplished clinical response. The efficacy of Infliximab in the treatment of fistulizing CD was first demonstrated in a study published in the NEJM in 1999 [9]. The primary efficacy analysis showed that 68 % of patients treated with Infliximab 5 mg/kg at weeks 0, 2, and 6 achieved the primary endpoint of a greater than 50 % reduction in fistulae, while only 26 % of patients taking placebo accomplished the same endpoint.

But Infliximab was only the first of a new generation of revolutionary medicines for CD patients. Adalimumab, for instance, a human recombinant DNA anti-TNFα antibody that can be given subcutaneously [10], became also available and was approved by the U.S. Food and Drug Administration (FDA) in 2002.

These medications are very effective, but also very expensive. Yearly patient costs of infliximab and adalimumab average $25–35,000 in the U.S.

In addition, there are significant risks associated with the use of these new biological agents. Morbidity and even mortality may result from infections, lymphatic/hematopoietic cancers, septicemia and respiratory diseases that may be related to the use of these immunomodulatory medications. A relatively recent systematic review estimated a 1-year incidence of death from serious infection of 0.4 % and a rate of lymphoma of 0.2 % among patients with moderate to severe CD unresponsive to conventional therapy who received infliximab [11]. Another study investigated the risk of opportunistic infections in patients with IBD [12] and the results in terms of odds ratio (OR) were the following: in univariate analysis, use of corticosteroids—OR, 3.4; 95 % CI, 1.8–6.2—, azathioprine/6-mercaptopurine—OR, 3.1; 95 % CI, 1.7–5.5—, and infliximab—OR, 4.4; 95 % CI, 1.2–17.1—were associated individually with significantly increased odds for opportunistic infection; multivariate analysis indicated that use of any of these drugs yielded an OR of 2.9 (95 % CI, 1.5–5.3), whereas use of two or three simultaneously yielded an OR of 14.5 (95 % CI, 4.9–43) for opportunistic infection. Other side effects of Crohn's medications include severe agranulocytosis (from sulfasalazine) [13], bone marrow suppression (from azathioprine, including life-threatening agranulocytosis in about 0.3 % of patients and leucopenia in up to 10 % of patients) [14] non-Hodgkin's lymphoma [15], tuberculosis (infliximab) and other serious severe or opportunistic infections (in up to 4 % of patients) [16], drug-induced lupus (infliximab) [17], and, very rarely, noncurable hepatosplenic T cell lymphoma (infliximab) [18] and progressive multifocal leukoencephalopathy (natalizumab) [19].

On the other hand, to not introduce these effective drugs when indicated may have a deleterious impact in patients' morbidity and mortality. And these are not negligible, in CD. Several long-term population-based studies have described increased mortality rates with CD [20]. A meta-analysis found 50 % increased mortality in the CD population [21]. The increased overall mortality may be attributed to death from gastrointestinal complications, gastrointestinal malignant neoplasms and some extraintestinal manifestations [22]. A population-based study done in the Olmsted county (MN, USA) found that 32 % of all deaths in the CD cohort related directly to the underlying disease. These deaths were related to severe fistulizing CD, post-surgical sepsis secondary to immunomodulator theraphy, etc. [20]. In another large population study, increased mortality in CD population was most strongly related to infections, septicemia and other digestive diseases other than CD.

These two aspects—(1) important cost and potential side effects from IBD drugs and (2) significant morbidity and mortality that can potentially be prevented with a judicious administration of such drugs—prompt the Gastroenterologists to try to acquire all the possible reliable information about the patients and their disease, in order to avoid the risks of not initiating immunosuppression in patients where it is indicated and the drawbacks associated with a delay in the diagnosis due to diagnostic uncertainty or underestimation of disease extent and severity. They need objective information about the presence of active inflammation, the extension of the disease, the existence of penetrating disease and the presence of complications that preclude medical therapy. Besides imaging, the main tools Gastroenterologists have at hand to decide their approach are the historical data, patient symptoms, endoscopic assessment and serum markers. These other sources of information are reflected in numerous scoring systems seeking to objectively quantify disease type and severity: the Crohn's Disease Activity Index (CDAI), the Harvey–Bradshaw Index (HBI), the Perianal Disease Activity Index, the Fistula Drainage Assessment, the Endoscopic Index of Severity, the Scoring System for CD mucosal biopsy specimens, etc. Unfortunately, these indices and the information they reflect are prone to interobserver variability and incorporate subjective terms like "well-being" or "abdominal pain". Moreover, it is known that both CDAI and HBI downgrade draining fistulae, and that histologic evaluation does not match other estimates of activity [23].

Given all these aspects, more objective measures of active disease and complications are needed, and this is why CTE and MRE, with all the evidence regarding their performance and clinical impact (discussed below), gained preponderance and became very frequently ordered by IBD-dedicated Gastroenterologists.

MRE Performance and Clinical Benefit

Another important factor contributing to the increase in the popularity of CTE was the rising body of evidence concerning CTE's performance and clinical benefit.

MRE Performance

A recent study evaluated 33 patients with suspected active ileal Crohn's disease that underwent CT enterography and ileo-colonoscopy, 30 of which subsequently underwent MR enterography [24]. The sensitivities of MR enterography and CT enterography for detecting small bowel disease were very similar (90.5 % vs. 95.2 %). In 8 patients (24 %) MR enterography and CT enterography identified inflammatory changes when endoscopy demonstrated normal ileal mucosa. This was due to the presence of bowel inflammation in the proximal small bowel in four patients (i.e. skipping of "terminal" TI), intramural disease in four patients (as manifested by mural hyperenhancement, wall thickening, or mural stratification on MRE and CTE at the TI or neoterminal ileum), and penetrating disease in one patient. Several important conclusions can be drawn from the results of this study: (1) CTE and MRE accuracy is very high; (2) there is a complementary role of cross-sectional imaging with endoscopy where mucosal assessment alone may underestimate the extent of transmural involvement (which also means ileocolonoscopy is not perfect as a reference standard for CTE/MRE); (3) CT and MR enterography perform similarly. This last point is important because it shows that the large body of evidence available for CTE (studies of the first decade of this century were largely on CTE rather than on MRE) applies to MRE.

As another example of a study on the performance of cross-sectional imaging of the small bowel, Solem et al. published in 2008 a head-to-head trial comparing CTE, CE, ileocolonoscopy and SBFT in 42 patients with suspected or known CD. The sensitivity of CTE was 82 % (almost identical to the sensitivity of CE, 83 %), and the specificity was 89 % (significantly higher than CE, 53 %; $p<0.02$) [25].

However prospective comparative studies of MR enteroclysis and CE have shown MR enteroclysis to be less sensitive than CE, although there was no statistically significant difference in diagnostic performance [26]. Consequently, in patients with strong underlying suspicion and markers for Crohn's disease, negative imaging should not deter assessment of mucosal involvement by endoscopic techniques, namely CE.

Clinical Benefit of MR Enterography

Sensitivity and specificity of a technique are especially important if they add to the information available to the clinician in a way that changes patients' clinical management. Having this consideration in mind, several studies have interrogated the clinical benefit of CTE and MRE.

It has been recently published a large prospective study where 273 patients with established (128) or suspected (145) CD were included [27]. The purpose was to prospectively evaluate the effect of CTE on patient's management and physician level of confidence (LOC) for various intestinal findings. Gastroenterologists ordering the CTEs were asked to state before and after patients underwent diagnostic procedures if they thought that active small bowel inflammation, fistulas, abscesses, and/or strictures were present. Their LOC for each of these four items was measured on a 5-point scale. After the CTE was performed, the clinicians were also asked whether the changes in their suggested clinical management plans were caused by the results of the CTE. Clinician's opinion on the existence of mural inflammatory activity, strictures, fistulas or abscesses changed in 28 %, 16 %, 8 %, and 5 %, respectively. Computed tomography enterography results altered the management plans in 139 patients (51 %), including 70 patients with established CD (48.3 %) and 69 patients with suspected IBD (54.9 %). The physicians' LOC changed in more than 90 % of cases. In multivariate models where each model included whether or not the Gastroenterologist described a change resulting from CTE findings, there was no laboratory or clinical feature (CRP≥8 mg/L, CDAI>150, Albumin<3.5 g/dL, low Hematocrit or active chronic ileitis/colitis on endoscopic biopsies) that was significantly associated with an actual change in management. However, in each of these models a patient with a physician-reported modification in management due to the CTE exam had a significantly greater OR (OR=4.0) of an alteration in their management ($p<0.001$).

These results emphasize both the clinical benefit of cross-sectional imaging of the small bowel and the physicians' lack of confidence regarding CD activity and complications based exclusively on history and physical examination.

Similar results, of course, have been published regarding MRE clinical benefit. For instance, Lang G et al. have recently published a study where a total of 347 small bowel MRI examinations were analyzed, with MRE and MRe having an average sensitivity/specificity of 82.5 % and 99.9 %, respectively, and in every second patient, new relevant diagnostic information was provided, frequently causing significant shifts in Montreal Classification [28].

These results have been acknowledged by most scientific committees on inflammatory bowel disease. For instance, the European Crohn's and Colitis Organization has published in 2010 the second European evidence-based consensus on the diagnosis and management of Crohn's disease: Definitions and diagnosis [29]. It is clearly stated that "*irrespective of the findings at ileocolonoscopy, further investigation is recommended to examine the location and extent of any CD in the upper gastrointestinal tract or small bowel*" and then, at the "*extent of disease*" section, ECCO statement 2G says that "*MR and CT enterography or enteroclysis is an imaging technique with the highest diagnostic accuracy for the detection of intestinal involvement and penetrating lesions in CD*". It also says that "*radiation exposure should be considered when selecting techniques*", which means that whenever possible, MR should be preferred to CT. And it also acknowledges that "*CT and MR have a similar diagnostic accuracy for the detection of small intestine inflammatory lesions*".

Computed Tomography vs Magnetic Resonance Enterography/Enteroclysis

Both CTE and MRE exquisitely image the small bowel. In terms of performance, there are no striking differences between the two techniques. In the already mentioned study of Siddiki et al. [24], despite the fact that the mean image quality scores of MRE were significantly lower when compared with CTE (MRE is occasionally compromised by idiosyncratic factors including motion, artefacts, and signal inhomogeneity), they found no statistically significant differences between the sensitivities and specificities of CTE and MRE in the diagnosis of CD. A meta-analysis of 33 studies [30] also found no statistically significant difference between MRI and CT in values for mean sensitivity or specificity on a per-patient basis. A recent systematic review as well concluded that MRI and CT have similar accuracy [31].

Performance is similar, but each technique has its own advantages and weaknesses. Computed tomography enterography is easily and quickly available (which is crucial when the patient is symptomatic or needs a fast diagnosis), has the highest temporal and spatial resolution, is very robust (it rarely fails to generate high-quality images) and it is cheaper than MRE, but uses ionizing radiation, which carries potential risks, particularly in patients with CD, that will probably need repeated studies throughout their lifetimes. On the other hand, MRE requires much longer acquisition time, has decreased temporal and spatial resolution and is less available for the symptomatic patient, but has a higher contrast resolution and, most importantly, does not use ionizing radiation.

Additionally, MRE differs from CTE in that a range of objective scores were developed to evaluate intestinal and perianal disease activity and severity, as well as postoperative recurrence. To the best of our knowledge, only one study reported a CT-scan based index of inflammatory severity for CD. This index is based on the presence of wall thickening, mucosal or mural enhancement, mural stratification, comb sign, and regional lymph nodes [32]. The same study proposed an index for assessment of stenotic lesions based on the identification of a thickened non-enhancing wall, luminal narrowing, and the presence of pre-stenotic dilation. Of the several MRI scores of severity proposed, only the Magnetic Resonance Index of Activity (MaRIA) has been externally validated, with nearly the same performance in the derivation and validation sets (vide infra) [33].

Taking into consideration the described aspects, when available MRE is probably preferable to CTE in most situations, particularly in asymptomatic patients, when the goal of imaging is to determine if inflamed bowel loops or fistulae have responded to therapy and in patients with suspicion of low-grade SBO (given the ability to perform *MR fluoroscopy* (cine-imaging) to observe bowel peristalsis in real time and dynamically characterize stenotic lesions [34].

MR Enteroclysis vs MR Enterography

Few studies compared MR enterography and MR enteroclysis. Neggard et al. [35], in 40 patients with Crohn's disease who underwent both MR enterography and MR enteroclysis, demonstrated that bowel distention was better with MR enteroclysis but that both methods enabled the diagnosis of Crohn's disease with high diagnostic accuracy and reproducibility. Schreyer et al. [36] did not find any significant difference in 21 patients with Crohn's disease who underwent both MR examinations. On the other hand, Masselli et al. [37] compared 22 patients with Crohn's disease who underwent MR enteroclysis with 18 patients with Crohn's disease who underwent MR enterography and demonstrated better bowel distention and better detection of superficial abnormalities with MR enteroclysis, particularly at the level of the jejunum.

MR enteroclysis has been proven to have better diagnostic performance for depiction of subtle mucosal abnormalities but similar results are obtained by both techniques when identifying stenoses and fistulas. Patient acceptance is greater when MR enterography is performed as compared with MR enteroclysis. Finally, the additional cost and time entailed by having to perform and schedule a fluoroscopic tube insertion lead most departments to perform MR enterography in preference for both logistic and technical reasons.

Very recently, a survey to the perceived indications for MR imaging of the small bowel by experts, when MR enteroclysis or MR enterography may be chosen, was conducted and published. Views were variable, but 79 % of the experts favoured MR enterography over enteroclysis to confirm/refute an initial diagnosis of Crohn's disease and 93 % prefer MR enterography over enteroclysis for the follow-up of patients with Crohn's.

In conclusion, there are several views on this topic. MR enterography is probably the best option for most departments, but if the logistics allow for the needed MR studies of the small bowel to be performed with enteroclysis technique, there is probably a small diagnostic benefit, as described.

Technique and Protocol

At a minimum we require a 4–6 h fast or preferably an overnight fast in this category of patients. Colonic loading with faecal matter is known to impair the transit of contrast material through the small bowel. In some institutions, the fasting is augmented by a low residue diet for between 3–5 days prior to the study. The rationale is also to minimize the number of false positives, which can be generated by stool particles masquerading as filling defects or polyps.

In terms of pulse sequences, individual protocols will be tailored depending on manufacturer and magnet strength. However, Table 18.1 gives a sample protocol used for both small and large bowel MRI. As a guideline, most sequences include a combination of T2-weighted and contrast enhanced gradient echo (GE) sequences. Steady state free precession sequences are also routine. The most important advantages and disadvantages of each pulse sequence are stated on the table.

The introduction of parallel imaging techniques, as well as improvements in coil technology, have contributed to the increased robustness of MRI as well as reduction in acquisition times. For instance, the recently introduced "CAIPIRINHA" (Controlled Aliasing In Parallel Imaging Results IN Higher Acceleration) sequence, which accelerates data acquisition in phase-encoding and slice-encoding directions with the additional advantage of using a non-standard sampling pattern, volumetric imaging can be acquired using higher acceleration factors, resulting in less image degradation, reduced acquisition times and superb spatial resolution. In our institution, we use 1.5 mm slice thickness CAIPIRINHA sequences routinely, which approaches the spatial resolution of CT (Fig. 18.1).

Diffusion-weighted imaging is also slowly being integrated in the protocols, and discussed below.

Preliminary data on magnetization transfer imaging has been published as useful for the assessment of fibrosis in strictures (Adler J et al., Radiology 229(1):275–81, 259(1), 127–135 2011), but more data is needed for full acceptance.

The ideal patient positioning is a theme of discussion. In many institutions these studies are performed prone to allow separation of pelvic small bowel loops. This position also allows maximum coverage on coronal images and decreases scanning volume. We prefer supine imaging for patient comfort in these patients, many of whom are slim and find prone imaging uncomfortable, in some cases due to prior surgical procedures.

Most institutions routinely administer an anti-peristaltic agent to minimize peristaltic artefact. This is of prime importance in maintaining image quality in sequences that are

Table 18.1 Protocol sample for MR enterography

Sequence	Plane	Number of sections	Section thickness (mm)	Field of view (mm)	Advantages	Limitations
HASTE/SSFSE	Coronal	1	50	512×512	Minimal susceptibility artefact	Prone to flow artefacts
SSFP (True-FISP/ FIESTA) With and without fat suppression	Coronal and axial	19–25	5/0	160–512×160–400	Useful for extra enteric visualization including mesentery and nodes when fat saturation absent In presence of fat suppression useful for enteric changes and subtle mural abnormality	Susceptibility artefact
HASTE with fat saturation	Coronal and axial	19–25	2–4	As above		Mesenteric evaluation impaired due to k-space filtering
2D and/or 3D fat-saturated dynamic T1-weighted GE (LAVA, VIBE, etc.)	Dynamic coronal with axial delayed	52–64	1.5–2.5	288–400×312–400	Mural assessment and evaluation of disease activity	3D better for spatial resolution and SNR but more prone to Misregistration artefact

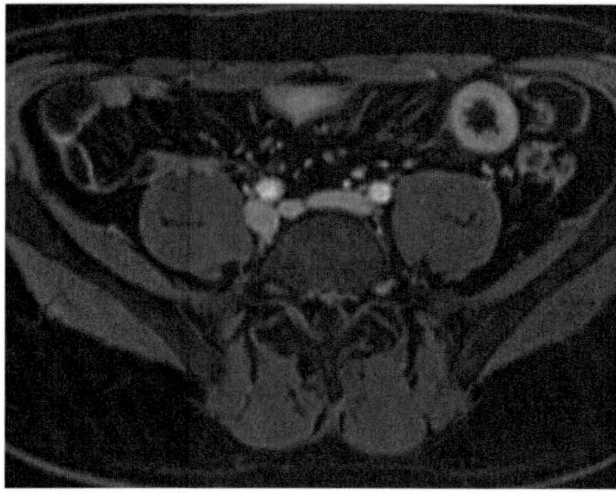
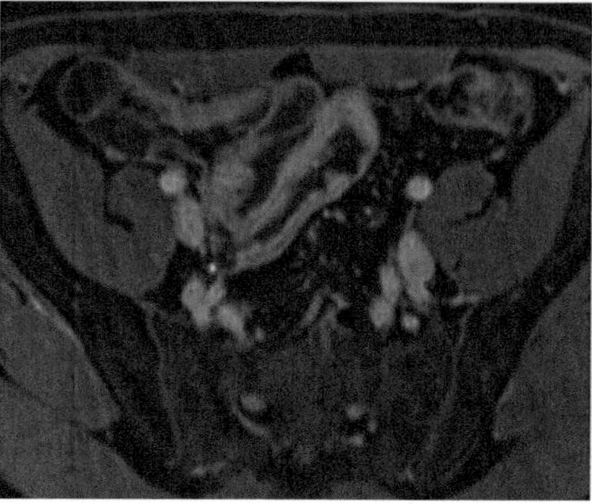
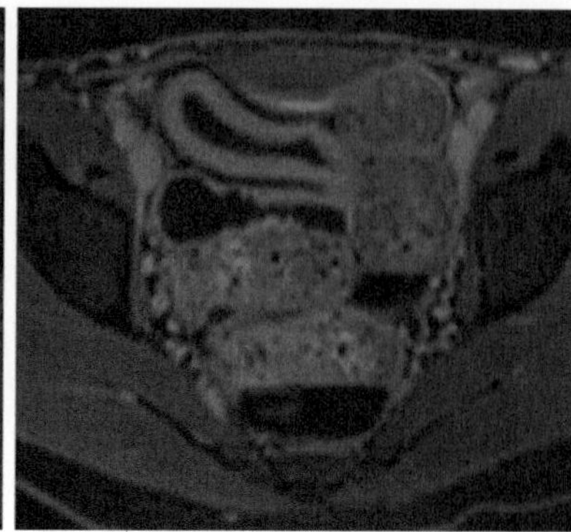

Fig. 18.1 Exquisite spatial resolution of "CAIPIRINHA" images. These fat-saturated T1 weighted GE images allow higher acceleration factors and, consequently, can be obtained within a breath hold and simultaneously have exquisite spatial resolution. The *arrows* point to subtle ulcers in inflamed ileal segments

prone to flow artefacts, such as the HASTE or SSFSE (Half Fourier single shot turbo spin echo and Single shot fast spin echo sequences). We usually administer a divided dose of an anti-peristaltic with the second aliquot being given prior to the gadolinium enhanced sequences. Depending on local availability this can either be obtained with 10 mg of hyoscine butylbromide (Buscopan®) or 0.2 mg of glucagon given intravenously. Buscopan is not licensed for use in the United States. To promote gastric emptying whilst ingesting oral contrast, either erythromycin or metaclopramide (20 mg) can be given once the first 500 mg of contrast has been drunk.

For MR enteroclysis X-ray fluoroscopic guidance is used to confirm catheter placement at or beyond the duodenojejunal flexure. Baseline imaging is then obtained prior to instillation of 1.5–2 L of fluid at a rate of 100–120 ml/min using an infusion pump. The progress of the contrast and the degree of distension can be monitored via thick slabs or dynamic MR fluoroscopic sequences. These are typically SSFP (Steady State Free Precession) 5 mm section images aligned parallel to the longitudinal axis of the segment of concern. The images are acquired at between 0.5–2 frames per second. When the contrast reaches the ileocecal junction, we administer antispasmodics (see below).

For MR enterography, patients are given 1–2 L of one of the several possibilities of oral contrast (see below) about 45 min before the acquisition of images.

Oral Contrast

In most institutions, the majority of MR studies are performed as an enterography rather than enteroclysis, as discussed.

Luminal distension with oral contrast is vital for detailed assessment of the bowel wall. Additional benefits include the displacement of air from the lumen by oral contrast. This is necessary as air produces susceptibility artefact and degrades image quality.

Oral contrast utilization will be determined by several factors including local availability, patient tolerance, cost and the effectiveness of distension. In addition to the choice of agent there is departmental variation in the volumes administered and the timing of image acquisition following ingestion of the contrast material. In some instances there may be rapid transit of contrast to the right colon but in the majority of individuals a delay of 40–60 min from the start of contrast ingestion is adequate to obtain small bowel distension.

Significant variance exists between the agents available and it is important to be cognizant of the differences. Agents can be stratified into several categories:

- *Negative contrast agents* are of low signal intensity on T1-weighted and T2-weighted imaging. These include super paramagnetic iron oxide agents such as ferumoxsil. It is rarely used.
- *Positive contrast agents* are of high signal intensity on T1-weighted and T2-weighted imaging. They are currently very rarely used.
- *Biphasic agents* are of variable signal intensity depending on the sequence that is applied (low signal intense on T1-weighted imaging and high signal intensity on T2-weighted imaging). In clinical practice, these are the most utilized and there is consequently a greater choice in this category. Table 18.2 provides more information regarding the characteristics of different contrast agents.

In our department we utilize a technique that is well reported in the literature and consists in a total volume of between 1–2 L of contrast being ingested in divided aliquots over a 45–60 min time period. Water is an undesirable biphasic contrast agent due to its rapid absorption and erratic distension of the distal small bowel. This can be problematic as the distal small bowel is most commonly involved in Crohn's disease. There are many commercially available biphasic contrast agents. In our practice we have utilized both dilute barium 0.1 % wt/vol solution with sorbitol as well as a bulk fibre

Table 18.2 Comparison of oral contrast agents

Agent category	Name	Benefits	Limitations	Practical issues
Positive (high T1 and high T2)	• Gadolinium chelates • Manganese • Milk with high fat content • Fruit juices (e.g. pineapple, blueberry)		Limit detection of subtle mucosal abnormality or wall enhancement	Cost, availability
Negative	• SPIO • Feruomoxsil oral	Improve conspicuity of wall oedema		Unpleasant taste, Cost
Biphasic (low T1 high T2)	• Water • Methylcellulose • Mannitol or mannitol with locust bean gum • PEG (polyethylene glycol) • VoLumen® (Sorbitol solution with low-density barium)	High intrinsic contrast between wall and lumen allows assessment of subtle fold thickening	Distension with agents such as water inconsistent The hyperosmolar agents may promote diarrhoea. Isosmolar agents should be used	Absorption, taste, diarrhoea. These are the most frequently used in today's practice

laxative, which helps luminal expansion by retaining water. High osmotic agents such as mannitol and sorbitol can have undesirable side effects depending on the sugar alcohol concentration. They can cause diarrhoea, excessive gas and cramping. This can be improved by keeping the concentration below 2.5 %.

An optional method for simultaneous large bowel assessment is administration of a rectal water enema. This allows the colonic wall to be examined for disease involvement (vide infra).

Intravenous Contrast Material

Gadolinium derivatives are typically administered intravenously at a dose of 0.2 mmol/kg body weight. Peak bowel enhancement is thought to occur between 70 and 75 s following contrast material administration but can vary between individuals [38]. It is therefore standard practice to perform multi-phasic MRI commencing in the arterial phase at 25 s and obtaining at least two further acquisitions. If patient is know to have strictures, the addition of a delayed (7 min) phase is a consideration, as it better allows the characterization of the presence/degree of wall fibrosis [39]. In circumstances where gadolinium usage is relatively or absolutely contra-indicated, unenhanced sequences usually suffice in demonstrated areas of mural abnormality as well as mesenteric hyperaemia in diseased segments.

MR Motility Imaging

MRE allows not only the static display of morphology but can be combined with ultrafast imaging techniques ("cine MRI" or "MR fluoroscopy") for analysis of bowel motility. Traditional X-ray fluoroscopic imaging confirms that involvement with Crohn's may result in motility disorders. Pathological changes in the bowel wall result in areas of aperistalsis or diminished motility. When used in conjunction with routine MRE it can improve lesion detection. In a study performed to assess if cine MRI improves additional lesion detection in patients with Crohn's, 40 patients with CD underwent cine MR enterography in addition to a standard MR protocol. Blinded reads were performed with and without cine MRI. Overall cine MRI detected more Crohn's specific findings than static MR enterography alone ($p=0.007$) and more patients with CD relevant MR findings ($p=0.03$) [40].

There is growing literature supporting the use of cine MR enterography. Froehlich et al. [40] showed that the addition of cine MR enterography identified more patients with MR findings of Crohn's disease compared to static MR enterography alone because altered motility on cine imaging highlighted abnormal bowel segments and may lead to increased diagnostic confidence and because Cine MR enterography can facilitate diagnosis in otherwise equivocal cases, especially if other sequences are motion-degraded. Abnormal motility on cine MR enterography in Crohn's disease has also been shown to correlate with inflammatory markers, biopsy results, and clinical disease activity scores [41, 42].

Multiphasic imaging can also be used to evaluate for adhesions or stenoses and helps distinguish true strictures from temporarily contracting or underdistended segments [43] (Fig. 18.2). Cine MR enterography has also been shown to increase visualization of the proximal small bowel compared to static MR enterography, simulating the benefits of enteroclysis [44].

Although still not widely used in routine clinical practice in most institutions, there is growing interest in cine MR enterography as a valuable technique for motility evaluation. The joint European Crohn's and Colitis Organisation (ECCO)/European Society of Gastrointestinal and Abdominal Radiology (ESGAR) guidelines in 2013 acknowledge that small bowel motility evaluation may increase lesion detection in Crohn's disease compared to

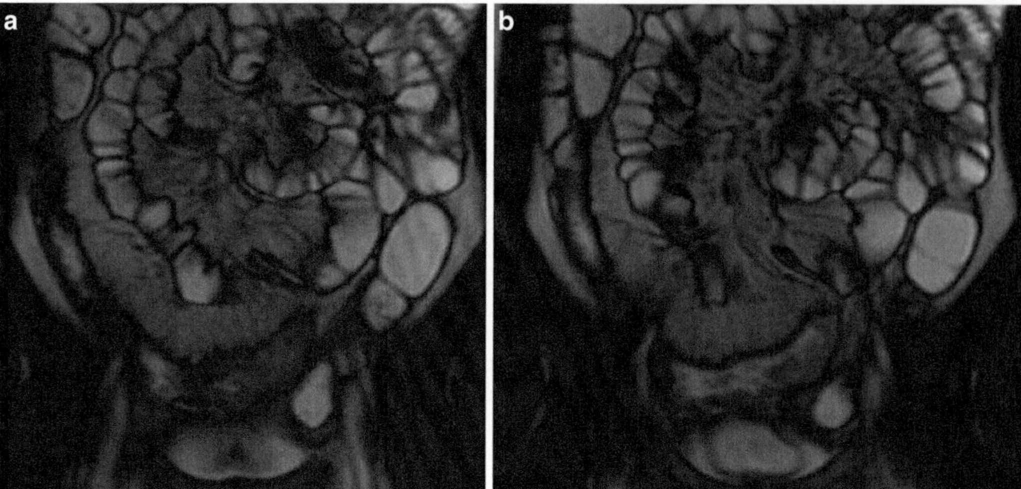

Fig. 18.2 Utility of cine-imaging to distinguish true stenosis from peristalsis. In (**a**) the loop involved with Crohn's disease seems to be strictured, but in (**b**), an image acquired just a few seconds later using a MR fluoroscopic technique (SSFP based), the loop is seen to distend, demonstrated that the first image was acquired during a peristaltic contraction

static MR enterography alone [45]. The consensus statement from the Society of Abdominal Radiology (SAR) Crohn's disease-focused panel published in 2015 includes multiphasic imaging as an optional additional sequence in MR enterography evaluation [46].

Cine MRI can be performed by single slice techniques, usually SSFP sequences, which are repeated at intervals of 0.5–1 s in the same plane but in a stepwise location from anterior to posterior. After the images are acquired, the cine loop function of the workstations allows visualization of bowel motility. Anti-spasmodics should not be administered until the cine MRI sequence is obtained, otherwise they will artificially reduce peristaltism. Consequently, the SSFP sequences that allow cine MRI are the first sequence in our protocol. Since with MR radiation is not utilized, potential sites of disease can be repeatedly evaluated without incurring any risk. It must be emphasized, however, that cine MRI does not have sufficient spatial resolution to be used in isolation when performing diagnostic MRI.

Role of Diffusion Weighted Imaging

Diffusion weighted imaging (DWI) relies on differences in the motion of water molecules between tissues to provide image contrast. It is more and more becoming a standard application in routine imaging and it has already been incorporated in two MRI scores (the Clermont score, which is very similar to the MaRIA score but replaces contrast enhancement by restricted diffusion), and the Nancy score [47], but DWI's low spatial resolution is a drawback compared with the anatomical details provided by the high-resolution post-gadolinium sequences. It remains to be determined whether DWI's low specificity for detecting activity [47], can be overcome by including it in an overall index. However, in the presence of other imaging findings of inflammation, DWI is associated with more severe disease [48] (Fig. 18.3).

In the future, if DWI is proven to be of benefit in larger patient groups, it may circumvent the need for gadolinium and potentially avoid issues related to cost and patient safety with this intravenous contrast media.

MR Colonography (MRC)

Conventional colonoscopy remains the gold standard for mucosal evaluation of the colon and allows biopsy performance for histological confirmation of a suspected diagnosis of inflammatory bowel disease. Entire colonic visualization and stepwise biopsies are considered mandatory and IBD is typically correctly classified in 80–90 % of cases at the time of initial examination. In specific circumstances, however, imaging is a suitable alternative for the establishment of disease extent and severity. These include the presence of a fulminant colitis when the patient is at higher risk of colonic perforation. Similarly, for both patient and technical reasons, incomplete colonoscopy may preclude colonic assessment in between 5–20 % of cases. Additionally, submucosal and mesenteric involvement, which is common in Crohn's disease, cannot be assessed with colonoscopy; consequently, the evaluation of the mucosa with colonoscopy alone may result in underestimation of the extent and activity of the disease, as when assessing small bowel involvement. Imaging is also invaluable for assessment of colonic anastomoses [49]. The assessment of an anastamosis can be challenging on endoscopy and is the most common site of disease recurrence.

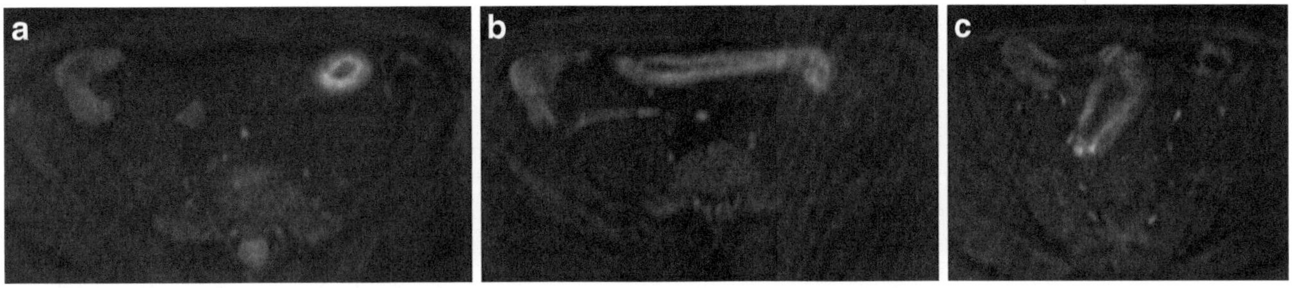

Fig. 18.3 Utility of DWI to discriminate segments with more severe disease. (**a**), (**b**) and (**c**) are from the same patient and with the same window and level parameters. Diffusion is significantly more restricted in the segment of image **a**, representing more severe disease

MRC Technique

Routine bowel cleansing is performed as for optical colonoscopy. Replacing standard cleansing with faecal tagging is not advocated in this patient subgroup as compared with those undergoing screening examinations for colorectal cancer [50].

Adequate colonic distension is a requisite in order to minimize false positive or false negative studies. MR colonography can also be performed with positive, negative or biphasic agents. A warm tap water enema has the ideal characteristics of a biphasic agent being of low signal intensity on T1-weighted and high signal on T2-weighted sequences. A volume of between 1.5–2.5 L is administered via a rectal catheter once the patient is on the table.

Routine utilization of an anti-peristaltic agent (Hyoscine 20 mg, or Glucagon 1 mg) produces reflex atonia that helps in retention of the water enema. In addition it minimizes peristaltic artefacts as well as achieving more optimal colonic distension.

When MR Colonography is performed, it is usually as part of a MR entero-colonography study and the pulse sequences performed are the ones obtained for regular MR enterography (previously described). Of note, the MaRIA score, defined previously, was deducted with a MR entero-colonography protocol.

MR colonography may also be performed without the enterography component. The obtained pulse sequences are similar to the ones obtained for the regular MR enterography: a combination of SSFP, T2 weighted and fat-suppressed T1 weighted post-gadolinium 3D sequences (e.g. VIBE, LAVA or similar). A SSFP sequence allows initial evaluation to see if there is adequate colonic distension. A multiphasic post-contrast acquisition is performed, as for the regular MR enterography.

Imaging Findings

Ulcerative Colitis

Classic findings on imaging include involvement of the rectosigmoid colon which extends proximally to involve the entire colon. Less commonly there is a sub-total colitis (usually right sided) and in 15 % of cases there may be a backwash ileitis.

Uniform thickening of the wall is a hallmark feature. The degree of thickening is usually less marked in UC than in CD with mean values of 7–8 mm as compared with 13 mm respectively. In more active disease however mural thickness can exceed 10 mm. Mural stratification is observed in 60 % of patients with UC versus 8 % of patients with CD [51]. This is due to the presence of fat or oedema in the submucosal layer as described in the small bowel above.

The outer contour of the colonic wall is typically smooth and regular in patients with UC whereas serosal and outer mural irregularity is seen in 80 % of patients with CD (Gore RM et al., AJR Am J Roentgenol, 158(1):59–61.). However, not infrequently, the two diseases are not distinguishable by imaging alone (Fig. 18.4).

As in Crohn's disease, there is frequently engorgement of the vasa recta and mucosal hyperenhancement, as well as enlargement of regional pericolonic nodes. The presence of small traces of peri-colonic fluid is usually a marker of focal serosal involvement and typically indicates the presence of severe disease.

In long standing disease there will be wall thickening, an absence of haustra and associated luminal narrowing. This is thought to be due to hypertrophy of the muscularis mucosa. Mesenteric fatty proliferation in UC is typically confined to the perirectal space.

Ulcerative colitis is much less frequently an indication for MRE or MRC than Crohn's disease. The most frequent indication for patients with UC is to rule out Crohn's disease.

Crohn's Disease

Involvement of the colon can be seen in more than 60 % of patients with CD and is exclusively limited to the colon in approximately 15–25 % of cases. The rectum may be involved in approximately 50 % of patients.

As in the small bowel, colonic wall thickening is present and post contrast enhancement is a good correlate of disease severity. The inner profile of the colonic wall may have an undulating configuration. This is thought to represent mucosal

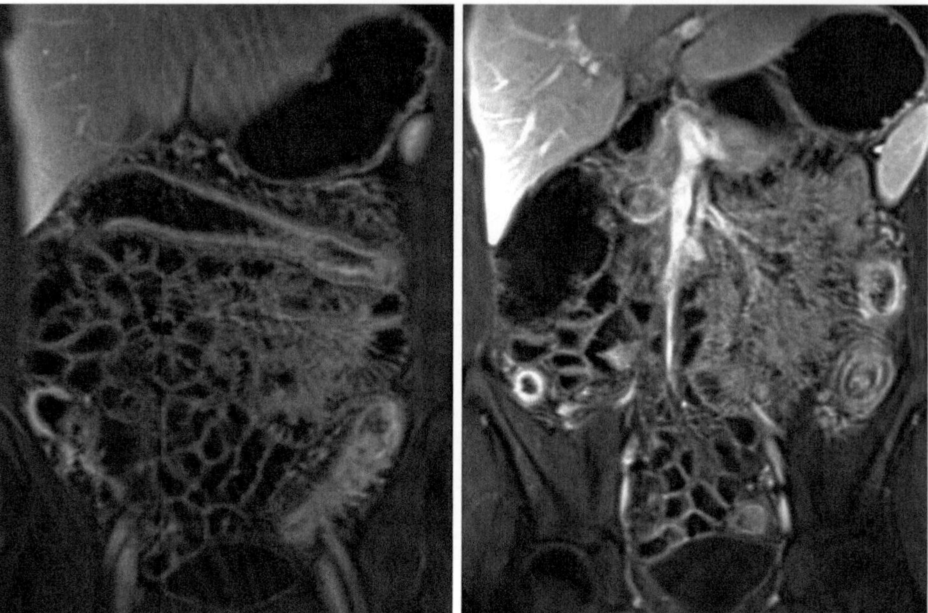

Fig. 18.4 Pancolitis could represent both Crohn's disease or UC. This particular patient had Crohn's disease

oedema and there may also be a relative absence of haustration for the same reason.

Other imaging findings that overlap with those in the small bowel include the presence of fistulae and sinus tracts.

Long standing quiescent disease may depict no abnormality on imaging. If however there is transmural fibrosis there is shortening of the bowel with ahaustration. This results in a relatively fixed and tubular configuration to the bowel. On post gadolinium sequences there is homogenous enhancement and absence of wall stratification.

Diagnostic Accuracy

A study by Ajaj et al. [49] assessed 23 patients with IBD on MR colonography. The imaging findings (MRC score) were correlated with histopathological specimens obtained on endoscopy. In this study group, MRC correctly identified 68 of 73 segments found to reveal IBD changes on pathology. The imaging score utilized four quantifiable criteria including colonic wall thickness, colonic wall enhancement, number of haustral folds and number of perienteric nodes. There were no false positive findings. MRC detected and characterized clinically relevant IBD of the large bowel with sensitivity and specificity values of 87 % and 100 %.

Rottgen et al. correlated bowel enhancement on MRC with inflammatory activity of Crohn's disease at colonoscopy in 42 patients and found a significant correlation between colonoscopic inflammatory activity and changes in signal intensity within the bowel wall. These relatively modest patient numbers need to be replicated in larger cohorts however the data suggests that MRC is a credible alternate to conventional colonoscopy in both monitoring activity as well as evaluating therapeutic response [52].

Characteristic Imaging Findings

The earliest changes of Crohn's disease such as erythema, superficial apthous ulcers and nodularity of the mucosa are difficult to appreciate on MR. An attempt to address this deficiency has been made by authors who have obtained high resolution thin section images (2–3 mm thick) aligned parallel to the bowel segment [53]. This allows a detailed depiction of the mucosa and provides in plane resolution of 1–2 mm.

However, there are several imaging findings that are characteristic of inflammatory bowel disease and they are discussed in some detail below.

Wall, Fold and Mucosal Abnormality

A normal bowel wall should be no more than 3 mm in thickness if it is optimally distended. In CD, wall thickness ranges between 5–10 mm. The degree of mural thickening correlates well with the Crohn's disease activity index (CDAI) [54]. In the absence of mural oedema, the bowel wall is usually low to moderate in signal intensity on T2-weighted MR sequences. The black boundary artefact seen on SSFP sequences can confound assessment of wall thickness. HASTE sequences are relatively insensitive to this artefact and more accurate at estimating bowel thickness (Fig. 18.5).

Fold abnormalities are more evident along the mesenteric border. They can manifest in several ways including diffuse fold thickening, ulceration or in more severe disease as areas of cobblestoning. Early areas of apthous ulceration are seen as small focus of high T2 signal intensity surrounded by a

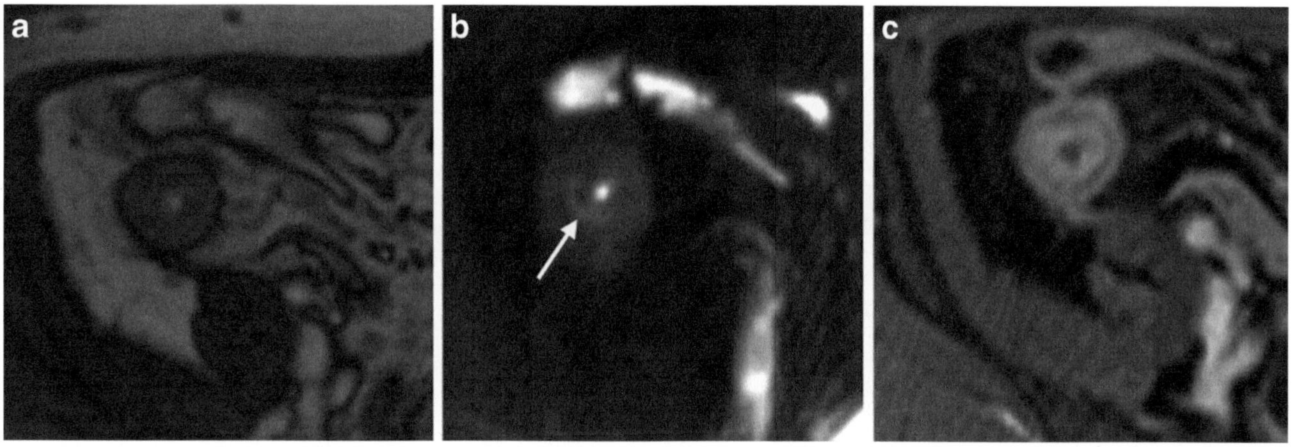

Fig. 18.5 Mural thickening. Distal ileal segment demonstrates wall thickening. Part (**a**) is a SSFP image and an India ink artefact at the interface with the mesenteric fat can be seen. Part (**b**) is a T2 fat-saturated image. The bright signal in the submucosa represents oedema and is in keeping with active disease (significant inflammatory component). The same segment is demonstrated in (**c**), a T1 weighted fat-saturated image post contrast administration

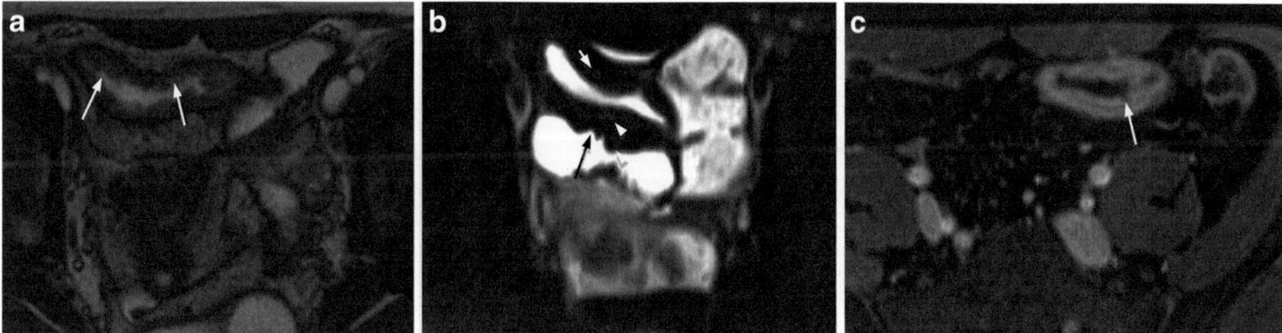

Fig. 18.6 Ulcers. Multiple ulcers can be seen in (**a**) (SSFP image). In (**b**), a T2 fat-saturated image, both superficial (*arrowheads*) and deep (*arrows*) can be identified. Subtle ulcers can also be seen in (**c**) (*arrow*), a CAIPIRINHA image

rim of oedema (seen as an area of moderate signal intensity), but these are usually difficult to see with MR. Deeper areas of penetrating ulcers are easier to appreciate than superficial ulcers. They are seen as areas of high T2 signal intensity within areas of segmental wall thickening (Fig. 18.6).

Strictures

These are seen as fixed, consistent areas of luminal narrowing. If there is upstream dilatation of bowel loops by greater than 3 cm, the stricture is considered to be functionally significant. If however there is no dilatation and a more than 10 % narrowing in the lumen as compared with subjacent bowel, the stricture is most likely functionally insignificant.

As recently proven by many studies, most stenotic lesions in CD have a mixed component: fibrosis plus inflammation [55, 56]. Differentiating the presence of significant inflammation, significant fibrosis and/or which component predominantes has important prognostic and management implications, and MRI can contribute significantly here.

The presence of ulcerations, acute mural oedema (areas of high T2-weighted signal intensity within thickened loops of small bowel on fat-saturated T2 weighted sequences) and mural thickening is associated with presence of inflammation. High submucosal T2 signal is also an independent correlate of disease activity [57, 58] (Fig. 18.7).

Fibrotic strictures tend to be hypointense on T1- and T2-weighted sequences and enhance inhomogenously following contrast. There is an absence of accompanying mesenteric hyperaemia or inflammatory change. They may cause bowel obstruction and MR fluoroscopic sequences can be helpful in locating the level and degree of obstruction. A recent publication from Rimola et al. demonstrated prospectively and with pathological correlation that the assessment of gadolinium enhancement over time allows the identification of segments with a high component of fibrosis, regardless of the degree of coexisting inflammation. In their publication, >24 % of enhancement from the 70 s acquisition to a 7 min delay acquisition was strongly associated with severe fibrosis [39] (Fig. 18.8).

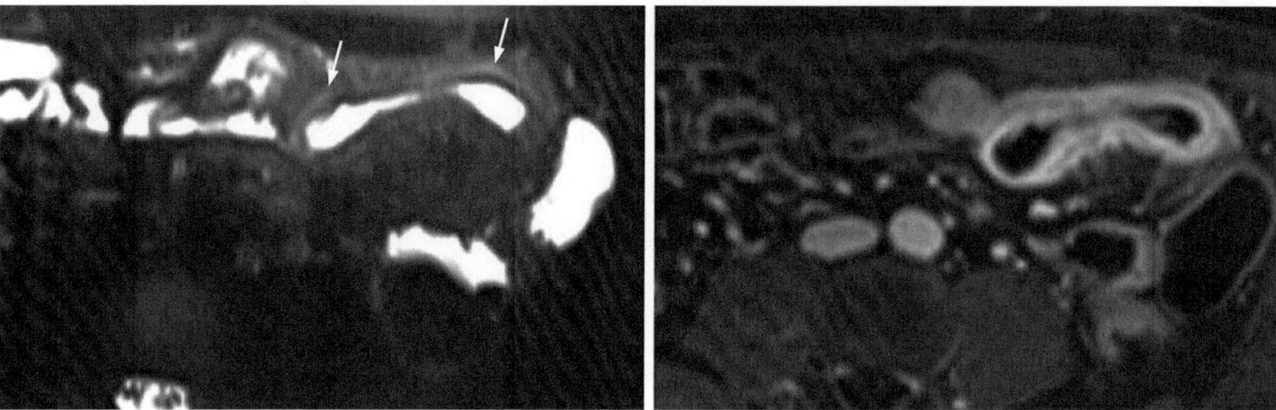

Fig. 18.7 Submucosal oedema, sign of active disease. A wall thickened and hyperenhancing ileal segment is demonstrated. In (**a**) several areas of high T2 signal in the submucosa are demonstrated, represent oedema. Findings are in keeping with active disease

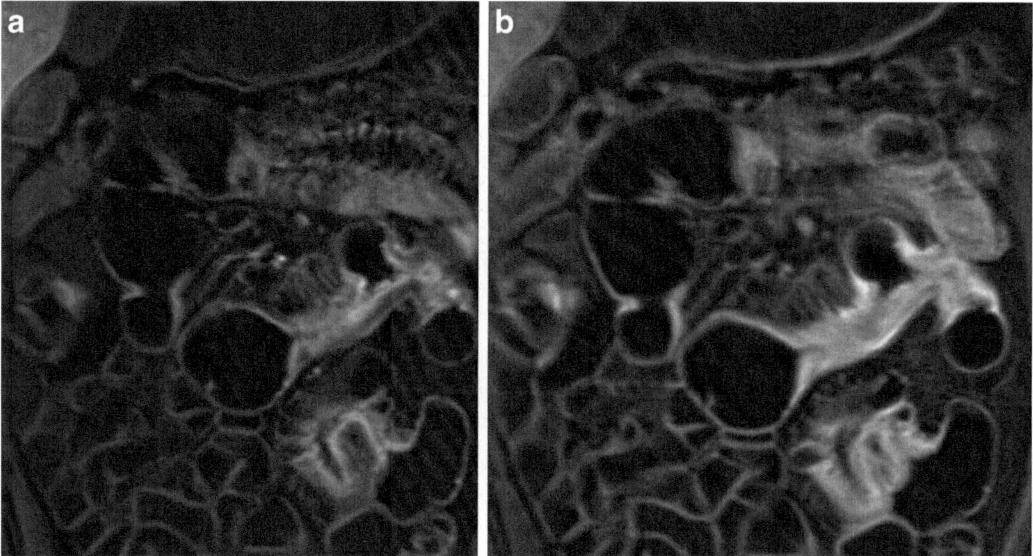

Fig. 18.8 Delayed enhancement, sign of significant fibrosis. Multiple stenotic segments with pseudosacculation are identified. Of note, there is progressive enhancement from image (**a**) (enteric phase) to image (**b**) (5 min delay), in keeping with presence of significant fibrosis

Multiple other investigators have analyzed numerous pulse sequences and imaging methods to estimate the degree of fibrosis in an effort to estimate the potential for medical response to therapy. Magnetization transfer MR imaging has been shown in animal studies to depict intestinal fibrosis [59], and initial experience in patients has shown that magnetization transfer ratios are elevated in patients with predominantly fibrotic strictures [60]. Zappa et al. examined inflammation and fibrosis at MRI by comparison with histopathologic scoring systems and found a high correlation between advanced inflammation and advanced fibrosis [55], so reliance on enhancement, so separation of these two processes was difficult when relying upon imaging findings such as wall thickness and hyperenhancement. Further investigation into reliable imaging markers for intestinal fibrosis such as magnetization transfer, diffusion-weighted imaging, and delayed enhancement is ongoing.

Fatty replacement of the sub-mucosa is also seen in long standing IBD and is seen as an area of high signal intensity on non-fat-saturated T1 and T2 sequences, which suppresses on fat-saturated sequences.

Wall Enhancement

Mural hyper-enhancement in diseased segments is usually seen in comparison with adjacent normal loops of small bowel, which act as a reference standard. The pattern of enhancement is also useful in determining the level of activity that exists:

– *Stratified* enhancement refers to enhancement of the mucosa exceeding that of the poorly enhancing submucosa. This is seen where there is active disease and

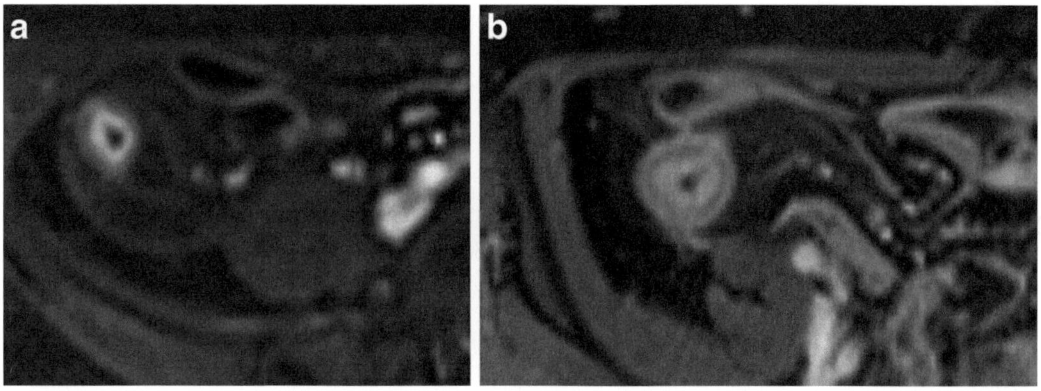

Fig. 18.9 Mural stratification. In (**a**), the mucosa is enhancing significantly more than the other wall layers, in keeping with mural stratification. In (**b**), the serosa is also hyperenhancing, creating a "target" appearance

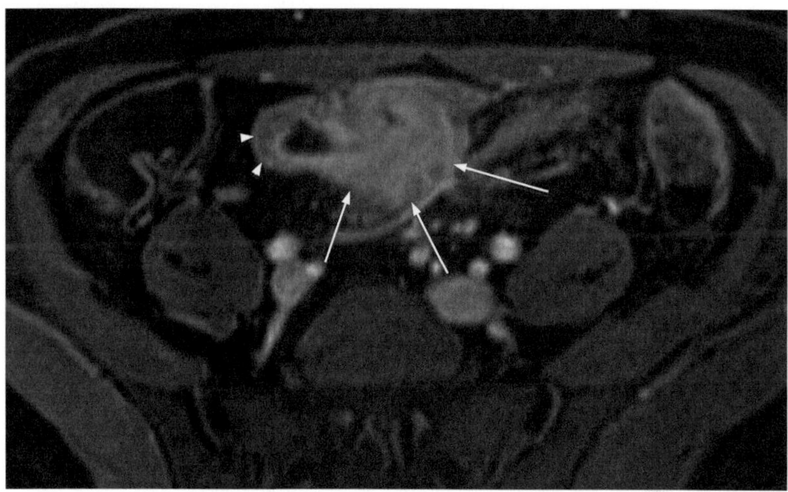

Fig. 18.10 Mural stratification, severe disease. Two different patterns of enhancement are seen in this image. The arrowheads point to an area of trilaminated stratification. The *arrows* point to an area of diffuse hyperenhancement, extending to the surrounding fat, in keeping with severe inflammation

submucosal oedema. When combined with areas of serosal hyper-enhancement the bowel wall may adopt a target like appearance (Fig. 18.9).

- *Diffuse* enhancement reflects transmural disease with uniform enhancement of the entire bowel wall (Fig. 18.10).
- *Minimal* and somewhat heterogeneous enhancement in the early phases (arterial and portal venous phases) is seen in areas where fibrosis predominates. Progressive enhancement can be seen in fibrotic areas if more delayed phases are acquired and this is specific for the presence of significant fibrosis [39] (Fig. 18.8).

The absolute level of enhancement has been suggested as a surrogate marker of disease activity but its value is inconsistent and there may be considerable inter- and intra-observer variation [61]. In particular inadequate distension of segments of bowel may result in false positive assessment of hyper-enhancement. Areas of relative sparing along the anti-mesenteric border of the bowel may result in redundancy and pseudo-sacculation (Fig. 18.8). In contradistinction the diseased mesenteric wall is often shortened and may be fibrotic.

Extra Enteric Manifestations

Mesenteric hyperaemia and vascular engorgement (vasa recta) are seen in conjunction with the *comb* sign. As its name implies it is seen as areas of parallel low signal intensity perpendicular to the long axis of the diseased segments of bowel on true FISP sequences and correspond to the engorged vasa recta. There is avid enhancement in these vessels following intravenous administration of contrast material. Mesenteric oedema like the comb sign may be an accompaniment of active disease and is seen as areas of high signal intensity on T2-weighted images tracking along a diseased segment [62] (Fig. 18.11).

Hypertrophy of the mesenteric fat also preferentially involves the mesenteric border and causes significant mass effect with separation of adjacent bowel as well as of the

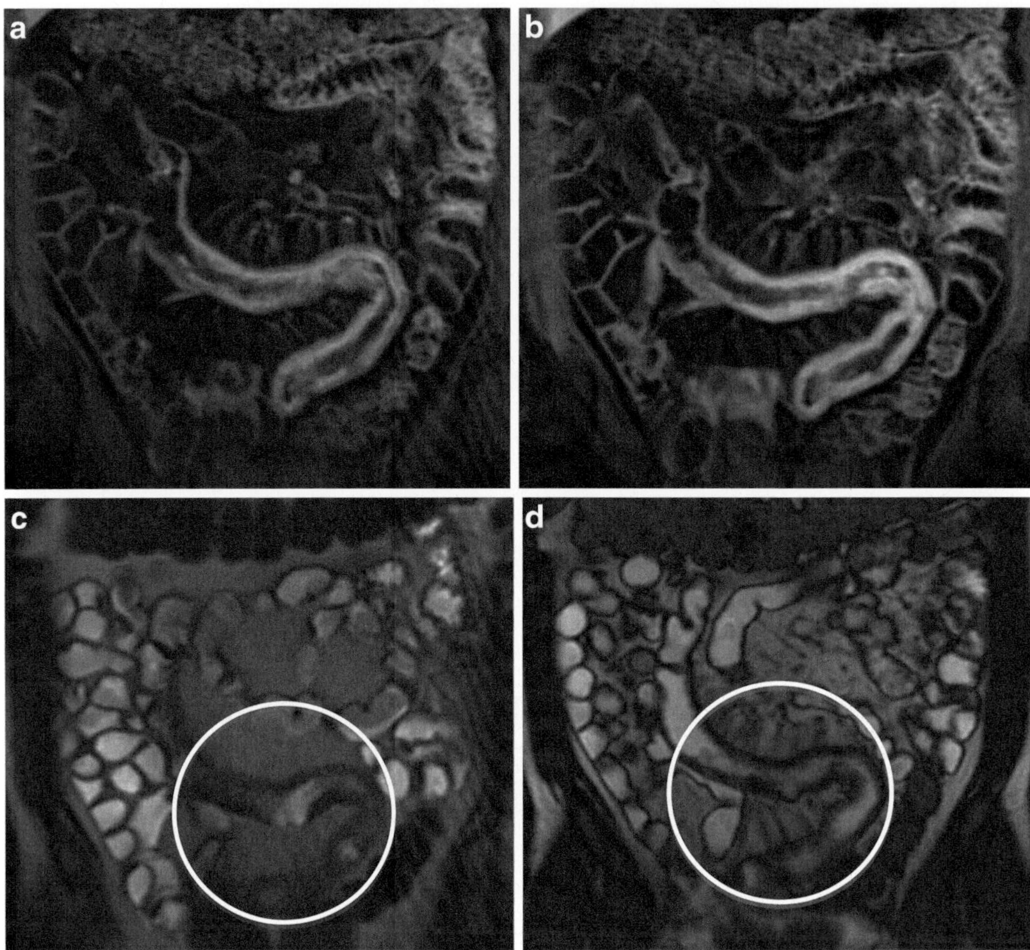

Fig. 18.11 Comb sign. A long segment of ileum demonstrates mural thickening and hyperenhancement. Additionally, engorgement of the vasa recta is noted (*comb sign*). Please note how the mesenteric structures (including the vasa recta) are much better seen in (**d**) (SSFP image) than in (**c**) (HASTE). Additionally, it can be seen that there is progressive enhancement from (**a**) to (**b**), suggesting presence of significant fibrosis

mesenteric vessels. It is commonly seen in the context of transmural disease and is specific to Crohn's disease (Fig. 18.12).

Nodal enlargement and enhancement in a specific vascular territory may be seen in areas of active disease and is well displayed on fat-saturated T2-weighted sequences. The degree of enhancement within a node relative to that of an adjacent vessel has been speculated as being predictive of disease activity [62].

Fistulas and Sinuses

Penetrating disease is a hallmark of Crohn's disease. Deep areas of transmural ulceration may communicate with adjacent epithelial surfaces resulting in formation of a fistula. The fluid containing tracts are seen as areas of high signal intensity on T2-weighted sequences and enhance following intravenous contrast material administration. If they are complex, they may have a more stellate appearance with multiple tracts emanating from a central point to adjacent bowel loops (Fig. 18.13). Imaging has high sensitivity for depiction of these fistulae ranging from 71–100 % for entero-enteric fistulae to those communicating with other viscera [62, 63].

Abscesses are seen as encapsulated fluid collections demonstrating peripheral enhancement. They may contain air but are often heterogeneous due to the presence of particulate content. Using negative enteric contrast agents may increase the conspicuity of smaller, subtle inter-loop abscesses. The presence of abscesses is an important contra-indication to the use of anti-tumour necrosis factor drugs and therefore, their detection on imaging is important.

MR Scoring Systems

Several indexes of activity have been proposed, three of them based on adequate external references: the Magnetic Resonance Index of Activity (MaRIA) score, the Nancy score and the Crohn's Disease MRI Index (CDMI) score.

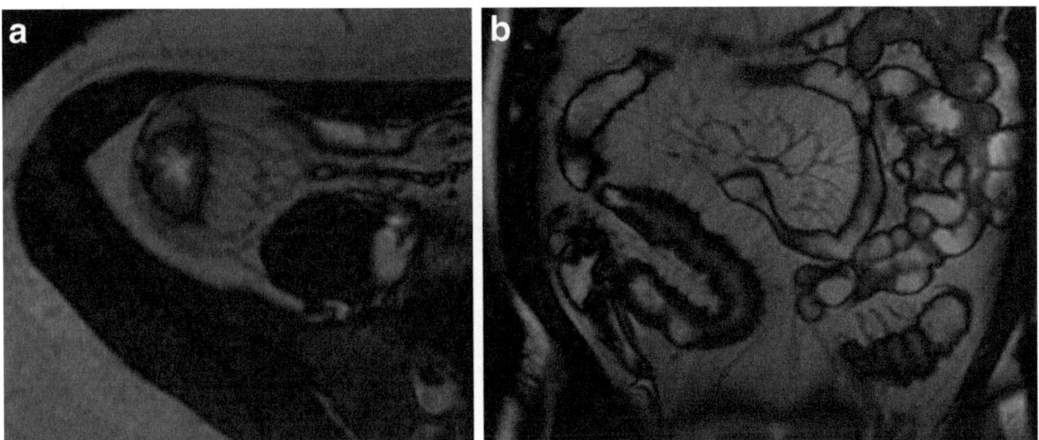

Fig. 18.12 Creeping fat. Both in (**a**) and (**b**), the inflamed ileal loop is surrounded by a thick layer of fat, which is a typical finding in chronic Crohn's disease. This is specific of Crohn's and is associated with ulcers on the mesenteric border of the small bowel, which can be seen in (**b**)

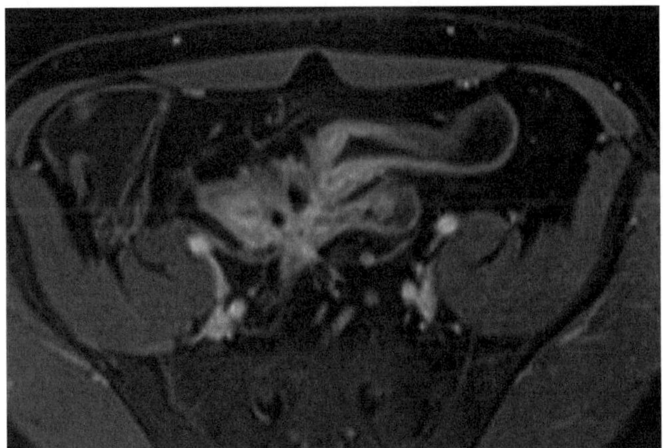

Fig. 18.13 Fistulas. Contrast enhanced T1 weighted image demonstrates at least three fistulous tracts between two adjacent bowel segments, creating a "stelate" appearance, typical of penetrating Crohn's disease. MRE can exquisitely identify and characterize these fistulas

Only two of these have been externally validated: the MaRIA score [33] and the CDMI [41]. The MaRIA score has additionally been used prospectively in a multicenter study to monitor medical treatment, which further validated the score, showing that it is reliable in assessing the response to therapy in patients with CD [64]. This is the score we will focus on with a little more detail on this chapter.

Rimola et al. have evaluated various parameters indicative of CD activity and severity using 3.0 T MRI and analyzed the data on a per-patient and per-bowel-segment basis. The MaRIA score has been derived and validated from these results. This score includes bowel wall thickening, the relative contrast-enhancement value (RCE), and presence of oedema and ulcers ($1.5 \times \text{wall thickness in mm} + 0.02 \times \text{RCE} + 5 \times \text{oedema} + 10 \times \text{ulceration}$). The authors propose the use of MaRIA as the reference index for measuring CD activity by MRI, with a cutoff point of ≥7 for determining presence of active disease and a cutoff point of ≥11 for assessment of presence of severe disease. The MaRIA score demonstrated a statistically significant correlation with clinical and endoscopic disease activity, and with C-reactive protein levels [31].

Only the MaRIA score provided a cutoff point defining severe inflammatory lesions (accuracy 0.96 when segmental MaRIA >11), increasing its clinical relevance for the optimization of medical treatment [33]. The accuracy of MRE using the MaRIA score in identifying mucosal healing was 0.83. No data are available regarding the accuracy of the other two indexes for predicting mucosal healing. Tielbeck et al. demonstrated that both the MaRIA and CDMI scores are reproducible between radiologist readers and have moderate correlation with standardized endoscopic assessment [65].

The Lémann Score

Until recently, the therapeutic goals in Crohn's disease focused on achieving control of symptoms. However, CD is increasingly seen as a progressive disease that conducts to irreversible bowel damage and intestinal resection in the large majority of patients. This concept is not new [66], but has become better recognized since the referral centre studies of Louis et al. [66] and Cosnes et al. [67] have been published. The results of these articles have then been confirmed in a large population-based cohort [68].

Today, complex scores (such as CDAI, HBI, Perianal Disease Activity Index, etc.) are used to estimate the severity of disease activity. While they are useful to evaluate the severity of CD activity at a specific time point, they do not assess the cumulative structural bowel damage. For instance, CDAI can be similar in one patient with recent onset CD and in another patient with a lengthy history of CD who has extensive irreversible bowel damage from inflammation or previous surgical resection.

Data from rheumatologic studies show that treating lesions as early as possible to prevent tissue damage might improve the long-term benefits of therapy and slow the disease progression [69]. On the other hand, studies investigating the influence of new therapeutic agents on the natural history of CD did not show a significant reduction in bowel damage over time. Intervention before the beginning of bowel damage may be necessary to change the natural history of CD, but a tool to measure cumulative structural damage to the bowel is needed. The International Program to develop New Indexes in Crohn's disease (IPNIC) group is at present developing the Crohn's Disease Digestive Damage Score, the Lémann Score [70]. The creation of this score aims to change the traditional treatment paradigm oriented by symptoms to a model driven by the amount of small bowel structural damage. The score is based on damage location, extent and severity, as assessed by abdominopelvic cross-sectional imaging (MRE or CTE), combined with the surgical history and findings from endoscopic studies (esophagogastroduodenoscopy and ileocolonoscopy) [70]. The score is expected to be able to depict a patient's disease course on a double-axis graph, with time as the x-axis, bowel damage severity as the y-axis, and the slope of the line connecting data points as a rate of disease evolution. This instrument could be used to evaluate the effect of medical therapies on the progression of bowel damage.

Cross-sectional imaging (CTE and MRE) is a keystone of this score. To be included in the study that is defining Lémann score, patients should undergo MRE or CTE. Crohn's disease is transmural, but current methods of determining disease activity, such as ileocolonoscopy, are not able to visualize the entire bowel wall. Looking beyond the mucosa and preventing bowel damage may be the only ways to change the natural history of the disease and to prevent surgery. As described previously in this chapter, CTE and MRE have greatly improved the detection of structural small bowel lesions in CD. These imaging methods permit the identification of the precise location of CD lesions, a better evaluation of bowel wall involvement, to visualize fat or mesenteric changes around segments of the gastrointestinal tract, as well as the presence of strictures, fistulas, or abscesses. Additionally, several imaging scores of disease activity and severity were developed, with the Magnetic Resonance Index of Activity (MaRIA) being externally validated. Magnetic resonance enterography is preferred over CTE when possible, since it can also be used for repeated examinations without radiation exposure, unlike CTE.

MR Imaging of Perianal Fistulas

Around 40 % of patient with Crohn's disease will develop a perianal fistula and this proportion increases in those with underlying anal strictures. Up to 36 % of patients with CD present with this entity as their presenting symptom. Adequate evaluation of the full extent of disease including its anatomic relations and degree of inflammation is vital to making management decisions. MRI is recognized as being the reference standard for the anatomical depiction of disease extent. Increased enhancement on T1-weighted sequences following gadolinium is considered a good correlate of active inflammation [71]. Prior to commencing treatment with immunosuppressive and anti-tumour necrosis antibodies it is imperative to exclude an abscess. Recurrence following surgery is a common concern in circumstances where pre-operative imaging has not been performed.

There may be irreversible functional consequences if a fistula is inappropriately managed. MRI is excellent at depiction of perianal fistulising disease and in particular can be used to track the relationship to the sphincter complex as well as the remainder of the pelvic floor.

Classification

A surgically based classification system by Parks utilizes the external anal sphincter as a reference point [72] and classifies the fistulae in (1) *trans-sphincteric* (with extension of the tract through the external sphincter), (2) *inter-sphincteric* (confined to the inter-sphincteric space and internal sphincter), (3) *supra-sphincteric* (the result of supralevator abscesses, they pass through the levator ani muscle, over the top of the puborectalis muscle) and (4) *extra-sphincteric* (bypass the anal canal and sphincter mechanism, passing through the ischiorectal fossa and levator ani muscle, opening high in the rectum).

There are also imaging (MR) based classification systems [71, 73]. A detailed description of these scores is beyond the scope of this chapter, but for a reference, the Van Assche score attributes a score to (1) the number of fistula tracks, (2) the location (anatomic classification of Parks), (3) presence/absence of supralevatoric extension, (4) intensity of T2 signal, (5) presence of collections and (6) rectal wall involvement. The assessment of all these items by the radiologists allows a better stratification of patients in terms of management.

In order to strategize patient management, fistulas can roughly be sub-divided into two main categories, simple or complex:

1. *Simple* fistulas are superficial, intersphincteric or low trans-sphincteric, with only one opening, not associated with an abscess and showing no communication with an adjacent structure such as the vagina or bladder.
2. *Complex* fistulas have greater involvement of the anal sphincter (high trans-sphincteric, extra-sphincteric or supra-sphincteric), have multiple openings or a complex course (horseshoe), or are associated with a perianal abscess and/or communicates with an adjacent structure such as the bladder or vagina.

Technique

Perianal MRI can be performed with an endoanal coil, or a phased array external coil. Wider availability, a non-invasive procedure and consequently better patient acceptance mean that the phased array coil is more commonly used in perianal imaging. In addition the larger field of view (FOV) allows accurate assessment of fistulas that may extend beyond the sphincter complex.

The higher spatial resolution of the endoanal coil does however improve visualization of the internal opening and smaller tracts particularly in the case of recto-vaginal fistulas. The average diameter of 12–19 mm for an endoluminal coil may preclude placement in patients with local pain or in the presence of anal strictures. In comparison with the phased array technique there is a limited field of view and it is more prone to motion artefact.

At our institution, high resolution T2-weighted images are acquired in the axial and coronal planes after aligning with the plane of the anal canal. In addition, fat suppressed sequences are routinely performed and are useful for depiction of smaller tracts. A T1-weighted post gadolinium sequence helps in distinguishing between fluid and granulation tissue.

MRI allows not just precise anatomical localization of disease extent but also permits an assessment of disease chronicity. On T2-weighted sequences, active tracts containing particulate material, pus or debris is hyperintense whereas more fibrotic tracts show low signal intensity. Post-gadolinium sequences show fluid as being non-enhancing whereas areas of fibrosis or granulation tissue show delayed enhancement. A study by Horsthuis et al. [74] demonstrated good correlation between maximum enhancement and the patient's CRP. In their study of 33 patients with perianal CD larger numbers of rapidly enhancing pixels were seen in patients who required changes in medication or developed new abscesses during follow up.

Efficacy

Multiple studies using both endoscopic ultrasound (EUS) and MRI have demonstrated persistent fistula activity long after the fistula has ceased draining. Ng et al. [75] assessed 26 patients treated with either infliximab or adalimumab. Complete cessation of drainage occurred in 46 % of patients whereas MRI demonstrated that there had been complete healing in only 28 %. As there is such disparity between the clinical "picture" and the imaging findings there is a compelling argument for obtaining imaging at baseline as well as to assess and monitor healing response.

Studies comparing examination under anaesthesia (EUA) with pelvic MRI or endoluminal ultrasonography (EUS) also suggest that in 10 % of cases EUA incorrectly classifies the disease. This leads to inappropriate management decisions or additional surgical procedures [76]. Another study showed MRI as adding additional information to EUA and led to additional surgery in 21 % of 56 patients with fistulizing disease [77].

Radiological input is also vital in providing prognostic information. Patients who show signs of persistent disease at a 10 week imaging evaluation were more likely to recur [78]. In the study by Ng MRI was used to decide how long to continue with anti-TNF therapy [75]. This need for imaging has been recognized by the American gastroenterological association and the European Crohn's and Colitis Organization who have issued guidelines recommending imaging for perianal disease.

Cancer in Perianal Disease

Patients with Crohn's disease have a 4- to 20-fold increase in the risk of colorectal carcinoma [79]. The incidence of colorectal cancer is 3.7 % and patients with perianal disease have a 0.7 % incidence of carcinoma [80]. This complication poses both a clinical and imaging challenge.

Early diagnosis is imperative to improve patient outcome and facilitate appropriate management.

A retrospective review of six patients with anorectal carcinoma and perianal CD at our institution was used to describe the MRI features of cancer [81]. Four of the patients had a mucinous adenocarcinoma, whereas the remainder had squamous malignancy. Typical features of malignancy included irregular wall contours, double layer enhancement and delayed internal tissue enhancement. The mucinous carcinomas displayed a lobulated pattern with fluid-filled cavities again showing delayed internal enhancement. This stresses the importance of post-gadolinium imaging in perianal disease not merely to assess activity of tracts but to exclude concomitant malignant transformation.

References

1. Appleyard M et al. A randomized trial comparing wireless capsule endoscopy with push enteroscopy for the detection of small-bowel lesions. Gastroenterology. 2000;119(6):1431–8.
2. Fletcher JG. CT enterography technique: theme and variations. Abdom Imaging. 2009;34(3):283–8.
3. Triester SL et al. A meta-analysis of the yield of capsule endoscopy compared to other diagnostic modalities in patients with non-stricturing small bowel Crohn's disease. Am J Gastroenterol. 2006;101(5):954–64.
4. Eliakim R et al. Wireless capsule video endoscopy compared to barium follow-through and computerised tomography in patients with suspected Crohn's disease—final report. Dig Liver Dis. 2004;36(8):519–22.

5. Hara AK et al. Crohn disease of the small bowel: preliminary comparison among CT enterography, capsule endoscopy, small-bowel follow-through, and ileoscopy. Radiology. 2006;238(1):128–34.
6. Cirillo LC et al. Accuracy of enteroclysis in Crohn's disease of the small bowel: a retrospective study. Eur Radiol. 2000;10(12):1894–8.
7. Van Deventer SJ. Tumour necrosis factor and Crohn's disease. Gut. 1997;40(4):443–8.
8. Targan SR et al. A short-term study of chimeric monoclonal antibody cA2 to tumor necrosis factor alpha for Crohn's disease. Crohn's Disease cA2 Study Group. N Engl J Med. 1997;337(15):1029–35.
9. Present DH et al. Infliximab for the treatment of fistulas in patients with Crohn's disease. N Engl J Med. 1999;340(18):1398–405.
10. Feldmann M et al. The rationale for the current boom in anti-TNFalpha treatment. Is there an effective means to define therapeutic targets for drugs that provide all the benefits of anti-TNFalpha and minimise hazards? Ann Rheum Dis. 1999;58 Suppl 1:I27–31.
11. Siegel CA et al. Risks and benefits of infliximab for the treatment of Crohn's disease. Clin Gastroenterol Hepatol. 2006;4(8):1017–24. quiz 976.
12. Toruner M et al. Risk factors for opportunistic infections in patients with inflammatory bowel disease. Gastroenterology. 2008;134(4):929–36.
13. Andersohn F, Konzen C, Garbe E. Systematic review: agranulocytosis induced by nonchemotherapy drugs. Ann Intern Med. 2007;146(9):657–65.
14. Juillerat P et al. Drug safety in Crohn's disease therapy. Digestion. 2007;76(2):161–8.
15. Kandiel A et al. Increased risk of lymphoma among inflammatory bowel disease patients treated with azathioprine and 6-mercaptopurine. Gut. 2005;54(8):1121–5.
16. Keane J et al. Tuberculosis associated with infliximab, a tumor necrosis factor alpha-neutralizing agent. N Engl J Med. 2001;345(15):1098–104.
17. Vermeire S et al. Autoimmunity associated with anti-tumor necrosis factor alpha treatment in Crohn's disease: a prospective cohort study. Gastroenterology. 2003;125(1):32–9.
18. Rosh JR et al. Hepatosplenic T-cell lymphoma in adolescents and young adults with Crohn's disease: a cautionary tale? Inflamm Bowel Dis. 2007;13(8):1024–30.
19. Van Assche G et al. Progressive multifocal leukoencephalopathy after natalizumab therapy for Crohn's disease. N Engl J Med. 2005;353(4):362–8.
20. Jess T et al. Risk of intestinal cancer in inflammatory bowel disease: a population-based study from Olmsted County, Minnesota. Gastroenterology. 2006;130(4):1039–46.
21. Canavan C, Abrams KR, Mayberry JF. Meta-analysis: mortality in Crohn's disease. Aliment Pharmacol Ther. 2007;25(8):861–70.
22. Danzi JT. Extraintestinal manifestations of idiopathic inflammatory bowel disease. Arch Intern Med. 1988;148(2):297–302.
23. Sandborn WJ, Targan SR. Biologic therapy of inflammatory bowel disease. Gastroenterology. 2002;122(6):1592–608.
24. Siddiki HA et al. Prospective comparison of state-of-the-art MR enterography and CT enterography in small-bowel Crohn's disease. AJR Am J Roentgenol. 2009;193(1):113–21.
25. Solem CA et al. Small-bowel imaging in Crohn's disease: a prospective, blinded, 4-way comparison trial. Gastrointest Endosc. 2008;68(2):255–66.
26. Albert JG et al. Diagnosis of small bowel Crohn's disease: a prospective comparison of capsule endoscopy with magnetic resonance imaging and fluoroscopic enteroclysis. Gut. 2005;54(12):1721–7.
27. Bruining DH et al. Benefit of computed tomography enterography in Crohn's disease: effects on patient management and physician level of confidence. Inflamm Bowel Dis. 2012;18(2):219–25.
28. Lang G et al. Impact of small bowel MRI in routine clinical practice on staging of Crohn's disease. J Crohns Colitis. 2015;9(9):784–94.
29. Van Assche G et al. The second European evidence-based Consensus on the diagnosis and management of Crohn's disease: definitions and diagnosis. J Crohns Colitis. 2010;4(1):7–27.
30. Horsthuis K et al. Inflammatory bowel disease diagnosed with US, MR, scintigraphy, and CT: meta-analysis of prospective studies. Radiology. 2008;247(1):64–79.
31. Panes J et al. Systematic review: the use of ultrasonography, computed tomography and magnetic resonance imaging for the diagnosis, assessment of activity and abdominal complications of Crohn's disease. Aliment Pharmacol Ther. 2011;34(2):125–45.
32. Chiorean MV et al. Correlation of CT enteroclysis with surgical pathology in Crohn's disease. Am J Gastroenterol. 2007;102(11):2541–50.
33. Rimola J et al. Magnetic resonance imaging for evaluation of Crohn's disease: validation of parameters of severity and quantitative index of activity. Inflamm Bowel Dis. 2011;17(8):1759–68.
34. Fidler JL, Guimaraes L, Einstein DM. MR imaging of the small bowel. Radiographics. 2009;29(6):1811–25.
35. Negaard A et al. A prospective randomized comparison between two MRI studies of the small bowel in Crohn's disease, the oral contrast method and MR enteroclysis. Eur Radiol. 2007;17(9):2294–301.
36. Schreyer AG et al. Abdominal MRI after enteroclysis or with oral contrast in patients with suspected or proven Crohn's disease. Clin Gastroenterol Hepatol. 2004;2(6):491–7.
37. Masselli G et al. Comparison of MR enteroclysis with MR enterography and conventional enteroclysis in patients with Crohn's disease. Eur Radiol. 2008;18(3):438–47.
38. Florie J et al. Dynamic contrast-enhanced MRI of the bowel wall for assessment of disease activity in Crohn's disease. AJR Am J Roentgenol. 2006;186(5):1384–92.
39. Rimola J et al. Characterization of inflammation and fibrosis in Crohn's disease lesions by magnetic resonance imaging. Am J Gastroenterol. 2015;110(3):432–40.
40. Froehlich JM et al. MR motility imaging in Crohn's disease improves lesion detection compared with standard MR imaging. Eur Radiol. 2010;20(8):1945–51.
41. Menys A et al. Quantified terminal ileal motility during MR enterography as a potential biomarker of Crohn's disease activity: a preliminary study. Eur Radiol. 2012;22(11):2494–501.
42. Guglielmo FF et al. Identifying decreased peristalsis of abnormal small bowel segments in Crohn's disease using cine MR enterography: the frozen bowel sign. Abdom Imaging. 2015;40(5):1150–6.
43. Heye T et al. CT and endoscopic ultrasound in comparison to endoluminal MRI: preliminary results in staging gastric carcinoma. Eur J Radiol. 2009;70(2):336–41.
44. Torkzad MR et al. Value of cine MRI for better visualization of the proximal small bowel in normal individuals. Eur Radiol. 2007;17(11):2964–8.
45. Panes J et al. Imaging techniques for assessment of inflammatory bowel disease: joint ECCO and ESGAR evidence-based consensus guidelines. J Crohns Colitis. 2013;7(7):556–85.
46. Grand DJ, Guglielmo FF, Al-Hawary MM. MR enterography in Crohn's disease: current consensus on optimal imaging technique and future advances from the SAR Crohn's disease-focused panel. Abdom Imaging. 2015;40(5):953–64.
47. Oussalah A et al. Diffusion-weighted magnetic resonance without bowel preparation for detecting colonic inflammation in inflammatory bowel disease. Gut. 2010;59(8):1056–65.
48. Kim KJ et al. Diffusion-weighted MR enterography for evaluating Crohn's disease: how does it add diagnostically to conventional MR enterography? Inflamm Bowel Dis. 2015;21(1):101–9.
49. Ajaj W et al. MR colonography in patients with incomplete conventional colonoscopy. Radiology. 2005;234(2):452–9.

50. Langhorst J et al. MR colonography without bowel purgation for the assessment of inflammatory bowel diseases: diagnostic accuracy and patient acceptance. Inflamm Bowel Dis. 2007;13(8):1001–8.
51. Gore RM et al. CT features of ulcerative colitis and Crohn's disease. AJR Am J Roentgenol. 1996;167(1):3–15.
52. Rottgen R et al. Bowel wall enhancement in magnetic resonance colonography for assessing activity in Crohn's disease. Clin Imaging. 2006;30(1):27–31.
53. Sinha R et al. Utility of high-resolution MR imaging in demonstrating transmural pathologic changes in Crohn disease. Radiographics. 2009;29(6):1847–67.
54. Sempere GA et al. MRI evaluation of inflammatory activity in Crohn's disease. AJR Am J Roentgenol. 2005;184(6):1829–35.
55. Zappa M et al. Which magnetic resonance imaging findings accurately evaluate inflammation in small bowel Crohn's disease? A retrospective comparison with surgical pathologic analysis. Inflamm Bowel Dis. 2011;17(4):984–93.
56. Tielbeek JA et al. Evaluation of conventional, dynamic contrast enhanced and diffusion weighted MRI for quantitative Crohn's disease assessment with histopathology of surgical specimens. Eur Radiol. 2014;24(3):619–29.
57. Punwani S et al. Mural inflammation in Crohn disease: location-matched histologic validation of MR imaging features. Radiology. 2009;252(3):712–20.
58. Masselli G et al. Crohn disease: magnetic resonance enteroclysis. Abdom Imaging. 2004;29(3):326–34.
59. Adler J et al. Magnetization transfer helps detect intestinal fibrosis in an animal model of Crohn disease. Radiology. 2011;259(1): 127–35.
60. Pazahr S et al. Magnetization transfer for the assessment of bowel fibrosis in patients with Crohn's disease: initial experience. MAGMA. 2013;26(3):291–301.
61. Miao YM et al. Ultrasound and magnetic resonance imaging assessment of active bowel segments in Crohn's disease. Clin Radiol. 2002;57(10):913–8.
62. Maccioni F et al. MR imaging in patients with Crohn disease: value of T2- versus T1-weighted gadolinium-enhanced MR sequences with use of an oral superparamagnetic contrast agent. Radiology. 2006;238(2):517–30.
63. Rieber A et al. MRI in the diagnosis of small bowel disease: use of positive and negative oral contrast media in combination with enteroclysis. Eur Radiol. 2000;10(9):1377–82.
64. Ordas I et al. Accuracy of magnetic resonance enterography in assessing response to therapy and mucosal healing in patients with Crohn's disease. Gastroenterology. 2014;146(2):374–82.e1.
65. Tielbeek JA et al. Grading Crohn disease activity with MRI: interobserver variability of MRI features, MRI scoring of severity, and correlation with Crohn disease endoscopic index of severity. AJR Am J Roentgenol. 2013;201(6):1220–8.
66. Louis E et al. Behaviour of Crohn's disease according to the Vienna classification: changing pattern over the course of the disease. Gut. 2001;49(6):777–82.
67. Cosnes J et al. Long-term evolution of disease behavior of Crohn's disease. Inflamm Bowel Dis. 2002;8(4):244–50.
68. Thia KT et al. Risk factors associated with progression to intestinal complications of Crohn's disease in a population-based cohort. Gastroenterology. 2010;139(4):1147–55.
69. St Clair EW et al. Combination of infliximab and methotrexate therapy for early rheumatoid arthritis: a randomized, controlled trial. Arthritis Rheum. 2004;50(11):3432–43.
70. Pariente B et al. Development of the Crohn's disease digestive damage score, the Lemann score. Inflamm Bowel Dis. 2011;17(6):1415–22.
71. Spencer JA et al. Dynamic contrast-enhanced MR imaging of perianal fistulas. AJR Am J Roentgenol. 1996;167(3):735–41.
72. Parks AG, Gordon PH, Hardcastle JD. A classification of fistula-in-ano. Br J Surg. 1976;63(1):1–12.
73. Van Assche G et al. Magnetic resonance imaging of the effects of infliximab on perianal fistulizing Crohn's disease. Am J Gastroenterol. 2003;98(2):332–9.
74. Horsthuis K et al. Perianal Crohn disease: evaluation of dynamic contrast-enhanced MR imaging as an indicator of disease activity. Radiology. 2009;251(2):380–7.
75. Ng SC et al. Prospective evaluation of anti-tumor necrosis factor therapy guided by magnetic resonance imaging for Crohn's perineal fistulas. Am J Gastroenterol. 2009;104(12):2973–86.
76. Schwartz DA et al. A comparison of endoscopic ultrasound, magnetic resonance imaging, and exam under anesthesia for evaluation of Crohn's perianal fistulas. Gastroenterology. 2001;121(5): 1064–72.
77. Beets-Tan RG et al. Preoperative MR imaging of anal fistulas: does it really help the surgeon? Radiology. 2001;218(1):75–84.
78. Ardizzone S et al. Imaging of perianal Crohn's disease. Dig Liver Dis. 2007;39(10):970–8.
79. Hamilton SR. Colorectal carcinoma in patients with Crohn's disease. Gastroenterology. 1985;89(2):398–407.
80. Winkler R, Wittmer A, Heusermann U. Cancer and Crohn's disease. Z Gastroenterol. 2002;40(8):569–76.
81. Lad SV et al. MRI appearance of perianal carcinoma in Crohn's disease. J Magn Reson Imaging. 2007;26(6):1659–62.

19 Computed Tomography Enterography and Inflammatory Bowel Disease

J.G. Fletcher

CT enterography is a high spatial and temporal resolution multidetector CT exam of the abdomen and pelvis, following the administration of a large volume of enteric contrast agent that distends the small bowel. It provides exquisite images of the small bowel wall, lumen, and perienteric tissues. It can be routinely performed in the outpatient setting in nearly all radiology departments to evaluate for inflammatory bowel disease and other small bowel diseases. Improvements in CT technology have enabled greater adaptation of CT technique to clinical questions and dramatically reduced radiation dose. Over the past decade, CT enterography has become a widely available test with interpreted with local expertise, and there is emerging standardization of acquisition techniques and image interpretation methods, especially with relation to the staging of Crohn's disease [1, 2]. CT enterography is complementary to other imaging modalities, and provides unique information that impacts clinical management of patients with inflammatory bowel disease.

Role of CT Enterography in Inflammatory Bowel Disease

CT enterography is used to image the small bowel to detect and stage inflammatory bowel disease and its complications, in addition to detecting alternative small bowel disorders (e.g., pancreatic disease, sprue, NSAID enteropathy, small bowel tumors). For known Crohn's disease patients, in particular, CT enterography is used to detect the location(s) and severity of enteric inflammation; the presence, location and type of penetrating disease (fistula, abscess, or phlegmon); and the location and degree of obstruction caused by inflammatory and fibrostenotic strictures. In ulcerative colitis, CT enterography is used to gauge the extent of colonic inflammation if a stricture precludes endoscopic assessment, but more frequently to exclude small bowel inflammation after ileocolonoscopy and prior to colectomy. Both Crohn's disease and ulcerative colitis also cause a variety of extraintestinal complications that can be visualized at CT enterography, such as primary sclerosing cholangitis, neoplasia, mesenteric thromboses, nephrolithiasis, cholelithiasis, and sacroiliitis. CT enterography also detects complications from surgical and medical therapy, such avascular necrosis, surgical leak, pancreatitis, etc.

Patient Preparation and Image Acquisition

Patients generally are requested to fast 4 h prior to CT enterography so that ingested materials are not in the stomach or small bowel. A neutral enteric contrast agent, which possesses a CT number similar to water, is then administered in multiple aliquots over 45–60 min prior to CT examination. Neutral enteric agents other than water distend the lumen better and provide a long temporal window over which imaging can occur and still provide adequate luminal distention. The low attenuation of the bowel lumen filled with a neutral enteric contrast agent facilitates visualization of hyperattenuating bowel wall, masses and inflamed bowel segments. Enteric contrast agents generally contain sugar alcohols or osmotic laxatives to prevent resorption of water along the course of the small bowel, thereby improving ileal distention [3, 4]. Commonly used enteric contrast agents include low-contrast barium solution (which contains sorbitol; Volumen®; Bracco Diagnostics, Princeton, NJ), other oral formulations that contain sugar alcohols such as sorbitol, polyethylene glycol electrolyte solution, methylcellulose solution, or water. Side effects from oral contrast are minimal but can include nausea, abdominal cramping or distension, time-limited diarrhea, and excess gas [3]. In the hospital and emergency room (ER) setting, water is typically given as an oral contrast agent, as patients typically have an underlying degree of bowel obstruction, and the predisposition to nausea

J.G. Fletcher (✉)
Mayo Clinic, Rochester, MN 55905, USA
e-mail: Fletcher.Joel@mayo.edu

D.C. Baumgart (ed.), *Crohn's Disease and Ulcerative Colitis*, DOI 10.1007/978-3-319-33703-6_19

is increased. Unlike MR enterography, glucagon or butylscopolamine is not needed at CT enterography because of the speed of imaging acquisition, and its use in CT has not been proven to improve test performance.

In addition to enteric contrast, intravenous iodinated contrast is given at a rapid rate (e.g., ≥4 cc/s) through an intravenous catheter in order to enhance the bowel wall, with CT enterography image acquisition typically initiated during an enteric phase of contrast enhancement, when small bowel enhancement is maximal, typically occurring 50 s after initiation of the injection of IV contrast [5]. Alternatively, imaging can be performed in the portal or hepatic phase (i.e., beginning at 65–70 s), when the radiologic imaging of solid organs is preferable, without decrement in the identification of mural inflammation [6]. Many groups now initiate image acquisition at 60 s after initiation of intravenous contrast injection to maximize visualization of the potential acute or chronic mesenteric thromboses or occlusions, which can be seen in Crohn's disease [7, 8].

CT parameters governing spatial resolution and imaging speed are chosen so that the entire abdomen and pelvis can be imaged in 20 s or less (i.e., within a single breath hold) and so that spatial resolution in non-axial planes is optimized. With multi-detector CT with 16 detector rows or more, a minimal detector configuration less than 1 mm is chosen so that isotropic or near-isotropic coronal images can be obtained. Automatic exposure control should be used to modulate the tube current as the X-ray tube travels around the patient and as the patient travels through the scanner, in order to adapt radiation dose to patient size, thereby reducing dose on the order of about 30 % [9]. Additionally, while imaging on older CT systems is often performed at a tube voltage of 120 kV [10], many radiology practices now use lower tube potentials (e.g., 80–100 kV) that simultaneously reduce radiation dose and increase the conspicuity iodine-containing structures such as inflamed bowel segments [11–13] (Fig. 19.1). Tube potential (kV) selection requires technique charts or vendor-supported software, but these are now widely available [13]. Alternatively, lower kV (80 or 100 kV) imaging may be chosen to improve iodine signal and contrast to compensate for reduced injection rate or amount of intravenous iodinated contrast (Fig. 19.2).

Generally, narrow slice thickness of 3 mm or less are reconstructed in the axial, coronal and sagittal planes for image review. Many practices also reconstruct thicker maximum intensity projection images to highlight the vasa recta and inflamed bowel segments (Fig. 19.3). Finally, because most CT enterography exams are now performed at lower radiation dose than in the past, routine filtered back projection images have increased image noise owing to the use of lower tube potentials and tube current in image acquisition. To compensate, images are generally reconstructed using a variety of CT noise techniques such as iterative reconstruction [1, 13–15]. Noise reduction techniques improve image quality by decreasing image noise so that images resemble routine-dose images (Fig. 19.4) [16, 17]. For small and medium-sized patients, radiation dose from CT enterography can approach that from annual background radiation [14]. Numerous author groups have demonstrated that there is no reduction in the performance of CT enterography using lower radiation doses, as the increase in image noise is offset by the high contrast of enhancing bowel loops and penetrating disease [18–20].

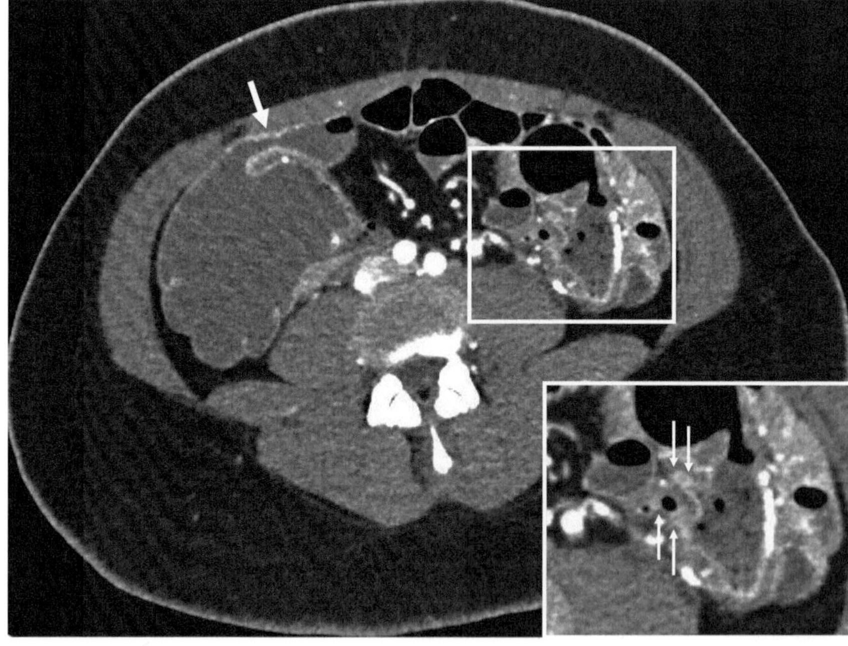

Fig. 19.1 Example of dose reduction at lower kV in a 43-year-old female with prior right hemicolectomy. CTDIvol lowered from 24 mGy (routine protocol) to 10 mGy after kV selection (80 kV). Note active ileitis in neoterminal ileum (*arrow*) and small fistulous tracts between descending colon and adjacent small bowel (*inset, arrows*)

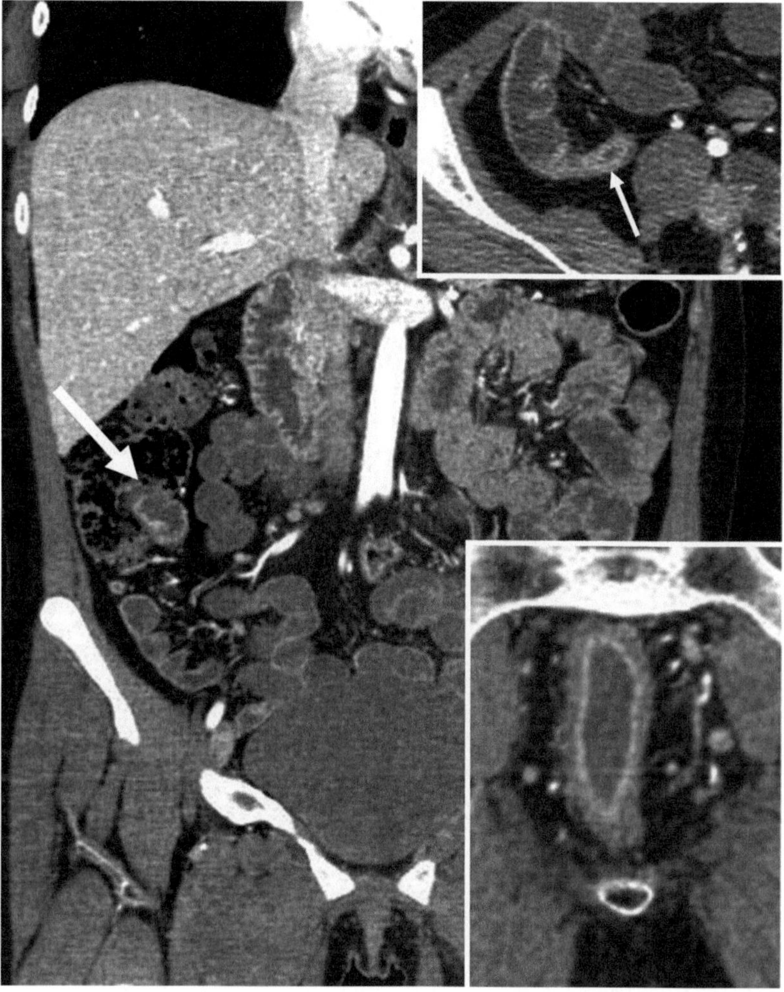

Fig. 19.2 CT enterography performed in a 32-year-old with indeterminate proctitis and poor intravenous access. To compensate, tube voltage was lowered to 100 kV with initiation of scanning delayed until 70 s. Large coronal image shows mild asymmetric hyperenhancement at terminal ileum reflecting mild inflammation (*large white arrow*), while *insets* show stratification and enhancement of the appendiceal tip (*upper inset, arrow*), and active proctitis with mural stratification, hyperenhancement, and reactive lymphadenopathy (*lower inset*)

Imaging Findings

Mural Inflammation

Mural hyperenhancement refers to segmentally increased attenuation of bowel loops compared to adjacent loops, and this correlates histologically with areas of active inflammation in Crohn's patients [21]. Mural hyperenhancement is the most sensitive sign of bowel inflammation, and it can be an isolated finding in mild inflammation. Hyperenhancement alone is a nonspecific finding in the small bowel, but asymmetric and patchy hyperenhancement, particularly along the mesenteric border, is indicative of Crohn's disease (Figs. 19.1 and 19.5).

Mural hyperenhancement is often accompanied by bowel wall thickening, which in the small bowel wall is greater than 3 mm in thickness in a bowel loop that is distended with luminal contrast. Wall thickening in Crohn's disease is often asymmetric and more prominent along the mesenteric border as well. As mural inflammation increases, wall thickening is often accompanied by mural stratification, which refers to a bilaminar and trilaminar appearance to the bowel wall (Fig. 19.5). The presence of both segmental mural hyperenhancement and wall thickening in the presence of asymmetric bowel involvement yields the best combination of imaging criteria for diagnosing mural inflammation in Crohn's disease [10, 22].

Several CT findings indicate more severe inflammation. Penetrating ulcers can also be seen in severely inflamed bowel loops, and they may appear as filling defects in the inflamed bowel wall; however, they are more frequently seen at MR enterography. Stranding in the perienteric fat is correlated with C-reactive protein elevation [23]. The "comb sign" refers to engorged vasa recta, which supply inflamed bowel loops and penetrate the gut wall perpendicular to the gut lumen, resembling the shape of a comb [24]. The comb sign is associated with increased serum C-reactive protein, length of hospitalization, and response to anti-inflammatory treatment (Fig. 19.5) [20, 23, 25]. Successful response to treatment following medical therapy is evidenced primarily by decreasing length of inflammatory bowel involvement along the length of the GI tract, but also a reduction in wall thickness and hyperenhancement [26].

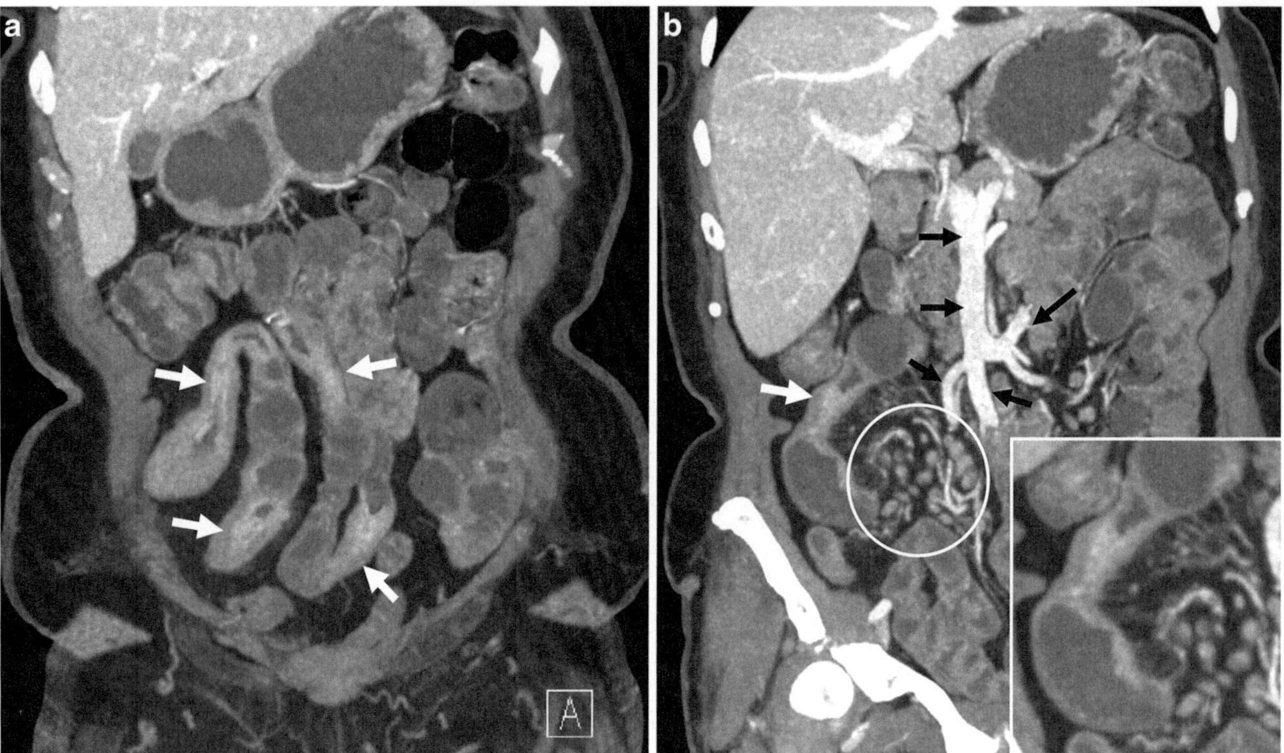

Fig. 19.3 Coronal 8 mm thick maximum intensity projection images in an asymptomatic 65 year-old female on adalimumab show multifocal Crohn's ileitis (*large arrows*), engorged vasa recta along the mesenteric border (**b**, *inset*), numerous reactive mesenteric lymph nodes (**b**, *circle*), and normal superior mesenteric vein and branches (**b**, *black arrows*)

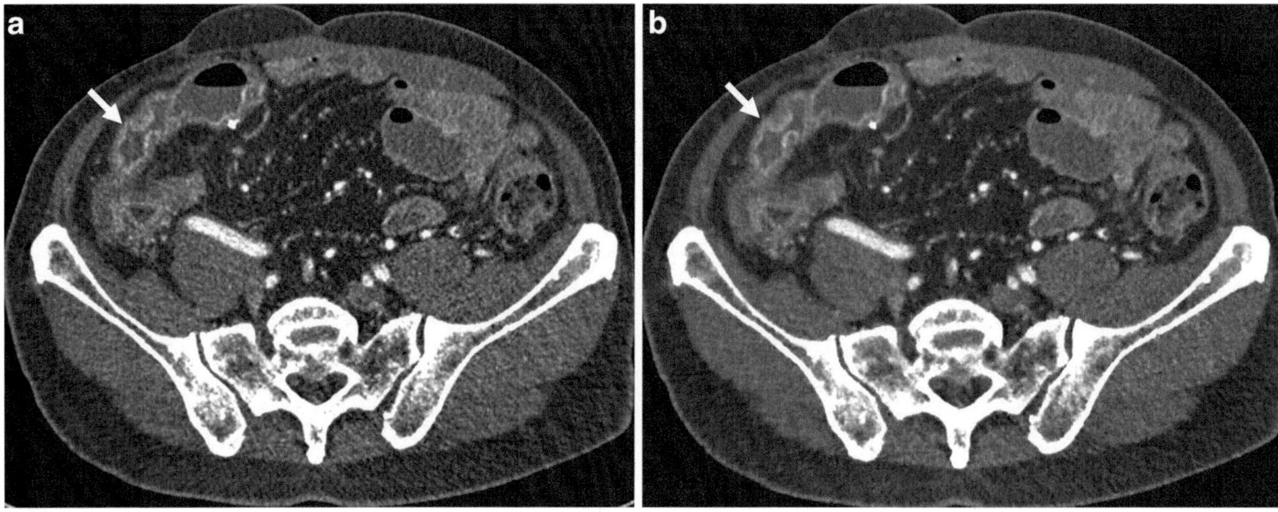

Fig. 19.4 Lower dose CTE in a 63-year-old male showing twofold reduction in image noise from routinely reconstructed image (**a**) to image reconstructed using image noise reduction techniques (**b**). Note that mural stratification and hyperenhancement indicating active ileitis in the terminal ileum (*arrow*) between ileoileostomy and ileocecal valve can be detected before image quality improvement with noise reduction

CT enterography can also display findings of chronic inflammation. Intramural fat can be seen in actively and uninflamed small bowel loops in the colon, indicating chronic inflammation, but intramural fat in the terminal ileum is a normal finding. Alternatively, pseudopolyps are frequently seen throughout the colon after healing of acute inflammation [27]. Fibrofatty proliferation is seen as proliferation of fat, usually allowing the mesenteric aspect of the bowel loop, displacing nearby abdominal loops; however, in the rectum fibrofatty proliferation is circumferential, mimicking pelvic lipomatosis, except that there are prominent perirectal vessels and reactive lymphadenopathy. Crohn's strictures generally possess both an inflammatory and fibrotic component [28, 29], and while CT findings of inflammation correlate histo-

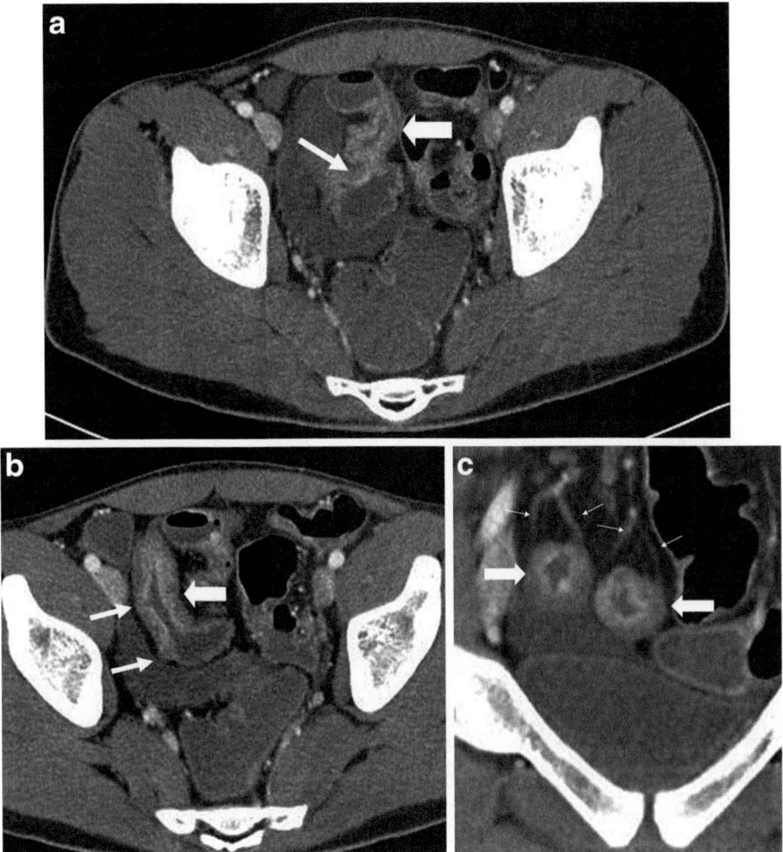

Fig. 19.5 Transverse CT enterography images in a 19-year-old Crohn's patient with "back pain." Images demonstrate mural thickening and stratification (*large arrows*, **a–c**), with a bilaminar appearance to the bowel wall. Note that mural thickening and luminal hyperenhancement are asymmetric (**a**, **c**), with one loop demonstrating mesenteric border thickening and hyperenhancement and antimesenteric border pseudosacculation (*small arrow*, **a**). One inflamed loop demonstrates small penetrating ulcers (*small arrow*, **b**), while another has prominent vasa recta, or "comb sign" (**c**, *small arrows*)

logically with inflammation in these strictures, the absence of CT findings of inflammation does not correlate with fibrosis [28]. CT enterography can be used to estimate the length of strictures to evaluate for potential endoscopic dilation or plan surgical treatment, and to evaluate for complications such as obstruction, enterolith, fistula, or malignancy.

Findings of intestinal inflammation in ulcerative colitis are similar to Crohn's colorectal involvement, but differ in some respects. The pattern of inflammation in ulcerative colitis that is most typical is continuous inflammation from the rectum proximally, whereas patchy inflammation will be typical of Crohn's colitis. Ulcerative colitis typically involves both the mesenteric and antimesenteric colonic wall to a similar degree, and does not cause penetrating complications. A patulous ileocecal valve is often seen when inflammation extends to the cecum (Fig. 19.6), as well as backwash ileitis, which involves the terminal ileum symmetrically without penetration. Inflammation can be mild to severe, often with loss of haustral markings. Rectal sparing can be seen when patients utilize steroid enemas. As inflammation becomes chronic, foreshortening of the colon is also often seen. As inflammation diminishes and becomes chronic, intramural fat is deposited throughout the colon, but this finding is not unique to ulcerative colitis. While surveillance of disease activity in ulcerative colitis is performed with endoscopy, CT enterography is often used to exclude small bowel inflammation in indeterminate colitis or symptomatic patients (that may have extraintestinal IBD manifestations) [30]. It is also used to evaluate for complications of severe acute colitis such as toxic megacolon, perforation or septic thrombosis (Fig. 19.7) [31, 32]. CT findings of toxic megacolon are only described in small retrospective series, but include marked colonic distension with loss of haustral markings and segmental colonic wall thinning [31].

Perienteric Inflammation and Penetrating Disease

The most subtle findings of perienteric inflammation in Crohn's disease are perienteric fat stranding [23]. Fistulas appear as hyperenhancing extraenteric tracts, which may or may not contain air and fluid [33], and are named by the structures that they connect (e.g., entero-enteric, entero-colic, entero-vesical, entero-cutaneous, and perianal). They generally arise from or proximal to an inflammatory stricture [34] or inflamed bowel segment, and cause tethering of the involved loops, frequently forming asterisk-shaped fistulae complexes (Fig. 19.8). Fistulas may extend to other bowel loops or organs and structures, e.g., the bladder and iliopsoas muscle. CT enterography has been shown to be highly accurate for the detection of penetrating complications such as

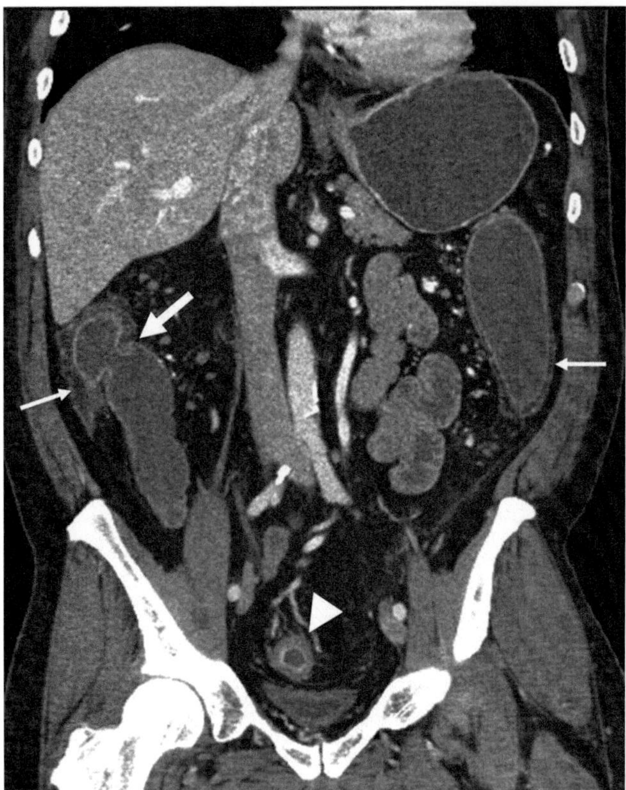

Fig. 19.6 A 58-year-old with 4-month history of altered bowel pattern. Coronal CT enterography images shows findings of chronic ulcerative colitis, including moderate sigmoid inflammation (*arrowhead*) and mild chronic proximal colitis in the descending colon and cecum (*small arrows*), as manifested by intramural fat, loss of haustration, and prominent pericolic vessels with reactive lymphadenopathy. The ileocecal valve is widely patulous (*large arrow*)

abscesses and fistulae [35]. CT enterography can be used for surgical planning in patients with known fistulizing disease, and several studies have shown that fistulizing Crohn's disease is often clinically unsuspected [33, 36], so the principal benefit of the enterography examination is often to identify unsuspected fistulas in symptomatic patients. Every CT enterography exam should image the perineum, as CT exam can identify an unsuspected perianal fistula or abscess in patients with indeterminate colitis, a key finding likely indicating that colonic inflammation is due to Crohn's disease. Fistulas may also arise from surgical anastomoses and leaks. Postoperative and some perianal fistulas are often not hyperenhancing due to their chronic nature.

Obstruction and Strictures

Mural inflammation often causes luminal narrowing of the small bowel. Luminal narrowing alone at CT enterography does not imply lack of distensibility or stricturing disease. Distensibility can be observed fluoroscopically, for example, using peroral pneumocolon. At CT enterography assessment, lack of distensibility is only indicated with certainty when proximally located small bowel loops are unequivocally dilated. Small bowel dilation can occur proximal to an inflamed bowel segment or stricture. At histopathologic assessment, most Crohn's strictures demonstrate a spectrum of inflammatory and fibrotic changes [29], and most Crohn's strictures will demonstrate some degree of hyperenhancement at imaging, consistent with the histopathologic observation that some degree of inflammation is present. In contradistinction, however, lack of is not a good indicator of fibrosis [28].

Extraintestinal Findings

CT enterography can detect Crohn's-related extra-enteric findings in addition to penetrating complications. In one retrospective series of over 300 Crohn's patients, nearly 20 % of Crohn's patients had extraintestinal IBD manifestations, and in about two-thirds of these patients, the findings were previously unknown [36]. Common extraintestinal, nonpenetrating complications detected at CT enterography include primary sclerosing cholangitis, mesenteric vascular thromboses or occlusions, cholelithiasis and nephrolithiasis, sacroiliitis, and avascular necrosis of the femoral heads. Chronic mesenteric venous occlusions, which are associated with Crohn's related inflammation (Fig. 19.9), are rarely seen in the acute setting, have recently been described and correlate with subsequent stricture and surgery [7, 8]. While acute portal and superior mesenteric vein thrombi typically resolve completely, peripheral chronic mesenteric vein thromboses often result in chronically narrowed mesenteric veins with dilated collateral veins and potentially varices.

CT Enterography Performance and Correlation with Clinical Symptoms

CT enterography has an estimated sensitivity for detecting ileal inflammation of approximately 75–90 % using mucosal inspection and biopsy as a reference standard [21, 22, 37, 38]. When clinical assessments additionally including surgery, serum, and clinical follow-up are integrated, the sensitivity of CT enterography for detecting ileal and inflammation improves to 90–95 % [10, 39, 40], as studies utilizing ileoscopic reference standards necessarily exclude patients with stenotic ileocecal valves, and misclassify patients with proximal ileal disease. In one retrospective study of 189 consecutive Crohn's patients, approximately half of the patients with a normal-appearing ileum at ileoscopy had either intramural or proximal small bowel inflammation at CT enterography, an observation they called "endoscopic skipping of the terminal ileum" [41]. Using

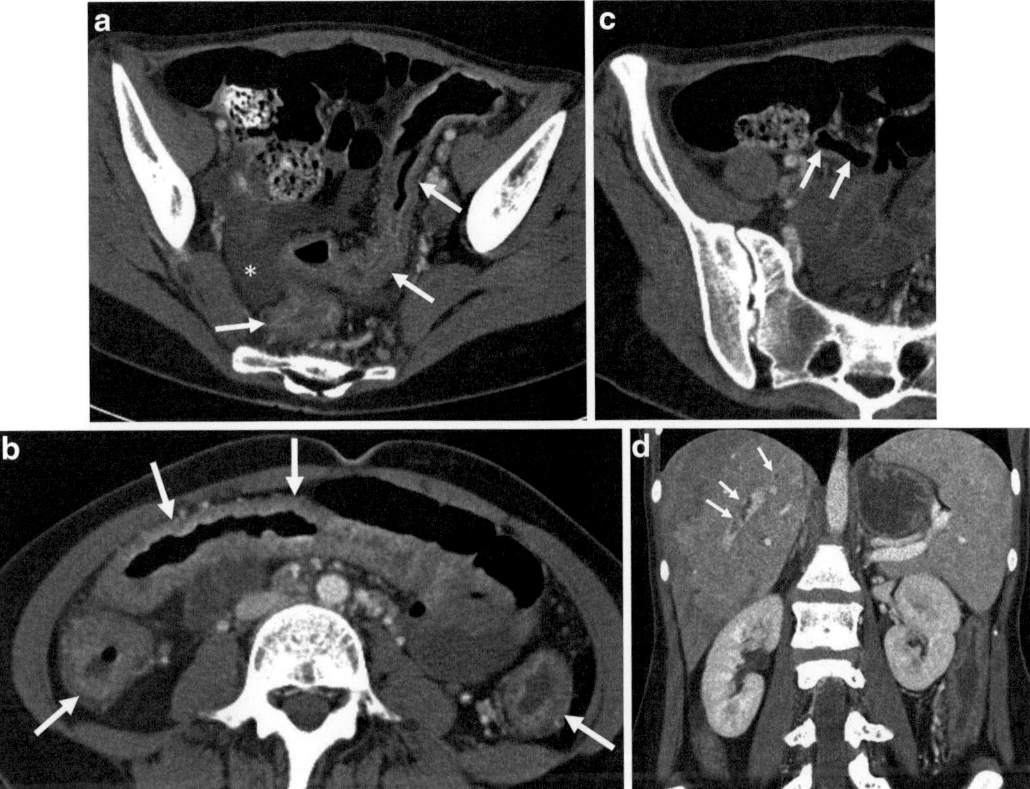

Fig. 19.7 CT enterography in a 21-year-old female with steroid-refractory ulcerative colitis with fever and normal plain film. Ulcerative colitis is manifest by continuous marked wall thickening, prominent vasa rectal and mild hyperenhancement extending from the rectum to the ascending colon (**a**, **b**, *arrows*). Exam was performed in part to exclude small bowel involvement, with a normal terminal ileum (**c**, *arrows*) and cecum noted on CT images. CT enterography images also demonstrated ascites (**a**, *asterisk*) and multifocal hepatic venous thromboses (**d**, *arrows*) and peripheral hepatic perfusion defects. At subsequent colectomy for fulminant colitis, severely active ulcerative colitis with numerous intravascular thrombi was found at histologic examination

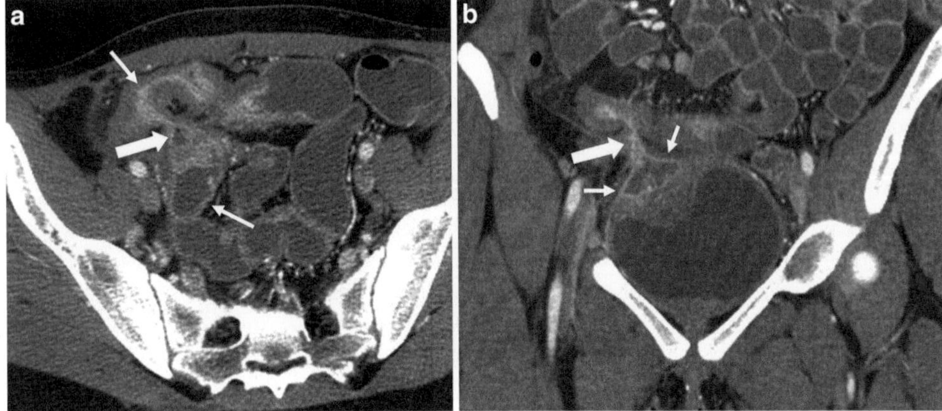

Fig. 19.8 CT enterography in a 23-year-old female demonstrating a complex fistula (large arrow, **a** and **b**) connecting two loops of ileum (*small arrows*, transverse image, **a**) in the right lower quadrant, with an inferior arm extending to the dome of the bladder, where there is a 3.2 cm abscess within the bladder wall (*small arrows*, coronal image, **b**)

CT enterography in conjunction with ileocolonoscopy also correlates with serum markers of inflammation better than ileocolonoscopy alone [42]. The performance of CT enterography for identifying active jejunal inflammation is likely decreased due to the greater enhancement of jejunal loops and the complexity of jejunal folds [37], and capsule endoscopy is often complementary to CT enterography because it can detect unsuspected or additional jejunal inflammation [38].

Like other objective measures of inflammation in Crohn's disease, CT enterography findings often do not correlate with symptomatology. In a retrospective study Higgins et al. found that CT enterography added unique information to clinical assessment and changed perception of steroid benefit

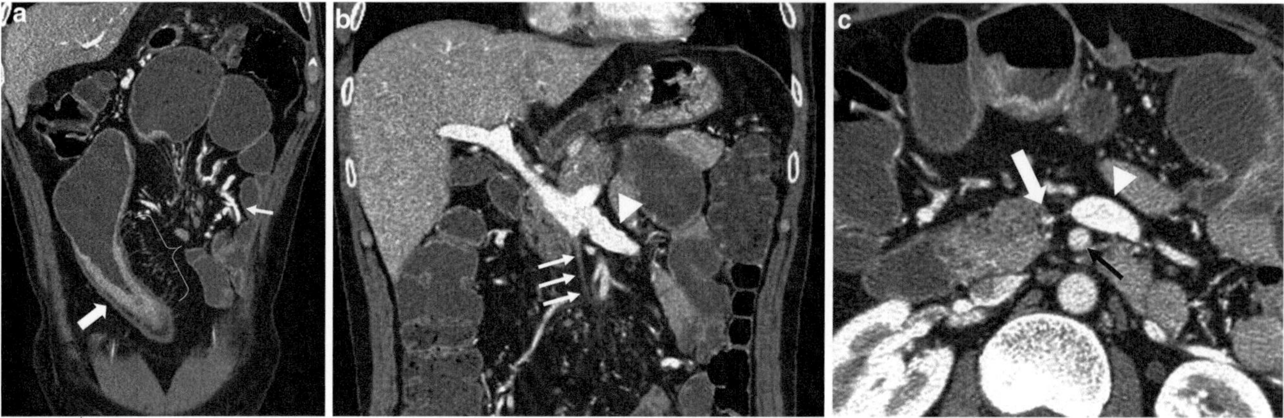

Fig. 19.9 Coronal CT enterography image in a 46-year-old Crohn's patient with obstructive symptoms demonstrates long segment inflammation (*large arrow*, **a**) with mural stratification, wall thickening and comb sign (*brackets*, **a**), with multiple loops of dilated proximal small bowel having prominent mesenteric veins (*small white arrow*, **a**). Coronal image slightly posteriorly (**b**) with corresponding transverse image (**c**) shows chronic occlusion and narrowing of the superior mesenteric vein (*small arrows*, **b**; *large arrow* **c**) and enlarged inferior mesenteric vein (*arrowhead*, **b**, **c**). (SMA = *black arrow*, **c**)

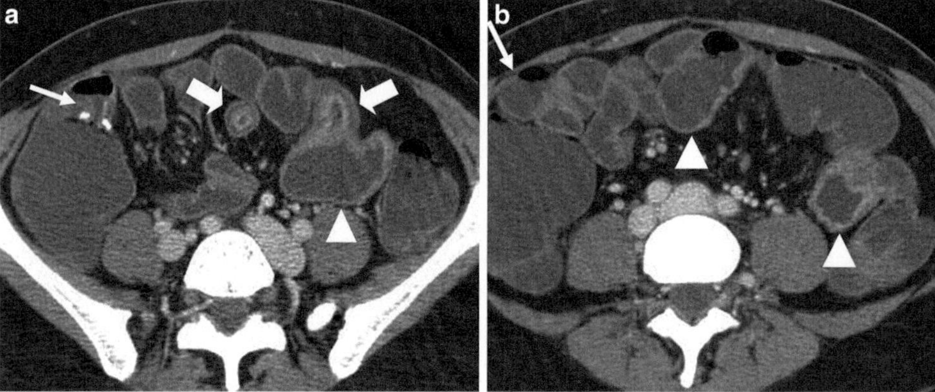

Fig. 19.10 A 46-year-old female with prior right hemicolectomy and frequent diarrhea thought to be without obstructive symptoms. CT enterography demonstrates two regions of luminal narrowing (*large arrows*, **a**) with proximally dilated loops (*arrowheads*, **a**, **b**). Luminal narrowing at anastomosis (*small arrow*, **a**) does not cause proximal dilation of neoterminal ileum (*small arrow*, **b**). At operative assessment the two strictures in the mid small bowel underwent strictureplasty, but ileocolic anastomosis was distensible

in nearly two-thirds of patients [43]. In a prospective study of 270 patients at Mayo Clinic, Bruining et al recorded management decision before and after CT enterography, and found that CT imaging changed management decisions in about half of Crohn's patients, and a similar portion of those with suspected Crohn's disease [25].

CT enterography is highly accurate in identifying penetrating disease, which is often unsuspected [33, 35, 36]. It has an estimated accuracy for identifying enteric fistulas of 86 %, with a per-patient sensitivity of 94 %, and 97–100 % in detecting patients with fistulas and phlegmon/abscesses, respectively [35]. Booya et al. found that nearly half the patients with penetrating disease had either no clinical suspicion or remote clinical suspicion of penetrating disease at pre-imaging clinical assessment [33].

While CT enterography has a high sensitivity for detecting obstructive strictures in one surgical series [35], it's performance is suboptimal in evaluating low grade obstruction. Nevertheless, many Crohn's patients with partial small bowel obstruction at CT enterography do not have obstructive symptoms. The fact that capsule endoscopy retention rates are higher in this cohort underscores the frequency of asymptomatic stenotic lesions in Crohn's [44]. In one prospective study, 17 % of patients without obstructive symptoms had an inflammatory stricture causing partial small bowel obstruction at CT enterography (Fig. 19.10) [38]. When CT enterography does not reveal partial obstruction associated with luminal narrowing, capsule endoscopy maybe useful in identifying additional enteric inflammation [38, 45].

Multimodality Imaging Assessment

Ileocolonoscopic assessment is generally considered complementary to cross-sectional enterography, as a colonoscopy is more sensitive for identifying mucosal inflammation, particularly in the colon, provides cancer surveillance not provided by CT imaging, and is usually performed with random biopsies, which also assist with risk stratification for cancer [38, 46]. While CT enterography is more sensitive than fluoroscopic analysis, particularly in identifying penetrating complications of Crohn's disease [40], fluoroscopy can provide functional information relating to luminal distensibility and partial obstruction that cannot be ascertained from volumetric CT imaging at a single time point. Capsule endoscopy is more sensitive at identifying mucosal inflammation than enterography (particularly in the jejunum), but is less specific and cannot identify perienteric complications, and usually requires preimaging assessment or use of a patency capsule [38, 47, 48]

MR enterography has an estimated performance for the detection of mural inflammation similar to CT enterography [39, 40], but is not available at all centers, requires much more imaging time, and is likely more prone to interobserver variability [49]. While the American College of Radiology recommends CT enterography as the most appropriate imaging test for patients with suspected Crohn's disease, or known Crohn's patients with fevers and abdominal pain [50], MR enterography is likely more appropriate for the follow-up of patients with known Crohn's disease for monitoring therapeutic response or those with obstructive symptoms [51]. Additionally, because MR utilizes a variety of pulse sequences that display different pathophysiologic properties, a variety of imaging findings have been shown to correlate with inflammatory severity (e.g., restricted diffusion [52]). Consequently, validated scoring systems have been developed to reflect Crohn's inflammation severity at MR imaging [53, 54], and potentially to reflect fibrosis [55]. Analogous validated measures of inflammation severity have not been developed for CT enterography. MR is also able to stage perianal fistulas when they are present. Because of the improved spatial and temporal resolution of CT compared to MR, CT enterography can be used a subsequent test when MR enterography demonstrates complex penetrating disease that may require surgical or interventional treatment.

In the Crohn's patient with acute symptoms, imaging with CT is almost always performed due to its widespread availability and speed. Imaging with MR enterography typically requires 30 min, for example, compared to 15 s for CT. It should be realized that hospitalized patients are generally poor candidates for CT enterography, as the oral contrast ingestion regimen will be poorly tolerated [1]. Similarly, postoperative patients are usually imaged with routine abdominopelvic CT with positive oral contrast, which will assist in the detection of anastomotic leaks [1]. Despite these limitations, abdominopelvic CT or CT enterography can be very useful in the emergent setting in evaluating symptomatic Crohn's patients, in which the incidence of penetrating and obstructive complications is high [56, 57].

Benefits and Risks

The principal benefits of CT enterography in Crohn's patients is to identify suspected and occult mural inflammation and penetrating complications that will change medical or interventional treatment. Protean patient symptomatology and the poor relationship between symptoms and biologic activity in Crohn's disease result in substantial benefit to patients from imaging [25]. However, CT utilizes low levels of ionizing radiation. While the low risk estimates of radiation induced malignancy are uncertain enough that the absence of risk cannot be excluded on a scientific basis for a single CT exam [58, 59], a small risk should be assumed to protect patients [60, 61], particularly for younger patients who are at greatest risk [62]. Ameliorating conditions which make CT a more appropriate compared to imaging alternatives include patient symptomatology, absence of prior imaging, contemplated surgical intervention, higher age, and contraindications to MRI. A principal advantage of CT enterography is its widespread availability at most medical institutions, being performed and interpreted with a high degree of local expertise.

Summary

CT enterography has become an accepted adjunctive test in the evaluation of patients with inflammatory bowel disease. Its role is to detect mural inflammation and penetrating complications of Crohn's disease which are clinically occult, and its routine use results in substantial impact on patient management decisions. It is complementary with other imaging tests, and is providing new insights into Crohn's disease and newer medical therapies in inflammatory bowel disease.

References

1. Baker ME, Hara AK, Platt JF, Maglinte DD, Fletcher JG. CT enterography for Crohn's disease: optimal technique and imaging issues. Abdom Imaging. 2015;40(5):938–52.
2. ACR-SAR-SPR practice parameter for the performance of computed tomography (CT) enterography; 2015. Available from: http://www.acr.org/~/media/ACR/Documents/PGTS/guidelines/CT_Enterography.pdf.
3. Young B, Fletcher J, Booya F, Paulsen S, Fidler J, Johnson CD, et al. Head-to-head comparison of oral contrast agents for

cross-sectional enterography: small bowel distention, timing, and side effects. J Comput Assist Tomogr. 2008;32:32–8.
4. Lauenstein T, Schneemann H, Vogt F, Herborn C, Ruhm S, Debatin J. Optimization of oral contrast agents for MR imaging of the small bowel. Radiology. 2003;228:279–83.
5. Schindera ST, Nelson RC, DeLong DM, et al. Multi-detector row CT of the small bowel: peak enhancement temporal window—initial experience. Radiology. 2007;243(2):438–44.
6. Vandenbroucke F, Mortele KJ, Tatli S, et al. Noninvasive multidetector computed tomography enterography in patients with small-bowel Crohn's disease: is a 40-second delay better than 70 seconds? Acta Radiol. 2007;48:1052–60.
7. Vietti Violi N, Fournier N, Duran R, et al. Acute mesenteric vein thrombosis: factors associated with evolution to chronic mesenteric vein thrombosis. AJR Am J Roentgenol. 2014;203(1):54–61.
8. Violi NV, Schoepfer AM, Fournier N, Guiu B, Bize P, Denys A. Prevalence and clinical importance of mesenteric venous thrombosis in the Swiss Inflammatory Bowel Disease Cohort. AJR Am J Roentgenol. 2014;203(1):62–9.
9. McCollough CH, Bruesewitz MR, Kofler Jr JM. CT dose reduction and dose management tools: overview of available options. Radiographics. 2006;26(2):503–12.
10. Siddiki H, Fletcher JG, Hara AK, et al. Validation of a lower radiation computed tomography enterography imaging protocol to detect Crohn's disease in the small bowel. Inflamm Bowel Dis. 2011;17(3):778–86.
11. Yu L, Liu X, Leng S, et al. Radiation dose reduction in CT: techniques and future perspective. Imaging Med. 2009;1(1):65–84.
12. Yu L, Primak AN, Liu X, McCollough CH. Image quality optimization and evaluation of linearly mixed images in dual-source, dual-energy CT (PMC2672422). Med Phys. 2009;36(3):1019–24.
13. Del Gaizo AJ, Fletcher JG, Yu L, et al. Reducing radiation dose in CT enterography. Radiographics. 2013;33(4):1109–24.
14. Kaza RK, Platt JF, Al-Hawary MM, Wasnik A, Liu PS, Pandya A. CT enterography at 80 kVp with adaptive statistical iterative reconstruction versus at 120 kVp with standard reconstruction: image quality, diagnostic adequacy, and dose reduction. AJR Am J Roentgenol. 2012;198(5):1084–92.
15. Ehman EC, Yu L, Manduca A, et al. Methods for clinical evaluation of noise reduction techniques in abdominopelvic CT. Radiographics. 2014;34(4):849–62.
16. Hara AK, Paden RG, Silva AC, Kujak JL, Lawder HJ, Pavlicek W. Iterative reconstruction technique for reducing body radiation dose at CT: feasibility study. AJR Am J Roentgenol. 2009;193(3):764–71.
17. Prakash P, Kalra MK, Kambadakone AK, et al. Reducing abdominal CT radiation dose with adaptive statistical iterative reconstruction technique. Invest Radiol. 2010;45(4):202–10.
18. Allen BC, Baker ME, Einstein DM, et al. Effect of altering automatic exposure control settings and quality reference mAs on radiation dose, image quality, and diagnostic efficacy in MDCT enterography of active inflammatory Crohn's disease. AJR Am J Roentgenol. 2010;195(1):89–100.
19. Kambadakone AR, Prakash P, Hahn PF, Sahani DV. Low-dose CT examinations in Crohn's disease: impact on image quality, diagnostic performance, and radiation dose. AJR Am J Roentgenol. 2010;195(1):78–88.
20. Lee S, Ha H, Yang S, et al. CT of prominent pericolic or perienteric vasculature in patients with Crohn's disease: correlation with clinical disease activity and findings on barium studies. AJR Am J Roentgenol. 2002;179:1029–36.
21. Bodily KD, Fletcher JG, Solem CA, et al. Crohn disease: mural attenuation and thickness at contrast-enhanced CT enterography—correlation with endoscopic and histologic findings of inflammation. Radiology. 2006;238(2):505–16.
22. Baker ME, Walter J, Obuchowski NA, et al. Mural attenuation in normal small bowel and active inflammatory Crohn's disease on CT enterography: location, absolute attenuation, relative attenuation, and the effect of wall thickness. AJR Am J Roentgenol. 2009;192(2):417–23.
23. Colombel JF, Solem CA, Sandborn WJ, et al. Quantitative measurement and visual assessment of ileal Crohn's disease activity by computed tomography enterography: correlation with endoscopic severity and C reactive protein. Gut. 2006;55(11):1561–7.
24. Meyers MA, McGuire PV. Spiral CT demonstration of hypervascularity in Crohn's disease: "vascular jejunization of the ileum" or the "comb sign". Abdom Imaging. 1995;20:327–32.
25. Bruining D, Siddiki H, Fletcher J, et al. Clinical benefit of CT enterography in suspected or established Crohn's disease: impact on patient management and physician level of confidence. 109th Annual Meeting of the American Gastroenterological Association Institute, San Diego, CA; 2008. p. A-202.
26. Bruining DH, Loftus Jr EV, Ehman EC, et al. Computed tomography enterography detects intestinal wall changes and effects of treatment in patients with Crohn's disease. Clin Gastroenterol Hepatol. 2011;9(8):679–83. e1.
27. Paulsen SR, Huprich JE, Fletcher JG, et al. CT enterography as a diagnostic tool in evaluating small bowel disorders: review of clinical experience with over 700 cases. Radiographics. 2006;26(3):641–57. discussion 57-62.
28. Adler J, Punglia DR, Dillman JR, et al. Computed tomography enterography findings correlate with tissue inflammation, not fibrosis in resected small bowel Crohn's disease. Inflamm Bowel Dis. 2012;18(5):849–56.
29. Chiorean MV, Sandrasegaran K, Saxena R, Maglinte DD, Nakeeb A, Johnson CS. Correlation of CT enteroclysis with surgical pathology in Crohn's disease. Am J Gastroenterol. 2007;102(11):2541–50.
30. Deepak P, Bruining DH. Radiographical evaluation of ulcerative colitis. Gastroenterol Rep. 2014;2:169–77.
31. Moulin V, Dellon P, Laurent O, Aubry S, Lubrano J, Delabrousse E. Toxic megacolon in patients with severe acute colitis: computed tomographic features. Clin Imaging. 2011;35:431–6.
32. Imbriaco M, Balthazar EJ. Toxic megacolon: role of CT in evaluation and detection of complications. J Clin Imaging. 2001;25:349–54.
33. Booya F, Akram S, Fletcher JG, et al. CT enterography and fistulizing Crohn's disease: clinical benefit and radiographic findings. Abdom Imaging. 2009;34(4):467–75.
34. Oberhuber G, Stangl PC, Vogelsang H, Schober E, Herbst F, Gasche C. Significant association of strictures and internal fistula formation in Crohn's disease. Virchows Arch. 2000;437(3):293–7.
35. Vogel J, da Luz MA, Baker M, et al. CT enterography for Crohn's disease: accurate preoperative diagnostic imaging. Dis Colon Rectum. 2007;50(11):1761–9.
36. Bruining DH, Siddiki HA, Fletcher JG, Tremaine WJ, Sandborn WJ, Loftus Jr EV. Prevalence of penetrating disease and extraintestinal manifestations of Crohn's disease detected with CT enterography. Inflamm Bowel Dis. 2008;14(12):1701–6.
37. Booya F, Fletcher JG, Huprich JE, et al. Active Crohn disease: CT findings and interobserver agreement for enteric phase CT enterography. Radiology. 2006;241(3):787–95.
38. Solem CA, Loftus Jr EV, Fletcher JG, et al. Small-bowel imaging in Crohn's disease: a prospective, blinded, 4-way comparison trial. Gastrointest Endosc. 2008;68(2):255–66.
39. Siddiki HA, Fidler JL, Fletcher JG, et al. Prospective comparison of state-of-the-art MR enterography and CT enterography in small-bowel Crohn's disease. AJR Am J Roentgenol. 2009;193(1):113–21.
40. Lee SS, Kim AY, Yang SK, et al. Crohn disease of the small bowel: comparison of CT enterography, MR enterography, and small-bowel follow-through as diagnostic techniques. Radiology. 2009;251(3):751–61.

41. Samuel S, Bruining DH, Loftus Jr EV, et al. Endoscopic skipping of the distal terminal ileum in Crohn's disease can lead to negative results from ileocolonoscopy. Clin Gastroenterol Hepatol. 2012;10(11):1253–9.
42. Faubion Jr WA, Fletcher JG, O'Byrne S, et al. EMerging BiomARKers in Inflammatory Bowel Disease (EMBARK) study identifies fecal calprotectin, serum MMP9, and serum IL-22 as a novel combination of biomarkers for Crohn's disease activity: role of cross-sectional imaging. Am J Gastroenterol. 2013;108(12): 1891–900.
43. Higgins PD, Caoili E, Zimmermann M, et al. Computed tomographic enterography adds information to clinical management in small bowel Crohn's disease. Inflamm Bowel Dis. 2007;13(3): 262–8.
44. Liao Z, Gao R, Xu C, Li ZS. Indications and detection, completion, and retention rates of small-bowel capsule endoscopy: a systematic review. Gastrointest Endosc. 2010;71(2):280–6.
45. Voderholzer WA, Beinhoelzl J, Rogalla P, et al. Small bowel involvement in Crohn's disease: a prospective comparison of wireless capsule endoscopy and computed tomography enteroclysis. Gut. 2005;54(3):369–73.
46. Johnson KT, Hara AK, Johnson CD. Evaluation of colitis: usefulness of CT enterography technique. Emerg Radiol. 2009;16(4): 277–82.
47. Dionisio PM, Gurudu SR, Leighton JA, et al. Capsule endoscopy has a significantly higher diagnostic yield in patients with suspected and established small-bowel Crohn's disease: a meta-analysis. Am J Gastroenterol. 2010;105(6):1240–8. quiz 9.
48. Goldstein JL, Eisen GM, Lewis B, Gralnek IM, Zlotnick S, Fort JG. Video capsule endoscopy to prospectively assess small bowel injury with celecoxib, naproxen plus omeprazole, and placebo. Clin Gastroenterol Hepatol. 2005;3(2):133–41.
49. Schmidt S, Lepori D, Meuwly JY, et al. Prospective comparison of MR enteroclysis with multidetector spiral-CT enteroclysis: interobserver agreement and sensitivity by means of "sign-by-sign" correlation. Eur Radiol. 2003;13(6):1303–11.
50. American College of Radiology. ACR appropriateness criteria: Crohn's disease. 2008. Available at http://www.acrorg/SecondaryMainMenuCategories/quality_safety/app_criteria/pdf/ExpertPanelonGastrointestinalImaging/CrohnsDiseaseDoc5aspx. Accessed 01 Nov 2010.
51. Guimaraes LS, Fidler JL, Fletcher JG, et al. Assessment of appropriateness of indications for CT enterography in younger patients. Inflamm Bowel Dis. 2010;16(2):226–32.
52. Kim KJ, Lee Y, Park SH, et al. Diffusion-weighted MR enterography for evaluating Crohn's disease: how does it add diagnostically to conventional MR enterography? Inflamm Bowel Dis. 2015;21(1):101–9.
53. Rimola J, Rodriguez S, Garcia-Bosch O, et al. Magnetic resonance for assessment of disease activity and severity in ileocolonic Crohn's disease. Gut. 2009;58(8):1113–20.
54. Tielbeek JA, Makanyanga JC, Bipat S, et al. Grading Crohn disease activity with MRI: interobserver variability of MRI features, MRI scoring of severity, and correlation with Crohn disease endoscopic index of severity. AJR Am J Roentgenol. 2013;201(6): 1220–8.
55. Rimola J, Planell N, Rodriguez S, et al. Characterization of inflammation and fibrosis in Crohn's disease lesions by magnetic resonance imaging. Am J Gastroenterol. 2015;110(3):432–40.
56. Kerner C, Carey K, Mills AM, et al. Use of abdominopelvic computed tomography in emergency departments and rates of urgent diagnoses in Crohn's disease. Clin Gastroenterol Hepatol. 2012;10(1):52–7.
57. Israeli E, Ying S, Henderson B, Mottola J, Strome T, Bernstein CN. The impact of abdominal computed tomography in a tertiary referral centre emergency department on the management of patients with inflammatory bowel disease. Aliment Pharmacol Ther. 2013;38(5):513–21.
58. Cohen BL. Cancer risk from low-level radiation. AJR Am J Roentgenol. 2002;179(5):1137–43.
59. Muirhead CR, O'Hagan JA, Haylock RG, et al. Mortality and cancer incidence following occupational radiation exposure: third analysis of the National Registry for Radiation Workers. Br J Cancer. 2009;100(1):206–12.
60. Committee to Assess Health Risks from Exposure to Low Levels of Ionizing Radiation, National Research Council. Health risks from exposure to low levels of ionizing radiation: BEIR VII Phase 2. Washington, DC: National Academies Press; 2006.
61. McCollough CH, Guimaraes L, Fletcher JG. In defense of body CT. AJR Am J Roentgenol. 2009;193(1):29–39.
62. Brenner DJ, Hall EJ. Computed tomography—an increasing source of radiation exposure. N Engl J Med. 2007;357(22):2277–84.

Ultrasound in Inflammatory Bowel Disease

20

A. Potthoff, C. Agné, and M. Gebel

Crohn's Disease

Crohn's disease (CD) is typically diagnosed in young patients and follows a course of chronic relapse. The risk of exposure to cumulative ionizing radiation must be taken into account when choosing the diagnostic means for managing these patients [1].

The exposure to diagnostic radiation for Crohn's patients recently increased from 12 millisievert (mSv) (1992–1997) to 32 mSv (2002–2007). An exposure of 75 mSv was calculated for up to 16 % of patients, which theoretically induces a lifetime cancer risk of 7.3 % [2]. According to a recent meta-analysis, the pooled prevalence of IBD patients receiving potentially harmful levels of radiation (defined as ≥50 mSv), was 8.8 % (11.1 % and 2 % for CD and UC, respectively). IBD-related surgery and corticosteroid use were significant risk factors, with pooled adjusted odds ratios of 5.4 (95 %; CI 2.6–11.2) and 2.4 (95 %; CI 1.7–3.4) respectively [3]. Other factors associated with a high cumulative effective dose were age <17 years at diagnosis, the first year after diagnosis, upper gastrointestinal tract disease, penetrating disease, use of infliximab, and multiple surgeries [4].

Therefore, gastroenterologists treating CD patients should aim to avoid diagnostic radiation. Other than MRT imaging, only ultrasound is radiation free. In addition, ultrasound is a real-time imaging technique that is noninvasive, risk-free, and highly accepted in everyday practice by CD patients.

A recent meta-analysis [5] indicated that there were no significant differences in diagnostic accuracy between CT, MR imaging, and US. In a study, Martinez et al. even demonstrated slight advantages in terms of diagnostic sensitivity and specificity for ultrasound compared to MRI (US 91 % vs. MRI 83 %; US 80 % vs. MRI 72 %, respectively) [6]. The commonly accepted ultrasound features of activity in CD—bowel wall thickness and mesenteric lymph node enlargement—showed high interobserver reproducibility [7]. Additionally, loss of stratification and hyperemia of the wall correlated well with severity and course of the disease [8–11].

The updated German S3 Guideline regarding the diagnosis of CD (implementation of radiological modalities) underlines the importance of ultrasound in the diagnostic management of CD [12]. According to the current joint ECCO and ESGAR evidence based consensus guidelines, ultrasound demonstrates high accuracy for the assessment of penetrating complications (i.e., fistula, abscess) and for monitoring disease progression. Ultrasound allows the detection of complications such as fistulas (and the early stage of fistula, transmural inflammation), abscesses, and ileus/subileus with high sensitivity and specificity [13].

Initial Diagnosis of Crohn's Disease via Transabdominal B-Mode Ultrasound

Ultrasound has been long-neglected as a diagnostic tool in patients with CD. The gaseous content and delicate anatomical structures of the bowel were believed to make reproducible diagnostic evaluation via ultrasound difficult. One of the first publications leading the way in this field hinted at the hidden possibilities associated with this technique [14]. Modern high frequency transducers (5–17 MHz) allow the differentiation of five layers of the bowel wall [15] (Figs. 20.1, 20.2, and 20.3):

First layer: hyperechoic, interface between the lumen and superficial mucosa.

Second layer: hypoechoic, interface between the deep and superficial mucosa.

Third layer: hyperechoic, interface between submucosa and the muscularis propria.

Fourth layer: hypoechoic, muscularis propria.

Fifth layer: hyperechoic, the superficial interface of the perivisceral serosa

A. Potthoff, M.D. • C. Agné, M.D. • M. Gebel, M.D. (✉)
Department of Gastroenterology, Hepatology and Endocrinology, Hannover Medical School, Hannover, Germany
e-mail: potthoff.andrej@mh-hannover.de; agne.clemens@mh-hannover.de; Gebel.Michael@mh-hannover.de

D.C. Baumgart (ed.), *Crohn's Disease and Ulcerative Colitis*, DOI 10.1007/978-3-319-33703-6_20

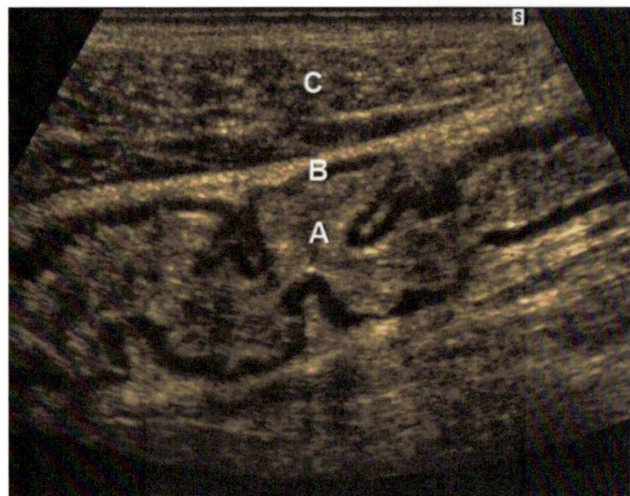

Fig. 20.1

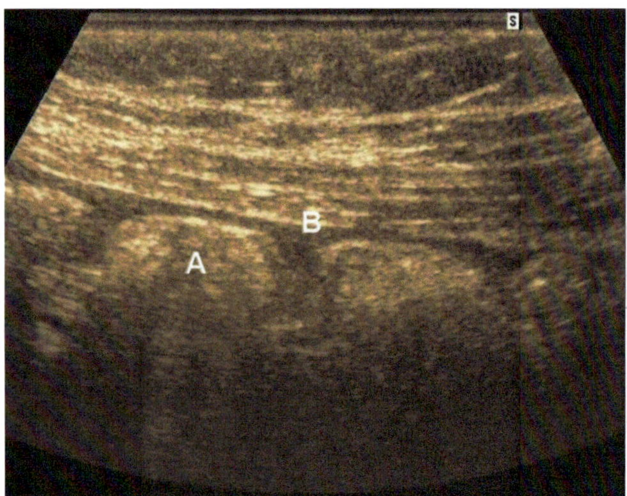

Fig. 20.2

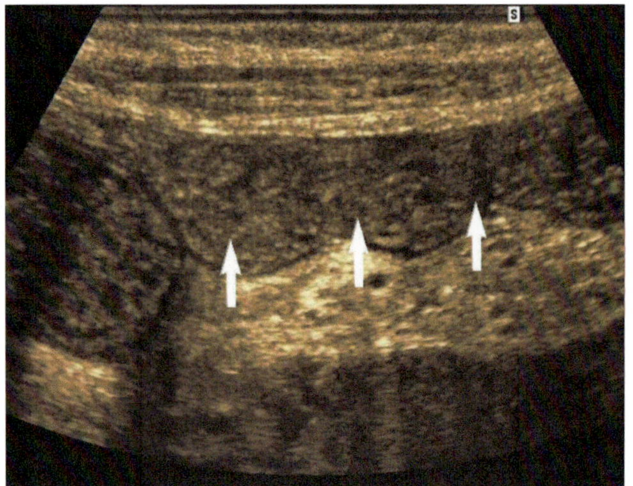

Fig. 20.3

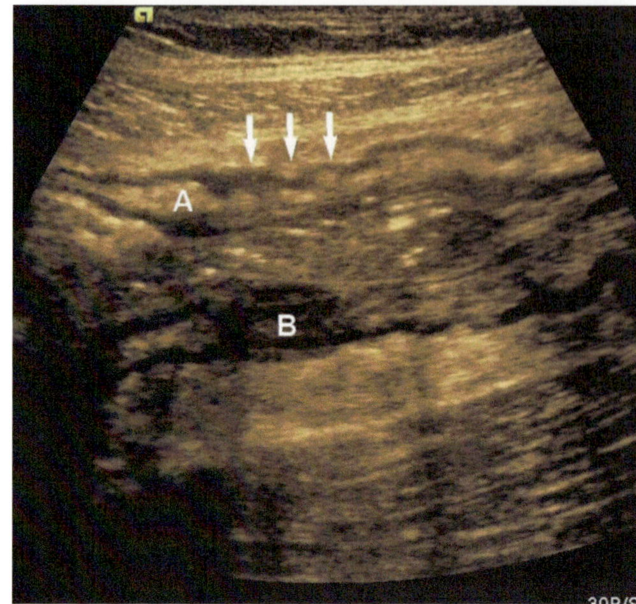

Fig. 20.4

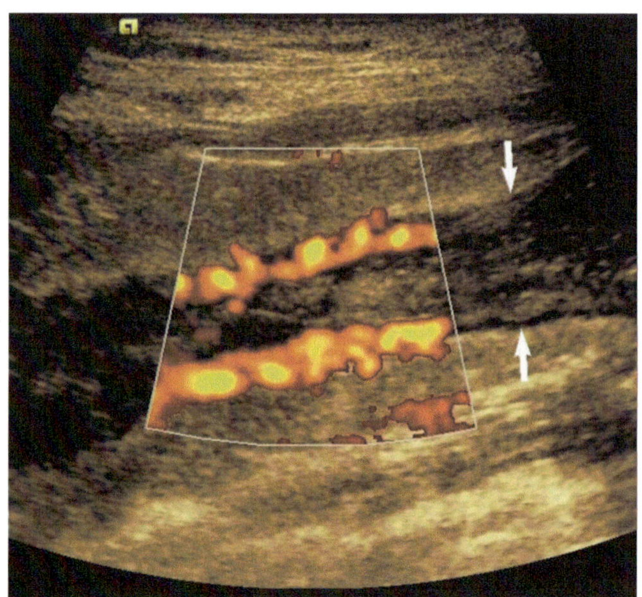

Fig. 20.5

The typical and constant features of CD revealed via B-mode ultrasound are the presence of thickened and stiff bowel wall, modification or disappearance of echo stratification of the bowel wall, loss of peristalsis in the small bowel, and loss of haustrae coli in the colon [16] (Figs. 20.4 and 20.5). Disease activity can be accompanied by mesenterial fat hypertrophy and enlargement of surrounding lymph nodes. B-mode ultrasound revealed a high sensitivity and specificity in the detection of CD (73–96 % and 90–100 %, respectively) compared with other methods such as endoscopy and/or radiological imaging [17]. The diagnostic accuracy and costs of noninvasive diagnostic strategies including magnetic resonance imaging, intestinal ultrasonography, ileocolonoscopy, and video-capsule endoscopy in suspected CD were analyzed in a recent study [18]. The authors found that both accuracy and costs depend on the pretest probability of CD and vary according to the first test used. Ileocolonoscopy plus ultrasonography was the most accurate and least expensive initial diagnostic strategy. Many studies differed in terms of study design, population characteristics, and reference standard, as did the accuracy of ultrasound as a diagnostic tool in CD. Fraquelli et al. demonstrated that raising the bowel wall thickness threshold from 3 to 4 mm increased specificity (93–97 %) at the extent of sensitivity (88–75 %) [19], without any differences between adults and children [20].

Assessment of Disease Activity

Several sonomorphological findings of disease activity in CD are commonly used in daily practice: degree of bowel wall thickening, echo pattern, luminal narrowing, fibro-fatty proliferation, and mesenteric lymphadenopathy.

A Japanese study established a strong correlation between the maximum bowel wall thickness and the histological findings of surgical specimens and also between the echo pattern and histopathological disease activity. A loss of stratification (hypoechoic echo pattern) predicted the prevalence of severe inflammation [21]. Another study described a blurred wall layer more frequently in active disease than in inactive disease (62.0 vs. 5 %; $p<0.05$) [17]. One of the first attempts to create a sonographic score to describe disease activity in CD was published by Futagami [22]. The sonographic score showed a good correlation to endoscopic findings, but the implemented sonomorphological features—bowel wall thickness and wall stratification—correlated weakly with CDAI or biological indices of inflammation (C-reactive protein, erythrocyte sedimentation rate). Many studies have demonstrated a marginal correlation between disease activity measured by CDAI and sonographic findings [23]. The CDAI is widely used as a reference standard, even if it mirrors the subjective complaints of the patient without necessarily reflecting sonomorphological abnormalities or endoscopic or histological findings [24].

Assessment of Disease Location

Several studies have compared the accuracy of bowel ultrasound to various radiological techniques in defining the anatomical location of CD [25–28]. One of the largest studies ($n=296$) demonstrated sensitivity and specificity according to the location of the affected bowel segment (overall: sensitivity 93 %, specificity 97 %). The highest accuracy was achieved when examining the terminal ileum (sensitivity 95 %). The upper small bowel was much more difficult to assess correctly (jejunum 72 %). In particular, the detection of lesions in the pelvic area via transabdominal ultrasound remained poor. Proctitis was diagnosed correctly in only 15 % of patients [25]. Alternative ultrasound techniques such as small bowel contrast ultrasound (SICUS) and perianal ultrasound (PAUS) enriched the noninvasive arsenal for evaluating the upper small bowel or pelvic region. These examination techniques are discussed later.

Detection of Complications

Pediatric patients with CD and adults with childhood onset CD are at increased risk of developing comorbidities and complications [29]. In approximately 50–70 % of cases, CD patients are affected by complications such as bowel strictures, fistulae, and abscesses during the course of their disease [30]. Complications of CD that effect further treatment can often be found even in asymptomatic patients. High-resolution transabdominal ultrasound has an excellent diagnostic accuracy in the diagnosis of complications in patients with Crohn's disease [31].

In a study by Hirche et al. [32], routine ultrasound detected transmural inflammation in 17 out of 255 patients without clinical signs of active disease (CD activity index 150). Eleven patients from this group had interenteric, enteromesenteric, or perirectal fistula, whereas six patients displayed a transmural mesenteric inflammation reaction without fistulae. In another series of 100 consecutive patients without active disease, fistulae were detected in 4 % of cases, mostly interenteric [17].

Detection of Abscesses

An abscess develops in 15–20 % of Crohn's patients during the course of their illness. Identifying this complication is essential for the right management choice. Abscesses require surgical or percutaneous drainage [16] and are seen as a contraindication for numerous modern medical approaches. Abscesses appear as hypoechoic lesions with an irregular wall in transabdominal ultrasound. Internal echoes are a sign of debris, and a posterior echo enhancement can show liquid compartments of the structure (Figs. 20.6 and 20.7). The detection of vascular signs in the lesion is a sign of inflammatory masses and allows it to be differentiated from an abscess [33, 34]. Most studies evaluating the accuracy of ultrasound in the detection of abscesses use computed tomography or surgico-pathological findings as the gold

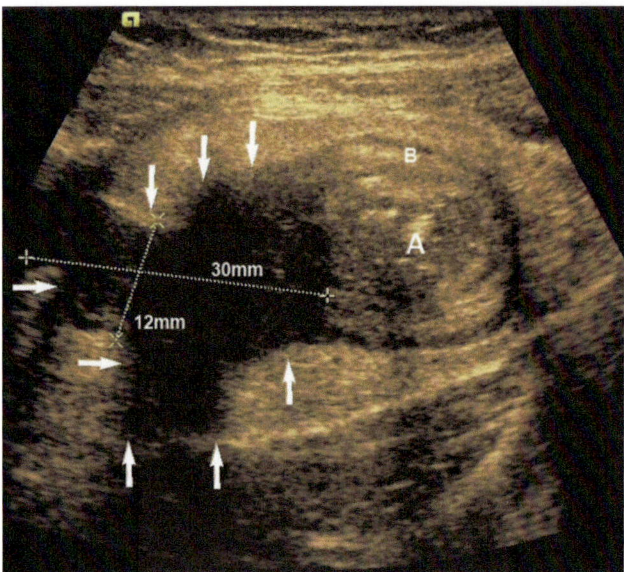

Fig. 20.6

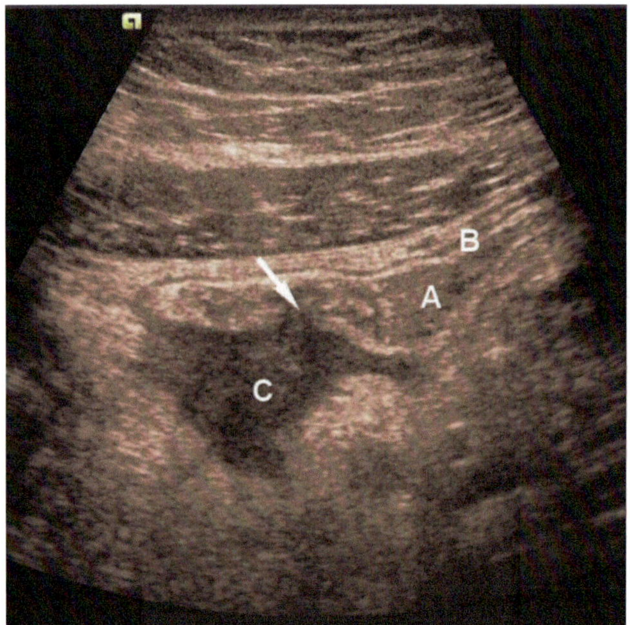

Fig. 20.7

standard. Sensitivity and specificity range between 90 % and 100 % [26, 31, 35, 36]. In a head-to-head comparison of ultrasound and CT scans, using only surgical findings as reference, no significant difference in sensitivity was detected (US 91 %, CT 86 %) [36]. Ultrasound lacks accuracy when detecting abdominal abscesses deep in the pelvis or retroperitoneal collections obscured by overlying bowel gas. One advantage of ultrasound is in the detection of small intraparietal or para-intestinal abscesses, which can be missed or misinterpreted as short fistulous tracts or hypoechoic lymph nodes in CT scans [37].

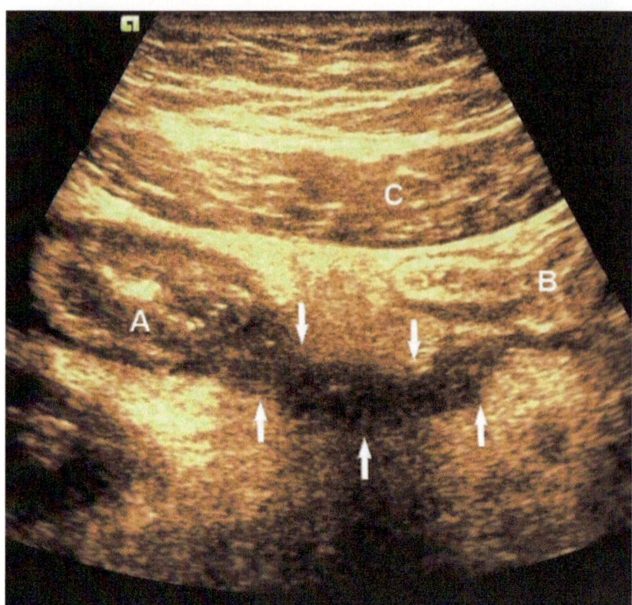

Fig. 20.8

Detection of Fistula

Fistulae either connect the gut with abdominal organs (e.g., enterovesical, enterovaginal, interenteric), reach the cutaneous surface (enterocutaneous), or end blindly in the mesentery (enteromensenteric). The most common fistulae are enteroenteric (50 %); these connect two bowel loops and often develop in the presence of stenosis (Fig. 20.8). Fistulae appear as hypoechoic ducts or hypoechoic areas arising from a thickened bowel wall.

Fistulae can show signs of air, debris, or intestinal material in the form of stationary or moving echoic spots [26, 35] (Fig. 20.9). The gold standard in fistulae detection is a surgical specimen. CT scan miss fistulae in up to 40 % of cases. Therefore, CT scans cannot be recommended as a reference standard in clinical trials [38]. The sensitivity and specificity of ultrasound in the detection of surgically proven fistulae varies between 70 and 87 % and 90 and 96 %, respectively [35, 39]. Fistulae connecting bowel segments often show a greater wall thickness and the wall stratification appears blurred with a loss of layer architecture [17].

Detection of Strictures

Strictures are a common cause of surgery in CD and develop in 21 % of patients with ileal disease and 8 % of those with ileocolic disease [40]. Significant strictures are marked by prestenotic bowel dilatation above 3 cm. The stricture itself shows a thickened bowel wall with an associated narrowed lumen (Fig. 20.10). Peristalsis in the prestenotic bowel loop is often increased [41]. The accuracy of the detection of bowel

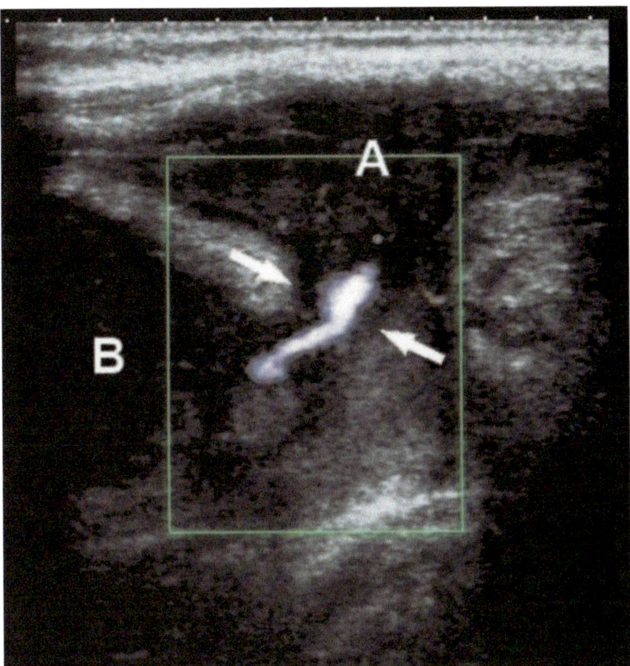

Fig. 20.9

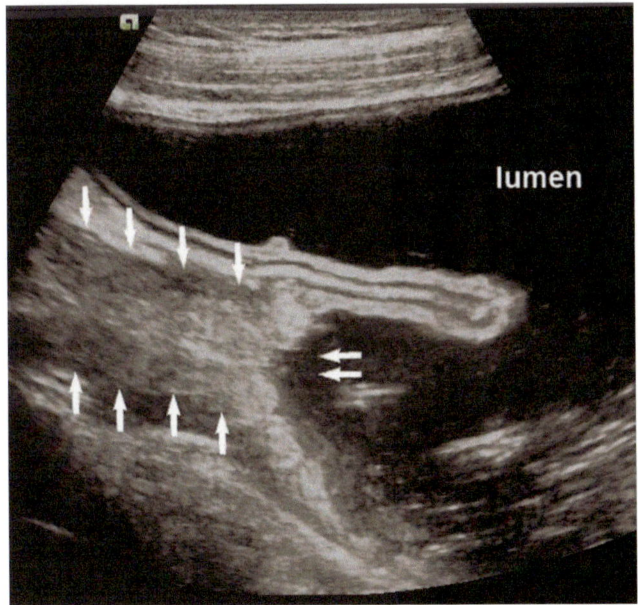

Fig. 20.10

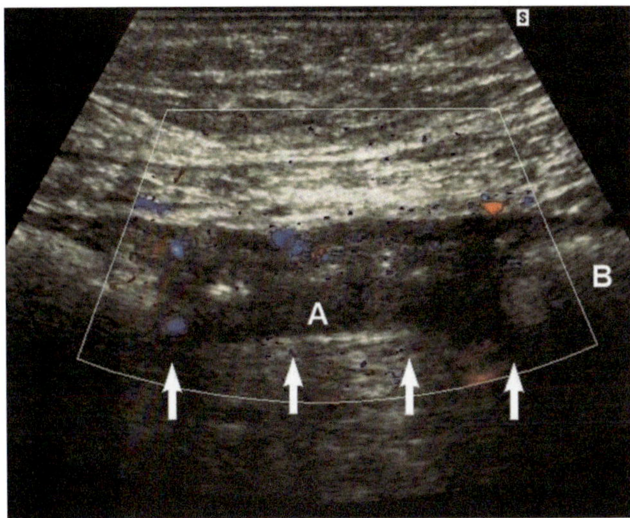

Fig. 20.11

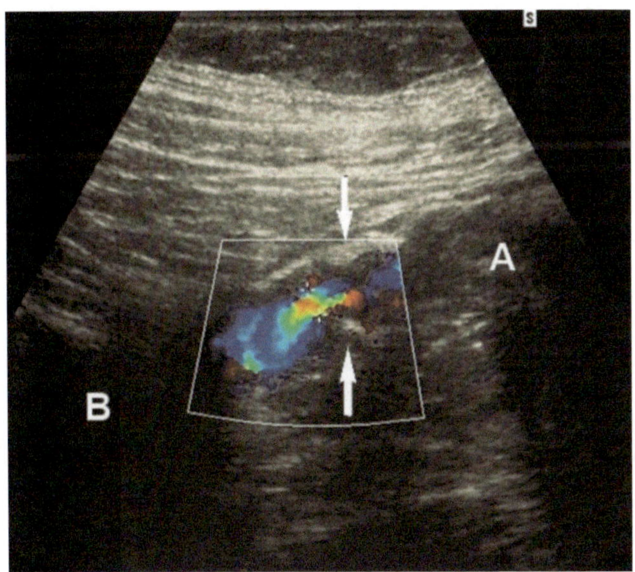

Fig. 20.12

wall strictures via transabdominal ultrasound varies between 74 and 91 % sensitivity and 93 and 100 % specificity compared to radiological or surgical findings [26, 28, 31, 35, 42]. The differentiation between inflammatory and fibrotic strictures is of major interest in clinical practice. Inflammatory changes can be targeted by anti-inflammatory agents, whereas fibrotic strictures are treated surgically or via endoscopic intervention. A stricture length of >30 mm increases the chance of inflammation [43]. The loss of stratification of the affected bowel wall has also been associated with inflammatory stenosis. The hypoechoic echo pattern is due to hyperemia and neovascularization related to the inflammatory response [39] (Fig. 20.11). Conversely, preserved bowel wall layers, especially with a pronounced third layer (submucosa), suggest that the stricture is fibrotic (Fig. 20.12). An increase in bowel wall thickness within the third layer seems to represent increased collagen deposition in the submucosa [44].

Extraluminal Findings

The extraluminal findings of CD which can be seen via ultrasound are ascites, lymphadenopathy, and mesenteric fat hypertrophy. Enlarged lymph nodes and free fluid are commonly seen in active CD but it has not been possible to show a correlation with disease activity [17]. Abnormalities of fat in the mesentery including adipose tissue hypertrophy and fat wrapping have long been recognized as characteristic features of Crohn's disease on surgical specimens. Mesenteric fat hypertrophy appears in transabdominal ultrasound as a hyperechoic area surrounding the bowel wall, predominantly along the mesenteric side of the bowel [45, 46]. Different studies have shown that mesenteric fatty alterations, as evaluated by CT scan or MRI, correlate with biological activity [47–49]. One of the few studies into mesenteric fatty alterations found via ultrasound showed a significant correlation to biochemical/clinical CD activity, the presence of internal fistulae, and increased bowel wall thickness [50]. However, prediction of clinical relapse based on the presence of mesenteric fat hypertrophy was not successful. There are few studies into extraluminal findings of CD via ultrasound. The clinical significance and implication of these findings need further investigation.

Detection of Postsurgical Recurrence

Postoperative recurrence after ileocolonic resection is a common feature of CD. The recurrence rates evaluated by endoscopy after 1 and 3 years are 73 % and 90 %, respectively [51–54]. The diagnostic gold standard for the detection of early signs of recurrence is conventional ileocolonoscopy, with the severity of the lesions graded using Rutgeert's score [54]. Numerous studies have evaluated noninvasive techniques for the detection of postoperative recurrence in CD. One approach is to measure the bowel wall thickness of the anastomosis after bowel resection via ultrasound. It has been shown that an increase in bowel wall thickness is not due to physiological healing of the anastomosis, because cancer patients did not show any increase in bowel wall thickness of the anastomosis [55]. Similar to the ultrasound findings in active CD, an increase in bowel wall thickness (>3–5 mm) can be interpreted as a recurrence of the disease. The sensitivity and specificity of ultrasound in the detection of postsurgical recurrence of CD is about 80 % and 85–100 %, respectively [55, 56]. A more recent study by Rispo et al. [57] used a cutoff level in bowel wall thickness of 5 mm to differentiate between mild and severe disease recurrence. A bowel wall thickness above 5 mm predicted a severe postsurgical recurrence with sensitivity and specificity of 94 % and 100 %, respectively. The author concluded that these methods were sufficiently accurate to detect a clinically significant postsurgical recurrence that would need specific treatment. Different studies have already stressed the value of ultrasound in the prediction of postsurgical recurrence in CD. In a study of 127 consecutive patients, 90 % of patient in the group with an unchanged or worsened bowel wall thickness in month 12 after the operation measured by transabdominal ultrasound developed clinical recurrence within 5 years [58]. Only 33 % of patients with improved bowel wall thickness relapsed over this same period. Similar data were shown a few years earlier by Maconi et al., evaluating bowel wall thickness before and 6 months after bowel resection [59].

Color/Power Doppler Ultrasound

As stated in current guidelines, color Doppler imaging increases the sensitivity and specificity of transabdominal ultrasound, in particular for CD limited to the ileum [60]. In particular, disease activity has been studied by visualizing the extent of bowel wall vascularity. The examination techniques using color/power Doppler ultrasound are:

- Semi quantitative documentation of the intensity of color signals and/or the analysis of Doppler curves obtained from the vessels detected within the bowel wall.
- Quantitative measurement of flow parameters of the superior and inferior mesenteric arteries.

Studies correlating clinical (CDAI) or biochemical (e.g., CRP/ESR) parameters with color/power Doppler ultrasound findings did not produce conclusive results. Numerous studies have described increased bowel wall vascularity more often in active than in quiescent CD, but these results rarely reached clinical significance [61–63]. On the other hand, recent studies have shown a significant correlation between endoscopic and color/power Doppler ultrasound activity scores in CD [64, 65]. The prognostic significance of color/power Doppler ultrasound findings was demonstrated by Ripolles [66]. Patients in clinical remission after treatment with residual hyperemia on sonographic examination (week 4) had an unfavorable clinical course compared with patients with no or barely visible residual hyperemia. In a prospective study by Paredes et al. ultrasound was used to assess changes (thickness and Doppler flow grade of the bowel wall) caused by biological therapy and its relationship with the clinical-biological response in 23 patients with CD. They found that sonographic changes were significantly more marked in patients who achieved clinical and biological response compared to those patients who did not respond to treatment [67].

In order to achieve optimal results in daily practice, it is essential to use the right color Doppler ultrasound settings. The settings should be optimized for slow flow detection (pulse repetition frequencies of 800–1500 Hz, wall filter of 40–50 Hz, maximal color signal gain immediately below the noise threshold). Color Doppler flow is considered present when color pixels persist throughout the examination. The blood flow can be confirmed by visualizing an arterial or venous flow pattern at the location of the color pixel on spectral analysis. Vascularity is graded subjectively as absent

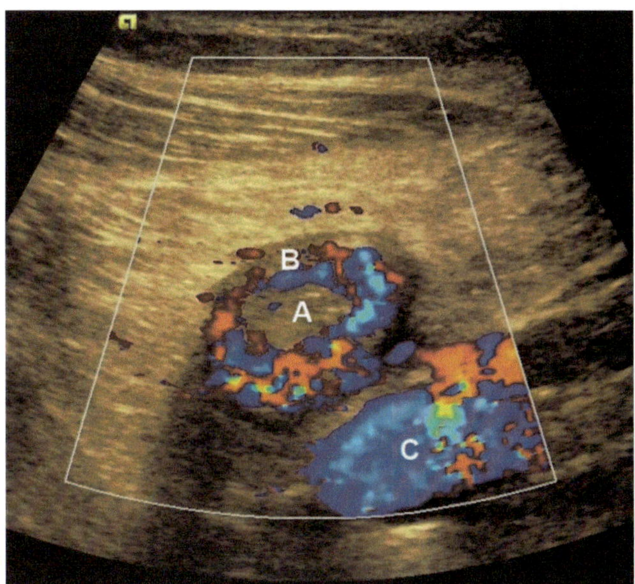

Fig. 20.13

(grade 0), barely visible (grade 1), or marked (grade 3) (Fig. 20.13). Another access to disease activity via color/power Doppler ultrasound is the analysis of quantitative parameters. In active disease, the end-diastolic blood flow in bowel wall vessels disproportionately increases, which leads to a drop in the resistance index. Power Doppler ultrasound has been suggested to improve the diagnostic accuracy of transabdominal ultrasound in discriminating inflammatory from fibrotic strictures [5, 19, 65].

The decreased resistance index in active CD has been described several times in the literature [61, 63, 68] (Fig. 20.14a and b). CD manly affects bowel segments supplied by the superior mesenteric artery (SMA). In active CD, the SMA flow volume was found to be greater than 500 ml/min and the resistance index was significantly lower than in the reference group with quiescent disease [69]. The pulsatility index of the SMA can also help predict a relapse in CD when it is repeatedly evaluated [70, 71]. The decrease in the pulsatility index of the SMA is associated with remission in CD. However, measuring the quantitative pulsed Doppler indices is time-consuming and highly demanding. Therefore, it still is not established in daily practice.

Special Ultrasound Method in Crohn's Disease

Small Bowel Contrast Ultrasound

The extent of Crohn's lesions, especially in the upper small bowel, is sometimes underestimated by transabdominal ultrasound because of the insufficient distention of the bowel lumen. An isosmolar solution containing a nondigestible, nonabsorbable, and non-fermentable hydrophilic macro molecule, such as polyethylene glycol (PEG), was used to distend the small bowel walls, which allowed for a more detailed assessment of the wall thickness and lumen diameter [72]. A follow-up study showed that the entire small intestine could be visualized on ultrasonography about 45 min after the ingestion of 600 ml or less of contrast solution without any significant side effects [73]. In daily practice, 300–500 ml of PEG is sufficient to achieve an optimal distention of the small bowel walls (Fig. 20.15). If stenosis is absent, the examination will be completed in 10–20 min. In comparison to small bowel follow through, SICUS reached a sensitivity of 72–100 % and specificity of 97–100 % in the detection of small bowel pathologies [3, 74–76]. False negative findings in the study by Cittadini et al. were mainly due to lymphoid hyperplasia, which is a feature of unknown significance in adults. As expected, the advantage of SICUS over conventional ultrasound was particularly clear in the detection of pathologies in the upper small bowel (jejunum: conventional ultrasound 80 % vs. SICUS 100 % detection rate) [77]. The sensitivity of identifying multiple strictures increased from 55 % to 78 % using SICUS [78] (Fig. 20.16a and b). In a recently published study, SICUS was able to detect all fistulae and stenosis initially diagnosed via CT [3]. Other convincing features of SICUS are a good interobserver agreement [72, 77, 79, 80] and ease of use for inexperienced ultrasound users, reaching even higher accuracy rates than those of an experienced examiner using conventional ultrasound [78]. SICUS has been the topic of several studies evaluating accuracy in predicting postsurgical recurrence [81–83]. A study on 40 patients with CD with previous bowel resection showed a sensitivity and specificity of 77 % and 94 % for transabdominal ultrasound and 82 % and 94 % for SICUS [81].

Endoanal and Perianal Ultrasound

Perianal disease is a common manifestation in complicated CD, occurring in 20–40 % of patients in the course of their disease [84]. Pelvic magnetic resonance imaging (MRI) and endoanal ultrasound are the established methods for the assessment of perianal inflammatory lesions in patients with CD. MRI and EAUS are especially recommended by German S3 Guidelines for CD in patients with perianal disease [85]. The combination of MRI and EAUS is capable of detecting perianal fistulae with a sensitivity of 100 % [86, 87]. These methods require specialized and fairly expensive equipment and experienced investigators. Furthermore, MRI is not applicable in patients with metallic clips or suffering from claustrophobia, and EAUS can be painful or impossible to perform in patients with anal stenosis. PAUS was introduced into clinical practice as an alternative. It can be performed using regular ultrasound probes [3.5–7.5 MHz]. The ultra-

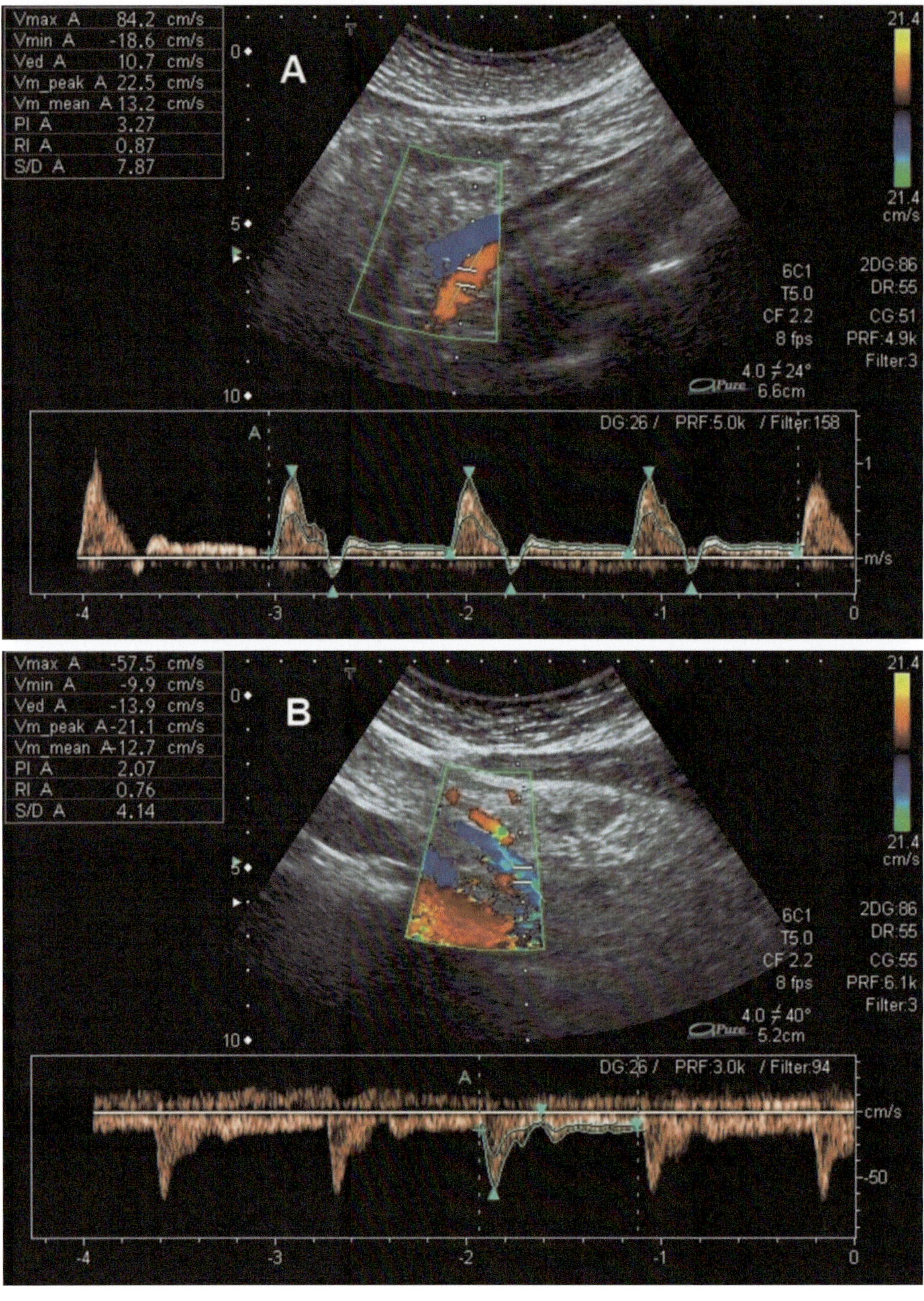

Fig. 20.14

sound probe is wrapped with a latex glove after applying contact gel on the surface of the probe. No patient preparation is required prior to the examination. Patient lies down in the left lateral decubitus position, and the ultrasound probe is then placed near the anal opening.

Further advantages of PAUS include its unproblematic use in patients with anal stenosis and the ability to examine the gluteal region, which is restricted in EAUS. PAUS is comparable in sensitivity and specificity to MRI and EAUS in the detection of perianal fistulae and/or abscesses [88–91].

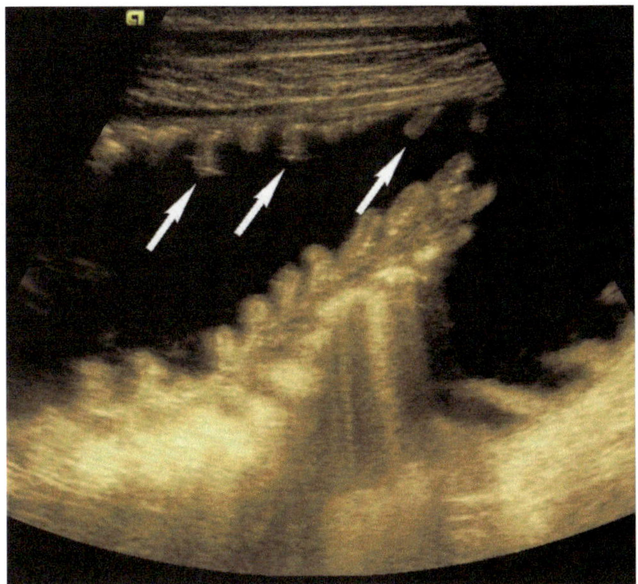

Fig. 20.15

Contrast Enhanced Ultrasound

Contrast enhanced ultrasound (CEUS) is the next logical step after color Doppler ultrasound in the assessment of bowel wall vascularization. The accuracy of power Doppler ultrasound is limited by tissue motion artifacts and a possible transmural vessel perfusion below the detection threshold [92]. CEUS combines second-generation ultrasound contrast-enhancing agents with low mechanical index real-time harmonic ultrasound. It permits a real-time visualization of the small vessels in the bowel wall with image contrast similar to that of computed tomography and MRI [93]. The absence of established CEUS parameters has led to the development of different semi quantitative and quantitative approaches to predict disease activity in CD. One study by Migaleddu et al. was highly recommended by the medical community [94]. It defined three major enhancement patterns: submucosal enhancement or transmural enhancement with an outward or inward flow direction. Using endoscopic and histologic findings as reference standards, CEUS showed higher performance than conventional ultrasound or color Doppler ultrasound in the detection of active disease (93.5 % sensitivity, 93.7 % specificity, and 93.6 % overall accuracy). Despite the impact of the study, the enhancement pattern remained a semi quantitative approach that is highly influenced by the subjective assessment of the ultrasound examiner. Using the increase in bowel wall enhancement after contrast application in relation to the baseline enhancement showed promising results. In a population of 61 patients, the sensitivity and specificity to predict moderate and severe disease were 96 % and 73 %, respectively [9].

Dynamic quantitative CEUS is currently the subject of scientific investigations in patients with CD. Three studies indicated that the time to peak in CEUS examinations could be a parameter worth measuring to evaluate disease activity. An increase in time to peak was connected to a decrease in clinical activity [10, 95]. Furthermore, Bataille et al. [96] found a negative correlation between histopathological score and the time to peak [97]. A more recent study quantitatively assessed microvascular activation in the thickened ileal walls of 54 patients with CD by using CEUS and evaluated its correlation with CDAI [98]. The authors analyzed the maximum peak intensity (MPI) and the wash-in slope coefficient (beta) and evaluated their correlation with the composite index of CD activity (CICDA), the CD activity index (CDAI), and the simplified endoscopic score for CD (SES-CD) for the terminal ileum. The sensitivity/specificity to detect active CD were 97 %/83 % for MPI and 86 %/83 % for beta coefficients. Both parameters significantly correlated with the CDAI ($p=0.0005, 0.0011$) and the endoscopic SES-CD ($p=0.0052, 0.0011$).

The differentiation of fibrotic and inflammatory strictures could be a beneficial application of CEUS in clinical practice, but there is still no established approach to solving this puzzle. One study focused on this question and evaluated the accuracy of several ultrasound parameters, especially of contrast-enhanced ultrasound, for evaluation of mural inflammation versus fibrostenonic changes in 25 patients with CD undergoing elective bowel resection [99]. Histopathology was used as reference. When the pathology score was dichotomized into two groups (inflammatory and fibrostenotic) 23 out of 28 stenoses were correctly classified via ultrasound, with substantial agreement (kappa=0.632). There was a good correlation between the sonographic and pathology scores, both inflammation (Spearman's rank, $r=0.53$) and fibrostenosis (Spearman's rank, $r=0.50$). Thus, ultrasound, including CEUS is a useful tool for distinguishing inflammatory lesions from fibrostenotic ones in CD and small bowel follow-through (SBFT) is regarded obsolete due to the high radiation exposure, particularly in children with IBD Sauer CG, Inflamm Bow dis 2011.

CEUS was also evaluated in the context of postoperative recurrence of CD [100]. Classic ultrasound parameters, such as wall thickness >3 mm and color Doppler flow revealed an accuracy of 88.3 % for recurrence detection compared to the endoscopic results. A sonographic score of 2, including thickness >5 mm or contrast enhancement >46 %, improved the diagnosis of endoscopic recurrence a sensitivity, specificity and accuracy of 98 %, 100 % and 98.3 %, respectively. The use of CEUS in the detection and localization of fistulae and abscesses [101] needs further studies (Fig. 20.17a and b).

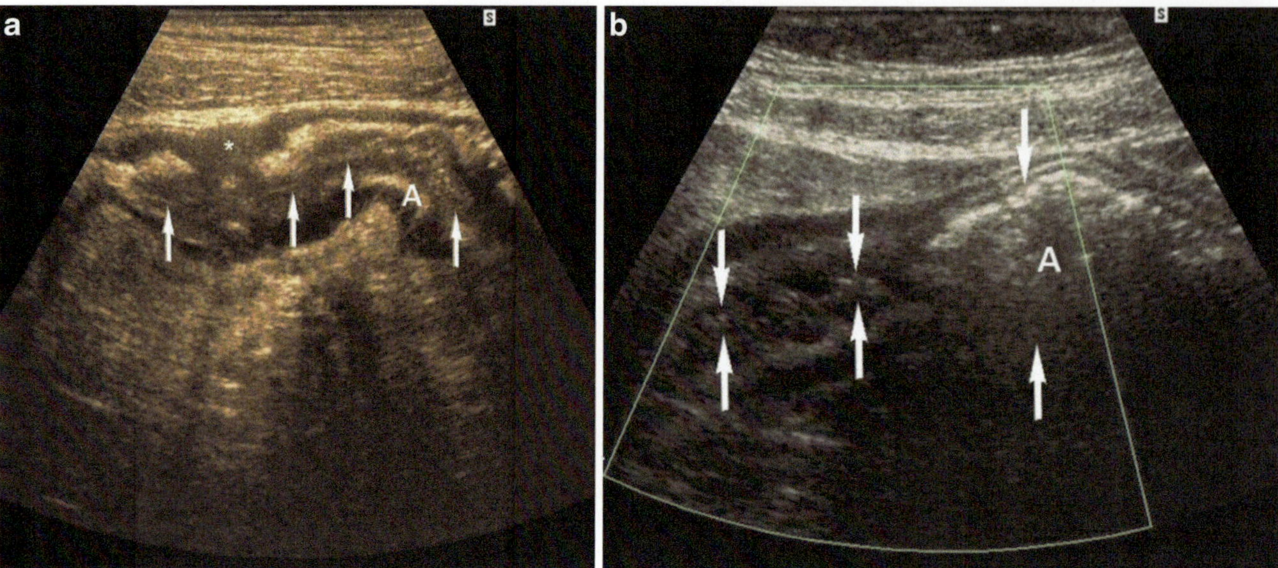

Fig. 20.16

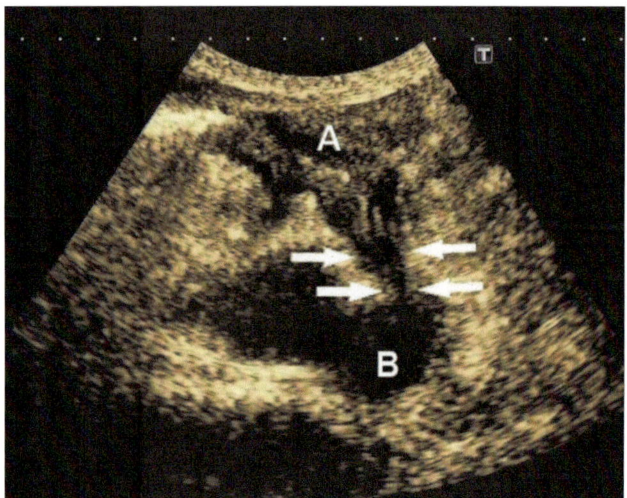

Fig. 20.17

Ulcerative Colitis

The regions of interest in patients with ulcerative colitis (UC) are far more accessible via endoscopy than in patients with CD. Most cases see a continuous inflammation from the anus that can extend up to the cecum. Rectal sparing and backwash ileitis can be detected in rare cases of UC. Early and mild cases of UC can show unspecific signs of an inner hypoechoic layer. It has been postulated that the hypoechoic layer represents the endoscopic findings of the swollen mucosa. In more severe to fulminant cases, a transmural bowel wall thickening similar to CD has been described. Normally the bowel wall stratification is preserved [17]. In active UC, the thickened mucosa can be explained by the round cell infiltration in the lamina propria, whereas the submucosa swells with oedema development. Unfortunately, no correlation between sonographic activity parameters of UC (wall thickness, symmetry of thickness, transmural reaction, and extraluminal findings, e.g., more than two lymph nodes) and endoscopic disease activity (Colitis activity index, CAI) has been found [17]. Two studies from Parente et al. [102, 103] contradict these common findings. These studies suggest that an ultrasound score based on bowel wall thickness and intramural blood flow, graded via color Doppler ultrasound, can be used as a surrogate of colonoscopy in assessing the short-term response of severe forms of UC to therapy. Furthermore, it was possible to using three-month ultrasound results to predict the outcome at 15 months after steroid treatment. These are very interesting data which need to be reproduced in further studies before transabdominal ultrasound can be recommended more strongly in the management of UC. Two studies have evaluated the extent of the inflammation in UC measured via ultrasound. The sensitivity varied according to the bowel segment. The best results were achieved in the left colon (>95 %) [104, 105].

A more recent study evaluated the usefulness of colonic ultrasonography in assessing the extent and activity of disease in 60 pediatric ulcerative colitis cases with suspected disease flare-up and compared ultrasound findings with clinical and endoscopic features [106]. Multiple regression analysis revealed that ultrasound measurements with an independent predictive value of severity at endoscopy were increased bowel wall thickness ($p<0.0008$), increased vascularity ($p<0.002$), loss of haustrae ($p=0.031$), and loss of stratification of the bowel wall ($p=0.021$). The ultrasound score strongly correlated with clinical ($r=0.94$) and endoscopic activity ($r=0.90$) of disease ($p<0.0001$).

A quantitative assessment of power Doppler indices can help distinguish between active and inactive disease or can be used as a parameter to evaluate the response to treatment. The mean blood flow volume, mean peak systolic and end diastolic velocity in the inferior mesenteric artery were significantly higher in patients with active rather than inactive UC [107].

Contrast-enhanced ultrasound (CEUS) in combination with perfusion assessment using specific quantification software was evaluated in 15 patients with ulcerative colitis and results were compared with endoscopic findings [108]. The study revealed a strong negative correlation between the ratio TTP (s)/Peak (%) ($r=-0.761$, $p<0.01$). There was no significant relationship between CRP and the histopathological scoring or CEUS parameters. Thus, quantitative evaluation with CEUS may provide a simple method for assessment of inflammatory activity in UC.

Detection of Primary Sclerosing Disease via Ultrasound

Primary sclerosing cholangitis (PSC) is a chronic liver disease that is characterized by inflammation, fibrosis, and the destruction of intrahepatic and extrahepatic bile ducts. PSC is the most common form of chronic inflammatory liver disease in IBD patients, with a prevalence of up to 8% [109, 110]. The vast majority of PSC patients (70–90%) have, or subsequently will develop, an inflammatory bowel disease [109, 111]. The detection of enlarged perihilar lymph nodes has been identified as a highly predictive indicator for the presence of PSC [112, 113]. Ultrasound has been proposed as a screening tool for PSC in IBD patients. In combination with serological makers, ultrasound allows a better selection of patients for invasive procedures than ERC.

Perspective

The transmural aspect of CD in imaging is only partially understood. This kind of "extra" information is available via ultrasound and MRI and should have an impact on daily treatment decisions. A lot of questions have to be unraveled, e.g., which bowel wall findings predict Crohn's complications or response to treatment? A cooperation of experts in gastroenterology, radiology, and pathology will hopefully resolve this.

Quantification of CEUS findings will be an important step in the development of ultrasound techniques in inflammatory bowel disease. An objective assessment with clear findings will replace interobserver error. Studies are currently taking place and the primary clinical and prognostic data are still under investigation. Although the quantitative CEUS is a promising tool in monitoring patients with IBD, echo contrast agents are costly and quantitative evaluation of CEUS is time consuming. In contrast, Doppler techniques (PW, CDI, and PDI) are cost-effective and well established, but have some limitations with the evaluation of micro vessels.

A novel ultrasound Doppler technique that captures the extraordinarily slow velocity flow characteristic of tiny blood vessels, the so-called "Superb Micro-Vascular Imaging" (SMI), captures the flow at high resolution, high frame rates with minimal motion artifact and may contribute to the assessment und monitoring of inflammatory bowel activity in patients with IBD (Fig. 20.18a and b).

Conclusion

Ultrasound is crucial in the detection and management of patients with CD. It is the only noninvasive, risk-free, and real-time method for assessing the important features in CD patients, from intestinal activity to postsurgical recurrence. In the hands of an experienced investigator, ultrasound is a

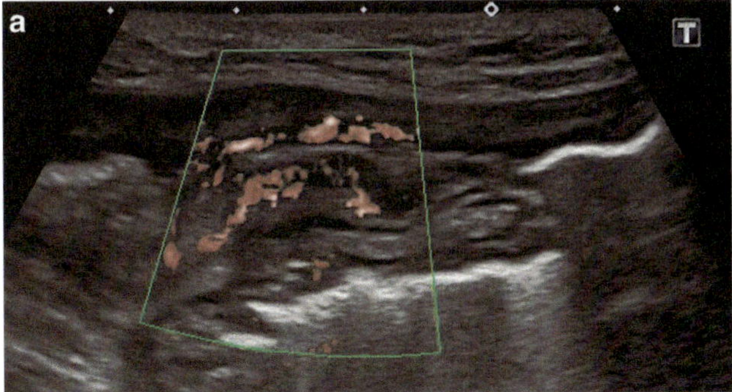

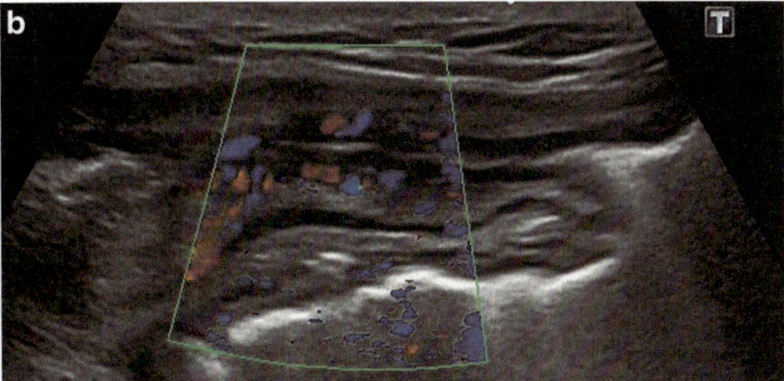

Fig. 20.18

powerful technique to guide the treatment of CD directly from the patient's bedside. Modern high frequency transducers offer the highest local resolution in bowel imaging today. Ultrasound can be used to assess extraluminal findings and complications in CD that can be missed by endoscopy or other imaging techniques. Limitations of the normal transabdominal B-mode ultrasound can be overcome by the use of extended ultrasound features (e.g., color Doppler ultrasound) or special ultrasound methods (e.g., CEUS or SICUS). Intestinal inflammatory activity can be visualized via color Doppler ultrasound or CEUS. Abscess demarcation can also be supported by these ultrasound techniques. SICUS is a useful tool in the detection of pathologies in the upper small bowel region. In addition SICUS, offers a real-time assessment and grading of intestinal stenosis. Endoanal and PAUS have a comparable accuracy to MRI in the detection of perianal inflammatory pathologies in CD. Thus far, mucosal healing has been defined endoscopically as the absence of ulcers. Ultrasound findings include transmural and extramural events indicating the state of the disease independent of clinical markers. For healing beyond superficial markers, ultrasound methods seem to be indispensable for the development and evaluation of actual and future effective treatment regimens.

In order to support the use of modern ultrasound techniques in the clinical practice and to sustain the quality of the examinations, the ultrasound simulator (Schallware GmbH, Berlin, *Germany*) has been introduced into the teaching routine. The ultrasound simulator is a patient dummy, which can be examined through a dummy ultrasound probe. The ultrasound images are read out of 3D-volumes recorded from true patients according to the probe position and displayed onto a screen. The 3D color Doppler recordings are also used and support the diagnostic purpose, accordingly. Even CEUS examinations can be simulated by the recordings of different contrast phases. Special teaching modules for chronic inflammatory bowel diseases have been prepared. Training on these modules (e.g., CD) is helpful for acquiring specific ultrasound skills in IBD, especially to detect IBD associated complications and to monitor therapeutic response to treatment [114, 115]. In order to achieve the best quality in bowel sonography, the investigator should be taught those specified sonographic techniques.

In conclusion, transabdominal ultrasound is a cost-effective, noninvasive tool in patients with IBD and is recommended as diagnostic first line tool in the assessment of patients with IBD, irrespective of their clinical symptoms and disease activity [12]. Important advantages of IBD ultrasonography are that it avoids unnecessary exposure to the radiation (CT and MRT) and can be performed uncritically in patients with renal and liver insufficiency or contrast agent allergy. It has a high diagnostic accuracy in detection of fistulae and abscesses, furthermore, monitoring disease progression and treatment response. Techniques such as color Doppler imaging and CEUS are helpful imaging maneuvers determining the disease activity and its associated complications. Other special ultrasound methods including SICUS, EUS, PAUS, and REUS are also helpful in determining the disease course and identifying complications in patients with IBD.

References

1. Jaffe TA, Gaca AM, Delaney S, Yoshizumi TT, Toncheva G, Nguyen G, et al. Radiation doses from small-bowel follow-through and abdominopelvic MDCT in Crohn's disease. AJR Am J Roentgenol. 2007;189(5):1015–22.
2. Desmond AN, O'Regan K, Curran C, McWilliams S, Fitzgerald T, Maher MM, et al. Crohn's disease: factors associated with exposure to high levels of diagnostic radiation. Gut. 2008;57(11): 1524–9.
3. Chatu S, Pilcher J, Saxena SK, Fry DH, Pollok RC. Diagnostic accuracy of small intestine ultrasonography using an oral contrast agent in Crohn's disease: comparative study from the UK. Clin Radiol. 2012;67(6):553–9.
4. Levi Z, Fraser E, Krongrad R, Hazazi R, Benjaminov O, Meyerovitch J, et al. Factors associated with radiation exposure in patients with inflammatory bowel disease. Aliment Pharmacol Ther. 2009;30(11–12):1128–36.
5. Horsthuis K, Bipat S, Bennink RJ, Stoker J. Inflammatory bowel disease diagnosed with US, MR, scintigraphy, and CT: meta-analysis of prospective studies. Radiology. 2008;247(1):64–79.
6. Martinez MJ, Ripolles T, Paredes JM, Blanc E, Marti-Bonmati L. Assessment of the extension and the inflammatory activity in Crohn's disease: comparison of ultrasound and MRI. Abdom Imaging. 2009;34(2):141–8.
7. Fraquelli M, Sarno A, Girelli C, Laudi C, Buscarini E, Villa C, et al. Reproducibility of bowel ultrasonography in the evaluation of Crohn's disease. Dig Liver Dis. 2008;40(11):860–6.
8. Kratzer W, Foeller T, Kaechele V, Reinshagen M, Tirpitz CV, Haenle MM. Intestinal wall vascularisation in Crohn's disease. Z Gastroenterol. 2004;42(9):973–8.
9. Ripolles T, Martinez MJ, Paredes JM, Blanc E, Flors L, Delgado F. Crohn disease: correlation of findings at contrast-enhanced US with severity at endoscopy. Radiology. 2009;253(1):241–8.
10. Quaia E, Migaleddu V, Baratella E, Pizzolato R, Rossi A, Grotto M, et al. The diagnostic value of small bowel wall vascularity after sulfur hexafluoride-filled microbubble injection in patients with Crohn's disease. Correlation with the therapeutic effectiveness of specific anti-inflammatory treatment. Eur J Radiol. 2009;69(3): 438–44.
11. Rigazio C, Ercole E, Laudi C, Daperno M, Lavagna A, Crocella L, et al. Abdominal bowel ultrasound can predict the risk of surgery in Crohn's disease: proposal of an ultrasonographic score. Scand J Gastroenterol. 2009;44(5):585–93.
12. Preiss JC, Bokemeyer B, Buhr HJ, Dignass A, Hauser W, Hartmann F, et al. Updated German clinical practice guideline on "Diagnosis and treatment of Crohn's disease" 2014. Z Gastroenterol. 2014;52(12):1431–84.
13. Panes J, Bouhnik Y, Reinisch W, Stoker J, Taylor SA, Baumgart DC, et al. Imaging techniques for assessment of inflammatory bowel disease: joint ECCO and ESGAR evidence-based consensus guidelines. J Crohns Colitis. 2013;7(7):556–85.
14. Holt S, Samuel E. Grey scale ultrasound in Crohn's disease. Gut. 1979;20(7):590–5.

15. Migaleddu V, Quaia E, Scano D, Virgilio G. Inflammatory activity in Crohn disease: ultrasound findings. Abdom Imaging. 2008; 33(5):589–97.
16. Parente F, Greco S, Molteni M, Anderloni A, Bianchi Porro G. Imaging inflammatory bowel disease using bowel ultrasound. Eur J Gastroenterol Hepatol. 2005;17(3):283–91.
17. Dietrich CF. Significance of abdominal ultrasound in inflammatory bowel disease. Dig Dis. 2009;27(4):482–93.
18. Maconi G, Bolzoni E, Giussani A, Friedman AB, Duca P. Accuracy and cost of diagnostic strategies for patients with suspected Crohn's disease. J Crohns Colitis. 2014;8(12):1684–92.
19. Fraquelli M, Colli A, Casazza G, Paggi S, Colucci A, Massironi S, et al. Role of US in detection of Crohn disease: meta-analysis. Radiology. 2005;236(1):95–101.
20. Chiorean L, Schreiber-Dietrich D, Braden B, Cui X, Dietrich CF. Transabdominal ultrasound for standardized measurement of bowel wall thickness in normal children and those with Crohn's disease. Med Ultrason. 2014;16(4):319–24.
21. Hata J, Haruma K, Yamanaka H, Fujimura J, Yoshihara M, Shimamoto T, et al. Ultrasonographic evaluation of the bowel wall in inflammatory bowel disease: comparison of in vivo and in vitro studies. Abdom Imaging. 1994;19(5):395–9.
22. Futagami Y, Haruma K, Hata J, Fujimura J, Tani H, Okamoto E, et al. Development and validation of an ultrasonographic activity index of Crohn's disease. Eur J Gastroenterol Hepatol. 1999; 11(9):1007–12.
23. Allgayer H, Braden B, Dietrich CF. Transabdominal ultrasound in inflammatory bowel disease. Conventional and recently developed techniques—update. Med Ultrason. 2011;13(4):302–13.
24. Minderhoud IM, Samsom M, Oldenburg B. What predicts mucosal inflammation in Crohn's disease patients? Inflamm Bowel Dis. 2007;13(12):1567–72.
25. Parente F, Greco S, Molteni M, Cucino C, Maconi G, Sampietro GM, et al. Role of early ultrasound in detecting inflammatory intestinal disorders and identifying their anatomical location within the bowel. Aliment Pharmacol Ther. 2003;18(10): 1009–16.
26. Maconi G, Parente F, Bollani S, Cesana B, Bianchi Porro G. Abdominal ultrasound in the assessment of extent and activity of Crohn's disease: clinical significance and implication of bowel wall thickening. Am J Gastroenterol. 1996;91(8):1604–9.
27. Brignola C, Belloli C, Iannone P, De Simone G, Corbelli C, Levorato M, et al. Comparison of scintigraphy with indium-111 leukocyte scan and ultrasonography in assessment of X-ray-demonstrated lesions of Crohn's disease. Dig Dis Sci. 1993;38(3): 433–7.
28. Parente F, Maconi G, Bianchi Porro G. Bowel ultrasound in Crohn disease: current role and future applications. Scand J Gastroenterol. 2002;37(8):871–6.
29. Chiorean L, Schreiber-Dietrich D, Braden B, Cui XW, Buchhorn R, Chang JM, et al. Ultrasonographic imaging of inflammatory bowel disease in pediatric patients. World J Gastroenterol. 2015; 21(17):5231–41.
30. Farmer RG, Whelan G, Fazio VW. Long-term follow-up of patients with Crohn's disease. Relationship between the clinical pattern and prognosis. Gastroenterology. 1985;88(6):1818–25.
31. Neye H, Ensberg D, Rauh P, Peitz U, Monkemuller K, Treiber G, et al. Impact of high-resolution transabdominal ultrasound in the diagnosis of complications of Crohn's disease. Scand J Gastroenterol. 2010;45(6):690–5.
32. Hirche TO, Russler J, Schroder O, Schuessler G, Kappeser P, Caspary WF, et al. The value of routinely performed ultrasonography in patients with Crohn disease. Scand J Gastroenterol. 2002;37(10):1178–83.
33. Maconi G, Sampietro GM, Russo A, Bollani S, Cristaldi M, Parente F, et al. The vascularity of internal fistulae in Crohn's disease: an in vivo power Doppler ultrasonography assessment. Gut. 2002;50(4):496–500.
34. Tarjan Z, Toth G, Gyorke T, Mester A, Karlinger K, Mako EK. Ultrasound in Crohn's disease of the small bowel. Eur J Radiol. 2000;35(3):176–82.
35. Gasche C, Moser G, Turetschek K, Schober E, Moeschl P, Oberhuber G. Transabdominal bowel sonography for the detection of intestinal complications in Crohn's disease. Gut. 1999;44(1):112–7.
36. Maconi G, Sampietro GM, Parente F, Pompili G, Russo A, Cristaldi M, et al. Contrast radiology, computed tomography and ultrasonography in detecting internal fistulas and intra-abdominal abscesses in Crohn's disease: a prospective comparative study. Am J Gastroenterol. 2003;98(7):1545–55.
37. Cybulsky IJ, Tam P. Intra-abdominal abscesses in Crohn's disease. Am Surg. 1990;56(11):678–82.
38. Michelassi F, Stella M, Balestracci T, Giuliante F, Marogna P, Block GE. Incidence, diagnosis, and treatment of enteric and colorectal fistulae in patients with Crohn's disease. Ann Surg. 1993;218(5):660–6.
39. Maconi G, Carsana L, Fociani P, Sampietro GM, Ardizzone S, Cristaldi M, et al. Small bowel stenosis in Crohn's disease: clinical, biochemical and ultrasonographic evaluation of histological features. Aliment Pharmacol Ther. 2003;18(7):749–56.
40. Maconi G, Radice E, Greco S, Bianchi Porro G. Bowel ultrasound in Crohn's disease. Best Pract Res Clin Gastroenterol. 2006;20(1): 93–112.
41. Ko YT, Lim JH, Lee DH, Lee HW, Lim JW. Small bowel obstruction: sonographic evaluation. Radiology. 1993;188(3):649–53.
42. Kohn A, Cerro P, Milite G, De Angelis E, Prantera C. Prospective evaluation of transabdominal bowel sonography in the diagnosis of intestinal obstruction in Crohn's disease: comparison with plain abdominal film and small bowel enteroclysis. Inflamm Bowel Dis. 1999;5(3):153–7.
43. Dietrich CF, Jedrzejczyk M, Ignee A. Sonographic assessment of splanchnic arteries and the bowel wall. Eur J Radiol. 2007;64(2): 202–12.
44. Geboes KP, Cabooter L, Geboes K. Contribution of morphology for the comprehension of mechanisms of fibrosis in inflammatory enterocolitis. Acta Gastroenterol Belg. 2000;63(4):371–6.
45. Di Mizio R, Maconi G, Romano S, D'Amario F, Bianchi Porro G, Grassi R. Small bowel Crohn disease: sonographic features. Abdom Imaging. 2004;29(1):23–35.
46. Sarrazin J, Wilson SR. Manifestations of Crohn disease at US. Radiographics. 1996;16(3):499–520. discussion -1.
47. Colombel JF, Solem CA, Sandborn WJ, Booya F, Loftus Jr EV, Harmsen WS, et al. Quantitative measurement and visual assessment of ileal Crohn's disease activity by computed tomography enterography: correlation with endoscopic severity and C reactive protein. Gut. 2006;55(11):1561–7.
48. Maccioni F, Viscido A, Broglia L, Marrollo M, Masciangelo R, Caprilli R, et al. Evaluation of Crohn disease activity with magnetic resonance imaging. Abdom Imaging. 2000;25(3):219–28.
49. Booya F, Fletcher JG, Huprich JE, Barlow JM, Johnson CD, Fidler JL, et al. Active Crohn disease: CT findings and interobserver agreement for enteric phase CT enterography. Radiology. 2006;241(3):787–95.
50. Maconi G, Greco S, Duca P, Ardizzone S, Massari A, Cassinotti A, et al. Prevalence and clinical significance of sonographic evidence of mesenteric fat alterations in Crohn's disease. Inflamm Bowel Dis. 2008;14(11):1555–61.
51. Rutgeerts P. Strategies in the prevention of post-operative recurrence in Crohn's disease. Best Pract Res Clin Gastroenterol. 2003;17(1):63–73.
52. Olaison G, Smedh K, Sjodahl R. Natural course of Crohn's disease after ileocolic resection: endoscopically visualised ileal ulcers preceding symptoms. Gut. 1992;33(3):331–5.

53. Rutgeerts P, Geboes K, Vantrappen G, Kerremans R, Coenegrachts JL, Coremans G. Natural history of recurrent Crohn's disease at the ileocolonic anastomosis after curative surgery. Gut. 1984; 25(6):665–72.
54. Rutgeerts P, Geboes K, Vantrappen G, Beyls J, Kerremans R, Hiele M. Predictability of the postoperative course of Crohn's disease. Gastroenterology. 1990;99(4):956–63.
55. Andreoli A, Cerro P, Falasco G, Giglio LA, Prantera C. Role of ultrasonography in the diagnosis of postsurgical recurrence of Crohn's disease. Am J Gastroenterol. 1998;93(7):1117–21.
56. DiCandio G, Mosca F, Campatelli A, Bianchini M, D'Elia F, Dellagiovampaola C. Sonographic detection of postsurgical recurrence of Crohn disease. AJR Am J Roentgenol. 1986;146(3): 523–6.
57. Rispo A, Bucci L, Pesce G, Sabbatini F, de Palma GD, Grassia R, et al. Bowel sonography for the diagnosis and grading of postsurgical recurrence of Crohn's disease. Inflamm Bowel Dis. 2006;12(6):486–90.
58. Parente F, Sampietro GM, Molteni M, Greco S, Anderloni A, Sposito C, et al. Behaviour of the bowel wall during the first year after surgery is a strong predictor of symptomatic recurrence of Crohn's disease: a prospective study. Aliment Pharmacol Ther. 2004;20(9):959–68.
59. Maconi G, Sampietro GM, Cristaldi M, Danelli PG, Russo A, Bianchi Porro G, et al. Preoperative characteristics and postoperative behavior of bowel wall on risk of recurrence after conservative surgery in Crohn's disease: a prospective study. Ann Surg. 2001;233(3):345–52.
60. Van Assche G, Dignass A, Reinisch W, van der Woude CJ, Sturm A, De Vos M, et al. The second European evidence-based consensus on the diagnosis and management of Crohn's disease: special situations. J Crohns Colitis. 2010;4(1):63–101.
61. Heyne R, Rickes S, Bock P, Schreiber S, Wermke W, Lochs H. Non-invasive evaluation of activity in inflammatory bowel disease by power Doppler sonography. Z Gastroenterol. 2002;40(3):171–5.
62. Spalinger J, Patriquin H, Miron MC, Marx G, Herzog D, Dubois J, et al. Doppler US in patients with Crohn disease: vessel density in the diseased bowel reflects disease activity. Radiology. 2000;217(3):787–91.
63. Esteban JM, Maldonado L, Sanchiz V, Minguez M, Benages A. Activity of Crohn's disease assessed by colour Doppler ultrasound analysis of the affected loops. Eur Radiol. 2001;11(8): 1423–8.
64. Neye H, Voderholzer W, Rickes S, Weber J, Wermke W, Lochs H. Evaluation of criteria for the activity of Crohn's disease by power Doppler sonography. Dig Dis. 2004;22(1):67–72.
65. Drews BH, Barth TF, Hanle MM, Akinli AS, Mason RA, Muche R, et al. Comparison of sonographically measured bowel wall vascularity, histology, and disease activity in Crohn's disease. Eur Radiol. 2009;19(6):1379–86.
66. Ripolles T, Martinez MJ, Barrachina MM. Crohn's disease and color Doppler sonography: response to treatment and its relationship with long-term prognosis. J Clin Ultrasound. 2008; 36(5):267–72.
67. Paredes JM, Ripolles T, Cortes X, Martinez MJ, Barrachina M, Gomez F, et al. Abdominal sonographic changes after antibody to tumor necrosis factor (anti-TNF) alpha therapy in Crohn's Disease. Dig Dis Sci. 2010;55(2):404–10.
68. Nuernberg D, Ignee A, Dietrich CF. Current status of ultrasound in gastroenterology—bowel and upper gastrointestinal tract—part 2. Z Gastroenterol. 2008;46(4):355–66.
69. Yekeler E, Danalioglu A, Movasseghi B, Yilmaz S, Karaca C, Kaymakoglu S, et al. Crohn disease activity evaluated by Doppler ultrasonography of the superior mesenteric artery and the affected small-bowel segments. J Ultrasound Med. 2005;24(1):59–65.
70. Ludwig D. Doppler sonography in inflammatory bowel disease. Z Gastroenterol. 2004;42(9):1059–65.
71. Ludwig D, Wiener S, Bruning A, Schwarting K, Jantschek G, Stange EF. Mesenteric blood flow is related to disease activity and risk of relapse in Crohn's disease: a prospective follow-up study. Am J Gastroenterol. 1999;94(10):2942–50.
72. Pallotta N, Tomei E, Viscido A, Calabrese E, Marcheggiano A, Caprilli R, et al. Small intestine contrast ultrasonography: an alternative to radiology in the assessment of small bowel disease. Inflamm Bowel Dis. 2005;11(2):146–53.
73. Pallotta N, Baccini F, Corazziari E. Small intestine contrast ultrasonography. J Ultrasound Med. 2000;19(1):21–6.
74. Pallotta N, Baccini F, Corazziari E. Small intestine contrast ultrasonography (SICUS) in the diagnosis of small intestine lesions. Ultrasound Med Biol. 2001;27(3):335–41.
75. Cittadini G, Giasotto V, Garlaschi G, de Cicco E, Gallo A, Cittadini G. Transabdominal ultrasonography of the small bowel after oral administration of a non-absorbable anechoic solution: comparison with barium enteroclysis. Clin Radiol. 2001;56(3): 225–30.
76. Pallotta N, Civitelli F, Di Nardo G, Vincoli G, Aloi M, Viola F, et al. Small intestine contrast ultrasonography in pediatric Crohn's disease. J Pediatr. 2013;163(3):778–84.e1.
77. Parente F, Greco S, Molteni M, Anderloni A, Sampietro GM, Danelli PG, et al. Oral contrast enhanced bowel ultrasonography in the assessment of small intestine Crohn's disease. A prospective comparison with conventional ultrasound, X ray studies, and ileocolonoscopy. Gut. 2004;53(11):1652–7.
78. Calabrese E, La Seta F, Buccellato A, Virdone R, Pallotta N, Corazziari E, et al. Crohn's disease: a comparative prospective study of transabdominal ultrasonography, small intestine contrast ultrasonography, and small bowel enema. Inflamm Bowel Dis. 2005;11(2):139–45.
79. Levine A, Koletzko S, Turner D, Escher JC, Cucchiara S, de Ridder L, et al. ESPGHAN revised porto criteria for the diagnosis of inflammatory bowel disease in children and adolescents. J Pediatr Gastroenterol Nutr. 2014;58(6):795–806.
80. Migaleddu V, Quaia E, Scanu D, Carla S, Bertolotto M, Campisi G, et al. Inflammatory activity in Crohn's disease: CE-US. Abdom Imaging. 2011;36(2):142–8.
81. Castiglione F, Bucci L, Pesce G, De Palma GD, Camera L, Cipolletta F, et al. Oral contrast-enhanced sonography for the diagnosis and grading of postsurgical recurrence of Crohn's disease. Inflamm Bowel Dis. 2008;14(9):1240–5.
82. Pallotta N, Giovannone M, Pezzotti P, Gigliozzi A, Barberani F, Piacentino D, et al. Ultrasonographic detection and assessment of the severity of Crohn's disease recurrence after ileal resection. BMC Gastroenterol. 2010;10:69.
83. Biancone L, Calabrese E, Petruzziello C, Onali S, Caruso A, Palmieri G, et al. Wireless capsule endoscopy and small intestine contrast ultrasonography in recurrence of Crohn's disease. Inflamm Bowel Dis. 2007;13(10):1256–65.
84. Sandborn WJ, Fazio VW, Feagan BG, Hanauer SB. American Gastroenterological Association Clinical Practice C. AGA technical review on perianal Crohn's disease. Gastroenterology. 2003;125(5):1508–30.
85. Schreyer AG, Ludwig D, Koletzko S, Hoffmann JC, Preiss JC, Zeitz M, et al. Updated German S3-guideline regarding the diagnosis of Crohn's disease—implementation of radiological modalities. Rofo. 2010;182(2):116–21.
86. Orsoni P, Barthet M, Portier F, Panuel M, Desjeux A, Grimaud JC. Prospective comparison of endosonography, magnetic resonance imaging and surgical findings in anorectal fistula and abscess complicating Crohn's disease. Br J Surg. 1999;86(3):360–4.
87. Schwartz DA, Wiersema MJ, Dudiak KM, Fletcher JG, Clain JE, Tremaine WJ, et al. A comparison of endoscopic ultrasound,

magnetic resonance imaging, and exam under anesthesia for evaluation of Crohn's perianal fistulas. Gastroenterology. 2001;121(5):1064–72.

88. Wedemeyer J, Kirchhoff T, Manns MP, Gebel MJ, Bleck JS. Transcutaneous perianal ultrasound (PAUS) for the imaging of fistulas and abscesses in Crohn's disease. Z Gastroenterol. 2004;42(11):1315–20.
89. Wedemeyer J, Kirchhoff T, Sellge G, Bachmann O, Lotz J, Galanski M, et al. Transcutaneous perianal sonography: a sensitive method for the detection of perianal inflammatory lesions in Crohn's disease. World J Gastroenterol. 2004;10(19):2859–63.
90. Maconi G, Ardizzone S, Greco S, Radice E, Bezzio C, Bianchi Porro G. Transperineal ultrasound in the detection of perianal and rectovaginal fistulae in Crohn's disease. Am J Gastroenterol. 2007;102(10):2214–9.
91. Dietrich CF, Barreiros AP, Nuernberg D, Schreiber-Dietrich DG, Ignee A. Perianal ultrasound. Z Gastroenterol. 2008;46(6):625–30.
92. Schlottmann K, Kratzer W, Scholmerich J. Doppler ultrasound and intravenous contrast agents in gastrointestinal tract disorders: current role and future implications. Eur J Gastroenterol Hepatol. 2005;17(3):263–75.
93. Pauls S, Gabelmann A, Schmidt SA, Rieber A, Mittrach C, Haenle MM, et al. Evaluating bowel wall vascularity in Crohn's disease: a comparison of dynamic MRI and wideband harmonic imaging contrast-enhanced low MI ultrasound. Eur Radiol. 2006; 16(11):2410–7.
94. Migaleddu V, Scanu AM, Quaia E, Rocca PC, Dore MP, Scanu D, et al. Contrast-enhanced ultrasonographic evaluation of inflammatory activity in Crohn's disease. Gastroenterology. 2009;137(1): 43–52.
95. Romanini L, Passamonti M, Navarria M, Lanzarotto F, Villanacci V, Grazioli L, et al. Quantitative analysis of contrast-enhanced ultrasonography of the bowel wall can predict disease activity in inflammatory bowel disease. Eur J Radiol. 2014;83(8):1317–23.
96. Bataille F, Klebl F, Rummele P, Straub RH, Wild P, Scholmerich J, et al. Histopathological parameters as predictors for the course of Crohn's disease. Virchows Arch. 2003;443(4):501–7.
97. Girlich C, Jung EM, Huber E, Ott C, Iesalnieks I, Schreyer A, et al. Comparison between preoperative quantitative assessment of bowel wall vascularization by contrast-enhanced ultrasound and operative macroscopic findings and results of histopathological scoring in Crohn's disease. Ultraschall Med. 2011;32(2):154–9.
98. De Franco A, Di Veronica A, Armuzzi A, Roberto I, Marzo M, De Pascalis B, et al. Ileal Crohn disease: mural microvascularity quantified with contrast-enhanced US correlates with disease activity. Radiology. 2012;262(2):680–8.
99. Ripolles T, Rausell N, Paredes JM, Grau E, Martinez MJ, Vizuete J. Effectiveness of contrast-enhanced ultrasound for characterisation of intestinal inflammation in Crohn's disease: a comparison with surgical histopathology analysis. J Crohns Colitis. 2013; 7(2):120–8.
100. Paredes JM, Ripolles T, Cortes X, Moreno N, Martinez MJ, Bustamante-Balen M, et al. Contrast-enhanced ultrasonography: usefulness in the assessment of postoperative recurrence of Crohn's disease. J Crohns Colitis. 2013;7(3):192–201.
101. Ripolles T, Martinez-Perez MJ, Paredes JM, Vizuete J, Garcia-Martinez E, Jimenez-Restrepo DH. Contrast-enhanced ultrasound in the differentiation between phlegmon and abscess in Crohn's disease and other abdominal conditions. Eur J Radiol. 2013; 82(10):e525–31.
102. Parente F, Molteni M, Marino B, Colli A, Ardizzone S, Greco S, et al. Bowel ultrasound and mucosal healing in ulcerative colitis. Dig Dis. 2009;27(3):285–90.
103. Parente F, Molteni M, Marino B, Colli A, Ardizzone S, Greco S, et al. Are colonoscopy and bowel ultrasound useful for assessing response to short-term therapy and predicting disease outcome of moderate-to-severe forms of ulcerative colitis?: a prospective study. Am J Gastroenterol. 2010;105(5):1150–7.
104. Maconi G, Ardizzone S, Parente F, Bianchi Porro G. Ultrasonography in the evaluation of extension, activity, and follow-up of ulcerative colitis. Scand J Gastroenterol. 1999;34(11): 1103–7.
105. Pascu M, Roznowski AB, Muller HP, Adler A, Wiedenmann B, Dignass AU. Clinical relevance of transabdominal ultrasonography and magnetic resonance imaging in patients with inflammatory bowel disease of the terminal ileum and large bowel. Inflamm Bowel Dis. 2004;10(4):373–82.
106. Civitelli F, Di Nardo G, Oliva S, Nuti F, Ferrari F, Dilillo A, et al. Ultrasonography of the colon in pediatric ulcerative colitis: a prospective, blind, comparative study with colonoscopy. J Pediatr. 2014;165(1):78–84.e2.
107. Sigirci A, Baysal T, Kutlu R, Aladag M, Sarac K, Harputluoglu H. Doppler sonography of the inferior and superior mesenteric arteries in ulcerative colitis. J Clin Ultrasound. 2001;29(3):130–9.
108. Girlich C, Schacherer D, Jung EM, Klebl F, Huber E. Comparison between quantitative assessment of bowel wall vascularization by contrast-enhanced ultrasound and results of histopathological scoring in ulcerative colitis. Int J Colorectal Dis. 2012;27(2):193–8.
109. Biancone L, Petruzziello C, Calabrese E, Zorzi F, Naccarato P, Onali S, et al. Long-term safety of Infliximab for the treatment of inflammatory bowel disease: does blocking TNFalpha reduce colitis-associated colorectal carcinogenesis? Gut. 2009;58(12):1703.
110. Sokol H, Beaugerie L. Inflammatory bowel disease and lymphoproliferative disorders: the dust is starting to settle. Gut. 2009; 58(10):1427–36.
111. Lewis JD, Bilker WB, Brensinger C, Deren JJ, Vaughn DJ, Strom BL. Inflammatory bowel disease is not associated with an increased risk of lymphoma. Gastroenterology. 2001;121(5):1080–7.
112. Caspersen S, Elkjaer M, Riis L, Pedersen N, Mortensen C, Jess T, et al. Infliximab for inflammatory bowel disease in Denmark 1999–2005: clinical outcome and follow-up evaluation of malignancy and mortality. Clin Gastroenterol Hepatol. 2008;6(11): 1212–7. quiz 176.
113. Cortot A, Maetz D, Degoutte E, Delette O, Meunier P, Tan G, et al. Mesalamine foam enema versus mesalamine liquid enema in active left-sided ulcerative colitis. Am J Gastroenterol. 2008; 103(12):3106–14.
114. Terkamp C, Kirchner G, Wedemeyer J, Dettmer A, Kielstein J, Reindell H, et al. Simulation of abdomen sonography. Evaluation of a new ultrasound simulator. Ultraschall Med. 2003;24(4): 239–44.
115. Holtmann MH, Barreiros AP, Mudter J, Atreya R, Galle PR, Terkamp C, et al. Ultrasound education by simulator training—analysis of the largest simulator-based training in Germany. Z Gastroenterol. 2010;48(11):1279–84.

21 Laboratory Evaluation, Including Novel Diagnostic Markers

M. Flamant and X. Roblin

Abbreviations

IBD	Inflammatory bowel disease
CRP	C-reactive protein
IL-6	Interleukin 6
IL-1ß	Interleukin-1 beta
TNF	Tumor necrosis factor
CD	Crohn's disease
UC	Ulcerative colitis
CDAI	Crohn's disease activity index
HBI	Harvey–Bradshaw index
CDEIS	Crohn's disease endoscopic score index
TLs	Trough levels
IFX	Infliximab
FC	Fecal calprotectin
LF	Lactoferrin
IBS	Irritable bowel syndrome
PPV	Positive predictive value
NPV	Negative predictive value
ASCA	Anti-*Saccharomyces cerevisiae* antibodies
ANCA	Antineutrophil cytoplasmic antibodies
anti-OmpC	Anti-outer membrane porin C
anti-I2	Anti-Pseudomonas fluorescence-associated sequence I2
anti-CBir1	Anti-bacterial flagellin
AMCA	Anti-mannobioside carbohydrate antibodies
ACCA	Anti-chitobioside carbohydrate antibodies
ALCA	Anti-laminariobioside carbohydrate antibodies
6-MP	6-mercaptopurine
AZA	Azathioprine
TPMT	Thiopurine S-methyltransferase
XO	Xanthine oxidase
6-MMP	6-methylmercaptopurine
6TU	6-thiouric acid
HPRT	Hypoxanthine phosphoribosyltransferase
6-TGN	6-thioguanine
RBC	Red blood cell
ADA	Anti-drug antibody
IMM	Immunosuppressive therapy

M. Flamant
Institut des Maladies de l'Appareil Digestif (IMAD), Hotel Dieu, CHU de Nantes, 44093 Nantes cedex, France

X. Roblin (✉)
CHU de Saint Etienne, Hopital Nord, Service de Gastroentérologie, 42277 Saint-Priest-en-Jarez, France
e-mail: xavier.roblin@chu-st-etienne.fr

C-Reactive Protein

Increased serum concentrations of acute-phase proteins can be found in active inflammatory bowel disease (IBD). The production of C-reactive protein (CRP) occurs almost exclusively in the liver by the hepatocytes upon stimulation by interleukin-6 (IL-6), which is increased in patients with IBD [1], and to a lesser extent by IL-1β and tumor necrosis factor (TNF) [2]. CRP tests are widely available, relatively inexpensive and allow for a regular monitoring of IBD patients.

At Diagnosis

CRP levels are raised in both Crohn's disease (CD) and ulcerative colitis (UC), but many studies have demonstrated that CRP levels are significantly higher in CD than UC for all categories of disease severity. Although the reason is unknown, an explanation could be that UC is limited to the mucosa whereas CD involves a transmural inflammation of the gut wall. At IBD diagnosis, 25 % of patients with CD and 71 % with ulcerative colitis have CRP levels within the normal range. Indeed, CRP generation is extremely variable between individuals and may be related to variation in CRP genotype; a recent study demonstrated that elevated CRP levels could be associated with nucleotide polymorphisms in CRP genotype (rs1205, rs1130864, and rs1417938) at IBD

D.C. Baumgart (ed.), *Crohn's Disease and Ulcerative Colitis*, DOI 10.1007/978-3-319-33703-6_21

diagnosis [3]. Hence, in the case of nonspecific digestive symptoms, CRP alone is not a good biological marker to differentiate IBD from functional disorders.

Correlation with IBD Activity and Location

Measurement of clinical activity in IBD using the Crohn's disease activity index (CDAI) or the Harvey–Bradshaw index (HBI) can suffer from subjective interpretation. Some studies have evaluated whether noninvasive markers such as CRP could be tools to help clinicians to measure disease activity objectively in CD patients. Solem et al. aimed to correlate CRP with clinical, endoscopic, histologic, and radiographic activity in CD: in this retrospective analysis of 104 patients, moderate-to-severe clinical activity, as well as active lesions at colonoscopy or histologically active inflammation, were significantly associated with elevated CRP levels. Conversely, abnormal radiologic findings in the small bowel were not significantly correlated with elevated CRP levels [4]. These results add weight to those of studies finding low CRP levels for an ileal location of CD in comparison to an ileocolonic or colonic location [5, 6].

A recent meta-analysis (19 studies) evaluated the diagnostic accuracy of CRP and other biological markers for the assessment of endoscopically detectable activity in symptomatic IBD patients. This study, which included 2499 IBD patients, showed that CRP ≥5 mg/L has a relatively high specificity (92 %) but poor sensitivity (49 %) for endoscopic activity. This result means that a negative value did not reliably exclude the possibility of active inflammation [7]. Similarly, Denis et al. found that in CD patients with clinically active disease (CDAI >150) and normal CRP levels (<5 mg/L), colonoscopy revealed endoscopic lesions, although these lesions were only mild (CDEIS ≤6) [8].

A Factor Predictive of Response to Treatment

A high-level systemic inflammation in CD patients treated with anti-TNF alpha is associated with a positive clinical response to infliximab (IFX). Louis et al. found that the response rate was significantly higher in patients with an elevated (>5 mg/L) than a normal (<5 mg/L) CRP value before treatment (76 % versus 46 %; $P=0.004$) [9], and the authors suggested that CRP level may help to identify better candidates for IFX treatment. In the same way, Jürgens et al. demonstrated that more patients with high baseline CRP levels responded to IFX than those with normal levels ($P=0.014$). Moreover, early normalization of CRP levels correlated with sustained long-term response ($P<0.001$) [10] without the need for a therapeutic adjustment [11].

A Factor Predictive of Disease Outcome

Some studies have shown an increased risk of relapse in CD patients with elevated CRP during follow-up [12, 13]. Moreover, in a prospective study, Henriksen et al. demonstrated that high CRP levels at diagnosis were significantly associated with increased risk of subsequent surgery in IBD patients, especially those with ileal location (L1) and CRP >53 mg/L (OR = 6.0; $P=0.03$) for CD patients and with extensive colitis and CRP >23 mg/L (OR = 4.8; $P=0.02$) for UC patients [14].

A recent study indicated that following initiation of infliximab therapy, CRP could be predictive of loss of response in CD patients. Indeed, at week 22 of initiation, a CRP level >5 mg/L and a trough level (TL) >5.5 μg/mL, and the presence of anti-drug antibody (ADA) could predict a loss of response in 50 % of patients within 20 months [15].

CRP has been identified as a predictive factor for relapse in CD patients after anti-TNF withdrawal. Louis et al., in the prospective STORI study conducted by the GETAID group, investigated anti-TNF withdrawal in CD patients with longstanding remission of at least 6 months treated with combination therapy for at least 12 months (i.e., anti-TNF plus azathioprine or methotrexate). In this study, relapse occurred in 50 % of these patients within 18 months of IFX withdrawal. Based on multivariate analysis, the study demonstrated that a CRP level ≥5 mg/L before anti-TNF discontinuation was one of the risk factors for subsequent relapse [16]. In a post hoc analysis of this study, Meuwis et al. also found that the median CRP level, measured every 2 months until follow-up or relapse, was higher in relapsers compared with nonrelapsers (3.9 vs 2.8 mg/L; $P=0.07$) [17].

Fecal Biomarkers

Fecal calprotectin (FC) and lactoferrin (LF) are the two most commonly used fecal markers in IBD. FC is a calcium- and zinc-binding protein found in large amounts in neutrophil granulocytes and, by consequence, increased in the presence of intestinal inflammation, with a high sensitivity. However, FC is not a specific marker of IBD and can also be increased in neoplasia, infections, gastritis with Helicobacter pylori, NSAID use, polyps…

In patients with a clinical suspicion of IBD (with symptoms of abdominal pain, diarrhea…) the main interest of FC is due to its high negative predictive value to detect intestinal inflammation. The prospective study of Tibble et al. reported in 2000 demonstrated that at levels <30 mg/L, FC had 100 % sensitivity and 97 % specificity to discriminate between active CD and irritable bowel syndrome (IBS) [18]. A meta-analysis published by Van Rhennen et al. that included 13 studies (670 adults, 371 children) confirmed that high FC levels can differentiate IBD from IBS, with a pooled sensitivity of 93 % and a pooled specificity of 96 % [19]. In this meta-analysis, the authors concluded that screening by measuring FC levels helps to avoid a colonoscopy. This aspect was reported in an economic study that estimated a 50 % reduction in colonoscopies after pre-endoscopic screening with FC, using a cutoff level of 50 μg/g [20]. FC measurement can also be helpful in children, but a level over 100 μg/g has been calculated as the cutoff that can distinguish between active inflammatory disorders and functional bowel disorders [21].

Correlation with Endoscopic Activity

Although some studies did not find a good correlation between FC and IBD clinical activity [22, 23], others have reported a significant correlation between FC levels and endoscopic activity in IBD. In CD patients, in a prospective study, Schoepfer et al. demonstrated that FC >70 μg/g was the most predictive marker of endoscopic activity (based on Simple Endoscopic Score for CD) with 80 % sensitivity and 60 % specificity, rather than CRP, blood leukocytes or the CDAI. In this study, FC was also the only marker that reliably discriminated inactive from mild, moderate, and highly active disease [24]. In the same way, Langhorst et al. demonstrated that FC was able to differentiate active IBD from inactive IBD and was consistently superior to CRP in its ability to reflect endoscopic inflammation [25].

In UC patients, Schoepfer et al. reported from a large study that FC more accurately reflects endoscopic activity (Spearman's rank correlation coefficient, $r=0.821$) and Nancey et al. also demonstrated a good correlation ($r=0.75$) between FC and endoscopic activity, with levels above 250 μg/g associated with active disease ($P<0.001$) [26, 27]. A recent meta-analysis evaluated the diagnostic accuracy of FC for the assessment of endoscopically defined disease activity in IBD. Including 2499 patients, this meta-analysis confirmed that FC is more sensitive than CRP to predict endoscopic activity (pooled sensitivity: 0.88 vs 0.49, respectively), both in UC and CD [7]. These data are particularly interesting in IBD patients with abdominal symptoms but with a lower clinical suspicion of active disease or relapse, in helping to decide who should be referred for further investigation.

Mucosal healing has become a therapeutic goal in IBD patients as it is associated with longstanding remission. D'Haens et al. demonstrated that FC levels ≤250 μg/g predicted endoscopic remission (defined by CDEIS ≤3) with 94.1 % sensitivity and 62.2 % specificity (PPV=48.5 %, NPV=96.6 %) [28]. Roseth et al. demonstrated that mucosal healing can be determined by a normalization of FC in IBD patients, showing that all patients with normal FC (median of 18 mg/L, range 1–50) had an appearance of both the colon and the terminal ileum that was completely normal endoscopically [29]. Moreover, in a recent study assessing IBD patients both in clinical remission and with mucosal healing, an elevated FC level alone was found in patients who relapsed compared to those without relapse (284 mg/kg vs 37 mg/kg; $P<0.01$) suggesting the added value of FC over mucosal healing in the prediction of clinical remission [30].

A Factor Predictive of Response to Treatment and Disease Outcome

Many studies have studied the interest of FC measurement to predict IBD outcome in clinical practice. Molander et al. demonstrated in a cohort of 60 IBD patients that a normalization of FC (<100 μg/g) after induction therapy with TNFα blocking agents was predictive of sustained clinical remission after 12 months compared to an elevated post-induction FC level (88 % vs 38 %; $P<0.0001$) [31]. In addition, in acute, severe UC, Ho et al. found that FC concentrations remained significantly higher in patients requiring colectomy compared to those responding to medical therapy (1200 μg/g vs 887 μg/g; $P=0.04$) [32].

Studies have also evaluated whether FC measurement for IBD patients in clinical remission could be helpful to predict disease outcome over time or to evaluate a possible de-escalation of treatment. Mao et al. reported a meta-analysis demonstrating that in quiescent IBD patients, the pooled sensitivity and specificity of FC to predict relapse were 78 % and 73 %, respectively, and comparable between CD and UC. Similarly, de Vos et al. studied the interest of repeated FC measurement in UC patients in remission under IFX maintenance therapy, and demonstrated that two consecutive FC measurements >300 μg/g with a 1-month interval were the best predictor of flare during a 52-week follow-up (61.5 % sensitivity and 100 % specificity) [33]. For CD patients with longstanding remission of at least 6 months (STORI study), Louis et al. demonstrated that an FC level ≥250 μg/g before anti-TNF discontinuation was a risk factor for subsequent relapse [16]. In the same way, in a recently published study, Ben Horin et al. found that after anti-TNF discontinuation (both IFX and adalimumab), an abnormal CRP and/or FC ≥50 μg/g was predictive of risk of relapse even in patients with endoscopic mucosal healing [34]. Thus, regarding these studies, discontinuation of medical therapy for patients with high FC levels appears to be a risk for relapse.

In the special situation of surgery, a recent study evaluated the accuracy and usefulness of FC to identify asymptomatically operated patients in postoperative endoscopic remission or recurrence; at a level of 100 μg/g, FC distinguished between endoscopic remission and recurrence with 95 % sensitivity and 54 % specificity. Due to an excellent negative predictive value (93 %), the authors concluded that 30 % of colonoscopies could be replaced by a simple FC measurement to exclude postoperative recurrence [35].

Lactoferrin (LF) is an iron-binding protein expressed by activated neutrophils and secreted by mucosal membranes. Some studies have reported similar performance of FC and LF tests [25, 36]. The mean sensitivity and specificity of fecal LF determination for the diagnosis of IBD are 80 % and 82 %, respectively [37]. Regarding Langhorst's study, fecal markers (LF and FC) were able to differentiate IBD patients with endoscopically assessed inflammation from IBD patients without inflammation, and from IBS. In this study, neither of the two stool markers investigated was clearly superior in the ability to reflect endoscopic inflammation but they were both superior to CRP in diagnostic accuracy [25].

Serological Markers

Although incompletely understood, an abnormal immune response to the commensal intestinal flora (various microbial antigens) could generate the production of a panel of antibodies in IBD. Blaser et al. demonstrated for the first time in 1984 an increase in serum antibodies to seven bacterial pathogens in a group of CD patients [38]. Anti-*Saccharomyces cerevisiae* antibodies (ASCA) and atypical perinuclear antineutrophil cytoplasmic antibodies (ANCA) have been the most widely investigated. However, knowledge of newly discovered antibodies directed against specific microbial antigens has expanded, such as anti-outer membrane porin C (anti-OmpC)—which is directed against the OmpC transport protein of *Escherichia coli*, anti-I2, anti-CBir1, and antiglycan antibodies (AMCA, ACCA, and ALCA). The clinical significance of these antibodies is being actively investigated, however an increasing number of studies have suggested that patients expressing serological markers at high titers are more likely to have complicated disease [39, 40].

Serological markers have been studied in a "prediagnostic IBD phase." Indeed, some studies have assessed the presence of serological markers many years before the diagnosis of IBD, suggesting that individuals at risk of IBD could be identified using a combination of serological markers (ANCA, ASCA, anti-CBir1, and anti-OmpC) [41, 42].

At diagnosis, ASCA are more frequently detected in CD patients (50–80 %) than in UC patients (2–14 %) or normal healthy subjects (1–7 %) [43, 44]. Conversely, ANCA have been reported in 60–80 % of UC patients but in only 30 % of CD patients [45]. In clinical practice, combination of ASCA and ANCA has been described as a valuable serological tool to differentiate CD from UC, especially for indeterminate colitis, which represents 10 % of IBD patients. Indeed, a very high specificity was obtained using a combination of both parameters (92 % for CD patients with ASCA+/ANCA− and 98 % for UC patients with ANCA+/ASCA−) [44, 46].

Correlation with Disease Location

Recently, some studies have demonstrated that these antibodies can be associated with disease location. Indeed, ASCA+ is more frequent in CD patients with upper disease or with a pure small bowel involvement compared with CD patients with a pure colonic location (81 % and 68 % vs 38 %) or ileocolonic location [44, 47, 48]. In the same way, Targan et al. found that CBir1 was associated with small bowel disease (OR = 2.16; $P=0.009$) [49].

Correlation with Disease Severity

Some studies have shown that serological markers, and hence high-level immune responses towards microbial antigens, are associated with a more severe disease course. Numerous studies indicate that ASCA positivity is correlated with an earlier disease onset [50, 51], which is a recognized factor of disease aggressivity. Moreover, ASCA positivity in CD is associated with a higher risk of complicated disease, such as stricturing or penetrating disease, and of small bowel resection [39, 52, 53]. Indeed, Vasiliauskas et al. demonstrated that all patients with a high ASCA level (>50 U/mL) and the ANCA negative immune marker subprofile developed fibrostenosis (14/14, 100 %) and most of them experienced internal penetrating complications (11/14, 79 %). In this study, taking into account the prevalence and number of surgical procedures per patient with small bowel involvement, analysis revealed that surgery was required by 86 % (12/14) of the high-level-ASCA/ANCA-negative subgroup [53]. By contrast, in patients with UC, the increased frequency of ANCA in treatment-resistant left-sided ulcerative colitis suggests a possible association between these antibodies and relative resistance to medical therapy [52]. Moreover, patients with very high levels of ANCA had a much greater risk of developing pouchitis following ileal pouch-anal anastomosis [52, 54].

In the same way, it has been demonstrated that the newly discovered antibodies could also be associated with disease severity. In the study of Targan et al., CBir1 was associated with complicated CD (internal-penetrating, fibrostenosing disease features) in 61 %, compared to 42 % of patients with inflammatory-only CD ($P=0.002$) [49]. Anti-OmpC antibody has been detected in 55 % of CD patients [55] and its measurement could be useful at diagnosis in ASCA-negative patients; Mow et al. demonstrated that CD patients with anti-OmpC antibody were more likely to have internal perforating disease (50.0 % vs 30.7 %; $P=0.001$) and to require small bowel surgery (61.4 % vs 44.2 %; $P=0.003$), whereas anti-I2 is an independent marker of fibrostenosis (64.4 % vs 40.7 %; $P<0.001$) and is also associated with small bowel surgery (62.2 % vs 37.4 %; $P<0.001$) [39].

A very recent study by Paul et al. confirmed the usefulness of anti-glycan antibodies (AMCA, ACCA, and ALCA), alone or combined with ASCA or ANCA, for determination of the course of IBD. Measuring a large panel of anti-glycans in a cohort of 195 IBD patients (107 CD, 85 UC), (1) a severe CD course was significantly more likely in the case of high levels of AMCA, ASCA, and ACCA (OR = 4.3, 3.5, and 2.8, respectively), and (2) a severe UC course was significantly associated with AMCA and ACCA (OR = 3.4 and 3.0, respectively) [40]. However, tests for these anti-glycan antibodies are not widely available in clinical practice.

Thiopurine Metabolites

Thiopurines in CD are mainly represented by 6-mercaptopurine (6-MP) and its prodrug azathioprine (AZA). AZA and 6-MP have proven efficacy to induce remission in active CD, to maintain remission and spare steroid treatment in quiescent, steroid-dependent CD, and to prevent recurrence after surgery. The clinical efficacy of thiopurines in IBD is related to the production of active metabolites. Three key enzymes are involved in 6-MP metabolism: thiopurine S-methyltransferase (TPMT) and xanthine oxidase (XO), which catalyze the production of the inactive metabolites, 6-methyl-mercaptopurine (6-MMP) and 6-thiouric acid (6TU), respectively; and hypoxanthine phosphoribosyltransferase (HPRT), which is the only enzyme that catalyzes the production of the active metabolite, 6-thioguanine nucleotide (6-TGN) that is responsible for thiopurine efficacy.

Monitoring thiopurine metabolites can help to predict treatment efficacy. Dubinski et al. demonstrated, in a prospective study of pediatric IBD patients, that a threshold 6-TGN level above 235 pmol/8 × 10^8 red blood cells (RBC) was predictive of a therapeutic response ($P<0.001$) [56]. Numerous prospective studies have subsequently found a correlation between 6-TGN and clinical response [57–59] and a meta-analysis by Osterman et al. in 2006 confirmed that more patients with 6-TGN levels above 230–260 pmol/8 × 10^8 RBC were in remission than those with levels below this threshold value (62 % vs 36 %; $P<0.001$) [60]. A meta-analysis by Moreau et al. also supported the same 6-TGN level, between 230–260 pmol/8 × 10^8 RBC, as a therapeutic threshold for clinical remission (pooled OR = 3.1) [61].

Metabolite measurement is particularly useful in patients with inadequate response at the initiation or during the course of thiopurine treatment. In the case of nonresponse to treatment, measurement of 6-TGN can easily identify noncompliant patients (total absence of both 6-TGN and 6-MMP levels), for whom a therapeutic education should be considered. For the others, metabolite measurement may help to understand the mechanism of the inadequate response: (1) low levels of both 6-TGN and 6-MMP can be related to a subtherapeutic dosing, for which an increased dose and a level recheck will be considered; (2) a low 6-TGN level with a high 6-MMP level could indicate that the patient preferentially metabolizes the 6-MP to 6-MMP, rather than to therapeutically active 6-TGN, by a phenomenon of thiopurine hypermethylation. In this particular case, some studies have demonstrated that it could be possible to optimize thiopurine treatment by reducing the thiopurine dose to 25–33 % but adding a low dose of allopurinol (50 mg), which is an inhibitor of the xanthine oxidase enzymatic pathway [62]. Conversely, (3) high levels of both 6-TGN and 6-MMP are the consequence of supratherapeutic dosing and a decreased dose will be proposed.

The measurement of thiopurine metabolites also allows the risk of treatment-related toxicity to be reduced. High 6-TGN levels (>450 pmol/8 × 10^8 RBC) can result in myelotoxicity [56, 63, 64]. In particular, high levels can be observed in patients with very low activity of the enzyme TPMT, and result in leukopenia observed early in the course of thiopurine treatment. Indeed, several polymorphisms have been described in the TMPT gene (chromosome 6) leading to different TPMT enzyme activities. Homozygous mutation of the TPMT gene, present in 0.3 % of patients, is associated with very low TPMT activity and a particular risk of myelotoxicity. Thus it is current practice to determine TPMT phenotype/genotype before prescribing AZA/6-MP, in order to predict those patients at risk of accumulating high levels of 6-TGN.

Dubinsky et al. described for the first time an association of 6-MMP levels above 5700 pmol/8 × 10^8 RBC with a threefold risk of hepatotoxicity [56, 65]. For these patients, who are preferential 6-MMP metabolizers, a study demonstrated that splitting the daily dose of thiopurine (switch from once daily to *BID*) can result in the reduction of 6-MMP metabolites (5955 vs 11,879 pmol/8 × 10^8 RBC; $P<0.0001$) while maintaining 6-TGN levels (227 vs 250 pmol/8 × 10^8; $P>0.05$) [66].

Therapeutic Drug Monitoring of Anti-TNF Alpha

Anti-TNF alpha drugs have revolutionized IBD treatment since their approval in the last decade. However, some patients do not respond to treatment or may lose clinical remission over time. Two meta-analyses found a loss of response in 37 % and 18.2 % for IFX and adalimumab, respectively, with annual risk calculated to be 13 % and

24.4 % per patient year, respectively [67, 68]. In clinical practice, a loss of response requires either anti-TNF dose escalation or a switch to another anti-TNF therapy. In this refractory category of patients, therapeutic drug monitoring of anti-TNF, represented by anti-TNF trough levels (TLs) and anti-drug antibody (ADA) concentrations, could be helpful to guide therapeutic decisions. TLs correspond to the serum concentration of the anti-TNF just before a next administration and depend on different pharmacokinetic parameters of the drug. Conversely, therapeutic drug monitoring may also be interesting in patients under long-term immunosuppressive therapy with long-standing remission and for whom a therapeutic de-escalation or discontinuation may be considered.

TLs and Clinical Outcome

In 2006, Maser et al. confirmed the link between pharmacokinetics and clinical outcome by demonstrating that in CD patients treated with scheduled maintenance infusions the rate of clinical remission was higher for those with detectable IFX levels than for patients in whom TLs were undetectable (82 % vs 6 %; $P<0.001$) [69]. In the same way for UC, Seow et al. reported that detectable levels of IFX at week 54 after IFX initiation were associated with higher rates of clinical remission (69 % vs 15 %; $P<0.001$) and endoscopic improvement (76 % vs 28 %; $P<0.001$). Conversely, undetectable serum IFX was predictive of an increased risk of colectomy (55 % vs 7 %, RR = 9.3; $P<0.001$) [70].

Many studies have subsequently attempted to identify an IFX TL cutoff that can predict a favorable clinical outcome after IFX initiation. TL cutoff levels have differed between studies according to the definition of the time of clinical remission [71, 72], but a minimum of 3 μg/mL is recognized to be considered beneficial during maintenance therapy.

Some studies have considered therapeutic drug monitoring as the basis for a "personalized medicine" by treating patients on the basis of TL concentrations rather than according to a standard dose regimen. A recent prospective study evaluated the clinical benefit of proactive therapeutic drug monitoring in IBD patients with a stable response to IFX during maintenance therapy. A TL target range of 3–7 μg/mL IFX was established (on the basis of previous studies) and a dose escalation or reduction was performed depending on the level measured. In this study, which included 76 patients, more than 90 % of patients achieved the 3–7 μg/mL IFX target range. Achievement of the target range in patients with prior low levels resulted in a higher proportion of patients in remission than before dose escalation (88 % vs 65 %; $P=0.02$). Conversely, for patients with on-treatment TLs measured >7 μg/mL, achievement of the target range by de-escalation resulted in a 28 % reduction in drug cost from before dose reduction ($P<0.0011$) without affecting clinical outcome [73].

TLs have been less well evaluated for patients treated with adalimumab. However, Karmiris et al. demonstrated that high TLs in CD patients treated with adalimumab were associated with a lower risk of loss of response. Moreover, where there was loss of response, dose escalation to 40 mg weekly resulted in an increase in TLs (from 4.8 to 9.4 μg/mL ($P=0.001$)) and was correlated with a new clinical response ($P<0.0001$) [74]. Roblin et al. demonstrated that high adalimumab TLs were also associated with clinical remission and mucosal healing in CD and UC patients [75].

Influence of ADA

In 2003, Baert et al. reported the influence of immunogenicity on the long-term efficacy of IFX. The development of antibodies against IFX occurs in up to 61 % of CD patients and represents the main factor of immunogenicity [76]. Other patient-related characteristics could also interfere with anti-TNF TLs, increasing drug clearance independently of ADA production: male sex, high body weight, low albumin, or endoscopic lesions [77, 78].

ADA production in IBD patients treated with anti-TNF drugs is linked with a reduced duration of treatment response and also an increased risk of infusion reactions. In particular, it has been demonstrated that CD patients treated episodically with IFX and having an ADA above the threshold of 8 μg/mL were at significant risk of infusion reactions (RR = 2.4; 95 % CI, 1.65–3.66; $P<0.001$) [76]. A recent meta-analysis by O'Meara et al. confirmed this increased risk of infusion reactions in patients with the presence of ADA compared to those without (RR = 2.4; 95 % CI, 1.5–3.8; $P<0.001$) [79].

Concomitant immunosuppressive therapy reduced ADA formation and influenced the pharmacokinetics of IFX. Vermeire et al. indicated that concomitant immunosuppressive therapy (IMM) was predictive of low titers of anti-IFX antibodies regardless of the type of immunosuppressor used (i.e., azathioprine or methotrexate). This study determined that a level of ADA above 8 μg/mL at week 4 of initiation was predictive of a low IFX serum level during follow-up [80]. In their meta-analysis, O'Meara et al. confirmed that patients on immunomodulators during maintenance with IFX therapy had a reduced risk for ADA formation (RR = 0.6; 95 % CI, 0.4–0.9; $P=0.02$), and hence for infusion reactions (RR = 0.6; 95 % CI, 0.4–0.8; $P<0.001$) [79].

A recently published, retrospective analysis suggested that anti-TNF monitoring could be helpful to guide therapeutic decisions according to TLs and ADA concentrations.

In particular, depending on pharmacokinetic measurements, this could help in the case of a loss of response to decide whether to perform an anti-TNF dose escalation or to switch to another anti-TNF therapy. Indeed, dosage increases were more effective for patients with no or low ADA titers ($P=0.02$) whereas a switch to another anti-TNF drug rather than dose escalation could be advised in patients with high ADA levels (>4 μg/mL for adalimumab and >9 μg/mL for IFX) ($P=0.03$, log rank test) [81].

Discontinuation of Anti-TNF Drugs

Therapeutic drug monitoring may also be useful for CD patients in clinical remission for whom a withdrawal of anti-TNF is considered. The prospective STORI study conducted by the GETAID group investigated anti-TNF withdrawal in Crohn's disease patients with long-standing remission of at least 6 months treated with combination therapy for at least 12 months (i.e., anti-TNF plus immunosuppressors). Among the predictive factors identified for risk of relapse (which occurs in 50 % within 18 months of IFX withdrawal) was a TLs >4.5 μg/mL prior to IFX cessation. In the same way, Papamichael et al. also demonstrated, in a retrospective study including 84 CD patients treated with anti-TNF and IMM, that patients presenting high TLs (TL >6 μg/mL) had a significant risk of relapse whilst sustained clinical remission was likely for patients with TLs <6 μg/mL ($P=0.031$) at the time of IFX discontinuation. Furthermore, low or undetectable anti-TNF levels predict a relapse-free survival over time [82]. This suggests that patients with higher TLs at the time of IFX discontinuation are more prone to relapse and probably require continued anti-TNF administration in order to maintain an adequate drug concentration, and therefore a clinical remission. These data were strengthened by the study of Ben-Horin, where a relapse occurred in 80 % of patients with measurable drug levels compared to 32 % of patients with undetectable drug levels at anti-TNF cessation (OR = 8.4; $P=0.002$). This suggests that clinical remission in these patients is perhaps no longer dependent on anti-TNF treatment, which may be stopped [34].

In the TAXIT trial, Vande Casteele et al. implemented a drug de-escalation in CD patients with clinical remission and high TLs (>7 μg/mL) by one of two means: (1) reduction of the dose to 5 mg/kg (if previously on 10 mg/kg), (2) extension of the interval between two infusions, each time by 2 weeks (to a maximum interval of 12 weeks). Of 72 patients with TLs >7 μg/mL, 93 % achieved a normal range after dose reduction without affecting clinical outcome [73]. Return to a normal TL range could be of benefit in considering potential, but not demonstrated, increased risk of adverse events related to high TLs.

Discontinuation of Immunosuppressive Drugs

Stopping IMM in IBD patients treated with combination therapy may be considered. In a controlled trial performed by Van Assche et al., the influence of immunosuppressive drug discontinuation in patients in remission treated with combination therapy was studied. Continuation of IMM beyond 6 months offered no clear benefit over scheduled IFX monotherapy, but was associated with a higher median IFX TL and decreased CRP levels. Indeed, CRP was lower and IFX TLs higher in the "continuation" group compared with the "discontinuation" group (CRP: 1.6 mg/L vs 2.8 mg/L and TLs: 2.87 μg/mL vs 1.65 μg/mL for continuation vs discontinuation, respectively; $P<0.0001$) [83]. In the same way, Drobne et al. reported the results of a retrospective cohort of CD patients in remission under combination therapy who stopped their IMM. Patients with an IFX TLs >5 μg/mL at baseline were the best candidates for IMM discontinuation without altering the natural history of the disease. In the subgroup of patients with detectable IFX TLs <5 μg/mL, the cumulative risk of relapse during follow-up was 12 % in this cohort [84].

In conclusion, in recent years many retrospective studies have demonstrated the interest of therapeutic anti-TNF drug monitoring in inflammatory bowel disease, both in the case of loss of response and for therapeutic de-escalation or discontinuation. The results from an ongoing randomized controlled study, TAILORIX (NCT01442025), which aims to compare the management of IBD patients according to pharmacological and clinical criteria versus clinical criteria only, could be useful in this context in the near future.

References

1. Gross V, Andus T, Caesar I, Roth M, Scholmerich J. Evidence for continuous stimulation of interleukin-6 production in Crohn's disease. Gastroenterology. 1992;102(2):514–9.
2. Vermeire S, Van Assche G, Rutgeerts P. Laboratory markers in IBD: useful, magic, or unnecessary toys? Gut. 2006;55(3):426–31.
3. Henderson P, Kennedy NA, Van Limbergen JE, Cameron FL, Satsangi J, Russell RK, et al. Serum C-reactive protein and CRP genotype in pediatric inflammatory bowel disease: influence on phenotype, natural history, and response to therapy. Inflammatory bowel diseases. 2015;21(3):596–605.
4. Solem CA, Loftus Jr EV, Tremaine WJ, Harmsen WS, Zinsmeister AR, Sandborn WJ. Correlation of C-reactive protein with clinical, endoscopic, histologic, and radiographic activity in inflammatory bowel disease. Inflammatory bowel diseases. 2005;11(8):707–12.
5. Yang DH, Yang SK, Park SH, Lee HS, Boo SJ, Park JH, et al. Usefulness of C-reactive protein as a disease activity marker in Crohn's disease according to the location of disease. Gut and liver. 2015;9(1):80–6.
6. Florin TH, Paterson EW, Fowler EV, Radford-Smith GL. Clinically active Crohn's disease in the presence of a low C-reactive protein. Scandinavian journal of gastroenterology. 2006;41(3):306–11.

7. Mosli MH, Zou G, Garg SK, Feagan SG, MacDonald JK, Chande N, et al. C-Reactive Protein, Fecal Calprotectin, and Stool Lactoferrin for Detection of Endoscopic Activity in Symptomatic Inflammatory Bowel Disease Patients: A Systematic Review and Meta-Analysis. The American journal of gastroenterology. 2015.
8. Denis MA, Reenaers C, Fontaine F, Belaiche J, Louis E. Assessment of endoscopic activity index and biological inflammatory markers in clinically active Crohn's disease with normal C-reactive protein serum level. Inflammatory bowel diseases. 2007;13(9):1100–5.
9. Louis E, Vermeire S, Rutgeerts P, De Vos M, Van Gossum A, Pescatore P, et al. A positive response to infliximab in Crohn disease: association with a higher systemic inflammation before treatment but not with -308 TNF gene polymorphism. Scandinavian journal of gastroenterology. 2002;37(7):818–24.
10. Jurgens M, Mahachie John JM, Cleynen I, Schnitzler F, Fidder H, van Moerkercke W, et al. Levels of Creactive protein are associated with response to infliximab therapy in patients with Crohn's disease. Clinical gastroenterology and hepatology : the official clinical practice journal of the American Gastroenterological Association. 2011;9(5):421–7. e1.
11. Magro F, Rodrigues-Pinto E, Santos-Antunes J, Vilas-Boas F, Lopes S, Nunes A, et al. High C-reactive protein in Crohn's disease patients predicts nonresponse to infliximab treatment. Journal of Crohn's & colitis. 2014;8(2):129–36.
12. Boirivant M, Leoni M, Tariciotti D, Fais S, Squarcia O, Pallone F. The clinical significance of serum C reactive protein levels in Crohn's disease. Results of a prospective longitudinal study. Journal of clinical gastroenterology. 1988;10(4):401–5.
13. Consigny Y, Modigliani R, Colombel JF, Dupas JL, Lemann M, Mary JY, et al. A simple biological score for predicting low risk of short-term relapse in Crohn's disease. Inflammatory bowel diseases. 2006;12(7):551–7.
14. Henriksen M, Jahnsen J, Lygren I, Stray N, Sauar J, Vatn MH, et al. C-reactive protein: a predictive factor and marker of inflammation in inflammatory bowel disease. Results from a prospective population-based study. Gut. 2008;57(11):1518–23.
15. Roblin X, Marotte H, Leclerc M, Del Tedesco E, Phelip JM, Peyrin-Biroulet L, et al. Combination of C-reactive Protein, Infliximab Trough Levels, and Stable but Not Transient Antibodies to Infliximab Are Associated With Loss of Response to Infliximab in Inflammatory Bowel Disease. Journal of Crohn's & colitis. 2015;9(7):525–31.
16. Louis E, Mary JY, Vernier-Massouille G, Grimaud JC, Bouhnik Y, Laharie D, et al. Maintenance of remission among patients with Crohn's disease on antimetabolite therapy after infliximab therapy is stopped. Gastroenterology. 2012;142(1):63–70. e5-quiz e31.
17. Meuwis MA, Vernier-Massouille G, Grimaud JC, Bouhnik Y, Laharie D, Piver E, et al. Serum calprotectin as a biomarker for Crohn's disease. Journal of Crohn's & colitis. 2013;7(12): e678–83.
18. Tibble J, Teahon K, Thjodleifsson B, Roseth A, Sigthorsson G, Bridger S, et al. A simple method for assessing intestinal inflammation in Crohn's disease. Gut. 2000;47(4):506–13.
19. van Rheenen PF, Van de Vijver E, Fidler V. Faecal calprotectin for screening of patients with suspected inflammatory bowel disease: diagnostic meta-analysis. Bmj. 2010;341:c3369.
20. Mindemark M, Larsson A. Ruling out IBD: estimation of the possible economic effects of pre-endoscopic screening with F-calprotectin. Clin Biochem. 2012;45(7-8):552–5.
21. Berni Canani R, Rapacciuolo L, Romano MT. Tanturri de Horatio L, Terrin G, Manguso F, et al. Diagnostic value of faecal calprotectin in paediatric gastroenterology clinical practice. Dig Liver Dis. 2004;36(7):467–70.
22. Gaya DR, Lyon TD, Duncan A, Neilly JB, Han S, Howell J, et al. Faecal calprotectin in the assessment of Crohn's disease activity. QJM. 2005;98(6):435–41.
23. Jones J, Loftus Jr EV, Panaccione R, Chen LS, Peterson S, McConnell J, et al. Relationships between disease activity and serum and fecal biomarkers in patients with Crohn's disease. Clinical gastroenterology and hepatology : the official clinical practice journal of the American Gastroenterological Association. 2008;6(11):1218–24.
24. Schoepfer AM, Beglinger C, Straumann A, Trummler M, Vavricka SR, Bruegger LE, et al. Fecal calprotectin correlates more closely with the Simple Endoscopic Score for Crohn's disease (SES-CD) than CRP, blood leukocytes, and the CDAI. The American journal of gastroenterology. 2010;105(1):162–9.
25. Langhorst J, Elsenbruch S, Koelzer J, Rueffer A, Michalsen A, Dobos GJ. Noninvasive markers in the assessment of intestinal inflammation in inflammatory bowel diseases: performance of fecal lactoferrin, calprotectin, and PMN-elastase, CRP, and clinical indices. The American journal of gastroenterology. 2008;103(1): 162–9.
26. Nancey S, Boschetti G, Moussata D, Cotte E, Peyras J, Cuerq C, et al. Neopterin is a novel reliable fecal marker as accurate as calprotectin for predicting endoscopic disease activity in patients with inflammatory bowel diseases. Inflammatory bowel diseases. 2013;19(5):1043–52.
27. Schoepfer AM, Beglinger C, Straumann A, Safroneeva E, Romero Y, Armstrong D, et al. Fecal calprotectin more accurately reflects endoscopic activity of ulcerative colitis than the Lichtiger Index, C-reactive protein, platelets, hemoglobin, and blood leukocytes. Inflammatory bowel diseases. 2013;19(2):332–41.
28. D'Haens G, Ferrante M, Vermeire S, Baert F, Noman M, Moortgat L, et al. Fecal calprotectin is a surrogate marker for endoscopic lesions in inflammatory bowel disease. Inflammatory bowel diseases. 2012;18(12):2218–24.
29. Roseth AG, Aadland E, Grzyb K. Normalization of faecal calprotectin: a predictor of mucosal healing in patients with inflammatory bowel disease. Scandinavian journal of gastroenterology. 2004;39(10):1017–20.
30. Mooiweer E, Severs M, Schipper ME, Fidder HH, Siersema PD, Laheij RJ, et al. Low fecal calprotectin predicts sustained clinical remission in inflammatory bowel disease patients: a plea for deep remission. Journal of Crohn's & colitis. 2015;9(1):50–5.
31. Molander P. af Bjorkesten CG, Mustonen H, Haapamaki J, Vauhkonen M, Kolho KL, et al. Fecal calprotectin concentration predicts outcome in inflammatory bowel disease after induction therapy with TNFalpha blocking agents. Inflammatory bowel diseases. 2012;18(11):2011–7.
32. Ho GT, Lee HM, Brydon G, Ting T, Hare N, Drummond H, et al. Fecal calprotectin predicts the clinical course of acute severe ulcerative colitis. The American journal of gastroenterology. 2009;104(3):673–8.
33. De Vos M, Louis EJ, Jahnsen J, Vandervoort JG, Noman M, Dewit O, et al. Consecutive fecal calprotectin measurements to predict relapse in patients with ulcerative colitis receiving infliximab maintenance therapy. Inflammatory bowel diseases. 2013;19(10): 2111–7.
34. Ben-Horin S, Chowers Y, Ungar B, Kopylov U, Loebstein R, Weiss B, et al. Undetectable anti-TNF drug levels in patients with long-term remission predict successful drug withdrawal. Alimentary pharmacology & therapeutics. 2015.
35. Boschetti G, Laidet M, Moussata D, Stefanescu C, Roblin X, Phelip G, et al. Levels of Fecal Calprotectin Are Associated With the Severity of Postoperative Endoscopic Recurrence in Asymptomatic Patients With Crohn's Disease. The American journal of gastroenterology. 2015;110(6):865–72.
36. Joishy M, Davies I, Ahmed M, Wassel J, Davies K, Sayers A, et al. Fecal calprotectin and lactoferrin as noninvasive markers of pediatric inflammatory bowel disease. J Pediatr Gastroenterol Nutr. 2009;48(1):48–54.

37. Gisbert JP, McNicholl AG, Gomollon F. Questions and answers on the role of fecal lactoferrin as a biological marker in inflammatory bowel disease. Inflammatory bowel diseases. 2009;15(11):1746–54.
38. Blaser MJ, Miller RA, Lacher J, Singleton JW. Patients with active Crohn's disease have elevated serum antibodies to antigens of seven enteric bacterial pathogens. Gastroenterology. 1984;87(4):888–94.
39. Mow WS, Vasiliauskas EA, Lin YC, Fleshner PR, Papadakis KA, Taylor KD, et al. Association of antibody responses to microbial antigens and complications of small bowel Crohn's disease. Gastroenterology. 2004;126(2):414–24.
40. Paul S, Boschetti G, Rinaudo-Gaujous M, Moreau A, Del Tedesco E, Bonneau J, et al. Association of Antiglycan Antibodies and Inflammatory Bowel Disease Course. Journal of Crohn's & colitis. 2015;9(6):445–51.
41. van Schaik FD, Oldenburg B, Hart AR, Siersema PD, Lindgren S, Grip O, et al. Serological markers predict inflammatory bowel disease years before the diagnosis. Gut. 2013;62(5):683–8.
42. Israeli E, Grotto I, Gilburd B, Balicer RD, Goldin E, Wiik A, et al. Anti-Saccharomyces cerevisiae and antineutrophil cytoplasmic antibodies as predictors of inflammatory bowel disease. Gut. 2005;54(9):1232–6.
43. Quinton JF, Sendid B, Reumaux D, Duthilleul P, Cortot A, Grandbastien B, et al. Anti-Saccharomyces cerevisiae mannan antibodies combined with antineutrophil cytoplasmic autoantibodies in inflammatory bowel disease: prevalence and diagnostic role. Gut. 1998;42(6):788–91.
44. Peeters M, Joossens S, Vermeire S, Vlietinck R, Bossuyt X, Rutgeerts P. Diagnostic value of anti-Saccharomyces cerevisiae and antineutrophil cytoplasmic autoantibodies in inflammatory bowel disease. The American journal of gastroenterology. 2001;96(3):730–4.
45. Ruemmele FM, Targan SR, Levy G, Dubinsky M, Braun J, Seidman EG. Diagnostic accuracy of serological assays in pediatric inflammatory bowel disease. Gastroenterology. 1998;115(4):822–9.
46. Joossens S, Reinisch W, Vermeire S, Sendid B, Poulain D, Peeters M, et al. The value of serologic markers in indeterminate colitis: a prospective follow-up study. Gastroenterology. 2002;122(5):1242–7.
47. Vermeire S, Peeters M, Vlietinck R, Joossens S, Den Hond E, Bulteel V, et al. Anti-Saccharomyces cerevisiae antibodies (ASCA), phenotypes of IBD, and intestinal permeability: a study in IBD families. Inflammatory bowel diseases. 2001;7(1):8–15.
48. Walker LJ, Aldhous MC, Drummond HE, Smith BR, Nimmo ER, Arnott ID, et al. Anti-Saccharomyces cerevisiae antibodies (ASCA) in Crohn's disease are associated with disease severity but not NOD2/CARD15 mutations. Clinical and experimental immunology. 2004;135(3):490–6.
49. Targan SR, Landers CJ, Yang H, Lodes MJ, Cong Y, Papadakis KA, et al. Antibodies to CBir1 flagellin define a unique response that is associated independently with complicated Crohn's disease. Gastroenterology. 2005;128(7):2020–8.
50. Nakamura RM, Matsutani M, Barry M. Advances in clinical laboratory tests for inflammatory bowel disease. Clin Chim Acta. 2003;335(1-2):9–20.
51. Vasiliauskas EA, Plevy SE, Landers CJ, Binder SW, Ferguson DM, Yang H, et al. Perinuclear antineutrophil cytoplasmic antibodies in patients with Crohn's disease define a clinical subgroup. Gastroenterology. 1996;110(6):1810–9.
52. Sandborn WJ, Landers CJ, Tremaine WJ, Targan SR. Association of antineutrophil cytoplasmic antibodies with resistance to treatment of left-sided ulcerative colitis: results of a pilot study. Mayo Clinic proceedings. 1996;71(5):431–6.
53. Vasiliauskas EA, Kam LY, Karp LC, Gaiennie J, Yang H, Targan SR. Marker antibody expression stratifies Crohn's disease into immunologically homogeneous subgroups with distinct clinical characteristics. Gut. 2000;47(4):487–96.
54. Vecchi M, Gionchetti P, Bianchi MB, Belluzzi A, Meucci G, Campieri M, et al. p-ANCA and development of pouchitis in ulcerative colitis patients after proctocolectomy and ileoanal pouch anastomosis. Lancet. 1994;344(8926):886–7.
55. Landers CJ, Cohavy O, Misra R, Yang H, Lin YC, Braun J, et al. Selected loss of tolerance evidenced by Crohn's disease-associated immune responses to auto- and microbial antigens. Gastroenterology. 2002;123(3):689–99.
56. Dubinsky MC, Lamothe S, Yang HY, Targan SR, Sinnett D, Theoret Y, et al. Pharmacogenomics and metabolite measurement for 6-mercaptopurine therapy in inflammatory bowel disease. Gastroenterology. 2000;118(4):705–13.
57. Cuffari C, Hunt S, Bayless T. Utilisation of erythrocyte 6-thioguanine metabolite levels to optimise azathioprine therapy in patients with inflammatory bowel disease. Gut. 2001;48(5):642–6.
58. Wright S, Sanders DS, Lobo AJ, Lennard L. Clinical significance of azathioprine active metabolite concentrations in inflammatory bowel disease. Gut. 2004;53(8):1123–8.
59. Roblin X, Serre-Debeauvais F, Phelip JM, Faucheron JL, Hardy G, Chartier A, et al. 6-tioguanine monitoring in steroid-dependent patients with inflammatory bowel diseases receiving azathioprine. Alimentary pharmacology & therapeutics. 2005;21(7):829–39.
60. Osterman MT, Kundu R, Lichtenstein GR, Lewis JD. Association of 6-thioguanine nucleotide levels and inflammatory bowel disease activity: a meta-analysis. Gastroenterology. 2006;130(4):1047–53.
61. Moreau AC, Paul S, Del Tedesco E, Rinaudo-Gaujous M, Boukhadra N, Genin C, et al. Association between 6-thioguanine nucleotides levels and clinical remission in inflammatory disease: a meta-analysis. Inflammatory bowel diseases. 2014;20(3):464–71.
62. Curkovic I, Rentsch KM, Frei P, Fried M, Rogler G, Kullak-Ublick GA, et al. Low allopurinol doses are sufficient to optimize azathioprine therapy in inflammatory bowel disease patients with inadequate thiopurine metabolite concentrations. Eur J Clin Pharmacol. 2013;69(8):1521–31.
63. Hanai H, Iida T, Takeuchi K, Arai O, Watanabe F, Abe J, et al. Thiopurine maintenance therapy for ulcerative colitis: the clinical significance of monitoring 6-thioguanine nucleotide. Inflamm Bowel Dis. 2010;16(8):1376–81.
64. Dubinsky MC, Yang H, Hassard PV, Seidman EG, Kam LY, Abreu MT, et al. 6-MP metabolite profiles provide a biochemical explanation for 6-MP resistance in patients with inflammatory bowel disease. Gastroenterology. 2002;122(4):904–15.
65. Cuffari C, Theoret Y, Latour S, Seidman G. 6-Mercaptopurine metabolism in Crohn's disease: correlation with efficacy and toxicity. Gut. 1996;39(3):401–6.
66. Shih DQ, Nguyen M, Zheng L, Ibanez P, Mei L, Kwan LY, et al. Split-dose administration of thiopurine drugs: a novel and effective strategy for managing preferential 6-MMP metabolism. Alimentary pharmacology & therapeutics. 2012;36(5):449–58.
67. Gisbert JP, Panes J. Loss of response and requirement of infliximab dose intensification in Crohn's disease: a review. The American journal of gastroenterology. 2009;104(3):760–7.
68. Billioud V, Sandborn WJ, Peyrin-Biroulet L. Loss of response and need for adalimumab dose intensification in Crohn's disease: a systematic review. The American journal of gastroenterology. 2011;106(4):674–84.
69. Maser EA, Villela R, Silverberg MS, Greenberg GR. Association of trough serum infliximab to clinical outcome after scheduled maintenance treatment for Crohn's disease. Clinical gastroenterology and hepatology : the official clinical practice journal of the American Gastroenterological Association. 2006;4(10):1248–54.
70. Seow CH, Newman A, Irwin SP, Steinhart AH, Silverberg MS, Greenberg GR. Trough serum infliximab: a predictive factor of clinical outcome for infliximab treatment in acute ulcerative colitis. Gut. 2010;59(1):49–54.

71. Hanauer SB, Feagan BG, Lichtenstein GR, Mayer LF, Schreiber S, Colombel JF, et al. Maintenance infliximab for Crohn's disease: the ACCENT I randomised trial. Lancet. 2002;359(9317):1541–9.
72. Reinisch W, Colombel JF, Sandborn WJ, Mantzaris GJ, Kornbluth A, Adedokun OJ, et al. Factors associated with short- and long-term outcomes of therapy for Crohn's disease. Clinical gastroenterology and hepatology : the official clinical practice journal of the American Gastroenterological Association. 2015;13(3):539–47. e2.
73. Vande Casteele N, Ferrante M, Van Assche G, Ballet V, Compernolle G, Van Steen K, et al. Trough concentrations of infliximab guide dosing for patients with inflammatory bowel disease. Gastroenterology. 2015;148(7):1320–9. e3.
74. Karmiris K, Paintaud G, Noman M, Magdelaine-Beuzelin C, Ferrante M, Degenne D, et al. Influence of trough serum levels and immunogenicity on long-term outcome of adalimumab therapy in Crohn's disease. Gastroenterology. 2009;137(5):1628–40.
75. Roblin X, Marotte H, Rinaudo M, Del Tedesco E, Moreau A, Phelip JM, et al. Association between pharmacokinetics of adalimumab and mucosal healing in patients with inflammatory bowel diseases. Clinical gastroenterology and hepatology : the official clinical practice journal of the American Gastroenterological Association. 2014;12(1):80–4. e2.
76. Baert F, Noman M, Vermeire S, Van Assche G. G DH, Carbonez A, et al. Influence of immunogenicity on the long-term efficacy of infliximab in Crohn's disease. The New England journal of medicine. 2003;348(7):601–8.
77. Dotan I, Ron Y, Yanai H, Becker S, Fishman S, Yahav L, et al. Patient factors that increase infliximab clearance and shorten half-life in inflammatory bowel disease: a population pharmacokinetic study. Inflammatory bowel diseases. 2014;20(12):2247–59.
78. Fasanmade AA, Adedokun OJ, Ford J, Hernandez D, Johanns J, Hu C, et al. Population pharmacokinetic analysis of infliximab in patients with ulcerative colitis. Eur J Clin Pharmacol. 2009;65(12):1211–28.
79. O'Meara S, Nanda KS, Moss AC. Antibodies to infliximab and risk of infusion reactions in patients with inflammatory bowel disease: a systematic review and meta-analysis. Inflammatory bowel diseases. 2014;20(1):1–6.
80. Vermeire S, Noman M, Van Assche G, Baert F, D'Haens G, Rutgeerts P. Effectiveness of concomitant immunosuppressive therapy in suppressing the formation of antibodies to infliximab in Crohn's disease. Gut. 2007;56(9):1226–31.
81. Yanai H, Lichtenstein L, Assa A, Mazor Y, Weiss B, Levine A, et al. Levels of drug and antidrug antibodies are associated with outcome of interventions after loss of response to infliximab or adalimumab. Clinical gastroenterology and hepatology : the official clinical practice journal of the American Gastroenterological Association. 2015;13(3):522–30. e2.
82. Papamichael K, Vande Casteele N, Gils A, Tops S, Hauenstein S, Singh S, et al. Long-term outcome of patients with Crohn's disease who discontinued infliximab therapy upon clinical remission. Clinical gastroenterology and hepatology : the official clinical practice journal of the American Gastroenterological Association. 2015;13(6):1103–10.
83. Van Assche G, Magdelaine-Beuzelin C, D'Haens G, Baert F, Noman M, Vermeire S, et al. Withdrawal of immunosuppression in Crohn's disease treated with scheduled infliximab maintenance: a randomized trial. Gastroenterology. 2008;134(7):1861–8.
84. Drobne D, Bossuyt P, Breynaert C, Cattaert T, Vande Casteele N, Compernolle G, et al. Withdrawal of immunomodulators after co-treatment does not reduce trough level of infliximab in patients with Crohn's disease. Clinical gastroenterology and hepatology : the official clinical practice journal of the American Gastroenterological Association. 2015;13(3):514–21. e4.

Pathology of Inflammatory Bowel Disease

22

Nora E. Joseph and Christopher R. Weber

The diagnosis of inflammatory bowel disease (IBD) depends as much on pathologic findings as it does on clinical presentation and endoscopic appearance. This chapter focuses on the gross and microscopic features used to diagnose IBD. As the clinical course for many IBD patients is often complicated by surgical and medical interventions it is important to relay diagnostically important information between team members, particularly the pathologist and gastroenterologist. Emphasis is placed on the written pathology report to provide a framework for future communication. Starting with a discussion on general features of IBD, subsequent sections focus on unique criteria required to differentiate Crohn's disease (CD) from ulcerative colitis (UC). A major hurdle in rendering a diagnosis of IBD can be excluding other chronic disease processes. Therefore, the final segment of this chapter delineates the differential diagnosis of IBD in detail. Relevant aspects of disease etiology, pathogenesis, epidemiology, and management are only briefly addressed when pertinent to the diagnostic process, as these aspects of IBD are extensively reviewed elsewhere in this book.

General Features of IBD

IBD is a disease characterized by relapsing and remitting episodes of diarrhea, which can be further subdivided into CD and UC based on unique clinical, endoscopic, and pathologic features. Prior to rendering a diagnosis of IBD, careful inspection of macroscopic and microscopic features are required to rule out other disease processes. To that end, three key histologic features must be closely evaluated: chronic injury, disease distribution, and disease activity. Chronic injury to gastrointestinal mucosa is established following months to years of repeated damage rather than days to weeks. As such, the characteristic histologic features of chronic injury must be present in order to render a diagnosis of inflammatory bowel disease. Next, the extent of active disease, or the degree of neutrophilic inflammation, is assessed to determine the severity of disease at the time of biopsy. Finally, to subclassify IBD into either Crohn's disease or ulcerative colitis, the distribution of both chronic and active inflammation must be taken into consideration. We now explore each of these measures in greater detail.

Chronic Injury

Chronic injury is not synonymous with IBD, as other chronic intestinal diseases may show similar features of cyclical injury and regeneration. However, once histologic evidence of chronic injury is indentified, self-limited processes, such as most forms of infectious colitis, can essentially be ruled out. Mimics of IBD are discussed in detail in the last section of this chapter. Chronic mucosal injury occurs during periods of regeneration following repeated episodes of crypt destruction and is defined by three hallmark histologic features: architectural distortion, basal lymphoid hyperplasia, and metaplastic epithelial changes.

Architectural distortion: Crypts are irregularly spaced, branched, and/or reduced in number (Fig. 22.1) Crypts in normal mucosa extend to the muscularis mucosae; however, in IBD, crypts are of variable lengths.

Metaplasia: Defined as "a reversible change in which one differentiated cell type (epithelial or mesenchymal) is replaced by another cell type" [1]. In intestinal chronic injury there are two common types of metaplasia: Paneth cell (Fig. 22.2) and pyloric cell. While Paneth cells normally

N.E. Joseph, M.D.
Department of Pathology and Laboratory Medicine, NorthShore University Health System, 2650 Ridge Ave, Evanston, IL 60201, USA
e-mail: njoseph@northshore.org

C.R. Weber, M.D., Ph.D. (✉)
Department of Pathology, The University of Chicago, 5841 South Maryland, MC 1089, Chicago, IL 60637, USA
e-mail: christopher.weber@uchospitals.edu

D.C. Baumgart (ed.), *Crohn's Disease and Ulcerative Colitis*, DOI 10.1007/978-3-319-33703-6_22

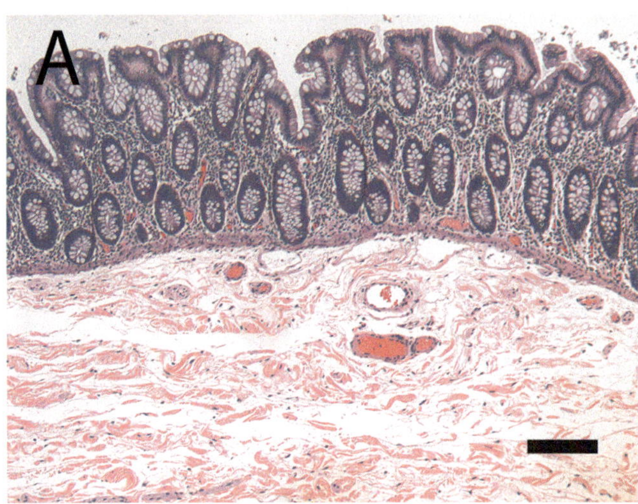

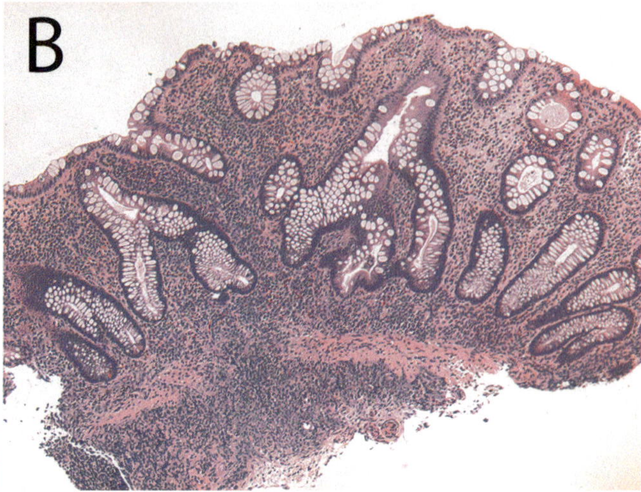

Fig. 22.1 Architectural distortion is a feature of chronic injury. (**a**) Normal colonic mucosa displays evenly spaced non-branched crypts that line up along the muscularis mucosa. Lamina propria contains sparse infiltrate of inflammatory cells. (**b**) Crypt branching and basal lymphoplasmacytic infiltrate are features of chronic injury in CD

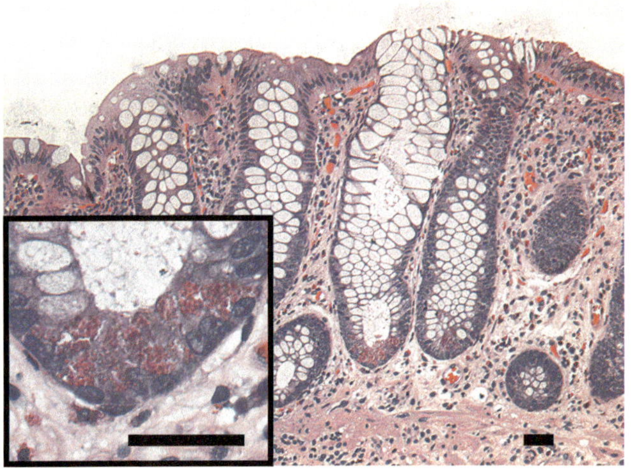

Fig. 22.2 Metaplasia is a feature of chronic injury. Paneth cells are normally present in the small intestine and variably in the right colon. When identified in the left colon, as in this biopsy, Paneth cells are considered to result from a metaplastic process secondary to chronic injury (scale bars: 40 μm)

reside throughout the small intestine and in colonic mucosa close to the ileocecal valve, the mucosa distal to the splenic flexure should have none [2]. Similarly, the presence of pyloric glands, normally restricted to gastric epithelium, signifies chronic injury when observed in ileal or colonic mucosa (e.g., as in Fig. 22.4b).

Basal lymphoid hyperplasia: (Fig. 22.1b) In IBD, an increase in lymphocytes and plasma cells are characteristically seen in the basal portion of the lamina propria where they form a band-like infiltrate. Increased eosinophils and mast cells may also be occasionally observed in this location; however, abundance of neutrophils should raise the suspicion of active inflammation.

Disease Activity

Disease activity refers to the presence of neutrophils within the epithelium. By definition IBD occurs on a background of chronic injury; however, activity can occur without evidence of chronic injury. Therefore a diagnosis of "chronic active colitis" describes the histologic findings of intraepithelial neutrophils superimposed on features of chronic injury. This diagnosis differs from "active colitis," which is present in acute self-limited inflammatory processes devoid of chronic injury. No system for grading of disease activity is universally accepted since studies show poor correlation between microscopic appearance, endoscopic impression, and clinical symptomology [3–6]. However, knowledge of disease severity is important clinically, and many pathologists use scales such as the one below to quantify activity (Fig. 22.3).

1. Quiescent: Features of chronic injury are present, but intraepithelial neutrophils are not observed (Fig. 22.3a).
2. Mildly active: Scattered neutrophils are seen within the epithelium (Fig. 22.3b).
3. Moderately active: Neutrophils have migrated across the epithelium to collect within crypts and form microabscesses referred to as "crypt abscesses" (Fig. 22.3c). Crypt rupture and destruction can also be observed.
4. Severely active: Crypt abscesses have evolved into erosions and/or ulcerations (Fig. 22.3d).

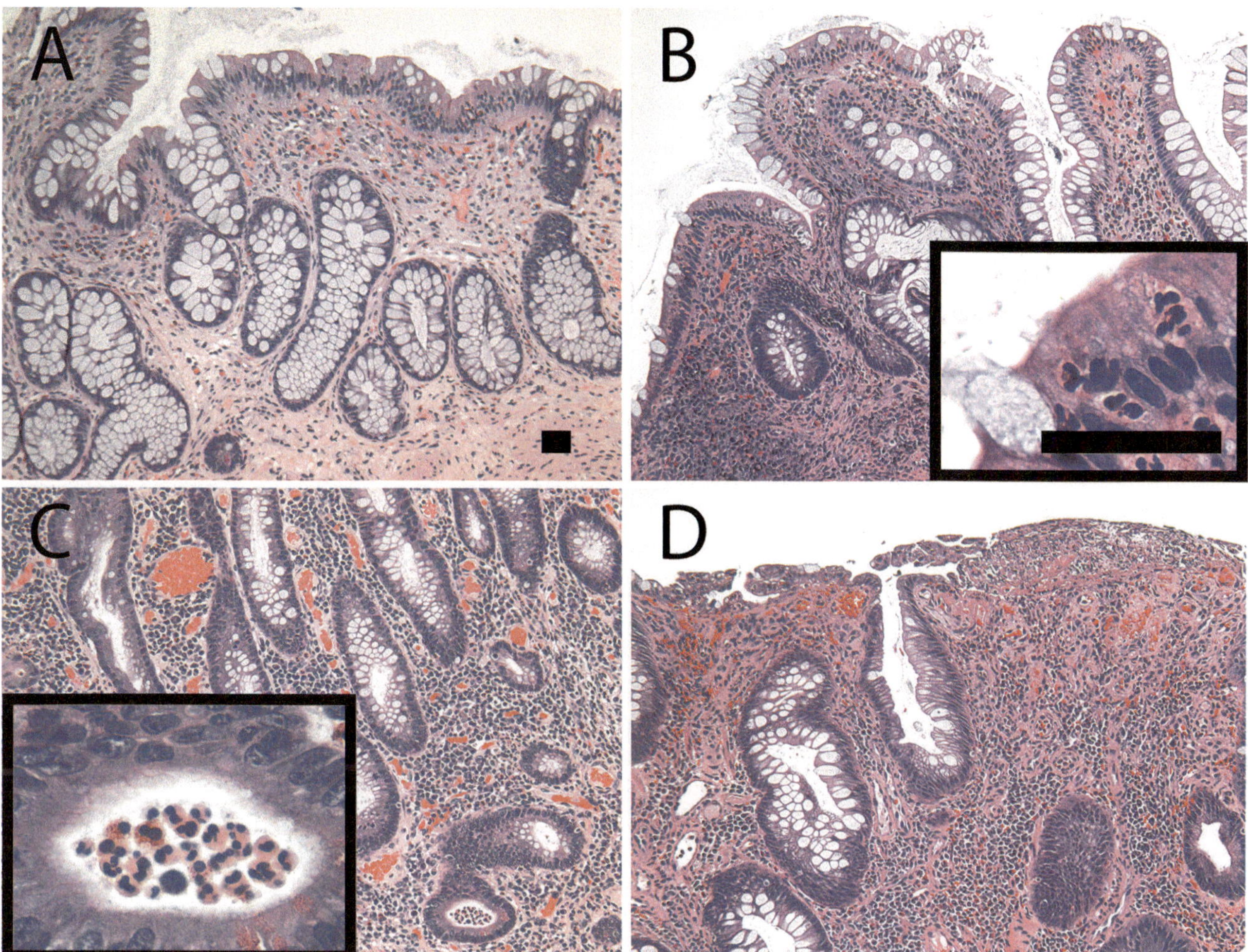

Fig. 22.3 The acute, neutrophilic component of inflammation is graded as activity. (**a**) Quiescent IBD displays chronic injury, but no intraepithelial neutrophils. (**b**) The presence of intraepithelial neutrophils indicates mild active inflammation. (**c**) Crypt abscesses indicate moderate activity. (**d**) Ulcerations or erosions are a feature of severely active IBD. (**a**–**d**: scale bars: 40 μm)

Mucin depletion, decreased numbers of goblet cells, and increased mitotic activity are additional regenerative features that are commonly present in IBD but these are not diagnostic, as they may also be present in active disease without chronic features. Although UC and CD share many of these key aspects of injury, unique details define each entity, which are elucidated in the subsequent sections.

Disease Distribution

In the pathology report descriptive words such as "patchy," "focal," and "diffuse" are used to describe distribution of chronic injury. These terms are avoided in descriptions of active inflammation as specific patterns of chronic, but not active, injury have diagnostic implications in IBD. To accurately assess distribution of disease the pathologist must rely on the endoscopist to both sample endoscopically normal and abnormal areas of mucosa and submit the biopsies in separate containers clearly labeled with anatomic location. A thorough treatment history should accompany the endoscopy report as therapeutic interventions can alter disease distribution and create diagnostic confusion, as detailed below [7].

Ulcerative Colitis

UC is characterized by diffuse chronic injury starting in the rectum and extending proximally to involve sequential segments of colon. Ulcerative proctitis refers to disease limited to the rectum, whereas ulcerative pancolitis describes disease involving the entire colon and rectum. In addition to a diffuse pattern of distribution, untreated UC inflammation is limited to the mucosa and submucosa in most cases.

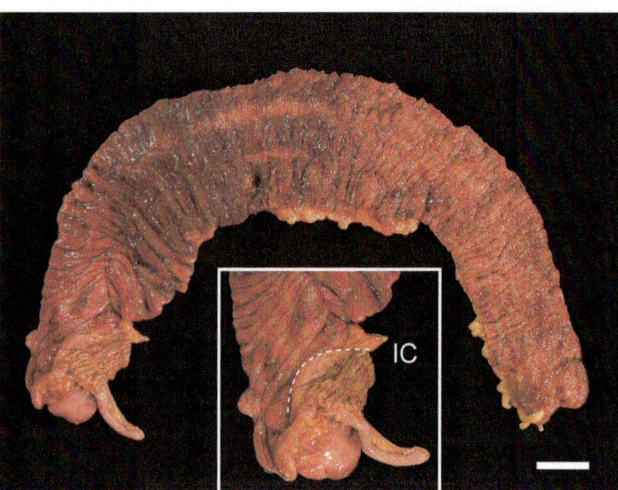

Fig. 22.4 Features of UC are evident on gross examination. In this total colectomy specimen, the entire mucosa from distal rectum to the cecum is hemorrhagic and friable. The specimen lies flat because of the absence of full thickness inflammation. There is a sharp transition to normal tan colored small intestinal mucosa at the ileocecal valve (IC; *dashed line*). (Scale bar: 5 cm)

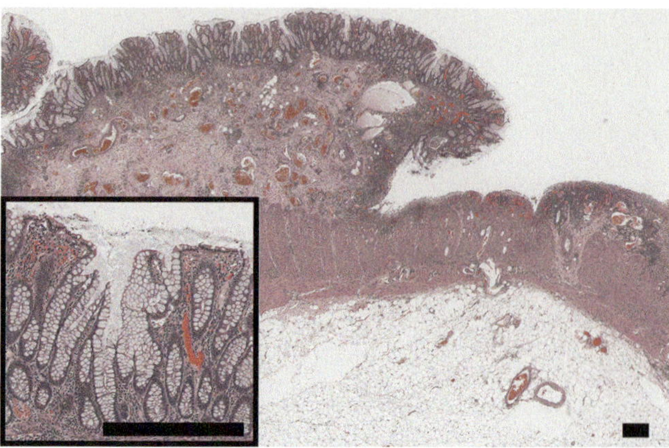

Fig. 22.5 Inflammation in UC is limited to the mucosa and superficial submucosa. In this case of severely active disease, a broad based area of ulceration is present in the right portion of the image. Inflammation does not extend deeply into the muscularis propria, there is no fibrosis, and there are no granulomas present. In an area of epithelium away from the ulcer, architectural distortion is present and is indicative of chronic injury (scale bars 0.6 mm)

Gross Appearance

Key aspects defining UC as a distinct entity are observed macroscopically. Typically, the diffusely affected UC resection specimen lies flat when opened on the pathologist's bench, in contrast to the rigid CD specimen (Fig. 22.4). Further inspection reveals a smooth external surface (serosa) and bowel wall of normal thickness, devoid of strictures and fistulas. These simple observations reflect two characteristic pathologic features of UC: diffuse superficial mucosal inflammation and absence of fibrosis. Inflamed mucosal surfaces appear red, granular and friable with areas of hemorrhage and ulceration in severe cases. The following histologic correlates provide explanation for these macroscopic features.

Microscopic Appearance

Diffuse chronic injury: Histologic features of chronic injury described above are seen diffusely throughout the affected colon and rectum. Caveats to this distribution of disease are discussed at the end of this section.

Depth of disease: In differentiating UC from CD, it is important to consider depth of disease. Active UC shows varying degrees of neutrophilic inflammation; usually limited to the mucosa and superficial submucosa, superimposed on chronic injury (Fig. 22.5). Significant mural fibrosis is not usually present. However, in severe cases with extensive ulceration (i.e., severely active disease), inflammation may extend to the muscularis propria or even the subserosal tissues.

Type of ulcer formation: UC ulcers are morphologically distinct from those observed in CD. Broad based superficial ulcers (Fig. 22.5), typical of UC, markedly contrast with the deep knife-like ulcerations associated with CD (below). These different types of ulcers reflect the superficial and transmural extent of active disease in UC and CD, respectively.

Inflammatory polyps: Also known as pseudopolyps, inflammatory polyps are believed to form during repeated cycles of ulceration and regeneration in both UC and CD. Pseudopolyps are not associated with an increased risk for neoplastic transformation; however, they may be extensive (Fig. 22.6) and are frequently biopsied to rule out polypoid dysplasia. Although not a premalignant lesion, the presence of pseudopolyps, in general, indicates long duration of severe disease, a factor which increases overall risk for dysplasia or frank malignancy anywhere in the affected colorectum [8].

Microscopic Features of UC That Can Mimic CD

Continuous distribution and superficial extent of disease are hallmarks of UC; however, overlapping features with CD may arise and are discussed in this section. *Backwash ileitis* [9, 10]: Activity and even low grade chronic injury may extend into the distal ileum, particularly in severe UC pan-colitis. In contrast to Crohn's ileitis, which typically shows a patchy pattern throughout the ileum, involvement in UC is distal, diffuse, and predominately limited to the ileocecal valve. As ileal involvement by UC resolves following totally colectomy, the inflammation is believed to be caused by proximal extension of colonic disease through an incompetent ileocecal valve. Thus, the

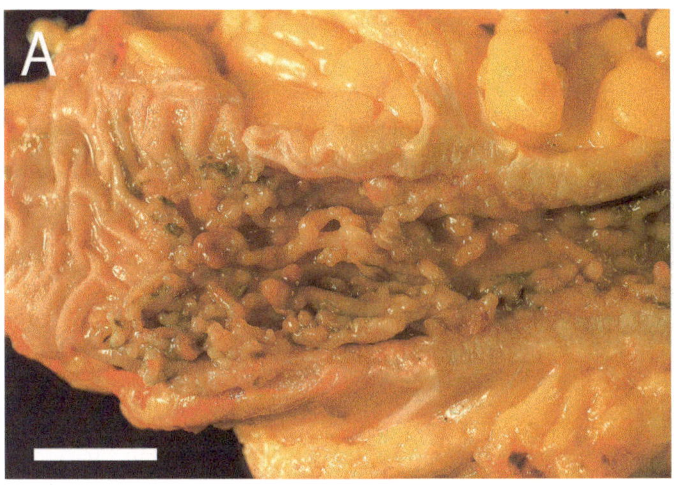

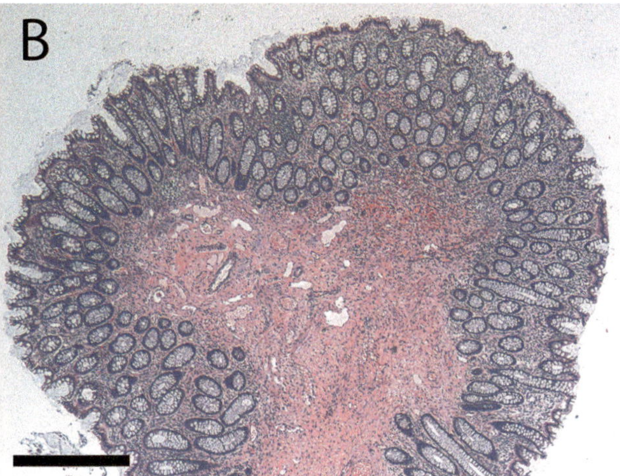

Fig. 22.6 Inflammatory polyps may be numerous. (**a**) In this total colectomy specimen, the cecum displays numerous filiform polyps in the descending colon and rectum (scale bar: 2.5 cm). (**b**) Histologic examination of one of the polyps from (**a**) reveals quiescent IBD, and no evidence of dysplasia. (Scale bar: 1 mm)

clever name "backwash ileitis" is a diagnosis which should be only made if cecal disease is severe. It can be a challenge to make a definitive diagnosis of backwash ileitis and completely rule out CD, therefore a detailed diagnostic comment should be added to the pathology report to facilitate clear communication amongst the clinical team.

Cecal red patch [11–13]: Disease localized to the appendix and periappendiceal cecal mucosa, or "cecal red patch," and can be seen in up to one third of patients with UC. Histologically, these biopsies resemble mildly active ulcerative colitis (i.e., evidence of chronic injury and intraepithelial neutrophils) and should not be interpreted as patchy CD-like distribution.

Transitional areas: Biopsies from the immediate transition between normal and the most proximal extent of diseased mucosa may create a patchy, CD-like, appearance of disease distribution to the pathologist. Therefore, if possible, the endoscopist should focus on sampling, and submitting in separate containers, representative regions of diseased and normal mucosa to provide an accurate map for the pathologist.

True rectal sparing: Although rectal involvement is one of the key features of UC, pediatric patients may present with rectal sparing [14, 15]. This unconventional distribution of disease is considered a normal variant in the pediatric UC population.

False rectal sparing: UC patients receiving long-term therapeutic enemas may completely resolve rectal disease but still show proximal involvement. The pathologist will be able to explain the significance of normal rectal biopsies in this clinical context. However, if the treatment history is withheld, an incorrect diagnosis of CD is possible.

Granuloma formation: Presence or absence of granulomas is a common histologic feature used to differentiate UC from CD. Well or poorly formed granulomas, characteristic of CD, appear as pale compact aggregates of histiocytes surrounded by lymphocytes, discussed in detail below. Diagnostic confusion may arise when similar features are seen in UC patients. Although well-formed granulomas are not associated with UC pathogenesis, loose aggregates of histiocytes, or macrophages, may be seen in UC patients. Histiocytes function to clear cellular debris and foreign material following injury. Therefore, during episodes of active inflammation, crypts may rupture, releasing mucin into the lamina propria. The extracellular mucin signals histiocytes to the affected area, and results in formation of the so-called "mucin granulomas." Additionally, multinucleated histiocytes, known as "foreign body type giant cells" can cluster near areas of ulceration and mimic granuloma formation. Thus, it is essential to carefully inspect the quality of the histiocytic reaction in respect to the associated background features to determine the significance of granuloma formation in IBD patients.

Crohn's Disease

The first microscopic description of what is now known as Crohn's disease was made by Crohn, Ginzburg, and Oppenheimer in 1932, although autopsy and clinical case reports of patients with CD-like symptoms have existed for centuries (e.g., Louis XIII of France) [16]. In the description by Crohn et al., the term, "regional ileitis" was used to describe full-thickness inflammation of the bowel wall, fibrosis, stricture formation, well-formed granulomas, and a tendency to form fistula tracts [17]. Today, we recognize a similar spectrum of findings anywhere in the gastrointestinal tract as CD.

Gross Appearance

Unique gross and microscopic features of CD and UC are shown in Table 22.1. CD occurs in a patchy or segmental distribution anywhere in the gastrointestinal tract in contrast to UC which is diffuse and limited to the colon and rectum. Segmental distribution is illustrated in Fig. 22.7. Here the involved external serosa reveals "creeping fat" or "fat wrapping" due to fibrous adhesions and increased fat deposition (Fig. 22.7 inset). The affected area in this resection specimen is characteristically narrowed from stricture formation and flanked by discrete regions of normal appearing intestine. Most notably, the opened specimen does not lay flat (compare Fig. 22.7 CD specimen to Fig. 22.4 UC specimen), a result of extensive fibrosis and transmural disease. On closer inspection, a markedly thickened bowel wall and strikingly narrowed luminal diameter can be appreciated in the strictured segment. The mucosa takes on a cobblestone appearance due to alternating areas of ulcerated and preserved mucosa. Deep, knife-like ulcerations, which give rise to fistula tracts, are common but not easily appreciated in this image. When examining a severely active CD specimen such as this, it is not difficult to understand how stricture and fistula formation carry a high risk of perforation and abscess formation, both indicators for segmental resection. Pseudopolyps (e.g., Fig. 22.6), created by cycles of regeneration and injury, are identical to those observed in UC (see above discussion).

Table 22.1 Key gross and microscopic features of UC and CD

	Ulcerative colitis	Crohn's disease
Gross features		
Distribution	Continuous extending proximally from rectum	Segmental, involving any part of the GI tract
Thickness	Superficial, limited to mucosa and submucosa	Full thickness, often extending through muscularis propria
Microscopic features		
Ulcerations	Broad and shallow	Knife-like and fissuring
Granulomas	Associated with ruptured crypts and areas of ulceration	Compact and well formed
Distribution	Diffuse throughout biopsy	Patchy, alternating areas of normal and injured mucosa in single biopsy

Microscopic Appearance

As CD may involve any part of the gastrointestinal tract classic histologic features can be observed in the oral cavity (Fig. 22.8a), esophagus, stomach (Fig. 22.8b), and small (Fig. 22.8c) and large intestines (Fig. 22.8d). Along with distribution and depth of disease, several additional histologic features define CD: type of ulcer, fibrosis, granuloma formation and neuronal hyperplasia.

Patchy chronic injury: Analogous to the gross morphologic features described in the previous discussion, histologic

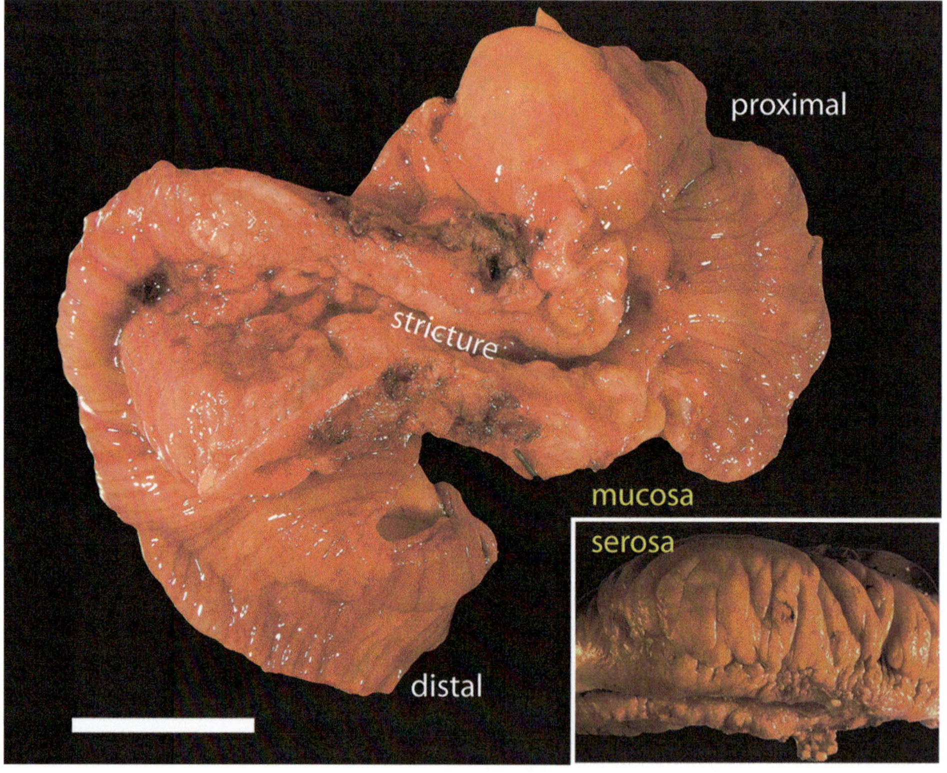

Fig. 22.7 Features of Crohn's colitis are evident on gross examination. In this segmental resection of colon, the resection margins have a normal pink tan appearance. The lumen in the center portion of the specimen is narrowed, and the walls are thickened. In contrast to what is observed in UC, the specimen will not lay flat. The serosal surface (*inset*) displays evidence of fat wrapping, or creeping fat. (Scale bar: 5.0 cm)

discontinuous disease distribution is illustrated by distinct areas of normal and diseased mucosa within a single biopsy (Fig. 22.8d), as well as separate affected and non affected biopsies from sequential segments of small and large intestine. Please refer to the to the UC section on caveats to disease distribution.

Depth of disease: Similar to UC, active neutrophilic inflammation ranging from quiescent to severely active is superimposed on chronic injury (Fig. 22.4). However, in CD, inflammation may extend transmurally to form strictures and fistula tracts, features not present in UC. Limited superficial mucosal inflammation without full thickness involvement can occur and should not rule out a diagnosis of CD.

Type of ulcer: Small aphthous ulcers and deep, knifelike, fissuring ulcers are characteristic of CD. Aphthous ulcers seen endoscopically correlate with small collections of intraepithelial neutrophils overlying lymphoid aggregates histologically (Fig. 22.9). These are believed to coalesce, resulting in deep ulceration which eventually can extend into the muscularis propria. Fistula formation likely develops from these large deep fissuring, knife-like, ulcers extending through the serosa and into pericolonic fibroadipose tissue (Fig. 22.10).

Fibrosis: In CD, transmural lymphoid aggregates along with diffuse lymphoplasmacytic and variable neutrophilic inflammatory infiltrates are observed within a markedly thickened, fibrotic stroma. Proliferation of inflammatory cells, fibroblasts

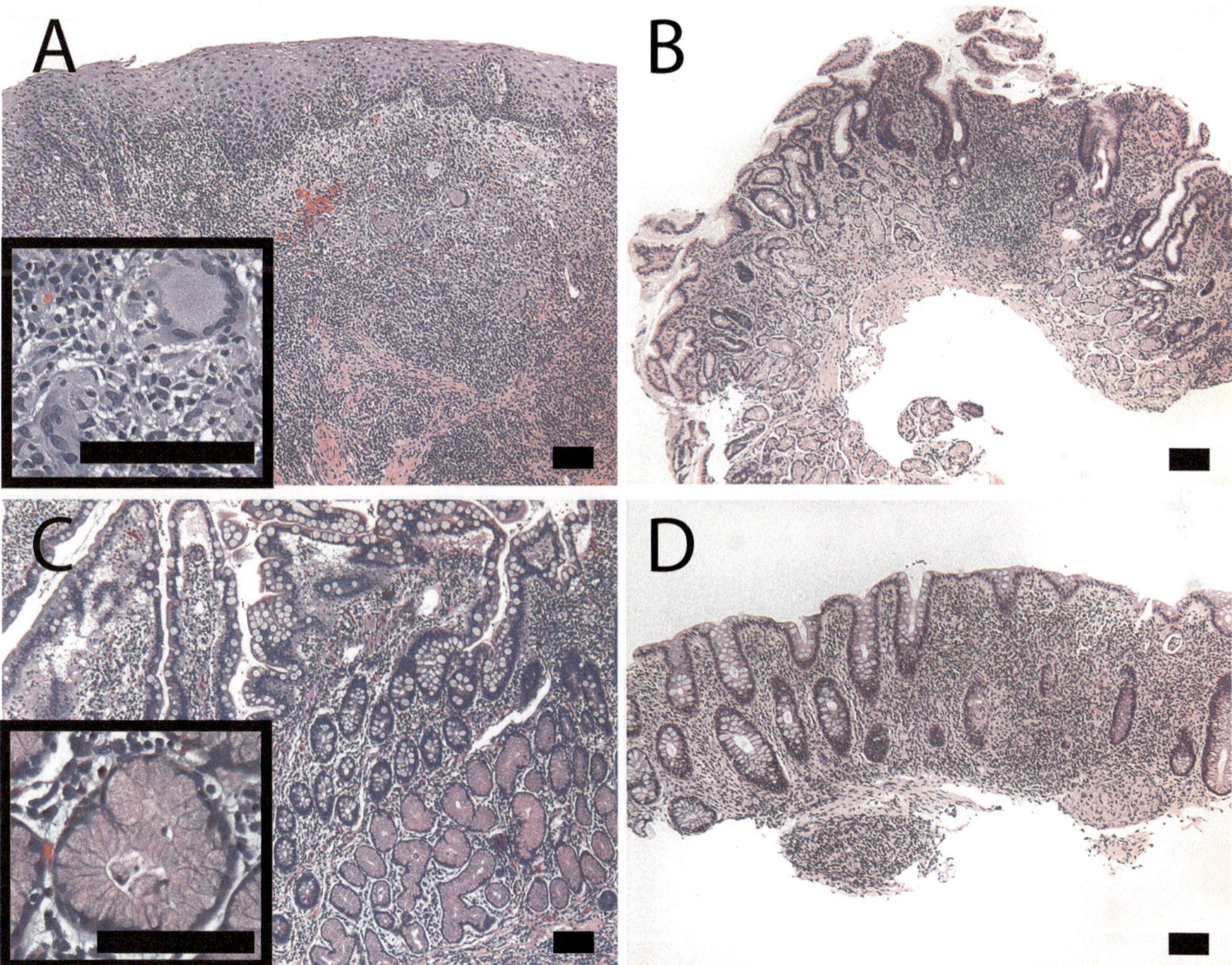

Fig. 22.8 CD may occur anywhere in the gastrointestinal tract. (**a**) Squamous mucosa has increased intraepithelial lymphocytes and numerous inflammatory cells are present in the lamina propria. Epithelial cells are reactive, and mild basal cell layer hyperplasia is present. A granuloma is present in the lamina propria (*inset*). (**b**) Antral mucosa in the left portion of the image appears normal with clear mucous and bicarbonate secreting foveolar cells, which normally line the entire gastric mucosa. Focal active CD with ulceration is present in the right portion of image. The regenerating foveolar epithelial cells appear mucin depleted and the lamina propria has a dense lymphoplasmacytic infiltrate. Antral glands have been destroyed in this area. *Helicobacter pylori* organisms were not present. (**c**) Ileal villus architectural distortion and pyloric metaplasia (*inset*) are present in this patch of ileal mucosa involved by CD. (**d**) Focal chronic active colitis is present in this biopsy from a patient with CD. (All scale bars: 60 μm)

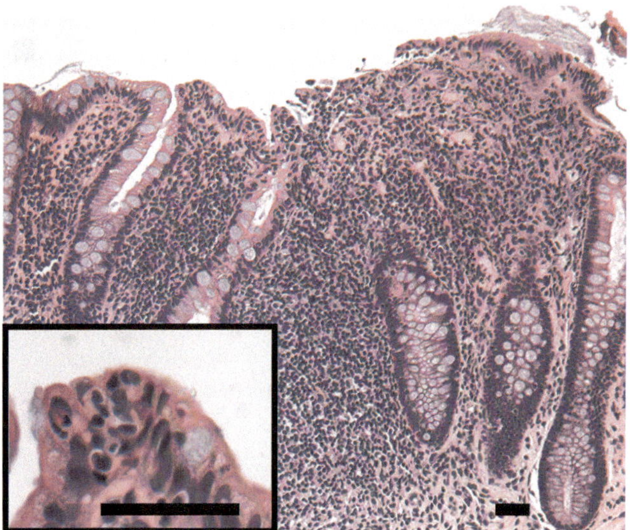

Fig. 22.9 Aphthous ulcerations are early lesions of CD. These occur over lymphoid follicles and are associated with the presence of intraepithelial neutrophils (*inset*) (scale bars: 40 μm)

and myofibroblasts along with increased collagen deposition can extend into the serosa and pericolonic fibroadipose tissues culminating in stricture formation.

Granulomas: The granulomas of CD may be poorly or tightly formed and can be found in any layer in the bowel wall. As described in the UC section, mucin granulomas and foreign body type reactions secondary to epithelial injury must be differentiated from well-formed granulomas diagnostic of CD. Sarcoidosis and tuberculosis are other granuloma forming processes to be considered and ruled out prior to rendering a diagnosis of CD.

Neuronal hyperplasia: Parasympathetic ganglia in the submucosa (Meissner's plexus) and muscularis propria (myenteric, or Auerbach's, plexus) can become hypertrophic in CD, displaying irregularly shaped nerve bundles and increased ganglion cells.

Although many cases of CD will display some or all of the above morphologic features, there is often significant histologic and clinical overlap between CD and UC. Therefore, it is important to include detailed descriptions in the pathology report to properly assess future biopsy material in order to render a definitive diagnosis.

Complications of IBD

Management of the IBD patient is complicated by the natural progression of the disease process, as well as the therapeutic interventions themselves. The pathology of commonly encountered complications in IBD is addressed below.

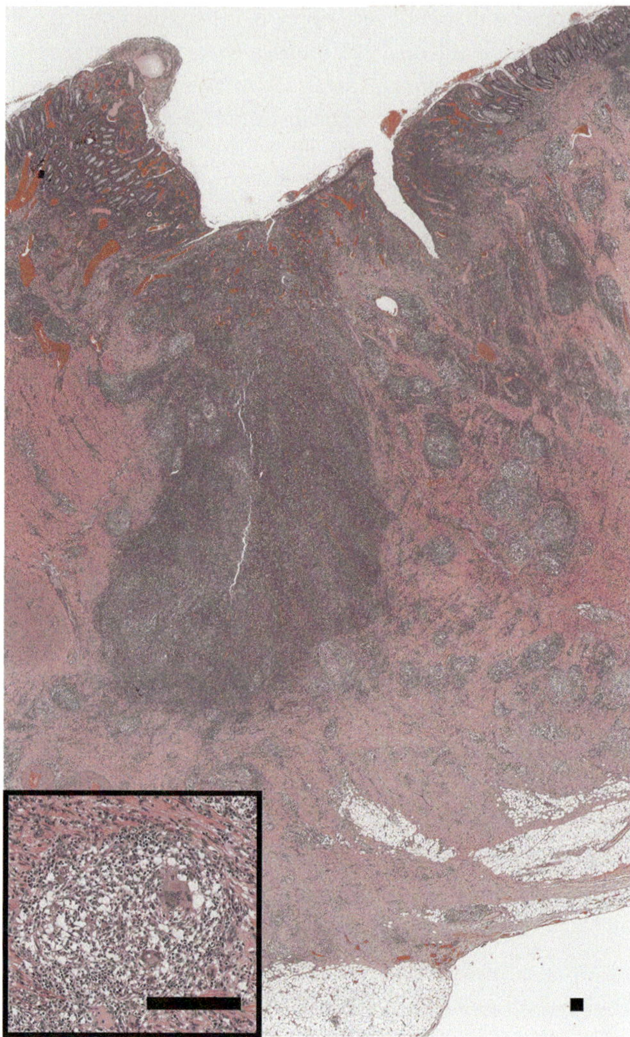

Fig. 22.10 Inflammation in CD may be transmural. In this case of severely active disease in the colon, a knife-like fissuring ulcer is present, there is fibrosis of the submucosa and serosa, and numerous granulomas (*inset*) are present (scale bars 0.4 mm)

Complications of Severe IBD

Obstruction, fissures, and fistulas: As discussed above, CD is associated with stricture and fistula formation necessitating segmental resection. Strictures seen in UC patients can also be associated with obstruction from diverticular disease, but can represent an advanced adenocarcinoma.

IBD associated dysplasia: IBD is linked to an increased risk of colorectal carcinoma. IBD-associated dysplasia, a precursor lesion, and carcinoma occur at a younger age than the general population [18]. Endoscopic screening allows for the detection of dysplastic lesions and early carcinomas, thereby decreasing the risk of developing invasive and metastatic disease, respectively [19]. Guidelines for screening and management are discussed in Chap. 9.

In patients with IBD dysplasia may present with an endoscopically apparent lesion or mass (dysplasia-associated lesion/mass; DALM), or may be flat, which can be difficult to detect. Therefore, random biopsies of both suspicious and normal appearing mucosa are critical in IBD associated dysplasia. In addition, sporadic adenomas occur in IBD patients in the same frequency as non-IBD patients. As treatment for a sporadic adenoma is simple polypectomy versus aggressive follow-up and often resection for IBD associated dysplasia [19], much effort is given to differentiate the two. This can be quite a difficult task as there are currently no highly specific guidelines to follow [20]. However, the key feature favoring IBD-associated dysplasia is the presence of chronic injury in the mucosa surrounding the area of dysplasia. Patient age and duration of disease are essential clinical features to consider as well. For instance a patient under the age of 40 is less likely to have developed a sporadic adenoma. Similarly, IBD associated dysplasia would be unusual in a patient with new-onset IBD.

Microscopically dysplasia is categorized as either low or high grade. An important feature in both grades of dysplasia is the lack of maturation of epithelial cells towards the surface epithelium. Low grade dysplasia is characterized by tall columnar epithelial cells with pseudo-stratified, basally oriented, hyperchromatic and elongated nuclei (Fig. 22.11a). In contrast, high grade dysplasia (Fig. 22.11b) displays more severe cytologic features such as loss of epithelial polarity, pleomorphic nuclei, and bizarre mitotic figures, as well as architectural abnormalities, i.e., back to back, or cribriform glands. To complicate a diagnosis of IBD-associated dysplasia further, during active disease states, the non-dysplastic mucosa is quite inflamed which can result in atypical histologic features referred to as "reactive epithelial atypia." Reactive epithelial atypia can sometimes be difficult to differentiate from high grade dysplasia as there may be overlapping abnormal cytologic features. However, the most critical histologic feature to assess in differentiating high grade dysplasia from reactive epithelial atypia is epithelial polarity. As epithelial cells demonstrating high grade dysplasia display loss of apicobasolateral polarity the cells no longer line up uniformly on the basement membrane. The higher the grade of dysplasia, the more severe loss of polarity. Epithelial cells displaying features of reactive atypia secondary to inflammation should always maintain polarity, lining up evenly and regularly on the basement membrane (Fig. 22.12).

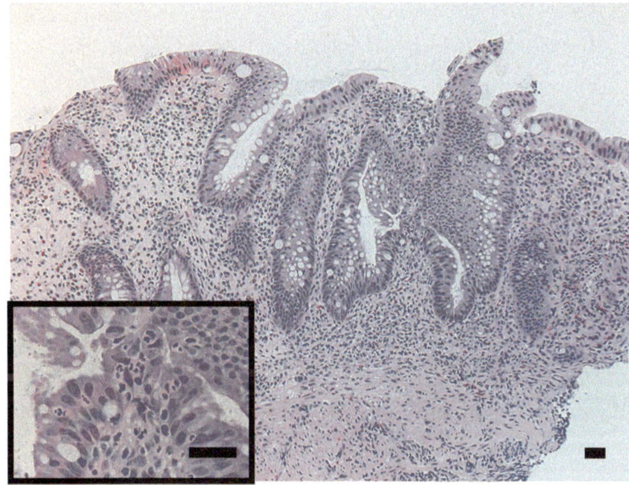

Fig. 22.12 Indefinite for dysplasia. This biopsy from a patient with ulcerative colitis was called, "indefinite for dysplasia." The biopsy shows some hyperchromatic enlarged nuclei and loss of polarity extending to the surface epithelium. In this setting of moderate active inflammation (*inset*), it was felt that this was most likely not dysplastic, and this was expressed in a diagnostic comment. The clinical plan was to follow this patient closely and to re-biopsy at a later time once the active inflammation was brought under control (scale bar 40 μm)

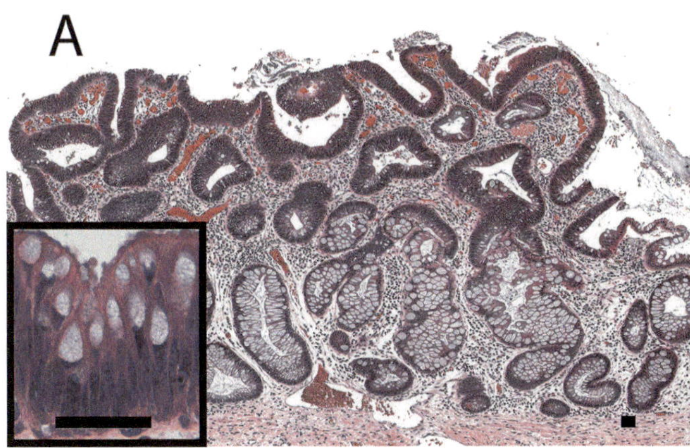

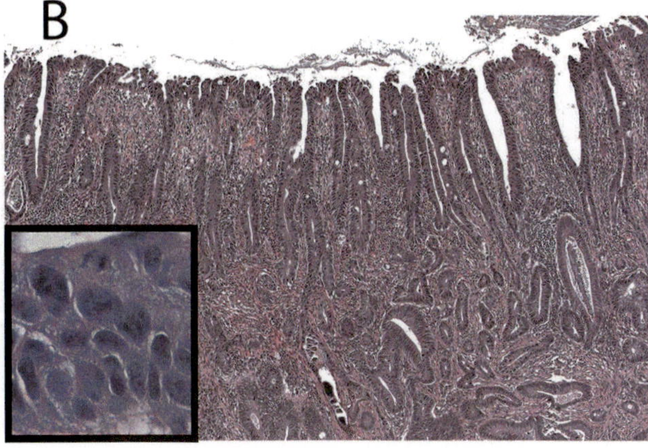

Fig. 22.11 Patients with inflammatory bowel disease have an increased risk of developing premalignant, dysplastic epithelial lesions. Low grade dysplasia (**a**) is characterized by the presence of hyperchromatic, enlarged nuclei, with some stratification (*inset*), but all dysplastic cells are similar in shape and oriented in the same direction. (**b**) Cells of high grade dysplasia are markedly pleomorphic and nuclei are haphazardly oriented with respect to the basement membrane. Cribiforming, or formation of back to back glands, is present, and a desmoplastic (fibrotic) response indicates invasion in the lower part of the image (scale bar 40 μm)

In addition, if the biopsy material is limited or poorly processed, it may be impossible to differentiate dysplasia from histologic artifact. Therefore, a third category of "indefinite for dysplasia" may be used sparingly to communicate to the clinician that a firm diagnosis of dysplasia cannot be made on the current biopsy material submitted for review. In these situations it is critical to write a comment in the pathology report detailing the reason behind a diagnosis "indefinite for dysplasia." For example if the mucosa revealed severe inflammation, additional biopsy material should be obtained after the patient is treated and active inflammation reduced. On the other hand, if the biopsies were too small or crushed, or the tissue processing was poor, then the clinician may re-biopsy right away given the high risk for invasive carcinoma in IBD patients with dysplasia.

Toxic Megacolon: Several inflammatory conditions, most commonly UC, can involve rapid dilation and loss of contractility within a colonic segment. Inflammation and or stretching causes increased wall tension and subsequent damage to the muscularis propria and myenteric plexus. Nonfunctional muscle and nerve results in extreme bowel wall thinning that, when subjected to increased luminal pressure, is at high risk for perforation. This process, known as "toxic megacolon" is associated with a high mortality rate and is an indication for immediate colectomy.

Complications of Therapy

Diversion Colitis: Segments of bowel surgically isolated from the normal fecal stream can develop extensive mucosal follicular hyperplasia, a condition known as diversion colitis (Fig. 22.13). Inflammation can also extend more deeply and

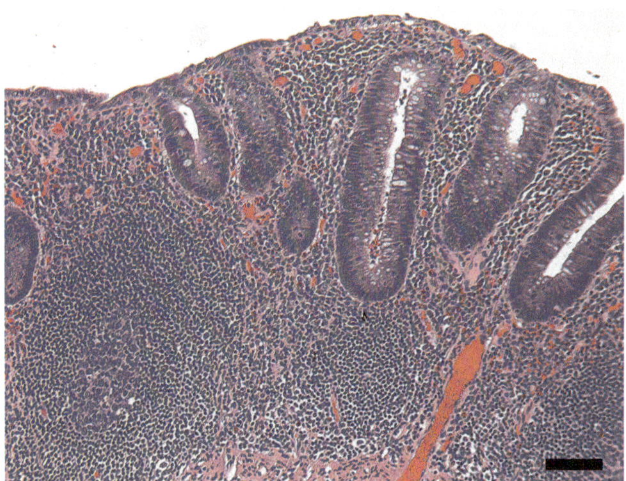

Fig. 22.13 Histologic features of diversion colitis are seen in segments of bowel removed from the normal intestinal flow. In this biopsy, the typical diversion colitis features (i.e., lymphoid hyperplasia) are seen in a background of chronic injury of UC

resemble CD. Knowledge of the surgical anatomy is critically important in differentiating diversion colitis from CD.

Pouchitis: Total abdominal colectomy with ileal-anal anastomosis is the surgical treatment of choice for uncontrolled UC. An ileal pouch can be created to serve as a fecal reservoir in selected patients; however, as small bowel does not normally perform colonic functions, the pouch mucosa is subject to irritation and inflammation, a complication termed pouchitis (Fig. 22.14). Chronic and active injury in the small bowel mucosa of the pouch in a UC patient can create diagnostic confusion by raising the possibility of a missed CD diagnosis. Differentiating pouchitis from CD is critically important. Features favoring a diagnosis of pouchitis include:

1. Prior biopsy and colectomy specimens that do not display macroscopic or microscopic features of CD (Table 22.1).
2. Preserved mucosal architecture in pre-pouch ileal biopsies (Fig. 22.14a vs. 22.14b).
3. Absence of clinical and radiographic evidence of CD elsewhere in the body.
4. A positive family history of Crohn's disease and/or HLA genotypes.

Cytomegalovirus infection: IBD patients are considered at baseline to be immunocompromised compared to the general population. With the standard use of immunosuppressive agents for therapy, treated patients will become even further immunosuppressed. As such, they are at increased risk for many infections, including cytomegalovirus (CMV). Unsuspected CMV infection during treatment is of particular importance because it can mimic therapeutic failure and worsen symptoms. The classic eosinophilic cytoplasmic and intranuclear inclusions (Fig. 22.15) are present in enlarged endothelial and epithelial cells. When surrounded by a clear halo, the nuclear inclusions are referred to as "owl's eyes." As these inclusions can be difficult to find, multiple H&E levels must be examined and, when suspicion is high, as in severe active disease states, immunohistochemical stains and or PCR for CMV DNA can be utilized to highlight viral proteins.

Pseudomembranous Colitis: After antibiotic therapy, infection with Clostridium difficile, or other toxigenic bacteria may lead to severe diarrhea in IBD and non IBD patients. White to yellow pseudomembranes seen on endoscopy correlate with supraepithelial lamellated layers of fibrin, mucin, neutrophils, and necrotic cells histologically. Eruptions of the lamellated layers streaming out of crypts, are referred to as "volcano lesions." When the active inflammatory component is not obvious, epithelial withering and other features of ischemia can provide clues to a diagnosis of pseudomembranous colitis. All of the above features can be seen on a

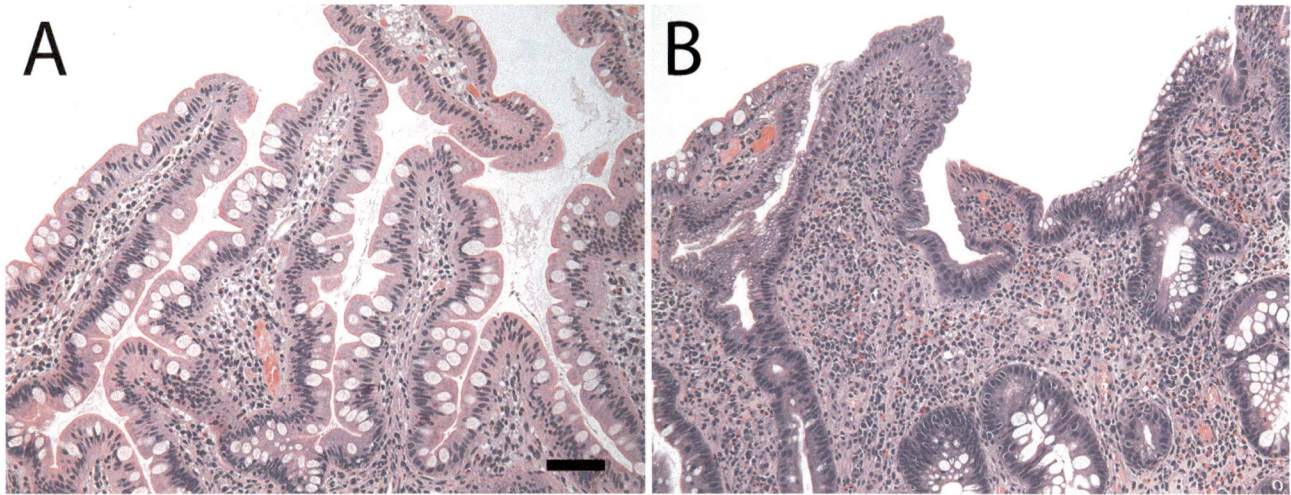

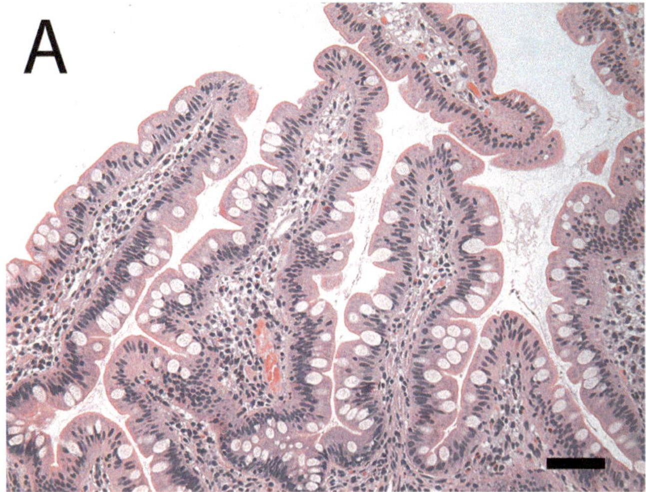

Fig. 22.14 Pouchitis may be associated with features of chronic injury that should not be confused with recurrent CD. (**a**) The pre-pouch biopsy shows relatively normal small intestinal architecture. (**b**) Diffuse chronic mucosal injury with active inflammation is seen in the pouch, but there are no features specific for CD

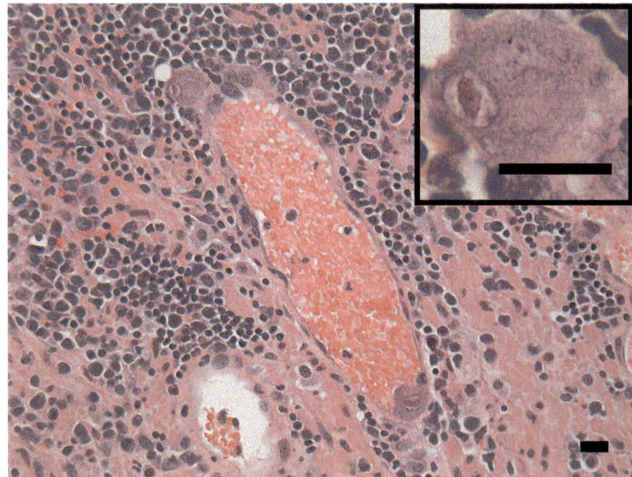

Fig. 22.15 Cytomegalovirus superinfection is a feature that should not be overlooked in any immunosuppressed patient. Endothelial cells contain intranuclear viral inclusions (scale bar 20 μm)

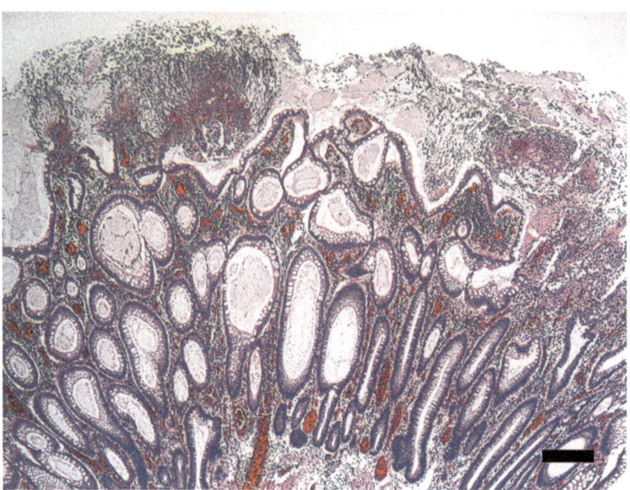

Fig. 22.16 Pseudomembranous colitis may coexist with IBD. A pseudomembrane composed of fibrin and inflammatory cells is a typical feature of pseudomembranous colitis. Several "volcano lesions" are notable in the upper left portion of the image (scale bar: 300 μm)

background of chronic injury (Fig. 22.16), so IBD patients with a history of extensive antibiotic use should be assessed for the presence of fecal C. difficile toxin.

Extraintestinal Manifestations of IBD

IBD manifests in many other organs besides the gastrointestinal tract, including the pancreas, skin, and the musculoskeletal system. Detailed discussions of these entities are beyond the scope of this chapter (see Chap. 5), but a few clinically important manifestations will be briefly addressed here.

Primary Sclerosing Cholangitis: Primary Sclerosing Cholangitis (PSC) is a chronic cholestatic disease characterized by inflammation, fibrosis and strictures of extra and intrahepatic bile ducts ultimately leading to cirrhosis. PSC is strongly associated with UC and affected patients carry a threefold increased risk of developing colonic dysplastic lesions [21]. The hallmark histologic features in liver specimens include "onion-skinning" fibrosis and lymphocytic inflammation surrounding large, mainly extra-hepatic, bile ducts (Fig. 22.17).

Mucocutaenous lesions: Skin and oral lesions have been reported in up to 20% of IBD patients [22]. These lesions may be direct manifestations of the primary inflammatory process or secondary to nutritional deficiency.

Pyoderma gangrenosum [23]: More common in UC than CD, pyoderma gangrenosum is seen exclusively in the IBD patient population. These lesions occur during times of active disease but can also herald a diagnosis of IBD. Clinically, the lesions appear most commonly in the pretibial region, as ulcers with dark necrotic centers surrounded by bright erythematous skin. Histologic features of necrosis, vasculitis, thrombosis and dense neutrophilic infiltrates are nonspecific. These lesions become important clinically when ulcerations extend into the bone resulting in osteomyelitis, an infection requiring intensive medical treatment.

Cutaneous Crohn's Disease: Inflammation can extend directly from perianal and ostomy sites to the skin, and rarely can involve areas of skin without direct spread from the gastrointestinal tract. Lesions can be raised or flat, with or without ulcerations [24]. Histologically, noncaseating granulomatous inflammation is observed predominantly in the dermis. Since several other inflammatory and infectious processes result in granulomatous inflammation in the skin, it is important to be aware of cutaneous manifestations of CD.

Oral Lesions

Recurrent oral aphthous ulcers are the most common extraintestinal manifestation of IBD. These well-defined, "punched-out" superficial ulcerations may indicate primary IBD or result from nutritional deficiencies secondary to gastrointestinal pathology. Occurring most often during active disease, aphthous ulcers are often associated with other extraintestinal demonstrations of IBD.

Eye Lesions

A variety of eye lesions involving not only the conjunctiva and retina but also periorbital skin and muscle are observed in approximately 10% of IBD patients.

Mimics of IBD

Many diseases characterized by ongoing active inflammation for an extended period of time are included in the clinical differential diagnosis of IBD. Therefore entities lacking features of chronic injury such as acute self-limited infectious colitis, lymphocytic colitis, and collagenous colitis are frequently biopsied, but can usually be differentiated from IBD. However, when chronic injury is present, as seen in association with radiation, ischemia, mucosal prolapse, diverticular disease, autoimmune disease and medication, knowledge of unique histologic features is required to differentiate IBD from these entities.

Infectious colitis: Infectious colitis due to bacterial infections, such as Yersinia, Campylobacter, Salmonella, and Shigella, are self-limited, and therefore, the causative agent is frequently not determined. Inflammation is predominantly neutrophilic, similar to active IBD; however, chronic injury is absent (Fig. 22.18). Interestingly, several bacterial species can create granulomatous inflammation, a feature not to be

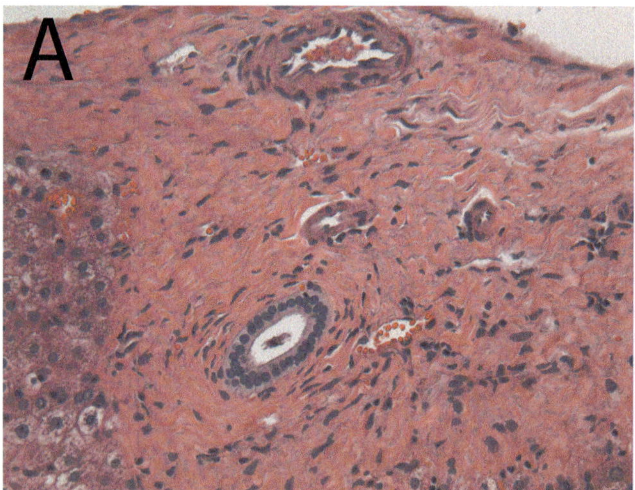

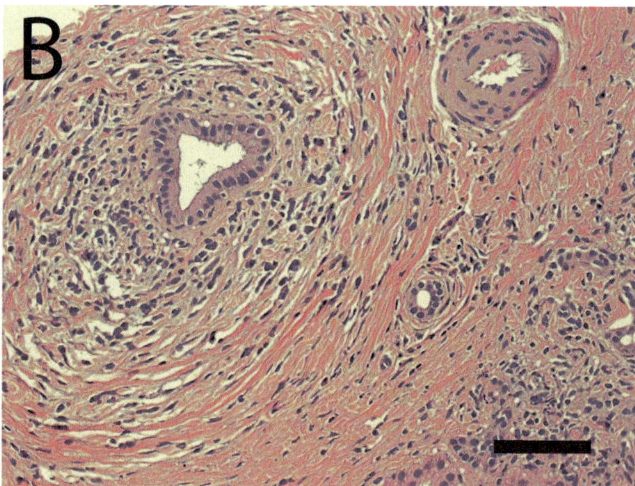

Fig. 22.17 Primary Sclerosing Cholangitis affects extrahepatic and larger intrahepatic bile ducts. (**a**) Several layers of hypocellular collagen surround normal intralobular bile ducts, which are lined by simple cuboidal epithelium. (**b**) The bile duct of a patient with UC and primary sclerosing cholangitis demonstrates "onion-skinning" fibrosis and prominent periductal lymphocytic infiltrate (scale bars: 150 μm)

confused with CD [25]. Parasitic infections such as *Entamoeba histolytica* can produce deep ulcerations resembling CD. While uncommon in most Western nations, these infections must be considered in the differential diagnosis of any patient who may have lived or recently visited tropical countries where such diseases are endemic.

Microscopic colitis: Microscopic colitis manifests as chronic diarrhea appearing endoscopically normal but histologically abnormal. The term microscopic colitis actually describes two main pathologic entities: collagenous colitis (Fig. 22.19a) and lymphocytic colitis (Fig. 22.19b). Both collagenous and lymphocytic colitis are defined by increased intraepithelial lymphocytes. Mild active inflammation may be present, but is not a principle histologic feature. Increased numbers of mononuclear cells are observed in the lamina propria; however, this tends to be more superficial and not the characteristic basal, band-like infiltrate of IBD. Some chronic regenerative features such as Paneth cell metaplasia and mild crypt architectural distortion can also be seen, but [26] severe architectural irregularities should raise the possibility of IBD. Collagenous colitis is differentiated from lymphocytic colitis by the presence of a thickened, eosinophilic, collagenous table located directly beneath the epithelial layer, classically entrapping small capillaries and cellular debris.

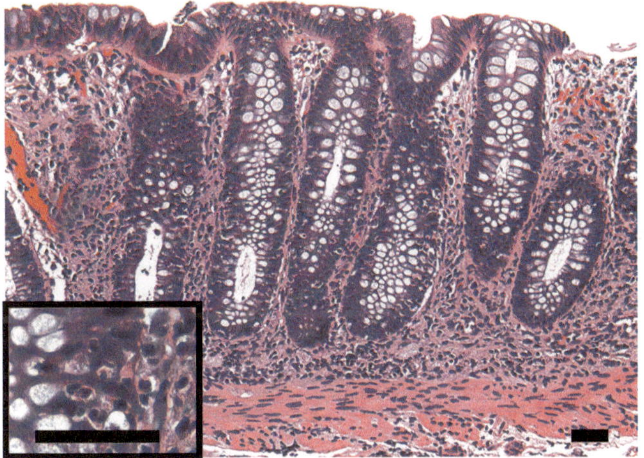

Fig. 22.18 Self-limiting infectious colitis is associated with active inflammation, but the absence of chronic injury. Mild to moderately active inflammation is present within this colonic biopsy (*inset*). There is no evidence of crypt architectural distortion (scale bar: 80 μm)

Chronic Radiation Colitis: When provided with proper clinical history, radiation damage is usually not a diagnostic challenge; however, chronic mucosal injury sustained from radiation may remain clinically silent for years [27]. Biopsies reveal marked architectural distortion along with regenerative cytological atypia beyond what can be attributed to chronic injury in IBD (Fig. 22.20a). Extreme cellular and nuclear enlargement in unusually shaped, flattened epithelial and endothelial cells and fibroblasts are atypical cytologic clues to previous radiation therapy. Additionally, extensive hyalinization can be seen in connective tissue and within blood vessel walls, the latter of which may result in vascular occlusion and superimposed ischemic injury (below).

Ischemia: Causes of ischemic injury may be primarily vascular or hematologic, may occur secondary to intrinsic intestinal obstruction causing vascular compression, infection, or drugs [28]. The characteristic features of ischemia are a withered or

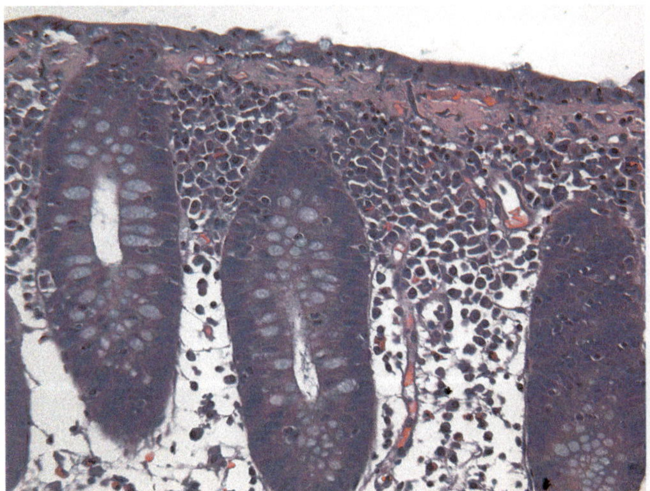

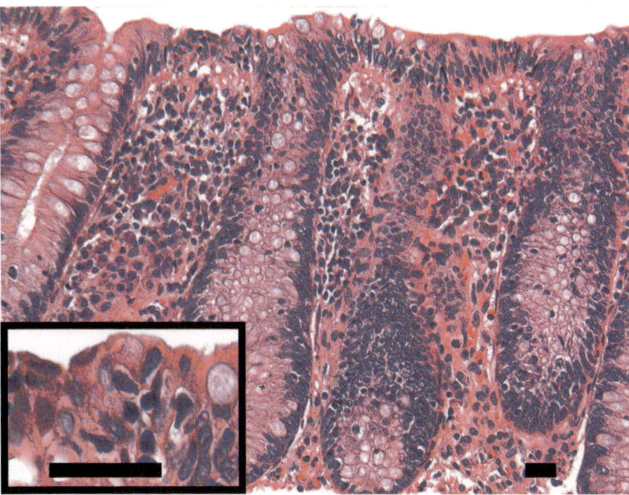

Fig. 22.19 Microscopic findings in two patients with watery diarrhea and normal endoscopy. (**a**) Collagenous colitis is associated with a thickened and irregular subepithelial fibrous band present beneath the surface epithelium. Overall crypt architecture is preserved. Lamina propria plasma cells are numerous towards the surface. (**b**) Intraepithelial lymphocytes are numerous in this biopsy from a patient with lymphocytic colitis. Absence of a thickened collagen band differentiates lymphocytic from collagenous colitis. Again, overall crypt architecture is preserved (scale bars: 20 μm)

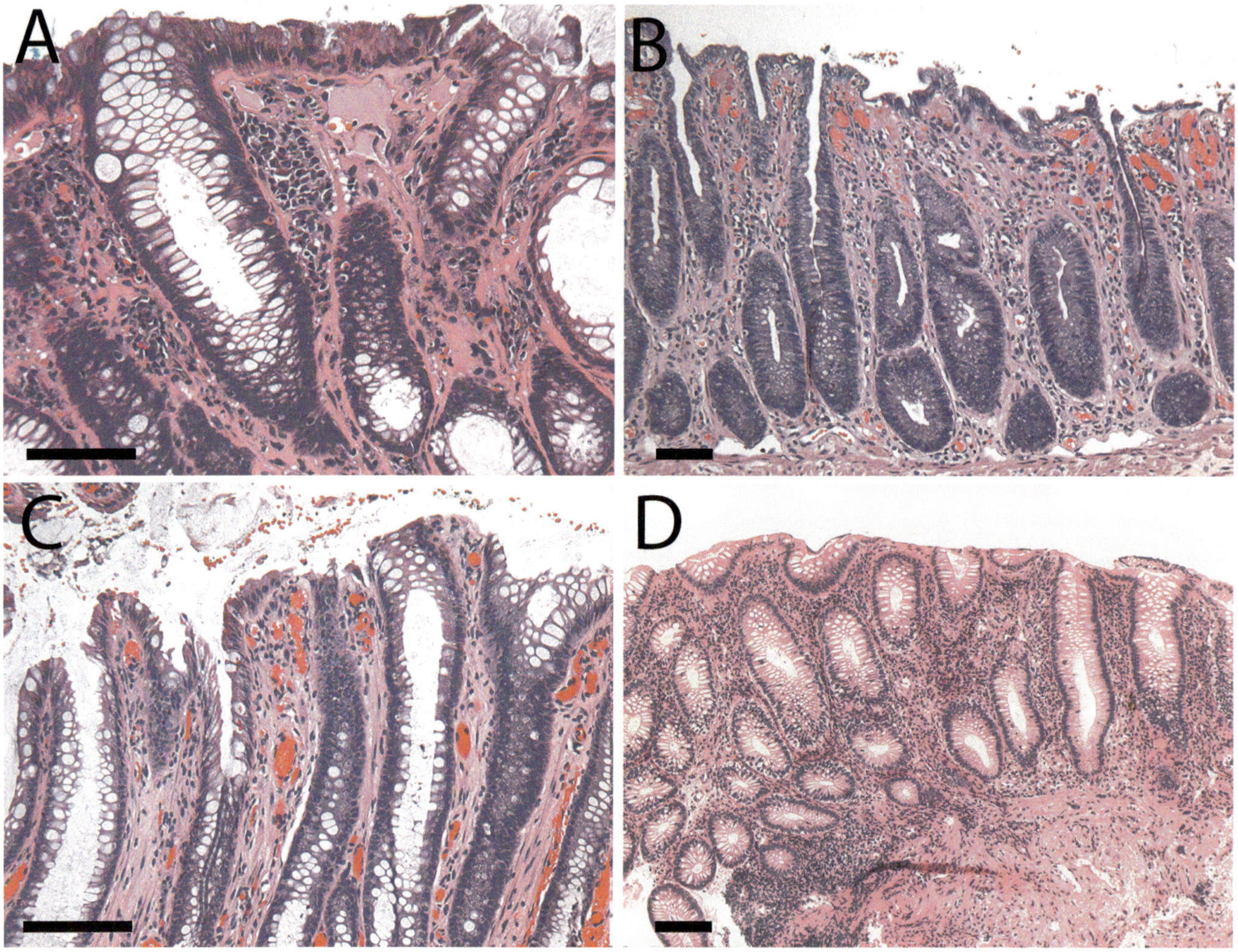

Fig. 22.20 Features of chronic injury are seen in disorders other than inflammatory bowel disease. In each of these situations, clinicopathological correlations are essential. (**a**) Chronic colonic injury may occur secondary to radiation therapy. Fibrosis of the basement membrane and surface cytological atypia are features consistent with a known history of radiation injury. (**b**) Ischemia is associated with withering of surface epithelial cells and mild fibrosis of the lamina propria. Basally located crypt epithelial cells appear relatively well preserved. (**c**) In solitary rectal ulcer syndrome smooth muscle fibers extend upward from into the lamina propria. (**d**) Diverticular associated colitis may similarly resemble IBD (all scale bars: 80 μm)

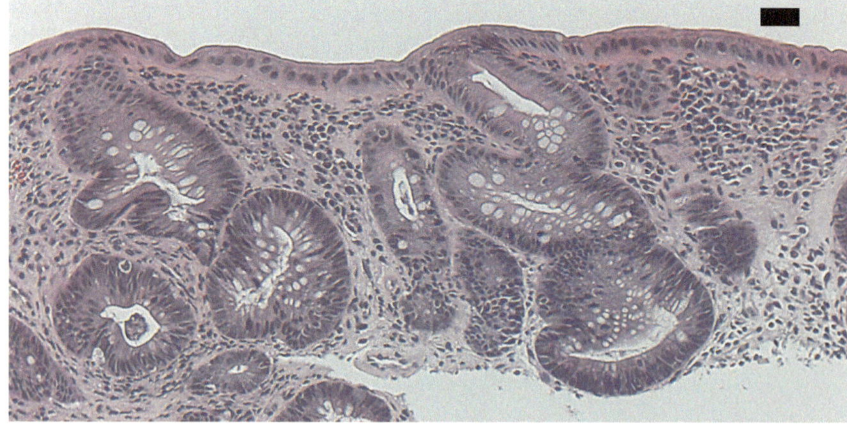

Fig. 22.21 Chronic active colitis may occur secondary to drugs. This is an example of ipilimumab colitis in a patient with melanoma (scale bars: 40 μm)

attenuated surface epithelium, increasing in severity towards the luminal surface, in association with relatively preserved crypt epithelium. This appearance reflects low oxygen tension towards the lumen while crypt epithelial cells remain close to the lamina propria vasculature (Fig. 22.20b). In severe cases the entire mucosa may display intense active inflammation with crypt abscesses formation and ulceration or show complete mucosal necrosis. The lamina propria is hemorrhagic and edematous early in the disease process, becoming increasingly fibrotic after repeated ischemic episodes (Fig. 22.20c). As ischemia is dictated by vascular supply, injury is usually focal or segmental, a pattern of distribution similar to CD. Careful examination of submucosal vessels may reveal diagnostic clues such as vessels with fibrin thrombi or amyloid deposition; however, the etiology of ischemia is often unknown.

Solitary Rectal Ulcer/Mucosal Prolapse: Solitary rectal ulcer syndrome typically occurs in the anterior rectal wall, and, ironically, may be neither solitary nor ulcerated. The histological features reflect injury due to prolapse of mucosa into the fecal stream, including epithelial hyperplasia with mucosal ischemic changes. Prolapsed strands of smooth muscle can be seen in a hyalinized lamina propria running perpendicular to the muscularis mucosa (Fig. 22.20c). Depending on severity and duration of prolapse, the mucosa may become markedly inflamed and architecturally distorted and the lamina propria fibrotic, mimicking IBD.

Diverticular disease [29–31]: Biopsies taken from the immediate area of an inflamed diverticulum may display similar features of CD; crypt architectural distortion, crypt abscesses, and foreign body type giant cell reactions. Furthermore, IBD patients can manifest disease within segments of colon containing diverticula, most often the sigmoid colon. This is termed diverticular disease-associated colitis (Fig. 22.20d) and is not limited to patients with IBD [29]. Thus, knowledge of diverticular disease is essential information to relay to the pathologist.

Drugs and Toxins: Chemotherapeutic agents, NSAIDS, or other drugs (Fig. 22.21) cause a variety of nonspecific active and chronic injury throughout the GI tract that can appear identical to IBD. Therefore in evaluating erosions, ulcerations and diffuse inflammation, knowledge of medication history is extremely helpful as new onset IBD would be very rare in an immunosuppressed patient on chemotherapy.

Behçet's disease [25, 32]: Although rare in Europe and North America, Behçet's disease should be considered in individuals with a history of iritis and oral and genital ulcers. Gastrointestinal involvement manifests preferentially in the ileocecal mucosa as transmural, patchy Crohn's-like, inflammation. However, Behçet's disease is defined by prominent vasculitis involving veins in varying stages of activity, a feature which may or may not be seen as a minor component in IBD.

Summary

An exhaustive review of IBD pathology in this short chapter is not possible, so emphasis is intentionally placed on diagnostically and clinically relevant macroscopic and microscopic manifestations of UC and CD. Difficulty in providing a definitive diagnosis of UC or CD can be due to many factors, as classic features are not present in every patient. Furthermore, the majority of IBD patients have an extensive treatment history, thus providing additional complexity to the diagnostic process. Therefore, strong communication between the pathologist and the clinician is essential in caring for the IBD patient.

References

1. Kumar V, Abbas AK, Fausto N, Aster J. Robbins and Cotran pathologic basis of disease. 8th ed. Philadelphia, PA: Elsevier Saunders; 2009.
2. Paterson JC, Watson SH. Paneth cell metaplasia in ulcerative colitis. Am J Pathol. 1961;38:243–9.
3. Kleer CG, Appelman HD. Ulcerative colitis: patterns of involvement in colorectal biopsies and changes with time. Am J Surg Pathol. 1998;22(8):983–9.
4. Binder V. A comparison between clinical state, macroscopic and microscopic appearances of rectal mucosa, and cytologic picture of mucosal exudate in ulcerative colitis. Scand J Gastroenterol. 1970;5(7):627–32.
5. Gomes P, du Boulay C, Smith CL, Holdstock G. Relationship between disease activity indices and colonoscopic findings in patients with colonic inflammatory bowel disease. Gut. 1986;27(1):92–5.
6. Geert D'haens, William J. Sandborn, Brian G. Feagan, Karel Geboes, Stephen B. Hanauer, E. Jan Irvine et al. A review of activity indices and efficacy end points for clinical trials of medical therapy in adults with ulcerative colitis. Gastroenterology. 2007;132(2):763–86.
7. Joo M, Odze RD. Rectal sparing and skip lesions in ulcerative colitis: a comparative study of endoscopic and histologic findings in patients who underwent proctocolectomy. Am J Surg Pathol. 2010;34(5):689–96.
8. Velayos FS, Loftus Jr EV, Jess T, et al. Predictive and protective factors associated with colorectal cancer in ulcerative colitis: a case-control study. Gastroenterology. 2006;130(7):1941–9.
9. Haskell H, Andrews Jr CW, Reddy SI, et al. Pathologic features and clinical significance of "backwash" ileitis in ulcerative colitis. Am J Surg Pathol. 2005;29(11):1472–81.
10. Okita Y, Miki C, Araki T, et al. Ulcerative colitis with severe backwash ileitis successfully treated by staged operation without sacrificing any involved ileum. J Pediatr Surg. 2009;44(1):e37–9.
11. D'Haens G, Geboes K, Peeters M, Baert F, Ectors N, Rutgeerts P. Patchy cecal inflammation associated with distal ulcerative

colitis: a prospective endoscopic study. Am J Gastroenterol. 1997;92(8):1275–9.
12. Ladefoged K, Munck LK, Jorgensen F, Engel P. Skip inflammation of the appendiceal orifice: a prospective endoscopic study. Scand J Gastroenterol. 2005;40(10):1192–6.
13. Yang SK, Jung HY, Kang GH, et al. Appendiceal orifice inflammation as a skip lesion in ulcerative colitis: an analysis in relation to medical therapy and disease extent. Gastrointest Endosc. 1999;49(6):743–7.
14. Washington K, Greenson JK, Montgomery E, et al. Histopathology of ulcerative colitis in initial rectal biopsy in children. Am J Surg Pathol. 2002;26(11):1441–9.
15. Markowitz J, Kahn E, Grancher K, Hyams J, Treem W, Daum F. Atypical rectosigmoid histology in children with newly diagnosed ulcerative colitis. Am J Gastroenterol. 1993;88(12):2034–7.
16. Baron JH. Inflammatory bowel disease up to 1932. Mt Sinai J Med. 2000;67(3):174–89.
17. Crohn BB, Ginzburg L, Oppenheimer GD. Regional ileitis; a pathologic and clinical entity. JAMA. 1932;99:1323–8.
18. Bernstein CN, Blanchard JF, Kliewer E, Wajda A. Cancer risk in patients with inflammatory bowel disease: a population-based study. Cancer. 2001;91(4):854–62.
19. Rubin DT, Turner JR. Surveillance of dysplasia in inflammatory bowel disease: the gastroenterologist-pathologist partnership. Clin Gastroenterol Hepatol. 2006;4(11):1309–13.
20. Odze RD. Adenomas and adenoma-like DALMs in chronic ulcerative colitis: a clinical, pathological, and molecular review. Am J Gastroenterol. 1999;94(7):1746–50.
21. Brentnall TA, Haggitt RC, Rabinovitch PS, et al. Risk and natural history of colonic neoplasia in patients with primary sclerosing cholangitis and ulcerative colitis. Gastroenterology. 1996;110(2):331–8.
22. Veloso FT, Carvalho J, Magro F. Immune-related systemic manifestations of inflammatory bowel disease. A prospective study of 792 patients. J Clin Gastroenterol. 1996;23(1):29–34.
23. Mir-Madjlessi SH, Taylor JS, Farmer RG. Clinical course and evolution of erythema nodosum and pyoderma gangrenosum in chronic ulcerative colitis: a study of 42 patients. Am J Gastroenterol. 1985;80(8):615–20.
24. Tavarela VF. Review article: skin complications associated with inflammatory bowel disease. Aliment Pharmacol Ther. 2004;20 Suppl 4:50–3.
25. Fenoglio-Preiser CM. Gastrointestinal pathology: an atlas and text. 3rd ed. Philadelphia, PA: Wolters Kluwer/Lippincott Williams & Wilkins; 2008.
26. Ayata G, Ithamukkala S, Sapp H, et al. Prevalence and significance of inflammatory bowel disease-like morphologic features in collagenous and lymphocytic colitis. Am J Surg Pathol. 2002;26(11):1414–23.
27. Oya M, Yao T, Tsuneyoshi M. Chronic irradiation enteritis: its correlation with the elapsed time interval and morphological changes. Hum Pathol. 1996;27(8):774–81.
28. Gandhi SK, Hanson MM, Vernava AM, Kaminski DL, Longo WE. Ischemic colitis. Dis Colon Rectum. 1996;39(1):88–100.
29. Makapugay LM, Dean PJ. Diverticular disease-associated chronic colitis. Am J Surg Pathol. 1996;20(1):94–102.
30. Gledhill A, Dixon MF. Crohn's-like reaction in diverticular disease. Gut. 1998;42(3):392–5.
31. Goldstein NS, Leon-Armin C, Mani A. Crohn's colitis-like changes in sigmoid diverticulitis specimens is usually an idiosyncratic inflammatory response to the diverticulosis rather than Crohn's colitis. Am J Surg Pathol. 2000;24(5):668–75.
32. Lehner T. Pathology of recurrent oral ulceration and oral ulceration in Behcet's syndrome: light, electron and fluorescence microscopy. J Pathol. 1969;97(3):481–94.

Objective Assessment of Clinical Disease Activity

23

Edouard Louis, Catherine Van Kemseke, and Catherine Reenaers

Inflammatory bowel diseases (IBD) are characterized by a chronic relapsing inflammation of the gastrointestinal tract. This inflammation may lead to complications, including intestinal strictures and fistulas in Crohn's disease (CD) and fulminant colitis, microrectum, and microcolon in ulcerative colitis (UC). Assessment and quantification of disease activity by indices is important to distinguish remission from flares and to determine different degrees of disease activity and severity. These indices are particularly important in clinical trials where an objective and reproducible quantification of disease activity is mandatory to clearly establish the effect of a new drug or to compare treatment strategies. They also tend to be more frequently used than in the past in routine practice. This is linked to the availability of new treatment options, which have been associated with an upgrading of treatment objectives and the expanding use of treatment optimization in incomplete responders to a given therapy. The currently available indices assess either clinical activity using simple scores or intestinal healing using cross-sectional imaging and endoscopy. In UC, the importance of mucosal healing and its good correlation to clinical activity of the disease has been recognized for a long time [1, 2], and endoscopic assessment has been integrated in several composite scores of activity. In CD, the correlation between clinical and endoscopic activity, albeit significant, was usually weak [3]. The clinical activity of the disease has long been considered as the only relevant end point of treatments [4, 5]. It is only recently that the significance of the persistence of endoscopic lesions in patients with clinical remission has been questioned. Particularly, the disappearance of significant endoscopic lesions, also called "mucosal healing," has been associated with a better outcome in a few clinical trials, cohort or population based studies [6, 7]. Cross-sectional imaging and stool or blood biomarkers are also more frequently used to better characterize disease activity and the simple clinical assessment has been very much challenged and often considered as inadequate for an objective assessment of disease activity, particularly in CD. These biomarkers, as well as endoscopic and medical imaging scores, are reviewed elsewhere in this book. Meanwhile, much emphasis is put on the importance of patients' reported outcomes and the necessity to collect them in a standardized and validated format. These patients' reported outcomes are also reviewed elsewhere in this book. The simple clinical assessment of the disease has thus lost a bit of its relevance between the necessity of collecting objective markers of disease activity and the one of collecting patients reported outcomes. Hence for clinical trial, a decision of the FDA in 2014 indicates that judgement criteria in CD clinical trials should be based on both endoscopic assessment of the disease and patients reported outcomes, leaving aside the classical clinical activity indexes like the Crohn's disease activity index (CDAI) [8]. Nevertheless, these clinical scores still represent an important part of the patient's assessment, particularly in routine practice, where the clinician still needs reliable, reproducible, and easy-to-use tools to assess clinical activity.

Activity Indices in Ulcerative Colitis

UC activity indices have been recently reviewed by the task force of the International Organization of Inflammatory Bowel Disease (IOIBD) [9]. Truelove and Witts first attempted to quantify disease activity and defined mild, moderate and severe colitis in 1955 [10]. In 1978, Powell-Tuck transformed these definitions into a continuous point scale based on ten clinical variables (the Powell-Tuck Index also called St Mark's Index) [11]. In 1990, Lichtiger et al. modified the Truelove and Witts severity index and described a Lichtiger Index based on eight clinical items [12]. Other authors tried to create simplified versions. Schroeder et al. developed the Mayo disease activity index and Sutherland et al. developed the ulcerative colitis disease activity index (UCDAI), both of which have four components and include endoscopy [13, 14]. Seo et al.

E. Louis (✉) • C. Van Kemseke • C. Reenaers
Department of Gastroenterology, University Hospital CHU of Liège, 4000 Liège, Belgium
e-mail: edouard.louis@ulg.ac.be

D.C. Baumgart (ed.), *Crohn's Disease and Ulcerative Colitis*, DOI 10.1007/978-3-319-33703-6_23

proposed an index only based on symptoms and laboratory variables [15]. Walmsley and colleagues developed the simple clinical colitis activity index (SCCAI), a survey of six questions about symptoms [16]. Rachmilewitz et al. reported in 1989 a score based on six clinical variables and one laboratory finding named Clinical Activity Index (CAI) [17]. In 2002, Levine at al. described another composite score based on five clinical items and endoscopic evaluation while Feagan et al. developed in 2005 the Ulcerative Colitis Clinical Score (UCSS), a modification of the Mayo Score [18, 19]. Recently more emphasis has been put on patients reported outcomes beside objective assessment using mainly sigmoidoscopy and fecal calprotectin.

Truelove and Witts, Lichtiger (Also Called Modified Truelove and Witts Severity Index, MTWSI) and Seo index

In 1955, in a placebo-controlled trial of oral cortisone in ulcerative colitis, Truelove and Witts first described an instrument to measure disease activity: the Truelove and Witts Severity Index based on the six following criteria: number of stools per day, blood in stools, temperature, pulse, hemoglobin, and erythrocyte sedimentation rate (ESR). The main drawback of this score is that it is not quantitative (i.e., no disease severity score is generated). Furthermore, it has not been validated.

In 1990, Lichtiger et al. described a modified Truelove and Witts Severity Index (MTWSI), also named Lichtiger Index, in a pilot trial of intravenous cyclosporine for the treatment of severely active steroid-refractory UC [12]. Eight variables composed the Lichtiger Index: diarrhea (number of daily stools), nocturnal stools, visible blood in stools (% of movements), fecal incontinence, abdominal pain or cramping, general well-being, abdominal tenderness and need for antidiarrheal drugs. Total score ranges from 0 to 21 points. Clinical response was initially defined as score reduction 50 % from baseline. A score of less than 10 on two consecutive days was considered to indicate a clinical response in a subsequent study [20]. Neither the Lichtiger Index nor the definitions of clinic response have been validated.

In 1992, Seo et al. collected prospectively 18 clinical, laboratory and endoscopic parameters from 72 patients during 85 clinical relapses [15]. A multiple regression analysis was done according to Truelove and Witts' classification with disease severity (mild, moderate, severe) as dependent variable and 18 clinical, laboratory and endoscopic parameters as independent variables [15]. Results showed that disease severity was significantly influenced by five factors: bloody stool, bowel movements per day, erythrocyte sedimentation rate (ESR), hemoglobin (Hg), and serum albumin (g/dl). The Activity Index (AI) was expressed as follows: $AI = 60 \times \text{bloody stool} + 13 \times \text{bowel movements} + 0.5 \times ESR - 4 \times Hb - 15 \times \text{albumin} + 200$. Activity index scores <150 points correspond to mild disease, 150–200 points to moderate disease, and >200 points to severely active disease. In two subsequent study performed by Seo in patients with active ulcerative colitis, AI was able to predict remission or colectomy: an AI score <180 points after 2 weeks of intravenous corticosteroids predicted remission [21] and, on the contrary, a score >200 predicted colectomy [22]. In a randomized controlled trial on infliximab as rescue therapy in severe and moderately severe ulcerative colitis, AI significantly predicted response to medical therapy or need for colectomy [23]. The AI also correlated significantly with endoscopic findings [2].

These three indexes are currently mainly used to assess patients with acute severe colitis. In routine practice, it is the Truelove and Witts criteria that are used. Acute severe colitis is defined by the presence of at least 6 bloody bowel movements per day, associated with at least one objective sign of systemic inflammation (low blood pressure, fever, tachycardia, elevated ESR or CRP…) [24]. In clinical trials, those are mainly Lichtiger and Seo scores which are used [23, 25].

Powell-Tuck Index (Also Called St. Mark's Index)

In 1978, Powell-Tuck et al. reported a disease activity measure (the Powell-Tuck Index) in a randomized controlled trial on oral prednisolone given as single or multiple daily doses for the treatment of active UC [11]. This disease activity index included ten clinical variables: general health ("Well-being," range 0–3), abdominal pain (range 0–2), bowel frequency (range 0–2), stool consistency (range 0–2), bleeding (range 0–2), anorexia (range 0–2), nausea or vomiting (range 0–1), abdominal tenderness (range 0–2), extraintestinal complications (eye, mouth, joint, skin) (range 0–2) and temperature (range 0–2). The Powell-Tuck index ranges from 0 to 20 points. One variation of the Powell-Tuck Index includes sigmoidoscopic appearance (0–2 points) increasing the total maximum score to 22 points. This endoscopic evaluation was mainly based on bleeding. "Remission" was defined as a symptom score of zero, "improvement" as a reduction in the baseline score by 2 or more points, "no change" as a fluctuation of the total score by one point or less and "worse" as an increase of 2 or more. Neither the Powell-Tuck Index nor the definitions of remission and improvement have been validated. Each of the ten clinical variables was correlated with the sigmoidoscopic appearance in a 74 patients "cohort" [26]. The sigmoidoscopic appearance contributes little to the variation of the index score (only 2 points of the maximum 22 points). This was confirmed by Higgins et al. who suggested that clinical practice of treating patients based on reported symptoms without endoscopic evaluation might be appropriate [27].

Simple Clinical Colitis Activity Index, Mayo Score and Other Simplified Indexes

Walmsley et al. evaluated 57 patients during 63 assessments of disease activity. They collected all items required to calculate the Powell-Tuck index including sigmoidoscopic assessment and added two additional clinical criteria: nocturnal bowel movement and urgency of defection [16]. The general well-being score from the Harvey–Bradshaw simple index of Crohn's disease activity was substituted for the general health question in the Powell-Tuck Index [28]. The category of extracolonic features incorporated arthritis, pyoderma gangrenosum, erythema nodosum, and uveitis. A multiple regression analysis was done according to Powell-Tuck Index as dependent variable and authors developed an equation with six variables which best predicted this index: bowel frequency (day) (range 0–3), urgency of defecation (range 0–3), blood in stool (range 0–3), general well-being (range 0–4) and extracolonic manifestations (score 1 per manifestation). Total score ranges from 0 to 19 points. This new index was further evaluated in a different group of patients and it showed a highly significant correlation with the Powell-Tuck index as well as with laboratory data (albumin, hemoglobin, platelet count, hematocrit, ESR). Walmsley also showed that this Simple Clinical Colitis Activity Index (SCCAI) correlated well with the Seo Index and IBDQ. Clinical remission and response criteria were not defined in the initial study. Nevertheless, a cutoff value below 2.5 points has been shown to correlate with patient-defined remission and a decrease of >1.5 points from baseline correlated with patient-defined significant improvement [29].

Schroeder et al. developed an instrument to measure disease activity (the Mayo Score) in a placebo-controlled trial on 5-aminosalicylic acid therapy for mildly to moderately active ulcerative colitis [13]. This score is a composite of clinical and endoscopic parameters. Mayo Score consists of four items: stool frequency (range 0–3), rectal bleeding (range 0–3), findings of flexible proctosigmoidoscopy (range 0–3), and physician's global assessment (range 0–3) (Table f). Total score ranges from 0 to 12 points. In addition, a patient's functional assessment representing a general sense of well-being was also measured and participated to evaluation of physician's general assessment. It was not included in the 12-point index calculation. A complete response (remission) was defined as complete resolution of all symptoms (all assessment scores were zero). A partial response was defined as substantial but incomplete improvement in the assessment scores. If any assessment score was noted to worsen, despite improvement in other scores, the patients were excluded from this category and considered to have had a treatment failure. Neither the Mayo Score nor the definitions of complete or partial responses have been validated. Subsequent studies have modified the definitions of remission or clinical response. A remission has been defined in the majority of the studies by a global score of zero, while clinical response has been defined different ways. The definition of response ranged from an improvement in the baseline physician's global assessment score and improvement in at least one other clinical assessment without worsening in any other clinical assessment [30] to a decrease in the disease activity index of at least three points [31] or two points [32]. More recently, the definition of remission has been extended to a score of 1 for either stool frequency or global physician's assessment while the endoscopic and bleeding subscore had to be zero [33, 34] or a total score no greater than 2 with a maximum of 1 for each subscore [35]. In this last study, a mucosal healing was defined by an endoscopic subscore not greater than 1. Despite the lack of formal validation, the clinical relevance of these last definitions was demonstrated by correlation between these definitions and significant improvement in quality of life as measured by the Inflammatory Bowel Disease Questionnaire (IBDQ) and by the Short Form-36 (SF-36) questionnaire [36–38].

Sutherland et al. described another simple disease assessment tool named the Sutherland Index (also called Disease Activity Index—DAI and the UC Disease Activity Index—UCDAI) in a placebo-controlled trial of mesalamine enema in the treatment of distal ulcerative colitis, proctosigmoiditis, and proctitis [14]. This index is very close to the Mayo score. It consists of four items: stool frequency (range 0–3), rectal bleeding (range 0–3), mucosal appearance (range 0–3), and physician's rating of disease activity (range 0–3). Total score ranges from 0 to 12 points. Efficacy was defined as a statistically significant reduction in the Sutherland Index Score and a significant reduction in the individual subscores (both calculated individually for each patient). Neither the Sutherland Score nor the definitions of complete or partial responses have been validated. Subsequent studies have modified the definitions of remission and clinical improvement. Remission was defined as Sutherland score of ≤1 point with a score of 0 for rectal bleeding and stool frequency, while clinical improvement was defined as a reduction in the Sutherland score ≥3 points from baseline [39, 40]. Despite the lack of formal validation, the Sutherland Index has been shown to correlate with an index based on patient's opinion developed by Higgins et al. [29].

Feagan et al. described the Ulcerative Colitis Clinical Score in a double-blind placebo-controlled trial on a humanized α4β7 integrin-antibody for the treatment of ulcerative colitis [19]. This instrument was a modification of the Mayo Score and consisted on four items which were scored from 0 (normal) to 3 (severe): stool frequency (referring to the usual normal number of stools per day when the patient was in remission), rectal bleeding, functional assessment by the patient, and global assessment by the physician. To define clinical remission and response it was used with a modified

Table 23.1 Mayo Score (Mayo Clinic Score or Disease Activity Index—DAI)

Stool frequency[a]
0: Normal
1: Number of stools for this patient 1–2 stools more than normal
2: 3–4 stools more than normal
3: 5 or more stools more than normal
Rectal bleeding[b]
0: No blood seen
1: Streaks of blood with stool less than half the time
2: Obvious blood with stool most of the time
3: Blood alone passed
Findings of flexible proctosigmoidoscopy
0: Normal or inactive disease
1: Mild disease (erythema, decreased vascular pattern, mild friability)
2: Moderate disease (marked erythema, absent vascular pattern, friability, erosions)
3: Severe disease (spontaneous bleeding, ulceration)
Physician's global assessment[c]
0: Normal
1: Mild disease
2: Moderate disease
3: Severe disease

[a]Each patient served as his or her own control to establish the degree of abnormality of the stool frequency

[b]The daily bleeding score represented the most severe bleeding of the day

[c]The physician's global assessment acknowledged the three other criteria, the patient's daily record of abdominal discomfort and general sense of well-being (patient's functional assessment [Patient's functional assessment was not included in the 12-point index calculation but represented a general sense of well-being; it was also measured (score 0 = generally well, score 1 = fair, score 2 = poor, score 3 = terrible) and participated to evaluation of physician's general assessment]) and other observations such as physical findings and the patient's performance status. Score of 0 meant there were no symptom of colitis, the patient felt well and the flexible proctosigmoidoscopy score was 0. A score of 1 indicated mild symptoms and proctoscopic findings that were mildly abnormal. A score of 2 reflected more serious abnormalities and proctosigmoidoscopic and symptom scores of 1 to 2. A score of 3 indicated that proctosigmoidoscopic and symptom scores were 2–3 and the patient probably required corticosteroid therapy and possibly hospitalization

version of a previously described endoscopic index: the Baron score [41]. This score consisted of a four-point scale mainly based on the severity of bleeding and not including ulceration. The modified Baron score was based on a five-point scale (0–4). Clinical remission was defined as a UCCS score of 0 or 1 without rectal bleeding and with a normal mucosa or only granular mucosa with an abnormal vascular pattern on sigmoidoscopy. Clinical response was defined as an improvement of three points or more on the UCCS and endoscopic response (defined by a Baron score of zero or a decrease of at least two points). Neither the UCSS nor the definitions of clinical remission and clinical response have been validated.

Rachmilewitz et al. reported an instrument subsequently named the Clinical Activity Index (CAI) in a randomized trial comparing coated mesalamine versus sulfasalazine in the treatment of active ulcerative colitis [17]. This index was composed of seven variables: number of stools (range 0–3), blood in stools (range 0, 2, or 4), investigator's global assessment of symptomatic state (range 0–3), abdominal pain or cramps (range 0–3), temperature due to colitis (range 0 or 3), extraintestinal manifestations (range 0, 3, 6, or 9), and laboratory findings (range 0, 1, 2, or 4). Total score ranges from 0 to 29 points. It has been validated in one study in which remission was defined as a CAI score ≤4 points [42].

Towards More Emphasis on Patients Reported Symptoms to Complement Endoscopic Assessment

In 2002, Levine et al. reported an instrument to measure disease activity in a randomized, double-blind controlled trial on balsalazide versus mesalamine treatment in active mild to moderate ulcerative colitis [18]. This instrument was based on individual symptom scores including rectal bleeding, patient functional assessment, stool frequency, abdominal pain, but also on sigmoidoscopic grade, and physician global assessment. The scores of each item were graded from 0 to 3 points (0 = normal, 1 = mild, 2 = moderate, 3 = severe). Improvement was defined as a reduction from baseline of ≥1 point in rectal bleeding and at least one of the other individual symptoms. This instrument has not been validated. More recently, it was showed that a score based on the six-point

MayoEndoscopic assessment (stool frequency and rectal bleeding) and a general well-being question (from the SCCAI) correlated well with more complete activity indexes and was able to determine remission status [43].

Clinical Scores in Crohn's Disease

Assessment of Crohn's disease (CD) activity and monitoring for treatment response require the establishment of reliable and reproducible tools. The development of instruments that would accurately reflect the activity of CD has been more complex than in ulcerative colitis (UC) due to the heterogeneity of the disease and the unreliable translation of intestinal lesions into clinical symptoms. Hence, these complicated scores tend to be abandoned for a dual assessment of the disease based on objective markers (mainly endoscopy and cross sectional imaging associated with blood and stool biomarkers) and patients reported symptoms.

Crohn's Disease Activity Index

In 1970, the National Cooperative Crohn's Disease Study (NCCDC) was initiated to test the efficacy of prednisone, sulfasalazine, and azathioprine in clinical controlled trials. The Crohn's Disease Activity Index (CDAI) was developed to investigate the efficacy of these drugs [44]. It was published in 1976 and, has remained the most suitable instrument to evaluate CD activity in clinical trials for more than 30 years [45–50]. CDAI was initially developed from 112 patients and then later reanalyzed on a larger group with the same conclusions. Eighteen variables were first tested and eight were finally retained for the regression equation, out of which seven variables are purely clinical and one is biological (hematocrit). Moreover, four of them (liquid stools, well-being, use of loperamide, and abdominal pain) should be determined prospectively by keeping a 7-day patient diary; CDAI is therefore considered as a prospective index. In order to establish threshold cutoff value that indicates the disease activity, the global assessment of physicians was confronted to CDAI score. A value less than 150 was defined as remission and over 450 as a severe active disease. The clinical response to a treatment has generally been defined as a reduction of 70 or 100 points of the CDAI. The use of 100 points in CDAI decrease instead of 70 has been promoted to have more stringent criteria to differentiate between active drugs and placebo in clinical trials. However, the superiority of these judgment criteria has not been fully demonstrated [51]. CDAI has a good interobserver reproducibility. This index has been used to assess the efficacy of mesalamine, azathioprine, corticosteroid, methotrexate, cyclosporine, and more recently the biological therapies [47–50]. It has also been demonstrated recently that a retrospectively assisted evaluation of the CDAI was as accurate as the traditional prospective evaluation [52]. Although CDAI has been considered for a long time as the gold standard for the evaluation of CD activity, it may not reflect all the aspects of the disease and has some limitations. For instance, CDAI is not suitable for pediatric patients whose disease presentation differs from that of adults. Therefore, a Pediatric Crohn's Disease Activity Index (PCDAI) has been developed [53]. Moreover, CDAI does not take into account symptoms linked to predominant perianal CD and refers to unsuitable parameters in case of previous surgery or stoma, like the use of loperamide or stool frequency, which can be affected by biliary salt malabsorption or short bowel syndrome. Therefore, CDAI is not applicable for the assessment of perianal or operated CD. A prospective cohort study has also showed the inability of CDAI to differentiate between active CD and irritable bowel syndrome, both diseases giving rise to similar levels of CDAI increase [54]. Studies comparing CDAI and serum or stool biomarkers, mainly CRP and fecal calprotectin, have demonstrated only weak correlations [3, 55]. Poor correlation between CDAI and endoscopic examination has also been demonstrated [3, 56, 57]. For these different reasons, FDA decided in 2014, no longer to recommend CDAI as a primary judgement criteria for the assessment of the efficacy of new drugs in CD and to prefer a composite evaluation including endoscopic assessment and patients reported symptoms [8].

Harvey–Bradshaw Index

Because the CDAI has been reported to be difficult to use in daily clinical practice, other scores have been developed. The more practical one is the Harvey–Bradshaw Index (HBI), also known as the Simple Index or the Modified CDAI (Table 23.2) [28]. The HBI is based on subjective and clinical factors. It reduced the original eight items of the CDAI to five, removing the use of antidiarrheal drugs, the hematocrit and the body weight. It looks only at symptoms over the preceding 24 h which makes the measurement of severity easy and quick at an outpatient visit. However, it could be less reliable and its value could significantly change from one day to another. The original prospective study of 112 patients demonstrated a good correlation (r=0.93) between HBI and CDAI. More recently, one study compared the CDAI and HBI in the assessment of CD activity in two large clinical trials, PRECISE 1 and PRECISE 2 and confirmed a good correlation between the two scores [58]. This suggests that HBI might permit simpler CD activity assessment, particularly for routine practice. To this end, a study showed that a patient-based HBI index correlated well with the physician-based HBI and that the discordances rarely translated into a change in the remission vs active dis-

Table 23.2 Harvey–Bradshaw index

Patient's general well-being (for the previous day)
0 = well
1 = slightly below par
2 = poor
3 = very poor
4 = terrible
Abdominal pain (for the previous day)
0 = none
1 = mild
2 = moderate
3 = severe
Number of liquid stools per day (for the previous day; score 1 per movement)
Abdominal mass
0 = none
1 = dubious
2 = definite
3 = definite and tender
Complications (score 1 per item)
Arthralgia, uveitis, erythema nodosum, aphthous ulcers, pyoderma gangrenosum, anal fissure, new fistula, abscess
Harvey–Bradshaw index score: remission <5; mild disease 5–7; moderate disease 8–16, severe disease > 16

ease status of the patient [59]. This would allow the patient to monitor disease activity more regularly and communicate more proactively with the physician.

Van Hees Index

In order to overcome the disadvantages and the potential subjectivity of the CDAI, Van Hees et al. elaborated in 1980 an activity index, the Van Hees Index (VHI), based on entirely objective variables of which albumin serum level contributed the most [60]. A score of less than 100 is considered as clinical remission and over 210 as a severe disease. Its correlation with the CDAI is poor, which is due to an absence of consideration of clinical symptoms. This score calculation is more complex and has not supplanted the CDAI in clinical practice.

Focus on Patients Reported Outcomes

While the insufficient correlation between CDAI and tissue healing has been confirmed [61, 62], standardized symptoms-based assessment is still meaningful to describe the disease state and is particularly relevant and important for the patients. As a matter of fact, simple clinical disease activity still very significantly correlates with self-reported disability index [63]. However, as highlighted here above, there was a perceived necessity for simpler scores or indexes, mainly reflecting patients' perceptions. Khanna et al. showed that a simple symptoms assessment by the patient correlated well with CDAI [64]. The investigators could build two patient-reported outcome scales based on two or three symptoms (abdominal pain, liquid stools frequency, well-being) and, using database from previous clinical trials, determined cut-off values for remission and response to therapy. This kind of simple symptoms assessment could even be transferred to a web-platform to facilitate patient–physician communication. This was tested in a Korean study where the five items of the HBI were recorded online by the patients before the consultation [65]. A very good correlation was found with CDAI. Another study tried to further simplify the patient-based assessment using a simple numeric rating scale [66]. This showed an encouraging correlation with both CDAI and the health related quality of life score IBDQ.

Conclusions

In IBD, disease activity can be measured in different ways. For a long time it has been mainly based on the assessment of the clinical activity of the disease, mainly based on symptoms collected by the physician at the consultation or by the patient and the physician through diaries. This clinical assessment of the disease is considered as too subjective and correlating poorly with objective markers of disease activity, including biomarkers and endoscopic or medical imaging assessment. This is particularly the case in CD, while in UC the symptoms still reflect reasonably well the endoscopic activity of the disease. That is why complex clinical activity scores like the CDAI are progressively abandoned in clinical trials and are replaced by a combination of endoscopic or cross-sectional imaging assessment with symptoms-based patient reported outcomes.

Nevertheless, for routine practice, the increase in the number of drugs available to treat these illnesses and the increasing complexity of therapeutic strategies and algorithms require some quantitative clinical activity assessment to allow optimal patients management. To this end, simple and reproducible scoring systems, even potentially recorded by the patient him/herself like the HBI for CD or the clinical part of the Mayo for UC, seem well adapted.

References

1. Wright R, Truelove SR. Serial rectal biopsy in ulcerative colitis during the course of a controlled therapeutic trial of various diets. Am J Dig Dis. 1966;11:847–57.
2. Seo M, Okada M, Maeda K, Oh K. Correlations between endoscopic severity and the clinical activity index in ulcerative colitis. Am J Gastroenterol. 1998;93:2124–9.
3. Cellier C, Sahmoud T, Froguel E, Adenis A, Belaiche J, Bretagne JF, et al. Correlations between clinical activity, endoscopic severity, and biological parameters in colonic or ileocolonic Crohn's disease. A prospective multicentre study of 121 cases. The Groupe d'Etudes Thérapeutiques des Affections Inflammatoires Digestives. Gut. 1994;35:231–5.
4. Modigliani R, Mary JY, Simon JF, Cortot A, Soule JC, Gendre JP, et al. Clinical, biological, and endoscopic picture of attacks of Crohn's disease. Evolution on prednisolone. Groupe d'Etude Thérapeutique des Affections Inflammatoires Digestives. Gastroenterology. 1990;98:811–8.
5. Landi B, Anh TN, Cortot A, Soule JC, Rene E, Gendre JP, et al. Endoscopic monitoring of Crohn's disease treatment: a prospective, randomized clinical trial. The Groupe d'Etudes Therapeutiques des Affections Inflammatoires Digestives. Gastroenterology. 1992;102:1647–53.
6. Baert F, Moortgat L, Van Assche G, Caenepeel P, Vergauwe P, De Vos M, et al. Mucosal healing predicts sustained clinical remission in patients with early-stage Crohn's disease. Gastroenterology. 2010;138:463–8.
7. Frøslie KF, Jahnsen J, Moum BA, Vatn MH. Mucosal healing in inflammatory bowel disease: results from a Norwegian population-based cohort. Gastroenterology. 2007;133:412–22.
8. Williet N, Sandborn WJ, Peyrin-Biroulet L. Patient-reported outcomes as primary end points in clinical trials of inflammatory bowel disease. Clin Gastroenterol Hepatol. 2014;12:1246–56.
9. D'Haens G, Sandborn WJ, Feagan BG, Geboes K, Hanauer SB, Irvine EJ, et al. A review of activity indices and efficacy end points for clinical trials of medical therapy in adults with ulcerative colitis. Gastroenterology. 2007;132:763–86.
10. Truelove SC, Witts LJ. Cortisone in ulcerative colitis. Final report on a therapeutic trial. BMJ. 1955;2:1041–8.
11. Powell-Tuck J, Bown RL, Lennard-Jones JE. A comparison of oral prednisolone given as single or multiple daily doses for active proctocolitis. Scand J Gastroenterol. 1978;13:833–7.
12. Lichtiger S, Present DH. Preliminary report: cyclosporin treatment of severe active ulcerative colitis. Lancet. 1990;336:16–9.
13. Schroeder KW, Tremaine WJ, Ilstrup DM. Coated oral 5-aminosalicylic acid therapy for mildly to moderately active ulcerative colitis. A randomized study. N Engl J Med. 1987;317:1625–9.
14. Sutherland LR, Martin F, Greer S, Robinson M, Greenberger N, Saibil F, et al. 5-Aminosalicylic acid enema in the treatment of distal ulcerative colitis, proctosigmoiditis and proctitis. Gastroenterology. 1987;92:1894–8.
15. Seo M, Okada M, Yao T, Ueki M, Arima S, Okumura M. An index of disease activity in patients with ulcerative colitis. Am J Gastroenterol. 1992;87:971–6.
16. Walmsley RS, Ayres RC, Pounder RE, Akkan RN. A simple clinical colitis activity index. Gut. 1998;43:29–32.
17. Rachmilewitz D. Coated mesalazine (5-aminosalicylic acid) versus sulphasalazine in the treatment of active ulcerative colitis: a randomized trial. BMJ. 1989;298:82–6.
18. Levine DS, Riff DS, Pruitt R, Wruble L, Koval G, Sales D, et al. A randomized, double-blind, dose-response comparison of balsalazide (6.75 g), balsalazide (2.25 g) and mesalamine (2.4 g) in the treatment of active, mild-to-moderate ulcerative colitis. Am J Gastroenterol. 2002;97:1398–407.
19. Feagan BG, Greenberg GR, Wild G, Fedorak R, Pare P, McDonald JWD, et al. Treatment of ulcerative colitis with a humanized antibody to the a4b7 integrin. N Engl J Med. 2005;352:2499–507.
20. Lichtiger S, Present DH, Kornbluth A, Gelernt I, Bauer J, Galler G, et al. Cyclosporine in severe ulcerative colitis refractory to steroid therapy. N Engl J Med. 1994;330:1841–5.
21. Seo M, Okada M, Yao T, Okabe N, Matake H, Oh K. Evaluation of disease activity in patients with moderately active ulcerative colitis: comparison between a new activity index and Truelove and Witts classification. Am J Gastroenterol. 1995;90:1759–63.
22. Seo M, Okada M, Yao T, Matake H, Maeda K. Evaluation of the clinical course of acute attacks in patients with ulcerative colitis through the use of an activity index. J Gastroenterol. 2002;37:29–34.
23. Järnerot G, Hertervig E, Friis-Liby I, Blomquist L, Karlen P, Grännö C, et al. Infliximab as a rescue therapy in severe to moderately severe ulcerative colitis: a randomized, placebo-controlled study. Gastroenterology. 2005;128:1805–11.
24. Dignass A, Lindsay JO, Sturm A, Windsor A, Colombel JF, Allez M, et al. Second European evidence-based consensus on the diagnosis and management of ulcerative colitis. Part 2: Current management. J Crohns Colitis. 2012;6:991–1030.
25. Laharie D, Bourreille A, Branche J, Allez M, Bouhnik Y, Filippi J, et al. Ciclosporin versus infliximab in patients with severe ulcerative colitis refractory to intravenous steroids: a parallel, open-label randomised controlled trial. Lancet. 2012;380:1909–15.
26. Powell-Tuck J, Day DW, Buckell NA, Wadsworth J, Lennard-Jones JE. Correlations between defined sigmoidoscopic appearances and other measures of disease activity in ulcerative colitis. Dig Dis Sci. 1982;27:533–7.
27. Higgins PD, Schwartz M, Mapili J, Zimmerman EM. Is endoscopy necessary for the measurement of disease activity in ulcerative colitis? Am J Gastroenterol. 2005;100:355–61.
28. Harvey RF, Bradshaw JM. A simple index of Crohn's disease activity. Lancet. 1980;1:514.
29. Higgins PDR, Schwartz M, Mapili J, Krokos I, Leung J, Zimmerman EM. Patient defined dichotomous end points for remission and clinical improvement in ulcerative colitis. Gut. 2005;54:782–8.
30. Hanauer SB, Sandborn WJ, Kornbluth A, Katz S, Safdi M, Woogen S, et al. Delayed-release oral mesalamine at 4.8 g/day (800 mg tablet) for the treatment of moderately active ulcerative colitis: the ASCEND II trial. Am J Gastroenterol. 2005;100:2478–85.
31. Sandborn WJ, Tremaine WJ, Schroeder KW, Batts KP, Lawson GM, Steiner BL, et al. A placebo-controlled trial of cyclosporine enemas for mildly to moderately active left-sided ulcerative colitis. Gastroenterology. 1994;106:1429–35.
32. Sandborn WJ, Tremaine WJ, Hurt RD. Transdermal nicotine for ulcerative colitis. Ann Intern Med. 1997;127:491–3.
33. Sandborn WJ, Sands BE, Wolf DC, Valentine JF, Safdi M, Katz S, et al. Repifermin (keratinocyte growth factor-2) for the treatment of active ulcerative colitis: a randomized, double-blind, placebo-controlled, dose-escalation trial. Aliment Pharmacol Ther. 2003;17:1355–64.
34. Van Assche G, Sandborn WJ, Feagan BG, Salzberg BA, Silvers D, Monroe PS, et al. Daclizumab, a humanized monoclonal antibody to the interleukin-2 receptor (CD25), for the treatment of moderately to

severely active ulcerative colitis: a randomized, double-blind, placebo-controlled, dose-ranging trial. Gut. 2006;55:1568–74.
35. Rutgeerts P, Sandborn WJ, Feagan BG, Reinisch W, Olson A, Johanns J, et al. Infliximab induction and maintenance therapy for ulcerative colitis. N Engl J Med. 2005;353:2462–76.
36. Irvine EJ, Feagan B, Rochon J, Archambault A, Fedorak RN, Groll A, et al. Quality of life: a valid and reliable measure of therapeutic efficacy in the treatment of inflammatory bowel disease. Canadian Crohn's Disease Relapse Prevention Trial Study Group. Gastroenterology. 1994;106:287–96.
37. Ware Jr JE, Sherbourne CD. The MOS 36-item short-form health survey (SF-36). I. Conceptual framework and item selection. Med Care. 1992;30:473–83.
38. Sandborn WJ, Feagan BG, Reinisch W, Yan S, Eisenberg D, Bala M, et al. Response and remission are associated with improved quality of life in patients with ulcerative colitis. Gut. 2005;54(Suppl VII):A58.
39. Lichtenstein G, Kamm M, Sandborn W, Boddu P, Gubergrits N. SPD476 is a novel, once-daily, effective and well-tolerated 5-ASA formulation for the induction of remission of mild-to-moderate ulcerative colitis: a phase III study. Am J Gastroenterol. 2005;100(Suppl):S291.
40. Kamm M, Sandborn W, Gassull M, Schreiber S, Jackowski L, Mikhailova T. Comparison of the efficacy of SPD476, a novel, once-daily formulation of mesalamine, and Asacol with placebo for the induction of remission of mild-moderate ulcerative colitis: a phase III study. Am J Gastroenterol. 2005;100(Suppl):S291.
41. Baron JH, Connell AM, Lennard-Jones JE. Variation between observers in describing mucosal appearances in proctocolitis. BMJ. 1964;1:89–92.
42. Rutgeerts P. Comparative efficacy of coated, oral 5-aminosalicylic acid (Claversal) and sulphasalazine for maintaining remission in ulcerative colitis. International study group. Aliment Pharmacol Ther. 1989;3:183–91.
43. Bewtra M, Brensinger CM, Tomov VT, Hoang TB, Sokach CE, Siegel CA, et al. An optimized patient-reported ulcerative colitis disease activity measure derived from the Mayo score and the simple clinical colitis activity index. Inflamm Bowel Dis. 2014;20:1070–8.
44. Best W, Becktel JM, Singleton JW, Kern Jr F. Development of a Crohn's disease activity index. Gastroenterology. 1976;70:439–44.
45. Summers RW, Switz DM, Sessions Jr JT, Becktel JM, Best WR, Kern Jr F, et al. National Cooperative Crohn's Disease Study: results of drug treatment. Gastroenterology. 1979;77:847–69.
46. Singleton JW, Summers RW, Kern Jr F, Becktel JM, Best WR, Hansen RN, et al. A trial of sulfasalazine as adjunctive therapy in Crohn's disease. Gastroenterology. 1979;77:887–97.
47. Greenberg GR, Feagan BG, Martin F, Sutherland LR, Thomson AB, Williams CN, et al. Oral budesonide for active Crohn's disease. Canadian Inflammatory Bowel Disease Study Group. N Engl J Med. 1994;331:836–41.
48. Feagan BG, Rochon J, Fedorak RN, Irvine EJ, Wild G, Sutherland L, et al. Methotrexate for the treatment of Crohn's disease. The North American Crohn's Study Group Investigators. N Engl J Med. 1995;332:292–7.
49. Willoughby JM, Beckett J, Kum. Controlled trial of azathioprine in Crohn's disease. N Engl J Med. 1995;332:292–7.
50. Targan SR, Hanauer SB, van Deventer SJ, Mayer L, Present DH, Braakman T, et al. A short-term study of chimeric monoclonal antibody cA2 to tumor necrosis factor alpha for Crohn's disease. Crohn's Disease cA2 Study Group. N Engl J Med. 1997;337:1029–35.
51. Su C, Lichtenstein GR, Krok K, Brensinger CM, Lewis JD. A meta-analysis of the placebo rates of remission and response in clinical trials of active Crohn's disease. Gastroenterology. 2004;126:1257–69.
52. Frenz MB, Dunckley P, Camporota L, Jewell DP, Travis SP. Comparison between prospective and retrospective evaluation of Crohn's disease activity index. Am J Gastroenterol. 2005;100:1117–20.
53. Harms HK, Blomer R, Bertele-Harms RM, Shmerling DH, König M, Spaeth A. A pediatric Crohn's disease activity index (PCDAI). Is it useful? Study Group on Crohn's Disease in Children and Adolescents. Acta Paediatr Suppl. 1994;83:22–6.
54. Lahiff C, Safaie P, Awais A, Akbari M, Gashin L, Sheth S, et al. The Crohn's disease activity index (CDAI) is similarly elevated in patients with Crohn's disease and in patients with irritable bowel syndrome. Aliment Pharmacol Ther. 2013;37:786–94.
55. Garrett JW, Drossman DA. Health status in inflammatory bowel disease. Biological and behavioral considerations. Gastroenterology. 1990;99:90–6.
56. Gomes P, du Boulay C, Smith CL, Holdstock G. Relationship between disease activity indices and colonoscopic findings in patients with colonic inflammatory bowel disease. Gut. 1986;27:92–5.
57. Denis MA, Reenaers C, Fontaine F, Belaïche J, Louis E. Assessment of endoscopic activity index and biological inflammatory markers in clinically active Crohn's disease with normal C-reactive protein serum level. Inflamm Bowel Dis. 2007;13:1100–5.
58. Vermeire S, Schreiber S, Sandborn WJ, Dubois C, Rutgeerts P. Correlation between the Crohn's disease activity and Harvey-Bradshaw indices in assessing Crohn's disease severity. Clin Gastroenterol Hepatol. 2010;8:357–63.
59. Evertsz FB, Hoeks CC, Nieuwkerk PT, Stokkers PC, Ponsioen CY, Bockting CL, et al. Development of the patient Harvey Bradshaw index and a comparison with a clinician-based Harvey Bradshaw index assessment of Crohn's disease activity. J Clin Gastroenterol. 2013;47:850–6.
60. van Hees PA, van Elteren PH, van Lier HJ, van Tongeren JH. An index of inflammatory activity in patients with Crohn's disease. Gut. 1980;21:279–86.
61. Peyrin-Biroulet L, Reinisch W, Colombel JF, Mantzaris GJ, Kornbluth A, Diamond R, et al. Clinical disease activity, C-reactive protein normalisation and mucosal healing in Crohn's disease in the SONIC trial. Gut. 2014;63:88–95.
62. Falvey JD, Hoskin T, Meijer B, Ashcroft A, Walmsley R, Day AS, et al. Disease activity assessment in IBD: clinical indices and biomarkers fail to predict endoscopic remission. Inflamm Bowel Dis. 2015;21:824–31.
63. van der Have M, Fidder HH, Leenders M, Kaptein AA, van der Valk ME, van Bodegraven AA, et al. Self-reported disability in patients with inflammatory bowel disease largely determined by disease activity and illness perceptions. Inflamm Bowel Dis. 2015;21:369–77.
64. Khanna R, Zou G, D'Haens G, Feagan BG, Sandborn WJ, Vandervoort MK, et al. A retrospective analysis: the development of patient reported outcome measures for the assessment of Crohn's disease activity. Aliment Pharmacol Ther. 2015;41:77–86.
65. Kim ES, Park KS, Cho KB, Kim KO, Jang BI, Kim EY, et al. Development of a Web-based, self-reporting symptom diary for Crohn's Disease, and its correlation with the Crohn's Disease Activity Index: Web-based, self-reporting symptom diary for Crohn's Disease. J Crohns Colitis. 19 Sep 2014. pii:S1873-9946(14)00268-2. doi:10.1016/j.crohns.2014.09.003 [Epub ahead of print].
66. Surti B, Spiegel B, Ippoliti A, Vasiliauskas EA, Simpson P, Shih DQ, et al. Assessing health status in inflammatory bowel disease using a novel single-item numeric rating scale. Dig Dis Sci. 2013;58:1313–21.

Objective Assessment of Endoscopic Disease Activity and Mucosal Healing

24

Britt Christensen and David T. Rubin

Introduction

Historically the goal of therapy when treating patients with inflammatory bowel disease (IBD) has been to achieve and maintain symptomatic remission. This has been accomplished using a step-up approach, in which therapies were commenced and their efficacy evaluated based on symptom-based metrics, followed by adjustments of therapy occurring until the patient achieved clinical remission. Clinical remission usually was defined as normal stool frequency, no abdominal pain and no rectal bleeding. By achieving this goal short-term respite was provided to patients with the hope of improving their quality of life and avoiding disease-related complications such as hospitalizations and surgeries. However, recently it has been demonstrated that despite frequently achieving symptomatic remission in our patients and despite access to many new therapies over the years, the course of IBD has not been successfully or substantially modified in the modern era [1, 2].

It is now known that relying on a patient's clinical symptoms to assess the inflammatory response to treatment is unreliable. Up to 40 % of patients in clinical remission will have endoscopic disease activity [3–8] and patients who feel unwell often have no endoscopic findings of disease activity [5]. In addition, although a patient may present in symptomatic (clinical) remission, many patients do not have stable disease control, with over 37 % of patients having frequent intermittent symptom over time [9] and only 10 % of patients experiencing prolonged clinical remission [9, 10] making a single time point assessment of clinical response unreliable. Therefore, this puts a significant proportion of patients at risk of either disease progression due to inadequate treatment, or at risk of overtreatment with unnecessary medications if one only relies on symptoms to choose treatments.

The recognition of these facts has led to a paradigmatic change in the therapeutic approach of IBD. Frequent evaluation of objective markers of disease activity are increasingly being incorporated into treatment algorithms to allow for timely changes of therapy. Thus, achievement of mucosal healing has emerged as a major treatment goal in IBD. Although mucosal healing does not have a standardized or validated definition in IBD, it is most often defined as the absence of friability, blood, erosions, and ulcers in all visual segments of the gut in UC [11] and the absence of ulceration in CD [12]. Therefore assessment of mucosal healing continues to require endoscopic assessment.

This chapter discusses the importance and prognostic role of endoscopic assessment of disease activity and mucosal healing in IBD, summarizes the major endoscopic indices of activity in CD and UC including their strengths, limitations, and application to both clinical trials and clinical practice, and finally, highlights the integration of endoscopic disease activity utilizing a "treat-to-target" algorithm that incorporates endoscopic mucosal healing as a target.

Prognostic Role of Endoscopic Disease Activity and Mucosal Healing in IBD

Historically, clinical evaluation and treating to clinical remission was the objective of treatment in IBD. However it was found that despite advances in medical therapies that improved symptoms, patients still required hospitalization and surgery and the natural history of the disease was unchanged [1, 2]. Therefore increasingly there has been a move to objective assessment of disease activity, and endoscopic assessment has been the gold standard. Endoscopy can be used both at diagnosis to prognosticate the disease course and to determine response to therapy.

B. Christensen, M.B.B.S., F.R.A.C.P., M.P.H.
Department of Medicine, University of Chicago Medicine Inflammatory Bowel Disease Center, 5841 S. Maryland Avenue, MC4076, Chicago, IL 60637, USA

Department of Gastroenterology, Alfred Hospital and Monash University, Melbourne, Australia

D.T. Rubin, M.D. (✉)
Department of Medicine, University of Chicago Medicine Inflammatory Bowel Disease Center, 5841 S. Maryland Avenue, MC4076, Chicago, IL 60637, USA
e-mail: drubin@uchicago.edu

D.C. Baumgart (ed.), *Crohn's Disease and Ulcerative Colitis*, DOI 10.1007/978-3-319-33703-6_24

Table 24.1 Benefits of mucosal healing and unresolved challenges to the incorporation of routine endoscopic assessment of mucosal healing into clinical practice

Benefits of mucosal healing	Unresolved issues of mucosal healing
Decreased clinical relapse	How much mucosal healing is required to impact outcomes?
Decreased hospitalizations	Can mucosal healing be achieved in most patients?
Decreased rate of surgery	What is the incremental benefit achieved from dose escalation or switching therapies?
Increased quality of life	What is the time interval between changes in therapy and subsequent endoscopic reassessment?
Less incidence of neoplasia	Can de-escalation occur after deep remission is sustained for some time?
Decreased incidence of fistula's	Will patients agree to therapy changes based only on endoscopic findings even if they are in clinical remission?

Endoscopic severity has been shown to predict the future clinical aggressiveness of IBD, specifically non-response to medical therapy and need for surgery. In UC severe lesions increase the odds ratio of colectomy by 41 compared to those without severe lesions [13] and severe endoscopic lesions predict non-response to therapy, with only 34 % of patients with severe endoscopic lesions responding to medical therapy, compared to 91 % of those who have less severe endoscopic disease (OR>20) [14]. Therefore, an endoscopic assessment is indicated in a newly symptomatic patient or in severe flares of disease to guide appropriate medical or surgical intervention required. In CD, severe endoscopic ulcerations are associated with a 31 % risk of colectomy, compared to a 6 % risk in those without severe endoscopic lesions [15]. In addition, endoscopic assessment within 12 months of ileocolonic resection in Crohn's disease can be used to predict the postoperative clinical disease course [16].

Once a patient has had a baseline colonoscopy to prognosticate their disease course and commence an appropriate therapeutic regimen, there is increasing evidence that assessing for mucosal healing provides further prognostic information regarding future disease course. This is because once a patient is on treatment, achievement of mucosal healing in both UC and CD has been found to be independently associated with improved outcomes including prolonged remission, fewer hospitalizations, reduced surgical procedures, fewer fistulas, less immunosuppression therapy, a lower risk of colorectal cancer, and improved quality of life (Table 24.1) [3, 5, 9, 13, 17–32].

It is now known that whilst treating to clinical symptoms in IBD is important to aid a patient's immediate quality of life, adjustments to therapy frequently are delayed and long-term disability is not prevented [33]. Although no prospective study has demonstrated that treating to achieve mucosal healing rather than clinical symptoms alone changes outcomes, preliminary retrospective studies have demonstrated that repeated endoscopic assessment of disease activity with adjustment of medical therapy to the target of mucosal healing is feasible in clinical practice and is of benefit [34, 35]. In addition one can extrapolate the experience from other chronic diseases, where reaching an objective target does improve long-term outcomes. This is the case for lowered blood pressure in hypertension [36], lowered glycosylated hemoglobin in diabetes [37–39], and most relevant, reduced joint inflammation in rheumatoid arthritis [40–42]. If we take this experience and apply it to IBD, strict disease control with an assessment of the mucosa and an aim to achieve mucosal healing should lead to improved outcomes.

Endoscopic Assessment of Disease Activity in Ulcerative Colitis

Ulcerative colitis involves inflammation of only the large intestine, starting in the rectum and extending proximally, with clear demarcation of normal and abnormal mucosa. At endoscopy, the mucosa is edematous, granular and has a change in vascular pattern [43]. In more severe disease easy friability and bleeding, ulceration, and pseudopolyps can occur [43]. Despite the fact that it has been more than 50 years since the first report on endoscopic lesions and mucosal healing by Truelove and Witts [44], it is not until recently that attempts have been made to validate any of the many subsequent systems (Table 24.2). As there are many scoring systems available, this chapter focuses specifically on the most common endoscopic scoring system used in clinical trials, the Mayo Clinic endoscopy sub-score, and the newer scoring systems currently undergoing validation, the ulcerative colitis endoscopic index of severity (UCEIS) and the ulcerative colitis colonoscopic index of severity (UCCIS).

Currently the most widely used endoscopic scoring system to quantify mucosal disease activity in UC in clinical trials is the Mayo Clinic endoscopy sub-score (Fig. 24.1) [54]. This score assesses vascular pattern, erythema, friability, bleeding, erosions, and ulceration. It is a four-point scale ranging from 0 to 3, with 0 being inactive disease and 3 being severe disease. It is a simple score that is easy to calculate. In most trials, mucosal healing is defined as a Mayo score of either 0 or 1 [11]. Evidence for the appropriateness of this definition was found in a post hoc analysis of the Active Ulcerative Colitis Trials (ACT)-1 that demonstrated that patients with an 8-week post-treatment Mayo score of 0 or 1 had a lower risk of undergoing colectomy and had better clinical outcomes at 1 year compared to those with higher

Table 24.2 Endoscopic disease activity scoring systems in ulcerative colitis

Endoscopic scores	Variables	Score range	Definition of remission and response	Strengths	Weaknesses
Truelove and Witts sigmoidoscopic assessment [44]	Hyperemia, granularity and change in overall appearance of the mucosa	No description	Not defined	Possibility to stratify patients by their disease severity	Not validated High inter-observer variability No definition of mucosal healing
Baron score [45]	Severity of mucosal bleeding and friability	0–3	Remission: 0–1 (NV) Response: Not defined	Easy to use Good inter-observer correlation	Not validated No assessment of ulcers No definition of mucosal healing
Modified Baron score [46]	Friability, vascular pattern, granularity, bleeding and ulceration	0–4	Remission: 0–1 (NV) Response: Not defined	Easy to use Good inter-observer correlation	Not validated No definition of mucosal healing
Powell-Tuck sigmoidoscopic assessment [47, 48]	Severity of mucosal bleeding and friability	0–2	Not defined	Easy to use	Not validated No definition of mucosal healing Ulceration not included
Rachmilewitz endoscopic index [48]	Granulation, vascular pattern, vulnerability of mucosa, mucosal damage	Four items rated 0–3. Total of 0–12 points	Remission: 0–4 (NV) Response: Not defined		Not validated Complex and subjective descriptive terms
Sigmoidoscopic index [49]	Erythema, friability, ulceration, mucous, vascular pattern	Five items rated 0–3. Total 0–16 points	Remission: 0–4 (NV) Response: Not defined		Not validated Complex
Sigmoidoscopic inflammation grade score [50]	Edema, vascular pattern Granularity, friability, bleeding, ulcers	0–4	Not defined		Not validated No definition of mucosal healing
Sutherland mucosal appearance assessment [51]	Friability, exudation, bleeding	0–3	Not defined		Not validated Subjective No definition of mucosal healing Easy to use
Endoscopic activity index [52]	Ulcers (size and depth), erythema, bleeding, mucosal edema, mucosal exudate	0–3	Not defined		Complex Not validated No definition of mucosal healing Closely correlated with clinical activity
Matts Index [53]	Granularity, bleeding, edema, ulceration	1–4	Not defined		Not validated No definition of mucosal healing Easy to use Good inter- and intra-observer agreement
Mayo endoscopic sub-score [54]	Erythema, vascular pattern, friability, bleeding, erosions, ulcerations	0–3	Remission: 0 or 0–1 (PV) Response: Not defined		Not validated Extensive use in clinical trials and RCT's
Ulcerative colitis colonoscopy index of severity (UCCIS) [55, 56]	Vascular pattern, granularity, ulceration, bleeding/friability	Four items rated 0–2 for vascular pattern, granularity, bleeding/friability and 0–4 for ulcerations. To total 0–10 points	Not defined	Preliminary validation Based on rigorous methodology Provides pan-colonic assessment	Includes subjective parameters and complex scale No definition of mucosal healing Requires post-procedure time to be scored

(continued)

Table 24.2 (continued)

Endoscopic scores	Variables	Score range	Definition of remission and response	Strengths	Weaknesses
Ulcerative colitis endoscopic index of severity (UCEIS) [57]	Vascular pattern, bleeding, erosions/ ulceration	Three items rated 0–3 for vascular pattern and 0–4 for bleeding and ulceration. Total of 0–11 points	Not defined	Preliminary validation Easy to use Based on rigorous methodology Accounts for 94 % of variance between endoscopists for the overall assessment of severity Independent of clinical symptoms	Limited to rectosigmoid Low agreement for normal appearing mucosa Sensitivity to change and mucosal healing remain undefined

NV not validated
PV partially validated
This table was adapted from Current Gastroenterology Reports. Christensen B et al. Understanding Endoscopic Disease Activity in IBD: How to Incorporate It into Practice. 2016; 8:5; with permission from Springer

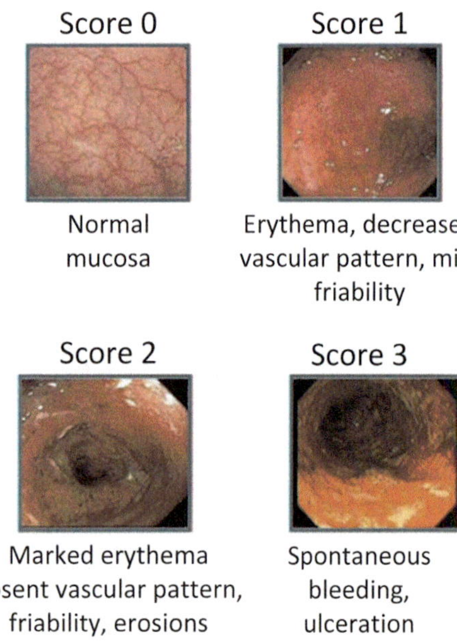

Fig. 24.1 Mayo endoscopic sub-score [54]. This figure was adapted from Current Gastroenterology Reports. Christensen B et al. Understanding Endoscopic Disease Activity in IBD: How to Incorporate It into Practice. 2016; 8:5; with permission

scores [3]. Of note, however, is that patients achieving a Mayo score of 0 also had higher rates of symptomatic remission, corticosteroid-free remission and subsequent mucosal healing at weeks 30 and 54 compared to those with a score of 1 but did not have lower rates of colectomy [3]. Despite its ease of use and frequent uptake in clinical trials, the Mayo endoscopic sub-score is hampered by a lack of validation and a high inter-observer discrepancy, particularly in regard to the inclusion of friability in the score of 1, which has been found to be so subjective as to lead to inconsistent results [58]. To overcome this, some studies have adapted the index and made the presence of friability an automatic Mayo sub-score of 2 [59–61].

Until recently, no endoscopic score to assess disease activity in UC was prospectively or completely validated. To overcome these limitations the ulcerative colitis endoscopic index of severity (UCEIS) [57, 62] and the ulcerative colitis colonoscopic index of severity (UCCIS) [55, 56] have recently been developed as the first prospectively validated scoring systems for UC. The UCEIS was a collaborative effort between 40 IBD specialists from 13 counties and evaluates three variables that were determined to be the most discriminating; vascular pattern, bleeding and erosions and ulcers (Table 24.3) [62]. The worst segment of the colon is given a score of 0–2 or 0–3 for each variable to give a total score of 0–8 and the scoring system has demonstrated excellent intra and inter-observer agreement [57, 58]. Limiting its use currently is the fact that cutoff scores to define disease severity or mucosal healing have not yet been determined and the sensitivity of the scoring system to change in disease activity and mucosal improvement remains unknown. However, validation of thresholds for defining mucosal healing and response are anticipated in the near future. With this in mind, this scoring system is likely to be increasingly adopted in clinical trials and applied to clinical practice.

Unlike the previously mentioned scores, which assess only the recto-sigmoid area of the colon, the UCCIS grades mucosal changes throughout the entire colon, which may provide further important prognostic data. The score examines vascular pattern, granularity, ulceration, bleeding/friability, and severity of damage in each colon segment and overall using a four-point scale and a 10-cm visual analogue scale [55]. As with the UCEIS, the UCCIS has excellent inter-observer agreement apart from the included variable of friability and has been found to have moderate correlation

Table 24.3 The ulcerative colitis endoscopic index of severity (UCEIS)

Descriptor	Score	Definition
Vascular pattern	Normal (0)	Normal vascular pattern with arborization of capillaries clearly defined, or with blurring or patchy loss of capillary margins
	Patchy obliteration (1)	Patchy obliteration of vascular pattern
	Obliterated (2)	Complete obliteration of vascular pattern
Bleeding	None (0)	No visible blood
	Mucosal (1)	Some spots or streaks of coagulated blood on the surface of the mucusa ahead of the scope, which can be washed away
	Luminal mild (2)	Some free liquid blood in the lumen
	Luminal moderate or severe (3)	Frank blood in the lumen ahead of endoscope or visible oozing from mucosa after washing intraluminal blood, or visible oozing from a hemorrhagic mucosa
Erosions and ulcers	None (0)	Normal mucosa no visible erosions or ulcers
	Erosions (1)	Tiny defects in the mucosa, of a white or yellow color with a flat edge
	Superficial ulcer (2)	Larger (>5 mm) defects in the mucosa which are discrete fibrin-covered ulcers when compared with erosion, but remain superficial
	Deep ulcer (3)	Deeper excavated defects in the mucosa with a slightly raised edge

The three descriptors are scored for the worst affected area of the colon to give a score of 0–8

[This table was adapted from Travis S et al. Reliability and initial validation of the Ulcerative Colitis Endscopic Index of Severity. Gastroenterology. 2013; 145:987–95; with permission.]

with laboratory markers of disease activity including CRP and albumin and patient-defined remission [55, 56]. However, as with the UCEIS, there is no validation or definition of response or remission and its future use may be limited due to the need for full colonoscopy limiting its practical application [59].

Endoscopic Disease Activity Assessment in Crohn's Disease

Crohn's disease can affect any part of the gastrointestinal tract from the mouth through to the anorectum and inflammation occurs in a patchy pattern. On endoscopy, findings in CD typically consist of segmental erythema, strictures and apthoid ulceration that can progress to stellate, longitudinal, tortuous, or serpiginous ulcers and a cobblestone appearance [43]. The terminal ileum can be involved and anal or perianal disease is suggestive of CD over UC. There are two validated endoscopic indices for evaluating CD disease activity and a further index that is routinely used to assess postoperative recurrence in CD (Table 24.4).

The Crohn's disease endoscopic index of severity (CDEIS) [12] and the simple endoscopic score for Crohn's disease (SES-CD) [63] have been prospectively validated and been shown to be reproducible, have good inter-observer agreement, have good correlation with the Crohn's disease activity index (CDAI) and are sensitive to changes in endoscopic mucosal appearance and healing [26, 64–66]. The CDEIS was the first endoscopic scoring system developed for CD (Table 24.5) and is the most commonly used endoscopic tool to assess disease activity in clinical trials. The score ranges from 0–44 and examines superficial ulcers, deep ulcers, ulcerated stenosis, and non-ulcerated stenosis in addition to the percentage of ulcerated and affected colonic surface in all five bowel segments (terminal ileum, right colon, transverse colon and rectum). Despite the CDEIS score being reliable and reproducible, its use is limited due to the fact that it is a complex scoring system that is time-consuming and not practical for routine clinical use [58]. To overcome these shortcomings, a simplified index, the simple endoscopic score for CD (SES-CD) was developed and consists of measuring ulcer size, ulcerated and affected surfaces and stenosis in each of the five intestinal segments to give a total score range of 0–56 (Table 24.6). The SES-CD correlates highly with the CDEIS and is a faster and more practical tool [63].

As with the UC endoscopic scoring systems, the CDEIS and the SES-CD do not have validated thresholds for mucosal disease severity, remission or response. In trials utilizing the CDEIS, a score < 6 [67] has been used to define partial endoscopic healing or endoscopic remission and <3 [67], 4 [68], ≤4 [69] or 0 [70] to define complete mucosal healing. In trials utilizing the SES-CD a score of <3 [69, 71, 72, 73] or equal to 0 [24, 70, 74–76] has previously been used to define endoscopic remission or minimal endoscopic activity although a study by Moskovitz et al. [77] validated the cut-off values as 0–2 for endoscopic remission, 3–6 for mild endoscopic disease, 7–15 for moderate endoscopic disease activity and ≥16 for severe endoscopic disease activity. In regard to defining endoscopic response to treatment, Ferrante et al. [78] demonstrated that a decrease from baseline of both the CDEIS and the SES-CD score of at least 50 % was most predictive of corticosteroid free remission by week 50.

Table 24.4 Crohn's disease endoscopic disease activity scoring systems

Score	Variables	Score range	Definition response/ Remission	Strengths	Weakness
Crohn's disease endoscopic index of severity (CDEIS) [12]	Deep ulceration, superficial ulceration, inflammation	0–44	Complete remission: 0, <3, <4 or <6 Response: Decrease from baseline of 50–75 % or decrease from baseline of 3–5 points	Validated Reproducible Extensive use in clinical trials	Complex Many variables Requires training and experience No validated definition of mucosal healing or response
Simple endoscopic score for Crohn's disease (SES-CD) [63]	Ulcers, inflammation, stenosis	0–60	Remission: 0 or <3 points. Response: Decrease from baseline of 50 % or decrease from baseline of ≥5 points	Validated Score correlates well with CDEIS Reproducible	Complex Not practical for clinical setting Validated against CDEIS in only one study No validated definition of mucosal healing or response
Rutgeerts score [16]	Apthoid lesions, ulcers, inflammation, nodules and stenosis	i0–i4	Score of i0–i1 low risk of clinical recurrence Score of i2 = intermediate risk of clinical recurrence Score of i3 = high risk of clinical recurrence	Gold Standard for assessment of postoperative recurrence Extensive use in clinical trials Validated cutoff values for clinical recurrence	No formal validation Only useful for ileal or ileal-colonic surgery

Table 24.5 The Crohn's disease endoscopic index of severity (CDEIS)

Endoscopic variable	Score (range 0–44)
Deep ulcerations	0 if absent or 12 if present
Superficial ulcerations	0 if absent or 6 if present
Length of ulcerated mucosa (0–10 cm)	0–10 according to length in cm
Length of diseased mucosa (0–10 cm)	0–10 according to length in cm

Four variables are scored for each of the following locations: rectum; sigmoid and left colon; transverse colon; right colon; and ileum. Total score is divided by the number of locations explored (1–5). An additional three points are given if ulcerated stenosis is present and a further three points are given if non-ulcerated stenosis is present

[This table was adapted from Mary JY et al. Development and validation of an endoscopic index of severity for Crohn's disease: a prospective multicenter study. Groupe d'Etude Therapeutique des Affections Inflammatoires du Tube Digestif (GETAID). Gut 1989;30:983–9; with permission]

Table 24.6 The simple endoscopic score for Crohn's disease (SES-CD)

Variable	Score 0	Score 1	Score 2	Score 3
Size of ulcers (cm)	None	Apthous ulcers (diameter 0.1–0.5 cm)	Large ulcers (diameter 0.5–2 cm)	Very large ulcers (diameter > 2 cm)
Ulcerated surface (%)	None	<10	10–30	>30
Affected surface (%)	Unaffected segment	<50	50–75	>75
Presence of narrowing	None	Single, can be passed	Multiple, can be passed	Cannot be passed

The SES-CD: sum of the values of the four variables for the five bowel segments. Values are given to each variable and for every examined bowel segment (rectum, left colon, transverse colon, right colon and ileum)

[This table was adapted from Daperno M et al. Development and validation of a new, simplified endoscopic activity score for Crohn's disease: the SES-CD. Gastrointest Endosc 2004;60:505–12; with permission from Elsevier]

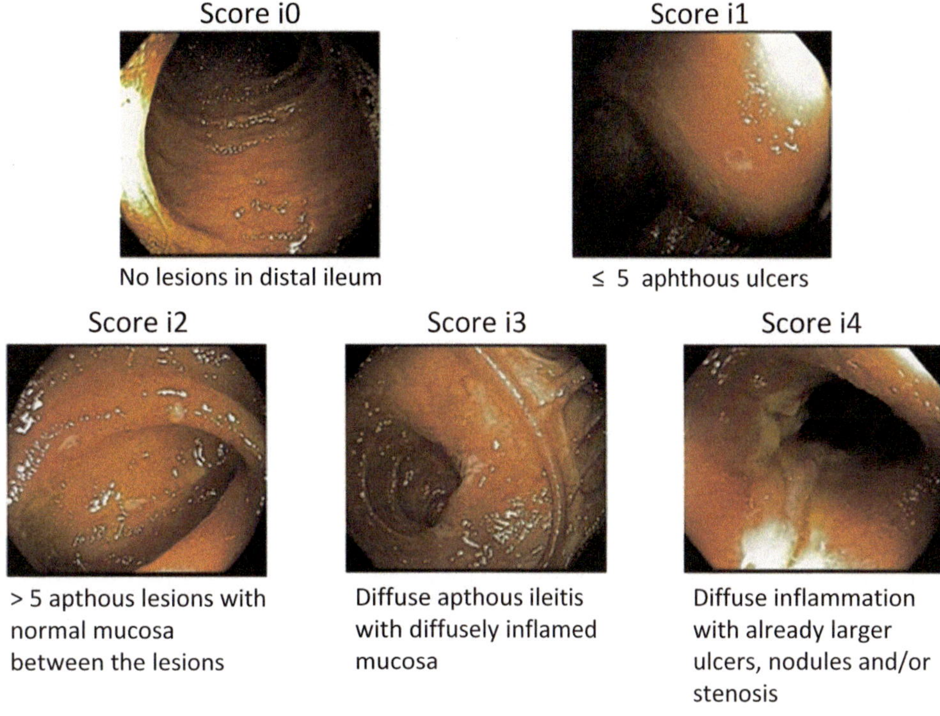

Score i0
No lesions in distal ileum
Score i1
≤ 5 aphthous ulcers
Score i2
> 5 apthous lesions with normal mucosa between the lesions
Score i3
Diffuse apthous ileitis with diffusely inflamed mucosa
Score i4
Diffuse inflammation with already larger ulcers, nodules and/or stenosis

Fig. 24.2 Rutgeerts' score for postoperative endoscopic recurrence [16]. This figure was adapted from Current Gastroenterology Reports. Christensen B et al. Understanding Endoscopic Disease Activity in IBD: How to Incorporate It into Practice. 2016; 8:5; with permission

Many CD patients undergo surgical resection and endoscopic disease recurrence may be as high as 90 % by 1 year [16]. To assess and score this recurrence in the neo-terminal ileum after ileal or ileocolonic resection in CD the so-called "Rutgeert's score" is commonly used (Fig. 24.2) [16, 79]. The score ranges from i0–i4 (where "i" stands for "ileum") and is a quick and easy score to calculate but has not been fully validated. A score of i0 or i1 is commonly classified as endoscopic postoperative remission due to the finding that grade i0 or i1 recurrence is associated with a low risk of clinical recurrence (20 % at 3 years follow-up) compared to those who have a score of i3 or i4 (92 % at 3 years follow-up) [16]. Those with a Rutgeert's score of i2 have an intermediate risk of symptomatic recurrence.

Central Reading of Endoscopic Scoring

The currently available endoscopic disease activity scoring systems are subject to error and bias. To address this, in 2009, a study of delayed-release mesalamine in moderately active UC (as determined using the Mayo scoring system) [80] utilized a central endoscopy reader to determine endoscopic severity and response to therapy with many further studies now following suit. The advantages of a central reader of endoscopy are clearly evident with Feagan et al. [61] demonstrating on a post hoc analysis of a placebo controlled trial of delayed release mesalamine for the treatment of mild to moderate UC that 31 % of participants who had met the inclusion criteria of a Ulcerative Colitis Disease Activity Index (UCDAI) sigmoidoscopy score of ≥2 per a site-investigator were considered ineligible when the images were reviewed by a central-reader of endoscopy. In addition, by comparing the results including all patients originally entered into the trial by the site investigators and just those that met the inclusion criteria per the central reader, the authors demonstrated a greater treatment effect in the mesalamine group and reduced placebo rates when analyzing patients only included by the central reader. In part because of this proof-of-concept analysis, central reading of endoscopy is playing an increasing role in the trial setting and may eventually gain regulatory support in both Europe and the US as a measure for endpoint assessment as well as assessing baseline disease severity as a means to decrease placebo response rates and increase the reliability of trial end-points [81].

Surrogate Markers of Endoscopic Healing

Currently, endoscopic evaluation of the mucosa is the gold standard to determine endoscopic disease activity and mucosal healing. However endoscopy is an invasive test, is not popular with patients and entails a risk to the patient. Therefore several surrogate markers are emerging that may be useful in assessing for smoldering endoscopic inflammation in the setting of minimal clinical symptoms, most of which have been discussed in more detail in other chapters.

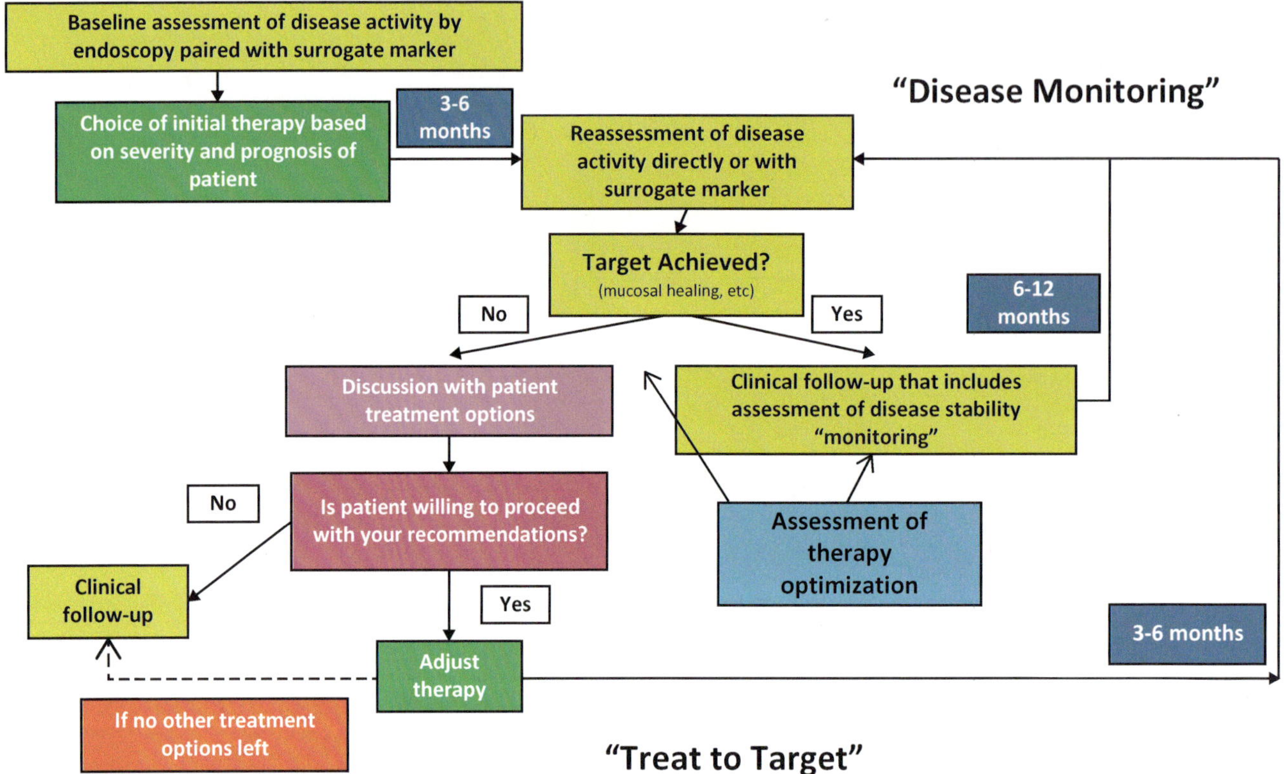

Fig. 24.3 Proposed "Treat to target" algorithm in IBD

Surrogate markers that may have some use in monitoring mucosal activity include the laboratory markers C-reactive protein and albumin, imaging studies including small bowel ultrasound and MRI and the most promising, fecal biomarkers including calprotectin and lactoferrin. All these modalities have their strengths and weaknesses to help in the assessment of mucosal healing however thus far none of these markers have been able to completely replace endoscopic assessment of disease activity in regard to predicting clinical course and response to therapy with complete certainty. Therefore, until further evidence is available, these tools should only be used in conjunction with endoscopic assessment of disease activity.

Incorporation of Endoscopic Assessment of Disease Activity and a "Treat to Target" Algorithm into Clinical Practice

To conclude the chapter, we propose an endoscopic assessment and "treat to target" algorithm incorporating endoscopic mucosal healing as an outcome acknowledging the fact that evidence for this approach in IBD is currently limited (Fig. 24.3). There are still many unresolved challenges in regard to incorporating mucosal healing into the treatment algorithm (Table 24.1); however, recently a group of IBD experts published a consensus summary of which targets should be used in UC and CD. They concluded that the endoscopic therapeutic target when treating patients with UC should be a Mayo endoscopic sub-score of 0–1 and in CD it should be resolution of all ulceration at ileocolonoscopy [82].

The incorporation of a "treat to target" approach to patient care first requires baseline disease assessment by endoscopy to assess disease activity and prognosticate the disease course. Initial therapy should be based on this prognosis and the severity of the findings with the aim to achieve early disease remission and limit bowel damage. Pairing this baseline assessment with a surrogate marker (C-reactive protein or fecal markers) may enable future assessments with the same marker. To quantify response to therapy, this should be followed by an endoscopy or use of surrogates between 3 to 6 months following treatment initiation depending on the type and speed of action of the treatment commenced (earlier if the faster acting anti-TNF therapies are utilized and later if the slower acting antimetabolite medications are used). If, on reassessment, the patient is symptomatic and has endoscopic inflammation, then escalation of medical therapies should occur. If, however, the patient is found to have mucosal activity and is in clinical remission, then the goals of treatment that occur when mucosal healing is achieved including prolonged remission and decreased disability and the risks of treatment escalation including possible higher rates of malignancy and infection should be discussed. If the patient is agreeable, medication intensification should occur and following this up-titration reassessment should occur every 3–6 months with medical therapies further optimized until the mucosal healing target is reached. Once mucosal healing is achieved then frequent clinical and objective monitoring with surrogate markers of mucosal healing should occur to assess for disease drift or early relapse every 6–12 months and endoscopic evaluation of the mucosa should be considered every 1–2 years [83]. Finally it is important to have an "exit strategy" if treatment escalation is unsuccessful and to maintain clear and open communication with the patient to maximize patient safety and satisfaction and increase the likelihood that the patient will adhere to the agreed on treatment strategy [70].

Conclusion

Endoscopic assessment in IBD is used as a diagnostic tool, to aid in the initial evaluation of disease severity and to prognosticate the disease course and for ongoing assessment of mucosal response and healing once treatment has been initiated. Repeat endoscopic assessment of disease activity with a target to achieve mucosal healing following treatment is increasingly being incorporated into both trial and clinical settings due to the fact that patients who achieve mucosal healing have longer periods of clinical remission, reduced hospitalizations and surgery and are less likely to develop colorectal neoplasia. With modern therapies, mucosal healing is obtainable and as physicians we should increasingly embrace a "treat to target" strategy to decrease the risk of future disability in our patients. Currently restricting this is a lack of consensus on the definition of mucosal healing in IBD and the lack of a single accepted and validated endoscopic scoring system for either CD or UC. Studies are currently underway to overcome these limitations. It is our hope that treating to achieve mucosal healing will help prevent permanent bowel damage in our patients and that utilizing this strategy that we will change the natural history of this disease.

References

1. Bouguen G, Peyrin-Biroulet L. Surgery for adult Crohn's disease: what is the actual risk? Gut. 2011;60(9):1178–81.
2. Filippi J, Allen PB, Hebuterne X, Peyrin-Biroulet L. Does anti-TNF therapy reduce the requirement for surgery in ulcerative colitis? A systematic review. Curr Drug Targets. 2011;12(10):1440–7.
3. Colombel JF, Rutgeerts P, Reinisch W, Esser D, Wang Y, Lang Y, et al. Early mucosal healing with infliximab is associated with improved long-term clinical outcomes in ulcerative colitis. Gastroenterology. 2011;141(4):1194–201.
4. Modigliani R, Mary JY, Simon JF, Cortot A, Soule JC, Gendre JP, et al. Clinical, biological, and endoscopic picture of attacks of Crohn's disease. Evolution on prednisolone. Groupe d'Etude Therapeutique des Affections Inflammatoires Digestives. Gastroenterology. 1990;98(4):811–8.
5. Rutgeerts P, Sandborn WJ, Feagan BG, Reinisch W, Olson A, Johanns J, et al. Infliximab for induction and maintenance therapy for ulcerative colitis. N Engl J Med. 2005;353(23):2462–76.
6. Baars JE, Nuij VJ, Oldenburg B, Kuipers EJ, van der Woude CJ. Majority of patients with inflammatory bowel disease in clinical remission have mucosal inflammation. Inflamm Bowel Dis. 2012;18(9):1634–40.
7. Gomes P, du Boulay C, Smith CL, Holdstock G. Relationship between disease activity indices and colonoscopic findings in patients with colonic inflammatory bowel disease. Gut. 1986;27(1):92–5.
8. Rubin DT, Pramoda K, Bonnie LS, Ningqi H. Frequency of subclinical disease activity in ulcerative colitis patients. Gastroenterology. 2011;140(5):S-423.
9. Solberg IC, Lygren I, Jahnsen J, Aadland E, Høie O, Cvancarova M, et al. Clinical course during the first 10 years of ulcerative colitis: results from a population-based inception cohort (IBSEN Study). Scand J Gastroenterol. 2009;44(4):431–40.
10. Munkholm P, Langholz E, Davidsen M. Binder V.l. Disease activity courses in a regional cohort of Crohn's disease patients. Scand J Gastroenterol. 1995;30(7):699–706.
11. D'Haens G, Sandborn WJ, Feagan BG, Geboes K, Hanauer SB, Irvine EJ, et al. A review of activity indices and efficacy end points for clinical trials of medical therapy in adults with ulcerative colitis. Gastroenterology. 2007;132(2):763–86.
12. Mary JY, Modigliani R. Development and validation of an endoscopic index of the severity for Crohn's disease: a prospective multicentre study. Groupe d'Etudes Therapeutiques des Affections Inflammatoires du Tube Digestif (GETAID). Gut. 1989;30(7):983–9.
13. Carbonnel F, Lavergne A, Lemann M, Bitoun A, Valleur P, Hautefeuille P, et al. Colonoscopy of acute colitis. A safe and reliable tool for assessment of severity. Dig Dis Sci. 1994;39(7):1550–7.
14. Daperno M, Sostegni R, Scaglione N, Ercole E, Rigazio C, Rocca R, et al. Outcome of a conservative approach in severe ulcerative colitis. Dig Liver Dis. 2004;36(1):21–8.
15. Allez M, Lemann M, Bonnet J, Cattan P, Jian R, Modigliani R. Long term outcome of patients with active Crohn's disease exhibiting extensive and deep ulcerations at colonoscopy. Am J Gastroenterol. 2002;97(4):947–53.
16. Rutgeerts P, Geboes K, Vantrappen G, Beyls J, Kerremans R, Hiele M. Predictability of the postoperative course of Crohn's disease. Gastroenterology. 1990;99(4):956–63.
17. Neurath MF, Travis SP. Mucosal healing in inflammatory bowel diseases: a systematic review. Gut. 2012;61(11):1619–35.
18. Sandborn WJ, Rutgeerts P, Feagan BG, Reinisch W, Olson A, Johanns J, et al. Colectomy rate comparison after treatment of ulcerative colitis with placebo or infliximab. Gastroenterology. 2009;137(4):1250–60.
19. Froslie KF, Jahnsen J, Moum BA, Vatn MH, Group I. Mucosal healing in inflammatory bowel disease: results from a Norwegian population-based cohort. Gastroenterology. 2007;133(2):412–22.
20. Feagan BG, Reinisch W, Rutgeerts P, Sandborn WJ, Yan S, Eisenberg D, et al. The effects of infliximab therapy on health-related quality of life in ulcerative colitis patients. Am J Gastroenterol. 2007;102(4):794–802.
21. Meucci G, Fasoli R, Saibeni S, Valpiani D, Gullotta R, Colombo E, et al. Prognostic significance of endoscopic remission in patients with active ulcerative colitis treated with oral and topical mesalazine: a prospective, multicenter study. Inflamm Bowel Dis. 2012;18(6):1006–10.
22. Ardizzone S, Cassinotti A, Duca P, Mazzali C, Penati C, Manes G, et al. Mucosal healing predicts late outcomes after the first course

of corticosteroids for newly diagnosed ulcerative colitis. Clin Gastroenterol Hepatol. 2011;9(6):483–9.e3.
23. Solem CA, Loftus Jr EV, Tremaine WJ, Harmsen WS, Zinsmeister AR, Sandborn WJ. Correlation of C-reactive protein with clinical, endoscopic, histologic, and radiographic activity in inflammatory bowel disease. Inflamm Bowel Dis. 2005;11(8):707–12.
24. Baert F, Moortgat L, Van Assche G, Caenepeel P, Vergauwe P, De Vos M, et al. Mucosal healing predicts sustained clinical remission in patients with early-stage Crohn's disease. Gastroenterology. 2010;138(2):463–8. quiz e10–1.
25. D'Haens G, Baert F, van Assche G, Caenepeel P, Vergauwe P, Tuynman H, et al. Early combined immunosuppression or conventional management in patients with newly diagnosed Crohn's disease: an open randomised trial. Lancet. 2008;371(9613):660–7.
26. Rutgeerts P, Feagan BG, Lichtenstein GR, Mayer LF, Schreiber S, Colombel JF, et al. Scheduled maintenance treatment with infliximab is superior to episodic treatment for the healing of mucosal ulceration associated with Crohn's disease. Gastrointest Endosc. 2006;63(3):433–42. quiz 64.
27. Schnitzler F, Fidder H, Ferrante M, Noman M, Arijs I, Van Assche G, et al. Mucosal healing predicts long-term outcome of maintenance therapy with infliximab in Crohn's disease. Inflamm Bowel Dis. 2009;15(9):1295–301.
28. Rutgeerts P, Feagan BG, Lichtenstein GR, Mayer LF, Schreiber S, Colombel JF, et al. Comparison of scheduled and episodic treatment strategies of infliximab in Crohn's disease. Gastroenterology. 2004;126(2):402–13.
29. Rutter M, Saunders B, Wilkinson K, Rumbles S, Schofield G, Kamm M, et al. Severity of inflammation is a risk factor for colorectal neoplasia in ulcerative colitis. Gastroenterology. 2004;126(2):451–9.
30. Rutter MD, Saunders BP, Wilkinson KH, Rumbles S, Schofield G, Kamm MA, et al. Thirty-year analysis of a colonoscopic surveillance program for neoplasia in ulcerative colitis. Gastroenterology. 2006;130(4):1030–8.
31. Gupta RB, Harpaz N, Itzkowitz S, Hossain S, Matula S, Kornbluth A, et al. Histologic inflammation is a risk factor for progression to colorectal neoplasia in ulcerative colitis: a cohort study. Gastroenterology. 2007;133(4):1099–105.
32. Rubin DT, Huo D, Kinnucan JA, Sedrak MS, McCullom NE, Bunnag AP, et al. Inflammation is an independent risk factor for colonic neoplasia in patients with ulcerative colitis: a case-control study. Clin Gastroenterol Hepatol. 2013;11(12):1601–8.e1–4.
33. Jess T, Riis L, Vind I, Winther KV, Borg S, Binder V, et al. Changes in clinical characteristics, course, and prognosis of inflammatory bowel disease during the last 5 decades: a population-based study from Copenhagen. Denmark Inflamm Bowel Dis. 2007;13(4): 481–9.
34. Bouguen G, Levesque BG, Pola S, Evans E, Sandborn WJ. Feasibility of endoscopic assessment and treating to target to achieve mucosal healing in ulcerative colitis. Inflamm Bowel Dis. 2014;20(2):231–9.
35. Bouguen G, Levesque BG, Pola S, Evans E, Sandborn WJ. Endoscopic assessment and treating to target increase the likelihood of mucosal healing in patients with Crohn's disease. Clin Gastroenterol Hepatol. 2014;12(6):978–85.
36. Weber MA, Julius S, Kjeldsen SE, Brunner HR, Ekman S, Hansson L, et al. Blood pressure dependent and independent effects of antihypertensive treatment on clinical events in the VALUE Trial. Lancet. 2004;363(9426):2049–51.
37. Intensive blood-glucose control with sulphonylureas or insulin compared with conventional treatment and risk of complications in patients with type 2 diabetes (UKPDS 33). UK Prospective Diabetes Study (UKPDS) Group. Lancet. 1998;352(9131):837–53.
38. Effect of intensive blood-glucose control with metformin on complications in overweight patients with type 2 diabetes (UKPDS 34). UK Prospective Diabetes Study (UKPDS) Group. Lancet. 1998;352(9131):854–65.
39. Reichard P, Nilsson BY, Rosenqvist U. The effect of long-term intensified insulin treatment on the development of microvascular complications of diabetes mellitus. N Engl J Med. 1993;329(5): 304–9.
40. Fransen J, Moens HB, Speyer I, van Riel PL. Effectiveness of systematic monitoring of rheumatoid arthritis disease activity in daily practice: a multicentre, cluster randomised controlled trial. Ann Rheum Dis. 2005;64(9):1294–8.
41. Stenger AA, Van Leeuwen MA, Houtman PM, Bruyn GA, Speerstra F, Barendsen BC, et al. Early effective suppression of inflammation in rheumatoid arthritis reduces radiographic progression. Br J Rheumatol. 1998;37(11):1157–63.
42. Symmons D, Tricker K, Roberts C, Davies L, Dawes P, Scott DL. The British Rheumatoid Outcome Study Group (BROSG) randomised controlled trial to compare the effectiveness and cost-effectiveness of aggressive versus symptomatic therapy in established rheumatoid arthritis. Health Technol Assess. 2005;9(34):iii–iv. ix–x, 1–78.
43. Fefferman DS, Farrell RJ. Endoscopy in inflammatory bowel disease: indications, surveillance, and use in clinical practice. Clin Gastroenterol Hepatol. 2005;3(1):11–24.
44. Truelove SC, Witts LJ. Cortisone in ulcerative colitis; final report on a therapeutic trial. Br Med J. 1955;2(4947):1041–8.
45. Baron JH et al. Variation between observers in describing mucosal appearances in proctocolitis. Br Med J. 1964;1(5375):89–92.
46. Feagan BG et al. Treatment of ulcerative colitis with a humanized antibody to the alpha4beta7 integrin. N Engl J Med. 2005;352(24): 2499–507.
47. Powell-Tuck J et al. A comparison of oral prednisolone given as single or multiple daily doses for active proctocolitis. Scand J Gastroenterol. 1978;13(7):833–7.
48. Rachmilewitz D. Coated mesalazine (5-aminosalicylic acid) versus sulphasalazine in the treatment of active ulcerative colitis: a randomised trial. BMJ. 1989;298(6666):82–6.
49. Hanauer S, Schwartz J, Robinson M, Roufail W, Arora S, Cello J, et al. Mesalamine capsules for treatment of active ulcerative colitis: results of a controlled trial. Pentasa Study Group Am J Gastroenterol. 1993;88(8):1188–97.
50. Hanauer SB, Robinson M, Pruitt R, Lazenby AJ, Persson T, Nilsson LG, et al. Budesonide enema for the treatment of active, distal ulcerative colitis and proctitis: a dose-ranging study. U.S. Budesonide enema study group. Gastroenterology. 1998;115(3): 525–32.
51. Sutherland LR, Martin F, Greer S, Robinson M, Greenberger N, Saibil F, et al. 5-Aminosalicylic acid enema in the treatment of distal ulcerative colitis, proctosigmoiditis, and proctitis. Gastroenterology. 1987;92(6):1894–8.
52. Naganuma M, Ichikawa H, Inoue N, Kobayashi T, Okamoto S, Hisamatsu T, et al. Novel endoscopic activity index is useful for choosing treatment in severe active ulcerative colitis patients. J Gastroenterol. 2010;45(9):936–43.
53. Matts SG. The value of rectal biopsy in the diagnosis of ulcerative colitis. Q J Med. 1961;30:393–407.
54. Schroeder KW, Tremaine WJ, Ilstrup DM. Coated oral 5-aminosalicylic acid therapy for mildly to moderately active ulcerative colitis. A randomized study. N Engl J Med. 1987;317(26):1625–9.
55. Neumann H, Neurath MF. Ulcerative colitis: UCCIS—a reproducible tool to assess mucosal healing. Nat Rev Gastroenterol Hepatol. 2012;9(12):692–4.
56. Samuel S, Bruining DH, Loftus Jr EV, Thia KT, Schroeder KW, Tremaine WJ, et al. Validation of the ulcerative colitis colonoscopic index of severity and its correlation with disease activity measures. Clin Gastroenterol Hepatol. 2013;11(1):49–54.e1.

57. Travis SP, Schnell D, Krzeski P, Abreu MT, Altman DG, Colombel JF, et al. Reliability and initial validation of the ulcerative colitis endoscopic index of severity. Gastroenterology. 2013;145(5): 987–95.
58. Walsh A, Palmer R, Travis S. Mucosal healing as a target of therapy for colonic inflammatory bowel disease and methods to score disease activity. Gastrointest Endosc Clin N Am. 2014;24(3):367–78.
59. D'Haens G, Feagan B, Colombel JF, Sandborn WJ, Reinisch W, Rutgeerts P, et al. Challenges to the design, execution, and analysis of randomized controlled trials for inflammatory bowel disease. Gastroenterology. 2012;143(6):1461–9.
60. Samaan MA, Mosli MH, Sandborn WJ, Feagan BG, D'Haens GR, Dubcenco E, et al. A systematic review of the measurement of endoscopic healing in ulcerative colitis clinical trials: recommendations and implications for future research. Inflamm Bowel Dis. 2014;20(8):1465–71.
61. Kamm MA, Sandborn WJ, Gassull M, Schreiber S, Jackowski L, Butler T, et al. Once-daily, high-concentration MMX mesalamine in active ulcerative colitis. Gastroenterology. 2007;132(1):66–75. quiz 432–3.
62. Feagan BG, Sandborn WJ, D'Haens G, Pola S, McDonald JW, Rutgeerts P, et al. The role of centralized reading of endoscopy in a randomized controlled trial of mesalamine for ulcerative colitis. Gastroenterology. 2013;145(1):149–57.e2.
63. Travis SP et al. Developing an instrument to assess the endoscopic severity of ulcerative colitis: the Ulcerative Colitis Endoscopic Index of Severity (UCEIS). Gut. 2012;61(4):535–42.
64. Daperno M, D'Haens G, Van Assche G, Baert F, Bulois P, Maunoury V, et al. Development and validation of a new, simplified endoscopic activity score for Crohn's disease: the SES-CD. Gastrointest Endosc. 2004;60(4):505–12.
65. Annese V, Daperno M, Rutter MD, Amiot A, Bossuyt P, East J, et al. European evidence based consensus for endoscopy in inflammatory bowel disease. J Crohns Colitis. 2013;7(12):982–1018.
66. Daperno M, Castiglione F, de Ridder L, Dotan I, Farkkila M, Florholmen J, et al. Results of the 2nd part Scientific Workshop of the ECCO. II: Measures and markers of prediction to achieve, detect, and monitor intestinal healing in inflammatory bowel disease. J Crohns Colitis. 2011;5(5):484–98.
67. Tontini GE, Bisschops R, Neumann H. Endoscopic scoring systems for inflammatory bowel disease: pros and cons. Expert Rev Gastroenterol Hepatol. 2014;8(5):543–54.
68. Hebuterne X, Lemann M, Bouhnik Y, Dewit O, Dupas JL, Mross M, et al. Endoscopic improvement of mucosal lesions in patients with moderate to severe ileocolonic Crohn's disease following treatment with certolizumab pegol. Gut. 2013;62(2):201–8.
69. Laharie D, Reffet A, Belleannee G, Chabrun E, Subtil C, Razaire S, et al. Mucosal healing with methotrexate in Crohn's disease: a prospective comparative study with azathioprine and infliximab. Aliment Pharmacol Ther. 2011;33(6):714–21.
70. Rutgeerts P, Van Assche G, Sandborn WJ, Wolf DC, Geboes K, Colombel JF, et al. Adalimumab induces and maintains mucosal healing in patients with Crohn's disease: data from the EXTEND trial. Gastroenterology. 2012;142(5):1102–11.e2.
71. Lemann M, Mary JY, Colombel JF, Duclos B, Soule JC, Lerebours E, et al. A randomized, double-blind, controlled withdrawal trial in Crohn's disease patients in long-term remission on azathioprine. Gastroenterology. 2005;128(7):1812–8.
72. Colombel JF, Rutgeerts PJ, Sandborn WJ, Yang M, Camez A, Pollack PF, et al. Adalimumab induces deep remission in patients with Crohn's disease. Clin Gastroenterol Hepatol. 2014;12(3): 414–22.e5.
73. Sipponen T, Bjorkesten CG, Farkkila M, Nuutinen H, Savilahti E, Kolho KL. Faecal calprotectin and lactoferrin are reliable surrogate markers of endoscopic response during Crohn's disease treatment. Scand J Gastroenterol. 2010;45(3):325–31.
74. Sipponen T, Karkkainen P, Savilahti E, Kolho KL, Nuutinen H, Turunen U, et al. Correlation of faecal calprotectin and lactoferrin with an endoscopic score for Crohn's disease and histological findings. Aliment Pharmacol Ther. 2008;28(10):1221–9.
75. Louis E, Mary JY, Vernier-Massouille G, Grimaud JC, Bouhnik Y, Laharie D, et al. Maintenance of remission among patients with Crohn's disease on antimetabolite therapy after infliximab therapy is stopped. Gastroenterology. 2012;142(1):63–70.
76. Aomatsu T, Yoden A, Matsumoto K, Kimura E, Inoue K, Andoh A, et al. Fecal calprotectin is a useful marker for disease activity in pediatric patients with inflammatory bowel disease. Dig Dis Sci. 2011;56(8):2372–7.
77. Dignass A, Stoynov S, Dorofeyev AE, Grigorieva GA, Tomsova E, Altorjay I, et al. Once versus three times daily dosing of oral budesonide for active Crohn's disease: a double-blind, double-dummy, randomised trial. J Crohns Colitis. 2014;8(9):970–80.
78. Moskovitz D, Deaperno M, Van Assche G. Defining and validating cut-off's for the simple endosocpic score for Crohn's disease. Gastroenterology. 2007;132(4):A173–S1097.
79. Ferrante M et al. Validation of endoscopic activity scores in patients with Crohn's disease based on a post hoc analysis of data from SONIC. Gastroenterology. 2013;145(5):978–86.e5.
80. Rutgeerts P et al. Natural history of recurrent Crohn's disease at the ileocolonic anastomosis after curative surgery. Gut. 1984;25(6): 665–72.
81. Sandborn WJ et al. Delayed-release oral mesalamine 4.8 g/day (800-mg tablet) is effective for patients with moderately active ulcerative colitis. Gastroenterology. 2009;137(6):1934–43. e1–3.
82. Adult inflammatory bowel disease (IBD). Presented at the Gastroenterology regulatory endopoints and the advancement of therapeutics (GREAT) workshop; Maryland: http://www.Regulations.Gov/-!Documentdetail;d=fda-2012-n-0001-0093.
83. Peyrin-Biroulet L et al. Selecting Therapeutic Targets in Inflammatory Bowel Disease (STRIDE): determining therapeutic goals for treat-totarget. Am J Gastroenterol. 2015;110:1324–38.
84. Bouguen G et al. Treat to target: a proposed new paradigm for the management of Crohn's disease. Clin Gastroenterol Hepatol. 2015;13:1042–50.e2.

Evaluation of Quality of Life in Crohn's Disease and Ulcerative Colitis: What Is Health-Related Quality of Life?

25

Katrine Carlsen, Pia Munkholm, and Johan Burisch

> *"We should not worry about how long we live but rather how satisfactorily;*
> *For in order to live a long time, you only require fate,*
> *But living satisfactorily requires understanding. Life is long if it is full."*
>
> Lucius Annaeus Seneca (4BC–65 AD)

History

While good Quality of Life (QoL) has long been a policy goal in the treatment of inflammatory bowel disease (IBD), adequate definition and measurement of it have remained elusive. The term "quality of life" is used to describe the general well-being of individuals in the field of healthcare. QoL should not be confused with "standard of living," a term defined primarily by income. Instead, standard indicators of QoL include not only wealth and employment, but also the built environment, physical and mental health, education, recreation and leisure time, and social belonging. Health-related quality of life (HRQoL) is a subjective measure of a person's physical and psychological well-being and represents a patient's assessment of how a particular disease or intervention has affected their life.

Crohn's disease (CD) and ulcerative colitis (UC) affect patients not only physically but also through limitations on social, educational, professional, and emotional activities due to their chronicity, unpredictable disease course, young age of onset, and their medical and surgical therapies [1]. Both adult and pediatric patients with IBD experience an impaired perception of HRQoL compared with a healthy age- and sex-matched background population [2–11], with disease course and disease activity [12–15], the perceived quality of care delivered, the individual's psychological status and social support [16, 17] emerging as important factors affecting HRQoL [18] (Fig. 25.1).

While most studies of HRQoL in the literature assess adult patients with IBD, several validated and reliable HRQoL questionnaires have been developed for pediatric IBD (P-IBD) patients in recent decades [19–21]. Measuring HRQoL in pediatric patients is challenging when compared to adult patients, as both the age-specific natural development and "life-concerns"—which differ significantly during childhood and adolescence [22, 23]—influence a patient's perception of HRQoL. Furthermore, a child may be unable (e.g., children <5 years old) [24] or unwilling to respond to questions. To overcome this challenge a *parent-proxy concept* is used where the parents answer questions on behalf of the child. Reviews examining the concordance between child self-reported and parent-proxy-reported HRQoL have shown that the best concordance concerns physical (objective) conditions while the least concordance relates to emotional and social items (subjective) [25]. However, parent-proxy answers for children with chronic diseases had a higher concordance than with those for healthy children. P-IBD patients are rarely younger than 5 years at diagnosis [26], nevertheless these patients often present with more severe or extensive disease [27], thereby underscoring the need to accurately measure HRQoL.

Clinicians and policymakers are increasingly cognizant of the importance of measuring HRQoL to inform patient management and policy decisions [28]. Patient-reported outcomes (PROs) capture the patient's illness experience in a structured format and may help physicians better understand symptoms from the patient's perspective [29]. PROs measure

K. Carlsen, M.D.
Department of Pediatrics, Hvidovre Hospital, Hvidovre, Denmark
e-mail: kcarlsen@gmail.com

P. Munkholm, M.D. (✉) • J. Burisch, M.D., Ph.D.
Danish Centre for eHealth & Epidemiology,
Department of Gastroenterology, North Zealand Hospital,
Frederikssund, Denmark
e-mail: pia_munkholm@mail.dk; Burisch@dadlnet.dk

D.C. Baumgart (ed.), *Crohn's Disease and Ulcerative Colitis*, DOI 10.1007/978-3-319-33703-6_25

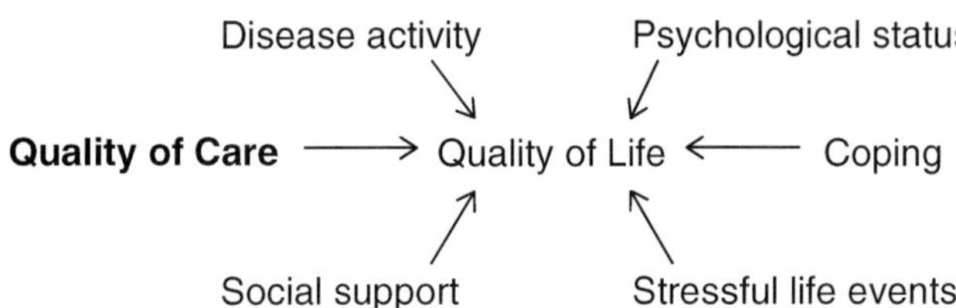

Fig. 25.1 Conceptual model of variables influencing quality of life in inflammatory bowel disease (reprinted from ref. [16] with permission from John Wiley & Sons, Inc.)

any aspect of health directly reported by the patient (e.g., physical, emotional, or social symptoms) and may help to direct care and improve clinical outcomes [30]. The ultimate PRO is improvement in HRQoL. In the U.S. Food and Drug Administration (FDA) and European Medicines Agency (EMA) guidelines [31, 32] for new drugs in IBD-validated HRQoL measurements, such as the inflammatory bowel disease questionnaire (IBDQ), are part of the secondary endpoint section among other considerations such as steroid sparing effect, treatment of abscess, endoscopic remission, and treatment of obstruction. Currently, the FDA is moving away from using disease activity indices as clinical trial endpoints and towards PROs when assessing the patient's experience of symptoms and objective measures of disease [33]. Recently, the first professorship in PROs has been established in Denmark [34].

Quality of Life Indices and Questionnaires

Several different instruments exist for the assessment of HRQoL in IBD, as described in Table 25.1. Disease-specific questionnaires for HRQoL—derived from, and validated in, the relevant disease groups—are the most sensitive indicators of change over time or with treatment. Generic instruments, on the other hand, are used to show similarities or differences among groups or populations; however, they may not be sensitive to changes over time or subsequently to treatment in groups of patients with specific diseases [35].

Disease-Specific Questionnaires

Inflammatory Bowel Disease Questionnaire (IBDQ)

In 1989, a group of doctors, together with sociologist Guyatt G at Hamilton University, Canada, developed and validated the disease-specific Inflammatory Bowel Disease Questionnaire (IBDQ) [36, 37]. To date the questionnaire has been translated into 37 languages by forward and backward translation and can be purchased from Hamilton University (www.mcmaster.flintbox.com).

The questionnaire comprises 32 items which measure the following broad domains: physical health, psychological health, social relationships, and environment. Responses are scored on a 7-point Likert scale, in which 7 corresponds to the highest level of functioning. Cumulative scoring above 170 points represents a good quality of life, with a possible range of 32–224. When compared with the general population, IBD patients have impaired quality of life in all four categories. The most frequent concerns of UC patients are having an ostomy bag, developing cancer, side effects, the uncertain nature of their disease, and the need for surgery. The most frequent concerns of CD patients are the uncertain nature of their disease, impaired energy level, side effects of medication, the need for surgery, and having an ostomy bag [35]. Surgical quality of life with inflammatory bowel disease has not been well examined and the IBDQ is not applicable to patients with stoma.

The short Inflammatory Bowel Disease Questionnaire (s-IBDQ) is a shorter version of the original instrument. It consists of ten items from the IBDQ covering all four dimensions where scoring above 50 points (range 10–70) indicates good quality of life [8] and may be more convenient for use in the office, for use in large research studies, or in clinical trials [38]. The s-IBDQ has recently been used for web-based treatment applications, where patients score their HRQoL at home using a validated eHealth tool [39–41].

In 1992 a questionnaire to determine the subjective health status of patients with inflammatory bowel disease was developed and verified. To examine the quality of life in a group of "healthy" outpatients with IBD, the group from Edmonton, Canada developed a self-administered form of this questionnaire comprising 36 questions across five dimensions: systemic symptoms, bowel symptoms, functional impairment, social impairment, and emotional function. Scores ranging between 36 and 252 points are possible, with scores above 180 indicative of a good quality of life [42].

Short Health Scale (SHS)

The Short Health Scale (SHS) was developed in Sweden, initially designed as part of a network strategy to describe various aspects of the concept of health [43]. It is a self-administered questionnaire comprised of four items, each addressing a subjective health dimension: symptoms, functional status, worry, and general well-being (Tables 25.1 and 25.2). Responses are graded on a 100-mm visual analogue scale. The results, presented as an individual score for each of the four items, form a profile. The questions are open-ended so that patients can take into account any or all aspects of their life that they feel are important when completing the questionnaire [44]. The SHS correlates with the IBDQ and has been validated in adult Swedish and Norwegian IBD patients [44–46], and has been evaluated in adult IBD patients in the UK [47] as well as Croatian pediatric-onset patients [48].

Table 25.1 Overview of disease-specific quality of life and generic rating systems in IBD

Quality of life	Items	Domains	Level (range)
Disease specific			
Inflammatory Bowel disease Questionnaire (IBDQ) [36]	32	4	Above 170 (32–224)
	10	Bowel symptoms	
	5	Systemic symptoms	
	5	Social function	
	12	Emotional function	
Short Inflammatory Bowel disease Questionnaire (sib) [38]	10	4	Above 50 good (10–70)
	3	Bowel symptoms	
	2	Systemic symptoms	
	2	Social function	
	3	Emotional function	
Inflammatory Bowel disease Questionnaire outpatients [42]	36	5	(36–252)
		Systemic symptoms	
		Bowel symptoms	
		Functional impairment	
		Social impairment	
		Emotional function	
Short Health Scale (SHS) [44, 45]	100-mm VAS	4	Less than 25 mm (0–400 mm)
		Symptoms	
		Functional status	
		Worry	
		General well-being	
Rating Form of IBD Patient Concern (RFIPC) [49]	100-mm VAS	25	0 mm represents "not at all"
IMPACT III Age 9–17 [22, 57]	35 7 3 7 12 3 3	6 Bowel symptoms Systemic symptoms Emotional functioning Social functioning Body image Treatment/interventions	(35–175)
Generic			
Short Form 36 (SF-36) [62]	36	8	(0, worst–100, best)
	10	Physical functioning	
	2	Social function	
	4	Role limitations due to physical problems	
	3	Role limitations due to emotional problems	
	4	Energy/vitality level	
	5	Mental health	
	2	Bodily pain	
	5	General health perception	
	1	Health transition over time	
Short Form 12 (SF-12) [63]	12	8	(0, worst–100, best)
	2	Physical functioning	
	1	Social function	
	2	Role limitations due to physical problems	
	2	Role limitations due to emotional problems	
	1	Vitality level	
	2	Mental health	
	1	Bodily pain	
	1	General health perception	

(continued)

Table 25.1 (continued)

Quality of life	Items	Domains	Level (range)
Psychological General well-being Index (PGWBI) [64]	22		Lower values—negative response (22–232)
	5	Anxiety	
	3	Depressed mood	
	4	Positive well-being	
	3	Self-control	
	3	General health	
	4	Vitality	
Pediatric Quality of Life Inventory™, Version 4.0 (PedsQL 4.0) [73] Child: age 5–18 Parent-proxy: age 2–18	23	2	Linear transformation (0–100)
	8	Physical functioning subscale	
		Psychosocial health:	
	5	Emotional functioning	
	5	Social functioning	
	5	School functioning	
TNO AZL Child Quality Of Life (TACQOL) Child: age 8–15 Parent-proxy: age 6–15 [76] Preschool Quality of life (TAPQOL) Parent-proxy: age 1–5 [77]	56	7	0–32 in each scale (0–224) Linear transformation (0–100)
	8 8 8 8 8 8 8	Physical complaints Motor functioning Autonomous functioning Cognitive functioning Social functioning Positive moods Negative moods	
	43 4 3 3 3 3 4 3 7 4 3 3 3	21 Sleeping Appetite Lungs Stomach Skin Motor functioning Social functioning Problem behavior Communication Anxiety Positive mood Liveliness	

Table 25.2 Short Health Scale (SHS) with the four dimensions and four questions presented as 100 mm in VAS scale

1. How severe symptoms do you suffer from your bowel disease?	
No symptoms ______________________	Very severe symptoms
2. Does your bowel disease interfere with your activities in daily life?	
Not at all ______________________	Interferes to a very high degree
3. How much worry does your bowel disease cause?	
No worry ______________________	Constant worry
4. What is your general sense of well-being?	
Very well ______________________	Dreadful
Based on data from refs. [44, 45].	

Rating Form of IBD Patient Concern (RFIPC)

The Rating Form of IBD Patient Concern (RFIPC), a 25-item disease-specific questionnaire, rates worries and concerns of patients with IBD on a 100-mm VAS scale (range, 0–100 mm) [49]. Zero mm represents "not at all" and 100 "a great deal." The sum score is the mean average of the scores across all 25 items. The RFIPC has been found to be reliable and valid [50–53]; while it is not applicable to patients with stoma, it has been validated in patients with pouch after proctocolectomy [54].

IMPACT

The most regularly used disease-specific HRQoL for P-IBD is IMPACT [55], which is also recommended by the pediatric committee of the European Crohn's and Colitis Organization (P-ECCO) as a secondary outcome measure in clinical trials [56]. The IMPACT questionnaire originates in Canada and was developed after item-generated and item-reduction interviews with 82 P-IBD patients (8–17 years) [22]. To mirror the adult IBDQ, it was decided beforehand to arrive at a 33-item questionnaire in the item-reduction phase. Responses to each question are recorded on a 10 cm VAS (with increments of 0.7 cm, for comparison to the IBDQ score). The 33 items are divided according to six dimensions: bowel symptoms; body image; emotional functioning; social functioning; tests/treatments; and systemic symptoms. A higher score represents a better quality of life (with a range of 0–231).

IMPACT has been validated and found reliable in Canada [57]. It was further tested in Europe, among British and Dutch children, where it was found that some of the questions were inappropriate and/or too difficult to understand. Subsequently a simpler wording of the questionnaire was introduced and some of the questions were replaced, resulting in IMPACT II (35 items, VAS score, same six dimensions, score range of 0–245) [58]. IMPACT III consists of the same questions as IMPACT II, but with a 5-point Likert scale (score range of 35–175) instead of VAS [59]. IMPACT III has been validated and evaluated in children [58, 60] as well as in a parent-proxy setting, showing overall good concordance—except with regard to emotional functioning, where parents scored emotional functioning lower than did their children [61]. IMPACT III has been translated through cross-cultural adaptation into 40 languages [56].

Generic Questionnaires

Short Form-36 (SF-36)

The SF-36 is a generic questionnaire containing 36 items [62]. Thirty-five of the items are grouped into eight multi-item scales. The eight domains of the SF-36 are as follows: physical function (ten items); social function (two items); role limitations due to physical problems (four items); role limitations due to emotional problems (three items); energy/vitality (four items); mental health (five items); bodily pain (two items); and general health perception (five items). In addition, it contains a one-item measure of self-evaluated change in health status (health transition) over the previous year. For each question, a raw score is coded and transformed into a percentage, with 0 indicating the least favorable possible health status and 100 indicating the most favorable.

The 12-item Short Form Health Survey (SF-12) was developed for the Medical Outcomes Study (MOS), a multi-year study of patients with chronic conditions [63]. The resulting short-form survey instrument provides a solution to the problem faced by many investigators who must restrict survey length. It consists of 12 questions grouped into a physical and a mental component summary score (PCS and MCS) and eight multi-item scales. The instrument was designed to reduce respondent burden while achieving minimum standards of precision for purposes of group comparisons involving multiple health dimensions.

Psychological General Well-Being Index (PGWBI)

The Psychological General Well-Being Index (PGWBI) is a generic 22-item questionnaire measuring subjective feelings of well-being and distress [64]. Responses are graded on a 6-point Likert scale. Lower values correspond to more negative responses and higher values to more positive responses. The overall score is the summation of the item responses, ranging from 22–132. The questionnaire has been used alone and in combination with other generic and disease-specific questionnaires, both in general populations and in studies of chronic illness. The PGWBI has been translated and culturally adapted into at least 36 languages.

Pediatric Quality of Life Inventory (PedsQL)

PedsQL [65] is a regularly used generic HRQoL for assessing those with P-IBD [10, 48, 66–72]. It is valid and reliable [73–75] and exists in several languages [19]. The updated version, PedsQL 4.0 Generic Core Scales [73], consists of 23 items covering the following dimensions: (1) physical functioning, (2) emotional functioning, (3) social functioning, and (4) school functioning. The questionnaire consists of parallel versions, with child self-reported (ages 5–7, 8–12, and 13–18) and parent-proxy-reported (age 2–18) scores. The child self-reported and parent-reported versions are essentially identical but differ in the wording of the questions (i.e., first or third person, respectively). Furthermore, the school-related items differ depending on the age of the child. Answers are given on a 5-point (0–4) scale or a 3-point (0, 2, and 4) scale, expressed as corresponding faces to ease the process for the youngest patients (age 5–7). Items are reverse-scored and linearly transformed to a 0–100 scale divided by the number of items answered. Higher scores represent a better HRQoL. The score can be evaluated as a total

HRQoL score and two summary scores: physical health (dimension 1) and psychosocial health (dimensions 2–4). A PedsQL family information form is used to collect demographic data and information about missing days of school and work (for the parents) caused by the child's ill health.

Another generic HRQoL measure is the Netherlands Organization for Applied Scientific Research Academic Medical Centers (TNO AZL) Child Quality Of Life (TACQOL) and Preschool Children Quality of Life (TAPQOL) [76, 77]. TACQOL and TAPQOL have been used in Dutch P-IBD publications [14, 58, 78]; while other pediatric generic HRQoL questionnaires used in pediatric populations exist [19, 20], they appear less regularly in P-IBD publications.

Evaluation of QoL in IBD Patients

The role of extrinsic factors—the characteristics of the social surroundings (e.g., family, social network, QoC, social security, infrastructure, occupation, cultural, and religious values)—in patients' perception of HRQoL is well studied in IBD. The significance of family and social support has been described in both adult and pediatric studies [71, 79–84]. Regarding HRQoL among parents of children with IBD, scores decrease with worsening disease activity in the child [85].

The aforementioned European Collaborative Study on IBD (EC-IBD) was able to show that HRQoL is influenced by a variety of factors in the community setting [16, 86]. A moderate correlation between patient-reported IBD-related concerns and adverse national parameters has been found [52]. Ethnic and religious differences have also been put forward as predictors of HRQoL outcome in IBD [87, 88].

Intrinsic factors refer to mental and physical aspects of the respondent dependent of respectively (1) gender, age, personality, preference, life goals, coping strategy, experience, knowledge, education, psychiatric disorder and (2) comorbidity, disease severity and duration, complication, general physical health status.

Being female has, in the majority of studies of adult IBD patients, been associated with a poorer HRQoL in CD, in other diseases, and in the general population [89–91]. However in P-IBD, results have shown no disparity in HRQoL among girls and boys [74, 78, 92, 93]. In some P-IBD studies, poorer HRQoL was associated with higher age (i.e., adolescents) [14, 15] while other studies showed no significant effect [74, 92]. While the elderly have a poorer generic HRQoL in general population health surveys, particularly regarding physical domains [89], in several studies on HRQoL in IBD age was shown to have little or no effect [3, 94, 95].

Personality traits, coping strategies and mental illness have been found to influence HRQoL in adult and pediatric IBD populations [93, 96–101]. Furthermore, an individual's ability to cope with ill-health can change over time. Health impairments may elicit a process of accommodation in which the internal standards, values, and conceptualization of subjective health evaluations are changed. This phenomenon, known as "response," is an important factor in HRQoL over time and an important contributor to HRQoL outcome, possibly explaining improvements of HRQoL in the long term, and also counterintuitive findings of enhanced HRQoL in patients with severe disease [102]. Despite this phenomenon, and the widely described mitigating long-term disease course [103–105], HRQoL seems not to be affected by disease duration in CD [2, 95, 99, 100, 106].

A higher educational level has been associated with better IBD-related HRQoL [49, 95], but specific IBD educational programs have not been shown to improve HRQoL in adult IBD patients [107, 108]. However, among P-IBD patients HRQoL was found to improve after attending a camp sponsored by the Crohn's and Colitis Foundation of America, suggesting a normalizing of the chronic illness experience [109].

Low socioeconomic status and smoking have also been linked to a poorer HRQoL among those with CD [5, 110]. Disease activity and severity has in many studies been a strong predictor of adult and pediatric HRQoL in IBD [10, 14, 15, 98, 101, 111, 112], even though a disease phenotype (as classified by age at diagnosis, location, and behavior) was found to have no effect on HRQoL in a 2005 study by Casella's [4]. Finally, comorbidity has been found to be detrimental to HRQoL, in both physical and mental terms, when assessing patients using IBD-specific instruments [3, 106].

In a comprehensive analysis of 22 studies of quality of life in CD [113], HRQoL was better in healthy controls and UC patients (except pre-colectomy ones) than in CD patients. Health-related quality of life was similar to, or worse than, that among those with a variety of other chronic medical conditions. Health-related quality of life was directly correlated with CD activity and was worse among those with active disease than among those in remission. In P-IBD studies, the HRQoL was comparable to that found in other chronic or acute illnesses, but worse than that among healthy children [10, 11]. Finally, HRQoL studies have found a high representation of depressive symptoms and disorders in P-IBD patients [82, 114–116].

Health-related quality of life was found to improve for a short time after surgical resection [117]. In addition, active IBD had a negative impact on labor force participation [118] and relationship and sexual health [119]. In P-IBD, patients receiving an ideal J-pouch anal anastomosis were reported to be satisfied with the surgical procedure [120] and HRQoL scores were similar to those among healthy children [72, 121]. As such, physicians should not necessarily avoid surgery when striving for the most important goal of medical therapy, which is to make the patient well [122, 123].

Perspectives

Health-related quality of life is a useful metric when assessing the efficacy of medication in trials and has been validated in several different disease activity scoring systems. Short form questionnaires for disease-specific and generic HRQoL are recommended in the everyday clinical setting. The most established HRQoL measures described in the literature are the IBDQ (adult) and IMPACT III (pediatric). PROs are emerging as important endpoints in drug trials as treatment targets for IBD that in the future could be used in treat-to-target strategies in routine clinical practice.

In recent year's eHealth, including self-management tools, has been introduced as an important "adjuvant" to medical therapy. This approach can improve adherence to medication among IBD patients [39], time in remission [39, 41], as well as HRQoL [39, 124] by involving patients in their own treatment and disease course. Two recent meta-analyses showed that distance management was able to decrease the number of clinic visits and improve HRQoL, adherence to therapies, knowledge about the disease, reduction of health care costs for IBD, and shorter time to remission [125, 126]. eHealth instruments in pediatric settings are currently under evaluation in Holland, the USA and Denmark [127–129].

New technologies and digital solutions continue to impact on health care, including IBD care, with telemedicine being increasingly studied for follow-up and treatment especially in young, busy, and rural patients with limited time or reduced access to standard care providers. Based on the evidence to date, eHealth technology is a tool that could potentially enhance long-term prognosis of gastrointestinal diseases, as well as improve the HRQoL of IBD patients.

References

1. Burisch J, Jess T, Martinato M, et al. The burden of inflammatory bowel disease in Europe. J Crohns Colitis. 2013;7:322–37. doi:10.1016/j.crohns.2013.01.010.
2. Canavan C, Abrams KR, Hawthorne B, et al. Long-term prognosis in Crohn's disease: factors that affect quality of life. Aliment Pharmacol Ther. 2006;23:377–85. doi:10.1111/j.1365-2036.2006.02753.x.
3. Hjortswang H, Järnerot G, Curman B, et al. The influence of demographic and disease-related factors on health-related quality of life in patients with ulcerative colitis. Eur J Gastroenterol Hepatol. 2003;15:1011–20. doi:10.1097/00042737-200309000-00012.
4. Casellas F, Arenas JI, Baudet JS, et al. Impairment of health-related quality of life in patients with inflammatory bowel disease: a Spanish multicenter study. Inflamm Bowel Dis. 2005;11:488–96.
5. Rubin GP, Hungin APS, Chinn DJ, et al. Quality of life in patients with established inflammatory bowel disease: a UK general practice survey. Aliment Pharmacol Ther. 2004;19:529–35. doi:10.1111/j.1365-2036.2004.1873.x.
6. Casellas F, López-Vivancos J, Badia X, et al. Influence of inflammatory bowel disease on different dimensions of quality of life. Eur J Gastroenterol Hepatol. 2001;13:567–72.
7. Nordin K, Påhlman L, Larsson K, et al. Health-related quality of life and psychological distress in a population-based sample of Swedish patients with inflammatory bowel disease. Scand J Gastroenterol. 2002;37:450–7. doi:10.1080/003655202317316097.
8. Burisch J, Weimers P, Pedersen N, et al. Health-related quality of life improves during one year of medical and surgical treatment in a European population-based inception cohort of patients with Inflammatory Bowel Disease—an ECCO-EpiCom study. J Crohns Colitis. 2014;8:1030–42. doi:10.1016/j.crohns.2014.01.028.
9. Bernklev T, Jahnsen J, Lygren I, et al. Health-related quality of life in patients with inflammatory bowel disease measured with the short form-36: psychometric assessments and a comparison with general population norms. Inflamm Bowel Dis. 2005;11:909–18. doi:10.1097/01.mib.0000179467.01748.99.
10. Kunz JH, Hommel KA, Greenley RN. Health-related quality of life of youth with inflammatory bowel disease: a comparison with published data using the PedsQL 4.0 generic core scales. Inflamm Bowel Dis. 2010;16:939–46. doi:10.1002/ibd.21128.
11. Ingerski LM, Modi AC, Hood KK, et al. Health-related quality of life across pediatric chronic conditions. J Pediatr. 2010;156:639–44. doi:10.1016/j.jpeds.2009.11.008.
12. Lix LM, Graff L, Walker JR, et al. Longitudinal study of quality of life and psychological functioning for active, fluctuating, and inactive disease patterns in inflammatory bowel disease. Inflamm Bowel Dis. 2008;14:1575–84. doi:10.1002/ibd.20511.
13. Bernklev T, Jahnsen J, Schulz T, et al. Course of disease, drug treatment and health-related quality of life in patients with inflammatory bowel disease 5 years after initial diagnosis. Eur J Gastroenterol Hepatol. 2005;17:1037–45. doi:10.1097/00042737-200510000-00006.
14. Loonen HJ, Grootenhuis MA, Last BF, et al. Quality of life in pediatric inflammatory bowel disease measured by a generic and a disease-specific questionnaire. Acta Paediatr. 2002;91:348–54. doi:10.1080/08035250252834049.
15. Otley AR, Griffiths AM, Hale S, et al. Health-related quality of life in the first year after a diagnosis of pediatric inflammatory bowel disease. Inflamm Bowel Dis. 2006;12:684–91.
16. Van der Eijk I, Vlachonikolis IG, Munkholm P, et al. The role of quality of care in health-related quality of life in patients with IBD. Inflamm Bowel Dis. 2004;10:392–8. doi:10.1097/00054725-200407000-00010.
17. Elkjaer M, Moser G, Reinisch W, et al. IBD patients need in health quality of care ECCO consensus. J Crohns Colitis. 2008;2:181–8. doi:10.1016/j.crohns.2008.02.001.
18. Van der Have M, van der Aalst KS, Kaptein AA, et al. Determinants of health-related quality of life in Crohn's disease: a systematic review and meta-analysis. J Crohns Colitis. 2014;8:93–106. doi:10.1016/j.crohns.2013.04.007.
19. Raat H, Mohangoo AD, Grootenhuis MA. Pediatric health-related quality of life questionnaires in clinical trials. Curr Opin Allergy Clin Immunol. 2006;6:180–5. doi:10.1097/01.all.0000225157.67897.c2.
20. Matza LS, Swensen AR, Flood EM, et al. Assessment of health-related quality of life in children: a review of conceptual, methodological, and regulatory issues. Value Heal. 2004;7:79–92. doi:10.1111/j.1524-4733.2004.71273.x.
21. Turner D, Otley AR, Mack D, et al. Development, validation, and evaluation of a pediatric ulcerative colitis activity index: a prospective multicenter study. Gastroenterology. 2007;133:423–32. doi:10.1053/j.gastro.2007.05.029.
22. Griffiths AM, Nicholas D, Smith C, et al. Development of a quality-of-life index for pediatric inflammatory bowel disease:

dealing with differences related to age and IBD type. J Pediatr Gastroenterol Nutr. 1999;28:S46–52.
23. Jenney ME, Campbell S. Measuring quality of life. Arch Dis Child. 1997;77:347–50.
24. Varni JW, Limbers CA, Burwinkle TM. How young can children reliably and validly self-report their health-related quality of life?: an analysis of 8,591 children across age subgroups with the PedsQL 4.0 Generic Core Scales. Health Qual Life Outcomes. 2007;5:1. doi:10.1186/1477-7525-5-1.
25. Eiser C, Morse R. Can parents rate their child's health-related quality of life? Results of a systematic review. Qual Life Res. 2001;10:347–57. doi:10.1023/A:1012253723272.
26. Balzola F, Bernstein C, Van Assche G. Paediatric inflammatory bowel disease during a 44-year period in Copenhagen County: occurrence, course and prognosis—a population-based study from the Danish Crohn Colitis Database. Commentary Inflamm Bowel Dis Monit. 2010;10:90. doi:10.1097/MEG.0b013e32832a4ed6.
27. Van Limbergen J, Russell RK, Drummond HE, et al. Definition of phenotypic characteristics of childhood-onset inflammatory bowel disease. Gastroenterology. 2008;135:1114–22. doi:10.1053/j.gastro.2008.06.081.
28. Guyatt GH, Feeny DH, Patrick DL. Measuring health-related quality of life. Ann Intern Med. 1993;118:622–9. doi:10.7326/0003-4819-118-8-199304150-00009.
29. Spiegel BMR. Patient-reported outcomes in gastroenterology: clinical and research applications. J Neurogastroenterol Motil. 2013;19:137–48. doi:10.5056/jnm.2013.19.2.137.
30. Wagner EH, Austin BT, Von Korff M. Organizing care for patients with chronic illness. Milbank Q. 1996;74:511–44.
31. European Medicines Agency. Pre-authorisation evaluation of medicines for human use. London: 2008.
32. U.S. Food and Drug Administration. Guidance for industry clinical trial endpoints for the approval of cancer drugs and biologics. 2007. doi:10.1089/blr.2007.9941.
33. Peyrin-Biroulet L, Sandborn W, Sands BE, et al. Selecting therapeutic targets in inflammatory bowel disease (STRIDE): determining therapeutic goals for treat-to-target. Am J Gastroenterol. 2015;110(9):1324–38. doi: 10.1038/ajg.2015.233. Epub 2015 Aug 25. Review.
34. Nielsen ML. New professor systematises patient data. Aarhus Univ News. 2015. http://newsroom.au.dk/en/news/show/artikel/ny-professor-saetter-patientdata-i-system/. Accessed 9 July 2015.
35. Irvine EJ. Quality of life issues in patients with inflammatory bowel disease. Am J Gastroenterol. 1997;92:18S–24.
36. Guyatt G, Mitchell A, Irvine EJ, et al. A new measure of health status for clinical trials in inflammatory bowel disease. Gastroenterology. 1989;96:804–10. doi:S0016508589000922 [pii].
37. Irvine E, Feagan B, Rochon J, et al. Quality of life: a valid and reliable measure of therapeutic efficacy in the treatment of inflammatory bowel disease. Canadian Crohn's Relapse Prevention Trial Study Group. Gastroenterology. 1994;106:287–96.
38. Jowett SL, Seal CJ, Barton JR, et al. The Short Inflammatory Bowel Disease Questionnaire is reliable and responsive to clinically important change in ulcerative colitis. Am J Gastroenterol. 2001;96:2921–8. doi:10.1016/S0002-9270(01)03244-0.
39. Elkjaer M, Shuhaibar M, Burisch J, et al. E-health empowers patients with ulcerative colitis: a randomised controlled trial of the web-guided 'Constant-care' approach. Gut. 2010;59:1652–61. doi:10.1136/gut.2010.220160.
40. Pedersen N, Elkjaer M, Duricova D, et al. EHealth: Individualisation of infliximab treatment and disease course via a self-managed web-based solution in Crohn's disease. Aliment Pharmacol Ther. 2012;36:840–9. doi:10.1111/apt.12043.
41. Pedersen N, Thielsen P, Martinsen L, et al. eHealth: Individualization of mesalazine treatment through a self-managed web-based solution in mild-to-moderate ulcerative colitis. Inflamm Bowel Dis. 2014;20:2276–85. doi:10.1097/MIB.0000000000000199.
42. Love J, Irvine E, Fedorak R. Quality of life in inflammatory bowel disease. J Clin Gastroenterol. 1992;14:15–9.
43. Hjortswang H, Almer S, Ström M. The network: a strategy to describe the relationship between quality of life and disease activity. The case of inflammatory bowel disease. Eur J Gastroenterol Hepatol. 1999;11:1099–104.
44. Hjortswang H, Järnerot G, Curman B, et al. The Short Health Scale: a valid measure of subjective health in ulcerative colitis. Scand J Gastroenterol. 2006;41:1196–203. doi:10.1080/00365520600610618.
45. Stjernman H, Grännö C, Järnerot G, et al. Short health scale: a valid, reliable, and responsive instrument for subjective health assessment in Crohn's disease. Inflamm Bowel Dis. 2008;14:47–52. doi:10.1002/ibd.20255.
46. Jelsness-Jørgensen LP, Bernklev T, Moum B. Quality of life in patients with inflammatory bowel disease: translation, validity, reliability and sensitivity to change of the Norwegian version of the Short Health Scale (SHS). Qual Life Res. 2012;21:1671–6. doi:10.1007/s11136-011-0081-7.
47. McDermott E, Keegan D, Byrne K, et al. The Short Health Scale: a valid and reliable measure of health related quality of life in English speaking inflammatory bowel disease patients. J Crohns Colitis. 2013;7:616–21. doi:10.1016/j.crohns.2012.07.030.
48. Abdovic S, Pavic AM, Milosevic M, et al. Short health scale: a valid, reliable, and responsive measure of health-related quality of life in children with inflammatory bowel disease. Inflamm Bowel Dis. 2015;21:818–23. doi:10.1097/MIB.0000000000000324.
49. Drossman DA, Leserman J, Li ZM, et al. The rating form of IBD patient concerns: a new measure of health status. Psychosom Med 1991;53:701–12. doi:0033-3174/91/5306-0701J03.00/0
50. Stjernman H, Tysk C, Almer S, et al. Worries and concerns in a large unselected cohort of patients with Crohn's disease. Scand J Gastroenterol. 2010;45:696–706. doi:10.3109/00365521003734141.
51. Hjortswang H, Ström M, Almeida RT, et al. Evaluation of the RFIPC, a disease-specific health-related quality of life questionnaire, in Swedish patients with ulcerative colitis. Scand J Gastroenterol. 1997;32:1235–40. doi:10.3109/00365529709028153.
52. Levenstein S, Li Z, Almer S, et al. Cross-cultural variation in disease-related concerns among patients with inflammatory bowel disease. Am J Gastroenterol. 2001;96:1822–30. doi:10.1016/S0002-9270(01)02441-8.
53. Moser G, Tillinger W, Sachs G, et al. Relationship between the use of unconventional therapies and disease-related concerns: a study of patients with inflammatory bowel disease. J Psychosom Res. 1996;40:503–9. doi:10.1016/0022-3999(95)00581-1.
54. Provenzale D, Shearin M, Phillips-Bute BG, et al. Health-related quality of life after ileoanal pull-through: evaluation and assessment of new health status measures. Gastroenterology. 1997;113:7–14. doi:10.1016/S0016-5085(97)70074-X.
55. Karwowski CA, Keljo D, Szigethy E. Strategies to improve quality of life in adolescents with inflammatory bowel disease. Inflamm Bowel Dis. 2009;15:1755–64. doi:10.1002/ibd.20919.
56. Ruemmele FM, Hyams JS, Otley A, et al. Outcome measures for clinical trials in pediatric IBD: an evidence-based, expert-driven practical statement paper of the pediatric ECCO committee. Gut. 2015;64:438–46. doi:10.1136/gutjnl-2014-307008.
57. Otley A, Smith C, Nicholas D, et al. The IMPACT questionnaire: a valid measure of health-related quality of life in pediatric inflammatory bowel disease. J Pediatr Gastroenterol Nutr. 2002;35:557–63. doi:10.1097/00005176-200210000-00018.
58. Loonen HJ, Grootenhuis MA, Last BF, et al. Measuring quality of life in children with inflammatory bowel disease: the impact-II (NL). Qual Life Res. 2002;11:47–56.
59. Ogden CA, Abbott J, Aggett P, et al. Pilot evaluation of an instrument to measure quality of life in British children with inflamma-

tory bowel disease. J Pediatr Gastroenterol Nutr. 2008;46:117–20. doi:10.1097/01.mpg.0000304467.45541.bb.

60. Ogden C, Akobeng A, Abbott J, et al. Validation of an instrument to measure quality of life in British children with inflammatory bowel disease. J Pediatr Gastroenterol Nutr. 2011;53:280–6. doi:10.1097/MPG.0b013e3182165d10.
61. Gallo J, Grant A, Otley AR, et al. Do parents and children agree? Quality-of-life assessment of children with inflammatory bowel disease and their parents. J Pediatr Gastroenterol Nutr. 2014;58:481–5. doi:10.1097/MPG.0000000000000236.
62. Ware JE, Sherbourne CD. The MOS 36-item short-form health survey (SF-36). I. Conceptual framework and item selection. Med Care. 1992;30:473–83. doi:10.1097/00005650-199206000-00002.
63. Ware J, Kosinski M, Keller SD. A 12-Item Short-Form Health Survey: construction of scales and preliminary tests of reliability and validity. Med Care. 1996;34:220–33. doi:10.2307/3766749.
64. Dupuy H. The psychological General Well-Being (PGWB) Index. In: Wenger N, Mattson M, Furburg C, et al., editors. Assessment of quality of life in clinical trials of cardiovascular therapies. Shelton CT: Le Jacq Publishing; 1984. Assessment of Quality of Life in Clinical Trials o.
65. Varni JW, Seid M, Rode CA. The PedsQL: measurement model for the pediatric quality of life inventory. Med Care. 1999; 37:126–39.
66. Perrin JM, Kuhlthau K, Chughtai A, et al. Measuring quality of life in pediatric patients with inflammatory bowel disease: psychometric and clinical characteristics. J Pediatr Gastroenterol Nutr. 2008;46:164–71. doi:10.1097/MPG.0b013e31812f7f4e.
67. Marcus SB, Strople J, Neighbors K, et al. Fatigue and health-related quality of life in pediatric inflammatory bowel disease. Clin Gastroenterol Hepatol. 2009;7:554–61. doi:10.1016/j.cgh.2009.01.022.
68. Gumidyala AP, Greenley RN. Correlates of health-related quality of life in pediatric inflammatory bowel disease: a cumulative risk model approach. J Pediatr Psychol. 2014;39:55–64. doi:10.1093/jpepsy/jst073.
69. Faus AL, Turchi RM, Polansky M, et al. Health-related quality of life in overweight/obese children compared with children with inflammatory bowel disease. Clin Pediatr (Phila). 2015;54:775–82. doi:10.1177/0009922814562555.
70. Ryan JL, Mellon MW, Junger KWF, et al. The clinical utility of health-related quality of life screening in a pediatric inflammatory bowel disease clinic. Inflamm Bowel Dis. 2013;19:2666–72. doi:10.1097/MIB.0b013e3182a82b15.
71. Kunz JH, Greenley RN, Howard M. Maternal, paternal, and family health-related quality of life in the context of pediatric inflammatory bowel disease. Qual Life Res. 2011;20:1197–204. doi:10.1007/s11136-011-9853-3.
72. Uchida K, Kawamata A, Hashimoto K, et al. Self-reported assessment of health-related quality of life in children who underwent restorative proctocolectomy with ileal J-pouch anal anastomosis for ulcerative colitis. Pediatr Surg Int. 2013;29:287–91. doi:10.1007/s00383-012-3224-1.
73. Varni JW, Seid M, Kurtin PS. PedsQL 4.0: reliability and validity of the Pediatric Quality of Life Inventory version 4.0 generic core scales in healthy and patient populations. Med Care. 2001; 39:800–12.
74. Upton P, Eiser C, Cheung I, et al. Measurement properties of the UK-English version of the Pediatric Quality of Life Inventory 4.0 (PedsQL) generic core scales. Health Qual Life Outcomes. 2005;3:22. doi:10.1186/1477-7525-3-22.
75. Varni JW, Burwinkle TM, Seid M, et al. The PedsQLTM 4.0 as a pediatric population health measure: feasibility, reliability, and validity. Ambul Pediatr. 2003;3:329–41. doi:10.1367/1539-4409(2003)003<0329:tpaapp>2.0.co;2.
76. Verrips E, Vogels T, Koopman H, et al. Measuring health-related quality of life in a child population. Eur J Public Health. 1999;9:188–93.
77. Fekkes M, Theunissen NC, Brugman E, et al. Development and psychometric evaluation of the TAPQOL: a health-related quality of life instrument for 1-5-year-old children. Qual Life Res. 2000;9:961–72.
78. De Boer M, Grootenhuis M, Derkx B, et al. Health-related quality of life and psychosocial functioning of adolescents with inflammatory bowel disease. Inflamm Bowel Dis. 2005;11:400–6. doi:10.1097/01.MIB.0000164024.10848.0a.
79. Sewitch MJ, Abrahamowicz M, Bitton A, et al. Psychological distress, social support, and disease activity in patients with inflammatory bowel disease. Am J Gastroenterol. 2001;96:1470–9. doi:10.1111/j.1572-0241.2001.03800.x.
80. Janke K-H, Klump B, Gregor M, et al. Determinants of life satisfaction in inflammatory bowel disease. Inflamm Bowel Dis. 2005;11:272–86.
81. Pihl-Lesnovska K, Hjortswang H, Ek A-C, et al. Patients' perspective of factors influencing quality of life while living with Crohn disease. Gastroenterol Nurs. 2010;33:37–44. doi:10.1097/SGA.0b013e3181d3d8db.
82. Engstrom I. Inflammatory bowel disease in children and adolescents: mental health and family functioning. J Pediatr Gastroenterol Nutr. 1999;28:S28–33. doi:10.1097/00005176-199904001-00004.
83. Tojek TM, Lumley MA, Corlis M, et al. Maternal correlates of health status in adolescents with inflammatory bowel disease. J Psychosom Res. 2002;52:173–9. doi:10.1016/S0022-3999(01)00291-4.
84. Herzer M, Denson LA, Baldassano RN, et al. Family functioning and health-related quality of life in adolescents with pediatric inflammatory bowel disease. Eur J Gastroenterol Hepatol. 2011;23:95–100. doi:10.1097/MEG.0b013e3283417abb.
85. Greenley RN, Cunningham C. Parent quality of life in the context of pediatric inflammatory bowel disease. J Pediatr Psychol. 2009;34:129–36. doi:10.1093/jpepsy/jsn056.
86. Huppertz-Hauss G, Høivik ML, Langholz E, et al. Health-related quality of life in inflammatory bowel disease in a European-wide population-based cohort 10 years after diagnosis. Inflamm Bowel Dis. Published Online First: 7 Jan 2015. doi:10.1097/MIB.0000000000000272.
87. Straus WL, Eisen GM, Sandler RS, et al. Crohn's disease: does race matter? The Mid-Atlantic Crohn's Disease Study Group. Am J Gastroenterol. 2000;95:479–83. doi:10.1111/j.1572-0241.2000.t01-1-01531.x.
88. Farrokhyar F, Marshall JK, Easterbrook B, et al. Functional gastrointestinal disorders and mood disorders in patients with inactive inflammatory bowel disease: prevalence and impact on health. Inflamm Bowel Dis. 2006;12:38–46. doi:10.1097/01.MIB.0000195391.49762.89.
89. Sullivan M, Karlsson J. The Swedish SF-36 Health Survey. III. Evaluation of criterion-based validity: results from normative population. J Clin Epidemiol. 1998;51:1105–13. doi:10.1016/S0895-4356(98)00102-4.
90. Sainsbury A, Heatley RV. Review article: psychosocial factors in the quality of life of patients with inflammatory bowel disease. Aliment Pharmacol Ther. 2005;21:499–508. doi:10.1111/j.1365-2036.2005.02380.x.
91. Cherepanov D, Palta M, Fryback DG, et al. Gender differences in health-related quality-of-life are partly explained by sociodemographic and socioeconomic variation between adult men and women in the US: evidence from four US nationally representa-

tive data sets. Qual Life Res. 2010;19:1115–24. doi:10.1007/s11136-010-9673-x.

92. Hill R, Lewindon P, Muir R, et al. Quality of life in children with Crohn disease. J Pediatr Gastroenterol Nutr. 2010;51:35–40. doi:10.1097/MPG.0b013e3181c2c0ef.
93. Van der Zaag-Loonen HJ, Grootenhuis MA, Last BF, et al. Coping strategies and quality of life of adolescents with inflammatory bowel disease. Qual Life Res. 2004;13:1011–9.
94. Blondel-Kucharski F, Chircop C, Marquis P, et al. Health-related quality of life in Crohn's disease: a prospective longitudinal study in 231 patients. Am J Gastroenterol. 2001;96:2915–20. doi:10.1111/j.1572-0241.2001.4681_b.x.
95. Casellas F, López-Vivancos J, Casado A, et al. Factors affecting health related quality of life of patients with inflammatory bowel disease. Qual Life Res. 2002;11:775–81.
96. Verissimo R, Mota-Cardoso R, Taylor G. Relationships between alexithymia, emotional control, and quality of life in patients with inflammatory bowel disease. Psychother Psychosom. 1998;67:75–80. doi:10.1159/10.1159/000012263.
97. Petrak F, Hardt J, Clement T, et al. Impaired health-related quality of life in inflammatory bowel diseases: psychosocial impact and coping styles in a national German sample. Scand J Gastroenterol. 2001;36:375–82.
98. Guthrie E, Jackson J, Shaffer J, et al. Psychological disorder and severity of inflammatory bowel disease predict health-related quality of life in ulcerative colitis and Crohn's disease. Am J Gastroenterol. 2002;97:1994–9. doi:10.1016/S0002-9270(02)04198-9.
99. Mussell M, Böcker U, Nagel N, et al. Predictors of disease-related concerns and other aspects of health-related quality of life in outpatients with inflammatory bowel disease. Eur J Gastroenterol Hepatol. 2004;16:1273–80. doi:10.1097/00042737-200412000-00007.
100. Moreno-Jiménez B, López Blanco B, Rodríguez-Muñoz A, et al. The influence of personality factors on health-related quality of life of patients with inflammatory bowel disease. J Psychosom Res. 2007;62:39–46. doi:10.1016/j.jpsychores.2006.07.026.
101. Nicholas DB, Otley A, Smith C, et al. Challenges and strategies of children and adolescents with inflammatory bowel disease: a qualitative examination. Health Qual Life Outcomes. 2007;5:28. doi:10.1186/1477-7525-5-28.
102. Sprangers MAG, Schwartz CE. Integrating response shift into health-related quality of life research: a theoretical model. Soc Sci Med. 1999: 1507–15. doi:10.1016/S0277-9536(99)00045-3.
103. Munkholm P, Langholz E, Davidsen M, et al. Disease activity courses in a regional cohort of Crohn's disease patients. Scand J Gastroenterol. 1995;30:699–706. doi:10.3109/00365529509096316.
104. Henriksen M, Jahnsen J, Lygren I, et al. Clinical course in Crohn's disease: results of a five-year population-based follow-up study (the IBSEN study). Scand J Gastroenterol. 2007;42:602–10. doi:10.1080/00365520601076124.
105. Solberg IC, Vatn MH, Høie O, et al. Clinical course in Crohn's disease: results of a Norwegian population-based ten-year follow-up study. Clin Gastroenterol Hepatol. 2007;5:1430–8. doi:10.1016/j.cgh.2007.09.002.
106. Pizzi LT, Weston CM, Goldfarb NI, et al. Impact of chronic conditions on quality of life in patients with inflammatory bowel disease. Inflamm Bowel Dis. 2006;12:47–52. doi:10.1097/01.MIB.0000191670.04605.e7.
107. Borgaonkar MR, Townson G, Donnelly M, et al. Providing disease-related information worsens health-related quality of life in inflammatory bowel disease. Inflamm Bowel Dis. 2002;8:264–9. doi:10.1097/00054725-200207000-00005.
108. Larsson K, Sundberg Hjelm M, Karlbom U, et al. A group-based patient education programme for high-anxiety patients with Crohn disease or ulcerative colitis. Scand J Gastroenterol. 2003; 38:763–9.
109. Shepanski MA, Hurd LB, Culton K, et al. Health-related quality of life improves in children and adolescents with inflammatory bowel disease after attending a camp sponsored by the Crohn's and Colitis Foundation of America. Inflamm Bowel Dis. 2005;11:164–70.
110. Russel MG, Nieman FH, Bergers JM, et al. Cigarette smoking and quality of life in patients with inflammatory bowel disease. South Limburg IBD Study Group. Eur J Gastroenterol Hepatol. 1996;8:1075–81.
111. Andersson P, Olaison G, Bendtsen P, et al. Health related quality of life in Crohn's proctocolitis does not differ from a general population when in remission. Color Dis. 2003;5:56–62. doi:10.1046/j.1463-1318.2003.00407.x.
112. Graff L, Walker JR, Lix L, et al. The relationship of inflammatory bowel disease type and activity to psychological functioning and quality of life. Clin Gastroenterol Hepatol. 2006;4:1491–501. doi:10.1016/j.cgh.2006.09.027.
113. Cohen RD. The quality of life in patients with Crohn's disease. Aliment Pharmacol Ther. 2002;16:1603–9. doi:10.1046/j.1365-2036.2002.01323.x.
114. Szigethy E, Levy-Warren A, Whitton S, et al. Depressive symptoms and inflammatory bowel disease in children and adolescents: a cross-sectional study. J Pediatr Gastroenterol Nutr. 2004;39:395–403. doi:10.1097/00005176-200410000-00017.
115. Mackner LM. Review: Psychosocial issues in pediatric inflammatory bowel disease. J Pediatr Psychol. 2004;29:243–57. doi:10.1093/jpepsy/jsh027.
116. Greenley RN, Hommel KA, Nebel J, et al. A meta-analytic review of the psychosocial adjustment of youth with inflammatory bowel disease. J Pediatr Psychol. 2010;35:857–69. doi:10.1093/jpepsy/jsp120.
117. Thirlby RC, Land JC, Fenster LF, et al. Effect of surgery on health-related quality of life in patients with inflammatory bowel disease: a prospective study. Arch Surg. 1998;133:826–32. doi:10.1001/archsurg.133.8.826.
118. Boonen A, Dagnelie PC, Feleus A, et al. The impact of inflammatory bowel disease on labor force participation: results of a population sampled case-control study. Inflamm Bowel Dis. 2002;8:382–9. doi:10.1097/00054725-200211000-00002.
119. Trachter AB, Rogers AI, Leiblum SR. Inflammatory bowel disease in women: impact on relationship and sexual health. Inflamm Bowel Dis. 2002;8:413–21. doi:10.1097/00054725-200211000-00006.
120. Wewer V, Hesselfeldt P, Qvist N, et al. J-pouch ileoanal anastomosis in children and adolescents with ulcerative colitis: functional outcome, satisfaction and impact on social life. J Pediatr Gastroenterol Nutr. 2005;40:189–93.
121. Stavlo PL, Libsch KD, Rodeberg DA, et al. Pediatric ileal pouch-anal anastomosis: functional outcomes and quality of life. J Pediatr Surg. 2003;38:935–9. doi:10.1016/S0022-3468(03)00127-1.
122. Sachar DB. Ten common errors in the management of inflammatory bowel disease. Inflamm Bowel Dis. 2003;9:205–9. doi:10.1097/00054725-200305000-00011.
123. Sachar DB. Indications for surgery in inflammatory bowel disease: a gastroenetrologists opinion. In: Kirsner JB, editor. Inflammatory bowel diseases. Philadelphia: WB Saunders; 2000. p. 611–5.

124. Elkjaer M. E-health: Web-guided therapy and disease self-management in ulcerative colitis. Impact on disease outcome, quality of life and compliance. Dan Med J. 2012;59:B4478.
125. Huang VW, Reich KM, Fedorak RN. Distance management of inflammatory bowel disease: systematic review and meta-analysis. World J Gastroenterol. 2014;20:829–42. doi:10.3748/wjg.v20.i3.829.
126. Knowles SR, Mikocka-Walus A. Utilization and efficacy of internet-based eHealth technology in gastroenterology: a systematic review. Scand J Gastroenterol. 2014;49:387–408. doi:10.3109/00365521.2013.865259.
127. Heida A, Dijkstra A, Groen H, et al. Comparing the efficacy of a web-assisted calprotectin-based treatment algorithm (IBD-live) with usual practices in teenagers with inflammatory bowel disease: study protocol for a randomized controlled trial. Trials. 2015;16:271. doi:10.1186/s13063-015-0787-x.
128. Hommel KA, Gray WN, Hente E, et al. The Telehealth Enhancement of Adherence to Medication in Pediatric IBD (TEAM) trial: design and methodology. Contemp Clin Trials. 2015;43:105–13. doi:10.1016/j.cct.2015.05.013.
129. Carlsen K, Christian J, Hansen LF, et al. P433. Is e-Health, web-based monitoring and treatment, useful for children and adolescents with inflammatory bowel disease?—a pediatric clinical trial. J Crohns Colitis. 2014;8:246.

Evaluation of Health Economics in Inflammatory Bowel Disease

26

Reena Khanna and Brian G. Feagan

Introduction

Crohn's disease (CD) and ulcerative colitis (UC) are chronic, inflammatory disorders of the gastrointestinal tract characterized by diarrhea, bleeding, and abdominal pain. Complications include formation of strictures, fistulae, and colorectal cancer. Cumulatively, the symptoms and complications of disease increase costs to both the individual and society, both related to provision of care and lost economic productivity. Patients with IBD are usually young, require a long duration of therapy, and no curative treatment is available. Accordingly the economic burden is large. Since medical therapy is directed against immune responses, treatment-related adverse events, specifically serious infection, also increase the cost of care [1]. In addition, many patients require hospitalization or surgery for management [1]. In summary, the cost of drugs and provision of other medical services are major contributors to the direct cost of managing these patients.

As new therapies emerge, pharmacoeconomic analyses will be used to determine which therapies are funded by payers. These analyses compare the relative monetary costs of therapy ("dollars") to achieve desirable outcomes, such as improved quality of life, reduced incidence of disease-related complications, or mortality. As an increasing numbers of high cost biologic drugs become available, public and private payers will rely on validated cost-effectiveness models to inform reimbursement decisions. Given that payment for drugs is now a major determinant in the choice of treatment for IBD, a basic understanding of pharmacoeconomic principles is helpful to clinicians.

R. Khanna, M.D.
Robarts Clinical Trials, University of Western Ontario, London, ON, Canada

Department of Medicine, Division of Gastroenterology, University of Western Ontario, London, ON, Canada

B.G. Feagan, M.D. (✉)
Robarts Clinical Trials, University of Western Ontario, London, ON, Canada

Department of Medicine, Division of Gastroenterology, University of Western Ontario, London, ON, Canada

Department of Epidemiology and Biostatistics, University of Western Ontario, London, ON, Canada
e-mail: brian.feagan@robartsinc.com

Methods of Economic Analysis

All economic analyses measure the monetary cost of an intervention to achieve or avoid a specific outcome. Four types of analyses are available.

Cost-Minimization

Cost-minimization [2] analysis compares the relative costs of two treatments under the dominant assumption that the relative difference in effectiveness and safety between the products is negligible. Therefore, the least expensive intervention is the preferred one. These types of analyses are straightforward if cost differences are large and no striking efficacy differences exist, however the real world is usually more complicated. A relevant example in IBD therapeutics would be the relative cost of the various 5-aminosalicylic acid (5-ASA) formulations to prevent a relapse of UC, given that no obvious differences in efficacy or safety exist [3], the preferred choice of product is simply the lowest cost formulation.

Cost-Effectiveness

In cost-effectiveness analysis [2], efficacy is defined by an objective clinical outcome whereas costs are measured in dollars. The specific outcome is selected on the basis of clinical relevance. For example in cardiovascular disease the relative cost of two treatments to prevent a death from myocardial infarction is a commonly used metric that is easily understood by clinicians, the public, and payers. However, a problem

D.C. Baumgart (ed.), *Crohn's Disease and Ulcerative Colitis*, DOI 10.1007/978-3-319-33703-6_26

exists in the application of this approach in IBD. The candidate "big ticket" outcomes in IBD that would be appropriate for use in these models such as need for surgery or hospitalization, development of major disease-related complications, or mortality occur infrequently within short to medium time horizons. Thus very large studies are needed to show statistically significant differences in these events. This circumstance is an important limitation for comparisons of drug therapies which usually specify shorter time horizons.

Cost–Benefit

In cost–benefit analysis [2] the efficacy of therapy is converted to monetary equivalents so that both costs and benefits can be expressed and directly compared in dollars. For example, according to the "Human Capital Approach" (HCA) [2] a patient with CD in remission is worth more to society than one with active disease because the former individual is more likely to participate in the work force and pay taxes and is less likely to require social assistance. Therefore, from a societal economic perspective remission is a more valuable health state than active disease. Although this approach is attractive because it facilitates comparisons in the common rubric of dollars, it has limited application to health care questions where it is problematic to evaluate differences in human health states in monetary terms both from logistical and moral perspectives.

Cost–Utility

Cost–utility [2] analysis uses health-related quality of life (HRQOL) as an outcome and costs are measured in dollars. Utility scores are global HRQ measures that generate scores ranging from 0 (death) to 1.0 (perfect health). These estimates provide the fundamental building blocks of cost–utility analyses. Quality adjusted life-years (QALYs) are derived by multiplying the time in a particular health state by the utility score. For example, if the utility of a patient with moderately severe UC is estimated to be 0.7, the number of QALYs associate with that state over 5 years would be $0.7 \times 5 = 3.5$. Relative costs per QALY gained following application of a new treatment can then be used to compare the relative value of the intervention. If treatment with a new monoclonal antibody increases the utility score from 0.7 to 0.9 the cumulative gain in QALYs would be 1.0 ($5 \times 0.9 = 4.5$ compared to 3.5). This gain in HRQL can then be expressed as a cost per QALY achieved. Simplistically, if the drug acquisition cost of 20,000 dollars per annum was considered over a time horizon of 5 years, the cost per QALY gained would be $5 \times 20{,}000 = 100{,}000$ dollars. These estimates can then be benchmarked against competing treatments or societal standards.

Measuring Costs in Inflammatory Bowel Disease

Direct Costs

The direct costs of chronic diseases, such as IBD, include health care related expenditures such as medications, hospitalizations, and investigations that are estimated using data from cohort studies, administrative/claims databases, or during conduct of controlled trials [4]. Although the latter approach enables accurate collection of all relevant variables, it is costly and usually produces estimates with limited generalizability. In contrast, administrative data bases provide convenient and inexpensive cost information, but are often limited by incomplete data and multiple biases inherent to insurance status. Expert opinion, which is often used to supplement other model estimates when no other data sources exist, has inherent validity limitations. In most circumstances models use all of these sources to overcome restrictions that are integral to individual sources. It should be recognized that cost estimates are highly jurisdiction specific due to differences in local economic circumstances and health care delivery models.

Indirect Costs

Indirect costs, which include impaired work productivity, "spillover" disutility to family caregivers, and provision of disability [5, 6] benefit provide greater challenges to accurately quantify than direct costs. However, capturing this component of the economic burden of IBD is critical in that these costs can be even greater than direct costs [7, 8].

Measuring Health Related Quality of Life in IBD

As noted previously major clinical outcomes (surgery hospitalization, complications, mortality) are not common enough that precise estimates can be easily derived in trials with durations of 1–2 years. Accordingly, HRQOL has been the primary outcome used for economic analyses in IBD. It is well established that HRQOL is worse in patients with IBD than healthy individuals and that administration of effective therapy improves HRQOL in patients with active disease [9–11].

HRQOL is a multidimensional concept that includes physical function, emotional and social well-being, ability to work productively, and freedom from disease-related symptoms [12]. In both clinical practice and clinical research, HRQOL can be used to assess for response to therapy. In addition, validated HRQL instruments provide unique insights into patient perceptions of disease, which may differ from that of health care providers. Both generic and disease-specific indices to assess HRQOL exist. Disease-specific measures are generally more sensitive to changes in health status than generic instruments, whereas the latter are useful for comparing the magnitude of treatment effects across different diseases.

Traditionally, two approaches have been employed to measure HRQL: psychometric questionnaires and utility analysis.

Psychometric Questionnaires

Both generic and disease-specific HRQOL instruments have been developed that range from a global assessment measured on a 10-point scale to complex inventories consisting of over 100 questions. Generic instruments, such as the Short Form-36 (SF-36) [13] and the McMaster Health Status Questionnaire measure HRQOL evaluate domains that are commonly effected during illness states, including physical, mental, and social health. These indices facilitate valuable comparisons between diseases. In contrast, disease-specific HRQOL instruments, such as the Inflammatory Bowel Disease Questionnaire (IBDQ) [14] emphasize condition-specific items. These indices may not address all domains of well-being, but are usually highly responsive to incremental changes in patient status for their specific disorder.

The IBDQ is a validated disease-specific measurement of quality of life comprising 32 items [14]. This questionnaire assesses bowel, systematic, social, and emotional function on a seven-point Likert scale and ranges between 32 (poor HRQOL) to 224 (very good HRQOL).

Despite the usefulness of these instruments in describing disease burden and quantifying treatment effects they are not sufficiently interpretable for clinicians and payers to accept them as meaningful outcomes in cost-effectiveness analyses. Therefore cost–utility evaluations remain the most important and widely used approach to quantify economic benefit in IBD.

Utility Analysis

Utility analysis [2] places a comprehensive value on a specific health state, which takes into account personal preferences [15].

Utility [2] is traditionally estimated using one of the following methods:

In the "Standard Gamble" patients determine whether they would accept their current health state or gamble with a varying probability (P) of returning to normal health associated with a complementary inverse probability ($1-P$) of sudden, painless death. Conceptually, patients with poor health states will be willing to accept high risk gambles in return for a chance to return to normal health than those with mild or quiescent disease. P is varied until the patient cannot decide whether to gamble or not. This point of ambivalence (equipoise) defines the utility score. Although this method, which comes from games theory [2] has been criticized for requiring abstract decision-making, advocates of this technique argue that is both simulates decisions in clinical settings and is backed by considerable empiric data to support its validity.

Time Trade-off (TTO) [2] is a standardized methodology that elicits the number of year of life a patient would exchange for a return to perfect health. While on first inspection this technique seems to resemble the Standard Gamble, it is intrinsically different in that the "trade" is not made under conditions of uncertainty, which is usually the case when treatment decisions are made in clinical medicine, i.e., even in a situation where a treatment is 95 % effective.

Utility in IBD

Both the Standard Gamble and the TTO have been validated as reliable measures of HRQOL in IBD [15]. Both measures correlate with, but are less responsive than, clinical assessments of disease severity. Generally, the Standard Gamble is considered the gold standard for utility elicitation.

Application of Utility Measurements

Utility scores allow comparison of HRQL impairment across chronic diseases. For example scores of 0.9 have been found in patients with class III/IV angina, 0.4 for chronic renal failure 0.4, and 0.82 for Crohn's disease in remission [13]. Patients with severely active Crohn's disease symptoms despite medical therapy have a score of approximately 0.5. Figure 26.1 displays utility score from patients with Crohn's disease and the general population [8].

Cost–Utility Analysis

In cost–utility analysis [2], utility scores are converted to quality adjusted life years (QALYs) to compare costs of therapies. An empiric value of approximately $60,000 US per QALY has been empirically determined to be an acceptable societal cost-effectiveness threshold using this paradigm. This approach is particularly useful in IBD, since therapies improve well-being rather than alter life-expectancy and both positive and negative aspects of competing treatments can be assessed by a single measure.

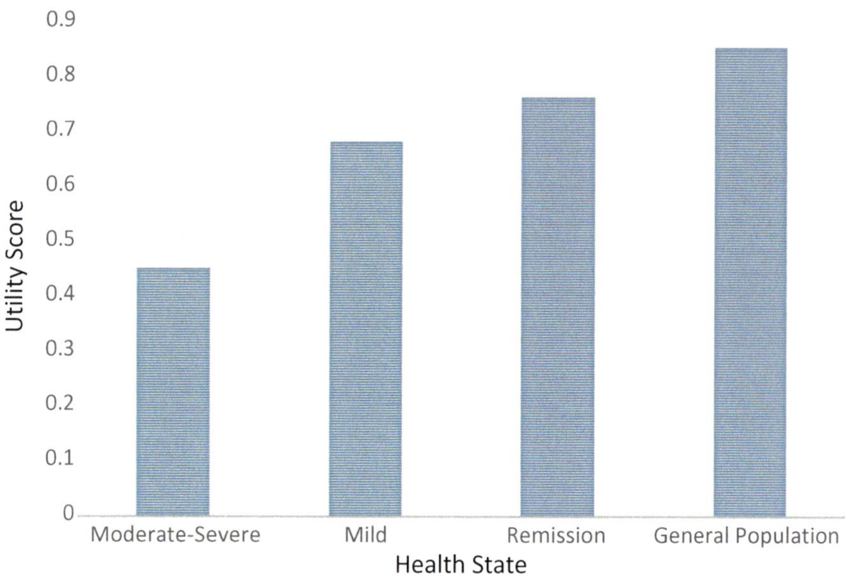

Fig. 26.1 Utility scores for Crohn's disease versus the general population. Adapted from Rocchi 2012 Nov;26(11):811–7

Examples of Economic Studies in IBD

The two most commonly performed types of economic studies in IBD are (1) cost of illness assessments that quantify the overall cost of the diseases and identify specific cost drivers and (2) cost–utility comparisons that evaluate the relative cost-effectiveness of treatment alternatives.

Cost of Illness Studies

A classic study performed by Hay and Hay in the 1990s, estimated the cost of IBD care in a cohort of patients registered with an American health maintenance organization [4, 16]. Cost modeling, based on a sample of 100 patients with CD, suggested the annual cost of disease was $6561 per person, with 70 % attributed to hospitalization and surgery, 11 % to medications, 18 % to testing and office visits, and 5.5 % to extra-intestinal manifestations. In UC, the annual cost of care was $1488. Importantly, 80 % of disease-related costs were generated by only 20 % of patients. Several valuable teachings came from this study. First, the overall economic burden of CD was greater than UC, Second, inpatient costs were paramount which suggested that interventions that kept patients well and out of hospital had the potential to be cost-effective even if drug acquisition costs were high. Finally, concentrating on delivering highly effective therapies to the sickest patients had the best chance of reducing overall costs. These data suggested that medical therapy that reduces surgery and hospitalization would have the highest likelihood of reducing the overall cost of IBD care.

In contrast to these historical data, modern studies have shown a dramatic shift away from the predominance of inpatient care costs to outpatient prescription drug costs as being responsible for the financial burden of the two diseases. Representative Canadian data are shown in Fig. 26.2.

The high cost of biologics drugs is directly responsible for this shift. In accordance with this change in treatment patterns, a number of studies indicate that surgery rates now appear to be falling, particularly in CD, likely as a consequence of the introduction of more effective biologic therapy for outpatient management [17–19]. Costa et al. [17] performed a meta-analysis that included 27 studies that evaluated the efficacy of infliximab-based treatment regimens for reducing surgery and hospitalization in both UC and CD. These investigators documented a substantial reduction in the rates risk of hospitalization overall [Odds Ratio (OR) 0.51; 95 % confidence interval (CI) 0.40, 9.65], that was not different between the two diseases. Surgical rates were similarly reduced [the effect was greater in CD (OR 0.31; 0.15, 0.64) than UC (OR 0.57; 0.37, 0.88)].

In summary, dramatic changes have taken place over the past three decades in the cost of managing IBD. Biologic drug costs have risen and there has been an associated drop in the rates of both surgery and hospitalization. Cost–utility studies are therefore needed to determine whether these changes in management have been cost-effective.

Cost–Utility Models in IBD

Performance of high quality cost–utility comparisons is not a small matter. Ideally these studies should be purpose built and randomize a large number of patients to standard therapy or the novel intervention. All important costs should be identified prospectively and collected meticulously. Relevant outcomes such as surgeries, hospitalizations, and complications should be collected for a fixed duration of time in both

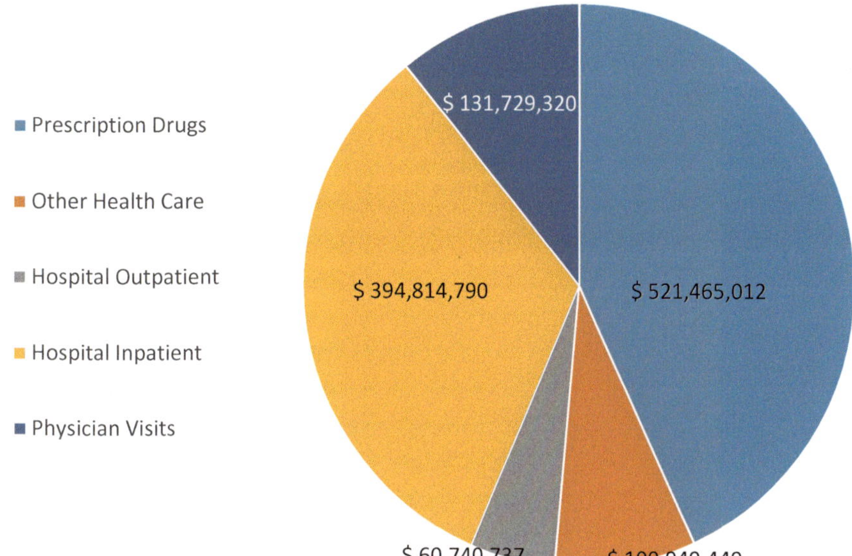

Fig. 26.2 Direct costs of inflammatory bowel disease in Canada, 2012

groups irrespective of whether patients continue to receive investigational drug. Utility assessments should be prospectively collected using validated instruments. The study should be of sufficient size and duration to collect clinically meaningful differences in costs and utility scores. Appropriate missing data conventions should be specified in the statistical analysis which should also state the expected cost per QALY estimate for the intervention (or incremental cost-effectiveness ratio or ICER). We are currently unaware of any comparative cost–utility study in IBD that meets these rigorous requirements. For a number of reasons, many of which arise from either operational and financial constraints, cost–utility models are often performed post-hoc by using trial outcome data to generate an economic model that draws in cost and utility data from other sources. The most common approach is to utilize Markov modeling. Markov models are based on the concept that a finite number of health states (Markov states) exist for any chronic disease and that the probability of transitioning between any one state and another during a defined period of time (a "cycle" often 3–6 months) can be estimated. These cycles can be rolled out computationally for various periods of time, depending on the specific question being addressed. And a descriptive picture of the probability of an individual being in any state at any specific time over the whole course of the disease from inception until death can be estimated. Assignment of costs and utilities to each state can be used to generate cost–utility estimates that can be differentially modeled to incorporate transition probability differences observed between placebo and active treatment in controlled clinical trials. To illustrate this concept, Fig. 26.3 shows a Markov stimulation of the natural history CD in Olmstead County Minnesota [20]. In this population, the portion of patients in remission decreases rapidly 5 years after diagnosis whereas the number of patients with mild disease increases. Patients transition into a prolonged remission following surgery, but fewer patients entered remission following therapy.

To illustrate the potential value of this approach, consider the following Markov model developed by Bodger and colleagues [21] who wished to evaluate the relative cost-effectiveness of TNF-antagonists for the treatment of CD from the perspective of the UK National health Service. The Olmstead County model previously described was used as the basis for a Markov model that described the usual course of the disease, however the number of health states were reduced to five (full response, partial response, non-response, surgery, and death). Efficacy estimates for the TNF-antagonists were derived from Phase III clinical trials [22, 23]. Costs were derived from UK specific sources, while utilities were estimated using an algorithm that translated differences in CDAI scores into EQ-5D [24] utilities. Both lifetime and 1 year time horizons were evaluated.

ICERs for 1-year of treatment with infliximab or adalimumab in comparison to conventional management were 19,050 pounds and 7190 pounds per QALY gained, respectively. Acceptable ICERs for these agents were observed when considering a lifetime horizon for treatment period of up to 4 years of continuous administration. These types of outputs are very valuable to decision-makers who have limited resources and many competing calls to provide reimbursement for new therapies.

Conclusion

In summary appropriate pharmacoeconomic techniques are available to assist decision makers in making informed decision regarding the allocation of health care resources for the

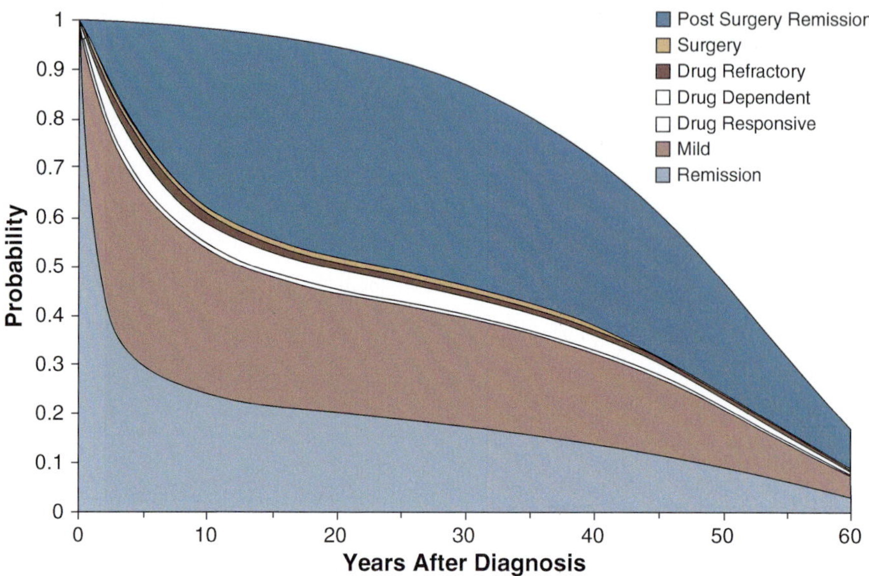

Fig. 26.3 Proportion of Crohn's disease patients in each treatment state by year since diagnosis of Crohn's disease. From Silverstein 1999 Clinical course and costs of care for Crohn's disease: Markov model analysis of a population-based cohort. Gastroenterology. July 1999;117(1):49–57

management of IBD. We have already observed a dramatic shift in costs from hospital-based care to ambulatory clinics which has been accompanied by higher drug acquisition costs. This trend is likely to continue. As multiple competing biologic drugs continue to arrive in the marketplace, pressure on payers will increase further. Consequently, the appropriate development and use of comparative economic models is likely to take on even greater importance.

Financial Disclosures *RK* has received honoraria from Takeda Pharma, AbbVie, Janssen, Pfizer.

BGF has received grant/research support from Millennium Pharmaceuticals, Merck, Tillotts Pharma AG, Abbott Labs, Novartis Pharmaceuticals, Centocor Inc., Elan/Biogen, UCB Pharma, Bristol-Myers Squibb, Genentech, ActoGenix, Wyeth Pharmaceuticals Inc.; Consulting fees from Millennium Pharmaceuticals, Merck, Centocor Inc., Elan/Biogen, Janssen-Ortho, Teva Pharmaceuticals, Bristol-Myers Squibb, Celgene, UCB Pharma, Abbott Labs, Astra Zeneca, Serono, Genentech, Tillotts Pharma AG, Unity Pharmaceuticals, Albireo Pharma, Given Imaging Inc., Salix Pharmaceuticals, Novonordisk, GSK, Actogenix, Prometheus Therapeutics and Diagnostics, Athersys, Axcan, Gilead, Pfizer, Shire, Wyeth, Zealand Pharma, Zyngenia, GiCare Pharma Inc. Sigmoid Pharma; Speakers Bureau for UCB, Abbott, J&J/Janssen.

References

1. Canada CsaCFo. The impact of inflammatory bowel disease in Canada. 2012 Final Report and Recommendations Toronto.
2. Morris S. Economic analysis in health care. West Sussex: John Wiley & Sons Ltd.; 2012.
3. Feagan BG, Macdonald JK. Oral 5-aminosalicylic acid for induction of remission in ulcerative colitis. Cochrane Database Syst Rev. 2012;10:CD000543.
4. Hay AR, Hay JW. Inflammatory bowel disease: medical cost algorithms. J Clin Gastroenterol. 1992;14:318–27.
5. Büsch K, Sonnenberg A, Bansback N. Impact of inflammatory bowel disease on disability. Curr Gastroenterol Rep. 2014;16(10):414.
6. Büsch K, da Silva SA, Holton M, Rabacow FM, Khalili H, Ludvigsson JF. Sick leave and disability pension in inflammatory bowel disease: a systematic review. J Crohns Colitis. 2014;8(11):1362–77.
7. Blomqvist P, Ekbom A. Inflammatory bowel diseases: health care and costs in Sweden in 1994. Scand J Gastroenterol. 1997; 32:1134.
8. Rocchi A, Benchimol EI, Bernstein CN, Bitton A, Feagan B, Panaccione R, et al. Inflammatory bowel disease: a Canadian burden of illness review. Can J Gastroenterol. 2012;26(11):811–7.
9. Bernklev T, Jahnsen J, Adland E, et al. Health-related quality of life in inflammatory bowel disease patients five years after the initial diagnosis. Scand J Gastroenterol. 2004;39:365–73.
10. Binder V. Prognosis and quality of life in patients with ulcerative colitis and Crohn's disease. Int Disabil Stud. 1988;10:172–4.
11. Turnbull GK, Vallis TM. Quality of life in inflammatory bowel disease: the interaction of disease activity with psychosocial function. Am J Gastroenterol. 1995;90:1450–4.
12. Fitzpatrick R, Fletcher A, Gore S, Jones D, Spiegelhalter D, Cox D. Quality of life measures in health care: I. Applications and issues assessment. Br Med J. 1992;305:74–7.
13. Coteur G1, Feagan B, Keininger DL, Kosinski M. Evaluation of the meaningfulness of health-related quality of life improvements as assessed by the SF-36 and the EQ-5D VAS in patients with active Crohn's disease. Aliment Pharmacol Ther. 2009;29(9):1032–41. doi: 10.1111/j.1365-2036.2009.03966.x.
14. Irvine EJ, Feagan B, Rochon J, et al. Quality of life: a valid and reliable measure of therapeutic efficacy in the treatment of inflammatory bowel disease. Gastroenterology. 1994;106:287–96.
15. Gregor JC, McDonald JWD, Klar N, et al. An evaluation of the utility measurement in Crohn's disease. Inflamm Bowel Dis. 1997;3:265–76.
16. Hay JW, Hay AR. Inflammatory bowel disease: costs-of-illness. Clin Gastroenterol. 1992;14:309–17.
17. Costa J, Magro F, Caldeira D, Alarcão J, Sousa R, Vaz-Carneiro A. Infliximab reduces hospitalizations and surgery interventions in patients with inflammatory bowel disease: a systematic review and meta-analysis. Inflamm Bowel Dis. 2013;19(10):2098–110.
18. Mandel MD, Balint A, Golovics PA, Vegh Z, Mohas A, Szilagyi B, et al. Decreasing trends in hospitalizations during anti-TNF therapy are associated with time to anti-TNF therapy: results from two referral centres. Dig Liver Dis. 2014;46(11):985–90.
19. Benchimol EI, Guttmann A, To T, Rabeneck L, Griffiths AM. Changes to surgical and hospitalization rates of pediatric

inflammatory bowel disease in Ontario, Canada (1994–2007). Inflamm Bowel Dis. 2011;17(10):2153–61.

20. Silverstein MD, Loftus EV, Sandborn WJ, Tremaine WJ, Feagan BG, Nietert PJ, et al. Clinical course and costs of care for Crohn's disease: Markov model analysis of a population-based cohort. Gastroenterology. 1999;117(1):49–57.
21. Bodger K, Kikuchi T, Hughes D. Cost-effectiveness of biological therapy for Crohn's disease: Markov cohort analyses incorporating United Kingdom patient-level cost data. Aliment Pharmacol Ther. 2009;30(3):265–74.
22. Hanauer SB, Feagan BG, Lichtenstein GR, Mayer LF, Schreiber S, Colombel JF, et al. Maintenance infliximab for Crohn's disease: the ACCENT I randomised trial. Lancet. 2002;359(9317):1541–9.
23. Colombel JF, Sandborn WJ, Rutgeerts P, Enns R, Hanauer SB, Panaccione R, et al. Adalimumab for maintenance of clinical response and remission in patients with Crohn's disease: the CHARM trial. Gastroenterology. 2007;132(1):52–65.
24. EuroQol Group. EuroQol—a new facility for the measurement of health-related quality of life. Health Policy. 1990;16(3): 199–208.

Part IV

Therapy: Crohn's Disease

The Natural History of Inflammatory Bowel Disease

27

Charles N. Bernstein

Introduction

In the first edition of this book in the Natural History chapter I made the argument that there was a short window of the 1950s through the 1960s where the natural evolution, the evolution of untreated inflammatory bowel disease (IBD) was recorded. Lennard-Jones identified diagnostic issues that would impact on the documentation of the natural history, such as mislabeling what we now call isolated Crohn's colitis as ulcerative colitis. Lennard-Jones also suggested that persons with imaging evidence of disease but no symptoms did not require treatment [1]. Modern writing about the natural history of IBD addresses the history of IBD as the practice of medicine has evolved through increasingly sophisticated diagnostics facilitating more accurate phenotyping of disease, as well as increasingly targeted and effective therapy. It is hoped that better diagnostics and better therapeutics would lead to better milestone outcomes as in the rates of death, surgery, and hospitalization. How these outcomes have changed over time and some factors that may impact on them are reviewed in this chapter. Further, I address the importance of the modern approach having progressed from treating symptoms to treating both symptoms and inflammatory disease. Summaries of outcomes in Crohn's disease and ulcerative colitis are provided in Tables 27.1 and 27.2, respectively.

Mortality

In ulcerative colitis (UC) mortality rates in the middle of the twentieth century were as high as 22 % but fell steadily to approximately 5 % in the 1960s. Rates had been the highest for those with a severe first attack, those operated on emergently compared to those operated on electively and among those over age 60 [2–4]. The magnitude of the rates of mortality have dramatically changed but the variables that pose risks for adverse outcomes have remained the same over the past 50 years. Being early in the disease course, undergoing surgery, particularly emergent surgery, and older age were all shown to be mortality risk factors in a recent population based analysis of mortality rates in Manitoba, Canada [5].

In this study assessing mortality in all persons in Manitoba with IBD between 1984 and 2012 Crohn's disease (CD) was associated with an increased risk for death [hazard ratio, HR of 1.26 (95 %, CI, 1.16–1.38)] but the HR for UC was 1.04 (95 % CI, 0.96–1.12). The lack of an increased death rate among persons with UC compared to controls suggests that either the disease is being diagnosed earlier, in less ill persons, or that it is being managed better, or both. Variables that increased the risk for death significantly compared to controls included the first year from diagnosis in both CD and UC, and the greatest risk for death in both CD and UC was within the first 30 days following GI surgery. Among IBD cases alone male sex, and older age at diagnosis, as well as increasing comorbidities significantly impacted on mortality in both CD and UC. The increase in mortality in CD compared to controls and the lack of increase in UC relative to controls generally mirror that reported elsewhere in the literature (reviewed in ref. [5]); however, there is heterogeneity by jurisdiction.

Surgery

While surgery can lead to prolonged disease free states for many with CD [6] and can enhance the quality of life for many with UC, it is, nonetheless, a disfiguring procedure accompanied by risks, a marked impact on daily activities and quality of life and as noted above, even in our modern era, occasionally death. So even while a well-timed surgery can be a critically important positive intervention to get a patient's life back on track, most of the time surgery is

C.N. Bernstein, M.D. (✉)
University of Manitoba IBD Clinical and Research Centre, Winnipeg, MB, Canada
e-mail: Charles.bernstein@umanitoba.ca

D.C. Baumgart (ed.), *Crohn's Disease and Ulcerative Colitis*, DOI 10.1007/978-3-319-33703-6_27

Table 27.1 Summary statements for disease course in Crohn's disease

1. Approximately one third of patients has chronically active disease or fluctuating disease and hence this is the cohort most likely to be treated by more aggressive immunomodulating therapy. However, treating beyond symptom remission to achieve mucosal healing as well, will very likely increase the use of immunomodulating medications
2. Mortality is increased in Crohn's disease compared to the general population. Surgery, especially the first 30 days from surgery, is associated with mortality
3. In general, at least from North America, there seems to be a recent trend toward reduced hospitalization rates. Hospitalization rates are dependent on the prevalence of disease, the approaches to settling disease in an outpatient setting and also the nature of the health care system and availability of access to inpatient therapy
4. In the pre biologic era, from population based studies, approximately 40–50 % of subjects will have undergone intestinal surgery within 10 years from diagnosis and the risk of postoperative recurrence may be about 50 % by 10 years. Surgery rates though are clearly falling. The drop in surgery rates began even before the introduction of biological therapy
5. In Crohn's disease the location of disease is mostly stable over time with 15–20 % having a change in disease location when followed over time. While ileitis has been a hallmark of Crohn's disease, in population based studies the colon (either alone or in combination with small bowel disease) is involved more often at a rate of up to 75 %. Data from some countries suggest that ileal disease location is more likely to be associated with complicated disease such as development of fibrostenosing or penetrating disease while data from other countries suggest that colonic disease is more likely to be associated with complicated disease. At diagnosis up to one third have evidence of fibrostenosing or penetrating disease but by 20 years half of all patients had these complications. Since there is a lack of uniformity in examining for disease behavior at all sites at time of diagnosis, the true incidence of evolution over time to complicated behavior is unknown
6. The main difference in pediatric onset disease versus adult onset disease is a higher prevalence of upper gastrointestinal disease in children; however, much of this may be related to the fact that pediatricians are more likely to pursue upper endoscopy in newly diagnosed children with Crohn's disease compared to the use of upper endoscopy in newly diagnosed adults. While it has been shown that disease onset prior to age 40 is more aggressive than after age 40 years it seems that pediatric onset disease (age less than 17 years of age at diagnosis) is in fact not more aggressive than adults presenting prior to age 40 years
7. Mucosal healing seems to be a desired effect of therapy and its presence may reduce some negative outcomes. Whether it can ultimately be associated with long term reduction in complications (strictures or fistulas), surgery, and other comorbidities remains to be proven. Symptoms may not always be associated with active inflammation; hence in the setting of increased symptoms it is important to document the presence of active inflammation either with endoscopy or surrogate markers before increasing anti-inflammatory or immunomodulating therapy

Table 27.2 Summary statements for disease course in UC

1. Mortality rate is not increased in UC compared to the general population, but surgery is associated with mortality in UC
2. Hospitalization in a hospital with low volume rates for colectomy in UC are associated with higher mortality rates
3. Surgery rates at 10 years from diagnosis are approximately 10 % from recent studies which is much lower than reported colectomy rates in studies completed prior to 1990
4. Short term colectomy rates in severe hospitalized UC have remained stable at 27 % for several years
5. Pancolitis is a risk factor over lesser disease extent for requiring surgery
6. Children seem to have higher rates of extensive colitis at diagnosis than adults. There also seems to be higher rates of colectomy in children than for adults (i.e., at least 20 % at 10 years) and perhaps this reflects a higher rate of extensive disease
7. While mucosal healing has become a study endpoint for clinical trials in UC it is unclear if treating an asymptomatic patient until mucosal healing is achieved will change prognosis and it would require treating a large number of persons who otherwise had no symptoms. However, many patients have symptoms that are unrelated to having active inflammation. Hence, when a patient presents with symptoms it is important to document active inflammation either with endoscopy or surrogate markers before increasing anti-inflammatory or immunomodulating therapy

considered a marker of failed therapy-failure to treat soon enough, or aggressively enough, or simply a failure of the available medical approaches in their effectiveness. Sometimes the person's disease just doesn't respond regardless of how timely and comprehensive the medical approach is that is taken.

CD: Surgery rates prior to 1970 were nearly 75 % [7, 8] which markedly influenced the long held view that surgery was a near inevitability at some time in the course of a patient's life. Even in a later era but prior to the availability of biologic therapy, approximately 40–50 % of subjects in population-based cohorts underwent intestinal surgery within 10 years from diagnosis. Reoperation rates were up to 50 % by 10 years [9]. The most recent data from Canada and the UK suggest that surgical rates were falling prior to the advent of biologic therapy, and continue to fall. For instance 5-year surgery rates by years of CD incidence were 59 % (1986–1991), 37 % (1992–1997), and 25 % (1998–2003) from Wales [10] and 30 % (1988–1995), 22 % (1996–2000), and 18 % (2001–2008) from Canada [11]. In Canada infliximab became available only in 2001 for CD and surgery rates were already falling before its availability.

Small bowel disease, perineal disease, penetrating disease, and fibrostenosing disease all increase the likelihood of requiring surgery. Reoperation rates are also impacted by disease phenotype, but studies extended out over years and that cover decades of biological therapy use may change some of these paradigms. As an example, it was always considered that persons with isolated CD colitis would have lower reoperation rates in those who have their entire colons removed and have an end ileostomy. However, when survival curves are extended far enough out, rates of reoperation among proctocolectomy patients may approach that of those treated with segmental resection [12].

UC: Surgery rates in UC were as high as high as 30 % at 10 years disease duration prior to 1990; however, in most modern studies at 10 years from diagnosis surgery rates are approximately 10 % [13]. The lower rates of colectomy in recent times might reflect improved therapy but might also reflect greater access to colonoscopy and greater diagnoses of subjects with milder disease. Interestingly, a population based study on colectomy rates in UC from Manitoba Canada found no reduction in early colectomy (within 90 days of diagnosis) by the era of diagnosis (different than overall colectomy rates which have been falling by era of diagnosis) [14]. One implication is that advances in medical therapy of acute severe colitis have not been widely experienced or have simply not been sufficiently effective. A recently published review of short term colectomy rates in severe hospitalized UC suggested that the short term colectomy rate has remained stable at approximately 27 % [15]. Acute severe colitis in patients with UC still represents a condition with a high early colectomy rate and a measurable mortality rate. However, overall colectomy rates have been declining by era in Manitoba. Ten-year colectomy rates decreased significantly over time (12.2 % [era of incident cases 1987–1991], 11.2 % [1992–1996], 9.3 % [1997–2001], $p=0.014$) [14].

Key predictors of colectomy in UC include age and disease extent [13]. Colectomy rates are higher in children than adults (i.e., at least 20 % at 10 years) perhaps reflecting a higher rate of extensive disease in children. Hospital volume has an impact on surgical outcomes. In a National Inpatient Survey study from the US hospitals with low volume colectomy rates were associated with an increased risk of death (adjusted OR relative to high-volume, 2.42; 95 % CI, 1.26–4.63), similar to medium-volume hospitals (OR, 2.02; 95 % CI, 1.02–4.01) [16]. Hence, centralizing IBD care in specialty centers may not only reduce surgery rates but also surgical mortality rates. It will also be of interest to determine how the introduction of therapy with monoclonal antibodies to tumor necrosis factor for moderate to severely active disease impacts on colectomy rates over the next 10 years.

Hospitalization

CD: Trends in hospitalization rates for CD from Europe and North America have been inconsistent, likely owing as much to differences in health systems as in disease incidence. For instance, in Copenhagen County, Denmark between 1962 and 1987, 83 % of patients with CD were admitted at least once within the first year after diagnosis, and then admissions decreased over the next 5 years to a steady rate of about 20 % per year [17]. However, the local treatment policy in effect at the time, encouraged hospitalization for more expeditious diagnosis and management, and so hospitalization in that era had a different implication than of a more recent era. In a European multi-country referral center prospective follow-up study over 10 years from 1991 (the EC-IBD), the cumulative risk of overall hospitalization was 52.7 % at 10 years from diagnosis, but with considerable differences between countries [18].

In a recent population-based study from In Manitoba, Canada where there is universal health care coverage for all residents for persons with CD diagnosed between 1988 and 2008, the highest hospitalization rates were within the first year of diagnosis and there were no differences among those diagnosed during 1988–1995, 1996–2000, or those diagnosed after 2001 [11].

In a population-based inception cohort from Olmsted County, Minnesota (diagnosed 1970–2004 and followed through mid-2009), with a median follow-up of 11.8 years, 71 % of CD patients were hospitalized at least once, and the cumulative risk of hospitalization was 62 % at 5 years and 71 % at 10 years after diagnosis [19]. Factors associated with time to first hospitalization included ileocolonic disease, small bowel, or upper gastrointestinal disease (relative to colonic only), and fibrostenotic or penetrating complications at baseline. Sonnenberg and colleagues analyzed the US Veterans Administration (VA) database for CD hospitalization patterns among US military veterans over a 32-year period [20]. The hospitalization rate peaked in the late 1980s, decreased through the 1990s, and remained relatively stable over the last 6 years of the study period. Trends in VA data are very dependent on American military activity and availability of heath care to veterans outside of the VA system.

In contrast to these studies, data from Kaiser Permanente Northern California (a health maintenance organization) suggested that hospitalization rates for CD decreased by 33 % between 1998 and 2005 [21]. The decrease in hospitalization rates in the Kaiser study and the stable rates in Manitoba (where disease prevalence rates are rising) support the possibility that more aggressive medical therapy accounts for these findings, or simply that better health care access for subjects in those health systems maintains their disease in a better state with a reduction in need for hospitalizations. These trends also may reflect health systems with greater incentives to capitate costs and control inpatient management. Hence, examining trends in hospitalizations requires an understanding of the individual health system, the prevalence of the disease within the population and management approaches (i.e., availability of different medical therapies and aggressiveness of using them).

UC: In a Manitoba population-based cohort of newly diagnosed persons with UC in 1987 followed for 15 years, 31 % were admitted at least once to hospital for an IBD-specific diagnosis, and, of those admitted, 51 % were readmitted at some point [22]. In the Kaiser Permanente of Northern California cohort 20 %, underwent colectomy during their initial hospitalization [23]. By 1 year after initial hospitalization, 29 % of those who had not undergone colectomy at first hospitalization, were rehospitalized for UC (most of which occurred within the first 3 months post discharge) and an additional 10 % required colectomy. By 5 years after initial hospitalization, 39 % of those who had not undergone colectomy after initial presentation, were rehospitalized for UC and an additional 15 % required colectomy. Hence, for patients with UC that is sufficiently severe such that they get hospitalized, for those that do not undergo colectomy there is nearly a one in two chance of being hospitalized again.

Superimposed infections remain a risk factor for hospitalizations and colectomy in UC patients. In a study from the Cleveland Clinic, patients with *Clostridium difficile* infection had significantly more UC-related emergency room visits in the year following initial infection (37.8 % vs. 4 %), and significantly higher rates of colectomy 1 year following the index infection admission (35.6 % vs. 9.9 %), than those without the infection [24]. Similar findings were reported from Mount Sinai, New York (2004–2005) where subsequent UC-related hospitalizations and colectomy rates 1 year after initial hospitalization were higher in patients with *Clostridium difficile* infection than those without infection [25].

Phenotype and Its Impact on Disease Course

Disease Localization

There is ample evidence that more extensive colon involvement in UC is associated with more aggressive disease and worse outcomes in terms of likelihood for developing colon cancer or having colectomy [26–31]. Further defining disease extent in UC is not a difficult ask especially with the widespread availability of colonoscopy. It is in CD where there is more discussion as to ways to define disease extent and its implications. The localization of disease in CD is divided as per the widely used Montreal Classification into ileal, colonic, ileocolonic and upper gastrointestinal disease [32]. The relative distributions of disease location vary by jurisdiction; however, in most studies ileocolonic is the most common site for disease. Whatever is reported as the relative distribution of disease by location remains relatively stable over time. The IBSEN study from Norway reported on changes in location over 5 years in 14 % [33]. This is not dissimilar from what Louis et al. reported in a referral population from Belgium where location changed in only 16 % by 10 years and 20 % changed overall [34]. Another oft reported finding is that of a high prevalence of upper gastrointestinal tract disease in pediatric CD. In a French population based cohort of children diagnosed between 1988 and 2002, at diagnosis, 63 % had ileocolonic disease and 36 % had upper gastrointestinal disease [35]. This is such a high prevalence of upper gastrointestinal tract disease that it suggests that perhaps they were considering any histologic inflammation as being pathological. The European guidelines on diagnostic evaluation for pediatric IBD includes an upper endoscopy for all which is much different than the approach in adults [36]. Has this practice biased what is perceived to be a higher rate of upper GI tract disease in children than adults?

Disease Behavior

In the Norwegian IBSEN cohort, at diagnosis, 28 % had fibrostenosing disease and 12 % had penetrating disease, leaving 61 % with inflammatory disease [33] with a change in behavior at 5 year follow-up of 14 %. Complicated disease (both fibrostenosing and penetrating disease) occurred in 86 % of those with isolated ileal disease, 30 % of those with colonic disease and in 60 % of those with ileocolonic disease. In the EC-IBD study at diagnosis 16 % had fibrostenosing disease and 8 % had penetrating disease and 2 % had both. Hence, 74 % had inflammatory disease, a higher proportion than the Norwegian cohort [37].

In a referral population from Belgium it was reported that 90 % of patients present with inflammatory disease but 69 % and 88 % had fibrostenosing or penetrating disease by 10 and 25 years, respectively [34]. In this study 46 % changed behavior over 10 years. Penetrating disease was more common from a colonic only or ileocolonic location than from an ileal only location [34] (the exact opposite from the IBSEN data). In a French referral cohort the 20 year actuarial rates of having inflammatory disease, fibrostenosing disease and penetrating disease were 12 %, 18 % and 70 %, respectively [38]. Fibrostenosing disease was associated with ileal disease (HR 2.5, 95 % CI 1.9–3.3) or jejunal disease (HR 3.2, 95 % CI 2.2–4.7) and penetrating disease with colonic disease on univariate but not multivariate analysis. In the Olmsted County cohort diagnosed between 1970 and 1993, 50 % had fistulas by 20 years [39] and fistulas were more likely to be seen in those with ileocolonic disease than in patients with disease at other sites. So how can we reconcile that studies from Belgium and France suggest that colonic disease location is the key to having penetrating disease and from Norway suggests that small bowel disease is associated with penetrating disease? To further complicate the issue the American study suggests that it is an ileocolonic site most associated with penetrating disease.

There is a notion that being diagnosed with CD in childhood is predictive of a more aggressive course of disease. In a Danish study of childhood onset Crohn's disease the mean yearly operation rate was 13 % with a cumulative probability of surgery at 20 years of disease of 47 %, which is not dissimilar to what is seen in adults [40]. In a French pediatric study complicated behavior occurred in 29 % at diagnosis (including 4 % with penetrating disease) and 59 % at follow-up (including 15 % with penetrating disease). What then has driven the notion that children have more aggressive disease and worse outcomes than persons diagnosed as adults?

The major flaw in all of these reports regarding phenotype regardless of the population being studied is a lack of uniformity in assessing the location and behavior of disease at diagnosis in most centers. Some patients have early surgery where previously undiagnosed fistulas are identified and hence early on are labeled as having penetrating disease whereas their diagnostic imaging studies may not have identified this. The lack of uniformity in methods used to establish the extent and behavior of disease limits the reliability of phenotype data established at time of diagnosis. The variation of disease behavior from even a single center is best reflected in a large French cohort of 2008 patients evaluated within 3 months of diagnosis between 1978 and 2002 [41]. In each 5 year period the prevalence of fibrostenosing disease ranged from 5–26 % with a high of 26 % in 1978–1982 and a low of 5 % in 1998–2002, likely accounted for because some with fibrostenosing disease either had surgery for stricture segment removal or evolved to penetrating disease. The prevalence of penetrating disease ranged from 29–54 %. Another example is an Olmsted County cohort where complicated disease behavior (fibrostenosing or penetrating disease) at diagnosis was noted for 18.6 % [42]. Within the first 90 days of follow-up an additional 4.6 % developed fibrostenosing complications and an additional 14.1 % developed penetrating complications. Hence, 37.3 % of the cohort were documented with complicated behavior at 90 days. There was no information in this study on which diagnostic tests were utilized at diagnosis or within this 90-day period of follow-up. It is likely that the doubling of complicated disease within 90 days reflected delayed testing that brought these complications to light. It is unlikely that advancement of phenotype occurred within such a short period.

With this in mind, Israeli et al. undertook a study where all charts were reviewed from a single referral center practice at a median disease duration of 11.1 years and an analysis was undertaken for the location and behavior patterns of disease at diagnosis and over time in children and adults [43]. Within 1 year of diagnosis, the proportion of patients with upper gastrointestinal involvement and ileocolonic location was higher in those diagnosed before age 17 (18.4 %) than those diagnosed between 17 and 40 years (10.2 %) or those diagnosed after age 40 (2.7 %). The rate of patients that underwent imaging with an upper endoscopy in the youngest group (37.4 %) was more than twice as high when compared to the other groups (those diagnosed over age 17, 14.3 %, $p<0.01$, and those diagnosed over age 40, 16.9 %, $p<0.01$). After adjusting for imaging testing, the difference in likelihood of having upper gastrointestinal disease between those diagnosed under age 17 and those diagnosed age 17–40 was no longer statistically significant (but regardless of imaging children had significantly more upper gastrointestinal disease than those diagnosed over age 40 years). Children had more extensive imaging than adults at the time of diagnosis. Despite more extensive imaging, complicated disease behavior (fibrostenosing or penetrating disease) was less prevalent in children particularly. At the last follow-up complicated disease behavior was similar regardless of age at diagnosis being under 17, under 40 or over 40 years. To further dispel the notion that being diagnosed in childhood carries a worse prognosis at final follow-up IBD-related abdominal surgery rates were significantly lower for children than those diagnosed after age 17 (OR = 0.63, 0.41–0.98) but not compared to those diagnosed after age 40 years (OR = 0.71, 0.40–1.27). The conclusions of this study were that studying the phenotype of CD among different cohorts has to account for the differing patterns of diagnostic imaging investigations. Further, while children are at increased risk of pan-enteric disease, this does not lead to them being more likely to have more complicated disease or surgery.

Can the Disease Phenotype Predict Outcomes?

In a large French cohort ileal location was associated with an increased risk for surgery (HR = 2.78, 95 % CI 2.19–3.15) [41] and absence of rectal involvement was associated with a decreased risk for surgery in this cohort (HR = 0.34, 95 % CI 0.27–0.43). In the Norwegian IBSEN cohort being less than 40 years at diagnosis, having fibrostenosing or penetrating disease and terminal ileum disease were associated with higher risk for surgery [44]. It was also shown that age less than 40 years at diagnosis and need for corticosteroids during the first presentation in IBSEN and age less than 40 years at diagnosis in the EC-IBD were associated with higher relapse rates [37, 44]. While it is useful to know that persons less than 40 years at diagnosis have more aggressive disease than older persons at presentation, since the peak age of incidence is the third decade and the majority of CD patients have presented by age 40, more refined predictors than age less than 40 years would be required to help identify those requiring earlier, more aggressive therapy. No studies have reported that sex impacts on disease outcome except for a Swedish study that suggested that females have a higher likelihood of postoperative recurrence [45].

Perianal disease is often debilitating and for sure impacts on quality of life. Patients with perianal fistulas in a Swedish study were at an increased risk for chronic continuous disease and also for surgery [46]. Patients with isolated colonic disease were more likely to have perianal disease in studies from both Sweden and Manitoba and elsewhere [46–48]. In a US referral population having penetrating disease (including both luminal and perianal fistulas) compared to fibrostenosing disease increased the risk for-postoperative recurrence [49].

Having small bowel disease seems to pose other disease outcome risks compared to colonic disease. Patients with small bowel only and ileocolonic disease have an increased risk of hospitalization compared to patients with isolated colonic disease [50, 51], an increased risk of evolution from inflammatory to fibrostenosing or penetrating disease [50], an increased risk for surgery [37] and an increased risk of post-operative recurrence [45].

In the Manitoba IBD Cohort Study a 15 year population based study following 182 participants with CD serially 65 % had complicated CD and 42 % underwent surgery [52]. To assess for predictors of adverse outcomes [complicated disease (fibrostenosing/penetrating disease) or surgery] the model included psychological parameters, phenotype, serological markers (antibodies from the Prometheus panel) and genotypes for the most common genetic mutations in CD. Multivariate analysis indicated that only ileal CD was predictive of fibrostenosing/penetrating behavior (OR = 2.2; 95 % CI: 1.07–4.54, $p = 0.03$); but in fact ASCA IgG seropositivity was more strongly predictive (OR = 3.01; 95 % CI: 1.28–7.09; $p = 0.01$). Complicated (fibrostenosing/penetrating) CD behavior was strongly associated with surgery (OR = 5.6; 95 % CI: 2.43–12.91; $p < 0.0001$) while in multivariate analysis, only positive serum ASCA IgG was associated (OR = 2.66; 95 % CI, 1.40–5.06, $p = 0.003$) [52]. Others have also found an association between antibodies to microbes as predictive including using quartile sum scores of all antibodies [37, 53–57]. Whether ASCA alone, as in this Manitoba study, is as good as a combination of antibodies, remains to be proven. The lack of predictive value of genetic mutations compared to other markers such as serological antibodies has been reported elsewhere [53, 58]. In the Manitoba study smoking was not predictive of an adverse outcome. This is contrary to what is widely considered in CD [59].

Disease Activity Over Time: Monitoring Both Symptoms and Mucosal Inflammation

In a Danish inception cohort of 373 CD patients diagnosed between 1962 and 1987, in the first year after diagnosis, 80 % had high disease activity, 15 % had low activity and 5 % were in remission. After the first year, only 30 % had high disease activity, and 55 % were in remission [17]. The relapse rate within the year of diagnosis and over the following 2 years correlated positively with relapse rate over the ensuing 5 years ($p = 0.00001$). Over years 3–7 after diagnosis 25 % had active disease every year, 22 % were in remission and 53 % had fluctuating courses. The probability of a relapse-free course decreased from 22 % over 5 years to 12 % over 10 years. Only 4 % at 5 years and 1 % at 10 years had continuously active disease and only 13 % had a relapse free course. So having some fluctuation of disease activity occurred in the majority. Approximately half of patients with active disease could expect to be in full remission by 3 years. These are not very promising data but they are also from an era with limited use of effective maintenance therapies. Even during that era of limited therapy, only 20 % of subjects in the first 7 years had active disease every year while 67 % of subjects had a fluctuating disease course. However, having active disease in one year predicted that 70–80 % would have active disease the next year, while being in remission in one year predicted that 80 % would be in remission the next year. Whether or not a person was in remission or had active disease was independent of age, sex, location of disease. The Norwegian IBSEN cohort provides some insight into CD patients diagnosed between 1990 and 1994 and followed for a median of 10 years. The cumulative relapse rates were 53 %, 85 %, and 90 % at 1, 5, and 10 years, respectively [44]. Sex, smoking status, disease location, and disease behavior at diagnosis did not predict relapse rates. In the second 5 years of follow-up 25 % did not use any medications and this was not significantly impacted on by age, disease location, or disease behavior at diagnosis. As many as 44 % were in clinical remission during the second 5 year follow-up period and the majority of them did not use any immunosuppressive therapy. Age at diagnosis over 40 years was associated with a greater likelihood of remission in years 6–10. Surgery for active Crohn's disease within the first 5 years from diagnosis did not influence the proportion in remission in the second 5 years. In the IBSEN cohort of persons with UC mucosal healing at 1 year was also associated with reduced colectomy rates (OR = 0.22, 95 % CI 0.06–0.79) [26].

In the European Inception Cohort (EC-IBD) of 358 subjects with CD enrolled in 1991–1993, at a median of 10 years follow-up, 27 % had no recurrence [37]. The cumulative recurrence rates at 1, 5, and 10 years, respectively were 34 %, 69 %, and 77 %, respectively, all somewhat lower than in the Norwegian study of the same era. In the EC-IBD Study ($n=358$) 27 % experienced no recurrence after diagnosis and 18 % had only one recurrence [37], although these may be underestimates since the study allowed for subjects to self-treat and not report if a mild flare of disease occurred. First recurrence rates occurred in 34 % by 1 year and 78 % by 10 years. For those who had surgery, recurrence rates were 6 % at 1 year and 63 % by 10 years. Within the first 5 years from diagnosis 25 % had undergone surgery. Of those who had surgery within 10 years from diagnosis, it occurred in the first year in 25 %. Of those who had surgery, second surgeries occurred in 18 %, 32 %, and 54 % by 1, 5, and 10 years, respectively. For each of first, second, and third recurrences the time interval between recurrences progressively shortened. Hence, relapse rates can positively influence further relapse rates. People who quit smoking were protected from first recurrence rates ($p=0.01$). Patients with upper gastrointestinal disease had an excess risk of disease recurrence (hazard ratio, HR = 1.54, 95 % confidence interval, CI 1.13–2.1) and nearly all of those patients had non-penetrating disease. Subjects with isolated colonic disease had a reduced risk for surgical resection (HR = 0.38, 95 % CI 0.21–0.69). Age greater than 40 years at diagnosis was protective against relapse of disease (HR = 0.82, 0.7–0.97).

It is difficult to summarize all of these population based studies in a uniform statement. Follow-ups are available to about 2004. Through the 1970s to the 1990s it could be estimated that 15 % of patients remain in long-lasting remission, while 50 % have mild disease, or rare or occasional relapse. At least two thirds of patients have easily managed disease from an era of no biological drugs and little use of immunosuppressives. It was only 10 % or so that had chronically active or difficult to manage disease. The remaining 25 % had fluctuating disease with substantive relapses interspersed with periods of remission. It is this one third of patients that may be most impacted by more aggressive therapy. However, a key caveat to interpreting these data is considering how active disease was defined. For the most part it was likely based on symptoms. We have learned from clinical trials that when active inflammation is not rigorously identified there is a risk either that the interventions will have minimal effect or that the interventions will have large effects but they will be no different than that seen with placebo [60, 61].

So while clinicians and clinical trials use noninvasive markers of inflammation such as fecal calprotectin and serum C reactive protein there has been increasing enthusiasm to treating patients until their mucosal inflammation is mostly or completely resolved. Surely clinicians are keen to see that their patient's symptoms are settled and they are in a symptomatic remission but terms such as deep remission have been invoked to describe when an asymptomatic state is matched by a lack of intestinal inflammation. The importance of a patient's psychological state driving their symptoms but not necessarily their inflammatory disease was underscored by two key studies from Manitoba [62, 63]. In a population based survey study of approximately 600 persons with IBD every 3 months for 1 year the only variable that was associated with a flare of symptoms 3 months later was a high perception of stress. Having an infection, using antibiotics, or using nonsteroidal anti-inflammatory drugs were not associated with symptomatic flares. In a subsequent study where approximately 480 persons completed surveys and sent in stool samples every 3 months for 6 months high stress was associated with a flare of symptoms but not with active inflammation (as measured by fecal calprotectin). In fact symptoms only weakly correlated with inflammation in UC and did not correlate with inflammation in CD. These studies highlight two key messages. One is that when patients are symptomatic it is critical to discuss their psychosocial health and how they are dealing with their life stress and secondly that before increasing anti-inflammatory or immunomodulating therapy in patients whose symptoms are increased it is important to document that their inflammation is at least partly driving their symptoms. While symptoms may exist in the absence of inflammation, inflammation may exist in the absence of symptoms. It is debatable as to the optimal approach whether it is in CD or UC when areas of intestinal inflammation are discovered in an asymptomatic patient. Firstly, how much inflammation is enough inflammation that is worth treating? Is the goal complete mucosal healing or can we settle for a marked reduction in ulceration and inflammation? It is easier to convince oneself as the clinician and also to convince the patient who is asymptomatic that enhanced treatment is worthwhile if for instance serological markers such as anemia or hypoalbuminemia coexist suggesting that the inflammation is having adverse impact.

Regardless, of whether the patient is prepared to "step up" therapy there is increasing evidence that patients whose mucosa gets healed have better outcomes in the long term. In a nested sample of the original "top down step up study" reported by D'Haens et al. [64], of the study cohort who underwent endoscopy at the end of 2 years ($n=49$), the presence of mucosal healing at 2 years significantly predicted a greater likelihood of steroid-free remission in those followed out to 3–4 years (OR = 4.35, 1.10–17.22) [65]. Of interest though when mucosal healing was diagnosed at 2 years only 52 % of those in clinical remission ($n=31$) had mucosal healing (reconfirming older information of the potential to feel clinically well while having active mucosal disease). Perhaps more perplexing was that of 11 patients without a clinical remission 73 % had mucosal healing. Hence do these patients have active mucosal disease out of the colonoscope's reach or do they have functional symptoms?

Another example showing the predictive value of mucosal healing was from the IBSEN Cohort from Norway. There were 141 patients with CD who underwent endoscopic evaluation at 0.5 and 1 years post diagnosis and 50 who underwent endoscopy at 5 years [66]. Mucosal healing at 0.5 years did not predict relapses, complications or surgery. Mucosal healing at 1 year, however, was associated with less endoscopic disease at 5 years and less need for subsequent corticosteroids. Corticosteroid use at diagnosis was associated with a significant reduction by 70 % of mucosal healing at 1 year. However, conclusions from this retrospective study are confounded by the issue as to whether corticosteroids per se reduce mucosal healing or that corticosteroids are used for more severe disease. Further, only 20 % of this cohort had isolated ileal involvement and assessment of predictability of mucosal healing for this subgroup was not undertaken [66].

Mucosal healing or by corollary mucosal recurrence can predict postoperative recurrence. The recent randomized trial in postoperative CD from Australia and New Zealand study showed that when patients' therapy is guided by routine endoscopic surveillance 6 months post-surgery in CD the outcomes are better than symptom based intervention [67]. All of this means that there is a need to continue to survey patients who are well with CD with noninvasive testing (such as fecal calprotectin, serum CRP) and with cross-sectional imaging and endoscopy to determine when active inflammatory disease is emerging. Surveillance intervals and the optimal therapy to achieve mucsal healing all need to be determined. However, this is the new frontier in terms of "natural history" in IBD. We cannot define the natural history of untreated IBD because we do not follow enough untreated IBD to understand or be able to predict outcomes in that scenario. However, we can accrue data on the "evolving history of treated IBD." Especially now that we are determining the effect of mucosal inflammation regardless of symptoms, we are gaining even further insights into the evolving history of both treated and undertreated IBD. In fact there are a substantive number of patients who are in a sufficiently deep remission that they do not use any IBD-specific medications [68]. An ultimate goal is to find how we can sufficiently heal the disease that patients can withdraw from medications altogether.

References

1. Lennard-Jones JE. Crohn's disease: natural history and treatment. Postgrad Med J. 1968;44:674–8.
2. Edwards FC, Truelove SC. The course and prognosis of ulcerative colitis. Gut. 1963;4:299–310.
3. Lennard-Jones JE, Vivian AB. Fulminating ulcerative colitis: Recent experience in management. Br Med J. 1960;2:96–102.
4. Goligher JC. Surgical treatment of ulcerative colitis. Br Med J. 1961;1:151–4.
5. Bernstein CN, Nugent ZN, Targownik LE, Singh H, Lix L. Predictors and risks for death in a population-based study of persons with IBD in Manitoba. Gut. 2015;64:1403–11.
6. Silverstein MD, Loftus EV, Sandborn WJ, et al. Clinical course and costs of care for Crohn's disease: Markov model analysis of a population-based cohort. Gastroenterology. 1999;117:49–57.
7. Truelove SC, Pena AS. Course and prognosis of Crohn's disease. Gut. 1976;17:192–201.
8. Farmer RG, Whelan G, Fazio VW. Long-term follow-up of patients with Crohn's disease. Relationship between the clinical pattern and prognosis. Gastroenterology. 1985;88:1818–25.
9. Bernstein CN, Loftus Jr EV, Ng SC, Lakatos PL, Moum B. Hospitalizations and surgery in Crohn's disease. Gut. 2012;61:622–9.
10. Ramadas AV, Gunesh S, Thomas GA, et al. Natural history of Crohn's disease in a population-based cohort from Cardiff (1986–2003): a study of changes in medical treatment and surgical resection rates. Gut. 2010;59:1200–6.
11. Nguyen GC, Nugent Z, Shaw S, et al. Outcomes of patients with Crohn's disease improved from 1988 to 2008 and were associated with increased specialist care. Gastroenterology. 2011;141:90–7.
12. Lewis JD, Schoenfeld P, Lichtenstein GR. An evidence-based approach to studies of the natural history of gastrointestinal disease: recurrence of symptomatic Crohn's disease after surgery. Clin Gastroenterol Hepatol. 2003;1:229–336.
13. Bernstein CN, Ng SC, Lakatos PL, et al. on behalf of the Epidemiology and Natural History Task Force of the International Organization of Inflammatory Bowel Disease (IOIBD). A review of mortality and surgery in ulcerative colitis: milestones of the seriousness of the disease. Inflamm Bowel Dis. 2013;19:2001–10.
14. Targownik LE, Nugent Z, Singh H, Bernstein CN. The epidemiology of colectomy in ulcerative colitis: results from a population-based cohort. Am J Gastroenterol. 2012;107:1228–35.
15. Turner D, Walsh CM, Steinhart AH, et al. Response to corticosteroids in severe ulcerative colitis: a systematic review of the literature and mega-regression. Clin Gastroenterol Hepatol. 2007;5: 103–10.
16. Kaplan GG, McCarthy EP, Ayanian JZ, et al. Impact of hospital volume on postoperative morbidity and mortality following a colectomy for ulcerative colitis. Gastroenterology. 2008;134(3): 680–7.
17. Munkholm P, Langholz E, Davidsen M, et al. Disease activity courses in a regional cohort of Crohn's disease patients. Scand J Gastroenterol. 1995;30:699–706.
18. Odes S, Vardi H, Friger M, et al. European Collaborative Study on Inflammatory Bowel Disease. Cost analysis and cost determinants in a European inflammatory bowel disease inception cohort with 10 years of follow-up evaluation. Gastroenterology. 2006;131:719–28.
19. Peyrin-Biroulet L, Loftus EV, Harmsen WS, et al. Emergency room visits and hospitalizations for Crohn's disease in a population-based cohort. Gastroenterology. 2010;138(5 Suppl 1):S-532.
20. Sonnenberg A, Richardson PA, Abraham NS. Hospitalizations for inflammatory bowel disease among U.S. military veterans 1975–2006. Dig Dis Sci. 2009;54:1740–5.
21. Herrinton L, Liu L, Fireman B, et al. Time trends in therapies and outcomes for adult inflammatory bowel disease, Northern California, 1998–2005. Gastroenterology. 2009;137:502–11.
22. Longobardi T, Bernstein CN. Health care resource utilization in inflammatory bowel disease. Clin Gastroenterol Hepatol. 2006;4: 731–43.
23. Allison J, Herrinton LJ, Liu L, et al. Natural history of severe ulcerative colitis in a community-based health plan. Clin Gastroenterol Hepatol. 2008;6:999–1003.
24. Navaneethan U, Mukewar S, Venkatesh PG, et al. Clostridium difficile infection is associated with worse long term outcome in patients with ulcerative colitis. J Crohns Colitis. 2012;6:330–6.
25. Jodorkovsky D, Young Y, Abreu MT. Clinical outcomes of patients with ulcerative colitis and co-existing Clostridium difficile infection. Dig Dis Sci. 2010;55(2):415–20.
26. Solberg IC, Lygren I, Jahnsen J, et al. Clinical course during the first 10 years of ulcerative colitis: results from a population-based inception cohort (IBSEN Study). Scand J Gastroenterol. 2009;44:431–40.

27. Henriksen M, Jahnsen J, Lygren I, et al. Ulcerative colitis and clinical course: results of a 5-year population-based follow-up study (The IBSEN Study). Inflamm Bowel Dis. 2006;12:543–50.
28. Ritchie JK, Powell-Tuck J, Lennard-Jones JE. Clinical outcome of the first ten years of ulcerative colitis and proctitis. Lancet. 1978;1:1140–3.
29. Sinclair TS, Brunt PW, Mowat NAG. Nonspecific proctocolitis in Northeastern Scotland; a community study. Gastroenterology. 1983;85:1–11.
30. Hendriksen C, Kreiner S, Binder V. Long term prognosis in ulcerative colitis-based on results from a regional patient group from the County of Copenhagen. Gut. 1985;26:158–63.
31. Höie O, Wolters F, Riis L, et al. Ulcerative colitis: patient characteristics may predict 10-yr disease recurrence in a European-wide population-based cohort. Am J Gastroenterol. 2007;102: 1692–701.
32. Silverberg M, Satsangi J, Ahmad T, et al. Toward an integrated clinical, molecular and serological classification of inflammatory bowel disease: Report of a Working Party of the 2005 Montreal World Congress of Gastroenterology. Can J Gastroenterol. 2005;19(Suppl A):5–36.
33. Henriksen M, Jahnsen J, Lygren I, et al. Clinical course in Crohn's disease: results of a 5-year population based follow-up study (the IBSEN Study). Scand J Gastroenterol. 2007;42:602–10.
34. Louis E, Collard A, Oger AF, et al. Behaviour of Crohn's disease according to the Vienna classification: changing pattern over the course of disease. Gut. 2001;49:777–82.
35. Vernier-Massouille G, Balde M, Salderon J, et al. Natural history of pediatric Crohn's disease: a population based cohort study. Gastroenterology. 2008;135:1106–13.
36. Levine A et al. ESPGHAN revised porto criteria for the diagnosis of inflammatory bowel disease in children and adolescents. JPGN. 2014;58:795–806.
37. Wolters FL, Russel MG, Sijbrandij J, et al. Phenotype at diagnosis predicts recurrence rates in Crohn's disease. Gut. 2006;55: 1124–30.
38. Cosnes JM, Cattan S, Blain A, et al. Long-term evolution of disease behavior of Crohn's disease. Inflamm Bowel Dis. 2002;8:244–50.
39. Schwartz DA, Loftus Jr EV, Tremaine WJ, et al. The natural history of fistulizing Crohn's disease in Olmsted County, Minnesota. Gastroenterology. 2002;132:875–80.
40. Langholz E, Munkholm P, Krasilnikoff PA, Binder V. Inflammatory bowel diseases with onset in childhood: clinical features, morbidity, and mortality in a regional cohort. Scand J Gastroenterol. 1997;32:139–47.
41. Cosnes J, Nion-Larmurier I, Beaugerie L, et al. Impact of the increasing use of immunosuppressants in Crohn's disease on the need for intestinal surgery. Gut. 2005;54:237–41.
42. Thia KT, Sandborn WJ, Harmsen WS, et al. Risk factors associated with progression to intestinal complications of Crohn's disease in a population-based cohort. Gastroenterology. 2010;139:1147–455.
43. Israeli E, Ryan JD, Shafer LA, Bernstein CN. Younger age at diagnosis is associated with a pan-enteric involvement but does not predict a more aggressive course of Crohn's disease. Clin Gastroenterol Hepatol. 2014;12:72–9.
44. Solberg IC, Vatn MH, Hoie O, et al. Clinical course in Crohn's disease results of a Norwegian population-based ten-year follow-up study. Clin Gastroenterol Hepatol. 2007;5:1430–8.
45. Bernell O, Lapidus A, Hellers G. Risk factors for surgery and postoperative recurrence in Crohn's disease. Ann Surg. 2000;231:38–45.
46. Lapidus A, Bernell O, Hellers G, et al. Clinical course of colorectal Crohn's disease: a 35 year follow-up study of 507 patients. Gastroenterology. 1998;114:1151–60.
47. Tang L, Rawsthorne P, Bernstein CN. Are perineal and luminal fistulas associated in Crohn's disease? A population-based study. Clin Gastroenterol Hepatol. 2006;4(9):1130–4.
48. Ingle SB, Loftus Jr EV. The natural history of perianal Crohn's disease. Dig Liver Dis. 2007;39:963–74.
49. Greenstein AJ, Lachman P, Sachar DB, et al. Perforating and non-perforating indications for repeated operations in Crohn's disease; evidence for two clinical forms. Gut. 1988;29:588–92.
50. Peyrin-Biroulet L, Loftus Jr EV, Colombel JF, Sandborn WJ. The natural history of adult Crohn's disease in population-based cohorts. Am J Gastroenterol. 2010;105:289–97.
51. Ingle SB, Loftus EV, Harmsen S. Hospitalization rates for Crohn's disease patients in Olmsted County, Minnesota, in the pre-biologic era. Am J Gastroenterol. 2007;102 Suppl 2:S487.
52. Ryan JD, Silverberg MS, Xu W, et al. Predicting complicated Crohn's disease and surgery: phenotypes, genetics, serology and psychological characteristics of a population based cohort. Aliment Pharmacol Ther. 2013;38:274–83.
53. Arnott ID, Landers CJ, Nimmo EJ, Drummond HE, Smith BK, Targan SR, et al. Sero-reactivity to microbial components in Crohn's disease is associated with disease severity and progression, but not NOD2/CARD15 genotype. Am J Gastroenterol. 2004; 99(12):2376–84.
54. Papadakis KA, Yang H, Ippoliti A, Mei L, Elson CO, Hershberg RM, et al. Anti-flagellin (CBir1) phenotypic and genetic Crohn's disease associations. Inflamm Bowel Dis. 2007;13(5):524–30.
55. Prideaux L, De Cruz P, Ng SC, Kamm MA. Serological antibodies in inflammatory bowel disease: a systematic review. Inflamm Bowel Dis. 2012;18(7):1340–55.
56. Rieder F, Schleder S, Wolf A, et al. Serum anti-glycan antibodies predict complicated Crohn's disease behavior: a cohort study. Inflamm Bowel Dis. 2010;16(8):1367–75.
57. Dubinsky MC, Kugathasan S, Mei L, et al. Increased immune reactivity predicts aggressive complicating Crohn's disease in children. Clin Gastroenterol Hepatol. 2008;6(10):1105–11.
58. Roberts RL, Gearry RB, Hollis-Moffatt JE, et al. IL23R R381Q and ATG16L1 T300A are strongly associated with Crohn's disease in a study of New Zealand Caucasians with inflammatory bowel disease. Am J Gastroenterol. 2007;102(12):2754–61.
59. Lakatos PL, Szamosi T, Lakatos L. Smoking in inflammatory bowel diseases: good, bad or ugly? World J Gastroenterol. 2007; 13:6134–9.
60. Schreiber S, Rutgeerts P, Fedorak RN, et al. A randomized, placebo-controlled trial of certolizumab pegol (CDP870) for treatment of Crohn's disease. Gastroenterology. 2005;129(3):807–18.
61. Sandborn WJ, Schreiber S, Feagan BG, et al. Certolizumab pegol for active Crohn's disease: a placebo-controlled, randomized trial. Clin Gastroenterol Hepatol. 2011;9(8):670–8.
62. Bernstein CN, Singh S, Graff LA, et al. A prospective population-based study of symptomatic triggers of flares in IBD. Am J Gastroenterol. 2010;105:1994–2002.
63. Targownik L, Sexton K, Bernstein MT, et al. The relationship among perceived stress, symptoms, and inflammation in persons with inflammatory bowel disease. Am J Gastroenterol. 2015;110:1001–12.
64. D'Haens G, Baert F, van Assche G, et al. Early combined immunosuppression or conventional management in patients with newly diagnosed Crohn's disease: an open randomised trial. Lancet. 2008;371:660–7.
65. Baert F, Moortgat L, Van Assche G, et al. Mucosal healing predicts sustained clinical remission in patients with early-stage Crohn's disease. Gastroenterology. 2010;138:463–8.
66. Froslie KF, Jahnsen J, Moum BA, et al. Mucosal healing in inflammatory bowel disease: results from a Norwegian population-based cohort. Gastroenterology. 2007;133:412–2276.
67. De Cruz P, Kamm MA, Hamilton AL, et al. Crohn's disease management after intestinal resection: a randomized trial. Lancet. 2015;38:1406–17.
68. Melesse DY, Targownik LE, Singh H, et al. Patterns and predictors of long term nonuse of medical therapy among persons with inflammatory bowel disease. Inflamm Bowel Dis. 2015;21:1615–22.

Conventional Medical Management of Crohn's Disease: Sulfasalazine

28

Miquel A. Gassull and Eduard Cabré

Introduction

Sulfasalazine (Salazosulfapyridine, SASP) is a prodrug composed of a molecule of 5-aminosalicylic acid (5-ASA) and sulfapyridine, linked by an azo bond. It was aimed to the treatment of rheumatic diseases such as rheumatoid arthritis and ankylosing spondylitis. When taken orally, anaerobic intestinal bacteria split the azo bond, releasing the two components 5-ASA and sulfapyridine, the former being the active anti-inflammatory component [1]. Because the lower G-I tract—terminal ileum and colon—are the areas of the gut with the highest commensal bacteria concentration (10^{10}–10^{14} cfu/mm^3), it was assumed that the 5-ASA moiety would exert its anti-inflammatory activity in the inflamed and ulcerated areas of the intestine where the active compound would be released [2, 3].

Mechanisms of Therapeutic Action

The mechanism of action of SASP and its metabolites is not well understood [4], especially their systemic effect on rheumatic diseases, since 5-ASA is poorly absorbed into the bloodstream [3]. The fact that the active molecule is particularly effective when administered topically into the rectum, as enema or suppository, supports this concept. It has been reported that SASP and its metabolites decrease eicosanoid synthesis [5–7], cytokine expression [8–10], and NF-kB activation [11, 12].

The antioxidant effects of SASP are well established which are probably due to its scavenging effects against reactive oxygen and nitrogen species (ROS and RNS), as well as metal chelating properties, and its inhibitory effects over neutrophil oxidative burst [13, 14]. A study compared the potential scavenging activity mediated by SASP and its metabolites 5-ASA and sulfapyridine on ROS and RNS, using validated in vitro screening systems [15]. SASP and its metabolite 5-ASA, but not sulfapyridine showed ROS- and RNS-scavenging effects which may be a contributing mechanism of its anti-inflammatory effects through the prevention of the oxidative/nitrative/nitrosative damages caused by these species [15].

Clinical Evidence

As mentioned, the fact that the effect of anaerobic bacteria is necessary to "activate" SASP explains why it has been used in ulcerative colitis where it has been shown to be effective in both inducing remission of active disease and preventing relapse in inactive patients. However, the role of SASP in the treatment of mild or moderate Crohn's disease is controversial still nowadays [16].

SASP was used in the treatment of active Crohn's disease on the belief that it would benefit of a treatment that has been effective in active ulcerative colitis, provided the similarity of mucosal lesions between both diseases. On the other hand, in the early sixties there were no other drugs available for such conditions, except for corticosteroids. Since Crohn's disease may affect independently the colon, the terminal ileum or both together, and both areas contain a high anaerobic bacteria concentration, it is logical to assume that the prodrug could be split by them in both locations and locally release 5-ASA. Some observational studies were published in the sixties and early seventies of the last century [17–19] to assess the effectiveness of SASP for both inducing and

M.A. Gassull, M.D., Ph.D. (✉)
Health Science Research Institute, Germans Trias i Pujol Foundation, Badalona, Catalonia, Spain

Gastroenterology and Hepatology Department, Germans Trias I Pujol University Hospital, Badalona, Catalonia, Spain
e-mail: gassull.ma@gmail.com

E. Cabré, M.D., Ph.D.
IBD/G-I Unit, Department of Gastroenterology, Hospital Universitari Germans Trias i Pujol, Badalona, Catalonia, Spain

CIBERehd, Barcelona, Catalonia, Spain

D.C. Baumgart (ed.), *Crohn's Disease and Ulcerative Colitis*, DOI 10.1007/978-3-319-33703-6_28

maintaining remission in Crohn's disease. Also in this decade, controlled trials were also performed with different designs to ascertain its effect as adjunctive therapy in active disease or as maintenance treatment, most of them with a small and heterogeneous group of patients [20, 21].

The first solid evaluation of the effect of SASP on Crohn's disease comes from two large studies: the American National Cooperative Crohn's Disease Study (NCCDS) [22] and the European Cooperative Crohn's Disease Study (ECCDS) [23].

The NCCDS compared the efficacy of SASP, prednisone and azathioprine with placebo, and showed that prednisone (0.25–0.75 mg/kg adjusted to disease activity) was superior to SASP (1 g/15 kg), and that SASP, but not azathioprine (2.5 mg/kg), was superior to placebo, in inducing 16-week clinical remission of Crohn's disease [22]. Subgroup analyses suggested that patients who had been treated with steroids previously failed to respond to SASP, while those who had not taken steroids at entry responded to SASP significantly better than placebo [22]. Patients with involvement limited to the colon responded to SASP better than to placebo, while those who had disease located only in small bowel were less likely to benefit from this therapy [22]. None of the treatments—including SASP—proved to be better than placebo for preventing clinical relapse in inactive disease [22].

The ECCDS randomized patients to treatment with 6-methylprednisolone (48 mg/day weekly, tapering to 8 mg/day) alone, 6-methylprednisolone in combination with SASP (3 g), SASP alone, or placebo. Effects on active disease where assessed at 6 weeks, whereas inactive patients were on therapy for 2 years or until relapse. 6-Methylprednisolone proved the most effective therapy for inducing remission [23]; in subgroup analyses it was significantly more effective than SASP for patients who had been previously treated with steroids, for those who had disease only in the small bowel, and for those with disease in the small bowel and colon [23]. The combination of the steroids plus SASP was most effective in previously untreated patients and when the disease was located in the colon [23]. SASP alone was the least effective active treatment regimen. No therapeutic regimen was better than placebo for inactive disease [23].

Other controlled trials in patients with active Crohn's disease have confirmed some of the conclusions of these subgroup analyses by demonstrating that SASP is not an effective adjunctive therapy to prednisone [21], whereas prednisolone is an effective adjunctive therapy to SASP [24], probably because corticosteroids are more effective therapies than SASP. In another small, comparative study of SASP (4–6 g/day) with placebo, van Hees et al. showed that 62 % of patients treated with SASP had a favorable response after 26 weeks compared with 8 % of placebo-treated patients [25].

In 2010, meta-analysis pooled the available data on the effect of different salicylates in mild-to-moderate active Crohn's disease [26]. SASP was more likely to induce remission (RR: 1.38; 95 % CI: 1.02–1.87; $n=263$) compared to placebo, with benefit confined mainly to patients with colitis, while it was less effective than corticosteroids (RR: 0.66; 95 % CI: 0.53–0.81; $n=260$) [26]. Interestingly, however, the performance of SASP was better than that of mesalazine, either at low or high dose. Low-dose mesalazine (1–2 g/day) was not superior to placebo (RR: 1.46, 95 % CI: 0.89–2.40; $n=302$) and was less effective than corticosteroids. High-dose mesalazine (3–4.5 g/day) was not superior to placebo for induction of remission (RR: 2.02; 95 %: CI 0.75–5.45) or response (Weighted mean difference: −19.8 points; 95 % CI: −46.2 to 6.7; $n=615$). The authors conclude that SASP shows modest efficacy for the treatment of active Crohn's disease [26]. In a more recent meta-analysis, Ford et al. [27] just showed a trend towards a benefit with sulfasalazine over placebo (two RCTs, RR of failure to achieve remission = 0.83; 95 % CI = 0.69–1.00), and also no definite benefit of mesalazine over placebo (four RCTs, RR = 0.91; 95 % CI = 0.77–1.06). Neither sulfasalazine nor mesalazine was effective in preventing quiescent CD relapse [27] However, a direct comparison between SASP and mesalazine in mild-to-moderate active Crohn's disease has never been performed.

Another setting where aminosalicylates have been assayed is the prevention of postoperative recurrence of Crohn's disease after resection and ileo-colonic anastomosis. A meta-analysis has pooled the data of 11 trials, five of them using SASP [20, 28–31], with a total of 1282 patients [32]. The RR of relapse of Crohn's disease in remission after surgery with aminosalicylates vs. placebo or no therapy was 0.86 (95 % CI: 0.74–0.99) (NNT = 13). As opposite to treatment of active disease, SASP was of no benefit in preventing relapse (RR: 0.97; 95 % CI: 0.72–1.31; $n=448$), whereas mesalazine was more effective than placebo or no therapy (RR: 0.80; 95 % CI: 0.70–0.92; $n=834$), with a NNT = 10 [32]. The authors conclude that mesalazine has only a modest effect in preventing postoperative recurrence in Crohn's disease and should be used in patients in whom immunosuppressive therapy is either not warranted or contraindicated [32].

Recommendations for Clinical Practice

On the light of the available evidence, both experts [33, 34] and consensus-based guidelines [16] recommend the use of high-dose (3–6 g/day) SASP in Crohn's disease only for patients with mild disease confined to the colon. Other authors, however, do not give any chance to SASP and its metabolites in the management of active Crohn's disease [35]. Anyway, SASP should be used in the short term, and active disease beyond 16 weeks of therapy should be considered a therapeutic failure. In addition, SASP are ineffective as maintenance therapy after both medically and surgically induced remission (in the latter setting, mesalazine may have a minor role).

In addition, SASP may have a role in the management of Crohn's disease patients with associated arthropathy. However, recent review of the available evidence indicates that its usefulness is confined to some patients with peripheral arthropathy, or in those with early ankylosing spondylitis (i.e., those with higher levels of ESR or active disease) [36]. Advanced disease does not benefit from this drug since no effect on physical function, pain, spinal mobility, or enthesitis has been observed [36].

Side effects of SASP include headache, epigastric pain, nausea, vomiting, skin rash, fever, hepatitis, autoimmune hemolysis, aplastic anemia, leucopenia, agranulocytosis, pancreatitis, pharmacological systemic lupus erythematosus, sulfonamide-induced toxic epidermal necrolysis, Stevens–Johnson syndrome, pulmonary dysfunction, and male infertility [37, 38]. Most of the side effects of SASP can be attributed to the systemic absorption of sulfapyridine and the adverse effects occur more frequently in patients who are genetically predisposed to "slow" acetylation of sulfapyridine to *N*-acetylsulfapyridine in the liver [37]. Some of the side effects (headache, nausea, vomiting, and epigastric pain) are dose related and can be minimized by gradual dose escalation [38]. It is well known than SASP reduces folate absorption [39, 40]. Thus, folate supplements should be administered in patients on SASP therapy. Nephrotoxicity, mainly as interstitial nephritis, has been reported in patients on aminosalicylate therapy. However, a systematic review of studies with regular monitoring of serum creatinine and creatinine clearance showed that its frequency is low, with a mean annual rate of only 0.26 % (95 % CI: 0.13–0.5 %) per patient-year [41]. The lack of relationship of this complication with dose suggests that it depends on idiosyncratic mechanisms [41]. Anyway, in spite of its low frequency, periodic monitoring of serum creatinine is advised [42].

References

1. Azad Khan AK, Piris J, Truelove SC. An experiment to determine the active therapeutic moiety of sulphasalazine. Lancet. 1977;2:892–5.
2. Goldman P, Peppercorn MA. Drug therapy: sulfasalazine. N Engl J Med. 1975;293:20–3.
3. Das KM, Dubin R. Clinical pharmacokinetics of sulphasalazine. Clin Pharmacokinet. 1976;1:406–25.
4. Rieder F, Karrasch T, Ben-Horin S, Schirbel A, Ehehalt R, Wehkamp J, et al. Results of the 2nd scientific workshop of the ECCO (III): basic mechanisms of intestinal healing. J Crohns Colitis. 2012;6:373–85.
5. Hawkey CJ, Boughton-Smith NK, Whittle BJ. Modulation of human colonic arachidonic acid metabolism by sulfasalazine. Dig Dis Sci. 1985;30:1161–5.
6. Ahnfelt-Ronne I, Nielsen OH, Bukhave K, Elmgreen J. Sulfasalazine and its anti-inflammatory metabolite, 5-aminosalicylic acid: effect on arachidonic acid metabolism in human neutrophils, and free radical scavenging. Adv Prostaglandin Thromboxane Leukot Res. 1987;17B:918–22.
7. Tornhamre S, Edenius C, Smedegard G, Sjoquist B, Lindgren JA Effects of sulfasalazine and a sulfasalazine analogue on the formation of lipoxygenase and cyclooxygenase products. Eur J Pharmacol. 1989;169:225–34.
8. Rachmilewitz D, Karmeli F, Schwartz LW, Simon PL. Effect of aminophenols (5-ASA and 4-ASA) on colonic interleukin-1 generation. Gut. 1992;33:929–32.
9. Stevens C, Lipman M, Fabry S, Moscovitch-Lopatin M, Almawi W, Keresztes S, et al. 5-Aminosalicylic acid abrogates T-cell proliferation by blocking interleukin-2 production in peripheral blood mononuclear cells. J Pharmacol Exp Ther. 1995;272:399–406.
10. Hasko G, Szabo C, Nemeth ZH, Deitch EA. Sulphasalazine inhibits macrophage activation: inhibitory effects on inducible nitric oxide synthase expression, interleukin-12 production and major histocompatibility complex II expression. Immunology. 2001;103:473–8.
11. Gan HT, Chen YQ, Ouyang Q. Sulfasalazine inhibits activation of nuclear factor-kappaB in patients with ulcerative colitis. J Gastroenterol Hepatol. 2005;20:1016–24.
12. Wahl C, Liptay S, Adler G, Schmid RM. Sulfasalazine: a potent and specific inhibitor of nuclear factor kappa B. J Clin Invest. 1998;101:1163–74.
13. Miles AM, Grisham MB. Antioxidant properties of aminosalicylates. Methods Enzymol. 1994;234:555–72.
14. Joshi R, Kumar S, Unnikrishnan M, Mukherjee T. Free radical scavenging reactions of sulfasalazine, 5-aminosalicylic acid and sulfapyridine: mechanistic aspects and antioxidant activity. Free Radic Res. 2005;39:1163–72.
15. Couto D, Ribeiro D, Freitas M, Gomes A, Lima JL, Fernandes E. Scavenging of reactive oxygen and nitrogen species by the prodrug sulfasalazine and its metabolites 5-aminosalicylic acid and sulfapyridine. Redox Rep. 2010;15:259–67.
16. Dignass A, van Assche G, Lindsay JO, Lemann M, Soderholm J, Colombel JF, et al. The second European evidence-based Consensus on the diagnosis and management of Crohn's disease: current management. J Crohns Colitis. 2010;4:28–62.
17. Jones JH, Lennard-Jones JE, Lockhart-Mummery HE. Experience in the treatment of Crohn's disease of the large intestine. Gut. 1966;7:448–52.
18. Goldstein F, Murdock MG. Clinical and radiologic improvement of regional enteritis and enterocolitis after treatment with salicylazosulfapyridine. Am J Dig Dis. 1971;16:421–31.
19. Anthonisen P, Barany F, Folkenborg O, Holtz A, Jarnum S, Kristensen M, et al. The clinical effect of salazosulphapyridine (Salazopyrin r) in Crohn's disease. A controlled double-blind study. Scand J Gastroenterol. 1974;9:549–54.
20. Lennard-Jones JE. Sulphasalazine in asymptomatic Crohn's disease. A multicentre trial. Gut. 1977;18:69–72.
21. Singleton JW, Summers RW, Kern Jr F, Becktel JM, Best WR, Hansen RN, et al. A trial of sulfasalazine as adjunctive therapy in Crohn's disease. Gastroenterology. 1979;77:887–97.
22. Summers RW, Switz DM, Sessions JT, Becketel JM, Best WR, Kern F, et al. National cooperative Crohn's disease study: results of drug treatment. Gastroenterology. 1979;77:847–69.
23. Malchow H, Ewe K, Brandes JW, Goebell H, Ehms H, Sommer H, et al. European Cooperative Crohn's Disease Study (ECCDS): results of drug treatment. Gastroenterology. 1984;86:249–66.
24. Rijk MC, Van Hogezand RA, van Lier HJ, van Tongeren JH. Sulphasalazine and prednisone compared with sulphasalazine for treating active Crohn disease. A double-blind, randomized, multicenter trial. Ann Intern Med. 1991;114:445–50.
25. Van Hees PA, van Lier HJ, Van Elteren PH, Driessen M, Van Hogezand RA, Ten Velde GP, et al. Effect of sulphasalazine in

patients with active Crohn's disease: a controlled double-blind study. Gut. 1981;22:404–9.
26. Lim WC, Hanauer S. Aminosalicylates for induction of remission or response in Crohn's disease. Cochrane Database Syst Rev. 2010;12:CD008870.
27. Ford AC, Kane SV, Khan KJ, Achkar JP, Talley NJ, Marshall JK, et al. Efficacy of 5-aminosalicylates in Crohn's disease: systematic review and meta-analysis. Am J Gastroenterol. 2011;106:617–29.
28. Bergman L, Krause U. Postoperative treatment with corticosteroids and salazosulphapyridine (Salazopyrin) after radical resection for Crohn's disease. Scand J Gastroenterol. 1976;11:651–6.
29. Ewe K, Holtermüller KH, Baas U, Eckhart V, Krieg H, Kutzner J, et al. Rezidivprophylaxe nach darmresektion wegen morbus Crohn durch salazosulfapyridin (Azulfidine): eine doppelblindstudie. Verh Dtsch Ges Inn Med. 1976;82:930–2.
30. Wenckert A, Kristensen M, Eklund AE, Barany F, Jarnum S, Worning H, et al. The long-term prophylactic effect of salazosulphapyridine (Salazopyrin) in primarily resected patients with Crohn's disease. A controlled double-blind trial. Scand J Gastroenterol. 1978;13:161–7.
31. Ewe K, Herfarth C, Malchow H, Jesdinsky HJ. Postoperative recurrence of Crohn's disease in relation to radicality of operation and sulfasalazine prophylaxis: a multicenter trial. Digestion. 1989; 42:224–32.
32. Ford AC, Khan KJ, Talley NJ, Moayyedi P. 5-Aminosalicylates prevent relapse of Crohn's disease after surgically induced remission: systematic review and meta-analysis. Am J Gastroenterol. 2011; 106:413–20.
33. Sandborn WJ, Feagan BG. Review article: mild to moderate Crohn's disease—defining the basis for a new treatment algorithm. Aliment Pharmacol Ther. 2003;18:263–77.
34. Gionchetti P, Calabrese C, Tambasco R, Brugnera R, Straforini G, Liguori G, et al. Role of conventional therapies in the era of biological treatment in Crohn's disease. World J Gastroenterol. 2011;17:1797–806.
35. Nielsen OH, Munck LK. Drug insight: aminosalicylates for the treatment of IBD. Nat Clin Pract Gastroenterol Hepatol. 2007; 4:160–70.
36. Chen J, Lin S, Liu C. Sulfasalazine for ankylosing spondylitis. Cochrane Database Syst Rev. 2014;11:CD004800.
37. Das KM, Eastwood MA, McManus JP, Sircus W. Adverse reactions during salicylazosulfapyridine therapy and the relation with drug metabolism and acetylator phenotype. N Engl J Med. 1973;289:491–5.
38. Taffet SL, Das KM. Sulfasalazine. Adverse effects and desensitization. Dig Dis Sci. 1983;28:833–42.
39. Franklin JL, Rosenberg HH. Impaired folic acid absorption in inflammatory bowel disease: effects of salicylazosulfapyridine (Azulfidine). Gastroenterology. 1973;64:517–25.
40. Halsted CH, Gandhi G, Tamura T. Sulfasalazine inhibits the absorption of folates in ulcerative colitis. N Engl J Med. 1981;305:1513–7.
41. Gisbert JP, Gonzalez-Lama Y, Mate J. 5-Aminosalicylates and renal function in inflammatory bowel disease: a systematic review. Inflamm Bowel Dis. 2007;13:629–38.
42. de Jong DJ, Tielen J, Habraken CM, Wetzels JF, Naber AH. 5-Aminosalicylates and effects on renal function in patients with Crohn's disease. Inflamm Bowel Dis. 2005;11:972–6.

29 Steroid Therapy for Crohn's Disease

A. Hillary Steinhart

Steroids are a class of hormones that are normally produced in a variety of organs in the human body. They have a number of different physiologic properties that are determined by the nature of the molecular substitutions at several points around the backbone ring structure that is common to all steroids. The steroid hormone cortisone is produced by the adrenal cortex and, in additional to promoting catabolic metabolism, it also demonstrates several anti-inflammatory properties. It is these properties that provide the potential for therapeutic use of steroids in Crohn's disease and a variety of other inflammatory and autoimmune disorders. Cortisone is rarely used clinically to treat Crohn's disease, but a number of synthetically altered forms of steroids are frequently utilized as therapeutic agents. These pharmacologic agents typically have modifications that enhance their potency by increasing their affinity for binding of the steroid receptor, that alter their excretion or elimination, or that change their relative glucocorticoid and mineralocorticoid effect. The most commonly used of the systemically administered and active steroids are prednisone, prednisolone, methylprednisolone, and hydrocortisone. Budesonide, a highly potent and topically active steroid, is also used as one of several controlled release preparations for treating Crohn's disease, particularly when inflammation is confined to the terminal ileum and the ascending colon.

Induction Therapy

Conventional Steroids

Steroids are very effective at reducing inflammation and alleviating symptoms in patients with active intestinal Crohn's disease. They have been in use for the treatment of Crohn's disease for well over half a century and generally have the advantage of being effective in treating active inflammation in a number of different locations throughout the gastrointestinal tract as well as treating some of the extraintestinal manifestations of Crohn's disease. Despite the widespread use of steroids there have been relatively few randomized controlled trials that have both demonstrated their effectiveness and provided clear guidance with respect to optimal dosing, duration of therapy and tapering regimens. The effectiveness of steroids in treating active Crohn's disease was confirmed by the first part of the National Cooperative Crohn's Disease Study (NCCDS) in the USA [1], and by the European Cooperative Crohn's Disease Study (ECCDS) [2].

In the NCCDS, Part 1, Phase 1 the effectiveness of prednisone, sulfasalazine, and azathioprine were compared to placebo in treating patients with symptoms of active Crohn's disease over a 17 week study period [1]. In the steroid treated arm the dose of prednisone was based upon the baseline disease activity with 0.5 mg/kg used for those patients with mild to moderate disease activity (Crohn's disease activity index score between 150 and 300) and 0.75 mg/kg for those with more severe disease activity (Crohn's disease activity index score greater than 300). The maximum daily dose of prednisone was 60 mg. A complex analysis of outcome rankings demonstrated superiority to placebo for both prednisone and sulfasalazine. Using that analytical method it appeared that prednisone was particularly effective in patients with small intestinal involvement but not terribly effective in patients with only colonic involvement. When the more conventional outcome assessment of the proportion of patients in remission by the end of the 17-week study period was used, only prednisone was found to be superior to placebo with approximately 62 % of patients in remission (Crohn's disease activity index below 150) compared with approximately 30 % in the placebo arm using life table analysis. Using simple proportional analysis 47 % of prednisone-treated patients and 26 % of placebo-treated patients were in remission at week 17.

A.H. Steinhart, M.D., M.Sc., F.R.C.P.(C) (✉)
IBD Centre, Mount Sinai Hospital and Department of Medicine, University of Toronto, Room 445, 600 University Avenue, Toronto, ON M5G 1X5, Canada
e-mail: hsteinhart@mtsinai.on.ca

D.C. Baumgart (ed.), *Crohn's Disease and Ulcerative Colitis*, DOI 10.1007/978-3-319-33703-6_29

In the induction phase of the European Cooperative Crohn's Disease Study (ECCDS) patients with active Crohn's disease were randomized to receive 6-methylprednisolone, sulfasalazine, combination 6-methylprednisolone and sulfasalazine, or placebo for 6 weeks [2]. The 6-methylprednisolone was initiated at 48 mg per day and tapered to a dose of 12 mg per day over the 6-week study period. Patients initially randomized to the steroid arm who were in remission at the end of the acute phase (CDAI < 150) were then continued on maintenance 6-methylprednisolone 8 mg per day. Two increases in steroid dose back to 48 mg per day followed by repeated attempts at tapering were permitted in the 6-methylprednisolone-treated patients who were not in remission by the end of 6 weeks. Treatment with 6-methylprednisolone was found to be effective in inducing remission and was superior to sulfasalazine when Crohn's disease was located in the small intestine or both small and large intestine. In patients with only colonic disease location the combination of 6-methylprednisolone and sulfasalazine was the most effective treatment. Overall, 83 % of patients in the steroid treated arm were in remission at the end of 18 weeks as compared with 32.9 % of patients in the placebo arm.

Pooled analysis of the steroid induction studies demonstrated a twofold increased likelihood of remission induction with steroids as compared with placebo and a number needed to treat of 3.33 [3].

Many potential side effects of prednisone were recognized and described within the context of the induction therapy phase (Part 1, Phase I) of the NCCDS with moon face reported in 47 % of patients, striae in 6 %, ecchymoses in 17 %, acne in 30 %, infection in 27 %, muscle weakness in 9 %, hirsutism in 7 %, and polyuria in 15 % [1]. However, the use of prednisone in that trial was not consistent with what would currently be considered to be standard practice in that no tapering of the dose was permitted over the 17-week trial period. The high cumulative steroid dose, particularly in patients with higher disease activity scores at baseline, may have contributed to the very high rate of steroid associated side effects. Combining the adverse event results of the NCCDS and ECCDS demonstrated an almost fivefold increased risk of adverse events in steroid-treated patients as compared to placebo [3]. Although most of these did not result in patient withdrawal from the studies, the use of steroids was associated with a trend toward greater withdrawal rates in steroid-treated patients.

The optimal form of systemically acting steroid therapy has not been determined and the choice of specific steroid preparation typically depends upon local experience. Steroids can also be administered intravenously (e.g., hydrocortisone, 6-methylprednisolone) to hospitalized patients with more severe disease or more acute presentations but the superiority of intravenous administration has not been proven. Its main advantage is that it can be given to patients who are not able to tolerate oral intake.

The optimal dose of steroids for the treatment of active Crohn's disease has not been established. In the National Cooperative Crohn's Disease Study, where a dose of prednisone of 0.5 mg/kg per day was used in patients with mild to moderate disease activity and 0.75 mg/kg per day (up to a maximum of 60 mg) was used in patients with moderate to severe disease activity, remission was achieved in 62 % of patients over 17 weeks of treatment [1]. However, in an unblinded single arm study from France, prednisolone was used at a dose of 1 mg/kg for between 3 and 7 weeks with induction of remission observed in 92 % [4]. This raises the possibility that the upper ranges of the steroid dose–response relationship has not been completely elucidated and that doses greater than the usual 40–60 mg per day of prednisone, or its equivalent, may provide additional benefit. Despite this possibility daily doses of steroid higher than the equivalent of 60 mg of prednisone are usually not recommended in the current environment when alternative induction therapies are available for Crohn's disease patients.

In the acutely ill patient it is important to sufficiently exclude the presence of an abscess or systemic sepsis before initiating any form of systemic steroid. In the European Cooperative Crohn's Disease Study, of the five deaths that occurred during or shortly after the study period, three occurred in patients treated with steroids who had a palpable abdominal mass prior to initiation of therapy [2]. No routine imaging was performed prior to study entry and, as a result, it is quite likely that these masses could have represented Crohn's related abscesses or collections that were not properly managed with drainage and antibiotic therapy prior to initiation of prednisolone.

Topical rectally administered steroids, in the form of liquid or foam enemas, can also be used as adjuvant therapy in controlling local symptoms in patients with distal colonic or rectal Crohn's disease. However, there is no evidence that this is an effective strategy and their use is based upon extension of the data from ulcerative colitis.

Budesonide

For patients with ileal or ileocolonic Crohn's disease the use of the controlled ileal release preparation of the topically active steroid budesonide is an effective treatment for controlling symptoms of active disease. When administered at a dose of 9 mg per day budesonide was shown to be more effective than placebo [5] and mesalamine [6]. Another placebo controlled trial demonstrated a trended towards higher remission rates on budesonide 9 mg once daily (46.2 %) and 4.5 mg twice daily (51.9 %) as compared with placebo (31.7 %) but this was not statistically significant [7]. A small Japanese trial showed a trend toward higher rate of clinical remission in patients receiving budesonide 9 mg per day compared with placebo (23.1 % versus 11.5 %) after 8 weeks of therapy in patients with ileal, ileocecal, or ascending colon involvement [8].

Doses greater than 9 mg per day do not appear to have any further therapeutic gain and may be associated with a greater incidence of steroid associated side effects and adrenal suppression [5, 8].

Another trial compared 16 weeks of budesonide 9 mg daily to mesalamine 2 g twice daily for control of active ileal or ileocolic Crohn's disease and demonstrated clear superiority for budesonide with 62 % of budesonide-treated patients and 36 % of mesalamine-treated patients in remission at the end of the study period [6]. Severe and serious adverse events were observed less often in budesonide-treated patients. Ten percent of budesonide-treated patients had abnormal ACTH stimulated cortisol testing at the end of 16 weeks of treatment.

Budesonide that is absorbed from the intestinal lumen into the portal circulation undergoes high first pass metabolism through the liver leading to the production of inactive metabolites. It is this high first pass metabolism that likely results in the favorable short term safety profile with steroid associated side effects seen no more frequently on a 9 mg daily dose as compared with patients receiving placebo. However, the 9 mg daily dose of budesonide resulted in a lowering of basal plasma cortisol levels in two trials [5, 6] and in another trial a smaller proportion of patients receiving budesonide had normal adrenal function after 8 weeks (53 % versus 83 %) [7]. Both placebo controlled trials demonstrated a reduction in ACTH stimulated plasma cortisol levels in patients treated with budesonide [5, 7]. Given the demonstrated subclinical degree of adrenal suppression the use of adrenal replacement therapy for patients undergoing surgery or other severe physiologic stresses should be considered in patients currently or recently on budesonide at a dose of 9 mg per day.

When compared directly to the use of conventional systemic steroids in patients with ileal and ileocolic Crohn's disease it appears that budesonide controlled ileal release formulation may produce somewhat less reduction in disease activity [9], although another study showed roughly equivalent efficacy [10]. In both studies, induction of remission was slightly less frequent with budesonide than with prednisolone, although the differences were not statistically significant [9, 10]. In the study of Rutgeerts and colleagues, fewer steroid associated side effects and less suppression of morning cortisol levels were observed on budesonide as compared with conventional steroids [9]. In the study of Campieri, steroid associated side effects were observed at similar frequencies in patients treated with budesonide and those treated with conventional steroids, although moon face was observed much more frequently on prednisolone [10]. Adrenal suppression, as measured by short ACTH stimulation test, was more frequent in patients treated with conventional systemic steroids [10].

A third small study of the controlled ileal release preparation of budesonide was carried out in pediatric patients with active Crohn's disease [11]. In that study the starting dose of prednisolone, the comparator conventional steroid, was adjusted between 20 and 40 mg per day according to the patient's body weight. All patients in the budesonide arm received 9 mg per day for 8 weeks. The proportion of patients who achieved clinical remission by the end of 8 weeks was higher in the prednisolone treated arm (71 % versus 55 %) but this was not statistically significant [11]. Possible steroid associated side effects were noted in 77 % of the prednisolone-treated patients compared with 50 % of the budesonide-treated patients. In particular, moon face and acne were much less frequent in the budesonide-treated patients. Similar to the adult studies, mean morning cortisol levels were higher in the budesonide-treated patients. Sixty-two percent of patients receiving budesonide had abnormal ACTH stimulated cortisol test results at the end of 8 weeks, indicating some degree of adrenal suppression, but this prevalence was less than the 89 % seen in prednisolone-treated patients.

Budesonide has also been formulated using a pH-dependent release mechanism and has been compared directly with mesalamine [12] and with conventional systemic steroids in patients with active Crohn's disease [13, 14]. The pH-dependent release budesonide was found to be noninferior to mesalamine 4.5 g per day in 309 patients with mild to moderately active Crohn's disease with 69.5 % of patients treated with budesonide 9 mg once daily or 3 mg tid achieving remission after 8 weeks of therapy compared with 62.1 % of patients treated with mesalamine 4.5 g per day [12]. However, in this study, patients with only colonic involvement, including the left side of colon and rectum, were included. In another study, the pH-dependent budesonide, given as 3 mg three times daily, resulted in remission almost as frequently as prednisone 40 mg per day followed by a tapering schedule after 2 weeks (51 % versus 52.5 %) [13]. In this study, patients with only colonic involvement, including distal disease, were included. In patients with only colonic involvement prednisone was much more effective than budesonide. Another smaller trial of pH-dependent budesonide 9 mg once daily found a nonsignificant trend toward higher response rates on the conventional steroid, 6-methylprednisolone given as 48 mg daily for 1 week followed by a tapering schedule over 8 weeks (72.7 % versus 55.9 %) [14].

One trial also examined the proportion of patients who achieved remission while not experiencing any side effects and found that 30 % of budesonide-treated patients met this goal whereas only 14 % of prednisone-treated patients did so [13].

Pooled analysis of the studies that have compared budesonide to conventional steroids for induction of remission demonstrates a likelihood of remission on budesonide that is approximately 85 % of that observed on conventional steroids [15].

Maintenance Therapy

Conventional Steroids

It is generally accepted that steroids are neither safe nor effective for maintenance of remission in Crohn's disease. Several controlled trials have shown no improvement in remission rates in patients treated with maintenance low dose steroids as compared with placebo [1, 2, 16]. Although these trials may have not demonstrated a statistically significant reduction in relapse rates on steroids, it is possible that this could have been due to inadequate sample size within the individual studies. The largest study to examine this question was the National Cooperative Crohn's Disease Study Part II in which patients with preexisting quiescent disease were randomly assigned to receive placebo, prednisone 0.25 mg/kg per day, sulfasalazine or azathioprine for up to 2 years [1]. However, this study included patients with both remission following medical therapy ($n=226$) and remission following surgical resection within the previous year ($n=48$). Of the total 274 patients participating in the trial, 101 were randomized to receive placebo, 61 to prednisone, 58 to sulfasalazine, and 54 to azathioprine. The heterogeneous patient population, with inclusion of patients with both medical and surgical induced remission may have diminished the trial's ability to find an overall treatment effect. However, combining the results of all three conventional steroid maintenance trials in a meta-analysis did not demonstrate any significant reduction in relapse rates in patients with quiescent Crohn's disease treated with steroids [17]. In addition to the fact that they do not appear to reduce relapse rates, chronic use of steroid therapy is associated with significant toxicity and potential adverse events. In the National Cooperative Crohn's Disease Study Part II in which patients were treated for up to 2 years, 26 % of patients experienced side effects that were rated as being moderate or severe. Moon face was observed in 25 %, hirsutism in 8 %, acne in 19 %, polyuria in 15 %, and muscle weakness in 3 % [1]. Although the deleterious effects of steroids on bone density are not measured in that trial, they are well known [18].

Although the major trials clearly showed no overall benefit of maintenance conventional steroids, there did appear to be a subset of patients within the ECCDS whose active disease was brought under control with a 6 week course of steroids who seemed to do better when they remained on low dose 6-methylprednisolone [2]. This seems to be consistent with the clinical experience of many physicians who find that there is a small proportion of patients who seem to be dependent on steroid therapy and, as such, are not able to reduce the dose below a certain threshold without recurrence of symptoms. In some cases, a proportion of symptoms are due to the adrenal suppression produced by chronic steroid use. However, in many cases it is clearly a recurrence of the Crohn's disease related symptoms. Nevertheless, the effect of low dose steroids on the course of Crohn's disease has not been shown to be beneficial and, given the potential long term side effects of steroids, even at low doses, other steroid sparing strategies and maintenance therapies are currently favored. These include the use of immunomodulators such as azathioprine, 6-mercaptopurine, or methotrexate and the use of biologic agents such as the anti-TNFα drugs infliximab, adalimumab, and certolizumab, the anti-integrin and anti-adhesion molecule drugs such as vedolizumab, and the anti-interleukin-23 drugs such as ustekinumab and briakinumab.

Budesonide

The side effect profile of the topically active steroid, budesonide, is more favorable than that of conventional systemically administered and available steroids but budesonide, at a maintenance dose of 6 mg per day, has been shown only to delay the recurrence of Crohn's disease symptoms in patients who achieved remission on an 8 week acute course of the ileal release form of budesonide [19]. Despite the fact that the occurrence of steroid associated side effects necessitating discontinuation of therapy was uncommon over 1 year of maintenance therapy, patients were no more likely to be in remission on budesonide by the end of 1 year of therapy than if they had received no active therapy. Other studies have confirmed the lack of efficacy of budesonide at doses of 3 or 6 mg per day in maintaining remission that has been achieved be an induction course of budesonide or conventional steroids [20–26]. A relatively small study compared the use of budesonide, 6–9 mg per day, to azathioprine for maintenance of remission in patients with steroid dependent ileocolonic Crohn's disease and found higher rates of endoscopic healing and histologic remission and a trend toward a higher rate of clinical remission in the azathioprine group [27]. Another relatively small study randomized patients with steroid dependent ileitis or ileocolitis or colitis who refused immunosuppressive therapy to receive either budesonide 6 mg per day or 5-aminosalicylic acid (5-ASA) 1 g tid for 1 year [28]. Relapse rates were lower in the budesonide-treated patients (55 % versus 82 %) and these patients also had higher quality of life scores [28].

Two other studies have determined that budesonide, given at doses of 3 or 6 mg daily, is not effective at preventing post-operative endoscopic recurrence of Crohn's disease [29, 30].

Meta-analysis of the budesonide maintenance trials did not provide any evidence for effectiveness of budesonide in maintaining remission, although heterogeneity among the included studies was high [31].

Although the side effect profile of budesonide is better than that of conventional steroids, with apparently less loss of bone mineral density [26], patients on budesonide were approximately 20–50 % more likely than patients on placebo to experience an adverse event deemed to be related to treatment [31]. In addition, an abnormal ACTH stimulation test was approximately two to three times more likely in patients on budesonide as compared with placebo [31].

References

1. Summers RW, Switz DM, Sessions Jr JT, Becktel JM, Best WR, Kern Jr F, et al. National Cooperative Crohn's Disease Study: results of drug treatment. Gastroenterology. 1979;77:847–69.
2. Malchow H, Ewe K, Brandes JW, Goebell H, Ehms H, Sommer H, et al. European Cooperative Crohn's Disease Study (ECCDS): results of drug treatment. Gastroenterology. 1984;86:249–66.
3. Benchimol EI, Seow CH, Steinhart AH, Griffiths AM. Traditional corticosteroids for induction of remission in Crohn's disease. Cochrane Database Syst Rev. 2008: CD006792.
4. Modigliani R, Mary JY, Simon JF, Cortot A, Soule JC, Gendre JP, et al. Clinical, biological, and endoscopic picture of attacks of Crohn's disease. Evolution on prednisolone. Groupe d'Etude Therapeutique des Affections Inflammatoires Digestives. Gastroenterology. 1990;98:811–8.
5. Greenberg GR, Feagan BG, Martin F, Sutherland LR, Thomson AB, Williams CN, et al. Oral budesonide for active Crohn's disease. Canadian Inflammatory Bowel Disease Study Group. N Engl J Med. 1994;331:836–41.
6. Thomsen OO, Cortot A, Jewell D, Wright JP, Winter T, Veloso FT, et al. A comparison of budesonide and mesalamine for active Crohn's disease. International Budesonide-Mesalamine Study Group. N Engl J Med. 1998;339:370–4.
7. Tremaine WJ, Hanauer SB, Katz S, Winston BD, Levine JG, Persson T, et al. Budesonide CIR capsules (once or twice daily divided-dose) in active Crohn's disease: a randomized placebo-controlled study in the United States. Am J Gastroenterol. 2002;97:1748–54.
8. Suzuki Y, Motoya S, Takazoe M, Kosaka T, Date M, Nii M, et al. Efficacy and tolerability of oral budesonide in Japanese patients with active Crohn's disease: a multicentre, double-blind, randomized, parallel-group Phase II study. J Crohns Colitis. 2013;7: 239–47.
9. Rutgeerts P, Lofberg R, Malchow H, Lamers C, Olaison G, Jewell D, et al. A comparison of budesonide with prednisolone for active Crohn's disease. N Engl J Med. 1994;331:842–5.
10. Campieri M, Ferguson A, Doe W, Persson T, Nilsson LG. Oral budesonide is as effective as oral prednisolone in active Crohn's disease. The Global Budesonide Study Group. Gut. 1997;41:209–14.
11. Escher JC. Budesonide versus prednisolone for the treatment of active Crohn's disease in children: a randomized, double-blind, controlled, multicentre trial. Eur J Gastroenterol Hepatol. 2004; 16:47–54.
12. Tromm A, Bunganic I, Tomsova E, Tulassay Z, Lukas M, Kykal J, et al. Budesonide 9 mg is at least as effective as mesalamine 4.5 g in patients with mildly to moderately active Crohn's disease. Gastroenterology. 2011;140:425–34.e1; quiz e13.
13. Bar-Meir S, Chowers Y, Lavy A, Abramovitch D, Sternberg A, Leichtmann G, et al. Budesonide versus prednisone in the treatment of active Crohn's disease. The Israeli Budesonide Study Group. Gastroenterology. 1998;115:835–40.
14. Gross V, Andus T, Caesar I, Bischoff SC, Lochs H, Tromm A, et al. Oral pH-modified release budesonide versus 6-methylprednisolone in active Crohn's disease. German/Austrian Budesonide Study Group. Eur J Gastroenterol Hepatol. 1996;8:905–9.
15. Seow CH, Benchimol EI, Griffiths AM, Otley AR, Steinhart AH. Budesonide for induction of remission in Crohn's disease. Cochrane Database Syst Rev. 2008: CD000296.
16. Smith RC, Rhodes J, Heatley RV, Hughes LE, Crosby DL, Rees BI, et al. Low dose steroids and clinical relapse in Crohn's disease: a controlled trial. Gut. 1978;19:606–10.
17. Steinhart AH, Ewe K, Griffiths AM, Modigliani R, Thomsen OO. Corticosteroids for maintaining remission of Crohn's disease. Cochrane Database Syst Rev. 2000: CD000301.
18. Schulte CM. Review article: bone disease in inflammatory bowel disease. Aliment Pharmacol Ther. 2004;20 Suppl 4:43–9.
19. Greenberg GR, Feagan BG, Martin F, Sutherland LR, Thomson AB, Williams CN, et al. Oral budesonide as maintenance treatment for Crohn's disease: a placebo-controlled, dose-ranging study. Canadian Inflammatory Bowel Disease Study Group. Gastroenterology. 1996;110:45–51.
20. Cortot A, Colombel JF, Rutgeerts P, Lauritsen K, Malchow H, Hamling J, et al. Switch from systemic steroids to budesonide in steroid dependent patients with inactive Crohn's disease. Gut. 2001;48:186–90.
21. de Jong DJ, Bac DJ, Tan G, de Boer SY, Grabowsky IL, Jansen JB, et al. Maintenance treatment with budesonide 6 mg versus 9 mg once daily in patients with Crohn's disease in remission. Neth J Med. 2007;65:339–45.
22. Ferguson A, Campieri M, Doe W, Persson T, Nygard G. Oral budesonide as maintenance therapy in Crohn's disease—results of a 12-month study. Global Budesonide Study Group. Aliment Pharmacol Ther. 1998;12:175–83.
23. Gross V, Andus T, Ecker KW, Raedler A, Loeschke K, Plauth M, et al. Low dose oral pH modified release budesonide for maintenance of steroid induced remission in Crohn's disease. The Budesonide Study Group. Gut. 1998;42:493–6.
24. Hanauer S, Sandborn WJ, Persson A, Persson T. Budesonide as maintenance treatment in Crohn's disease: a placebo-controlled trial. Aliment Pharmacol Ther. 2005;21:363–71.
25. Lofberg R, Rutgeerts P, Malchow H, Lamers C, Danielssonn A, Olaison G, et al. Budesonide prolongs time to relapse in ileal and ileocaecal Crohn's disease. A placebo controlled one year study. Gut. 1996;39:82–6.
26. Schoon EJ, Bollani S, Mills PR, Israeli E, Felsenberg D, Ljunghall S, et al. Bone mineral density in relation to efficacy and side effects of budesonide and prednisolone in Crohn's disease. Clin Gastroenterol Hepatol. 2005;3:113–21.
27. Mantzaris GJ, Christidou A, Sfakianakis M, Roussos A, Koilakou S, Petraki K, et al. Azathioprine is superior to budesonide in achieving and maintaining mucosal healing and histologic remission in steroid-dependent Crohn's disease. Inflamm Bowel Dis. 2009;15:375–82.
28. Mantzaris GJ, Petraki K, Sfakianakis M, Archavlis E, Christidou A, Chadio-Iordanides H, et al. Budesonide versus mesalamine for maintaining remission in patients refusing other immunomodulators for steroid-dependent Crohn's disease. Clin Gastroenterol Hepatol. 2003;1:122–8.
29. Ewe K, Bottger T, Buhr HJ, Ecker KW, Otto HF. Low-dose budesonide treatment for prevention of postoperative recurrence of Crohn's disease: a multicentre randomized placebo-controlled trial. German Budesonide Study Group. Eur J Gastroenterol Hepatol. 1999;11:277–82.
30. Hellers G, Cortot A, Jewell D, et al. Oral budesonide for prevention of postsurgical recurrence in Crohn's disease. The IOIBD Budesonide Study Group. Gastroenterology. 1999;116:294–300.
31. Kuenzig ME, Rezaie A, Seow CH, et al. Budesonide for maintenance of remission in Crohn's disease. Cochrane Database Syst Rev. 2014;8:CD002913.

Thiopurines in Crohn's Disease

30

Adi Lahat and Rami Eliakim

Abbreviations

CD	Crohn's disease
6-MP	6-mercaptopurine
AZA	Azathioprine
TPMT	Thiopurine-S-methyl transferase
Anti-TNFa	Anti-tumor necrosis factor a
6-MMPRs	6-methylmercaptopurine ribonucleotides
6-TGNs	6-thioguanine (6-TG) nucleotides
ECCO	European Crohn's and Colitis Organization
CDAI	Crohn's disease activity index
NNT	Number needed to treat
OR	Odds ratio
RR	Relative risk
SONIC	The study of biologic and immunomodulation naïve patient in Crohn's disease
NHR	Nodular regenerative hyperplasia
HLH	Hem phagocytic lymphohistiocytosis
EBV	Epstein–Barr virus
VOD	Veno-occlusive disease
HSTCL	Hepatosplenic T-cell lymphoma
CESAME	The European Commission's Clearing and Settlement Advisory and Monitoring Expert Group
HCV	Hepatitis c virus
HBV	Hepatitis B virus
HIV	Human immunodeficiency virus
VZV	Varicella zoster virus
TB	Tuberculosis
HPV	Human papilloma virus
CBC	Complete blood count
LFTs	Liver function tests
RBC	Red blood cells

A. Lahat, M.D. (✉) • R. Eliakim, M.D.
Department of Gastroenterology, Chaim Sheba Medical Center, Sackler School of Medicine, Tel-Aviv University, Tel Aviv, Israel
e-mail: zokadi@gmail.com

In the last few decades, the use of thiopurine agents has been one of the cornerstones in CD treatment. Both azathioprine (AZA) and 6-mercaptopurine (6-MP) are effective in maintaining remission and steroid sparing of CD patients refractory to or dependent of steroids [1, 2]. Purine analogs were also shown to prevent postoperative recurrence in CD [3, 4]. Even in the era of biologic treatment, the place of thiopurines in CD treatment is well established, and their use is widespread.

Purine metabolites were first synthesized in 1957 by Hitching and Elion, who hypothesized that the growth of rapidly dividing cells might be blocked with antimetabolites of nucleic acid bases [5]. Their work led to the development of thioguanine, 6-MP, and AZA—collectively named thiopurine analogs.

Thiopurine Metabolism

AZA and MP are prodrugs that undergo enzymatic metabolism. A simplified version of the metabolic pathway is shown in Fig. 30.1 [6]. First, the majority of AZA is metabolized to 6-MP. Notably, a small amount is metabolized to purine bases associated with hypersensitivity reactions [7]. Then, most of MP is metabolized by xanthine oxidase into an inactive metabolite—6-thiouric acid, which is excreted in the urine [8]. The remaining substrate is metabolized via two competing pathways. In one pathway, the enzyme thiopurine-S-methyl transferase (TPMT) methylates MP to form 6-methylmercaptopurine ribonucleotides (6-MMPRs), which are inactive metabolites. Alternatively, 6 MP is metabolized by a group of enzymes known as the purine salvage pathway to produce the pharmacologically active metabolites 6-thioguanine (6-TG) nucleotides (6-TGNs; the sum of 6-TG monophosphate (6-thio-GMP), 6-TG diphosphate (6-thio-GDP), and 6-TG triphosphate (6-thio-PTP)) [8]. Among the 6-TGNs, 6-thio-GTP is the main metabolite accounting for 80 % of the substrate, 6-thio-GDP accounts for 16 %, while only traces of 6-thio-GMP are present [9]. Schematic illustration of thiopurine metabolism is shown in Fig. 30.1.

D.C. Baumgart (ed.), *Crohn's Disease and Ulcerative Colitis*, DOI 10.1007/978-3-319-33703-6_30

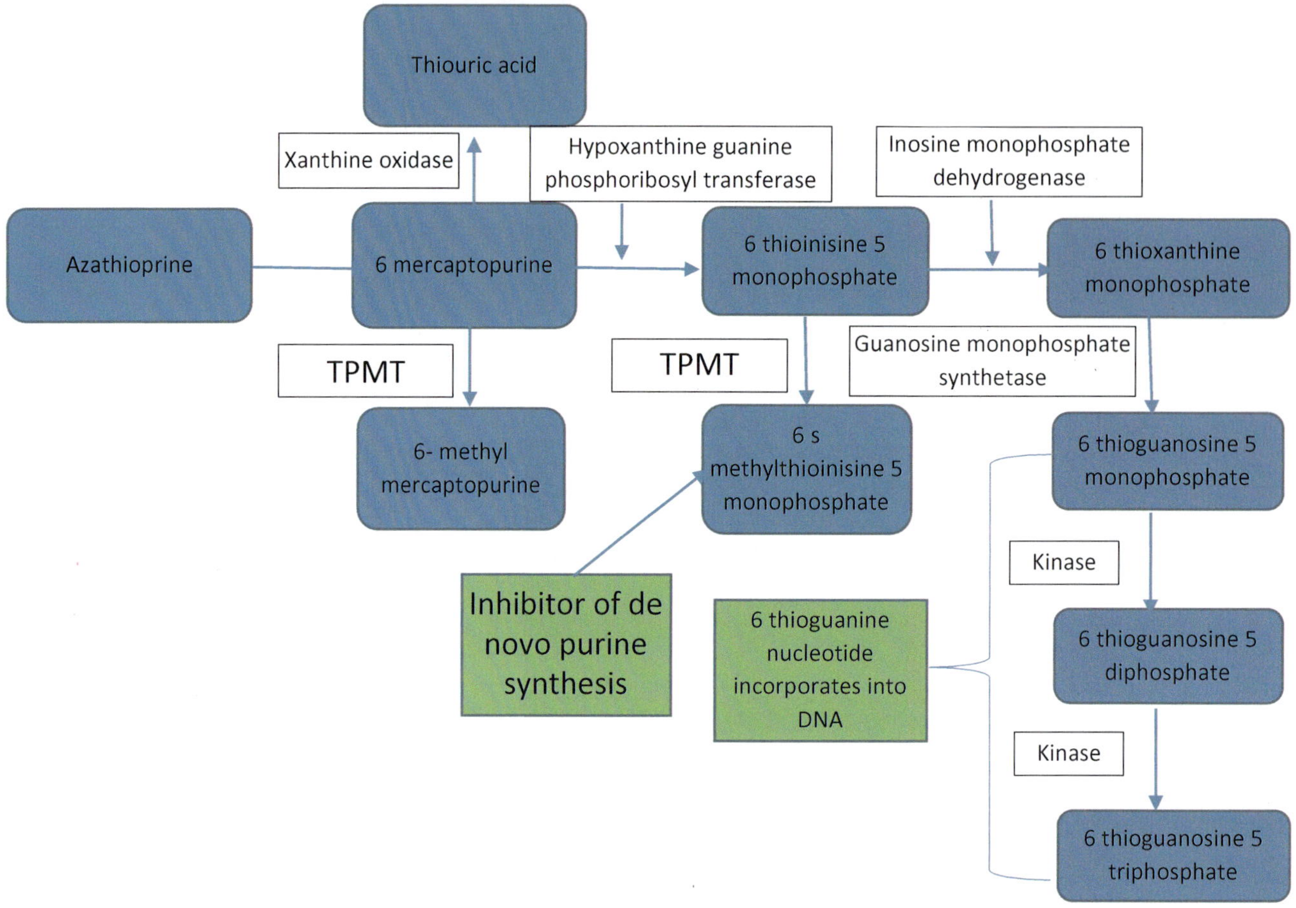

Fig. 30.1 Azathioprine metabolism. *TPMT* thiopurine-S-methyl transferase

Pharmacologic Mechanism of Thiopurines

6-TGNs affect the immune response via several potential mechanisms. They are incorporated into DNA, thereby inhibiting its synthesis and causing DNA strand breakage—and thus suppressing cell proliferation [10]. Other mechanisms include direct cytotoxicity, inhibition of de novo purine biosynthesis, and suppression of cytokine synthesis [8, 11–13].

Another important mechanism is by inducing T-cell apoptosis by modulating cell Rac 1 signaling. Rac 1 bounds to the metabolite 6-Thio-GTP instead of GTP, thus blocking the Rac1 activation pathway. Thus, Rac1 targeted genes as mitogen activated protein kinase, NF-kB, and bcl-x (L) are suppressed—leading to mitochondrial pathway of apoptosis [14, 15]. Defects in T cell apoptosis were identified as one of the triggers of gut inflammation in CD [16, 17].

Efficacy of Thiopurine Therapy in CD

The use of thiopurines for IBD treatment was initiated in the early 1960s [18, 19]. Since then, the effect of the medication on disease activity and symptoms has been intensively studied. AZA AND 6-MP were both shown to be effective in induction of remission of active CD with an odds ratio of up to 3.1 compared with placebo [20, 21].

Therapeutic onset after thiopurine initiation was shown to be between 12 and 17 weeks, the time needed for TGNs to be incorporated into DNA [22]. This Cochrane meta-analysis published in 2010 included eight randomized placebo-controlled trials in adults with active CD. The outcome measure was the proportion of patients with clinical improvement or remission (as defined by the Crohn's disease activity index (CDAI), the Harvey–Bradshaw Index, subjective evaluation, or steroid sparing effect). The pooled response rate was 54 % for the group with thiopurine analogs versus 34 % for the placebo treated patients.

The OR of response to azathioprine or 6-mercaptopurine therapy compared with placebo in active Crohn's disease was 2.43 (95 % CI 1.62–3.64). The number needed to treat (NNT) was 5 to observe an effect of therapy in one patient. Treatment of >17 weeks resulted in an OR of 2.61 (95 % CI 1.69–4.03). A steroid sparing effect was seen with an OR of 3.69 (95 % CI 2.12–6.42), with NNT of 3 to observe steroid sparing in one patient [22].

Another Cochrane meta-analysis including seven maintenance CD trials found that the OR for maintenance of remission was 2.32 with an NNT of 6. The OR for maintenance of remission with 6-MP was 3.32, with an NNT of 4 [2]. Overall remission rate was 71 % for AZA compared with 55 % for placebo.

However, a recent Cochrane database systematic review published in 2013 showed contradicting results [23]. This meta-analysis included 13 randomized controlled trials of thiopurine treatment compared to placebo or active therapy involving adult patients with active CD. One thousand two hundred and eleven patients were included in the study. The study found no statistically significant difference in clinical remission rates between thiopurines and placebo. Forty-eight percent (95/197) of patients receiving antimetabolites achieved remission compared to 37 % (68/183) of placebo patients (five studies, 380 patients; RR 1.23, 95 % CI 0.97–1.55). No statistically significant difference in clinical improvement rates were found between azathioprine or 6-mercaptopurine and placebo treated patients. Forty-eight percent (107/225) of patients receiving antimetabolites achieved clinical improvement or remission compared to 36 % (75/209) of placebo patients (eight studies, 434 patients; RR 1.26, 95 % CI 0.98–1.62). There was a statistically significant difference in steroid sparing (defined as prednisone dose < 10 mg/day while maintaining remission) between azathioprine and placebo. Sixty-four percent (47/163) of azathioprine patients were able to reduce their prednisone dose to <10 mg/day compared to 46 % (32/70) of placebo patients (RR 1.34, 95 % CI 1.02–1.77).

These results challenge the accepted concept regarding thiopurine treatment in CD patients that was accumulated in 6 decades of usage, and should be taken with excessive cautious.

Nevertheless, the second European evidence-based Consensus on the diagnosis and management of Crohn's disease from the European Crohn's and Colitis Organization (ECCO) states that AZA 1.5–2.5 mg/kg/day or 6-MP 0.75–1.5 mg/kg/day may be used in active CD as adjunctive therapy or steroid-sparing agent, and is also effective for the maintenance of remission in CD and has a steroid-sparing effect [24].

Mucosal Healing

Mucosal healing is an important indicator to evaluate the efficacy of treatment and serves as a predictor of delayed onset complications and a decreased need for surgery [25]. Therefore, mucosal healing is used as a therapeutic endpoint in many clinical trials [26–28].

Mucosal healing as a therapeutic goal in patients treated with thiopurines as a single agent was assessed in several studies [29–32]. A recent study from China assessed long-term mucosal healing in 36 patients with small bowel CD naïve to biologic therapy and to thiopurines using double balloon enteroscopy. After 6 months of treatment with an average dose of 61.8 ± 17.2 mg/day of AZA 26 patients (72.2 %) achieved clinical remission and the ten patients (27.8 %) had a clinical response. After 12 months of treatment, complete mucosal healing was achieved in seven patients (19.4 %), near-complete healing (defined as a marked endoscopic improvement, possible aphthous ulcers (<0.5 cm) or erosions in the absence of stenosis, the affected segment is less than 50 %) in 2 (5.6 %), partial healing (defined as less than 50 % affected areas and the size of the biggest ulcer of less than 2 cm, considerable numbers of ulcers still persisted and single luminal narrowing observed, but was passable by DBE) in 10 (27.8 %) and no healing in 17 (47.2 %). After 24 months of treatment complete healing was observed in 11 (30.6 %), near-complete healing in 9 (25.0 %), partial healing in 12 (33.3 %) and no healing in 4 (11.1 %) [29]. Another study compared AZA (2.0–2.5 mg/kg a day, $n = 38$) to Budesonide (BUD) (6–9 mg /day, $n = 39$) for 1 year [30]. Mucosal healing was assessed using ileocolonoscopy with regional biopsies. At the end of the study 32 and 25 patients in the AZA and BUD groups, respectively, were in clinical remission ($P = 0.07$). The Crohn's Disease Endoscopic Index of Severity (CDEIS) score fell significantly only in the AZA group ($P < 0.0001$). Complete or near complete healing of colonic mucosa was achieved in 83 % of AZA-treated patients compared to 24 % of BUD-treated patients ($P < 0.0001$). Histologic activity as assessed by an average histology score (AHS) fell significantly only in the AZA group ($P < 0.001$ versus baseline) and was significantly lower than in the BUD group at the end of the study ($P < 0.001$). In the terminal ileum complete healing was achieved in (59 %), near-complete healing in 4 of 19 (21 %) patients, partial healing in 16 %, and no change in 5 % of AZA-treated patients compared with 12 %, 18 %,24 %, and 35 % of BUD-treated patients, respectively ($P = 0.001$ and $P = 0.04$, for complete healing and worse/no change, respectively).

The SONIC trial [26] (The study of biologic and immunomodulation naïve patient in Crohn's disease) included 508 CD immunosuppressive and biologic naïve patients. At week 26, colonic mucosal healing was achieved in 16.5 % of patients on azathioprine monotherapy. Further colonoscopies after longer treatment period were not performed. However, week 26 is probably too early to assess mucosal healing on thiopurine therapy since as written above, therapeutic effect after treatment initiation only begins after 12–17 weeks [22].

Perianal Disease

Thiopurines were shown to be more effective than placebo for perianal fistula closure. In a prospective study conducted on 83 CD patients, the efficacy of 2 years 6-MP treatment compared to placebo was assessed. Thirty one percent of patients treated with 6-MP achieved closure of their fistula compared with only 6 % in the placebo group ($P<0.001$) [1]. Another observational study showed complete fistula closure in 39 % of patients and improvement in 26 % after >6 months of treatment [33].

In a meta-analysis of five clinical trials in which fistula closure served as a secondary end point, 54 % of patients treated with thiopurines had an improvement of their fistula status compared to 21 % of the placebo group (OR = 4.4 CI 1.5–13.2) [20].

Postoperative Recurrence

Postoperative endoscopic recurrence of CD has been reported to be as high as 73 % 1 year post surgery [34], and clinical relapse rates have been reported to range from 22–55 % 5 years post surgery [35]. Facing the high recurrence rate, preventive treatment post-surgery for maintaining remission is usually warned.

The role of thiopurines in postsurgical maintenance of disease remission was assessed in various clinical trials [36–41]. A recent Cochrane database meta-analysis summarizing the results of seven randomized controlled studies (584 CD patients post bowel resection) was published in 2014 [36]. The studies included in the analysis compared treatment with thiopurines to placebo, 5-ASA and anti-TNF agents. A pooled analysis of two studies ($n=168$ patients) showed 48 % relapse in thiopurine treated patients compared to 63 % relapse in the placebo group (RR 0.74, 95 % CI 0.58–0.94). A pooled analysis of five studies ($n=425$ patients) showed 63 % clinical relapse in patients treated with thiopurines, compared to 54 % of 5-ASA patients (RR 1.15, 95 % CI 0.99–1.34). One study ($n=33$) found decreased clinical (RR 5.18, 95 % CI 1.35–19.83) and endoscopic relapse (RR 10.35, 95 % CI 1.50). In summary, thiopurines are probably better than placebo for maintaining postsurgical remission. They might be less efficient than anti-TNFa agents—but data is scarce. Comparing their efficacy to 5-ASA agents is inconclusive.

Further research to assess their role in postoperative maintenance is warranted.

Timing of Treatment Initiation

Early data favors early commencing of immunomodulatory treatment in order to alter disease progression and avoid complications. Data from two studies in pediatric patients [42, 43] showed better outcome in patients treated with thiopurines within 3 months from diagnosis. Punati et al. [42] compared outcome in newly diagnosed CD pediatric patients treated within 0–3 months from diagnosis ($n=150$) (early) compared with patients treated within 3–12 months from diagnosis ($n=49$) (late). Twelfth months from diagnosis only 22 % of the early group had received corticosteroids in the preceding quarter, compared to 41 % from of late group ($P=0.013$). The number of hospitalizations per patient was significantly lower in the early group over the 2-year follow-up ($P=0.03$). No difference was noted in the rates of remission, infliximab use over time, or surgery.

A recent study from the Groupe d'Etude Thérapeutique des Affections Inflammatoires du Tube Digestif [44] compared early administration of AZA (within 6 months from diagnosis) with conventional management (AZA only in cases of corticosteroid dependency, chronic active disease with frequent flares, poor response to corticosteroids, or development of severe perianal disease). Patients were prospectively followed for 3 years. Primary end point was steroids and/or anti-TNFa-free remission during follow-up. During follow-up, 61 % of the conventional treatment group needed AZA initiation, at median time of 11 months. Remission rates did not differ between the groups (67 % in the early treatment group vs 56 % in the conventional) ($P=.69$). Among secondary outcomes, higher percentage of early treatment group was free of perianal surgery than in the conventional management group (96 % ± 3 % and 82 % ± 6 % at month 36, respectively; $P=.036$). The cumulative proportion of patients free of intestinal surgery and anti-TNF therapy did not differ between groups. The study conclusion was that early treatment with AZA had no benefit over conventional therapy in increasing time of clinical remission. A recent Spanish multicenter study reported similar results [45].

The conflicting results between these studies might be explained by the different patients' population (pediatric vs adults). However, the results of this prospective study challenge the common opinion regarding the yield of early treatment for all patients. Notably, almost 40 % of patients in the conventional treatment group were immunomodulators free for 3 years after diagnosis. Considering the drug adverse effects this is important data that should be taken into account while making decisions on treatment initiation. These data emphasize the importance of risk stratification and personalized—tailored—treatment while taking therapeutic decisions.

Duration of Treatment

The question of treatment duration after achieving long-term clinical remission was addressed in two multicenter randomized placebo-controlled trials. The first was published in 2005 [46] by Lemann et al. included 83 CD patients in clinical remission on AZA therapy for at least 42 months. Patients were randomized to maintenance therapy or placebo and were followed for 18 months. The primary end point was clinical relapse. At 18 months 8 % at the AZA group compared to 21 % in the placebo group relapsed. The difference did not reach statistical significance ($P=0.195$). C-reactive protein level >20 mg/L, time without steroids <50 months, and hemoglobin level <12 g/dL at baseline were found to be predictive of relapse in their multivariate analysis. The follow-up study published in 2009 [47] included 66 patients who stopped AZA treatment after median duration of 68 months treatment and 63 months remission. Thirty-two patients had a relapse after median follow-up of 54 months. The cumulative probabilities ± standard error of relapse at 1, 3, and 5 years were 14.0 % ± 4.3 %, 52.8 % ± 7.1 %, and 62.7 % ± 7.2 %, respectively. C-reactive protein concentration of 20 mg/L or greater, hemoglobin level less than 12 g/dL, and neutrophil count 4 × 10(9)/L or greater were associated increased risk of relapse. Retreatment with azathioprine alone achieved remission in 22/23 of the patients. A large retrospective multicenter study with 1176 IBD patients treated with AZA showed decreased disease exacerbations and need for steroid treatment within the first 4 years of AZA treatment ($P<0.001$). Treatment discontinuation after 3–4 years did not lead to immediate disease exacerbation; however continuation beyond 4 years decreased disease activity and steroid consumption [48]. A recent multicenter retrospective cohort study from the UK [49] included patients with at least 3 years thiopurine use that were in sustained clinical remission and with a minimum of 1 year of follow-up post drug withdrawal. Median duration of thiopurine use prior to withdrawal was 6.0 years. Relapse occurred in 23 % of patients at 12 months and 39 % at 24 months. Elevated CRP at withdrawal was again associated with higher relapse rates at 12 months.

According to the European Crohn's and Colitis Organization (ECCO) guidelines discontinuation of thiopurine maintenance therapy should be considered when the patient is 4 years in remission [50].

The conclusion driven from these studies is that if thiopurine treatment is well tolerated it should usually be continued for a long period. Risk factors for disease relapse as well as adverse events with long-term use as serious infections and risk of malignancy should be considered and discussed with the patient especially elderly patients, and decision should be individualized.

Combination Therapy with Anti-TNFa

The yield of combination therapy of thiopurines with anti-TNFa was assessed in several multicenter prospective studies. Baert et al. [51] showed that concomitant immunosuppressive therapy significantly lowers the titers of anti-infliximab antibodies, thus leading to improved pharmacokinetics as demonstrated by significantly higher concentrations of infliximab 4 weeks after drug infusion. The SONIC study that compared biologic therapy versus thiopurines alone or in combination in biologically and immunomodulation naïve and relatively newly diagnosed patients [26], included 508 CD patients. Fifty-seven percent of patients receiving combination therapy were in corticosteroid-free clinical remission at week 26 compared with 44.4 % of patients on infliximab monotherapy and 30.0 % of patients on azathioprine monotherapy. ($P<0.001$ for the comparison with combination therapy and $P=0.006$ for the comparison with infliximab.) Mucosal healing at week 26 was achieved in 44 % of patients receiving combination therapy, compared with 30 % of patients on infliximab monotherapy and 16.5 % of patients on azathioprine monotherapy ($P<0.001$ for the comparison with combination therapy and $P=0.02$ for the comparison with infliximab). At week 50 remission rates were 72 %, 61 % and 55 %, respectively.

Another study by Lémann et al. [52] assessed steroid-free remission at week 24 after combination therapy of thiopurines with infliximab or thiopurine monotherapy in patients naïve to immunomodulators and in patients that failed on a stable dose thiopurines In all patients group remission rates were higher on combination therapy; thus combination therapy was shown to be more effective than thiopurine monotherapy for induction of remission in steroid-dependent CD patients. However, at week 52 only 27 % of patients on combination therapy in the thiopurine failure group were still in remission off steroids, compared with 52 % in the naive group.

A recent meta-analysis assessed the yield of combination therapy of thiopurine with Adalimumab (ADA) [53]. Results showed that ADA monotherapy was inferior to combination therapy (OR = 0.78 CI 0.64–0.96, $P=0.02$) for induction of remission. However, there was no additional benefit of its addition for maintenance of remission or need for dose escalation over ADA monotherapy.

These evidence favors combination therapy in patients with moderate to severe CD, especially in immunosuppressive naïve patients. Combination therapy achieves higher rate of rapid disease control and limited tissue damage.

The superiority of combination therapy over monotherapy adds another therapeutic dilemma—whether and when to switch to monotherapy, and which of the treatments should be stopped. Van Assche et al. randomized 80 patients with at least 6 months of remission on combination therapy to infliximab monotherapy versus combination therapy [54]. After 104 weeks 60 % of the patients in the combination therapy group needed a change in infliximab doses or stopped therapy compared to 55 % of the infliximab monotherapy group (nonsignificant). CRP level were higher and the drug trough levels were lower, in the infliximab monotherapy group. They concluded that combination therapy beyond 6 months offers no clear benefit over scheduled infliximab monotherapy. The long-term implications of higher infliximab trough levels and decreased CRP levels in the combination group should be further studied. Predictors of relapse after azathioprine withdrawal were identified in a study by Oussalah et al. [55]. In this observational study patients were treated with combination therapy for at least 6 months before azathioprine was discontinued. At last follow-up (week 104), 35 out of 48 (73 %) patients were infliximab failure free. The disease-free probabilities were 85 % (±5 %) at 12 months and 41 % (±18 %) at both 24 and 32 months. Risk factor for disease relapse were in patients with duration of combination therapy of less than 27 months and/or the presence of biological inflammation (CRP>5 and platelets count>280,000).

Taken together, the decision whether and when to stop one of the medications on combination therapy should be taken individually, on the basis of disease history, side effects, personal preferences, and cost-effectiveness. Current data clearly indicates that combination therapy is more effective than monotherapy, and that thiopurine co-therapy is associated with higher infliximab trough levels.

Safety

Over 6 decades of thiopurine use in IBD provides a wide and very long-term safety profile. Generally, the medication is well tolerated. However, adverse events that require disease withdrawal occur in 10–18 % of patients. These include bone marrow toxicity, pancreatitis, and various allergic reactions as fever, flu-like illness, rash, and arthralgias [2, 20, 56–59]. Drug reaction may be related to drug metabolism and TPMT and TGN measurements can guide treatment (see below), but in 1–6.5 % of patients idiosyncratic reactions may occur [60]. Most of the nonspecific allergic reactions occur at treatment initiation, within 2–3 weeks, and tend to improve with time. Initiating treatment with 50 % of the optimal therapeutic dose can reduce the severity of the reaction and allow early intervention. Once tolerated, dose can be gradually increased with close monitoring of blood count, liver function tests, and TGN levels. Recent data suggests that dividing the optimal dose into two small daily doses can reduce some side effects as nausea [61, 62]. This treatment modification was also shown to improve long-term remission rate [63]. Patients who are intolerant to AZA may benefit from a switch to a metabolic descendant as 6-MP or TGN [64, 65]. Notably, post AZA/6-MP induced pancreatitis further treatment with 6-MP or AZA is contraindicated. However, tolerance and response to TGN was shown in these patients [66].

Hepatotoxicity may occur in 10–17 % of patients, and may be related to increased concentration of 6-MMPR [66]. Co-treatment with allopurinol was shown to shift the metabolic pathway to 6-TGN with normalization of liver enzymes [66, 67].

Rare disorders of the liver vasculature were described, including sinusoidal dilatation, nodular regenerative hyperplasia (NHR), fibrosis, peliosis hepatitis, and veno-occlusive disease (VOD) [68–70].

All immunomodulatory treatment carries an increased risk of infections. Thiopurines specifically increased susceptibility to viral infections [71]. In case of an acute infection, treatment with thiopurines can be withdrawn and renewed after recovery.

Risk of infections is accentuated in patients on combination therapy [71].

Mild leukopenia is observed in 5–25 % of patients treated with thiopurines and is associated with higher concentrations of 6 TGN metabolites. Leukopenia is most common at treatment initiation, but can occur at any time during treatment [57, 72].

Severe pancytopenia was reported in patients with TPMT deficiency. TPMT activity differs according to allelic polymorphism. In Caucasian population, 0.3 % is TPMT deficient with none or very little activity, 12.4 % have intermediate activity and 87.3 % have normal activity. Therefore, TPMT activity should be measured prior to therapy [73]. However, between 50 and 75 % of thiopurine related leukopenia occurs in patients with normal TPMT activity [74, 75]. Therefore, habitual monitoring during therapy is mandatory.

Most cases of myeloproliferative disorders in IBD patients on thiopurines are associated with EBV [76]. Recently, a few fatal cases have been reported in thiopurine treated young IBD EBV seronegative males associated with post-mononucleosis lymphoproliferation with or without hemophagocytic lymphohistiocytosis (HLH) [77]. Though the risk is very low, the ECCO Pathogenesis Scientific Workshop [78] recommends considering avoiding thiopurine treatment in IBD male patients less than 35 years who are EBV seronegative.

Increased risk of malignancy, specifically lymphoproliferative diseases is another concern during thiopurine therapy. The risk was shown to be ×4–×5 increased compared with the background population and is even more pronounced in elderly patients. Still, the absolute risk is low [79, 80].

Exposure to ultraviolet radiation was shown to increase the risk of non-melanoma skin cancer in thiopurine treated patients. A cohort study from South Africa [80] demonstrated an odds ratio of 5 for non-melanoma skin cancer. Among Caucasian patients the odds ratio was 12.4, and in non-Caucasians the risk was negligible.

Therefore, Caucasian patients on thiopurine therapy should be advised to avoid sun exposure and perform regular skin screening.

Recently, a large retrospective study assessed malignancy risk in patients treated with thiopurines and/or with anti-TNFa [81]. Data showed an increased risk of malignancy in IBD patients treated with thiopurines compared with patients treated with anti-TNF antibodies (hazard ratio 4.15; 95 % CI 1.82–9.44; $P=0.0007$; univariate Cox regression). Patients aged over 50 years treated with thiopurines had 18.2 % tendency to develop malignancy, compared with 3.8 % of patients under 50 years of age ($P=0.0008$). Treatment duration of more than 4 years was associated with an increased risk for skin cancer.

Table 30.1 Main side effects, prevalence, mechanism, and options to optimize treatment

Side effect	Symptoms	Prevalence	Onset	Mechanism	Optimizing treatment
Idiosyncratic reaction	Rash, arthralgia, hepatitis, myalgia, flu-like symptoms, GI complaints, fever, pancreatitis	1–6.5 %	Usually within 4 weeks from initiation	Immune mediated	Some reactions might be overcome with switch of AZA to 6-MP, or with split dose
Myelotoxicity	Leukopenia, anemia, thrombocytopenia	1.4–5 %	Usually within 8 weeks from initiation. However, it can develop throughout treatment	Dose dependent, caused by elevated 6-TGNs	Thiopurine treatment in TPMT deficient patients should be avoided. Habitual CBC throughout treatment
Hepatotoxicity	Variation from mildly elevated liver enzymes to liver fibrosis, nodular regenerative hyperplasia (NRH), veno-occlusive disease (VOD)	1–17 %	Dose independent within few weeks from initiation Dose dependent after months–years	Can be idiosyncratic (dose independent) or dose dependent. Dose-dependent histopathological changes	Habitual liver function tests throughout treatment
Malignancies	Mainly lymphomas and skin cancers	Rare	After years of treatment		Habitual skin screening, avoid sun exposure, avoid treatment in young EBV seronegative males

A recent prospective observational study from the CESAM study group [77] included 19,486 IBD patients with a total follow up of 49,736 patient-years, found that IBD patients with past exposure to thiopurines have a sevenfold increased risk to develop myeloproliferative disorders. The risk was not increased in IBD patients that stopped thiopurine treatment.

In the last decade a rare and aggressive extra-nodal form of non-Hodgkin's lymphoma—hepatosplenic T-cell lymphoma (HSTCL)—was reported in IBD patients, in association with immunosuppressive therapy [82–84]. Out of over 200 cases reported in the literature, less than 40 are IBD patients. The disease is often fatal.

All of the IBD patients were all treated with thiopurines alone or in combination therapy with anti-TNF a (more that 50 % of cases). Median thiopurine exposure was 6 years. Most patients were young (90 % were under 35 years) males (90 % of the cases). The ECCO Pathogenesis Scientific Workshop from 2014 [78] concluded that though the overall risk of HSTCL is very low, it is to be taken into account in young (<35 years) men treated with combination therapy with more than 2 years of thiopurine intake.

Table 30.1 summarizes the main side effects, their prevalence, and possible ways to optimize therapy.

Monitoring and Optimizing Thiopurine Therapy

There is a considerable diversity in drug absorption and metabolism among patients.

Thiopurine in vivo metabolism is influenced not only by the TPMT allelic polymorphism (see above) but also by the absorption, idiosyncratic reactions, and drug–drug interactions in each patient. The accepted AZA dose is 2–2.5 mg/kg/day and for 6-MP is 0.75–1.5 mg/kg/day [85]. The dose of TG is not related to body weight and is 20 mg/day. Since patients with TPMT deficiency are prone to severe pancytopenia upon thiopurine treatment, its levels should be measured prior to treatment initiation [73]. In addition to TPMT measurements, patients should be screened for infections and advised to be vaccinated accordingly.

Current European guidelines include [86] serological screening for the viruses: hepatitis c (HCV), hepatitis B (HBV), human immunodeficiency (HIV), varicella zoster (VZV). Screening for TB with chest X ray and interferon release assay should be considered. Screening for cervical cancer and human papilloma virus (HPV) in women is also advocated. Vaccinations that are indicated include: VZV, HPV, HBV, influenza (yearly), and pneumococcus (every 5 years). Live vaccines are contraindicated while on immunomodulatory treatment.

Upon treatment initiation, complete blood count (CBC) and liver function tests (LTTs) should be monitored every 2 weeks for the first 2 months and every 3 months thereafter. The purpose of monitoring is early detection of side effects, mainly pancytopenia, hepatitis, pancreatitis. As mentioned, most side effects tend to appear close to treatment initiation, but can appear at any time during treatment [74, 75].

TGN levels should be measured after 12–16 weeks, once the metabolite reached its steady state, in case of a flare to assure compliance and assess dose escalation, or in case of suspected toxicity. Early measurements, after 4 weeks, can

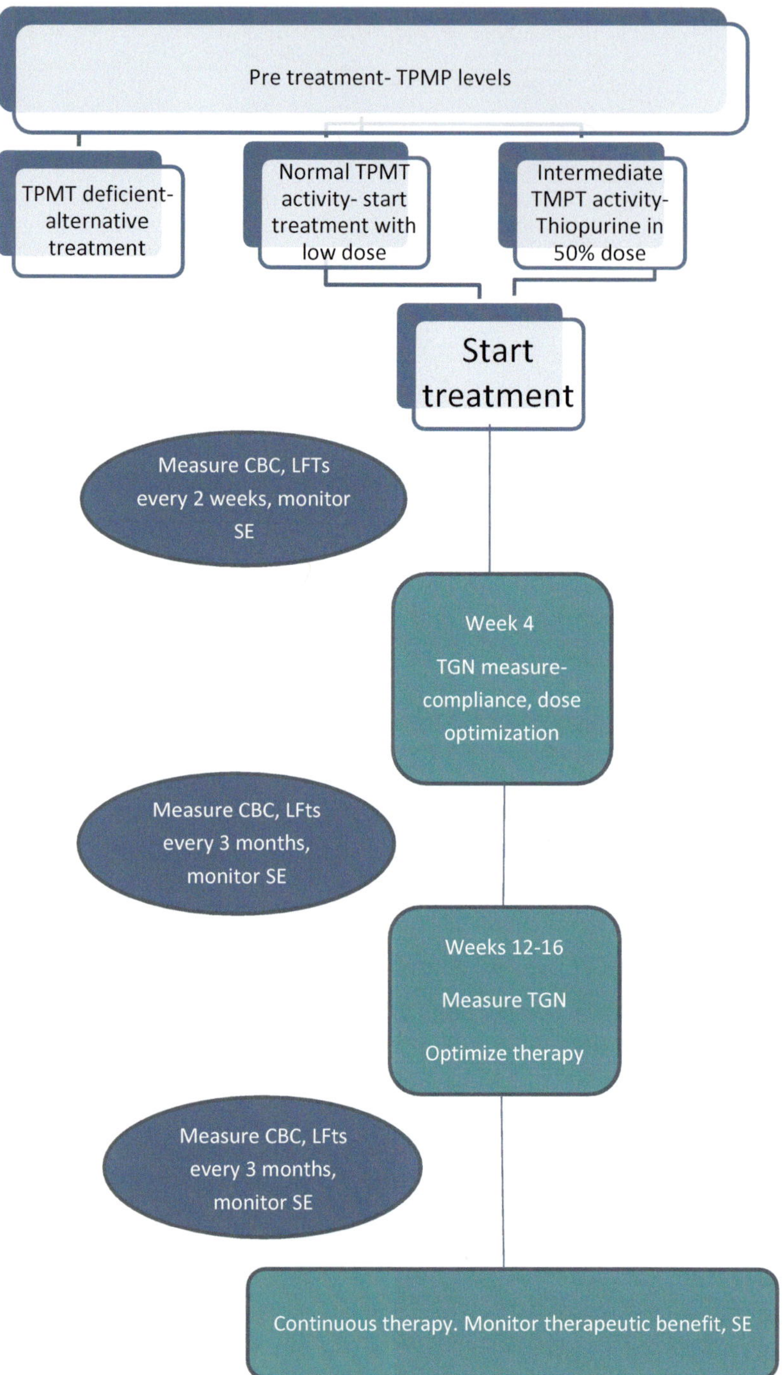

Fig. 30.2 Thiopurine monitoring algorithm. *CBC* complete blood count, *LFTs* liver function tests, *SE* side effects, *TPMT* thiopurine-s-methyl transferase, *TGN* thioguanine nucleotide

be taken to assess compliance and optimize dosing [87]. TGN levels >235 pmol/8 × 10⁸ red blood cells (RBC) were shown to correlate with clinical remission in 65 % of patients [85]. TGN levels above 450 pmol/8 × 10⁸ were shown to cause higher percentage of myelosuppression [67, 88]. A suggested algorithm for thiopurine monitoring is shown in Fig. 30.2.

Summary

Thiopurine therapy was shown to be effective in the management of CD for over 6 decades. Thiopurines were shown to be effective in inducing and maintaining remission, achieving mucosal healing, and treating complications. The combination therapy with anti-TNFa was shown to have a synergistic effect. Thus, even in the era of biologic therapy, and despite several side effects, it is still one of the cornerstones of CD treatment.

References

1. Present DH, Korelitz BI, Wisch N, Glass JL, Sachar DB, Pasternack BS. Treatment of Crohn's disease with 6-mercaptopurine. A long-term, randomized, double-blind study. N Engl J Med. 1980; 302:981–7.
2. Prefontaine E, Sutherland LR, Macdonald JK, Cepoiu M. Azathioprine or 6-mercaptopurine for maintenance of remission in Crohn's disease. Cochrane Database Syst Rev. 2009;1:CD000067.
3. Peyrin-Biroulet L, Deltenre P, Ardizzone S, D'Haens G, Hanauer SB, Herfarth H, et al. Azathioprine and 6-mercaptopurine for the prevention of postoperative recurrence in Crohn's disease: a meta-analysis. Am J Gastroenterol. 2009;104:2089–96.
4. Reinisch W, Angelberger S, Petritsch W, Shonova O, Lukas M, Bar-Meir S, et al. Azathioprine versus mesalazine for prevention of postoperative clinical recurrence in patients with Crohn's disease with endoscopic recurrence: efficacy and safety results of a randomised, double-blind, double-dummy, multicentre trial. Gut. 2010;59:752–9.
5. Elison G. The purine path to chemotherapy. Science. 1989; 244:41–7.
6. Blaker P, Arenas-Hernandez M, Marinaki A, Sanderson J. The pharmacogenetic basis of individual variation in thiopurine metabolism. J Pers Med. 2012;9:707–25.
7. McGovern D, Travis S, Duley J, Shobowale-Bakre E, Dalton H. Azathioprine intolerance in patients with IBD may be imidazole-related and is independent of TPMT activity. Gastroenterology. 2002;122:838–9.
8. Lennard L. The clinical pharmacology of 6-mercaptopurine. Eur J Clin Pharmacol. 1992;43:329–39.
9. Neurath MF, Kiesslich R, Teichgraber U, Fischer C, Hofmann U, Eichelbaum M, et al. 6-thioguanosine diphosphate and triphosphate levels in red blood cells and response to azathioprine therapy in Crohn's disease. Clin Gastroenterol Hepatol. 2005;3:1007–14.
10. Aarbakke J, Janka-Schaub G, Elion G. Thiopurine biology and pharmacology. Trends Pharmacol Sci. 1997;18:3–7.
11. Swann PF, Waters TR, Moulton DC, Xu YZ, Zheng Q, Edwards M, et al. Role of post replicative DNA mismatch repair in the cytotoxic action of thioguanine. Science. 1996;273:1109–11.
12. Thomas CW, Myhre GM, Tschumper R, Sreekumar R, Jelinek D, McKean DJ, et al. Selective inhibition of inflammatory gene expression in activated T lymphocytes: a mechanism of immune suppression by thiopurines. J Pharmacol Exp Ther. 2005;312:537–45.
13. Inamochi H, Higashigawa M, Shimono Y, Nagata T, Cao DC, Mao XY, et al. Delayed cytotoxicity of 6-mercaptopurine is compatible with mitotic death caused by DNA damage due to incorporation of 6-thioguanine into DNA as 6-thioguanine nucleotide. J Exp Clin Cancer Res. 1999;18:417–24.
14. Gomez M, Tybulewicz V, Cantrell DA. Control of pre-T cell proliferation and differentiation by the GTPase Rac-I. Nat Immunol. 2000;1:348–52.
15. Tiede I, Fritz G, Strand S, Poppe D, Dvorsky R, Strand D, et al. CD28-dependent Rac1 activation is the molecular target of azathioprine in primary human CD4+ T lymphocytes. J Clin Invest. 2003;111:1133–45.
16. Boirivant M, Marini M, DiFelice G, Pronio AM, Montesani C, Tersigni R, et al. Lamina propria T cells in Crohn's disease and other gastrointestinal inflammation show defective CD2 pathway-induced apoptosis. Gastroenterology. 1999;116:557–65.
17. Plevy SE, Landers CJ, Prehn J, Carramanzana NM, Deem RL, Shealy D, et al. A role for TNF-a and mucosal T helper-1 cytokines in the pathogenesis of Crohn's disease. J Immunol. 1997;159:6276–82.
18. Bean RH. The treatment of chronic ulcerative colitis with 6-mercaptopurine. Med J Aust. 1962;49:592–3.
19. Brooke BN, Hoffmann DC, Swarbrick ET. Azathioprine for Crohn's disease. Lancet. 1969;2:612–4.
20. Pearson DC, May GR, Fick GH, Sutherland LR. Azathioprine and 6-mercaptopurine in Crohn disease. A meta-analysis. Ann Intern Med. 1995;123:132–42.
21. Sandborn W, Sutherland L, Pearson D, May G, Modigliani R, Prantera C. Azathioprine or 6-mercaptopurine for inducing remission of Crohn's disease. Cochrane Database Syst Rev. 2000: CD000545.
22. Prefontaine E, Macdonald JK, Sutherland LR. Azathioprine or 6-mercaptopurine for induction of remission in Crohn's disease. Cochrane Database Syst. Rev. 2009: CD000545.
23. Chande N, Tsoulis DJ, MacDonald JK. Azathioprine or 6-mercaptopurine for induction of remission in Crohn's disease. Cochrane Database Syst Rev. 2013;4:CD000545.
24. Dignass A, Van Assche G, Lindsay JO, Lémann M, Söderholm J, Colombel JF, et al. European Crohn's and Colitis Organisation (ECCO) The second European evidence-based Consensus on the diagnosis and management of Crohn's disease: current management. J Crohns Colitis. 2010;4:28–62.
25. Frøslie KF, Jahnsen J, Moum BA, Vatn MH. IBSEN Group. Mucosal healing in inflammatory bowel disease: results from a Norwegian population-based cohort. Gastroenterology. 2007;133:412–22.
26. Colombel JF, Sandborn WJ, Reinisch W, Mantzaris GJ, Kornbluth A, Rachmilewitz D, et al. SONIC Study Group. Infliximab, azathioprine, or combination therapy for Crohn's disease. N Engl J Med. 2010;362:1383–95.
27. D'Haens G, Baert F, van Assche G, Caenepeel P, Vergauwe P, Tuynman H, et al. Belgian Inflammatory Bowel Disease Research Group; North-Holland Gut Club. Early combined immunosuppression or conventional management in patients with newly diagnosed Crohn's disease: an open randomised trial. Lancet. 2008;371:660–7.
28. Baert F, Moortgat L, Van Assche G, Caenepeel P, Vergauwe P, De Vos M, et al. Belgian Inflammatory Bowel Disease Research Group; North-Holland Gut Club. Mucosal healing predicts sustained clinical remission in patients with early-stage Crohn's disease. Gastroenterology. 2010;138:463–8.
29. Yu LF, Zhong J, Cheng SD, Tang YH, Miao F. Low-dose azathioprine effectively improves mucosal healing in Chinese patients with small bowel Crohn's disease. J Dig Dis. 2014;15:180–7.
30. Mantzaris GJ, Christidou A, Sfakianakis M, Roussos A, Koilakou S, Petraki K, et al. Azathioprine is superior to budesonide in achieving and maintaining mucosal healing and histologic remission in steroid-dependent Crohn's disease. Inflamm Bowel Dis. 2009;15:375–82.
31. D'Haens G, Geboes K, Ponette E, Penninckx F, Rutgeerts P. Healing of severe recurrent ileitis with azathioprine therapy in patients with Crohn's disease. Gastroenterology. 1997;112:1475–81.
32. D'Haens G, Geboes K, Rutgeerts P. Endoscopic and histologic healing of Crohn's (ileo-) colitis with azathioprine. Gastrointest Endosc. 1999;50:667–71.
33. Korelitz BI, Present DH. Favorable effect of 6-mercaptopurine on fistulae of Crohn's disease. Dig Dis Sci. 1985;30:58–64.
34. Rutgeerts P, Geboes K, Vantrappen G, Beyls J, Kerremans R, Hiele M. Predictability of the postoperative course of Crohn's disease. Gastroenterology. 1990;99:956–63.
35. Williams JG, Wong WD, Rothenberger DA, Goldberg SM. Recurrence of Crohn's disease after resection. Br J Surg. 1990;78:10–9.
36. Gordon M, Taylor K, Akobeng AK, Thomas AG. Azathioprine and 6-mercaptopurine for maintenance of surgically-induced remission in Crohn's disease. Cochrane Database Syst Rev. 2014;8:CD010233.

37. Savarino E, Bodini G, Dulbecco P, Marabotto E, Assandri L, Bruzzone L. Adalimumab is more effective than azathioprine and mesalamine at preventing postoperative recurrence of Crohn's disease—a randomized trial. Gastroenterology. 2013;144(5 Suppl 1):S21.
38. Angelberger S, Schaeffeler E, Teml A, Petritsch W, Shonova O, Lukas M, et al. Mucosal improvement in patients with moderate to severe postoperative endoscopic recurrence of Crohn's disease and azathioprine metabolite levels. Inflamm Bowel Dis. 2013;19:590–8.
39. Reinisch W, Angelberger S, Petritsch W, Herrlinger K, Shonova O, Lukas M, et al. A double-blind, double-dummy, randomized, controlled, multicenter trial on the efficacy and safety of azathioprine vs mesalamine for prevention of clinical relapses in Crohn's disease patients with postoperative moderate or severe endoscopic recurrence. Gastroenterology. 2008;134(4 Suppl 1):A70.
40. Savarino E, Bodini G, Dulbecco P, Assandri L, Bruzzone L, Mazza F, et al. Adalimumab is more effective than azathioprine and mesalamine at preventing postoperative recurrence of Crohn's disease: a randomized controlled trial. Am J Gastroenterol. 2013;108:1731–42.
41. Herfarth H, Obermeier F, Tjaden C, Lukas M, Serclova Z, Dignass AU, et al. Double-blind, double dummy, randomized, multicentre, comparative study on the efficacy and safety of azathioprine (AZA) versus mesalazine (5-ASA) for prevention of postoperative endoscopic recurrence in Crohn's disease. Gastroenterology. 2006;130(4 Suppl 2):A480–1.
42. Punati J, Markowitz J, Lerer T, Hyams J, Kugathasan S, Griffiths A, et al. Pediatric IBD Collaborative Research Group. Effect of early immunomodulation use in moderate to severe pediatric Crohn disease. Inflamm Bowel Dis. 2008;14:949–54.
43. Markowitz J, Grancher K, Kohn N, Lesser M, Daum F. A multicenter trial of 6-mercaptopurine and prednisone in children with newly diagnosed Crohn's disease. Gastroenterology. 2000;119:895–902.
44. Cosnes J, Bourrier A, Laharie D, Nahon S, Bouhnik Y, Carbonnel F, et al. Groupe d'Etude Thérapeutique des Affections Inflammatoires du Tube Digestif (GETAID). Early administration of azathioprine vs conventional management of Crohn's Disease: a randomized controlled trial. Gastroenterology. 2013;145:758–65.
45. Panés J, López-SanRomán A, Bermejo F, García-Sánchez V, Esteve M, Torres Y, et al. AZTEC Study Group: Early azathioprine therapy is no more effective than placebo for newly diagnosed Crohn's disease. Gastroenterology. 2013;145:766–74.
46. Lémann M, Mary J, Colombel J, Duclos B, Soule J, Lerebours E, et al. A randomized, double-blind, controlled withdrawal trial in Crohn's disease patients in long-term remission on azathioprine. Gastroenterology. 2005;128:1812–8.
47. Treton X, Bouhnik Y, Mary JY, Colombel JF, Duclos B, Soule JC, et al. Groupe D'Etude Thérapeutique Des Affections Inflammatoires Du Tube Digestif (GETAID). Azathioprine withdrawal in patients with Crohn's disease maintained on prolonged remission: a high risk of relapse. Clin Gastroenterol Hepatol. 2009;7:80–5.
48. Holtmann MH, Krummenauer F, Claas C, Kremeyer K, Lorenz D, Rainer O, et al. Long-term effectiveness of azathioprine in IBD beyond 4 years: a European multicenter study in 1176 patients. Dig Dis Sci. 2006;51:1516–24.
49. Kennedy NA, Kalla R, Warner B, Gambles CJ, Musy R, Reynolds S, et al. Thiopurine withdrawal during sustained clinical remission in inflammatory bowel disease: relapse and recapture rates, with predictive factors in 237 patients. Aliment Pharmacol Ther. 2014;40:1313–23.
50. Van Assche G, Dignass A, Reinisch W, van der Woude CJ, Sturm A, De Vos M, et al.; European Crohn's and Colitis Organisation (ECCO). The second European evidence-based Consensus on the diagnosis and management of Crohn's disease: Special situations. J Crohns Colitis. 2010;4: 63–101.
51. Baert F, Noman M, Vermeire S, Van Assche G, D' Haens G, Carbonez A, et al. Influence of immunogenicity on the long-term efficacy of infliximab in Crohn's disease. N Engl J Med. 2003;348:601–8.
52. Lémann M, Mary JY, Duclos B, Veyrac M, Dupas JL, Delchier JC, et al. Groupe d'Etude Therapeutique des Affections Inflammatoires du Tube Digestif (GETAID). Infliximab plus aza-thioprine for steroid-dependent Crohn's disease patients: a randomized placebo-controlled trial. Gastroenterology. 2006;130:1054–61.
53. Kopylov U, Al-Taweel T, Yaghoobi M, Nauche B, Bitton A, Lakatos PL, et al. Adalimumab monotherapy versus combination therapy with immunomodulators in patients with Crohn's disease: a systematic review and meta-analysis. J Crohns Colitis. 2014;8:1632–41.
54. van Assche G, Magdelaine-Beuzelin C, D'Haens G, Baert F, Noman M, Vermeire S, et al. Withdrawal of immunosuppression in Crohn's disease treated with scheduled infliximab maintenance: a randomized trial. Gastroenterology. 2008;134:1861–8.
55. Oussalah A, Chevaux JB, Fay R, Sandborn WJ, Bigard MA, Peyrin-Biroulet L. Predictors of infliximab failure after azathioprine withdrawal in Crohn's disease treated with combination therapy. Am J Gastroenterol. 2010;105:1142–9.
56. Timmer A, McDonald JW, Macdonald JK. Azathioprine and 6-mercaptopurine for maintenance of remission in ulcerative colitis. Cochrane Database Syst Rev. 2007;1:CD000478.
57. Gisbert JP, Gomollon F. Thiopurine-induced myelotoxicity in patients with inflammatory bowel disease: a review. Am J Gastroenterol. 2008;103:1783–800.
58. Present DH, Meltzer SJ, Krumholz MP, Wolke A, Korelitz BI. 6-Mercaptopurine in the management of inflammatory bowel disease: short- and long-term toxicity. Ann Intern Med. 1989;111:641–9.
59. Schwab M, Schaffeler E, Marx C, Fischer C, Lang T, Behrens C, et al. Azathioprine therapy and adverse drug reactions in patients with inflammatory bowel disease: impact of thiopurine S-methyl transferase polymorphism. Pharmacogenetics. 2002;12:429–36.
60. de Boer N, Zondervan P, Gilissen L, den Hartog G, Westerveld B, Derijks L, et al. Drug insight: pharmacology and toxicity of thiopurine therapy in patients with IBD. Nat Clin Gastroenterol Hepatol. 2007;4:686–94.
61. Shih D, Nguyen M, Zheng L, Ibanez P, Mei L, Kwan L, et al. Split-dose administration of thiopurine drugs: a novel and effective strategy for managing preferential 6-MMP metabolism. Aliment Pharmacol Ther. 2012;36:449–58.
62. Pavlidis P, Ansari A, Duley J, Oancea I, Florin T. Splitting a therapeutic dose of thioguanine may avoid liver toxicity and be an efficacious treatment for severe inflammatory bowel disease: a 2-center observational cohort study. Inflamm Bowel Dis. 2014;20:2239–46.
63. Shih D, Yoon J, Huang B, Karsan S, Melmed G, Ippoliti A, et al. Potential synergism between anti-TNF and thiopurine therapy: increased thiopurine metabolites by anti-TNF. Gastroenterology. 2013;144:S772.
64. Nagy F, Molnar T, Szepes Z, Farkas K, Nyari T, Lonovics J. Efficacy of 6-mercaptopurine treatment after azathioprine hypersensitivity in inflammatory bowel disease. World J Gastroenterol. 2008;14:4342–6.
65. Amin J, Huang B, Yoon J, Shih D. Update 2014: advances to optimize 6-mercaptopurine and azathioprine to reduce toxicity and improve efficacy in the management of IBD. Inflamm Bowel Dis. 2015;21:445–52.
66. Ansari A, Elliott T, Baburajan B, Mayhead P, O'Donohue J, Chocair P, et al. Long-term outcome of using allopurinol co-therapy as a strategy for overcoming thiopurine hepatotoxicity in treating inflammatory bowel disease. Aliment Pharmacol Ther. 2008;28:734–41.
67. Dubinsky MC, Yang H, Hassard PV, Seidman EG, Kam LY, Abreu MT, et al. 6MP metabolite profiles provide a biochemical explanation for 6MP resistance in patients with inflammatory bowel disease. Gastroenterology. 2002;122:904–15.
68. Reshamwala PA, Kleiner DE, Heller T. Nodular regenerative hyperplasia: not all nodules are created equal. Hepatology. 2006;44:7–14.

69. Haboubi NY, Ali HH, Whitwell HL, Ackrill P. Role of endothelial cell injury in the spectrum of azathioprine-induced liver disease after renal transplant: light microscopy and ultrastructural observations. Am J Gastroenterol. 1988;83:256–61.
70. Vernier-Massouille G, Cosnes J, Lemann M, Marteau P, Reinisch W, Laharie D, et al. Nodular regenerative hyperplasia in patients with inflammatory bowel disease treated with azathioprine. Gut. 2007;56:1404–9.
71. Toruner M, Loftus E, Scott Harmsen W, Zinsmeister A, Orenstein R, Sandborn W, et al. Risk factors for opportunistic infections in patients with inflammatory bowel disease. Gastroenterology. 2008;134:929–36.
72. Lewis JD, Abramson O, Pascua M, Liu L, Asakura LM, Velayos FS, et al. Timing of myelosuppression during thiopurine therapy for inflammatory bowel disease: implications for monitoring recommendations. Clin Gastroenterol Hepatol. 2009;7:1195–201.
73. Higgs J, Payne K, Roberts C, Newman W. Are patients with intermediate TPMT activity at increased risk of myelosuppression when taking thiopurine medications? Pharmacogenomics. 2010;11:177–88.
74. Colombel J, Ferrari N, Debuysere H, Marteau P, Gendre J, Bonaz B, et al. Genotypic analysis of thiopurine S-methyl transferase in patients with Crohn's disease and severe myelosuppression during azathioprine therapy. Gastroenterology. 2002;118:1025–30.
75. Ansari A, Hassan C, Duley J, Marinaki A, Shobowale-Bakre E, Seed P, et al. Thiopurine methyl transferase activity and the use of azathioprine in inflammatory bowel disease. Aliment Pharmacol Ther. 2002;16:1743–50.
76. Beaugerie L, Brousse N, Bouvier A, Colombel J, Lemann M, Cosnes J, et al. Lymphoproliferative disorders in patients receiving thiopurines for inflammatory bowel disease: a prospective observational cohort study. Lancet. 2009;374:1617–25.
77. Lopez A, Mounier M, Bouvier AM, Carrat F, Maynadié M, Beaugerie L, et al. Increased risk of acute myeloid leukemias and myelodysplastic syndromes in patients who received thiopurine treatment for inflammatory bowel disease. Clin Gastroenterol Hepatol. 2014;12:1324–29.
78. Magro F, Peyrin-Biroulet L, Sokol H, Aldeger X, Costa A, Higgins PD, et al. Extra-intestinal malignancies in inflammatory bowel disease: results of the 3rd ECCO Pathogenesis Scientific Workshop (III). J Crohns Colitis. 2014;8:31–44.
79. Kandiel A, Fraser A, Korelitz B, Brensinger B, Lewis J. Increased risk of lymphoma among inflammatory bowel disease patients treated with azathioprine and 6-mercaptopurine. Gut. 2005;54:1121–25.
80. Setshedi M, Epstein D, Winter T, Myer L, Watermeyer G, Hift R. Use of thiopurines in the treatment of inflammatory bowel disease is associated with an increased risk of non-melanoma skin cancer in an at-risk population: a cohort study. J Gastroenterol Hepatol. 2012;27:385–89.
81. Beigel F, Steinborn A, Schnitzler F, Tillack C, Breiteneicher S, John J, et al. Risk of malignancies in patients with inflammatory bowel disease treated with thiopurines or anti-TNF alpha antibodies. Pharmacoepidemiol Drug Saf. 2014;23:735–44.
82. Mackey AC, Green L, Liang LC, Dinndorf P, Avigan M. Hepatosplenic T cell lymphoma associated with infliximab use in young patients treated for inflammatory bowel disease. J Pediatr Gastroenterol Nutr. 2007;44:265–7.
83. Shale M, Kanfer E, Panaccione R, Ghosh S. Hepatosplenic T cell lymphoma in inflammatory bowel disease. Gut. 2008;57:1639–41.
84. Kotlyar DS, Osterman MT, Diamond RH, Porter D, Blonski WC, Wasik M, et al. A systematic review of factors that contribute to hepatosplenic T-cell lymphoma in patients with inflammatory bowel disease. Clin Gastroenterol Hepatol. 2011;9:36–41.
85. Mowat C, Cole A, Windsor A, Ahmad T, Arnott I, Driscoll R, et al. Guidelines for the management of inflammatory bowel disease in adults. Gut. 2010;60:571–607.
86. Rahier J, Ben-Horin S, Chowers Y, Conlon C, De Munter P, D'Haens G, et al. European evidence-based consensus on the prevention, diagnosis and management of opportunistic infections in inflammatory bowel disease. J Crohns Colitis. 2009;3:47–91.
87. Goel RM, Blaker P, Mentzer A, Fong SC, Marinaki AM, Sanderson JD. Optimizing the use of thiopurines in inflammatory bowel disease. Ther Adv Chronic Dis. 2015;6:138–4.
88. Dubinsky M, Lamothe S, Yang H, Targan S, Sinnett F, Theoret Y, et al. Pharmacogenomics and metabolite measurement for 6-mercaptopurine therapy in inflammatory bowel disease. Gastroenterology. 2000;118:705–13.

Conventional Medical Management of Crohn's Disease: Methotrexate

31

Grace Harkin and Laurence Egan

Introduction

Methotrexate (MTX) was first developed for use as a chemotherapeutic agent in cancers such as leukemia, lymphoma, and choriocarcinoma. Subsequently, it became well established in treating two chronic inflammatory diseases, rheumatoid arthritis [1, 2] and psoriasis [3, 4].

In 1989, Kozarek et al. reported the first use of MTX for the treatment of refractory Inflammatory Bowel Disease (IBD) [5]. This study involved 21 patients with IBD (7 with ulcerative colitis, 14 with Crohn's disease) and showed encouraging results with 16 of the 21 patients showing objective improvement. Since then there have been several randomized controlled trials showing MTX to be efficacious in the treatment of refractory Crohn's disease.

Pharmacology of Methotrexate

MTX is a folate analog originally synthesized in the 1940s which acts as an antimetabolite drug but also has anti-inflammatory properties, depending on the dose used. The principal cellular action of MTX is the reversible competitive inhibition of dihydrofolate reductase (DHFR) [6] . Parent MTX, polyglutamated MTX metabolites (MTXPG), and 7-hydroxymethotrexate (7-OH-MTX) are all folate analogs with inhibitory activity against many of the enzymes involved in the metabolic pathway of folate [7] (Fig. 31.1). These folate-dependent enzymes are vital for the de novo synthesis of purines, pyrimidines, and the transmethylation of DNA, RNA, phospholipids, and proteins [7]. Antiproliferative effects dominate with high dose MTX therapy [6, 8] while low dose MTX has an immunosuppressive role that may be independent of the inhibition of cell proliferation via DHFR blockade [7, 9, 10]. In cell culture systems, MTX has been shown to lead to the accumulation of adenosine, a lymphotoxic and immunosuppressive autocoid [11]. However, a putative mechanism of action of MTX relating to adenosine has not been supported in inflammatory bowel disease, where no rise in plasma or rectal levels of adenosine was found following administration of MTX [12].

At the cellular level, MTX has been observed to induce apoptosis and clonal deletion of activated T-lymphocytes in a mechanism that is independent of the APO-1/Fas (CD95) receptor/ligand system [13]. MTX also acts as a strong differentiation factor for immature monocytes which in vitro is associated with natural cytokine inhibitor release and a simultaneous down-regulation of interleukin (IL)-1β effects [14].

MTX decreases the production of the pro-inflammatory cytokines IL1, IL6 [15–17], IL2, interferon-γ [18], and tumor necrosis factor (TNF)-α [14] and increases IL4 and IL10 gene expression, both of which have anti-inflammatory effects [18]. MTX was shown to inhibit IL-1 activity by blocking the binding of IL-1 to its receptor [19]. There is evidence in patients with rheumatoid arthritis that MTX indirectly inhibits COX-2 synthesis [20] and neutrophil chemotaxis [21]. It is likely that the anti-inflammatory effects of MTX in IBD are underpinned to an extent by combinations of these different actions.

Methotrexate Use in Crohn's Disease

The treatment of steroid-dependent IBD is problematic. In a population-based study on the natural history of corticosteroid therapy for IBD [22], 58 % of patients with Crohn's disease treated with corticosteroids were in complete remission after 30 days of therapy and one year outcomes revealed that 28 % of patients were steroid dependent. Corticosteroids are not indicated in the maintenance of IBD because of their side effect profile with 32 % of patients on high dose and 26 % on

G. Harkin, M.B., M.R.C.P.I. • L. Egan, M.D., F.R.C.P.I. (✉)
Clinical Science Institute, University Hospital Galway, Galway, Ireland
e-mail: laurence.egan@nuigalway.ie

D.C. Baumgart (ed.), *Crohn's Disease and Ulcerative Colitis*, DOI 10.1007/978-3-319-33703-6_31

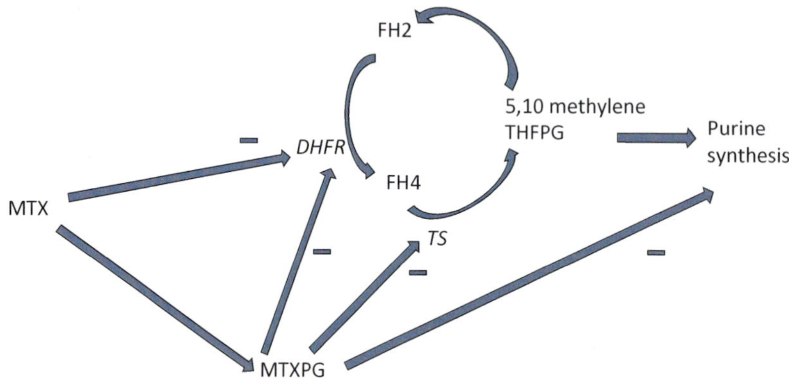

Fig. 31.1 Methotrexate (MTX) metabolism. MTX and its polyglutamate metabolites (MTXPG) potently inhibit dihydrofolate reductase (DHFR), impairing the conversion of dihydrofolate (FH2) to tetrahydrofolate (FH4). MTXPG also inhibit folate-dependent enzymes distal to DHFR such as thymidylate synthase (TS). 5,10, methylenetetrahydrofolate polyglutamate (5,10 methylene THFPG)

prophylactic dose requiring withdrawal or dose reduction of therapy secondary to side effects [23].

MTX has been studied for both induction and maintenance of remission in patients with chronic active Crohn's disease. There have been five randomized controlled trials reported on the use of MTX for induction of remission in refractory Crohn's disease.

Randomized Controlled Trials

The largest trial, by Feagan et al. in 1995, reported substantial benefit [24]. This trial used intramuscular administration of MTX 25 mg once weekly in patients with chronic active, steroid-dependent Crohn's disease. After 16 weeks, 39.4 % of patients were in clinical remission compared to 19.1 % with placebo. MTX also induced a substantial benefit in quality of life in these patients, as well as lower requirements for corticosteroid administration.

A study of 54 patients with chronic active Crohn's disease by Ardizzone et al. compared using intravenous MTX 25 mg once weekly for 3 months, followed by 3 months of oral therapy at the same dose, to therapy with oral azathioprine [25]. The study showed no significant difference in induction of remission between MTX and azathioprine [25]. Adverse reactions resulting in withdrawal of therapy were the same in both treatment groups (11 %) but more adverse effects that did not require withdrawal of therapy occurred in the MTX group (44 % versus 7 %).

Several trials have evaluated the oral administration of MTX at lower doses. Oren et al. compared oral MTX 12.5 mg once weekly to oral 6-mercaptopurine (6-MP) in chronic steroid-dependent Crohn's disease [26]. There was no statistically significant difference between the drugs for induction or maintenance of remission.

Mate-Jimenez et al. evaluated the efficacy and tolerance of oral MTX 15 mg once weekly to 6-MP and 5-aminosalicylic acid (5-ASA) [27]. This study similarly failed to show a benefit with oral MTX compared to 6-MP in inducing or maintaining remission in chronic active Crohn's disease. It did show a statistically significant benefit over therapy with 5-ASA. A study by Arora et al. which also investigated using 15 mg oral MTX once weekly in steroid-dependent Crohn's disease similarly failed to show a benefit [28]. This suggests that lower doses of 12.5–15 mg MTX per week and oral route of administration may be less effective than higher, parenterally administered doses. However, no firm conclusions can be drawn from these studies as the numbers involved were small and failure to respond may have been due to inadequate dose and oral route being utilized [26–28].

A randomized trial by Egan et al. investigated the optimum dose of MTX for induction of remission in patients with steroid-dependent IBD [29]. Of these patients, 80 % were refractory to corticosteroid therapy and 70 % had previously failed adequate therapy with 6-MP or azathioprine. Overall, 17 % of IBD patients investigated entered remission and there was no benefit to 25 mg over 15 mg of weekly subcutaneous MTX. The likely explanation for the low level of response seen in this group of IBD patients is the refractory nature of their disease. Interestingly, 11 of the patients who did not respond to treatment with 15 mg weekly after 16 weeks subsequently had their dose escalated to 25 mg weekly MTX and 36 % of these patients had an improvement in clinical status although there was no increase in the rate of remission. Toxicity was not different between the two groups [29].

A large trial by Feagan et al. in 2000 examined maintaining remission using intramuscular MTX 15 mg once weekly in patients with chronic active Crohn's disease who had already achieved remission after 14–24 weeks treatment with intramuscular MTX 25 mg once weekly [30]. This study showed that relapse occurred in 35 % after 40 weeks of therapy with MTX compared to 61 % with placebo. The number needed to treat to prevent one relapse was 4. The mean time to relapse was >40 weeks compared to 2 weeks with placebo [30]. This study followed on to treat 22 of the 36 patients who relapsed (14 in the MTX group and 22 in the placebo group) with 25 mg intramuscular MTX for 40 weeks. Of this group, 55 % were in remission at 40 weeks compared to 14 % of the remainder of the group not treated with MTX [30].

Concomitant immunosuppressive therapy has been shown to reduce the magnitude of the immunogenic response of infliximab (IFX) [31]. Feagan et al. compared MTX plus IFX to IFX monotherapy in a placebo controlled trial involving 126 patients to maintain remission in Crohn's disease [32]. Primary outcome was defined as treatment failure, i.e., lack of prednisone free remission at week 14, or failure to maintain remission by week 50. Steroid free remission was 76 % in the dual therapy group at week 14 as opposed to 78 % in the IFX monotherapy group. Remission was maintained in 56 % at week 50 in the dual therapy group verses 57 % with IFX alone. Combination therapy was well tolerated but not superior to IFX monotherapy in induction or maintenance of remission [32], indicating that MTX does not confer any additional benefit in IFX treated Crohn's disease patients. However, the remarkably high and prolonged remission rate in IFX monotherapy patients in this trial may have compromised the ability to detect any advantages of MTX.

For an overview of MTX clinical trials in Crohn's disease, see Table 31.1.

Published Clinical Data: Comparative Analysis of Methotrexate and Other Treatment Options

Harper et al. assessed dual therapy of azathioprine/6-MP or MTX in patients starting anti-TNF therapy for induction of disease remission. This study showed azathioprine/6-MP and MTX performed similarly in this treatment group with regard to maintaining response to infliximab [36]. Diaz-Saa et al. studied methotrexate monotherapy as a third line option after thiopurine and anti-TNF failure in Crohn's disease. They reported remission rates of 28 % at month four, and 22 % at month twelve of treatment. MTX was well tolerated in this difficult to treat group [37].

Margien et al. assessed the efficacy and tolerability of MTX use in Crohn's Disease. 63 % of patients discontinued MTX after a mean of 33 weeks for various reasons, primarily due to ineffectiveness (39 %) and side effects (35 %). At 12 months 59 % were maintained on MTX, while this number had fallen to 9 % after 5 years [38]. Similarly a study looking at tolerability of MTX monotherapy after thiopurine failure found a clinical benefit was maintained in 63 % at year 1. This number had fallen to 20 % at 5 years. 26 % stopped MTX due to intolerances primarily in the first 6 months of treatment but adverse events were generally minor suggesting this treatment is safe [39].

Methotrexate and Its Role in the Formation of Antibodies to Infliximab

Vermeire assessed the formation of antibodies to IFX when combined with azathioprine, MTX or placebo and reported a lower incidence of antibodies to IFX in the group receiving either azathioprine or MTX [40]. In the dual treatment groups (azathioprine/MTX plus IFX) 46 % of patients developed antibodies to IFX compared to 73 % on IFX alone. There was no significant difference in the incidence of antibodies between the MTX and azathioprine groups (44 % vs 48 % respectively). The formation of antibodies to IFX >8 μg/ml is associated with lower serum levels of IFX [40]. Feagan et al. measured serum antibody levels in their two study groups (IFX+MTX and IFX+placebo). Patients who received methotrexate were significantly less likely to develop antibodies to IFX than those who received IFX alone (4 % compared to 20 %). Serum trough IFX levels were higher in the MTX treatment group but were not significant. This was not explored beyond 50 weeks, and it is possible the effects of MTX on antibody formation would result in benefit in the long term however this would need to be studied further [32].

Administration of Methotrexate

Subcutaneous administration of MTX has been shown to have similar pharmacokinetics compared to the intramuscular route [41, 42]. Bioavailability approaches 100 % with parenteral administration in contrast to oral route which has shown 50–90 % bioavailability in other chronic inflammatory conditions [43–45]. The subcutaneous route has been shown to be well tolerated by patients and to have few local complications at the injection site [41, 46, 47].

Adverse Effects

Adverse effects experienced with MTX can be categorized as being due to bone marrow suppression [48], idiosyncratic reactions such as rash or pneumonitis [49]; or secondary to MTX-induced fibrosis, e.g., pulmonary fibrosis or hepatic fibrosis.

Table 31.1 Evidence base for MTX in Crohn's disease

Study	Methods	Patient selection	Category	Intervention	Primary endpoint	Outcome
Feagan (1995) [24]	Randomized, double-blind placebo-controlled, multicenter study	Chronic active CD despite minimum 3 months therapy with prednisone. $n = 141$	Induction of remission CD	IM MTX at 25 mg per week versus placebo for 16 weeks	Clinical remission at 16 weeks defined as off corticosteroids and CDAI < 150 [33]	39.4 % remission with MTX versus 19.1 % with placebo
Feagan (2000) [30]	Randomized, double-blind placebo-controlled, multicenter study	Chronic active CD previously achieving remission (CDAI ≤ 150) with MTX 25 mg per week IM for 16–24 weeks. $n = 76$	Maintenance of remission CD	IM MTX 15 mg per week versus placebo for 40 weeks. Relapsed patients subsequently treated with MTX 25 mg IM per week for 40 weeks	Occurrence of a relapse at 40 weeks (increase of 100 in CDAI above baseline or initiation of prednisone or an antimetabolite)	Relapse in 35 % MTX group, 61 % placebo group. Relapsed patients treated with 25 mg MTX per week, 55 % achieved remission versus 14 % in untreated group
Mate Jimenez (2000) [27]	Randomized, controlled unblind single center, three-arm study	Induction arm: Steroid-dependent CD and UC Maintenance arm: Achieved remission at 30 weeks on MTX from induction arm of study $n = 72$ (38 CD)	Induction and Maintenance of remission CD and UC	Oral MTX 15 mg per week 6-MP 1.5 mg/kg/day 5-ASA 3 g/day Induction: 30 weeks Maintenance: if achieved, MTX 10 mg once per week given for 76 weeks	Clinical remission at 30 weeks, CDAI < 150 Maintenance of remission at 76 weeks	Differences not statistically significant
Egan (1999) [29]	Randomized, single-blind study	Steroid-dependent IBD resistant to azathioprine and 6-MP $n = 32$ (22 CD)	Induction of remission CD and UC	Compared 25 and 15 mg once weekly subcutaneous MTX for 16 weeks. Non responders in 15 mg group escalated dose to 25 mg for 16 weeks	Compare clinical remission (IBDQ < 170 [34]) at 16 weeks between 15 and 25 mg once weekly dose of MTX	No significant difference between different doses of MTX. 17 % from each group achieved remission. Dose escalation did not improve remission or increase toxicity
Arora (1999) [28]	Randomized, double-blind placebo-controlled trial	Steroid-dependent CD $n = 33$	Induction and maintenance of remission CD	Oral MTX 15 mg once weekly for 1 year. Nonresponders had MTX titrated up to 22.5 mg/weekly	Remission (CDAI < 150) and reduction in corticosteroid use	Nonsignificant trend towards fewer flares and increased side effects in MTX group
Oren (1997) [26]	Randomized, double-blind placebo-controlled, multicenter trial	Chronic active, steroid-dependent CD (Harvey–Bradshaw Index ≥7 [35]) $n = 84$	Induction and maintenance of remission CD	Three arms: Oral MTX 12.5 mg weekly Oral 6-MP 50 mg daily Placebo	Induction of remission and not receiving corticosteroids	No statistically significant difference between the groups

Feagan (2014) [32]	Randomized, double-blind, placebo-controlled, multicenter trial	Active Crohn's disease on steroids $n = 126$	Induction and maintenance of remission of CD	IM MTX weekly, 10 mg initially uptitrating to 25 mg/week plus infliximab (5 mg/kg) at weeks 1, 3, 7, 14, and every 8 weeks thereafter for 50 weeks. Placebo plus infliximab (5 mg/kg) at weeks 1, 3, 7, 14, and every 8 weeks thereafter for 50 weeks. Prednisone was tapered to stop by week 14	Failure to enter prednisone free remission (CDAI < 150) at week 14, or failure to maintain remission at week 50	Combination therapy was well tolerated but not superior to infliximab monotherapy in induction or maintenance of remission

CD Crohn's disease, *UC* ulcerative colitis, *6-MP* 6-mercaptopurine, *5-ASA* 5-aminosalicylic acid, *IM* intramuscular, *MTX* methotrexate, *IFX* infliximab, *IBD* inflammatory bowel disease, *CDAI* Crohn's disease activity index, *IBDQ* inflammatory bowel disease questionnaire

There is evidence that the anti-inflammatory effect of MTX may be offset at higher doses by MTX-induced enterotoxicity [50, 51]. MTX causes morphological and functional abnormalities of the small intestinal mucosa [52, 53]. Two studies reporting on jejunal biopsies taken from children with acute lymphoblastic leukemia treated with MTX revealed striking structural abnormalities of the Paneth cells with marked vacuolar dilatation of the cytoplasm [51] and striking distension of the lateral basal intercellular spaces, cell vacuolation, and patchy necrosis [50]. This effect may have been due to a direct toxic effect of MTX therapy or interference with crypt cell generation [50]. There are also several case reports of MTX itself (or aminopterin, a related anti-folate compound) causing severe colitis [54–58].

Up to 18 % of patients in IBD trials discontinue the drug due to MTX related toxicity [24, 59]. In the largest study by Feagan et al., side effects were observed in similar frequency at 45 % in the MTX treated group versus 42 % in placebo group, however 17 % withdrew from treatment because of adverse events (including nausea and asymptomatic elevation in serum aminotransferase) compared to 2 % in the placebo group [24]. The patients who withdrew secondary to adverse effects improved after withdrawal of MTX.

The Oren 1997 study found that there was no statistically significant difference in withdrawals and adverse events between patients treated with MTX and 6-MP [26].

A similar small study looked at MTX use in patients who developed Azathioprine or 6 MP induced pancreatitis. Of the five patients who were started on MTX none had a recurrence of pancreatitis but in one patient MTX was stopped due to a rise in transaminases. Another patient developed a localized reaction at the site of drug administration but continued successfully on MTX after a brief course of antihistamines [60].

Chen et al. assessed frequency of adverse events (reactivation of Varicella Zoster Virus, Squamous Cell Carcinoma, non-dermatologic malignancies, and drug-induced pancreatitis) in patients on either MTX or Thiopurine monotherapy for their Crohn's disease. Of 852 patients, 105 had complications, 5.29 % in MTX group verses 13.77 % in the thiopurine group indicating adverse events were less numerous in the MTX group. Similarly being cognizant of gender, age, and length of treatment the probability of AEs were less in the MTX group. No notable differences were established between the groups with respect VZV reactivation and non dermatological malignancies [61].

Importantly, liver fibrosis and cirrhosis can develop in some patients that are treated chronically with weekly MTX. MTX polyglutamates accumulate in hepatocytes and hepatotoxicity with MTX is thought to be due to the direct toxic and steatogenic effects of MTX on the liver [62, 63].

Patients with psoriasis treated with MTX appear to be at the highest risk of developing hepatic toxicity. In that disease, liver biopsies are typically performed at cumulative MTX doses of 1.5 g [64, 65]. In contrast, patients with rheumatoid arthritis seem to be at a lower risk with the risk of cirrhosis after 5 years of continuous therapy estimated at only 1/1000 [63, 66].

Studies have suggested that patients with IBD appear to be at a lower risk of developing MTX induced hepatic toxicity than patients with psoriasis [67, 68]. Te et al. showed that cumulative doses of up to 5410 mg MTX given for up to 281 weeks in patients with IBD were associated with minimal hepatotoxicity, and that abnormal liver function tests did not identify patients with fibrosis [67]. They suggested that surveillance liver biopsies based on cumulative MTX doses are not warranted in patients with IBD [67]. However, it is the practice of other authors to perform biopsies at cumulative doses of 1.5 g MTX [29]. Whether or not IBD patients on chronic MTX should undergo liver biopsies remains controversial.

Monitoring for Toxicity

Ninety percent of MTX is excreted within 24 h of administration [46]. The remainder exists primarily as the pharmacologically active intracellular polyglutamate derivatives in many cell types, including erythrocytes. However, there is no evidence that therapeutic monitoring of erythrocyte or plasma MTX or 7-hydroxymethotrexate levels can be used to guide therapy [29].

Current guidelines advise routine monitoring of patients with complete blood counts and liver function tests to assess for bone marrow suppression and hepatic fibrosis. Persistently abnormal liver biochemistry tests above two times the upper limit of normal warrant discontinuation of the drug or liver biopsy [69]. For suggested guidelines regarding monitoring of patients receiving long-term MTX therapy, see Table 31.2.

In recent years less invasive tests have been assessed as a way of monitoring for hepatotoxicity and fibrosis when on long term MTX. The amino terminal of type III procollagen peptide (PIIINP) is produced during the synthesis of type III collagen and is released into the blood. PIIINP can function as a serum marker of hepatic fibrosis in patients on MTX for long periods. Using serum PIIINP as an indicator of hepatic fibrosis may reduce the need for liver biopsy if PIIINP levels are persistently normal. One such study found that up to 45 % fewer biopsies would be necessary using this practice [72].

Transient elastography (TE) is a noninvasive way of measuring liver stiffness to assess for fibrosis and a number of small studies have been undertaken to evaluate its usefulness in IBD patients on long term MTX. One such trial included 46 IBD patients with an accumulative dose of 1242 ± 1349 mg and average treatment period of 21 ± 24 months had liver stiffness

Table 31.2 Guidelines for monitoring of patients receiving long-term MTX therapy[a]

Baseline investigations
CBC, creatinine concentration, serum AST, ALT[b], alkaline phosphatase, albumin, bilirubin levels, Hepatitis B and C and HIV serologies, pregnancy test, chest X-ray
Consider liver biopsy if
Heavy alcohol consumption
Elevated serum liver enzyme activity
Type 2 diabetes mellitus
Toxicity monitoring during treatment
CBC and creatinine concentration weekly initially, with interval gradually increased to 2–3 monthly after therapy is stabilized
Serum ALT, AST, and albumin levels every 4–6 weeks
Liver Biopsy if:
More than half of regularly checked AST values are more than twice the upper limit of normal
Progressive increase in serum liver enzyme activity
Indications to discontinue use of MTX
Clinically evident liver disease
Fibrosis or cirrhosis on liver histology at biopsy

[a]Adapted from guidelines developed for rheumatoid arthritis and psoriasis [70, 71]
[b]*CBC* complete blood count, *ALT* alanine transaminase, *AST* aspartate transaminase

assessed by FibroScan®. The average liver stiffness finding was 4.7±6.9 kPa. (The threshold for significant liver fibrosis was a value of $F \geq 2$: 7.1 kPa.) Development of advanced liver fibrosis in IBD patients treated with methotrexate is uncommon. They concluded there was no variation in liver stiffness according to type of IBD or cumulative dose of MTX [73].

Another study involving 53 patients comparing liver stiffness in IBD patients on MTX ($n=30$) to a control group (MTX naïve $n=23$) did not show increased liver stiffness in the group treated with MTX [74]. Shah et al. looked at PIIINP and TE to assess for fibrosis in 34 patients on long term MTX for psoriasis and rheumatoid arthritis. Average accumulated dose of MTX was 5320 mg (SD 3682 mg) and average treatment duration of 427 weeks. The cut off for fibrosis was 7.1 kPa. Twenty-eight patients were included and they had an average hepatic stiffness was 7.4 kPa (SD 4.46), which correlated considerably with serum PIIINP. Thirty-three percent of treated patients developed liver fibrosis in this group [75]. These methods of monitoring need further evaluation in larger studies.

Recommendations for Clinical Practice

MTX has been proven to be effective for the induction of remission in patients with chronic active, steroid-dependent Crohn's disease. It should be started at a dose of 15 or 25 mg once weekly by subcutaneous injection for 12–16 weeks. An initial response after this period is unlikely. If there is failure to enter remission after this period on 15 mg once weekly, dose escalation to 25 mg once weekly for another 12–16 weeks may be considered if MTX is being well tolerated. There is no benefit in adding MTX to IFX to maintain remission; however studies looking at antibody formation in this group may show benefit of combination therapy [32].

Baseline investigations such as complete blood count, serum creatinine concentration and liver biochemistry tests should be performed as listed in Table 31.2.

Patients at risk for steatohepatitis, such as those with a prior history of high alcohol intake, increased weight, type 2 diabetes mellitus, or who have any chronic liver disease are at increased risk of developing hepatic fibrosis [62, 63]. We caution against starting MTX in such patients.

Contraindications to MTX therapy include known liver and renal disease, active infection, alcohol excess and obesity. Also, MTX is contraindicated in patients who are pregnant or lactating, and in women of childbearing age unless effective contraception is employed. Concomitant use of certain medications such as nonsteroidal anti-inflammatory drugs [76, 77] and trimethoprim-sulfamethoxazole is contraindicated and patients should avoid alcohol entirely.

Maintenance of remission with MTX in Crohn's disease patients is indicated for those who enter remission with this drug. Subcutaneous MTX therapy is continued at a dose of 15 mg once weekly. Regular monitoring of complete blood count as well as serum creatinine and liver function tests is indicated to detect cytopenias and patients developing hepatotoxicity.

Mild degrees of leukopenia or thrombocytopenia can be reversed by temporarily stopping MTX therapy and recommencing at a lower dose. Intravenous leucovorin is indicated in more serious or life threatening pancytopenia [49]. The administration of concomitant oral folic acid with MTX in patients with rheumatoid arthritis or psoriasis has been found to reduce hematological complications and gastrointestinal side effects such as stomatitis and gastrointestinal upset [78] without an apparent reduction in clinical efficacy [79]. Although this strategy has not been tested in patients with IBD, it is a common practice.

In a study of the tolerability of MTX, 50 % of IBD patients were considered intolerant, and 42 % of parents deemed their child to be intolerant of MTX. Intolerance was classified as behavioral symptoms (anticipatory/associative) pre MTX, gastrointestinal symptoms, or symptoms post MTX [80]. Empiric use of antiemetics such as metoclopramide or ondansetron may lessen post dose nausea or GI upset. Non-compliance should be considered in cases of treatment failure as one study found 53 % of patients had delayed and/or missed at least one dose or MTX when compliance was assessed. Age less than 44 was found to be the predominant risk factor related with non-compliance [81].

A phase 4 trial will shortly commence recruitment to evaluate if addition of MTX combined with full dose Infliximab can restore remission in pediatric patients [82] .

In summary, MTX has been proven to be effective for the induction of remission in patients with chronic active, steroid-dependent Crohn's disease and for the maintenance of remission in patients who enter remission with this drug.

References

1. Williams HJ et al. Comparison of low-dose oral pulse methotrexate and placebo in the treatment of rheumatoid arthritis. A controlled clinical trial. Arthritis Rheum. 1985;28:721–30.
2. Weinblatt ME et al. Efficacy of low-dose methotrexate in rheumatoid arthritis. N Engl J Med. 1985;312:818–22. doi:10.1056/NEJM198503283121303.
3. Lanse SB, Arnold GL, Gowans JD, Kaplan MM. Low incidence of hepatotoxicity associated with long-term, low-dose oral methotrexate in treatment of refractory psoriasis, psoriatic arthritis, and rheumatoid arthritis. An acceptable risk/benefit ratio. Dig Dis Sci. 1985;30:104–9.
4. Willkens RF et al. Randomized, double-blind, placebo controlled trial of low-dose pulse methotrexate in psoriatic arthritis. Arthritis Rheum. 1984;27:376–81.
5. Kozarek RA et al. Methotrexate induces clinical and histologic remission in patients with refractory inflammatory bowel disease. Ann Intern Med. 1989;110:353–6.
6. Jolivet J, Cowan KH, Curt GA, Clendeninn NJ, Chabner BA. The pharmacology and clinical use of methotrexate. N Engl J Med. 1983;309:1094–104.
7. Egan LJ, Sandborn WJ. Methotrexate for inflammatory bowel disease: pharmacology and preliminary results. Mayo Clin Proc. 1996;71:69–80.
8. Otterness IG, Chang YH. Comparative study of cyclophosphamide, 6-mercaptopurine, azathiopurine and methotrexate. Relative effects on the humoral and the cellular immune response in the mouse. Clin Exp Immunol. 1976;26:346–54.
9. Bianchi Porro G, Cassinotti A, Ferrara E, Maconi G, Ardizzone S. Review article: the management of steroid dependency in ulcerative colitis. Aliment Pharmacol Ther. 2007;26:779–94.
10. Herrlinger KR et al. The pharmacogenetics of methotrexate in inflammatory bowel disease. Pharmacogenet Genomics. 2005;15: 705–11.
11. Cronstein BN, Eberle MA, Gruber HE, Levin RI. Methotrexate inhibits neutrophil function by stimulating adenosine release from connective tissue cells. Proc Natl Acad Sci U S A. 1991;88: 2441–5.
12. Egan LJ, Sandborn WJ, Mays DC, Tremaine WJ, Lipsky JJ. Plasma and rectal adenosine in inflammatory bowel disease: effect of methotrexate. Inflamm Bowel Dis. 1999;5:167–73.
13. Genestier L et al. Immunosuppressive properties of methotrexate: apoptosis and clonal deletion of activated peripheral T cells. J Clin Invest. 1998;102:322–8.
14. Seitz M, Zwicker M, Loetscher P. Effects of methotrexate on differentiation of monocytes and production of cytokine inhibitors by monocytes. Arthritis Rheum. 1998;41:2032–8.
15. Crilly A et al. Interleukin 6 (IL-6) and soluble IL-2 receptor levels in patients with rheumatoid arthritis treated with low dose oral methotrexate. J Rheumatol. 1995;22:224–6.
16. Straub RH et al. Decrease of interleukin 6 during the first 12 months is a prognostic marker for clinical outcome during 36 months treatment with disease-modifying anti-rheumatic drugs. Br J Rheumatol. 1997;36:1298–303.
17. Thomas R, Carroll GJ. Reduction of leukocyte and interleukin-1 beta concentrations in the synovial fluid of rheumatoid arthritis patients treated with methotrexate. Arthritis Rheum. 1993;36: 1244–52.
18. Miossec P et al. Inhibition of the production of proinflammatory cytokines and immunoglobulins by interleukin-4 in an ex vivo model of rheumatoid synovitis. Arthritis Rheum. 1992;35: 874–83.
19. Brody M, Bohm I, Bauer R. Mechanism of action of methotrexate: experimental evidence that methotrexate blocks the binding of interleukin 1 beta to the interleukin 1 receptor on target cells. Eur J Clin Chem Clin Biochem. 1993;31:667–74.
20. Mello SB, Barros DM, Silva AS, Laurindo IM, Novaes GS. Methotrexate as a preferential cyclooxygenase 2 inhibitor in whole blood of patients with rheumatoid arthritis. Rheumatology (Oxford). 2000;39:533–6.
21. Kraan MC et al. Inhibition of neutrophil migration soon after initiation of treatment with leflunomide or methotrexate in patients with rheumatoid arthritis: findings in a prospective, randomized, double-blind clinical trial in fifteen patients. Arthritis Rheum. 2000;43:1488–95.
22. Faubion Jr WA, Loftus Jr EV, Harmsen WS, Zinsmeister AR, Sandborn WJ. The natural history of corticosteroid therapy for inflammatory bowel disease: a population-based study. Gastroenterology. 2001;121:255–60.
23. Singleton JW, Law DH, Kelley Jr ML, Mekhjian HS, Sturdevant RA. National Cooperative Crohn's Disease Study: adverse reactions to study drugs. Gastroenterology. 1979;77:870–82.
24. Feagan BG, Rochon J, Fedorak RN, Irvine EJ, Wild G, Sutherland L, et al. Methotrexate for the treatment of Crohn's disease. The North American Crohn's Study Group Investigators. N Engl J Med. 1995;332:292–7.
25. Ardizzone S et al. Comparison between methotrexate and azathioprine in the treatment of chronic active Crohn's disease: a randomized, investigator-blind study. Dig Liver Dis. 2003;35:619–27.
26. Oren R et al. Methotrexate in chronic active Crohn's disease: a double-blind, randomized. Israeli multicenter trial. Am J Gastroenterol. 1997;92:2203–9.
27. Mate-Jimenez J, Hermida C, Cantero-Perona J, Moreno-Otero R. 6-Mercaptopurine or methotrexate added to prednisone induces and

maintains remission in steroid-dependent inflammatory bowel disease. Eur J Gastroenterol Hepatol. 2000;12:1227–33.
28. Arora S et al. Methotrexate in Crohn's disease: results of a randomized, double-blind, placebo-controlled trial. Hepatogastroenterology. 1999;46:1724–9.
29. Egan LJ et al. A randomized dose-response and pharmacokinetic study of methotrexate for refractory inflammatory Crohn's disease and ulcerative colitis. Aliment Pharmacol Ther. 1999;13: 1597–604.
30. Feagan BG et al. A comparison of methotrexate with placebo for the maintenance of remission in Crohn's disease. North American Crohn's Study Group Investigators. N Engl J Med. 2000;342:1627–32. doi:10.1056/NEJM200006013422202.
31. Baert F, Noman M, Vermeire S, Van Assche G, D' Haens G, Carbonez A, et al. Influence of immunogenicity on the long-term efficacy of infliximab in Crohn's disease. N Engl J Med. 2003;348:601–8.
32. Feagan BG, McDonald JW, Panaccione R, Enns RA, Bernstein CN, Ponich TP, et al. Methotrexate in combination with infliximab is no more effective than infliximab alone in patients with Crohn's disease. Gastroenterology. 2014;146:681–8.
33. Best WR et al. Development of a Crohn's disease activity index. National Cooperative Crohn's Disease Study. Gastroenterology. 1976;70(3):439–44.
34. Guyatt G, Mitchell A, Irvine EJ, Singer J, Williams N, Goodacre R et al. A new measure of health status for clinical trials in inflammatory bowel disease. Gastroenterology. 1989;96(3):804–10.
35. Harvey RF, Bradshaw JM. A simple index of Crohn's-disease activity. Lancet. 1980;1(8167):514.
36. Harper J, Zisman T. Comparison of standard dose azathioprine versus low dose azathioprine when used as adjuvant therapy with infliximab in patients with inflammatory bowel disease. Am J Gastroenterol. 2012;107:S608–95.
37. Diaz-Saa W, Carpio-Lopez D, Fernandez-Salgado E, Alvarez-Sanchez MV, Vazquez-Rodriguez S, Gonzalez-Carrera V, et al. Methotrexate as a third-line therapy after thiopurine and anti-TNF failure in Crohn's Disease. J Crohns Colitis. 2012;6 Suppl 1: S104–5.
38. Seinen ML, de Boer NK, Mulder CJ, Bouma G, van Bodegraven AA. Effectiveness and tolerability of maintenance methotrexate therapy in Crohn's disease patient's; analysis of a referral hospital-based 10-years intercept cohort. Gastroenterology. 2011;140(5): S-280.
39. Seinen ML, Ponsioen C, de Boer NK, Oldenburg B, Bouma G, Mulder C, et al. Sustained clinical benefit and tolerability of methotrexate monotherapy after thiopurine therapy in patients with Crohn's disease. Clin Gastroenterol Hepatol. 2015;11(6):667–72.
40. Vermeire S, Noman M, Van Assche G, Baert F, D'Haens G, Rutgeerts P. Effectiveness of concomitant immunosuppressive therapy in suppressing the formation of antibodies to infliximab in Crohn's disease. Gut. 2007;56:1226–31.
41. Brooks PJ, Spruill WJ, Parish RC, Birchmore DA. Pharmacokinetics of methotrexate administered by intramuscular and subcutaneous injections in patients with rheumatoid arthritis. Arthritis Rheum. 1990;33:91–4.
42. Arthur V, Jubb R, Homer D. A study of parenteral use of methotrexate in rheumatic conditions. J Clin Nurs. 2002;11:256–63.
43. Jundt JW, Browne BA, Fiocco GP, Steele AD, Mock D. A comparison of low dose methotrexate bioavailability: oral solution, oral tablet, subcutaneous and intramuscular dosing. J Rheumatol. 1993;20:1845–9.
44. Oguey D, Kolliker F, Gerber NJ, Reichen J. Effect of food on the bioavailability of low-dose methotrexate in patients with rheumatoid arthritis. Arthritis Rheum. 1992;35:611–4.
45. Teresi ME, Crom WR, Choi KE, Mirro J, Evans WE. Methotrexate bioavailability after oral and intramuscular administration in children. J Pediatr. 1987;110:788–92.
46. Egan LJ et al. Systemic and intestinal pharmacokinetics of methotrexate in patients with inflammatory bowel disease. Clin Pharmacol Ther. 1999;65:29–39.
47. Balis FM et al. Pharmacokinetics of subcutaneous methotrexate. J Clin Oncol. 1988;6:1882–6.
48. al-Awadhi A, Dale P, McKendry RJ. Pancytopenia associated with low dose methotrexate therapy. A regional survey. J Rheumatol. 1993;20:1121–5.
49. Goodman TA, Polisson RP. Methotrexate: adverse reactions and major toxicities. Rheum Dis Clin North Am. 1994;20:513–28.
50. Gwavava NJ, Pinkerton CR, Glasgow JF, Sloan JM, Bridges JM. Small bowel enterocyte abnormalities caused by methotrexate treatment in acute lymphoblastic leukemia of childhood. J Clin Pathol. 1981;34:790–5.
51. Pinkerton CR, Cameron CH, Sloan JM, Glasgow JF, Gwevava NJ. Jejunal crypt cell abnormalities associated with methotrexate treatment in children with acute lymphoblastic leukemia. J Clin Pathol. 1982;35:1272–7.
52. Trier JS. Morphologic alterations induced by methotrexate in the mucosa of human proximal intestine. II. Electron microscopic observations. Gastroenterology. 1962;43:407–24.
53. Phelan MJ, Taylor W, van Heyningen C, Williams E, Thompson RN. Intestinal absorption in patients with rheumatoid arthritis treated with methotrexate. Clin Rheumatol. 1993;12:223–5.
54. Atherton LD, Leib ES, Kaye MD. Toxic megacolon associated with methotrexate therapy. Gastroenterology. 1984;86:1583–8.
55. Baker H. Intermittent high dose oral methotrexate therapy in psoriasis. Br J Dermatol. 1970;82:65–9.
56. Novak RA, Kessinger A. Methotrexate induced colitis. Nebr Med J. 1976;61:84–7.
57. Taylor SG, Hass GM, Crumrine JL, Slaughter DP. Toxic reactions of 4-amino-pteroylglutamic acid (aminopterin) in patients with far-advanced neoplastic disease. Cancer. 1950;3:493–503.
58. Uvizi J, Krajci A, Cerny K. Acute necrotizing colitis in a psoriatic treated by methotrexát (author's transl). Cesk Dermatol. 1977;52: 227–32.
59. Chong RY, Hanauer SB, Cohen RD. Efficacy of parenteral methotrexate in refractory Crohn's disease. Aliment Pharmacol Ther. 2001;15:35–44.
60. Patel N, Weatherly J, Abraham B. The role of methotrexate in azathioprine and 6-mercaptopurine-induced pancreatitis in inflammatory bowel disease patients. Am J Gastroenterol. 2013;108: S500–61.
61. Chen DD, Walijee AK, Govani SM, Higgins P, Stidham RW. Incident infectious and malignant adverse event risk is lower using methotrexate compared to thiopurines in Crohn's disease. Gastroenterology. 2015;148(4):S-234.
62. Kremer JM, Lee RG, Tolman KG. Liver histology in rheumatoid arthritis patients receiving long-term methotrexate therapy. A prospective study with baseline and sequential biopsy samples. Arthritis Rheum. 1989;32:121–7.
63. Lewis JH, Schiff E. Methotrexate-induced chronic liver injury: guidelines for detection and prevention. The ACG Committee on FDA-related matters. American College of Gastroenterology. Am J Gastroenterol. 1988;83:1337–45.
64. Newman M et al. The role of liver biopsies in psoriatic patients receiving long-term methotrexate treatment. Improvement in liver abnormalities after cessation of treatment. Arch Dermatol. 1989;125:1218–24.
65. Said S, Jeffes EW, Weinstein GD. Methotrexate. Clin Dermatol. 1997;15:781–97.
66. Walker AM et al. Determinants of serious liver disease among patients receiving low-dose methotrexate for rheumatoid arthritis. Arthritis Rheum. 1993;36:329–35.
67. Te HS et al. Hepatic effects of long-term methotrexate use in the treatment of inflammatory bowel disease. Am J Gastroenterol. 2000;95:3150–6.

68. Lemann M et al. Methotrexate in Crohn's disease: long-term efficacy and toxicity. Am J Gastroenterol. 2000;95:1730–4.
69. Lichtenstein GR, Abreu MT, Cohen R, Tremaine W. American Gastroenterological Association Institute medical position statement on corticosteroids, immunomodulators, and infliximab in inflammatory bowel disease. Gastroenterology. 2006;130:935–9.
70. Roenigk Jr HH et al. Methotrexate in psoriasis: revised guidelines. J Am Acad Dermatol. 1988;19(1 Pt 1):145–56.
71. Kremer JM et al. Methotrexate for rheumatoid arthritis. Suggested guidelines for monitoring liver toxicity. American College of Rheumatology. Arthritis Rheum. 1994;37(3):316–28.
72. Maurice PD, Maddox AJ, Green CA, Tatnall F, Schofield JK, Stott DJ. Monitoring patients on methotrexate: hepatic fibrosis not seen in patients with normal serum assays of aminoterminal peptide of type III procollagen. Br J Dermatol. 2005;152(3):451–8.
73. Barbero-Villares A, Mendoza Jiménez-Ridruejo J, Taxonera C, López-Sanromán A, Pajares R, Bermejo F, et al. Evaluation of liver fibrosis by transient elastography (Fibroscan®) in patients with inflammatory bowel disease treated with methotrexate: a multicentric trial. Scand J Gastroenterol. 2012;47(5):575–9.
74. Araujo Míguez A, Giráldez Gallego A, Leo Carnerero E, Trigo Salado C, De la Cruz Ramírez MD, HerreraJustiniano JM, et al. Assessment of liver fibrosis by transient elastography in patients with inflammatory bowel disease undergoing treatment with methotrexate. J Crohns Colitis. 2012;6 Suppl 1:S136.
75. Shah R, Petrova M, Redhead S, Berry P, Ala A. Liver fibrosis assessed by transient elastography in long-term methotrexate treated patients. United European Gastroenterol J. 2014:2(Suppl 1).
76. Frenia ML, Long KS. Methotrexate and nonsteroidal antiinflammatory drug interactions. Ann Pharmacother. 1992;26:234–7.
77. Baggott JE, Morgan SL, Ha T, Vaughn WH, Hine RJ. Inhibition of folate-dependent enzymes by non-steroidal anti-inflammatory drugs. Biochem J. 1992;282(Pt 1):197–202.
78. Duhra P. Treatment of gastrointestinal symptoms associated with methotrexate therapy for psoriasis. J Am Acad Dermatol. 1993;28:466–9.
79. Morgan SL et al. Supplementation with folic acid during methotrexate therapy for rheumatoid arthritis. A double-blind, placebo-controlled trial. Ann Intern Med. 1994;121:833–41.
80. Dupont-Lucas C, Grandiean-Blanchet C, Larocque C, Jantchou P, Amre DK, Deslandres C. Prevalence of methotrexate intolerance in paediatric inflammatory bowel disease. Gastroenterology. 2015;148(4, Suppl):S-235–6.
81. Laharie D, Billioud V, Roblin X, Filippi J, Ayroles A, Capdepont M, et al. Adherence to methotrexate (MTX) in inflammatory bowel disease (IBD) patients: an observational multicenter study. Gastroenterology. 2013;144(5, Suppl 1):S-778.
82. Salvage therapy with high/low methotrexate for loss of response to infliximab dose escalation. ClinicalTrials.gov Identifier: NCT02269358. ClinicalTrials.gov.

Adalimumab for the Treatment of Crohn's Disease

32

Remo Panaccione

Introduction

Crohn's disease (CD) is a chronic relapsing inflammatory disorder characterized by transmural inflammation, which can affect the gastrointestinal tract from mouth to anus. Common symptoms include abdominal pain, intestinal cramping, diarrhea, weight loss, and fatigue. The development of fibrostenosis of the intestinal lumen, fistulization, and the presence of significant extraintestinal manifestations may complicate the disease [1]. Many of the complications lead to the need for hospitalization and surgery. The ideal therapy for CD should be safe and effective. This therapy would effectively induce and maintain clinical remission without need for corticosteroids, halt the development of complications, and reduce hospitalizations and surgeries. This would lead to positive effects on quality of life (QoL) while enjoying a favorable safety profile [2]. Furthermore, demonstrating the ability to heal the mucosa is increasingly being appreciated as an important therapeutic endpoint with hopes that this may lead to a disease-modifying effect [3].

Advances in the understanding of the pathogenesis of IBD have led to the development of several agents specifically aimed at key elements of the inflammatory cascade. The development of antagonists to tumor necrosis factor-alpha (TNF-α) have played a major role in the advancement of therapy in CD. Infliximab (REMICADE®, Centocor Ortho Biotec Inc., Malvern, PA, USA) [4] and adalimumab (HUMIRA®, Abbott Laboratories, Abbott Park, IL, USA) [5] have been shown in pivotal clinical trials to induce and maintain clinical remission in patients with moderate-to-severe Crohn's disease (CD) [6–11], and certolizumab pegol (CIMZIA®, UCB Inc., Smyrna, GA, USA) [12] has been shown to reduce signs and symptoms of CD and maintain clinical response [13, 14]. In this chapter, the efficacy data from the major randomized controlled trials, open label studies, and safety data supporting the use of adalimumab in the treatment of CD are reviewed. The use of adalimumab in clinical practice will be put into context.

R. Panaccione, M.D., F.R.C.P.C. (✉)
Inflammatory Bowel Disease Clinic, Professor of Medicine, University of Calgary, Calgary, Canada
e-mail: rpanacci@ucalgary.ca

Background

Adalimumab (ADA) (Humira™, Abbott, USA) is a recombinant fully human IgG_1 monoclonal antibody that binds to TNF-α which can be self-administered subcutaneously (such). It consists of human-derived heavy and light chain variable regions and human IgG_1:k constant regions. TNF-α is a 51-kDa pro-inflammatory cytokine formed by three soluble 17-kDa monomer proteins. It is secreted by monocytes, macrophages, and T-cells [15–17]. The binding of TNF-α to its receptors leads to a number of intracellular events culminating in the activation of nuclear factor kB and the production of pro-inflammatory cytokines such as interleukin (IL)-1 and IL-6, activation of neutrophils, and promotion of leukocyte migration, all of which are key elements of the inflammatory cascade in Crohn's disease [18–20].

Pharmacodynamics

ADA binds with high affinity to TNF-α, thus blocking its interactions with its receptors. In binding both soluble and transmembrane TNF-α, ADA fixes complement, causes antibody-dependent cell-mediated cytotoxicity and induces T-cell apoptosis which is thought to be a key mechanism by which both infliximab and ADA exert their effect [21–23].

Pharmacokinetics

In a randomized, double-blind, placebo controlled trial of ADA for the induction of remission for Crohn's disease,

D.C. Baumgart (ed.), *Crohn's Disease and Ulcerative Colitis*, DOI 10.1007/978-3-319-33703-6_32

Clinical Assessment of Adalimumab Safety and Efficacy as Studied for the Induction of Crohn's Disease (CLASSIC-I), mean serum concentrations (microgram per milliliter) at week 4 were 2.79 ± 1.48 ($n=66$), 5.65 ± 3.06 ($n=65$), and 12.61 ± 5.25 ($n=67$) for the 40/20, 80/40, and 160/80 mg groups, respectively [9]. Concomitant use of 6-mercaptopurine or azathioprine was not associated with differences in mean serum concentrations [9]. In a randomized, double-blind, placebo-controlled trial of ADA for the induction of remission in patients who have had loss of response or intolerance to infliximab, Gauging Adalimumab Efficacy in Infliximab Non-Responders (GAIN), the median ADA concentration was 12.2 micrograms/ml following administration of 160 mg at week 0 and 80 mg at week 2 [11]. The bioavailability of ADA is 64% with a $T_{1/2}$ of approximately 2 weeks in healthy volunteers.

Immunogenicity

The immunogenicity of infliximab is a well-described phenomenon owing, in part, to its chimeric nature. In a study of ADA for the treatment of rheumatoid arthritis the development of anti-adalimumab antibodies (AAA) occurred in 5% of patients overall (1% for patients on concomitant methotrexate and 12% for patients on ADA monotherapy) [24]. No data was collected, in this study, on the influence of antibodies on ADA levels and clinical response. A later study in rheumatoid arthritis, however, demonstrated that 17% of patients developed AAA [25]. Moreover, the presence of AAA was associated with lack of clinical response and lower serum ADA levels. Patients with AAA had a median serum ADA concentration of 1.2 mg/l (range: 0.0–5.6) versus 11.0 mg/l (range: 2.0–33.0) for those with no antibodies. The presence of AAA and measurement of ADA levels in this study were assayed using a technique developed by the authors and is not performed in the context of an industry sponsored clinical trial so the assays may not be directly comparable. In the CLASSIC-II trial, a maintenance trial of adalimumab for CD, 2.6% of patients (7/269) for which data was available developed AAA. All AAAs occurred in patients on monotherapy as none of the 84 patients on concomitant antimetabolites developed antibodies [26].

Clinical Efficacy of Adalimumab in Crohn's Disease

Randomized Controlled Trials for the Induction of Remission and Response

In CLASSIC I [9], 299 patients with moderate-to-severe CD defined by a Crohn's Disease Activity Index (CDAI) score of 220–450 were randomized to one of three induction regimens of subcutaneous (such) ADA (ADA 160 mg week 0, 80 mg week 2; ADA 80 mg week 0, 40 mg week 2; ADA 40 mg week 0, 20 mg week 2) or placebo such at weeks 0 and 2. Primary endpoint was the proportion of patients who achieved clinical remission as defined by CDAI of less the 150 points at week 4 in the two highest dosing regimens compared to placebo. Secondary endpoints included responses as defined by both 70 and 100 point drops in the CDAI. Statistical differences were observed in the primary endpoint of remission between 160/80 mg ADA and combined (160/80 mg ADA and 80/40 mg ADA) groups compared to placebo. At the highest dosing group (160/80 mg ADA) 36% of patients achieved remission compared to 12% in the placebo group ($p=0.001$). Fifty percent of patients in the 160/80 mg group had a response defined by a 100 point decrease in CDAI and 59% had a response defined by a 70-point drop in the CDAI both superior and statistically significant to placebo.

In GAIN [11], 325 patients with moderate-to-severe CD who had previously been exposed to infliximab and lost response or became intolerant to infliximab were randomized to receive either ADA such 160 mg at week 0, followed by 80 mg at week 2 or placebo. The primary endpoint was remission as defined by the CDAI at week 4. Twenty-one percent of ADA treated at patients entered into remission, 52% had a decrease of 70 points in the CDAI, and 38% had a decrease of 100 points in the CDAI at week 4 (7%, 34%, 25% for placebo respectively; $p<0.05$). Based on the results of these studies ADA was granted expedited review by regulatory agencies in the USA, Canada, and the European Union.

Randomized Controlled Trials for the Maintenance of Remission and Response

Two hundred seventy-five patients from CLASSIC I enrolled in CLASSIC II and received open-label ADA 40 mg at Weeks 0 and 2 (Weeks 4 and 6 of CLASSIC I) [26]. Patients who were in remission at both Week 0 (end CLASSIC I/ beginning CLASSIC II) and Week 4 were re-randomized to 40 mg every other week (e.o.w.), weekly, or placebo through 56 weeks. In the re-randomized cohort, 79% who received ADA 40 mg e.o.w. and 83% who received 40 mg weekly maintained remission through Week 56, vs. 44% for placebo ($p<0.05$ for both ADA groups vs. placebo).

In CHARM (Crohn's Trial of the fully Human Antibody Adalimumab for Remission Maintenance), 854 patients with moderate-to-severe CD received open label ADA SC at doses of 80 mg at week 0 and 40 mg at week 2 [10]. Patients who had been exposed to IFX in the past and either lost response or had become intolerant to infliximab were eligible for this trial. Patients who responded, as defined by a drop in CDAI of 70 points, were then randomized to one of three treatment arms; ADA 40 mg e.o.w., ADA 40 mg weekly, or placebo. Approximately 60 % of patients responded to the initial 80/40 mg induction dose at week 4 and were randomized. At week 26, 40 % of the ADA 40 mg e.o.w., 47 % of the ADA 40 mg weekly and 17 % of the placebo group were in remission ($p=0.001$ for both groups compared to placebo, no difference between active groups). The benefit was maintained out to week 56 with 36 % ADA 40 mg e.o.w., 41 % ADA 40 mg weekly, and 12 % placebo group remaining in remission ($p=0.001$). A difference was not appreciated in the proportion of patients who were able to maintain remission or response according to their previous infliximab exposure.

Within the CHARM study population 117 patients had active perianal fistulizing disease. Although, the study was not specifically designed or powered to evaluate patients with fistula, one-third of patients treated with ADA had complete healing of fistula. Several open label cohorts from various parts of the world have substantiated this data with reported fistula closure rates between 30 and 50 % over the first year of therapy [27, 28].

Effect of Adalimumab on Quality of Life and Hospitalization

Quality of life in patients with CD is often assessed using the inflammatory bowel disease questionnaire (IBDQ); a validated measure of quality of life in patients with IBD assessing systemic features, bowel system, emotional and social function. Scores can range between 32 and 224 with a score of >170 on the IBDQ correlating with clinical remission as defined by a CDAI <150 [29]. In patients continued on ADA 40 mg SC every other week or weekly in CLASSIC-II, IBDQ >170 were maintained, whereas placebo-treated patients had IBDQ scores that rapidly declined demonstrating that sustained response to ADA was associated with improved QOL [30]. In patients in the GAIN study, scores in the ADA-treated patients were significantly higher in all four domains of the IBDQ than in placebo-treated patients again demonstrating improved quality of life associated with treatment with ADA [31].

An important measure of success with respect to managing patients with CD is an ability to reduce the rate of hospitalization for management of the disease. In a study evaluating patients enrolled in the CHARM study a secondary analysis evaluated rates of hospitalization in patients treated with placebo versus those treated with ADA [32]. At 56-weeks, the actuarial hospitalization rate in placebo- and ADA-treated patients was 13.9 % and 5.9 %, respectively ($p<0.01$) with treatment with ADA being the only independent factor associated with reduced risk [32].

Effect of Adalimumab on Mucosal Healing

In the 52-week EXTEND (*EXT*end the Safety and *E*fficacy of Adalimumab by E*ND*oscopic Healing) trial, mucosal healing (defined as absence of mucosal ulceration observed by endoscopy) at Weeks 12 and 52 was 27 % and 24 % ($p=0.056$), respectively, for the adalimumab maintenance group compared with 13 % and 0 % ($p<0.001$), respectively, for patients who received adalimumab 160-/80-mg for induction only followed by placebo [33]. A post-hoc analysis of mucosal healing rates by baseline disease duration showed a greater treatment effect (adalimumab vs. placebo) at Week 12 for patients with a disease duration <5 years versus ≥5 years ($p=0.029$) [34].

Safety and Tolerability

Safety of Anti-TNF Agents as a Class

With a few exceptions, the safety data with respect to anti-TNF agents falls into two broad categories: class specific and agent specific effects. For the most part, safety concerns are a class effect. The safety issues related to the use of anti-TNF agents includes infusion/injection reactions, infections, autoimmunity, malignancies (both hematological and solid organ) and other events such as demyelinating disease, congestive heart failure, hematologic and hepatic abnormalities including reactivation of hepatitis B.

Infusion reactions in infliximab-treated patients in clinical trials occurred in 2–16 % of cases [6–8] Premedication with corticosteroids and an antihistamine may prevent subsequent reactions [35]. Injection site reactions can occur with the subcutaneously administered anti-TNF agents at a rate of up to 6 % as reported in clinical trials [9–11, 24]. Delayed hypersensitivity reactions are well described in the setting of the administration of infliximab and can occur at any time point and are characterized by arthralgia, myalgias, fever, urticaria, and rash and generally occur several days after an infusion.

Infectious complications that occur with the use of anti-TNF agents can be thought of as minor infections and serious infections. Most minor infectious comprise of nonspecific upper respiratory tract infections or urinary tract infections and occur in approximately one third of patients and are comparable across all three agents in the class [36]. Generally, minor infections may delay a scheduled treatment, but do not lead to discontinuation of therapy. Serious infections have been reported with the use of anti-TNF agents and include pneumonia, cellulitis, and sepsis and abscess formation. In clinical trials of infliximab, serious infections occurred in 4–5 % of patients. Opportunistic infections, such as pneumocystis carinii pneumonia, listeriosis, histoplasmosis, and mucormycosis have been reported but are rare [37–40]. A recent meta-analysis did demonstrate that anti-TNF therapy doubled the risk of opportunistic infections [41]. However, it is important to recognize that patients using anti-TNF agents are often taking concomitant therapy with other potentially immune-suppressive medications including corticosteroids. Data from the TREAT registry (Crohn's disease Therapy, Evaluation and Assessment Tool), a large voluntary registry of patients with Crohn's disease treated with a variety of therapies, revealed that serious infections were linked more to the use of corticosteroids and narcotics than to the use of infliximab or immunosuppressive therapy when evaluated by multivariate logistic regression analysis [42]. The use of anti-TNF agents is known to be associated with reactivation of latent tuberculosis and appropriate screening in advance of administration is mandatory [43].

The development of antinuclear antibodies (ANAs) is known to be associated with the use of anti-TNF agents [44] in a cohort of 125 patients exposed to infliximab, the incidence of ANA at 24 months was 57 % [44]. Drug induced lupus with positive ANA and Anti-dsDNA has been described but is rare [45].

The potential for the development of a malignancy in association with anti-TNF therapy has always been a theoretical concern owing to their immunosuppressive nature. The majority of reported malignancies temporally associated with anti-TNF therapy have been non-Hodgkin's lymphomas. In the TREAT registry, 0.42 patients per 100 patient years in the infliximab-treated group developed malignancies compare to 0.51 patients per 100 patient years in those not treated with infliximab. With respect to lymphomas specifically, the incidence per 100 patient years was 0.062 in the infliximab-treated group compared to 0.057 in those not treated with infliximab [42]. The difference was not statistically significant between groups with either comparison. A meta-analysis of randomized trials examined the risk of serious infection and malignancy in patients with rheumatoid arthritis treated with infliximab and adalimumab [46]. This study concluded that the odds ratio for malignancy with anti-TNF therapy was 3.3 (95 % confidence interval, 1.2–9.1) compared to placebo. However, the study has been criticized with respect to how trials were selected for inclusion, the statistical methods employed, the lack of control for potential confounders and the inclusion of non-melanotic skin cancers into malignancy estimates. How this controversial data translates into the IBD population is unknown. There has been concern related to the reporting of a number of cases of a rare form of $\delta\gamma$ T cell lymphoma (hepatosplenic T cell lymphoma) in CD patients treated with anti-TNF agents [47]. These cases all occurred in younger patients between the ages of 12 and 31 with the majority being on or having recently received thiopurine therapy (6-MP/AZA). Given the rarity of the event, the true relevance of this as it pertains to the use of anti-TNF therapy in CD is unknown but remains an issue worthy of ongoing vigilance. There is however a recognition that anti-TNF therapy is associated with and increased risk of non-melanotic skin cancer (NMSC) and possibly even melanotic skin cancer (MSC) [48]. It is therefore recommended that patients receiving anti-TNF therapy have at least annual skin exams and employ proper skin protection [49].

Patients with preexisting New York Heart Congestive Heart Failure (CHF) Class III or IV, or those with a history of multiple sclerosis or optic neuritis should not receive anti-TNF therapy as worsening of CHF and demyelinating syndromes have been described [50–53].

Overall, however, the large experience from clinical trials in a variety of disease states over time with adalimumab has not shown an increase in adverse events which is reassuring [54].

Safety of Adalimumab in Open-Label and Controlled Studies

A recent study pooled all data from controlled trials of adalimumab in CD and assessed the rates of adverse events (AE) [45]. Data was available for 1459 patients with a total of 1506 patient years of ADA exposure. For those patients in induction studies, there was no difference in infectious AE at any dose of ADA versus placebo. For patients in maintenance studies, there was a significantly greater number of AE leading to discontinuation of therapy in the placebo-treated patients than in ADA exposed patients. In the total cohort of exposed patients, there were two cases of demyelinating disease, three cases of tuberculosis, one case of CHF, three cases of lupus like reaction and two deaths. The two deaths were due to pulmonary embolism in an elderly patient and acute myeloid leukemia in a patient on AZA.

With respect to autoimmunity, increases in titers of ANAs and Anti-dsDNA antibodies have been reported to occur in 5.3 % and 12.9 % of ADA-treated RA patients [55].

The Use of Adalimumab in Clinical Practice

For those patients who require biologic therapy, adalimumab is a very good option in both patients who are bio-naïve and those patients who have lost response to or become intolerant to infliximab. The efficacy of adalimumab with respect to both induction and maintenance of CD is comparable to that of infliximab. This is supported by data from the pivotal randomized controlled trials CLASSIC I, CHARM, and GAIN. Moreover, the safety concerns of the two agents are generally equivalent with the exception of agent-specific issues such as infusion vs. injection site reactions. For these reasons either agent is an acceptable choice as a first-line biologic agent for patients with luminal disease.

The induction dosing in the North American labels and Europe are slightly different. The approved induction dosing in North America is 160 mg/80 mg at weeks 0 and 2 as opposed to Europe where the 80 mg/40 mg dosing regimen is cited as the preferred induction except for patients with severe disease where the 160 mg/80 mg dosing is suggested. Of interest recent studies demonstrate that in large cohorts that the 160 mg/80 mg dosing is likely superior both short and long-term. A single-center analysis of adalimumab use for CD in 168 infliximab-exposed patients showed that the 160/80-mg induction dose was associated with more frequent CRP normalization ($p=0.04$), more frequent ($p=0.004$) and longer sustained clinical benefit ($p=0.04$), and less frequent primary nonresponse ($p<0.0001$) compared with the 80/40-mg regimen [56]. In addition, two real-world observational analyses found that patients who received the 160-/80-mg induction regimen were approximately half as likely to receive dosage intensification (i.e., weekly dosing) compared with other induction regimens ($p<0.0001$) [57, 58]. Based on the clinical trial data as well as these recent reports the author always uses the 160 mg/80 mg induction regimen.

In addition, it appears that a subgroup of patients may require longer than the "4 week induction period" to achieve full efficacy. Although many patients respond to ADA by Week 4, some may require a longer duration of therapy to achieve initial clinical response and remission. For nonresponders in CHARM and GAIN, defined as failure to achieve a ≥70-point decrease in CDAI at Week 4, more than 50 % achieved a response by Week 8 and at least 60 % achieved it by Week 12 [59]. Rates of clinical remission for the CHARM initial nonresponders were 26 % by Week 8 and 28 % by Week 12; the corresponding rates for the GAIN nonresponders were 19 % and 25 %, respectively [59]. Clinicians should consider continuing ADA 40-mg e.o.w. therapy for up to an additional 8 weeks after induction, before deeming the patient a treatment failure. Options for potential nonresponders include increasing the dosage to 40 mg weekly or switching to an alternative agent if symptoms persist after dosage adjustment.

The durability of response beyond 1 year may be a differentiating feature between the anti-TNF agents where it appears that ADA may have an advantage. ADA clinical trial data have demonstrated sustained clinical remission, improvements in quality of life, reductions in hospitalization, steroid-sparing effects, and fistula healing during long-term treatment for CD for up to 4 years [60–62].

Patient preference may play a large role in which anti-TNF agent is preferred by the patients [63]. In a young patient population such as CD, the every other week, subcutaneous administration of ADA may represent a significant potential advantage over the intravenous administration of infliximab. It allows for more flexibility regarding travel, work, and education [63].

ADA is the only biologic available for patients who have become intolerant to, or lost response to infliximab. This represents a significant proportion of patients after 1 year of therapy. Data from the GAIN study indicates that ADA has efficacy in this population. However, the expected response rate is approximately 8–15 % lower than in infliximab naïve patients.

An obvious temptation of both patients and physicians will be to consider switching from intravenously administered infliximab to subcutaneously administered adalimumab in those patients who have demonstrated and maintained a response to the former agent. It is worth noting that in the only study which systematically looked at this, elective switching from infliximab to adalimumab was associated with loss of tolerance and loss of efficacy within 1 year [64]. Therefore, adherence to the first anti-TNF agent is always recommended including proper dose optimization before switching.

Towards Earlier Use

Anti-TN therapy has been a significant advance in the treatment of Crohn's disease with the benefits that are outlined in this chapter. However, there has been a push towards earlier and earlier use. Most recently, the use of early combined adalimumab therapy (adalimumab plus an immunosuppressant) has been evaluated versus conventional management in a cluster randomization trial—REACT (Randomized Evaluation of an Algorithm for Crohn's Treatment) [65]. Although early combined therapy was not superior to conventional management with respect to controlling Crohn's disease symptoms, it did show significant differences in the reduction of complications, hospitalization, and surgery. The interpretation is that earlier use is associated with better long-term outcomes irrespective of symptoms.

In summary, adalimumab represents an important step in the evolution of anti-TNF therapy and is a welcome addition to our therapeutic armamentarium for CD. Its convenient subcutaneous administration coupled with its proven efficacy and safety will likely position it as the dominant biologic agent for luminal CD, especially if it delivers on other evolving areas of biologic therapy such as mucosal healing. Although the impact of anti-TNF therapy in the treatment of CD has been substantial, one-third of patients do not respond to these agents. This underscores the need for better defining not only which patients will best respond to these agents, but also which patients would benefit from earlier use of a biologic agent as well as the need to continue to develop novel biologic agents with alternate mechanisms of action.

References

1. Baumgart DC, Carding SR. Inflammatory bowel disease: cause and immunobiology. Lancet. 2007;369:1627–40. Review.
2. Panaccione R, Rutgeerts P, Sandborn WJ, Feagan B, Schreiber S, Ghosh S, et al. Treatment algorithms to maximize remission and minimize corticosteroid dependence in patients with inflammatory bowel disease. Aliment Pharmacol Ther. 2008;28:674–88.
3. Frøslie KF, Jahnsen J, Moum BA, et al. Mucosal healing in inflammatory bowel disease: results from a Norwegian population-based cohort. Gastroenterology. 2007;133:412–22.
4. REMICADE [prescribing information]. Malvern, PA: Centocor Otho Biotec Inc. (2010). Available at: http://www.remicade.com/remicade/global/hcp/hcp_pi.html. Accessed 2 Jan 2011.
5. HUMIRA [prescribing information]. North Chicago, IL: Abbott Laboratories. (2010). Available at: http://www.rxabbott.com/pdf/humira.pdf. Accessed 2 Jan 2011.
6. Targan SR, Hanauer SB, Sander JH, et al. A short-term study of chimeric monoclonal antibody cA2 to tumor necrosis factor α for Crohn's disease. N Engl J Med. 1997;337:1029–35.
7. Hanauer SB, Feagan BG, Lichtenstein GR, et al. Maintenance infliximab for Crohn's disease: the ACCENT I randomised trial. Lancet. 2002;359:1541–9.
8. Present DH, Rutgeerts P, Targan S, et al. Infliximab for the treatment of fistulas in patients with Crohn's disease. N Engl J Med. 1999;340:1398–405.
9. Hanauer SB, Sandborn WJ, Rutgeerts P, et al. Human anti-tumor necrosis factor monoclonal antibody (adalimumab) in Crohn's disease: the CLASSIC-I trial. Gastroenterology. 2006;130:323–33. quiz 591.
10. Colombel JF, Sandborn WJ, Rutgeerts P, et al. Adalimumab for maintenance of clinical response and remission in patients with Crohn's disease: the CHARM trial. Gastroenterology. 2007;132: 52–65.
11. Sandborn WJ, Rutgeerts P, Enns R, et al. Adalimumab induction therapy for Crohn disease previously treated with infliximab: a randomized trial. Ann Intern Med. 2007;146:829–38.
12. CIMZIA [prescribing information] UCB Inc., Smyrna, GA (2010). Available at: http://www.cimzia.com/pi.aspx#1ARbta4mCUE6. Accessed 2 Jan 2011.
13. Sandborn WJ, Feagan BG, Stoinov S, et al. Certolizumab pegol for the treatment of Crohn's disease. N Engl J Med. 2007;357: 228–38.
14. Schreiber S, Khaliq-Kareemi M, Lawrance IC, et al. Maintenance therapy with certolizumab pegol for Crohn's disease. N Engl J Med. 2007;357:239–50.
15. Aggarwal BB, Kohr WJ, Hass PE, et al. Human tumor necrosis factor. Production, purification, and characterization. J Biol Chem. 1985;260:2345–54.
16. Smith RA, Baglioni C. The active form of tumor necrosis factor is a trimer. J Biol Chem. 1987;262:6951–4.
17. Kozuch PL, Hanauer SB. General principles and pharmacology of biologics in inflammatory bowel disease. Gastroenterol Clin North Am. 2006;35:757–73.
18. Murch SH, Braegger CP, Walker-Smith JA, et al. Location of tumor necrosis factor alpha by immunohistochemistry in chronic inflammatory bowel disease. Gut. 1993;34:1705–9.
19. Reinecker HC, Steffen M, Witthoeft T, et al. Enhanced secretion of tumor necrosis factor-alpha, IL-6, and IL-1 beta by isolated lamina propria mononuclear cells from patients with ulcerative colitis and Crohn's disease. Clin Exp Immunol. 1993;94:174–81.
20. Ghezzi P, Cerami A. Tumor necrosis factor as a pharmacological target. Methods Mol Med. 2004;98:1–8.
21. Fosatti G, Nesbit AM. Effect of the anti-TNF agents, adalimumab, etanercept, infliximab, and certolizumab pegol on the induction of apoptosis in activated peripheral blood lymphocytes and monocytes. Am J Gastroenterol. 2005; 100.
22. Lugering A, Schmidt M, Lugering N, et al. Infliximab induces apoptosis in monocytes from patients with chronic active Crohn's disease by using a caspase-dependent pathway. Gastroenterology. 2001;121:1145–57.
23. Shen C, Assche GV, Colpaert S, et al. Adalimumab induces apoptosis of human monocytes: a comparative study with infliximab and etanercept. Aliment Pharmacol Ther. 2005;21:251–8.
24. Breedveld FC, Weisman MH, Kavanaugh AF, et al. The PREMIER study: a multicenter, randomized, double-blind clinical trial of combination therapy with adalimumab plus methotrexate versus methotrexate alone or adalimumab alone in patients with early, aggressive rheumatoid arthritis who had not had previous methotrexate treatment. Arthritis Rheum. 2006;54:26–37.
25. Bartelds GM, Wijbrandts CA, Nurmohamed MT, et al. Clinical response to adalimumab: relationship to anti-adalimumab antibodies and serum adalimumab concentrations in rheumatoid arthritis. Ann Rheum Dis. 2007;66:921–6.
26. Sandborn WJ, Hanauer SB, Rutgeerts P, et al. Adalimumab for maintenance treatment of Crohn's disease: results of the CLASSIC II trial. Gut. 2007;56:1232–9.
27. Panaccione R, Loftus Jr EV, Binion D, et al. Efficacy and safety of adalimumab in Canadian patients with moderate to severe Crohn's disease: results of the Adalimumab in Canadian SubjeCts with ModErate to Severe Crohn's DiseaSe (ACCESS) trial. Can J Gastroenterol. 2011;25:419–25.
28. Fortea-Ormaechea JI, González-Lama Y, Casis B, et al. Adalimumab is effective in long-term real life clinical practice in both luminal and perianal Crohn's disease. Madrid Exp Gastroenterol Hepatol. 2011;34:443–8.
29. Irvine EJ, Feagan B, Rochon J, et al. Quality of life: a valid and reliable measure of therapeutic efficacy in the treatment of inflammatory bowel disease. Canadian Crohn's Relapse Prevention Trial Study Group. Gastroenterology. 1994;106:287–96.
30. Rutgeerts PJ, Melilli LE, Li J, et al. Adalimumab maintains improvement in Inflammatory Bowel Disease Questionnaire (IBDQ) scores over 1 year following the initial attainment of remission in patients with moderately to severely active Crohn's disease: results of the Classic II Study. Gastroenterology. 2006;130:T1125.
31. Loftus EV, Feagan BG, Colombel JF, et al. Effects of adalimumab maintenance therapy on health-related quality of life of patients with Crohn's disease: patient-reported outcomes of the CHARM trial. Am J Gastroenterol. 2008;103:3132–41.
32. Feagan BG, Panaccione R, Sandborn WJ, D'haens GR, Schreiber S, Rutgeerts PJ, et al. Effect of adalimumab on the incidence of hospitalization and surgery in patients with Crohn's disease: results from the CHARM study. Gastroenterology. 2008;135:1493–9.
33. Rutgeerts P, D' Haens G, Colombel JF, et al. Adalimumab induces and maintains mucosal healing in patients with moderate to severe ileocolonic Crohn's disease—first results of the EXTEND trial. Gastroenterology. 2009;136(5 Suppl 1):A-116.
34. Sandborn WJ, Colombel JF, Rutgeerts P, et al. Crohn's disease mucosal healing in adalimumab-treated patients is affected by disease duration: results from EXTEND. Gastroenterology. 2010;138 Suppl 1:164.
35. Cheifetz A, Smedley M, Martin S, et al. The incidence and management of infusion reactions to infliximab: a large center experience. Am J Gastroenterol. 2003;98:1315–24.
36. Reddy JG, Loftus Jr EV. Safety of infliximab and other biologic agents in the inflammatory bowel diseases. Gastroenterol Clin North Am. 2006;35:837–55.
37. Colombel JF, Loftus Jr EV, Tremaine WJ, et al. The safety profile of infliximab in patients with Crohn's disease: the Mayo clinic experience in 500 patients. Gastroenterology. 2004;126:19–31.

38. Ricart E, Panaccione R, Loftus EV, et al. Infliximab for Crohn's disease in clinical practice at the Mayo Clinic: the first 100 patients. Am J Gastroenterol. 2001;96:722–9.
39. Cohen RD, Tsang JF, Hanauer SB. Infliximab in Crohn's disease: first anniversary clinical experience. Am J Gastroenterol. 2000;95: 3469–77.
40. Farrell RJ, Shah SA, Lodhavia PJ, et al. Clinical experience with infliximab therapy in 100 patients with Crohn's disease. Am J Gastroenterol. 2000;95:3490–7.
41. Ford AC, Peyrin-Biroulet L. Opportunistic infections with anti-tumor necrosis factor-α therapy in inflammatory bowel disease: meta-analysis of randomized controlled trials. Am J Gastroenterol. 2013;108(8):1268–76.
42. Lichtenstein GR, Feagan BG, Cohen RD, et al. Serious infections and mortality in association with therapies for Crohn's disease: TREAT registry. Clin Gastroenterol Hepatol. 2006;4:621–30.
43. Keane J, Gershon S, Wise RP, et al. Tuberculosis associated with infliximab, a tumor necrosis factor alpha-neutralizing agent. N Engl J Med. 2001;345:1098–104.
44. Vermeire S, Noman M, Van Assche G, et al. Autoimmunity associated with anti-tumor necrosis factor alpha treatment in Crohn's disease: a prospective cohort study. Gastroenterology. 2003;125:32–9.
45. Debandt M, Vittecoq O, Descamps V, et al. Anti-TNF-alpha-induced systemic lupus syndrome. Clin Rheumatol. 2003;22:56–61.
46. Bongartz T, Sutton AJ, Sweeting MJ, et al. Anti-TNF antibody therapy in rheumatoid arthritis and the risk of serious infections and malignancies: systematic review and meta-analysis of rare harmful effects in randomized controlled trials. JAMA. 2006;295:2275–85.
47. Shale M, Kanfer E, Panaccione R, et al. Hepatosplenic T cell lymphoma in inflammatory bowel disease. Gut. 2008;57(12):1639–41.
48. McKenna MR, Stobaugh DJ, Deepak P. Melanoma and non-melanoma skin cancer in inflammatory bowel disease patients following tumor necrosis factor-α inhibitor monotherapy and in combination with thiopurines: analysis of the Food and Drug Administration Adverse Event Reporting System. J Gastrointestin Liver Dis. 2014;23(3):267–71.
49. Annese V, Beaugerie L, Egan L, et al. European evidence-based consensus: inflammatory bowel disease and malignancies. J Crohns Colitis. 2015 Aug 20. pii: jjv141. [Epub ahead of print]. 2014; 23(3):267–71.
50. Kwon HJ, Cote TR, Cuffe MS, et al. Case reports of heart failure after therapy with a tumor necrosis factor antagonist. Ann Intern Med. 2003;138:807–11.
51. Chung ES, Packer M, Lo KH, et al. Randomized, double-blind, placebo-controlled, pilot trial of infliximab, a chimeric monoclonal antibody to tumor necrosis factor-alpha, in patients with moderate-to-severe heart failure: results of the anti-TNF Therapy Against Congestive Heart Failure (ATTACH) trial. Circulation. 2003;107:3133–40.
52. Mohan N, Edwards ET, Cupps TR, et al. Demyelination occurring during anti-tumor necrosis factor alpha therapy for inflammatory arthritides. Arthritis Rheum. 2001;44:2862–9.
53. Robinson WH, Genovese MC, Moreland LW. Demyelinating and neurologic events reported in association with tumor necrosis factor alpha antagonism: by what mechanisms could tumor necrosis factor alpha antagonists improve rheumatoid arthritis but exacerbate multiple sclerosis? Arthritis Rheum. 2001;44:1977–83.
54. Burmester GR, Panaccione R, Gordon KB, et al. Adalimumab: long-term safety in 23 458 patients from global clinical trials in rheumatoid arthritis, juvenile idiopathic arthritis, ankylosing spondylitis, psoriatic arthritis, psoriasis and Crohn's disease. Ann Rheum Dis. 2013;72(4):517–24.
55. Atzeni F, Turiel M, Capsoni F, Doria A, Meroni P, Sarzi-Puttini P. Autoimmunity and anti-TNF-alpha agents. Ann N Y Acad Sci. 2005;1051:559–69.
56. Karmiris K, Paintaud G, Noman M, et al. Influence of trough serum levels and immunogenicity on long-term outcome of adalimumab therapy in Crohn's disease. Gastroenterology. 2009;137(5): 1628–40.
57. Loftus EV, Pan X, Zurawski P, et al. Adalimumab real-world dosage pattern and predictors of weekly dosing: patients with Crohn's disease in the United States. J Crohns Colitis. 2011;238 Suppl 1:134.
58. Rubin DT, Uluscu O, Sederman R. Response to biologic therapy in Crohn's disease is improved with early treatment: an analysis of health claims data. Inflamm Bowel Dis. 2012;18(12):2225–31.
59. Panaccione R, Colombel JF, Sandborn WJ, et al. Response after 12 weeks of adalimumab therapy in patients with Crohn's disease who were nonresponders at week 4. Am J Gastroenterol. 2008;103 Suppl 1:S379.
60. Panaccione R, Colombel JF, Sandborn WJ, et al. Adalimumab sustains clinical remission and overall clinical benefit after 2 years of therapy for Crohn's disease. Aliment Pharmacol Ther. 2010;31: 1296–309.
61. Panaccione R, Colombel JF, Sandborn WJ, et al. Adalimumab maintains remission of Crohn's disease after up to 4 years of treatment: data from CHARM and ADHERE. Aliment Pharmacol Ther. 2013;38(10):1236–47.
62. Loftus EV, Rubin D, Mulani P, et al. Quality-of-life improvements in patients with Crohn's disease treated for 3 years with adalimumab in an open-label extension of CHARM. Gastroenterology. 2009;136 Suppl 1:179.
63. Allen PB, Lindsay H, Tham TC. How do patients with inflammatory bowel disease want their biological therapy administered? BMC Gastroenterol. 2010;10:1.
64. Van Assche G, Vermeire S, Ballet V, et al. Switch to adalimumab in patients with Crohn's disease controlled by maintenance infliximab: prospective randomised SWITCH trial. Gut. 2012;61(2): 229–34.
65. Khanna R, Bressler B, Levesque BG, et al. Early combined immunosuppression for the management of Crohn's disease (REACT): a cluster randomised controlled trial. Lancet. 2015;386(10006): 1825–34.

Biologic Therapy of Crohn's Disease: Certolizumab

33

Alessandro Armuzzi and Daniela Pugliese

Abbreviations

CD	Crohn's disease
CRP	C-reactive protein
CDAI	Crohn's disease activity index
HBI	Harvey–Bradshaw Index
CDEIS	Crohn's disease endoscopic index of severity
SD	Standard deviation
SCR	Steroid-free complete response
CI	Confidence interval

Introduction

Crohn's disease (CD) is a chronic inflammatory disorder characterized by a remitting–relapsing course, causing heavy morbidity and impairment of quality of life. The management of CD is mainly influenced by disease features that are mainly the extension and the behavior (inflammatory, penetrating, and stricturing), but also the presence of concomitant extraintestinal manifestations and/or poor prognostic factors at diagnosis [1, 2]. In the last years, the therapeutic aims of CD have moved from symptomatic control to the achievement of deep remission, with the ultimate goal of radically changing disease's natural history [3, 4]. This has been possible with the advent of "disease-modifying drugs," such as biological therapies, that work by curbing the underlying inflammatory cascade. Tumor necrosis factor (TNF)-alpha is a pro-inflammatory cytokine, responsible of the increased recruitment and adhesion of leukocytes into intestinal tissues, involved in the pathogenesis of CD [5]. Accordingly, monoclonal antibodies blocking TNF-alpha have shown to be effective therapies for patients with active CD, by inducing sustained steroid-free clinical and endoscopic remission [3, 6]. The present chapter focuses on certolizumab, the only PEGylated anti-TNF-alpha agent, developed for the treatment of CD patients.

Molecular and Pharmacological Characteristics

Certolizumab (CDP878) is an humanized PEGylated antigen-binding fragment (Fab) of anti-TNF-alpha monoclonal antibody. Certolizumab has been manufactured through recombinant DNA technology and protein engineering, with a two stages procedure: grafting of short, hypervariable complementarity-determining regions (CDRs) derived from the murine monoclonal antibody HTNF40 onto human antibody acceptor and then transfection in bacterial cells for a three days fermentation. Later on, Fab fragments are conjugated to two PEG chains (total molecular weight of 40 kDa) at a different site from TNF-alpha binding one. Figure 33.1 [7–9] PEGylation confer multiple pharmacological advantages, such as higher solubility, increased bioavailability and plasma half-life, but also lower toxicity and immunogenicity [10]. Certolizumab binds and neutralizes soluble and membrane-bound TNF-alpha, but lacking of Fc region, does not induce complement-dependent either antibody-dependent cell-mediated cytotoxicity. Furthermore, in vitro, certolizumab does not increase the proportion of apoptotic cells and the levels of polymorphonuclear cells degranulation [11]. For CD patients, the scheduled treatment includes an induction phase with three doses of subcutaneous certolizumab 400 mg at week 0, 2, and 4 and then a maintenance phase with one 400 mg dose every 4 weeks. After a subcutaneous administration, certolizumab is progressively absorbed and reach plasma peak concentrations (which is proportional to the dose administered) within maximum 7 days. The elimination

A. Armuzzi, M.D., Ph.D. (✉) • D. Pugliese
IBD Unit, Complesso Integrato Columbus, Gemelli Hospital Catholic University Foundation, Via G. Moscati 31, 00168 Rome, Italy
e-mail: alearmuzzi@yahoo.com

D.C. Baumgart (ed.), *Crohn's Disease and Ulcerative Colitis*, DOI 10.1007/978-3-319-33703-6_33

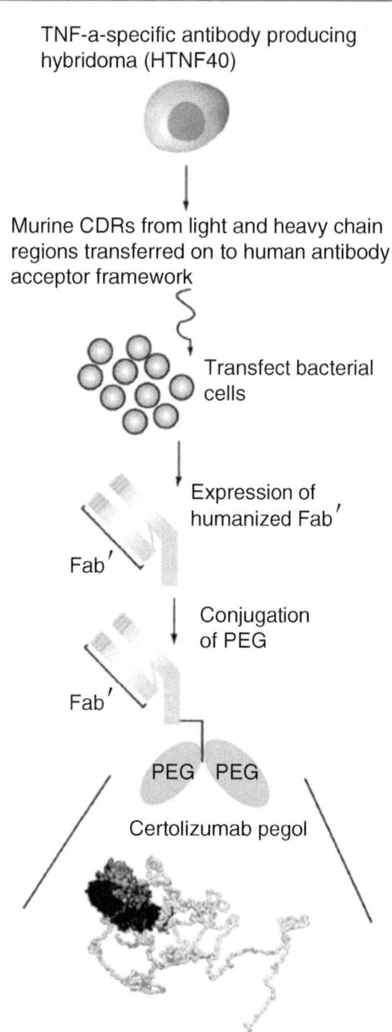

Fig. 33.1 The manufacturing process of certolizumab pegol

half-life is about 14 days and no dose adjustment are necessary for people with renal impairment [12]. Certolizumab is currently approved for the treatment of CD patients in the USA and Switzerland for patients with moderate-to-severe CD, failure to conventional treatments.

Effectiveness and Safety in Crohn's Disease: Randomized Controlled Trials

PRECISE Studies

Two randomized placebo-controlled double-blind Phase III studies, PRECISE 1 and 2 (Pegylated antibody fragment evaluation in Crohn's disease: safety and efficacy), evaluating the effectiveness of certolizumab against placebo, were the pivotal trials that led to regulatory approval for CD patients [13, 14]. Both these studies recruited in the same period (December 2003–May 2005), at different sites, patients with moderate-to-severe active disease (defined as a CDAI between 220 and 450) [15], despite the use of conventional drugs. Patients were eligible regardless disease's location or behavior, albeit those ones who presented symptomatic strictures or active abscess were excluded. In the first study, 662 patients were randomized to receive subcutaneous doses of certolizumab 400 mg or placebo at week 0, 2, and 4 and then every 4 weeks trough week 26. In both arms, patients were centrally stratified according to their basal C-reactive protein (CRP) serum level (< or >10 mg/l). This design was arranged taking in account to the certolizumab phase II dose-finding study, reporting higher rates of clinical response at week 12 in patients with baseline elevated CRP level treated with 400 mg of certolizumab every 4 weeks [16]. Thus, the primary endpoint was clinical response (defined as a reduction of at least 100 points in CDAI score) at week 6 and at both week 6 and 26 in the subgroups of patients with a baseline CRP level >10 mg/l. This endpoint was met by 37 % (54/145) of certolizumab treated patients versus 26 % (40/154) of control group (p-value = 0.04) and correspondingly, by 22 % (31/144) versus 12 % (19/154) (p-value = 0.05), respectively. Concerning to secondary aims, certolizumab was not more effective than placebo in inducing clinical remission (defined as a CDAI score of 150 points or less) at week 6 and at both week 6 and 26, in patients with baseline high level of CRP. Conversely, certolizumab was equally superior to placebo in inducing and maintaining clinical response in the overall population (regardless of the CRP level stratification) [13]. PRECISE 2 trial was specifically aimed to evaluate the efficacy of certolizumab as maintenance therapy. Therefore, 6-week responder patients to an open label induction with certolizumab (400 mg at week 0, 2, and 4), stratified according to their baseline CRP (< or >10 mg/l), were randomized to receive 400 mg of certolizumab or placebo every 4 weeks through week 26. After induction, 428 patients (64 %) achieved clinical benefit, of whom about 50 % had a baseline CRP >10 mg/l. The primary endpoint was clinical response (alike defined as in PRECISE 1) trough week 26 in 213 patients who responded to induction with a baseline CRP level >10 mg/l. This aim was reached by 62 % of patients (69/112) receiving certolizumab compared to 34 % on placebo treatment (34/101) ($p < 0.001$). Furthermore, in this specific population, patients on maintenance treatment with certolizumab were more likely to achieve clinical remission at week 26 (42 % in the certolizumab group versus 29 % of placebo one, $p < 0.001$). The differences between certolizumab and placebo were statistically significant, also considering clinical response and remission in all patients in the intention-to-treat population, regardless basal CRP level stratification (63 % versus 34 %, $p < 0.001$ and 48 % versus 29 %, $p < 0.001$, respectively). Moreover, the efficacy of certolizumab over placebo was confirmed in all subjects across subcategories, such as patients taking or not immunosuppressants or steroids and patients with or without previous experience with infliximab [14]. However, post hoc analysis showed that the likelihood of successful certolizumab treatment was increased when administered as first line biological therapy [17]. In PRECISE 2, continuous certolizumab treatment was associated with significant improvements in fistula closure. In particular, of 58 induction-responders (14 %) with an open draining fistula, 36 % of patients (10/28) treated with certolizumab achieved 100 % of fistula closure compared to 17 % (5/30) of the placebo ones [18]. After completing the PRECISE 1 and 2 studies, patients were eligible to enter into PRECISE 3, an open-label extension trials, in which a maintenance treatment with 400 mg of certolizumab every 4 weeks has been warranted for 7 years (362 weeks), aimed to evaluate long-term safety ([19], Fig. 33.2). Disease clinical activity was assessed at each available visit (every 4 weeks) with Harvey–Bradshaw Index (HBI) [20], defining clinical remission as an HBI score of 4 points or less. Patients, who experienced an exacerbation of disease and needed a dose-escalation or a rescue therapy, were considered to have treatment failure and were excluded from the efficacy analyses. Five hundred ninety-five patients entered the study, of whom 354 patients from PRECISE 1 and 241 from PRECISE 2. Patients were subdivided in three different categories, according to the drugs regimen received: (a) "First exposure" ($n = 166$): who were randomized to placebo in PRECISE 1; (b) "Re-exposure" ($n = 100$): who, after an open-label induction with certolizumab, were randomized to placebo in PRECISE 2; (c) "Continuous exposure group" (329): who were continuously treated with certolizumab in PRECISE 1 and 2. About 71 % of patients were treated with certolizumab for more than one year and the mean number of certolizumab doses was 41. During the years, 117 patients completed the follow-up, receiving certolizumab 400 mg every 4 weeks, while 478 patients discontinued from the study, mainly for adverse events (44.6 %) in the first year. Over 7 years, 88.2 % of patients experienced an adverse events and 40.3 % experienced a severe adverse event, without no significant differences among the three exposure groups. Opportunistic infections were reported in 114 patients (all of them concomitantly treated with steroids) and the malignant neoplasm incidence rate was 0.84 cases/100 patient-years. No new safety signals, no demyelinating disorders, congestive heart failure or lupus-like syndrome were reported. Clinical remission rates (secondary aim), assessed by observed cases analyses, and were 55 % (325/591) at

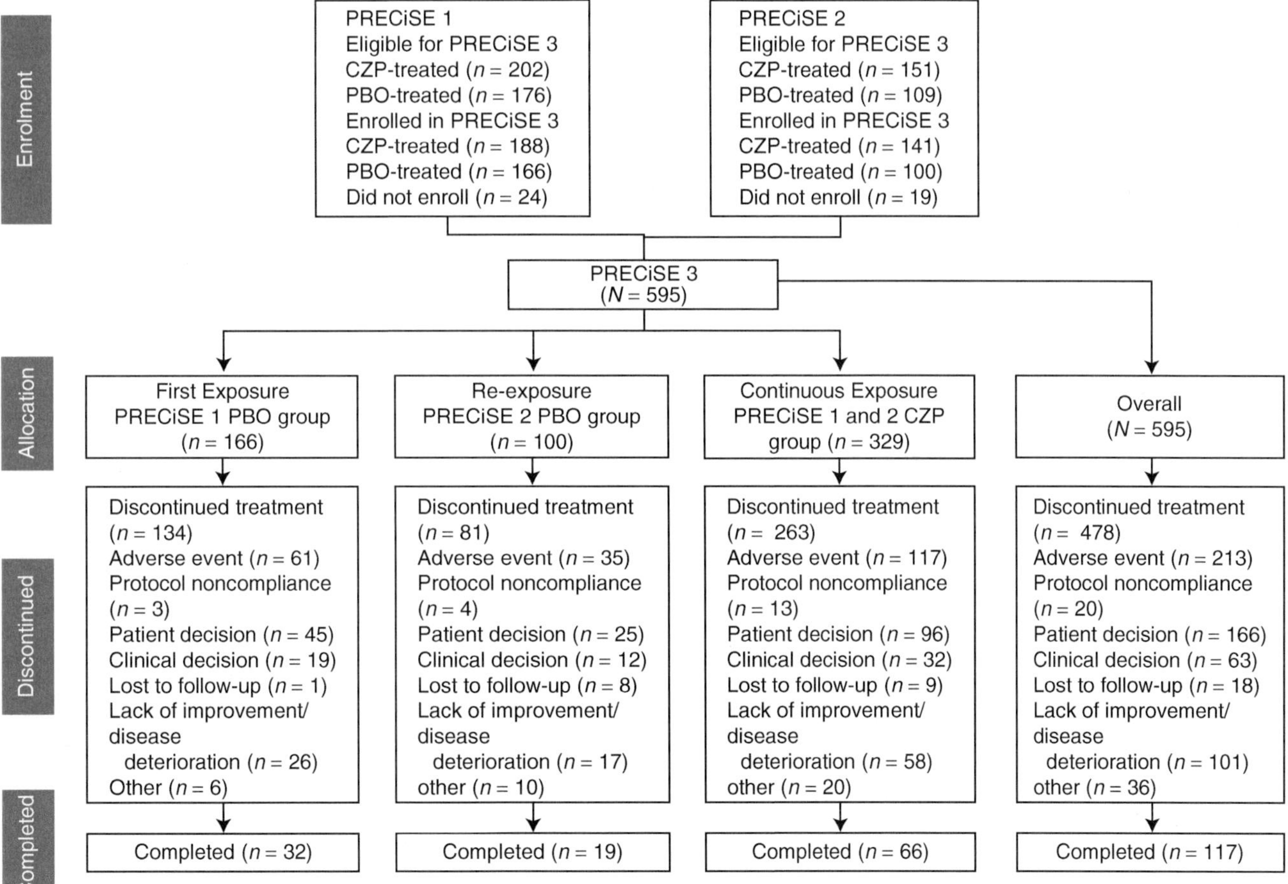

Fig. 33.2 Patient partecipation and allocation through 7 years of PRECISE 3 study

week 0 of PRECISE 3 and 75.5 % (78/103) at year 7. Remission rates for the first exposure group were generally lower than the re-exposure group or the continuous group throughout all the study. All patients enrolled in PRECISE 2, who relapsed before week 26 and withdrew from the study, could enter PRECISE 4 [21, 22]. In this open-label extension, patients were again subdivided in two groups according to different treatment received in PRECISE 2: Group A, "drug interruption" patients randomized to placebo after open-label induction, who were reinduced with three doses of certolizumab 400 mg at week 0, 2, and 4; Group B, "continuous group" patients, randomized to certolizumab 400 mg every 4 weeks, who were "recaptured" with an additional dose after two weeks (week 0, 2, and 4). As in PRECISE 3, HBI has been preferred for treatment efficacy assessments for its greater convenience, adopting the same definitions for clinical response and remission. Of 428 patients enrolled in PRECISE 2, 168 patients (39 %) withdrew prematurely from the study. One-hundred twenty-four patients entered PRECISE 4, 75 from "drug interruption" and 49 from "continuous group". The PRECISE 4 drop-out rate was 44 % (55 patients) within the first 52 weeks, (44 %). After week 4, 63 % of group A and 65 % of group B achieved clinical response that was maintained in 55 % and 59 % of them, respectively, through 52 weeks. No data are available beyond 52 weeks.

WELCOME Trial

The Welcome trial, a multicenter 26-week phase III-b, was the first study specifically aimed to evaluate the effectiveness and the tolerability of certolizumab in patients with moderate-to-severe CD with history of exposure to infliximab. Patients needed to have a well-documented history of loss of response (lack of improving or worsening after at least two infusions at standard dose) or intolerance (only mild-moderate infusion reactions) to infliximab. After an open-label induction with certolizumab 400 mg at week 0, 2, and 4, patients in clinical response (CDAI score lower of at least 100 points from baseline) were randomized to a maintenance treatment with certolizumab 400 mg either every 4 weeks or every 2 weeks. The primary outcome was clinical response at week 6 that was met in 62 % of patients (334/539). Moreover at week 6, 69.2 % of patients experienced a 70-point or greater CDAI reduction and 39.3 % clinical remission (CDAI <150 points). At week 6, 168 and 161 responders were randomized to certolizumab every 4 and 2 weeks, respectively. Of these, only 47 % (79 patients) and 44.1 % (71 patients) completed the 26-week study. Overall, 38 % (126/ 329) achieved clinical response at week 26, without any significant differences between two groups (39.9 % versus 36.6 %, $p=0.55$). Corresponding remission rates were 29.2 % and 30.4 %, respectively. After randomization, 38 % of patients relapsed and switched to open-label certolizumab every 2 weeks, with benefit in 71 % of them, who regained a 100-point CDAI reduction. Post hoc analysis showed relevant improvements in health-related quality of life and work productivity in both treatment groups as early as week 6, maintained through week 26 [23]. Certolizumab was well tolerated and serious drug-related adverse events were reported in 15 patients (2.8 %) during induction and 12 (3.2 %) during maintenance. A single case of malignant neoplasm occurred during the study [23].

Effectiveness and Safety in Crohn's Disease: Open Label Studies

MUSIC

This open-label multicenter single-arm study was the first aimed to evaluate the effectiveness of certolizumab in inducing and sustaining mucosal healing in patients with moderate-to-severe ileo-colonic CD. Eighty-nine patients with baseline active endoscopic disease (ulcers in at least two segments and a CDEIS score of 8 or greater) [24] were treated with certolizumab 400 mg at week 0, 2, and 4 and then every 4 weeks up to week 52. Endoscopic evaluations were performed at week 0, 10, and 54. Overall, 80 patients completed the 10-week period and 53 patients the 54-week one. The mean ± SD CDEIS score at baseline was 14.5 ± 5.3. At week 10, the mean change in CDEIS score (primary outcome) was 5.7 (95 % CI 4.6–6.8, $p<0.0001$). With regard to secondary aims: endoscopic response (decrease of CDEIS score > 5 points), endoscopic remission (CDEIS score < 6), complete endoscopic remission (CDEIS < 3), and mucosal healing (absence of ulcerations) at week 10 were 54 %, 37 %, 10 %, and 4 %, respectively. At week 54 the corresponding rates were 49 %, 27 %, 14 %, and 8 %, respectively. The safety profile was consistent with that of previous CZP trials [25]. At week 8 and 54, certolizumab plasma concentrations were measured and related to endoscopic activity. Higher plasma concentrations at week 8 were associated with endoscopic response (p-value = 0.0016) and remission (p-value = 0.0302) at week 10. At week 54, the rates of endoscopic remission correlated with plasma concentrations (p-value = 0.0206) [26].

Retrospective Cohort Studies

Stein et al. from Chicago retrospectively collected data of 87 certolizumab treated patients during a 3-year period (April 2008–May 2011). The majority of patients (75 %) had been previously exposed to another anti-TNF-alpha, discontinued in half of them for loss of response. Overall, 31 % (27/87) of patients achieved a sustained clinical response, including 13 ones who achieved remission (14.9 %). At last follow-up visit, 35.6 % (31 patients) were still on certolizumab treatment. A single reinduction dose of certolizumab 400 mg was administered to 31 patients (35.6 %) after a median of 29 weeks on therapy, but only five of them (16.1 %) maintained a sustained clinical response [27]. The largest retrospective cohort from clinical practice included 358 patients treated with certolizumab at Mayo Clinic during a 6-year period. The majority of patients (n=311, 86.9 %) had previously received one or more different anti-TNF-alpha, with a median of two agents per patient (112 one anti-TNF-alpha and 189 two) and most of them experienced one prior complication of CD and at least one bowel surgery. Certolizumab was administered to all patients with a standard induction regimen (400 mg at week 0, 2, and 4), but different maintenance regimens were adopted: 400 mg every 4 weeks (226 patients, 91.1 %), 400 mg every 2 weeks (8 patients, 2.2 %), 400 mg every 3 weeks (1 patient, 0.3 %) and 200 mg every 2 weeks (22 patients, 6.1 %), and 600 mg every 4 weeks (1 patient, 0.3 %). The median duration of certolizumab treatment was 13.2 months (range 0.5–75.1) and the median follow-up (after certolizumab starting) was 26.2 months (range 0.9–76.9). At last follow-up, 43 % of patients (154) remained on certolizumab treatment. The primary outcome assessment was steroid-free complete response (SCR), defined as cessation of diarrhea and abdominal pain and in patients with fistulae, cessation of fistula drainage and closure of all draining fistula without steroids. The cumulative probability of SCR at week 26 was 19.9 % (95 % CI, 15.9–24.5), lower for those one who received certolizumab as third line biological therapy. At a median of 8.7 weeks (range 2.4–25.3) 59 patients (16.8) achieved SCR, of whom 38 experienced a clinical relapse. The cumulative probability of survival free of loss of response was 65.3 % at 1 year and 45.7 % at 2 year. Younger patients, with perianal complicated CD and prior primary nonresponder to adalimumab were at higher to fail certolizumab therapy. Serious adverse events were reported in 23 patients (6.4 %) and 19 of these withdrew from certolizumab for this reason [28].

Conclusions

Certolizumab is both effective and well tolerated for the treatments of CD patients. Data from controlled trials revealed the effectiveness of certolizumab in inducing a durable clinical benefit, also in patients who had already experienced anti-TNF-alpha. Certolizumab showed also efficacy in inducing endoscopic improvements. The efficacy and safety of certolizumab outside clinical trials are not well-established, albeit a large cohort from real life confirmed the utility also in tough-to-treat patients.

References

1. Van Assche G, Dignass A, Panes J, Beaugerie L, Karagiannis J, Allez M, et al. European Crohn's and Colitis Organisation (ECCO). The second European evidence-based Consensus on the diagnosis and management of Crohn's disease: definitions and diagnosis. J Crohns Colitis. 2010;4(1):7–27. doi:10.1016/j.crohns.2009.12.003.
2. Beaugerie L, Sokol H. Clinical, serological and genetic predictors of inflammatory bowel disease course. World J Gastroenterol. 2012;18(29):3806–13. doi:10.3748/wjg.v18.i29.3806.
3. Colombel JF, Rutgeerts PJ, Sandborn WJ, Yang M, Camez A, Pollack PF, et al. Adalimumab induces deep remission in patients with Crohn's disease. Clin Gastroenterol Hepatol. 2014;12(3):414–22.e5. doi:10.1016/j.cgh.2013.06.019.
4. Panaccione R, Colombel JF, Louis E, Peyrin-Biroulet L, Sandborn WJ. Evolving definitions of remission in Crohn's disease. Inflamm Bowel Dis. 2013;19(8):1645–53. doi:10.1097/MIB.0b013e318283a4b3.
5. Abraham C, Cho J. Interleukin-23/Th17 pathways and inflammatory bowel disease. Inflamm Bowel Dis. 2009;15(7):1090–100. doi:10.1002/ibd.20894.
6. Colombel JF, Sandborn WJ, Reinisch W, Mantzaris GJ, Kornbluth A, Rachmilewitz D, et al. Infliximab, azathioprine, or combination therapy for Crohn's disease. N Engl J Med. 2010;362(15):1383–95. doi:10.1056/NEJMoa0904492.
7. Weir N, Athwal D, Brown D, Foulkes R, Kollias G, Nesbitt A, et al. A new generation of high-affinity humanized PEGylated Fab' fragment anti-tumor necrosis factor-alpha monoclonal antibodies. Therapy. 2006;3(4):535–45.
8. Dinesen L, Travis S. Targeting nanomedicines in the treatment of Crohn's disease: focus on certolizumab pegol (CDP870). Int J Nanomedicine. 2007;2(1):39–47.
9. Pasut G. Pegylation of biological molecules and potential benefits: pharmacological properties of certolizumab pegol. BioDrugs. 2014;28 Suppl 1:S15–23. doi:10.1007/s40259-013-0064-z.
10. Chapman AP. PEGylated antibodies and antibody fragments for improved therapy: a review. Adv Drug Deliv Rev. 2002;54(4):531–45.
11. Nesbitt A, Fossati G, Bergin M, Stephens P, Stephens S, Foulkes R, et al. Mechanism of action of certolizumab pegol (CDP870): in vitro comparison with other anti-tumor necrosis factor alpha agents. Inflamm Bowel Dis. 2007;13(11):1323–32.
12. CIMZIA® (certolizumab pegol) (prescribing information). Smyrna, GA: UCB, Inc.; 2012.
13. Sandborn WJ, Feagan BG, Stoinov S, Honiball PJ, Rutgeerts P, Mason D, et al. PRECISE 1 Study Investigators. Certolizumab pegol for the treatment of Crohn's disease. N Engl J Med. 2007;357(3):228–38.
14. Schreiber S, Khaliq-Kareemi M, Lawrance IC, Thomsen OØ, Hanauer SB, McColm J, et al. PRECISE 2 Study Investigators. Maintenance therapy with certolizumab pegol for Crohn's disease. N Engl J Med. 2007;357(3):239–50. Erratum in: N Engl J Med. 2007;357(13):1357.
15. Best WR, Becktel JM, Singleton JW, Kern Jr F. Development of a Crohn's disease activity index. National Cooperative Crohn's Disease Study. Gastroenterology. 1976;70(3):439–44.
16. Schreiber S, Rutgeerts P, Fedorak RN, Khaliq-Kareemi M, Kamm MA, Boivin M, et al. CDP870 Crohn's Disease Study Group. A randomized, placebo-controlled trial of certolizumab pegol (CDP870) for treatment of Crohn's disease. Gastroenterology. 2005;129(3):807–18.
17. Hanauer SB, Panes J, Colombel JF, Bloomfield R, Schreiber S, Sandborn WJ. Clinical trial: impact of prior infliximab therapy on the clinical response to certolizumab pegol maintenance therapy for Crohn's disease. Aliment Pharmacol Ther. 2010;32(3):384–93. doi:10.1111/j.1365-2036.2010.04360.x.

18. Schreiber S, Lawrance IC, Thomsen OØ, Hanauer SB, Bloomfield R, Sandborn WJ. Randomised clinical trial: certolizumab pegol for fistulas in Crohn's disease-subgroup results from a placebo-controlled study. Aliment Pharmacol Ther. 2011;33(2):185–93. doi:10.1111/j.1365-2036.2010.04509.x.
19. Sandborn WJ, Lee SD, Randall C, Gutierrez A, Schwartz DA, Ambarkhane S, et al. Long-term safety and efficacy of certolizumab pegol in the treatment of Crohn's disease: 7-year results from the PRECiSE 3 study. Aliment Pharmacol Ther. 2014;40(8):903–16. doi:10.1111/apt.12930.
20. Harvey RF, Bradshaw JM. A simple index of Crohn's-disease activity. Lancet. 1980;1(8167):514.
21. Sandborn WJ, Schreiber S, Hanauer SB, Colombel JF, Bloomfield R, Lichtenstein GR, et al. Reinduction with certolizumab pegol in patients with relapsed Crohn's disease: results from the PRECiSE 4 Study. Clin Gastroenterol Hepatol. 2010;8(8):696–702.e1. doi:10.1016/j.cgh.2010.03.024.
22. Sandborn WJ, Abreu MT, D'Haens G, Colombel JF, Vermeire S, Mitchev K, et al. Certolizumab pegol in patients with moderate to severe Crohn's disease and secondary failure to infliximab. Clin Gastroenterol Hepatol. 2010;8(8):688–95.e2. doi:10.1016/j.cgh.2010.04.021.
23. Feagan BG, Sandborn WJ, Wolf DC, Coteur G, Purcaru O, Brabant Y, et al. Randomised clinical trial: improvement in health outcomes with certolizumab pegol in patients with active Crohn's disease with prior loss of response to infliximab. Aliment Pharmacol Ther. 2011;33(5):541–50. doi:10.1111/j.1365-2036.2010.04568.x.
24. Mary JY, Modigliani R. Development and validation of an endoscopic index of the severity for Crohn's disease: a prospective multicentre study. Groupe d'Etudes Thérapeutiques des Affections Inflammatoires du Tube Digestif (GETAID). Gut. 1989;30(7):983–9.
25. Hébuterne X, Lémann M, Bouhnik Y, Dewit O, Dupas JL, Mross M, et al. Endoscopic improvement of mucosal lesions in patients with moderate to severe ileocolonic Crohn's disease following treatment with certolizumab pegol. Gut. 2013;62(2):201–8. doi:10.1136/gutjnl-2012-302262.
26. Colombel JF, Sandborn WJ, Allez M, Dupas JL, Dewit O, D'Haens G, et al. Association between plasma concentrations of certolizumab pegol and endoscopic outcomes of patients with Crohn's disease. Clin Gastroenterol Hepatol. 2014;12(3):423–31.e1.. doi:10.1016/j.cgh.2013.10.025.
27. Stein AC, Rubin DT, Hanauer SB, Cohen RD. Incidence and predictors of clinical response, re-induction dose, and maintenance dose escalation with certolizumab pegol in Crohn's disease. Inflamm Bowel Dis. 2014;20(10):1722–8. doi:10.1097/MIB.0000000000000146.
28. Moon W, Pestana L, Becker B, Loftus Jr EV, Hanson KA, Bruining DH, et al. Efficacy and safety of certolizumab pegol for Crohn's disease in clinical practice. Aliment Pharmacol Ther. 2015;42(4):428–40. doi:10.1111/apt.13288.

Biologic Therapy for Crohn's Disease: Infliximab

34

Jan-Michael A. Klapproth and Gary R. Lichtenstein

Infliximab Pharmacology in Crohn's Disease

Infliximab (initially called cA2) is a 149 kDa human–murine chimeric monoclonal IgG1 antibody, consisting to 25 % murine variable region and 75 % human constant region, linked by a disulfide bond [9]. In comparison to murine cA2, this chimeric antibody binds with higher specificity and affinity to soluble and membrane-bound TNF-α [10], the latter immunological interaction leading to complement activation and subsequent CD4+ macrophages and T cell cytotoxicity [11]. In addition, infliximab has been shown to increases the number of peripheral blood CD4+ and CD8+ T cells, preventing homing of Th1 lymphocytes into inflamed tissue [12]. This finding is reflected in clear histological evidence that infliximab successfully controls microscopic pathological findings [13]. This study compared histology specimen of patients exposed to infliximab and control subjects and revealed significant reduction of mucosal, submucosal inflammation, reduced formation of transmural lymphoid aggregates and increased prevalence of muscularis mucosae reduplication in the treatment group.

Standard induction therapy for the treatment of CD has been established at 5 mg/kg IV at week 0, 2, and 6, achieving stable median peak concentrations ranging from 158 to 195 μg/ml, with a terminal half-life of 9.5 days [14]. Interestingly, determination of serial infliximab serum concentrations post-infusion, and again at 2 and 4 weeks, did not differ in clinical responders vs. nonresponders. Following infusion of infliximab, the medication is exclusively found in the intravascular space with steady-state 4.5–6.0 L volume of distribution, primarily attributed to the low clearance, ranging from 9.8 to 15 ml/h. In all subjects, infliximab remains detectable up to week 8, but is cleared completely by week 12.

Early work suggested that a clinical response to a dosage of 5 mg/kg infliximab was linked to threshold serum concentrations above the limit of detection at 1.4 μg/ml [15], particularly in patients with an elevated C-reactive protein [7]. Independent of inflammatory or fistulizing CD, serum concentrations of C-reactive protein prior to therapy with infliximab were significantly higher in patients responding to infliximab (16.8 mg/L), versus nonresponders (9.6 mg/L; p 0.02). When using a cutoff concentration of 5 mg/L, C-reactive protein concentrations greater 5 mg/L and less than 5 mg/L resulted in clinical response in 76 % vs. 46 % of patients, respectively (p 0.004; OR: 0.26 (0.11–0.63)). Elevated concentrations off CRP indicate the presence of active inflammation. Those individuals with normal or low CRP may be unable to elevate serum response in response to inflammation or they may have non-inflammatory Crohn's (i.e., fibrotic disease), and thus they do not respond as well as those with active inflammation.

General Considerations, Indications, and Patient Selection

Criteria for the appropriate use of infliximab in patients with Crohn's disease have recently been reviewed by the European Panel on the Appropriateness of CD Therapy [16], the American College of Gastroenterology [17], The American Gastroenterological Association [18], The European Crohn's and Colitis Organization, and other societies. The general consensus agreement among experts is present for three specific clinical situations: (a) failure of azathioprine/6-mercaptoprine to control complex fistulizing disease, (b) steroid-dependent CD, and (c) for the maintenance of biologic-induced remission.

The need of biological therapy was further defined in the London Position Statement [19]. It was deemed appropriate in patients that have a virulent disease course. Specifically in

J.-M.A. Klapproth • G.R. Lichtenstein, M.D. (✉)
Division of Gastroenterology, Department of Medicine, University of Pennsylvania, 7th Floor South, Room 753, Perelman Center, 3400 Civic Center Boulevard, Philadelphia, PA 19104, USA
e-mail: gary.lichtenstein@uphs.upenn.edu

D.C. Baumgart (ed.), *Crohn's Disease and Ulcerative Colitis*, DOI 10.1007/978-3-319-33703-6_34

patients requiring two courses of steroids within a year, hospitalization, immunomodulators, or surgery within 5 years were associated with a disabling course of CD [20]. Additional factors associated with disabling disease include age <40 years, initial requirement for steroids and perianal disease, indications that have been confirmed independently [21]. Therapeutic intervention with a biologic agent has also been advocated for severe disease, defined by the requirement for colonic and more than two small bowel resections, definite stoma within 5 years of diagnosis and complex fistulizing disease [22]. Finally, stepwise logistic regression of 240 CD patients treated with infliximab identified young age, colonic inflammation and the use of immunosuppressive medications as factors for successful short term response to infliximab [23]. Whereas infliximab has been shown to play a significant role in the management of fistulizing and inflammatory CD, fibrostenotic disease is not controlled with this medication. The successful use of any therapeutic treatment in patients with Crohn's disease mandates the presence of inflammation. Hence the treatment of fibrostenotic disease mandates surgical intervention to manage the disease successfully. Results from an open pilot study showed that only a small number of patients were able to avoid surgery for fibrostenotic CD in response to infliximab [24].

Induction of Remission

The first randomized, placebo-controlled trial establishing infliximab as an agent for induction of remission was published in 1997 [2]. For this 12 week study, 108 patients with a Crohn's Disease Activity Index ranging from 220 to 450 were recruited to receive placebo, 5, 10, or 20 mg/kg as a single infusion. Primary endpoint was a reduction in CDAI of 70 points by week 4. A measurable effect was apparent after only 2 weeks in patients receiving infliximab vs. placebo, with a response rate of 61 % vs. 17 % and remission 27 % vs. 4 %, respectively. The primary endpoint at week 4 was met by 65 % of patients in the treatment groups, but only 17 % in the placebo group ($p<0.001$). This difference in clinical response rates remained statistically significant through week 12, with 41 % for infliximab treated patients vs. 12 % in the placebo group (p 0.008). Rates for remission rates were not different for all patients at week 12. These findings established infliximab as an agent for induction of remission for moderate to severe disease.

Subsequently, in 1995 an open label clinical trial with ten steroid-dependent patients with endoscopic evidence of active disease was published. Of these ten subjects, eight received 10 mg/kg and two were treated with 20 mg/kg as a single infusion [25]. With the exception of one, all subjects reported improvement as reflected in CDAI decrease from a mean score of 257 at baseline to 114 by week 4 and 69 by week 8. C-reactive protein returned to normal within 2 weeks in all patients and the anti-inflammatory effect of infliximab persisted for the duration of 4 months.

In a follow-up open label, multicenter, dose-escalating study, 20 steroid-refractory patients were subjected to a single infusion of 5, 10, or 20 mg/kg [26]. Clinical response and remission were defined as reduction of CDAI by 70 points from baseline and CDAI less than 150 at week 12, respectively. Even though not statistically significant, the highest response and remission rates of 80 % and 60 % were achieved for the 10 mg/kg subjects, respectively. These studies helped demonstrate the efficacy of infliximab for the induction of remission.

Maintenance of Remission and Mucosal Healing

Maintenance of Remission

Establishing the role for infliximab as an agent for the induction of remission left the question whether it would play a role in the maintenance of remission.

In a landmark trial, the efficacy of infliximab for the maintenance of remission was assessed. A total of 573 patients with a CDAI score of at least 220, consistent with mild to moderately active CD, received a single dose at week 0 [3] (ACCENT I). Subsequently, 335 responders at week 2 were then randomly assigned to one of three groups: I; placebo at week 2 and 6, followed by an infusion every 8 weeks: II, infliximab 5 mg/kg at week 2 and 6, continued at the same dosage every 8 weeks, and III, infliximab 5 mg/k at week 2 and 6, continued at 10 mg/kg every 8 weeks. The primary endpoint of the ACCENT I trial was the number of patients in remission at week 30 and time to loss of response by week 54. By week 30, the percentage of patients in remission was as follows: group I—21 %, group II—39 % ($p=0.003$), and group III—45 % ($p=0.0002$). The median time to loss of response was 19 weeks for group I, 38 weeks for group II and greater 54 weeks for group III. These findings highlight that patients responding to a single dose of infliximab are more likely to maintain remission at 1 year when treated with infliximab every 8 weeks.

Another study evaluated the efficacy of infliximab for the maintenance of remission in patients with Crohn's disease. Rutgeerts et al. [27] defined the primary endpoint as a reduction in CDAI by 70 points and response as CDAI less than 150, now determined at week 44. For this randomized, placebo controlled study, 73 patients were recruited and infused with 10 mg/kg infliximab, or albumin, the placebo arm of the study, every 8 weeks until week 36. Rates for remission increased from 37.8 % at week 12 to 52.9 % by week 44 in the treatment group, whereas rates went from 44.4 % at week

12 to 20 % in the placebo group (week 44: p 0.013). Interestingly, response rates were not statistically different comparing both groups.

At this point it is worth noting that a recent meta-analysis identified that there is a gap in knowledge regarding head-to-head trials comparing immunomodulator and biologic agents alone, and in combination [28]. There have been no large controlled trials yet performed to address these knowledge gaps. Analysis by the authors revealed that infliximab in combination azathioprine was superior to each medication alone for the maintenance of remission. The combination of infliximab and azathioprine, among other analyzed combinations, was estimated to have a 99 % probability of being superior in comparison to placebo.

Mucosal Healing

A follow-up subtrial investigated the rate of mucosal healing of the small and large bowel in a subset of 99 eligible participants of the ACCENT I trial with a total of 573 patients. The analysis was performed at baseline, week 10 and finally week 54 [27]. At week 10, mucosal healing was achieved in 31 % of participants that received three dosages of infliximab as opposed to 0 % of those treated with a single dose. At week 54, complete mucosal healing was observed in 50 % of subjects that received 5 or 10 mg/kg maintenance therapy, as opposed to 7 % of participants treated with episodic infliximab infusions. These results support the conclusion that scheduled maintenance therapy with infliximab is superior to episodic treatment to achieve mucosal healing. This study also identified a trend towards lower rates of hospitalization for patient with healed mucosa.

In lieu of repeat endoscopies to assess disease activity, C-reactive protein functions as a sensitive surrogate marker for intestinal inflammation. To evaluate for a maintained response or remission, a post hoc analysis of serum CRP concentrations in ACCENT I participants was performed [29]. This trial revealed a significant association of an elevated C-reactive protein at baseline ≥0.7 mg/dl with maintained remission in 45 % of participants at week 14, as opposed to 22 % in patients with C-reactive protein ≤0.7 mg/dl. Interestingly, normalization of C-reactive protein to <0.5 mg/dl in response to infliximab by week 14 was more likely to result in higher sustained response and remission (56 %) vs. concentrations >0.5 mg/dl (37.2 %, $p=0.005$).

Primary and Secondary Loss of Response

- Failure to control intestinal inflammation with infliximab can be immediate or delayed, after showing an effect initially, defined as primary and secondary loss of response, respectively. The clinical definition of primary nonresponse is lack of improvement of clinical signs and symptoms during induction therapy. Most clinicians assess treatment failure at 4 weeks. Recent data suggest that patients who initially respond may more gradually accrue remission over time Recognition that attainment of criteria for remission may require a longer period of time on therapy up to 6–12 weeks depending on agent.
- In contrast to primary response failure, some patients who meet the criteria for an initial clinical response eventually lose response to anti-TNF-α biopharmaceuticals. A major contributor to secondary response failure appears to be immunogenicity leading to production of antidrug antibodies with drug removal and/or neutralization of TNF-α antagonistic activity as a consequence.

Primary loss of response to anti-TNF-α induction therapy has been observed in 40 % of clinical trials and up to 20 % in clinical series [30]. Interestingly, choosing another antibody in the same class results in a clinical response in 50 % of patients, supporting the argument that the lack of response is dependent on a specific medication, not the immunological mechanism targeted.

Secondary loss of response has been managed by dose escalation, change to a different biologic agent in the same or different class, addition of an immunomodulator, or surgery [19, 31, 32]. These interventions take time and at a significant expense to patient and insurance companies [33].

Over time, patients on maintenance infliximab demonstrate a loss of response when infused every 8 weeks [34]. A prospective multicenter study assessed the efficacy of shortened infliximab infusion intervals in a cohort of patients with Crohn's Disease Activity Index, ranging from 220–400, that lost response by week 14, following induction and maintenance therapy at 8 weeks [35]. Increasing the frequency of infliximab 5 mg/kg infusions to every 4 weeks resulted in retrieval of clinical response and remission rates of 83.3 % and 55.6 % at week 54, respectively. Improvement regarding response and remission was paralleled by increased trough levels, ranging from 4.9 to 8.9 μg/ml.

In another, randomized, controlled, single-blinded 12 week study optimal management of secondary loss of response to infliximab was addressed [36]. Inclusion criteria were recurrent inflammation with a minimum CDAI score ≥220 while on standardized treatment with infliximab. Patients were equally divided in two groups, 36 patients receiving a fixed treatment at 5 mg/kg every 4 weeks and 33 patients receiving an individualized infliximab regimen based on (a) serum concentration (< or>3 μg/ml) and (b) the presence of antibodies (detectable or undetectable). The primary endpoint was defined as significant cost reduction for the individualized treatment group, without compromising control of CD.

Clinical response rates at week 12, defined as a ≥70 points CDAI reduction, were not different in the algorithm vs. intensification group, determined at 58 % and 53 %, respectively (RR 1.091, 0.731–1.673, 95 % CI, *p* 0.81). Quality of life assessment was similar for both groups. However, costs for the intensification group were 34 % lower in comparison to the algorithm treated group of patients ($p<0.001$). Therefore, the conclusion of this study, not without compromising treatment success, individualized dosing of infliximab based on therapeutic drug monitoring of trough levels affords a significant cost reduction.

Alternatively, a clinical trial directly compared whether doubling the dose of infliximab to 10 mg/kg or increasing the frequency of infusion was more effective [37]. Doubling the dose of infliximab was superior to increasing the infusion frequency, 77 % vs. 66 % (OR 1.7; 95 % CI 0.8–3.4). This increased therapeutic effect was sustained at 12 months, with 50 % of patients receiving 10 mg/kg showing a clinical response in comparison to 39 % (OR 1.5; 95 % CI 0.8–2.9) in group of patients that received infliximab at an increased frequency. It is worth mentioning that while on maintenance therapy, an observational, retrospective study identified specific single nucleotide polymorphisms in the TNF receptor superfamily were either associated with a loss of response and severe infusion reactions, or the maintenance of remission [38].

Given the concern of adverse outcomes, further increase in frequency and/or dosage of infliximab has not been studied systematically and it is worthwhile to consider alternative medications. In a multicenter, placebo-controlled, double-blinded study 325 patients, CDAI ranging from 220–450, becoming intolerant or lost their response to infliximab (secondary loss of response), were enrolled to receive adalimumab or placebo ([39], GAIN). Endpoints in this study were response and number of patients in remission at the end of adalimumab induction therapy at week 4. Remission was achieved in 21 % in the treatment group, as opposed to 7 % in the placebo group ($p<0.001$), a difference that became apparent by week 2. Even though not statistically significant, a 100 point reduction in the CDAI was higher in the treatment group at the end of the study, 38 % vs. 25 % placebo ($p>0.05$). Even though adalimumab presents a viable option treating infliximab loss of response, data regarding long-term outcome are not available. Thus, if a patient is intolerant to an anti-TNF-α agent or has a secondary loss of response there are two treatment strategies that can be used; treatment with another anti-TNF-α agent or treatment with a biologic agent from another class, such as an anti-integrin antibody.

Infliximab Serum Trough Concentrations and Antibodies

There is evidence that maintenance of infliximab trough levels is associated with clinical response, remission, and mucosal healing [15, 40, 41]. Even though initially successful, approximately 60 % of treated CD patients eventually lose response to infliximab [42]. Loss of response has been attributed to an increased clearance with a significantly shortened half-life and trough level or the development of antidrug antibodies.

Clearance of infliximab in patients with IBD is independent of disease type, CD or UC. However, antibody formation is associated with a 259 % increased clearance of infliximab from the circulation [43]. In addition, serum albumin concentrations <3 mg/dl and body mass index >30 lead to a decrease in half-life for this medication [8, 44].

In a recent prospective single center study (TAXIT study) it was demonstrated that screening patients with IBD on maintenance infliximab by measuring their trough infliximab serum concentrations, only 115 out of 263 (43 %) were found to be at target trough levels of 3 μg/ml to 7 μg/ml, with concentrations found to be <3 μg/ml in 76 (29 %) subjects [45]. At 1 year, dose escalation was successful in 69 CD patients out of 76 subjects, increasing the rate of remission from 66 % before dose adjustment to 85 % after correction, paralleled by a decrease in C-reactive protein from 4.3 to 3.2 mg/dl. Interestingly, 72 patients with infliximab trough level >7 mg/dl were treated with dose reduction, resulting in a 28 % reduction in drug costs. Whether adjustment of dosage was based on clinical features or trough level did not make a difference achieving remission (66 % vs. 69 %), but lead to a higher rate of relapse in the clinically adjusted group vs. subjects treated with concentration based dosing (17 % vs. 7 %; $p=0.018$).

Measurement of trough infliximab levels at week 14 following induction therapy with infliximab 5 mg/kg identified significantly lower serum concentrations in patients without sustained responses, as opposed to subjects with sustained response (1.9 μg/ml vs. 4.0 μg/ml) [41]. The authors concluded that trough level ≥3.5 μg/ml at week 14 of maintenance therapy with infliximab 5 mg/kg predict a durable sustained response in conjunction with a ≥60 % reduction in C-reactive protein in patient with a baseline C-reactive protein elevation ≥8 mg/L.

Infliximab for Perianal and Fistulizing Disease

Management of fistulizing CD continues to be a challenge, requiring a multidisciplinary approach, in particular perianal fistulae. Defining a primary endpoint of 50 % and greater decrease in drainage from enterocutaneous fistulas with gentle physical manipulation, infliximab at 5 mg/kg has been shown to be significantly more effective compared to placebo or 10 mg/kg (68 % $p=0.002$; 26 %; 56 %, $p=0.02$) [46]. Closure of all fistulas at 4 weeks duration when manipulated with gentle applied pressure of the fistulas, was observed in 55 % and 38 % of patients receiving 5 mg/kg and 10 mg/kg of infliximab, respectively, but only 13 % of the placebo group achieved this secondary endpoint.

In a multicenter, double blinded, placebo controlled trial the efficacy of infliximab to maintain fistula closure was assessed in 306 patients with CD (ACCENT II) and at least one active perianal or abdominal fistula [47]. All subjects received 5 mg/kg of infliximab intravenously at 0, 2, and 6 weeks. A total of 195 responders and 87 nonresponder to induction therapy, assessed at week 10 and 14, were randomly divided into groups receiving infliximab at 5 mg/kg or placebo every 8 weeks. Loss of response was defined as recurrence of draining fistulae and requirement for new or additional medications. For responders to induction therapy, at 54 weeks the median time to loss of response was 40 weeks in the treatment group, vs 14 weeks for placebo ($p<0.001$). Expressed differently, about 42 % in the treatment group experienced a loss of response, whereas 62 % of patients in the placebo group did. Response at week 54 was maintained in only 23 % of placebo treated patients, compared to 42 % in the infliximab group ($p=0.001$), without the identification of independent predictors for a sustained response. This study also revealed that cross over to 10 mg/kg in patients who lost response to 5 mg/kg might lead to recovery of a response. In summary, for patients responding to initiation therapy with infliximab at week 0, 2, and 6 for fistulizing CD, ongoing therapy maintained fistula closure.

Infliximab and Pregnancy

Data from a historical registry-based study revealed that the average birth weight of newborns to primaparas and multiparas mothers with CD was significantly reduced by 185 g and 134 g, respectively [48]. Managing induction and maintenance remission of CD during pregnancy is challenging, given the limited number of choices for medical therapy. Direct exposure to infliximab (category B) during pregnancy within 3 months of conception did not result in an increased adverse outcome when compared to a control population recruited from the National Center for Health Statistics [5]. Adverse outcomes for control vs. infliximab treatment during pregnancy was not significantly different when comparing live births (67 % vs. 67 % (95 % CI: 56.3, 76.0)), miscarriages (17 % vs. 15 % (95 % CI: 8.2, 23.2)), and therapeutic termination (16 % vs. 19 % (95 % CI: 11.5, 28.0)). These findings were confirmed in follow-up studies, finding no difference in the rate of preterm delivery, intensive care unit admission, low birth weight, congenital malformations, elective abortions, and intrauterine growth restriction [49, 50]. These results appear to hold true for the group of anti-TNF-α medications, regardless whether being started prior to or after conception [51, 52]. It is worth noting that sporadic case reports have described disseminated infection with Bacille Calmette-Guérin following vaccination of infants born to mothers treated with infliximab [53, 54]. However, immunization of infants born to mothers exposed to anti-TNF-α-α medications with non-live vaccines is considered safe without evidence of increased risk for infection of exposed children at 12 months [55] (PIANO).

Infliximab for the Treatment of Extraintestinal Manifestations in Crohn's Disease

A retrospective study of 10 years identified more than 5 % of patients with CD to be affected by at least one extraintestinal manifestation, with less than 1 % of patients having more than one disease [56]. In CD, prevalence rates of musculoskeletal, ocular, and dermatological diseases vary, depending on diagnosis and gender. Peripheral arthritis is a self-limited condition that parallels activity of intestinal inflammation, affecting large joints, like knee and ankle, being present in up to 15–20 % in CD patients [57]. With the exception of pyoderma gangrenosum, which occurred equally in women and men, 12.8 % vs. 12.6 %, ankylosing spondylitis was more common in men than women, 5.7 % vs. 4.3 %, and iritis/uveitis more common in women than men, 5.6 % vs. 3.4 %.

A large open label trial including 153 therapy refractory CD patients with peripheral arthritis showed that infliximab 5 mg/kg induction therapy at 0, 2 and 6 weeks lead to significant improvement in 61 % of cases at 12 weeks [58]. Interestingly, complete resolution of joint symptoms graded as none, mild, moderate and severe, and was observed in 46 % of patients. Similarly, another, smaller open label trial identified improvement in 7 out of 11 patients with IBD and arthralgia treated with a single infusion of infliximab, as assessed by questionnaire [59].

In a multicenter, retrospective study involving 13 therapy refractory patients with CD and pyoderma gangrenosum were tested for safety and efficacy of infliximab [60]. With a mean time to response of 111 days (range 7–210 days), all 13 patients experienced complete healing in response to treatments with 1–24 infusions and cessation of steroid use. In a related, randomized, placebo-controlled, double-blind placebo controlled study, 13 patients received infliximab and were compared to 17 control subjects with a diagnosis of pyoderma gangrenosum alone, but not CD [61]. At week 2, 46 % of subjects in the treatment group were considered improved, as opposed to 6 % in the placebo group ($p=0.025$).

Regarding ankylosing spondylitis and CD, only one controlled study has been published, so far [62]. In this study, infliximab induction therapy was followed by maintenance therapy every 5–8 weeks. Clinical response was measured by Bath Ankylosing Spondylitis Disease Activity Index at 12 months. In comparison to the control group, scores for the treatment group decreased rapidly and were maintained at 12 months (40.05 vs. 18.1, $p<0.05$), respectively.

Investigations of infliximab induction and maintenance therapy for treatment for ankylosing spondylitis without concomitant CD, showed significant differences in symptoms and global assessment of ankylosing spondylitis. At 12 weeks, 53 % of patients in the treatment group vs 9 % ($p<0.0001$) in the placebo group showed improvement of validated clinical criteria [63].

Finally, infliximab has proven successful in patients with refractory posterior uveitis [64]. A total of five patients were enrolled and at 6 months follow-up, all patients were weaned off immunosuppressive therapy. In a related study, 13 patients with uveitis were treated with infliximab 3 mg/kg, receiving between 1 and 24 infusions for up to 2 years [65]. Reduction of ocular inflammation and effect on visual acuity was observed in the majority of cases.

Postoperative Treatment with Infliximab

Up to 75 % of patients with CD will require surgical intervention at some point during the course of their disease with a cumulative rate for resection of 44 % at 1 year, 61 % at 5 years, and 71 % at 10 years [66]. Postoperative recurrence has been estimated at 33 % and 44 % at 5 and 10 years, respectively.

Infliximab has been shown to prevent endoscopic postoperative recurrence after ileo-colonic resection at 1 year when given within 4 weeks of surgery [6]. In comparison to placebo, recurrence was identified in 9.1 % of patient treated with infliximab vs. 84.6 % in the placebo group at 1 year ($p=0.0006$). Macroscopic findings were supported by microscopic examination of biopsy material with histological recurrence in the treatment group at 27.3 % and 84.6 % in the placebo group ($p=0.01$). A long-term follow-up study 5 years later showed that patients treated postoperatively with infliximab vs. placebo had a longer mean time to first endoscopic recurrence at 1231 ± 747 days, vs. 460 ± 121 days ($p=0.003$) and significantly longer mean time to surgery at 1798 ± 359 days vs. 1058 ± 529 days ($p=0.047$) [67]. The most recent study from the same group compared patients with a CDAI < 200 treated postoperatively with infliximab vs. placebo at week 76 and 104. Clinically, recurrence at week 76 was reported in 12.9 % of treated patients vs. 20.0 % in the placebo group, which did not reach statistical significance ($p=0.097$). However, endoscopic recurrence at week 76 and 104 was reported at 30.6 % vs 60 % ($p<0.001$) and 17.7 % vs. 25.3 % ($p=0.098$) for infliximab vs. placebo. This supports the consideration of infliximab for short and long term prevention of postoperative recurrence of CD.

Biosimilars of Infliximab

Over the past 60 years, the incidence of inflammatory bowel disease has increased worldwide, making this group of diseases a global problem, paralleled by an increase in patient eligibility for biologic therapy [68]. With the intention of lowering health care costs and improved affordability of medications, biosimilars were developed [69]. This includes CT-P13 (Remsima), which was approved by the European Medicines Agency and the Food and Drug Administration in 2013 for the treatment of CD [70]. CT-P13 is biochemically similar to infliximab, with identical binding affinities for monomeric and trimeric forms of TNF-α and Fcγ receptors. Immunogenicity of infliximab and CT-P13 is equally strong as all tested sera with antibodies against infliximab cross-react with CT-P13, too [71]. In vivo experiments have shown that pharmacokinetics at a dosing range of 10–50 mg/kg were similar to infliximab [72].

In a retrospective multicenter trial, CT-P13 was tested in anti-TNF-α naïve patient with CD [73]. Response and remission rates were 90.6 % and 68.8 % at week 2 and 87.5 % and 75 % at week 54. Remission was maintained in 25 out of 27 patients (92.6 %). These findings indicate that the effect of CT-P13 is comparable to infliximab regarding efficacy and interchangeability.

The safety profile for CT-P13 and infliximab are comparable, with adverse events reported at 63.9 % and 64.8 %, respectively [70]. The most significant adverse event was the reactivation of latent tuberculosis in patients that were treated with CT-P13 for rheumatoid arthritis.

Safety of and Contraindications for infliximab

As with other anti-TNF-α inhibitors, infliximab belongs to a class of medications for which the FDA has issued a black box warning, as its use can result in serious and life-threatening adverse events [74]. The three major components of this warning are increased risks for (a) serious infections (tuberculosis, histoplasmosis, listeriosis, Pneumocystis pneumonia), (b) the development of lymphoma and other malignancies, and even (c) fatal hepato-splenic T-cell lymphoma. While on treatment with infliximab, the estimated incidence for development of tuberculosis has been calculated at 52.5 cases per 100,000 patient years [75]. In addition, when prescribed for the control of draining fistulae, treatment with infliximab lead to infections requiring antibiotics in nearly one-third of patients, with 5 % of patients experiencing serious

Table 34.1 Summary of trials in infliximab-treated patients with Crohn's disease

Infliximab indication	Trial type	Outcome	Reference
Induction of remission	RPCT	CDAI ≥70 point reduction 65 % vs. 17 % placebo (p<0.001) at 12 weeks	Targan (1997)
Maintenance of remission	RPCT	CDAI ≤150 week 30: 21 % placebo, 39 % 5 mg/kg, 45 % 10 mg/kg TLTR week 54: 19 weeks placebo, 38 weeks 5 mg/kg, >54 weeks 10 mg/kg	Hanauer (2002)
		MH week 54: 50 % continuous IFX vs. 7 % sporadic IFX	Rutgeerts (2006)
Perianal/fistulizing CD	RPCT	TLTR week 54: 40 weeks 5 mg/kg vs. 14 weeks placebo	Sands (2004)
Pregnancy	CT	Live birth: 67 % IFX vs. 67 % ctrl (95 % CI: 56.3, 76.0) Miscarriage: 17 % IFX vs. 15 % (95 % CI: 8.2, 23.2) Termination: 16 % IFX vs. 19 % (95 % CI: 11.5, 28.0)	Katz (2004)
Extraintestinal manifestations	OLT	PA (153 pts steroid-refractory CD) 61 % improvement, 46 % resolution at 12 weeks	Herfarth (2002)
	RS	PG (13 therapy refractory): IFX mean response time 210 days, 100 % response	Regueiro (2003)
	RCT	AS: 18.1 IFX vs. 40.05 placebo BASDAI at 12 months	Generini (2004)
		PU: IFX improves visual acuity and controls ocular inflammation	Lindstedt (2005)
Postoperative management	PCT	Recurrence at 12 months: 9.1 % IFX vs. 84.6 % placebo	Regueiro (2009)
		First endoscopic recurrence: 1231 days IFX vs. 460 days placebo	Regueiro (2014)
Biosimilars	RT	Response/remission CT-P13: week 2 90.6 %/68.8 %; week 54 87.5 %/75 %	Jung (2015)

infections. In two patients the opportunistic infections were identified as cytomegalovirus and cutaneous Nocardia [47].

Common side effects during infusion with infliximab are hypersensitivity reactions as manifested by urticaria, dyspnea and hypotension, reactions usually encountered during the first 2 h of infusion (infliximab package insert). Type III hypersensitivity reaction in form of serum sickness usually occurs 1–3 weeks after infusion. It has been observed after reintroduction of infliximab and even as soon as with the second dose of induction therapy. Pathophysiologically, this type of hypersensitivity is characterized by antibodies towards infliximab with fixation and activation of complement and precipitation of immune complexes in joint tissue, blood vessels, and skin [76]. Symptoms consistent with this type of hypersensitivity include polyarthralgias, myalgias, sore throat, fever, edema, and dysphagia. In anticipation of these side effects, it is mandatory for the infusion center to have acetaminophen, antihistamines, corticosteroids, and epinephrine available for immediate use. Primary preventative measures for infusion reactions include the gradual increase of infusion rate, use of an immunomodulator, and possibly premedication. However, premedication with corticosteroids, antihistamines, and antipyretics has been shown to be of limited and inconclusive efficacy [76]. Recommended secondary preventative measures include the use of an immunomodulator, graded dose challenge, and desensitization (Table 34.1).

References

1. Richter JA, Bickston SJ. Infliximab use in luminal Crohn's disease. Gastroenterol Clin North Am. 2006;35(4):775–93.
2. Targan SR, Hanauer SB, van Deventer SJ, Mayer L, Present DH, Braakman T, et al. A short-term study of chimeric monoclonal antibody cA2 to tumor necrosis factor alpha for Crohn's disease. Crohn's Disease cA2 Study Group. N Engl J Med. 1997; 337(15):1029–35.
3. Hanauer SB, Feagen BG, Lichtenstein GR, Mayer LF, Schreiber S, Colomberl JF, et al. Maintenance infliximab for Crohn's disease: the ACCENT I randomised trial. Lancet. 2002;359(9317):1541–9.
4. Barrie A, Regueiro M. Biologic therapy in the management of extraintestinal manifestations of inflammatory bowel disease. Inflamm Bowel Dis. 2007;13(11):1424–9.
5. Katz JA, Antoni C, Keenan GF, Smith DE, Jacobs SJ, Lichtenstein GR. Outcome of pregnancy in women receiving infliximab for the treatment of Crohn's disease and rheumatoid arthritis. Am J Gastroenterol. 2004;99(12):2385–92.
6. Regueiro M, Schraut W, Baidoo L, Kip KE, Sepulveda AR, Pesci M, et al. Infliximab prevents Crohn's disease recurrence after ileal resection. Gastroenterology. 2009;136(2):441–50.e1. quiz 716.
7. Louis E, Vermeire S, Rutgeerts P, De Vos M, Van Gossum A, Pescatore P, et al. A positive response to infliximab in Crohn disease: association with a higher systemic inflammation before treatment but not with −308 TNF gene polymorphism. Scand J Gastroenterol. 2002;37(7):818–24.
8. Harper JW, Sinanan MN, Zisman TL. Increased body mass index is associated with earlier time to loss of response to infliximab in patients with inflammatory bowel disease. Inflamm Bowel Dis. 2013;19(10):2118–24.
9. Bell SJ, Kamm MA. Review article: the clinical role of anti-TNFalpha antibody treatment in Crohn's disease. Aliment Pharmacol Ther. 2000;14(5):501–14.

10. Knight DM, Trinh H, Le J, Siegel S, Shealy D, McDonough M, et al. Construction and initial characterization of a mouse-human chimeric anti-TNF antibody. Mol Immunol. 1993;30(16):1443–53.
11. Scallon BJ, Trinh H, Nedelman M, Brennan FM, Feldmann M, Ghrayeb J. Functional comparisons of different tumour necrosis factor receptor/IgG fusion proteins. Cytokine. 1995;7(8):759–70.
12. Maurice MM, van der Graaff WL, Leow A, Breedveld FC, van Lier RA, Verweij CL. Treatment with monoclonal anti-tumor necrosis factor alpha antibody results in an accumulation of Th1 CD4+ T cells in the peripheral blood of patients with rheumatoid arthritis. Arthritis Rheum. 1999;42(10):2166–73.
13. Schaeffer DF, Walsh JC, Kirsch R, Waterman M, Silverberg MS, Riddell RH. Distinctive histopathologic phenotype in resection specimens from patients with Crohn's disease receiving anti-TNF-alpha therapy. Hum Pathol. 2014;45(9):1928–35.
14. Cornillie F, Shealy D, D'Haens G, Geboes K, Van Assche G, Ceuppens J, et al. Infliximab induces potent anti-inflammatory and local immunomodulatory activity but no systemic immune suppression in patients with Crohn's disease. Aliment Pharmacol Ther. 2001;15(4):463–73.
15. Maser EA, Villela R, Silverberg MS, Greenberg GR. Association of trough serum infliximab to clinical outcome after scheduled maintenance treatment for Crohn's disease. Clin Gastroenterol Hepatol. 2006;4(10):1248–54.
16. Juillerat P, Pittet V, Vader JP, Burnand B, Gonvers JJ, de Saussure P, et al. Infliximab for Crohn's disease in the Swiss IBD Cohort Study: clinical management and appropriateness. Eur J Gastroenterol Hepatol. 2010;22(11):1352–7.
17. Lichtenstein GR, Hanauer SB, Sandborn WJ. Management of Crohn's disease in adults. Am J Gastroenterol. 2009;104(2):465–83. quiz 464, 484.
18. Melmed GY, Siegel CA, Spiegel BM, Allen JI, Cima R, Colombel JF, et al. Quality indicators for inflammatory bowel disease: development of process and outcome measures. Inflamm Bowel Dis. 2013;19(3):662–8.
19. D'Haens GR, Panaccione R, Higgins PD, Vermeire S, Gassull M, Chowers Y, et al. The London Position Statement of the World Congress of Gastroenterology on Biological Therapy for IBD with the European Crohn's and Colitis Organization: when to start, when to stop, which drug to choose, and how to predict response? Am J Gastroenterol. 2011;106(2):199–212. quiz 213.
20. Beaugerie L, Seksik P, Nion-Larmurier I, Gendre JP, Cosnes J. Predictors of Crohn's disease. Gastroenterology. 2006;130(3):650–6.
21. Loly C, Belaiche J, Louis E. Predictors of severe Crohn's disease. Scand J Gastroenterol. 2008;43(8):948–54.
22. Seksik P, Loftus LV, Beaugerie L. Validation of predictors of 5-year disabling CD in a population based-cohort from Olmsted County, Minnesota 1983–1996. Gastroenterology. 2007;132(A-17).
23. Vermeire S, Louis E, Carbonez A, Van Assche G, Noman M, Belaiche J, et al. Demographic and clinical parameters influencing the short-term outcome of anti-tumor necrosis factor (infliximab) treatment in Crohn's disease. Am J Gastroenterol. 2002;97(9): 2357–63.
24. Louis E, Boverie J, Dewit O, Baert F, De Vos M, D'Haens G. Treatment of small bowel subocclusive Crohn's disease with infliximab: an open pilot study. Acta Gastroenterol Belg. 2007;70(1): 15–9.
25. van Dullemen HM, van Deventer SJ, Hommes DW, Bijl HA, Jansen J, Tytgat GN, et al. Treatment of Crohn's disease with anti-tumor necrosis factor chimeric monoclonal antibody (cA2). Gastroenterology. 1995;109(1):129–35.
26. McCabe RP, Woody J, van Deventer SJ. A multicenter trial of cA2 anti-TNF chimeric monoclonal antibody in patients with active Crohn's disease. Gastroenterology. 1996;110 Suppl 4:A962.
27. Rutgeerts P, Diamond RH, Bala M, Olson A, Lichtenstein GR, Bao W, et al. Scheduled maintenance treatment with infliximab is superior to episodic treatment for the healing of mucosal ulceration associated with Crohn's disease. Gastrointest Endosc. 2006;63(3):433–42. quiz 464.
28. Hazlewood GS, Rezaie A, Borman M, Panaccione R, Ghosh S, Seow CH, et al. Comparative effectiveness of immunosuppressants and biologics for inducing and maintaining remission in Crohn's disease: a network meta-analysis. Gastroenterology. 2015;148(2): 344–54.e5. quiz e14–5.
29. Reinisch W, Van Assche G, Befrits R, Connell W, D'Haens G, Ghosh S, et al. C-reactive protein, an indicator for maintained response or remission to infliximab in patients with Crohn's disease: a post-hoc analysis from ACCENT I. Aliment Pharmacol Ther. 2012;35(5):568–76.
30. Ben-Horin S, Kopylov U, Chowers Y. Optimizing anti-TNF treatments in inflammatory bowel disease. Autoimmun Rev. 2014;13(1):24–30.
31. Dignass A, Van Assche G, Lindsay JO, Lémann M, Söderholm J, Colombel JF, et al. The second European evidence-based Consensus on the diagnosis and management of Crohn's disease: current management. J Crohns Colitis. 2010;4(1):28–62.
32. Mowat C, Cole A, Windsor A, Ahmad T, Arnott I, Driscoll R, et al. Guidelines for the management of inflammatory bowel disease in adults. Gut. 2011;60(5):571–607.
33. Blackhouse G, Assasi N, Xie F, Marshall J, Irvine EJ, Gaebel K, et al. Canadian cost-utility analysis of initiation and maintenance treatment with anti-TNF-alpha drugs for refractory Crohn's disease. J Crohns Colitis. 2012;6(1):77–85.
34. Chaparro M, Panes J, García V, Mañosa M, Esteve M, Merino O, et al. Long-term durability of infliximab treatment in Crohn's disease and efficacy of dose "escalation" in patients losing response. J Clin Gastroenterol. 2011;45(2):113–8.
35. Hibi T, Sakuraba A, Watanabe M, Motoya S, Ito H, Motegi K, et al. Retrieval of serum infliximab level by shortening the maintenance infusion interval is correlated with clinical efficacy in Crohn's disease. Inflamm Bowel Dis. 2012;18(8):1480–7.
36. Steenholdt C, Brynskov J, Thomsen OØ, Munck LK, Fallingborg J, Christensen LA, et al. Individualised therapy is more cost-effective than dose intensification in patients with Crohn's disease who lose response to anti-TNF treatment: a randomised, controlled trial. Gut. 2014;63(6):919–27.
37. Katz L, Gisbert JP, Manoogian B, Lin K, Steenholdt C, Mantzaris GJ, et al. Doubling the infliximab dose versus halving the infusion intervals in Crohn's disease patients with loss of response. Inflamm Bowel Dis. 2012;18(11):2026–33.
38. Steenholdt C, Enevold C, Ainsworth MA, Brynskov J, Thomsen OØ, Bendtzen K. Genetic polymorphisms of tumour necrosis factor receptor superfamily 1b and fas ligand are associated with clinical efficacy and/or acute severe infusion reactions to infliximab in Crohn's disease. Aliment Pharmacol Ther. 2012;36(7):650–9.
39. Sandborn WJ, Rutgeerts P, Enns R, Hanauer SB, Colombel JF, et al. Adalimumab induction therapy for Crohn disease previously treated with infliximab: a randomized trial. Ann Intern Med. 2007;146(12):829–38.
40. Seow CH, Newman A, Irwin SP, Steinhart AH, Silverberg MS, Greenberg GR. Trough serum infliximab: a predictive factor of clinical outcome for infliximab treatment in acute ulcerative colitis. Gut. 2010;59(1):49–54.
41. Cornillie F, Hanauer SB, Diamond RH, Wang J, Tang KL, Xu Z, et al. Postinduction serum infliximab trough level and decrease of C-reactive protein level are associated with durable sustained response to infliximab: a retrospective analysis of the ACCENT I trial. Gut. 2014;63(11):1721–7.

42. Gisbert JP, Panes J. Loss of response and requirement of infliximab dose intensification in Crohn's disease: a review. Am J Gastroenterol. 2009;104(3):760–7.
43. Dotan I, Ron Y, Yanai H, Becker S, Fishman S, Yahav L, et al. Patient factors that increase infliximab clearance and shorten half-life in inflammatory bowel disease: a population pharmacokinetic study. Inflamm Bowel Dis. 2014;20(12):2247–59.
44. Fasanmade AA, Adedokun OJ, Blank M, Zhou H, Davis HM. Pharmacokinetic properties of infliximab in children and adults with Crohn's disease: a retrospective analysis of data from 2 phase III clinical trials. Clin Ther. 2011;33(7):946–64.
45. Vande Casteele N, Ferrante M, Van Assche G, Ballet V, Compernolle G, Van Steen K, et al. Trough concentrations of infliximab guide dosing for patients with inflammatory bowel disease. Gastroenterology. 2015;148(7):1320–9.e3.
46. Present DH, Rutgeerts P, Targan S, Hanauer SB, Mayer L, van Hogezand RA, et al. Infliximab for the treatment of fistulas in patients with Crohn's disease. N Engl J Med. 1999;340(18):1398–405.
47. Sands BE, Anderson FH, Bernstein CN, Chey WY, Feagan BG, Fedorak RN, et al. Infliximab maintenance therapy for fistulizing Crohn's disease. N Engl J Med. 2004;350(9):876–85.
48. Fonager K, Sørensen HT, Olsen J, Dahlerup JF, Rasmussen SN. Pregnancy outcome for women with Crohn's disease: a follow-up study based on linkage between national registries. Am J Gastroenterol. 1998;93(12):2426–30.
49. Casanova MJ, Chaparro M, Domènech E, Barreiro-de Acosta M, Bermejo F, Iglesias E, et al. Safety of thiopurines and anti-TNF-alpha drugs during pregnancy in patients with inflammatory bowel disease. Am J Gastroenterol. 2013;108(3):433–40.
50. Arguelles-Arias F, Castro-Laria L, Barreiro-de Acosta M, García-Sánchez MV, Guerrero-Jiménez P, et al. Is safety infliximb during pregnancy in patients with inflammatory bowel disease? Rev Esp Enferm Dig. 2012;104(2):59–64.
51. Bortlik M, Machkova N, Duricova D, Malickova K, Hrdlicka L, Lukas M, et al. Pregnancy and newborn outcome of mothers with inflammatory bowel diseases exposed to anti-TNF-alpha therapy during pregnancy: three-center study. Scand J Gastroenterol. 2013;48(8):951–8.
52. Schnitzler F, Fidder H, Ferrante M, Ballet V, Noman M, Van Assche G, et al. Outcome of pregnancy in women with inflammatory bowel disease treated with antitumor necrosis factor therapy. Inflamm Bowel Dis. 2011;17(9):1846–54.
53. Cheent K, Nolan J, Shariq S, Kiho L, Pal A, Arnold J. Case report: fatal case of disseminated BCG infection in an infant born to a mother taking infliximab for Crohn's disease. J Crohns Colitis. 2010;4(5):603–5.
54. Heller MM, Wu JJ, Murase JE. Fatal case of disseminated BCG infection after vaccination of an infant with in utero exposure to infliximab. J Am Acad Dermatol. 2011;65(4):870.
55. van der Woude CJ, Kolacek S, Dotan I, Oresland T, Vermeire S, Munkholm P, et al. European evidenced-based consensus on reproduction in inflammatory bowel disease. J Crohns Colitis. 2010;4(5):493–510.
56. Bernstein CN, Blanchard JF, Rawsthorne P, Yu N. The prevalence of extraintestinal diseases in inflammatory bowel disease: a population-based study. Am J Gastroenterol. 2001;96(4):1116–22.
57. Gravallese EM, Kantrowitz FG. Arthritic manifestations of inflammatory bowel disease. Am J Gastroenterol. 1988;83(7):703–9.
58. Herfarth H, Obermeier F, Andus T, Rogler G, Nikolaus S, Kuehbacher T, et al. Improvement of arthritis and arthralgia after treatment with infliximab (Remicade) in a German prospective, open-label, multicenter trial in refractory Crohn's disease. Am J Gastroenterol. 2002;97(10):2688–90.
59. Kaufman I, Caspi D, Yeshurun D, Dotan I, Yaron M, Elkayam O. The effect of infliximab on extraintestinal manifestations of Crohn's disease. Rheumatol Int. 2005;25(6):406–10.
60. Regueiro M, Valentine J, Plevy S, Fleisher MR, Lichtenstein GR. Infliximab for treatment of pyoderma gangrenosum associated with inflammatory bowel disease. Am J Gastroenterol. 2003;98(8):1821–6.
61. Brooklyn TN, Dunnill MG, Shetty A, Bowden JJ, Williams JD, Griffiths CE, et al. Infliximab for the treatment of pyoderma gangrenosum: a randomised, double blind, placebo controlled trial. Gut. 2006;55(4):505–9.
62. Generini S, Giacomelli R, Fedi R, Fulminis A, Pignone A, Frieri G, et al. Infliximab in spondyloarthropathy associated with Crohn's disease: an open study on the efficacy of inducing and maintaining remission of musculoskeletal and gut manifestations. Ann Rheum Dis. 2004;63(12):1664–9.
63. Braun J, Brandt J, Listing J, Zink A, Alten R, Golder W, et al. Treatment of active ankylosing spondylitis with infliximab: a randomised controlled multicentre trial. Lancet. 2002;359(9313):1187–93.
64. Joseph A, Raj D, Dua HS, Powell PT, Lanyon PC, Powell RJ, et al. Infliximab in the treatment of refractory posterior uveitis. Ophthalmology. 2003;110(7):1449–53.
65. Lindstedt EW, Baarsma GS, Kuijpers RW, van Hagen PM. Anti-TNF-alpha therapy for sight threatening uveitis. Br J Ophthalmol. 2005;89(5):533–6.
66. Bernell O, Lapidus A, Hellers G. Risk factors for surgery and postoperative recurrence in Crohn's disease. Ann Surg. 2000;231(1):38–45.
67. Regueiro M, Kip KE, Baidoo L, Swoger JM, Schraut W. Postoperative therapy with infliximab prevents long-term Crohn's disease recurrence. Clin Gastroenterol Hepatol. 2014;12(9):1494–502.e1.
68. Molodecky NA, Soon IS, Rabi DM, Ghali WA, Ferris M, Chernoff G, et al. Increasing incidence and prevalence of the inflammatory bowel diseases with time, based on systematic review. Gastroenterology. 2012;142(1):46–54.e42. quiz e30.
69. Feldman SR. Inflammatory diseases: integrating biosimilars into clinical practice. Semin Arthritis Rheum. 2015;44(6 Suppl):S16–21.
70. McKeage K. A review of CT-P13: an infliximab biosimilar. BioDrugs. 2014;28(3):313–21.
71. Ben-Horin S, Yavzori M, Benhar I, Fudim F, Picard O, Ungar B, et al. Cross-immunogenicity: antibodies to infliximab in Remicade-treated patients with IBD similarly recognise the biosimilar Remsima. Gut. 2015;65(7):1132–8.
72. (CHMP), E.M.A.C.f.M.P.f.H.U., *Assessment report: Inflectra (Infliximab)*. http://www.ema.europa.eu/docs/en_GB/document_library/EPAR_-_Public_assessment_report/human/002778/WC500151490.pdf, 2013. EMA/402688/2013(EMEA/H/C/002778). p. 3.
73. Jung YS, Park DI, Kim YH, Lee JH, Seo PJ, Cheon JH, et al. Efficacy and safety of CT-P13, a biosimilar of infliximab, in patients with inflammatory bowel disease: a retrospective multicenter study. J Gastroenterol Hepatol. 2015;30(12):1705–12.
74. Seiderer J, Goke B, Ochsenkuhn T. Safety aspects of infliximab in inflammatory bowel disease patients. A retrospective cohort study in 100 patients of a German University Hospital. Digestion. 2004;70(1):3–9.
75. Wolfe F, Michaud K, Anderson J, Urbansky K. Tuberculosis infection in patients with rheumatoid arthritis and the effect of infliximab therapy. Arthritis Rheum. 2004;50(2):372–9.
76. Lichtenstein L, Ron Y, Kivity S, Ben-Horin S, Israeli E, Fraser GM, et al. Infliximab-related infusion reactions: systematic review. J Crohns Colitis. 2015;9(9):806–15.

Briakinumab and Ustekinumab: Anti-p40 Antibodies for Inflammatory Bowel Disease Treatment

35

Peter Mannon

Background

The introduction of IL-12/IL-23 anti-p40 antibodies as a novel therapy for Crohn's disease is a case study in basic immunologic observations derived from animal models of human disease translated to highly targeted treatment into the clinic. Based on the work of Mosmann and Coffman [1], effector T cell responses could be separated into two major types, the so-called Th1 T cells that produce interferon-gamma (IFNγ) and Th2 cells that produce IL-4, IL-5, and IL-13. The Th1 cells were implicated in Crohn's disease, with IFNγ produced in excess by lamina propria T cells in animal models of Crohn's disease as well as in Crohn's patients [2, 3]. Th1 cells are directly induced from naïve T cells after exposure to interleukin-12. IL-12 is secreted by antigen-presenting cells activated by particular microbial components. Naïve T cells encountering a cognate ligand presented by a monocyte in the presence of IL-12 develop into a Th1 cells. These Th1 cells secrete IFNγ as part of the inflammatory response after encountering the same ligand thereafter. Interleukin-12 is a heterodimeric protein composed of two covalently bound subunits, a p35 and p40 protein named for their relative molecular sizes (Fig. 35.1). Interleukin-12 binds to a specific cell surface receptor on T cells, the IL-12 receptor, another heterodimeric protein composed of the IL-12 receptor beta 1 (IL12Rβ1) and 2 (IL12Rβ2) subunits.

In the late 1990s, data from several studies using animal models of colitis confirmed an important role for IL-12 effects on Th1 T cells in the induction and maintenance of intestinal inflammation [4–6]. In a murine model of Crohn's disease, trinitrobenzene sulfonic acid (TNBS) colitis, administration of anti-IL-12 antibodies at Day 0 (before inflammation began) or Day 21 (after colitis is established) prevented or reversed the inflammation [4]. Another model of Crohn's disease, cell transfer colitis, also responded to anti-IL-12 antibodies when administered early or late in the induction of colitis [7]. Other studies showed that anti-IL-12 induced apoptosis in large numbers of lamina propria CD4 T cells, suggesting a mechanism of action for anti-IL-12 therapeutic effects. So the facts that patients with Crohn's disease have increased lamina propria IL-12 production coupled with the success of targeting IL-12 activity in animal models of disease (especially in treating established colitis) provided compelling evidence for trials of such an agent in Crohn's disease.

The discovery of IL-23 along with its role in IL-17 production, another cytokine appreciated for its emerging role in autoimmune inflammatory disease, forced a revision of the view that IL-12 and Th1 cells were solely responsible for Crohn's disease. In fact, these discoveries helped to explain some inconsistencies in the Th1-Th2 dichotomy of T cell inflammation (such as why some Th1 animal models of autoimmune disease get worse with blockade of interferon γ [8, 9]), and spurred interest in investigating the roles of IL-23 and IL-17 in IBD. IL-23 is related to IL-12 in that IL-23 is largely produced by cells of the innate immune system and, like IL-12, is a heterodimeric protein composed of a p19 subunit covalently bound to a p40 subunit, the subunit common to the IL-12 molecule (Fig. 35.1). While IL-12 induces Th1 T cells, IL-23 is more important for the maintenance and function of IL-17-secreting cells (Th17 cells) [10, 11]; Th17 T cells are induced by IL-6 and TGFβ, whereupon differentiation into Th17 cells is accompanied by expression of cell surface IL-23 receptor making them responsive to IL-23 stimulation. However, given the shared p40 subunit, an anti-p40 antibody would target both IL-12 and IL-23. Therefore it is easy to postulate that both IL-12- and IL-23-driven inflammation could be interrupted by administration of an anti-p40 antibody.

In fact, a role for IL-23 and IL-17 in human IBD, particularly Crohn's disease, was suggested by certain animal models.

P. Mannon (✉)
Professor of Medicine and Microbiology, University of Alabama at Birmingham, Birmingham, AL, USA
e-mail: pmannon@uab.edu

D.C. Baumgart (ed.), *Crohn's Disease and Ulcerative Colitis*, DOI 10.1007/978-3-319-33703-6_35

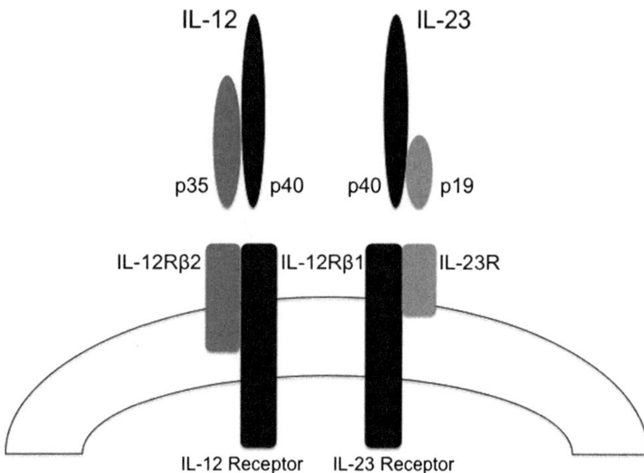

Fig. 35.1 Interleukin-12 is a heterodimeric protein composed of two covalently bound subunits, a p35 and p40 protein named for their relative molecular sizes

In the IL-10 deficient mouse model of spontaneous colitis, specifically eliminating IL-23 or IL-17 effects could successfully treat the colitis whereas eliminating IL-12 did not prevent inflammation [12]. In the cell transfer model of colitis, where colitogenic naïve CD4CD45RB^{high} T cells from wild type mice are infused into T cell-deficient mice (recombination activating gene (RAG) knockout or severe combined immunodeficiency (SCID) mice), the resulting gut inflammation displays a more pronounced dependency on IL-23. For instance in this transfer model, T cell-deficient recipient mice that also lacked IL-23 (RAG/p19 double knockout) were protected against developing severe colitis (which did not happen with IL-12-deficient RAG/p35 double knockout recipients) [13]. Similarly, mice that received CD4CD45RB^{high} T cells that also lacked the IL-23 receptor and therefore were defective in developing robust Th17 cells [14] were also protected from developing colitis. However, despite the important role of the IL-23/IL-17 axis in the transfer model of colitis, blockade of IFNγ activity (either by treating mice with an anti-IFNγ antibody [15] or transferring T cells defective in IFNγ production [16]) also prevented development of gut inflammation. Furthermore, there are data that show that an intact IL-23/IL-17 cytokine axis may limit inflammation in animal models since IL-17-deficient T cells used in the transfer model of colitis have earlier onset weight loss and higher expression of inflammatory cytokines in the gut while IL-23-deficient (p19 knockout) mice have more severe TNBS-induced colitis [17, 18].

In addition to the preclinical data, the IL-23/IL-17 axis is associated with human Crohn's disease since, like IL-12 and IFNγ, production of both IL-23 and IL-17 are significantly elevated [19, 20]. Moreover a low-prevalence polymorphism in the coding region of the IL-23 receptor gene confers protection from Crohn's disease, and although the mechanism of this effect is not clear it has been proposed that the polymorphism results in the production of a soluble receptor splice variant that acts to antagonize IL-23. These data have lead to clinical trials testing whether anti-IL-17 strategies can treat active Crohn's disease. Surprisingly, secukinumab (anti-IL-17A) treatment in Crohn's patients was no different than placebo and was associated with a 43 % infection rate compared to 0 % in placebo (and four patients had severe mucocutaneous Candidiasis) [21, 22]. Moreover, a trial of an antibody to an IL-17 receptor A subunit (Brodalumab, AMG 827) that could block activity of IL-17A, -E, and -F for the treatment of active Crohn's disease was stopped early when Crohn's disease symptoms worsened in the study drug treatment arm [23]. In summary, while animal models have provided guidance to inflammatory pathway aberrancies in Crohn's disease, namely the IL-12/INFγ and IL-23/IL-17 cascades, it is currently unclear whether there is a clear benefit to targeting one pathway over the other, but it is clear that an anti-p40 strategy has the potential to block important initiating and supporting cytokines that drive these pathways.

Clinical Trials with Briakinumab in Crohn's Disease

Briakinumab (ABT-874/J695) is a fully human $IgG_1\lambda$ antibody raised against the p40 subunit of IL-12/IL-23. This agent has been used in two completed Phase II trials in human Crohn's disease that tested efficacy and measured safety. The first trial enrolled 79 patients with active Crohn's disease and treated them with subcutaneous injections of placebo, 1 mg/kg, and 3 mg/kg [24]. Two cohorts received study drug as seven injections; the first treatment group was administered a single injection followed by six weekly injections and the other group was administered seven consecutive weekly injections. Patients were followed for 18 weeks after the final injection. The primary objective of this study was observation of safety endpoints. Overall the patients tolerated the anti-p40 well where 84 % of patients completed all seven injections and 87 % completed at least six injections. While there were a number of adverse events that occurred in more than 10 % of both briakinumab and placebo patients (nausea, vomiting, abdominal pain, arthralgia, urinary tract infection, bronchitis, cough, headache, fever, and fatigue), these were not significantly different between placebo and briakinumab, and there were no serious infections. However, 77–88 % of patients receiving 1 or 3 mg/kg and 25 % of placebo recipients reported local injection site reactions, the majority (88 %) of which was considered mild. Though nine severe adverse events occurred (seven briakinumab group, two placebo) none were adjudged related to the study drug.

For this study the secondary endpoints included rates of response (drop in the baseline Crohn's Disease Activity

Index (CDAI)≥100 points) and remission (CDAI≤150 points) at the end of treatment and at the end of follow-up (18 weeks after the final injection). The first treatment group showed response rates of 38 %, 63 %, and 56 % and remission rates at the end of treatment of 38 %, 31 % and 44 % for the placebo, 1 mg/kg, and 3 mg/kg groups respectively, without any significant differences among them. The first treatment group showed response rates of 25 %, 19 % and 50 % and remission rates at the end of follow-up of 13 %, 19 %, and 50 % for placebo, 1 mg/kg, and 3 mg/kg respectively, without any significant differences among them. In the second dose cohort, at the end of treatment the response rates were 25 %, 27 %, 75 % and the remission rates were 0 %, 8 % and 38 % for placebo, 1 mg/kg, and 3 mg/kg respectively, with significant differences seen between placebo and 3 mg/kg response rates ($p=0.03$). Furthermore, at the end of the 18 week follow-up period the response rates were 25 %, 19 %, 69 % and remission rates were 0 %, 13 % and 38 % for placebo, 1 mg/kg, and 3 mg/kg respectively, with differences seen between placebo and 3 mg/kg response rates that tended toward but did not reach significance ($p=0.08$). These data showed that clinical responses and remissions could be rapidly achieved (2–4 weeks) and could be durable after therapy was stopped.

Antidrug antibodies (ADAs) were identified in three patients from the 1 mg/kg dose (two in the first treatment group, and one who had them detected before receiving drug). These ADAs were associated with low serum levels of briakinumab and quick clearance but due to certain technical difficulties with this assay of measuring antidrug antibodies in the presence of anti-p40 drug, the actual rate of ADA formation may be underestimated, as they were not detected in three other subjects who also had unusually low briakinumab levels.

Changes in lamina propria mononuclear cell cytokine secretion and improvement in mucosal histology at the end of treatment were measured in a subset of nine patients. Of the eight patients who received briakinumab, seven reported a clinical response and all of these patients showed significantly decreased production of IL-12, IFNγ, and TNFα at the end of treatment; the sole primary nonresponder in this group had low pretreatment levels of IL-12, an increase in IFNγ production at the end of treatment and no change in TNFα. Similarly, primary responders to briakinumab had significantly decreased production of IL-23 and IL-17 at the end of treatment [20]. So these data show that anti-p40 was well tolerated by Crohn's patients. Additionally, there was efficacy at a higher dose and using a dosing strategy of uninterrupted administration.

With this data in hand, a second briakinumab Phase IIb, randomized, double-blind, parallel group, placebo-controlled dose ranging study was conducted. Using a 12 week induction phase and a 12 week maintenance phase, the objective was to test the efficacy and safety of inducing and maintaining remission in Crohn's disease [25]. Patients with active Crohn's disease (CDAI 220–450) received intravenous infusions of briakinumab (400, 700 mg) or placebo every 4 weeks for 12 weeks; at the end of treatment, responders (drop in CDAI of ≥70 points) were eligible for a maintenance extension phase at the same dose (only patients receiving 700 mg IV every 4 weeks in the induction phase were re-randomized to placebo, 200 mg, or 700 mg IV every 4 weeks) and treated for 12 weeks when clinical assessments were made at Week 24. Patients who were not in clinical response at week 12 were eligible for enrollment in open label treatment using 700 mg IV every 4 weeks (for up to 2 years from week 0) in addition to patients who were not in clinical remission at Week 24 (CDAI <150), and patients who relapsed during the maintenance treatment or follow-up. The primary endpoint was rate of remission at Week 6; secondary endpoints included remission rates at Week 12, Week 24 (among those responding at Week 12), and response rates (drop in CDAI of ≥100 points) at Weeks 6, 12, and 24. There were 48 patients receiving placebo, 45 receiving 400 mg, and 139 receiving 700 mg at the start of the study. The primary endpoint of remission at week 6 was not met, with no differences among rates for placebo (9 %), 400 mg (13 %), or 700 mg (17 %); however, at Week 12 there were significant differences among remission rates for briakinumab comparing placebo (11 %) to 400 mg (29 %, $p=0.03$) (but not versus 700 mg (22 %), $p=0.087$). At neither Weeks 6 nor 12 were there any significant differences among clinical response rates for placebo, 400 or 700 mg: 17 %, 36 %, 37 % and 20 %, 31 %, and 40 % respectively. At the end of the 12 week maintenance treatment, there were no significant differences between placebo and the 400 or 700 mg doses either for response (36 %, 62 %, and 71 %, respectively) or remission (29 %, 48 %, and 57 %). When looking at the subset of patients with elevated C reactive protein serum levels (CRP≥1 mg/dL), a group repeatedly seen to have lower placebo response rates across many trials, the six week remission rates showed a trend toward improved results without reaching significance: six week remission rates for placebo, 400 and 700 mg doses in the high CRP group were 5 %, 21 %, and 18 % compared to 11 %, 5 %, and 17 % respectively. Stratifying patients according to anti-TNFα experience (naïve, responder, nonresponder) did not show significant differences in remission rates at Week 6 either, although by this point the diminishing numbers in certain categories precluded adequate powering of the analysis. In terms of adverse events, there were no significant differences between rates in placebo or study drug groups; the infectious adverse events in both groups during induction and maintenance dosing were rather high (25–34 %), but the rate of serious infectious adverse events and opportunistic infections, specifically oroesophageal Candidiasis, were lower at less than 5 %. Injection site reactions were infrequent (0–6.5 %) consistent with the intravenous administration, and eight serious infusion reactions occurred in the open label extension phase.

In summary, the first of these two studies gave an indication that targeting the IL-12/IL-23 pathways could induce clinical improvement in Crohn's symptoms in patients with long-standing disease. Furthermore, this outcome was supported by significant decreases in the effector cytokines (IL-12, IFNγ, IL-23, and IL-17) thought to be specifically driving the gut inflammation in Crohn's disease. In contrast, the follow-up study using larger doses and long-interval intravenous infusion failed to show significant differences in early clinical benefit, however there were trends showing benefit at 12 weeks and beyond, even reaching rates of clinical response seen in the first trial. Briakinumab has subsequently been shown to be highly effective in psoriasis [26] but have more limited efficacy in multiple sclerosis [27].

It should be noted that briakinumab was primarily being developed as a treatment for psoriasis but was terminated during the approval process due to the need for further time-sensitive data required of the manufacturer and potential safety issues in the form of major cardiac events reported (in abstract) in one psoriasis trial may have contributed to this decision [28–30]. The issue of cardiovascular risk associated with psoriasis and biologic treatments has been subsequently reviewed [31].

Ustekinumab

Ustekinumab is a fully human monoclonal IgGκ antibody that can bind to IL-12, IL-23, and the p40 monomer [32]. Binding of ustekinumab to IL-12 or IL-23 interrupts coupling of the cytokines to the cell surface IL12 receptor (via the IL-12Rβ1 subunit) and prevents intracellular signaling and T cell activation. While this agent is currently approved for use in psoriasis, it has also been investigated for multiple sclerosis, psoriatic arthritis, and Crohn's disease [33]. The first published trial of ustekinumab in Crohn's disease randomized 104 patients to a double-blinded, cross-over, placebo-controlled Phase IIa induction study [34]. Patients were randomized to one of four dose regimens: (1) four weekly SC doses of placebo, then after a four week washout, four weekly doses of 90 mg ustekinumab SC ($n=25$), (2) four weekly SC doses of 90 mg ustekinumab SC, then after a four week washout, four weekly SC doses of placebo ($n=25$), (3) IV placebo followed by 4.5 mg/kg IV ustekinumab 8 weeks later ($n=27$), or (4) 4.5 mg/kg IV ustekinumab followed by IV placebo 8 weeks later ($n=26$). The primary endpoint was the rate of clinical response at Week 8 (overall decrease in CDAI by ≥70 representing a ≥25 % drop from the pretreatment score). Secondary endpoints included rates of clinical response at Weeks 4 and 6, and remission rates (CDAI ≤150 points) and "100-point response" rates at Weeks 4, 6, and 8 (there was also an endpoint assessment at Week 16 for those randomized to the third arm, so that response to the single dose of ustekinumab at Week 8 could be measured).

The Week 8 clinical response primary endpoint was not met in this study, but patients receiving the single intravenous dose of ustekinumab had a significantly higher response rate at Week 6 compared to placebo (54 % vs 22 %, $p=0.024$). Using the data combined from both routes of administration, rates of response were significantly higher at Weeks 4 and 6 (53 % versus 30 %, $p \le 0.02$), and a 100-point response was seen at Week 6 (49 % versus 25 %, $p=0.01$). There were no differences in rates of remission. Interestingly, when analyzing the subset of patients ($n=49$) who had previously been exposed to infliximab (regardless of response to infliximab), the clinical response rates for ustekinumab were significantly higher at every time point compared to placebo, 55–59 % versus 15–26 %, respectively. In an open label extension study of ustekinumab in patients who reported primary or secondary nonresponse to infliximab, the clinical response to either a single intravenous 4.5 mg/kg dose ($n=14$) or four weekly SC injections of 90 mg ($n=13$) was similar at Week 8 (54 % versus 43 %), but there were higher response rates for the IV administration at all the earlier time points perhaps reflecting a quicker onset of action related to the route of administration. Additional analyses based on changes in C reactive protein after treatment, show that ustekinumab administration is associated with decreased CRP serum levels, higher baseline CRP is associated with higher ustekinumab response rates, and prior infliximab experience may amplify these effects [35].

Safety results showed that while there were no significant differences in adverse event rates through week 8 between the blinded placebo and treatment groups, the total adverse event rates were rather high (68–85 %). However, of those adverse events reported more than 10 % of the time, the placebo patients reported more nausea, worsening of Crohn's symptoms, fatigue and pharyngolaryngeal pain. Placebo patients also reported higher rates of infection but no one had a serious or opportunistic infection or malignancy. Serious adverse events were mostly related to complications or worsening of Crohn's disease. During the follow-up phase, disseminated histoplasmosis was seen in an ustekinumab recipient who was taking azathioprine and prednisone concomitantly, and viral gastroenteritis occurred in another ustekinumab subject. A 54 year old male subject with an elevated prostate-specific antigen serum level at baseline was diagnosed with prostate cancer 2 months after intravenous ustekinumab. A female patient was diagnosed with basal cell carcinomas 6 months after her final ustekinumab injection.

A second trial tested the efficacy of ustekinumab in moderate-to-severe Crohn's disease patients who were resistant to anti-TNF drugs [36]. Eligible patients had active Crohn's disease (CDAI 220–450) and met specified criteria for anti-TNF primary nonresponse, secondary nonresponse, or side effect intolerance. For the 8 week induction phase, 526 patients randomly received 1, 3, or 6 mg/kg or placebo IV at week 0 and then 145 patients who had response to study drug (≥100 point drop in the CDAI) measured at week 6 were randomized to maintenance dose of 90 mg or placebo SC at weeks 8 and 16. Clinical response at week 6 was the primary end point and each dose level had a significantly higher rate (1 mg/kg 36.6 %, $p=0.02$; 3 mg/kg 34.1 % $p=0.06$; 6 mg/kf 39.7 % $p=0.005$) compared to placebo (23.5 %). However there were no differences in the remission rates (placebo 10.6 %, 1 mg/kg 16.0 %, 3 mg/kg 15.9 %, and 6 mg/kg 12.2 %). For those in the maintenance phase clinical response at week 22 occurred significantly more frequently in the treatment group (69.4 % vs 42.5 % $p<0.001$) including a significant achievement of remission (41.7 % vs 27.4 % $p=0.03$) and sustained clinical response (55.6 % vs 32.9 % $p=0.005$) compared to placebo. Patients who were primary nonresponders to the induction dose were unlikely to be responders to the maintenance dosing (20.2 % study drug vs 18.2 % placebo). Serious infections occurred in five patients in the 6 mg/kg induction group (*C. difficile*, viral gastroenteritis, urinary tract infection, anal abscess and vaginal abscess), in one 1 mg/kg patient (central line staphylococcal infection) and one placebo patient (anal abscess). There were no safety signals from the maintenance phase data. A survey of the supplemental data showed that baseline characteristics significantly associated with the primary outcome measures were above-median age, male gender, Caucasian race, the two lowest quartiles of weight, CDAI>300 and CRP>0.3 mg/dL. In addition secondary nonresponse and failure with at least two anti-TNF agents were significantly associated with the primary outcome. These data suggest additional biological effects that could affect outcome as endophenotypes of inflammatory bowel diseases and their susceptibility to more highly targeted therapies emerges.

In the interim, additional case reports have documented the utility of ustekinumab for similarly anti-TNF-refractory disease [37–40] as well as for treatment of pyoderma gangrenosum [41, 42] and even anti-TNF-induced alopecia and psoriasis [43, 44]. The long-term safety data show no characteristic predisposition to specific malignancies or infections and isolated reports document inexplicable central nervous system demyelinating inflammation coincident with ustekinumab use or appearance of melanoma (in a patient with dysplastic nevus syndrome) [45–48].

These ustekinumab trial data show that this agent can induce a clinical response in patients with active, established Crohn's disease, but this seems to be limited to patients who have a history of anti-TNF treatment either as primary or secondary nonresponders. This is counter to the experience with briakinumab where anti-TNF naïve Crohn's patients had significant response to treatment. The ustekinumab data also suggest that that there are subsets of disease that do respond better including the presence of an elevated CRP and anti-TNF exposure history.

Conclusions

The discovery of IL-12 and IL-23 and the key roles they play in inflammation in animal models of human disease have positioned them among the top targets for developing novel drugs for Crohn's disease. However, there is a notable gap between the success of blocking IL-12/IL-23 p40 in animal models of Crohn's disease and the reports of successful treatment of human disease. Obviously, an advantage of the animal model is that a more uniform inflammation is induced by the use of timed colitogenic exposures in genetically identical subjects to test the effects of a specific therapy. In human disease and therapeutic trials, subjects have various phenotypes of disease, with different durations of disease and have genetically disparate backgrounds. These factors can make blocking IL-12/IL-23 p40 of differential importance to early versus late disease, to recurrent versus persistent disease, or to one individual versus another independent of duration or course of disease. Unfortunately there are no biomarkers yet known that would predict which patient would derive the better outcome from IL-12/IL-23 p40 targeting.

Many other influences on the therapeutic effect of targeting IL-12/IL-23 p40 in Crohn's disease also have not been worked out. These include the differential pharmacologic effects of early, constant, prolonged high concentrations of IL-12/IL-23 p40 immunoneutralization on cytokine cell surface receptor and intracellular signaling as compared to peak and trough dosing. The results of the first briakinumab study in Crohn's disease would suggest this is important. In addition IL-12/IL-23 p40 is secreted in large amounts as a monomer and homodimer that can be recognized by antibodies, and ustekinumab recognizes the p40 monomer [32]. Binding to these molecules could act as a sink for the drug and leave the unbound IL-12 and IL-23 heterodimers still active; alternatively since p40 homodimers can act as an antagonist to IL-12, the differential binding of a therapeutic antibody to the p40 homodimer could alter what might have been a beneficial balance of homodimers and heterodimers even in an established inflammation [49]. Finally, it is not at all clear whether there is a hierarchy of cytokine targeting, e.g., IL-12/INFγ versus IL-23/IL-17, at various stages of Crohn's disease or among individuals; this is important in that INFγ, IL-17, and the regulatory cytokine IL-10 seem to exist in a balance, one that might be unpredictably disturbed with the use of anti-p40 antibody.

The data from animal models and human trials using anti-IL-12/IL-23 p40 antibodies in Crohn's disease suggest that there is a future for this targeted approach in establishing new therapies. Furthermore, because there are a large number of legitimate questions about how best to administer these drugs and monitor its activity, these trial results are only a first attempt at estimating efficacy. Additional knowledge about immunotypes and associated biomarkers that identify patients at highest probability for response as well as strategies that can position patients for improved response will ultimately fulfill the promise of targeting IL-12/IL-23 p40 in Crohn's disease.

References

1. Mosmann TR, Cherwinski H, Bond MW, Giedlin MA, Coffman RL. Two types of murine helper T cell clone. I. Definition according to profiles of lymphokine activities and secreted proteins. J Immunol. 1986;136(7):2348–57.
2. Fuss IJ, Neurath M, Boirivant M, Klein JS, de la Motte C, Strong SA, et al. Disparate CD4+ lamina propria (LP) lymphokine secretion profiles in inflammatory bowel disease. Crohn's disease LP cells manifest increased secretion of IFN-gamma, whereas ulcerative colitis LP cells manifest increased secretion of IL-5. J Immunol. 1996;157(3):1261–70.
3. Monteleone G, Biancone L, Marasco R, Morrone G, Marasco O, Luzza F, et al. Interleukin 12 is expressed and actively released by Crohn's disease intestinal lamina propria mononuclear cells. Gastroenterology. 1997;112(4):1169–78.
4. Neurath MF, Fuss I, Kelsall BL, Stuber E, Strober W. Antibodies to interleukin 12 abrogate established experimental colitis in mice. J Exp Med. 1995;182(5):1281–90.
5. Simpson SJ, Shah S, Comiskey M, de Jong YP, Wang B, Mizoguchi E, et al. T cell-mediated pathology in two models of experimental colitis depends predominantly on the interleukin 12/Signal transducer and activator of transcription (Stat)-4 pathway, but is not conditional on interferon gamma expression by T cells. J Exp Med. 1998;187(8):1225–34.
6. Wirtz S, Finotto S, Kanzler S, Lohse AW, Blessing M, Lehr HA, et al. Cutting edge: chronic intestinal inflammation in STAT-4 transgenic mice: characterization of disease and adoptive transfer by TNF- plus IFN-gamma-producing CD4+ T cells that respond to bacterial antigens. J Immunol. 1999;162(4):1884–8.
7. Liu Z, Geboes K, Heremans H, Overbergh L, Mathieu C, Rutgeerts P, et al. Role of interleukin-12 in the induction of mucosal inflammation and abrogation of regulatory T cell function in chronic experimental colitis. Eur J Immunol. 2001;31(5):1550–60.
8. Billiau A, Heremans H, Vandekerckhove F, Dijkmans R, Sobis H, Meulepas E, et al. Enhancement of experimental allergic encephalomyelitis in mice by antibodies against IFN-gamma. J Immunol. 1988;140(5):1506–10.
9. Ferber IA, Brocke S, Taylor-Edwards C, Ridgway W, Dinisco C, Steinman L, et al. Mice with a disrupted IFN-gamma gene are susceptible to the induction of experimental autoimmune encephalomyelitis (EAE). J Immunol. 1996;156(1):5–7.
10. Veldhoen M, Hocking RJ, Atkins CJ, Locksley RM, Stockinger B. TGFbeta in the context of an inflammatory cytokine milieu supports de novo differentiation of IL-17-producing T cells. Immunity. 2006;24(2):179–89.
11. McGeachy MJ, Chen Y, Tato CM, Laurence A, Joyce-Shaikh B, Blumenschein WM, et al. The interleukin 23 receptor is essential for the terminal differentiation of interleukin 17-producing effector T helper cells in vivo. Nat Immunol. 2009;10(3):314–24.
12. Yen D, Cheung J, Scheerens H, Poulet F, McClanahan T, McKenzie B, et al. IL-23 is essential for T cell-mediated colitis and promotes inflammation via IL-17 and IL-6. J Clin Invest. 2006;116(5): 1310–6.
13. Uhlig HH, McKenzie BS, Hue S, Thompson C, Joyce-Shaikh B, Stepankova R, et al. Differential activity of IL-12 and IL-23 in mucosal and systemic innate immune pathology. Immunity. 2006;25(2):309–18.
14. Ahern PP, Schiering C, Buonocore S, McGeachy MJ, Cua DJ, Maloy KJ, et al. Interleukin-23 drives intestinal inflammation through direct activity on T cells. Immunity. 2010;33(2):279–88.
15. Powrie F, Leach MW, Mauze S, Menon S, Caddle LB, Coffman RL. Inhibition of Th1 responses prevents inflammatory bowel disease in scid mice reconstituted with CD45RBhi CD4+ T cells. Immunity. 1994;1(7):553–62.
16. Neurath MF, Weigmann B, Finotto S, Glickman J, Nieuwenhuis E, Iijima H, et al. The transcription factor T-bet regulates mucosal T cell activation in experimental colitis and Crohn's disease. J Exp Med. 2002;195(9):1129–43.
17. Becker C, Dornhoff H, Neufert C, Fantini MC, Wirtz S, Huebner S, et al. Cutting edge: IL-23 cross-regulates IL-12 production in T cell-dependent experimental colitis. J Immunol. 2006;177(5): 2760–4.
18. O'Connor Jr W, Kamanaka M, Booth CJ, Town T, Nakae S, Iwakura Y, et al. A protective function for interleukin 17A in T cell-mediated intestinal inflammation. Nat Immunol. 2009;10(6):603–9.
19. Fujino S, Andoh A, Bamba S, Ogawa A, Hata K, Araki Y, et al. Increased expression of interleukin 17 in inflammatory bowel disease. Gut. 2003;52(1):65–70.
20. Fuss IJ, Becker C, Yang Z, Groden C, Hornung RL, Heller F, et al. Both IL-12p70 and IL-23 are synthesized during active Crohn's disease and are down-regulated by treatment with anti-IL-12 p40 monoclonal antibody. Inflamm Bowel Dis. 2006;12(1):9–15.
21. Hueber W, Sands BE, Lewitzky S, Vandemeulebroecke M, Reinisch W, Higgins PD, et al. Secukinumab, a human anti-IL-17A monoclonal antibody, for moderate to severe Crohn's disease: unexpected results of a randomised, double-blind placebo-controlled trial. Gut. 2012;61(12):1693–700.
22. Colombel JF, Sendid B, Jouault T, Poulain D. Secukinumab failure in Crohn's disease: the yeast connection? Gut. 2013;62(5):800–1.
23. Targan S, Feagan BG, Vermeire S, Panaccione R, Melmed G, Blosch C, et al. A randomized, double-blind, placebo-controlled study to evaluate the safety, tolerability, and efficacy of AMG 827 in subjects with moderate to severe Crohn's disease. Gastroenterology. 2012;143(3):e26.
24. Mannon PJ, Fuss IJ, Mayer L, Elson CO, Sandborn WJ, Present D, et al. Anti-interleukin-12 antibody for active Crohn's disease. N Engl J Med. 2004;351(20):2069–79.
25. Pannacione R, Sandborn W, Gordon G, Lee S, Safdi A, Sedghi S, et al. Briakinumab (anti-interleukin 12/23p40, ABT874) for treatment of Crohn's disease. Am J Gastroenterol. 2010;105:S457.
26. Kimball AB, Gordon KB, Langley RG, Menter A, Chartash EK, Valdes J. Safety and efficacy of ABT-874, a fully human interleukin 12/23 monoclonal antibody, in the treatment of moderate to severe chronic plaque psoriasis: results of a randomized, placebo-controlled, phase 2 trial. Arch Dermatol. 2008;144(2):200–7.
27. Vollmer TL, Wynn DR, Alam MS, Valdes J. A phase 2, 24-week, randomized, placebo-controlled, double-blind study examining the efficacy and safety of an anti-interleukin-12 and -23 monoclonal antibody in patients with relapsing-remitting or secondary progressive multiple sclerosis. Mult Scler. 2011.
28. Gordon K, Langley R, Gottlieb A, Papp K, Menter A, Krueger G, et al. Efficacy and safety results from a phase III, randomized controlled trial comparing two dosing regimens of ABT-874 to placebo

in patients with moderate to severe psoriasis. J Eur Acad Dermatol Venereol. 2010;24 Suppl 4:30.

29. Traczewski P, Rudnicka L. Briakinumab for the treatment of psoriasis. BioDrugs. 2012;26(1):9–20.
30. Tzellos T, Kyrgidis A, Zouboulis CC. Re-evaluation of the risk for major adverse cardiovascular events in patients treated with anti-IL-12/23 biological agents for chronic plaque psoriasis: a meta-analysis of randomized controlled trials. J Eur Acad Dermatol Venereol. 2013;27(5):622–7.
31. Hugh J, Van Voorhees AS, Nijhawan RI, Bagel J, Lebwohl M, Blauvelt A, et al. From the Medical Board of the National Psoriasis Foundation: the risk of cardiovascular disease in individuals with psoriasis and the potential impact of current therapies. J Am Acad Dermatol. 2014;70(1):168–77.
32. Luo J, Wu SJ, Lacy ER, Orlovsky Y, Baker A, Teplyakov A, et al. Structural basis for the dual recognition of IL-12 and IL-23 by ustekinumab. J Mol Biol. 2010;402(5):797–812.
33. Cingoz O. Ustekinumab. MAbs. 2009;1(3):216–21.
34. Sandborn WJ, Feagan BG, Fedorak RN, Scherl E, Fleisher MR, Katz S, et al. A randomized trial of Ustekinumab, a human interleukin-12/23 monoclonal antibody, in patients with moderate-to-severe Crohn's disease. Gastroenterology. 2008;135(4):1130–41.
35. Toedter GP, Blank M, Lang Y, Chen D, Sandborn WJ, de Villiers WJ. Relationship of C-reactive protein with clinical response after therapy with ustekinumab in Crohn's disease. Am J Gastroenterol. 2009;104(11):2768–73.
36. Sandborn WJ, Gasink C, Gao LL, Blank MA, Johanns J, Guzzo C, et al. Ustekinumab induction and maintenance therapy in refractory Crohn's disease. N Engl J Med. 2012;367(16):1519–28.
37. Heetun ZS, Keegan D, O'Donoghue D, Doherty GA. Report of successful use of ustekinumab in Crohn's disease refractory to three anti-TNF therapies. Ir J Med Sci. 2014;183(3):507–8.
38. Kopylov U, Afif W, Cohen A, Bitton A, Wild G, Bessissow T, et al. Subcutaneous ustekinumab for the treatment of anti-TNF resistant Crohn's disease—the McGill experience. J Crohns Colitis. 2014; 8(11):1516–22.
39. Rinawi F, Rosenbach Y, Assa A, Shamir R. Ustekinumab for resistant pediatric Crohn's disease. J Pediatr Gastroenterol Nutr. 2014;62:e34–5.
40. Martinez-Montiel M, Piedracoba-Cadahia P, Gomez-Gomez C, Gonzalo J. Ustekinumab is effective and safe in the treatment of Crohn's disease refractory to anti-TNFalpha in an orthotopic liver transplant patient. J Crohns Colitis. 2015;9(9):816–7.
41. Guenova E, Teske A, Fehrenbacher B, Hoerber S, Adamczyk A, Schaller M, et al. Interleukin 23 expression in pyoderma gangrenosum and targeted therapy with ustekinumab. Arch Dermatol. 2011;147(10):1203–5.
42. Fahmy M, Ramamoorthy S, Hata T, Sandborn WJ. Ustekinumab for peristomal pyoderma gangrenosum. Am J Gastroenterol. 2012;107(5):794–5.
43. Tillack C, Ehmann LM, Friedrich M, Laubender RP, Papay P, Vogelsang H, et al. Anti-TNF antibody-induced psoriasiform skin lesions in patients with inflammatory bowel disease are characterised by interferon-gamma-expressing Th1 cells and IL-17A/IL-22-expressing Th17 cells and respond to anti-IL-12/IL-23 antibody treatment. Gut. 2014;63(4):567–77.
44. Andrisani G, Marzo M, Celleno L, Guidi L, Papa A, Gasbarrini A, et al. Development of psoriasis scalp with alopecia during treatment of Crohn's disease with infliximab and rapid response to both diseases to ustekinumab. Eur Rev Med Pharmacol Sci. 2013; 17(20):2831–6.
45. Ehmann LM, Tillack-Schreiber C, Brand S, Wollenberg A. Malignant melanoma during ustekinumab therapy of Crohn's disease. Inflamm Bowel Dis. 2012;18(1):E199–200.
46. Scherl EJ, Kumar S, Warren RU. Review of the safety and efficacy of ustekinumab. Therap Adv Gastroenterol. 2010;3(5): 321–8.
47. Toussirot E, Michel F, Bereau M, Binda D. Ustekinumab in chronic immune-mediated diseases: a review of long term safety and patient improvement. Patient Prefer Adherence. 2013;7: 369–77.
48. Badat Y, Meissner WG, Laharie D. Demyelination in a patient receiving ustekinumab for refractory Crohn's disease. J Crohns Colitis. 2014;8(9):1138–9.
49. Ling P, Gately MK, Gubler U, Stern AS, Lin P, Hollfelder K, et al. Human IL-12 p40 homodimer binds to the IL-12 receptor but does not mediate biologic activity. J Immunol. 1995;154(1): 116–27.

Biological Therapy of Crohn's Disease: Natalizumab, Vedolizumab, and Anti-MadCAM

36

Pieter Hindryckx and Geert D'Haens

Intestinal inflammation is highly dependent on the recruitment of white blood cells out from the circulation to the mucosal immune system of the gut. Diapedesis and transmigration of activated lymphocytes to the site of inflammation is tightly regulated by a complex interaction between integrins on the leukocyte surface and cell adhesion molecules on microvascular endothelial cells of post-capillary venules (Fig. 36.1). Already in the early nineties, increased expression of vascular cell adhesion molecules was demonstrated in inflammatory bowel disease (IBD) [1–3]. This prompted investigation of anti-adhesion therapy as a therapeutic strategy in IBD. In 1993, Podolsky and coworkers showed that a monoclonal antibody targeting the leukocyte α4 integrin was effective in the treatment of colitis in the cotton-top tamarin [4]. Some years later, Hesterberg et al. found similarly beneficial effects in this model with an antibody against the gut-specific integrin dimer α4β7 [5]. These preclinical studies opened the gate for clinical pilot trials with anti-adhesion agents in IBD. Following a long developmental process, anti-adhesion molecules have now entered the therapeutic armamentarium of IBD. In this chapter, we summarize and discuss the evidence for the use of natalizumab, vedolizumab, and anti-MadCAM in CD.

Natalizumab

Natalizumab (Perrigo Company plc, Dublin, Ireland) is a recombinant humanized antibody (containing 5 % mouse-derived protein) against the human a4 integrin. In 2001, a first small-scale randomized, double-blind clinical trial was performed comparing a single dose of 3 mg/kg intravenous natalizumab with placebo in active CD patients [6]. Although the primary endpoint (change in the Crohn's disease activity index at week 2) was not met in this study, the results were promising enough to warrant a large-scale multicenter phase 2 trial with natalizumab in moderate-to-severe CD, published in 2003 [7]. Anti-TNF naïve CD patients were randomly assigned to four different treatment regimens (two IV infusions of placebo or one infusion natalizumab at 3 mg/kg and one infusion of placebo or two infusions of 3 mg/kg natalizumab or two infusions of 6 mg/kg natalizumab). The primary endpoint was clinical remission (CDAI < 150) at week 6. Patients receiving two infusions of 3 mg/kg natalizumab had a significantly higher rate of clinical remission at weeks 4, 6, 8, and 12 compared to the placebo group (27 % versus 44 % respectively at week 6) [7]. A few years later, these results were confirmed in the phase 3 "Efficacy of Natalizumab as Active Crohn's Therapy" (ENACT-1) [8]. In contrast to the previous studies, previous use of anti-TNF agents was allowed and natalizumab was given at a fixed dose of 300 mg at week 0, 4, and 8. The primary endpoint was clinical response (drop in CDAI of at least 70 points) at week 10 and was not reached in this study [8]. Patients who had a response both a week 10 and week 12 were eligible for the maintenance trial (ENACT-2) in which patients were re-randomized 1:1 to placebo or 300 mg of natalizumab every 4 weeks [8]. The primary endpoint in ENACT-2 was sustained response (with loss of response being defined by an increase in the CDAI score of at least 70 points after week 12 and by an absolute score of at least 220 or the need for intervention after week 12) at week 36 which was observed in 61 % of patients on natalizumab and 28 % on placebo ($P=0.003$) [8]. However, ENACT-2 was prematurely halted by the manufacturer because of three cases of JC virus-related progressive multifocal leukoencephalopathy (PML), which was considered to be associated with the study drug All published as case reports. PML was caused by reactivation of the ubiquitous JC virus in combination with impaired immune surveillance in the central nervous system due to blockade of α4

P. Hindryckx
Department of Gastroenterology, University Hospital of Ghent, Ghent, Belgium

G. D'Haens (✉)
Department of Gastroenterology, Academic Medical Centre, Amsterdam, The Netherlands
e-mail: g.dhaens@amc.uva.nl

D.C. Baumgart (ed.), *Crohn's Disease and Ulcerative Colitis*, DOI 10.1007/978-3-319-33703-6_36

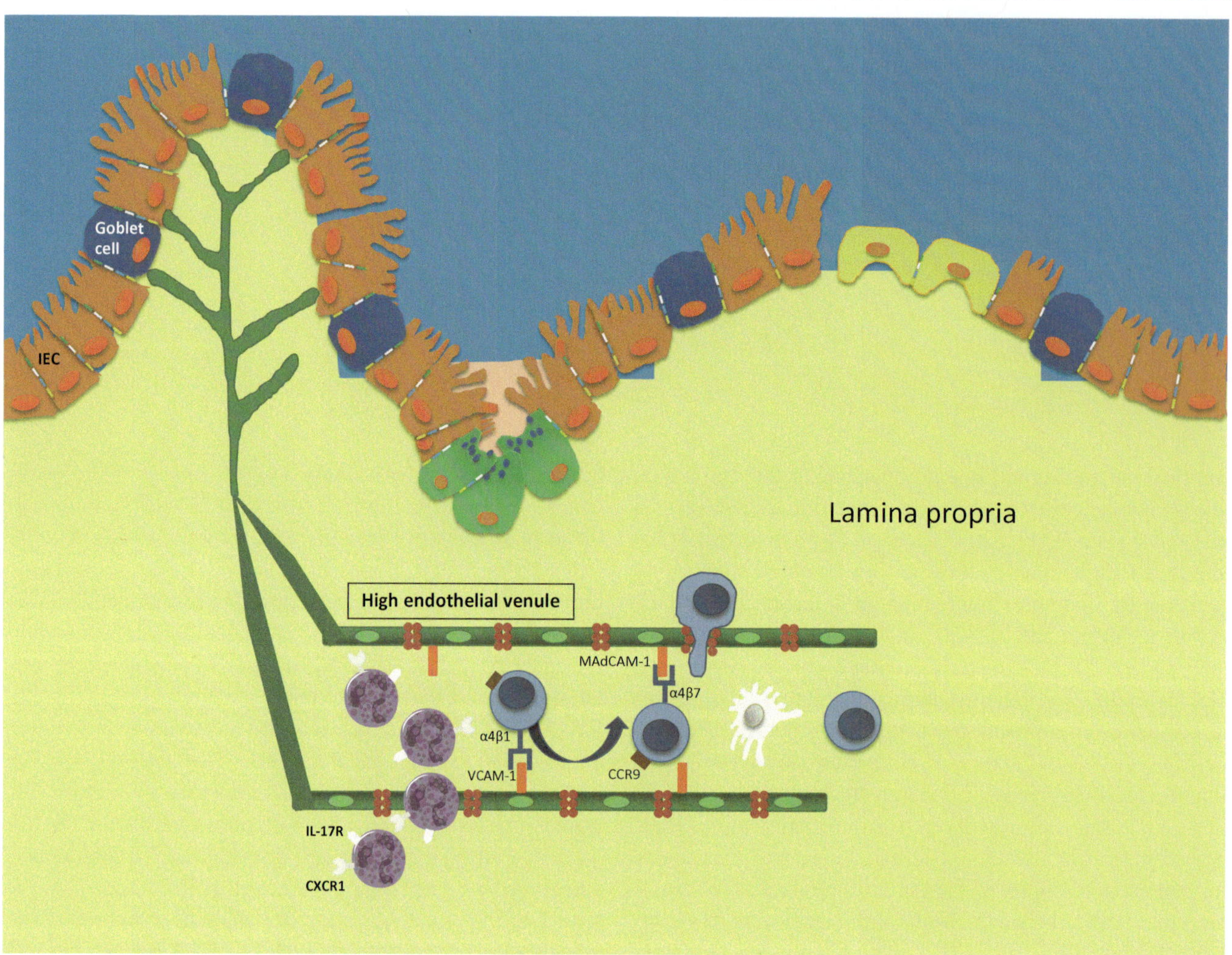

Fig. 36.1 Integrin heterodimers α4β1 and α4β7 on CCR9-expressing gut-homing T-lymphocytes form a stable binding complex with cell adhesion molecules (respectively VCAM-1 and MAdCAM-1) on the endothelium of postcapillary venules in the gut, allowing them to diapedesize into the lamina propria and feed the inflammatory process in IBD. Natalizumab is an anti-α4 antibody blocking both the α4β1-VCAM-1 interaction and the α4β7-MAdCAM-1 interaction. Vedolizumab and anti-MAdCAM-1 only inhibit the gut-specific α4β7-MAdCAM-1 interaction by respectively blocking the α4β7 dimer and MAdCAM-1

[9–11]. Retrospective analysis showed that an additional patient had died from JC virus-related PML during an open-label extension study of ENACT-2 [8]. As a result of this rare but life-threatening adverse event the European Medicine Agency (EMA) concluded that the benefits of natalizumab in the treatment of CD did not outweigh the risk [12] and refused marketing authorization in Europe for CD although the agent was approved for multiple sclerosis under the name Tysabri[R]. A later second induction trial, "Efficacy of Natalizumab in Crohn's Disease Response and Remission" (ENCORE), showed that natalizumab was also effective as an induction agent in patients with moderately to severely active CD with an elevated serum CRP as an objective marker of inflammation at baseline with the primary endpoint being induction of response (>70-point decrease from baseline in the Crohn's Disease Activity Index score at week 8), sustained through week 12 [13]. In 2008 the FDA approved natalizumab (Tysabri[R]) for the treatment of moderate-to-severe Crohn's disease not responding to, or not tolerating, conventional therapies for CD including inhibitors of TNF-α, albeit under a strict patient safety monitoring program [14, 15]. In the meantime, risk factors for PML have been identified: JCV seropositivity (in approximately 70 % of patients), previous exposure to immunosuppressive drugs, and exposure duration >2 years [16] leading to the recommendation to use the drug without concomitant immunosuppression However, the future of anti-integrin therapy was considered to lie in the development of more selective blockade of the integrin β7 or the combination α4β7 which would ensure higher gut-selectivity.

Vedolizumab

Vedolizumab is a recombinant humanized IgG1 monoclonal antibody targeting the alpha4beta7 integrin on leukocytes. In contrast to natalizumab, vedolizumab only inhibits adhesion of leukocytes to the relatively gut-selective MAdCAM-1 and not to VCAM-1, which is also expressed in the brain endothelium [17].

In 2008, a dose-finding trial with the anti-α4β7 antibody MLN0002 (Millennium, Boston, MA) in 185 moderately active anti-TNF-naïve CD patients [18] did not meet the primary endpoint (clinical response CDAI70 at 8 weeks although the results suggested a dose-dependent clinical benefit of MLN0002 therapy for the induction of remission, necessitating a larger clinical trial [18]. After humanizing the monoclonal antibody to "vedolizumab," a large phase 3 program was launched. In the GEMINI-2 study, 368 patients with moderately to severely active CD and at least one objective sign of active inflammation (significant endoscopic lesions, elevated CRP or elevated fecal calprotectin + positive findings on imaging) were randomly assigned to treatment with vedolizumab (300 mg IV at week 0 and week 2) or placebo at a 3:2 ratio [19]. The primary endpoints were clinical remission (CDAI < 150) and clinical response (CDAI drop of at least 100 points) as early as at week 6. In contrast to the previous trial, most of the patients were anti-TNF-experienced and concomitant use of corticosteroids and/or immunomodulators (in non-US patients) were allowed at stable dose. In addition, a significant proportion of patients had fistulizing disease and/or previous surgery for their CD. Patients receiving vedolizumab were twice as likely to be in clinical remission at week 6 as compared to patients who had received placebo, although the absolute numbers remained somewhat disappointing (14.5 % versus 6.8 % respectively) [19]. There was no statistically significant difference between vedolizumab- and placebo-treated CD patients with regard to the CDAI-100 response (one of the two primary endpoints) and there was surprisingly little effect of the treatment on serum CRP concentrations [19]. A later study (GEMINI 3) specifically investigated the efficacy of vedolizumab as an induction agent in CD patients with previous anti-TNF failure [20]. The primary efficacy outcome was clinical remission at week 6 (!). Again, vedolizumab treatment was not superior to placebo. However, these relatively poor "early" results may be explained by the slow mode of action, given the observation that vedolizumab significantly increased clinical response and remission rates beyond [20].

Also in GEMINI 2, 747 additional CD patients were treated with open label vedolizumab to in a feeder study for the maintenance study, in which patients with a clinical response (CDAI70) were re-randomized to placebo, vedolizumab 300 mg every 4 weeks or vedolizumab 300 mg every 8 weeks [19]. The primary endpoint was clinical remission at week 52. The effects of vedolizumab in this maintenance trial were quite robust, with 39 % of the patients in clinical remission on vedolizumab compared to 21.6 % on placebo and glucocorticoid-free remission in approximately one third of the vedolizumab-treated patients, irrespective of the dose interval (4 weeks or 8 weeks) [19]. The safety profile of vedolizumab was comparable to placebo and no single case of PML has been observed [19]. As a result, in 2014 both the FDA and the EMA approved vedolizumab (Entyvio^{R}) for the treatment of Crohn's disease (and ulcerative colitis) that is insufficiently controlled by conventional treatment and/or anti-TNF agents [20, 21]. Further data on mucosal healing, effects on fistula, postoperative recurrence, and pouchitis warrant further dedicated trials.

Anti-MAdCAM-1 Antibodies

The anti-MAdCAM monoclonal antibody PF-0547659 was investigated in a phase-2 dose-finding induction study (OPERA-1) in moderate—severe CD patients intolerant or refractory to anti-TNF and/or immunosuppressant therapy [22]. All patients had objective evidence of active disease (elevated (hs) CRP and mucosal ulcerations on endoscopy) and the primary efficacy parameter was a CDAI-70 response either by week 8 or week 12. Although the active treatment arms, in contrast to the placebo arm, were associated with increased circulating α4β7+ central memory T cells as a clear biological signal of the inhibitory effect of the active agent on MAdCAM-1, the primary endpoint was not met, most likely due to an unusually high placebo-response rate (41 % and 44 % at week 8 and 12, respectively) [22]. However, sub analysis revealed that a higher treatment effect was seen in CD patients with high hsCRP (>7.5 mg/dl) at baseline, with significantly more patients in the treatment arms being in remission at week 8 [22]. In addition, the safety profile was very reassuring. In a open-label induction study (Tosca) immune surveillance in the CNS was studied with repeated lumbar punctures. An induction course of anti-MAdCAM MAb did not affect the cellular determinants of immune surveillance in the central nervous system [22, 23]. In summary, the results with anti-MAdCAM for Crohn's disease are encouraging. The decision towards further development will depend on the results of the maintenance phase Opera-2 and the outcome of the UC study Turandot (Table 36.1).

Table 36.1 Characteristics and main outcome data of the major published trials on anti-adhesion therapy for Crohn's disease

Trial name	Year of publication	Number of study sites	Number of patients	Main outcome parameter	Concomitant drug exposure	Previous anti-TNF exposure allowed?	Placebo-controlled?	Open-label?	Study duration	Primary endpoint(s)	Placebo response (for primary endpoint)
Ghosh S et al. (natalizumab)	2003	35	248	CDAI	5-ASA Corticosteroids AZA/6-MP	No	Yes	No	12 weeks	Clinical remission at week 6: 44 %	27 %
ENACT-1 (natalizumab)	2005	142	905	CDAI	Corticosteroids 5-ASA AZA/6-MP Methotrexate Antibiotics	No	Yes	No	12 weeks	Clinical response at week 10: 56 %	49 %
ENACT-2 (natalizumab)	2005	142	339	CDAI	Corticosteroids 5-ASA AZA/6-MP Methotrexate Antibiotics	No	Yes	No	56 weeks	Maintenance of response through week 36: 61 %	28 %
ENCORE (natalizumab)	2007	114	509	CDAI	Corticosteroids 5-ASA AZA/6-MP Methotrexate Antibiotics	Yes	Yes	No	12 weeks	Clinical response at week 8 sustained through week 12: 48 %	32 %%
GEMINI-2 (vedolizumab)	2013	285	1115	CDAI	Corticosteroids 5-ASA AZA/6-MP Methotrexate Antibiotics	Yes	Yes	Until week 6 (cohort 2) and after week 6 in case of lack of clinical response to vedolizumab induction therapy (cohorte 1 and 2)	52 weeks	(1) clinical remission at week 6: 14.5 % (2) CDAI-100 response at week 6: 31.4 % (3) Clinical remission at week 52: 39 %	(1) 6.8 % (2) 25.7 % (3) 21.6 %

The Place Of Anti-adhesion Therapy in the Treatment Algorithm of Crohn's Disease

Currently, anti-adhesion molecules are being positioned as second line biologics (after anti-TNF) in the therapeutic armamentarium for CD (and IBD in general) in most jurisdictions. The phase 3 trials, however, suggest superior outcomes when the agent is given to patients who are naïve to anti-TNF agents and the mode of action suggests potentially better effects in earlier disease stages. This warrants further investigation and perhaps a head-to-head comparison with anti-TNF agents.

The question is indeed how we could implement this new class of drugs in the most effective way. Based on the results of the completed trials, some general conclusions can be drawn. Firstly, unlike most anti-TNF agents, the drugs seem to have a rather slow onset mode of action in CD [6–8, 13, 18, 19, 22], possibly because of the more pronounced transmural inflammatory infiltrate as compared to UC [24–26], where the inflammation is limited to the mucosa. For daily clinical practice, this means that anti-adhesion monotherapy may not be the ideal monotherapy in CD patients with severe disease that needs rapid remission. Combination with stronger "induction agents" such as corticosteroids and perhaps anti-TNF agents appears attractive. On the other hand, the integrin-inhibitors were shown to very effective maintenance drugs, with response and remission rates at least as high as with anti-TNF agents [8, 19, 27–30]. Future studies including real "strategy studies" will have to address where this novel class of biological should be positioned in the treatment algorithm of CD. Thus far, only one head-to-head trial is running, comparing vedolizumab IV with adalimumab SC in biological-naïve UC patients [31].

Is there still a place for natalizumab with the advent of the gut-selective integrin-inhibitor vedolizumab? In a recent editorial by Scott and Osterman in Clinical Gastroenterology and Hepatology, the authors state that natalizumab may remain a good option for patients that are JCV antibody negative (roughly one third of the patients) as there has never been a PML case described in this patient subgroup and seroconversion rates also seem to be low [32]. Nonetheless, natalizumab remains only registered without concomitant use of immunosuppressants.

Future studies will also have to address the immunogenicity of the anti-adhesion antibodies and whether combination therapy with immunosuppressant therapy is superior to monotherapy, as it is the case for infliximab [33].

The potential registration/indication of anti-Madcam antibodies in CD will depend on the maintenance phase 2 results and the phase 3 data if such studies will be set up in the future.

In summary, anti-adhesion antibodies are the second group of biologicals for the treatment of IBD. For CD, they seem to be slow-acting for induction but very effective for maintenance treatment. The advent of this new therapeutic option opens a completely new era of clinical trials in which therapeutic strategies will be compared in order to develop the best care for the patients.

References

1. Schuermann GM, Aber-Bishop AE, Facer P, Lee JC, Rampton DS, Doré CJ, et al. Altered expression of cell adhesion molecules in uninvolved gut in inflammatory bowel disease. Clin Exp Immunol. 1993;94:341–7.
2. Mishra L, Mishra BB, Harris M, Bayless TM, Muchmore AV. In vitro cell aggregation and cell adhesion molecules in Crohn's disease. Gastroenterology. 1993;104:772–9.
3. Koizumi M, King N, Lobb R, Benjamin C, Podolsky DK. Expression of vascular adhesion molecules in inflammatory bowel disease. Gastroenterology. 1992;103:840–7.
4. Podolsky DK, Lobb R, King N, Benjamin CD, Pepinsky B, Sehgal P, et al. Attenuation of colitis in the cotton-top tamarin by anti-alpha 4 integrin monoclonal antibody. J Clin Invest. 1993;92:372–80.
5. Hesterberg PE, Winsor-Hines D, Briskin MJ, Soler-Ferran D, Merrill C, Mackay CR, et al. Rapid resolution of chronic colitis in the cotton-top tamarin with an antibody to a gut-homing integrin alpha 4 beta 7. Gastroenterology. 1996;111:1373–80.
6. Gordon FH, Lai CW, Hamilton MI, Allison MC, Srivastava ED, Fouweather MG, et al. A randomized placebo-controlled trial of a humanized monoclonal antibody to alpha4 integrin in active Crohn's disease. Gastroenterology. 2001;121:268–74.
7. Ghosh S, Goldin E, Gordon FH, Malchow HA, Rask-Madsen J, Rutgeerts P, et al. Natalizumab for active Crohn's disease. N Engl J Med. 2003;348:24–32.
8. Sandborn WJ, Colombel JF, Enns R, Feagan BG, Hanauer SB, Lawrance IC, et al. Natalizumab induction and maintenance therapy for Crohn's disease. N Engl J Med. 2005;353:1912–25.
9. Kleinschmidt BK, Tyler KL. Progressive multifocal leukoencephalopathy complicating treatment with natalizumab and interferon beta-1a for multiple sclerosis. N Engl J Med. 2005;353:369–74.
10. Langer-Gould A, Atlas SW, Green AJ, Bollen AW, Pelletier D. Progressive multifocal leukoencephalopathy in a patient treated with natalizumab. N Engl J Med. 2005;353:375–81.
11. Van Assche G, Van Ranst M, Sciot R, Dubois B, Vermeire S, Noman M, et al. Progressive multifocal leukoencephalopathy after natalizumab therapy for Crohn's disease. N Engl J Med. 2005;353:362–8.
12. European Medicines Agency. Refusal CHMP assessment report for natalizumab Elan Pharma. Doc. Ref: EMEA/CHMP/8203/2008.
13. Targan SR, Feagan BG, Fedorak RN, Lashner BA, Panaccione R, Present DH, et al. Natalizumab for the treatment of active Crohn's disease: results of the ENCORE Trial. Gastroenterology. 2007;132:1672–83.
14. Honey K. The comeback kid: TYSABRI now FDA approved for Crohn disease. J Clin Invest. 2008;118:825–6.
15. Biogen Idec. Tysabri risk evaluation and mitigation strategy (REMS). http://www.fda.gov/downloads/Drugs/Drugsafety/postmarketdrugsafetyinformationforpatientsandproviders/.
16. Lichtenstein GR, Hanauer SB, Sandborn WJ. Risk of biologic therapy-associated progressive multifocal leukoencephalopathy: use of the JC virus antibody assay in the treatment of moderate-to-severe Crohn's disease. Gastroenterol Hepatol (NY). 2012;8:1–20.
17. Tilg H, Kaser A. Vedolizumab, a humanized mAb against the $\alpha 4\beta 7$ integrin for the potential treatment of ulcerative colitis and Crohn's disease. Curr Opin Investig Drugs. 2010;11:1295–304.

18. Feagan BG, Greenberg GR, Wild G, Fedorak RN, Paré P, McDonald JW, et al. Treatment of active Crohn's disease with MLN0002, a humanized antibody to the alpha4beta7 integrin. Clin Gastroenterol Hepatol. 2008;6:1370–7.
19. Sandborn WJ, Feagan BG, Rutgeerts P, Hanauer S, Colombel JF, Sands BE, et al. Vedolizumab as induction and maintenance therapy for Crohn's disease. N Engl J Med. 2013;369:711–21.
20. US Food and Drug Administration. BLA approval (BLA 125476/0). 2014. http://www.accessdata.fda.gov/drugsatfda_docs/appletter/2014/125476Orig1s000ltr.pdf.
21. Takeda. Takeda receives European commission marketing authorisation for Entyvio (vedolizumab) for the treatment of ulcerative colitis and Crohn's disease (media release); 28 May 2014. http://www.takeda.com/news/2014/20140528_6590.html.
22. D'Haens G, Lee S, Tarabar D, Louis E, Klopocka M, Park DI, et al. Anti-MAdCAM-1 antibody (PF-00547659) for active refractory Crohn's disease: results of the OPERA study. ECCO Congress Barcelona 2015;OP022.
23. D'Haens G, Vermeire S, Cataldi F, Vogelsang H, Allez M, Desreumaux P, et al. Anti-MAdCAM monoclonal antibody PF-00547659 does not affect immune surveillance in the central nervous system of anti-TNF and immunosuppressant experienced Crohn's disease patients who are anti-TNF inadequate responders: results from the TOSCA study. ECCO Congress Barcelona 2015;OP007.
24. Feagan BG, Greenberg GR, Wild G, Fedorak RN, Paré P, McDonald JW, et al. Treatment of ulcerative colitis with a humanized antibody to the alpha4beta7 integrin. N Engl J Med. 2005;352:2499–507.
25. Feagan BG, Rutgeerts P, Sands BE, Hanauer S, Colombel JF, Sandborn WJ, et al. Vedolizumab as induction and maintenance therapy for ulcerative colitis. N Engl J Med. 2013;369:699–710.
26. Vermeire S, Sandborn W, Danese S, Hebuterne X, Salzberg B, Klopocka M, et al. TURANDOT: a randomized, multicenter double-blind, placebo-controlled study of the safety and efficacy of Anti-MAdCAM Antibody PF-00547659 (PF) in patients with moderate to severe ulcerative colitis (UC). ECCO Congress Barcelona 2015;OP021.
27. Hanauer SB, Feagan B, Lichtenstein GR, Mayer LF, Schreiber S, Colombel JF, et al. Maintenance infliximab for Crohn's disease: the ACCENT I randomised trial. Lancet. 2002;359:1541–9.
28. Sandborn WJ, Hanauer SB, Rutgeerts P, et al. Adalimumab for maintenance treatment of Crohn's disease: results of the CLASSIC II trial. Gut. 2007;56:1232–9.
29. Colombel JF, Sandborn WJ, Rutgeerts P, et al. Adalimumab for maintenance of clinical response and remission in patients with Crohn's disease: the CHARM trial. Gastroenterology. 2007;132:52–65.
30. Schreiber S, Khaliq-Kareemi M, Lawrance IC, et al. Maintenance therapy with certolizumab pegol for Crohn's disease. N Engl J Med. 2007;357:239–50.
31. Takeda. An Efficacy and Safety Study of Vedolizumab Intravenous (IV) Compared to Adalimumab Subcutaneous (SC) in Participants With Ulcerative Colitis. https://clinicaltrials.gov/ct2/show/NCT02497469.
32. Scott FI, Osterman MT. Natalizumab for Crohn's disease: down but not out. Clin Gastroenterol Hepatol. 2015:S1542-3565(15)00979-9.
33. Colombel JF, Sandborn WJ, Reinisch W, Mantzaris GJ, Kornbluth A, Rachmilewitz D, et al. Infliximab, azathioprine, or combination therapy for Crohn's disease. N Engl J Med. 2010;362:1383–95.

Optimal Management of Fistulizing Crohn's Disease

37

Farhad Peerani and Bruce E. Sands

Abbreviations

CD	Crohn's disease
EUA	Examination under anesthesia
MRI	Magnetic resonance imaging
EUS	Endoscopic ultrasound
anti-TNF α	Anti-tumor necrosis factor α
pFCD	Perianal fistulizing Crohn's disease
CT	Computed tomography
PDAI	Perianal disease activity index
IFX	Infliximab
ADA	Adalimumab
6-MP	6-mercaptopurine
AZA	Azathioprine
CZP	Certolizumab pegol
LIFT	Ligation of the intersphincteric fistula tract
AF	Advancement flap
MTX	Methotrexate
AB	Antibiotics
D	Drainage
I	Incision
IS	Immunosuppressants

Optimal Management of Fistulizing Crohn's Disease

Transmural inflammation and stricturing predispose Crohn's disease (CD) patients to a fistulizing phenotype, which is associated with significant morbidity and predicts a more aggressive disease course [1]. In a population-based CD cohort from Olmsted County in the pre-biologic era, the cumulative risk of any fistula and more specifically perianal fistulas reached 50 % and 26 % respectively after 20 years [2]. Fistulas can be external or internal and are classified according to their location and their connection with adjacent organs. While the majority of Crohn's fistulas are perianal, other forms exist including enteroenteric, enterocutaneous, enterovesical, enterointra-abdominal, rectovaginal, and parastomal. Advances in imaging, medical treatment, and surgical techniques have improved our management of fistulizing disease; however, the majority of evidence-based recommendations are derived from small case series, secondary outcome analyses, or subgroup analyses from larger prospective studies. This chapter predominantly focuses on the management of perianal fistulizing Crohn's disease (pFCD), for which the evidence is most robust (Table 37.1).

Perianal Fistula Classification: Anatomical and Clinical

Fistulas may be classified based on whether they originate above (high) or below (low) the dentate line. The Parks classification describes fistulas anatomically as they relate to the external sphincter and includes five categories: superficial (low), intersphincteric (low or high), transsphincteric (low or high), suprasphincteric (high), and extrasphincteric (high) (Fig. 37.1) [3]. Unfortunately, Crohn's fistulas do not often follow the Parks classification nor does the Parks classification account for fistula association with adjacent organs, which can alter management.

F. Peerani, M.D., F.R.C.P.C.
Division of Gastroenterology, Department of Medicine, University of Alberta, Zeidler Ledcor Centre, Edmonton, AB T6G 2X8, Canada
e-mail: peerani@ualberta.ca

B.E. Sands, M.D., M.S. (✉)
Dr. Henry D. Janowitz Division of Gastroenterology and Department of Medicine, Icahn School of Medicine at Mount Sinai, New York, NY 10029, USA
e-mail: bruce.sands@mssm.edu

D.C. Baumgart (ed.), *Crohn's Disease and Ulcerative Colitis*, DOI 10.1007/978-3-319-33703-6_37

Table 37.1 Medical treatments available for perianal fistulizing Crohn's disease

Induction	Maintenance	Minimal evidence	Investigational	No role
IFX or ADA	IFX or ADA	CZP	Spherical carbon adsorbent	Steroids
[a]Antibiotics	[b]6-MP	Tacrolimus	Stem cells	Aminosalicylates
–	[b]AZA	Cyclosporine	–	–
–	–	Topical metronidazole or tacrolimus	–	–
–	–	MTX	–	–
–	–	Sargramostim	–	–
–	–	Local IFX or ADA injection	–	–
–	–	Thalidomide	–	–
–	–	Hyperbaric oxygen therapy	–	–

IFX infliximab, *ADA* adalimumab, *6-MP* 6-mercaptopurine, *AZA* azathioprine, *CZP* certolizumab pegol, *MTX* methotrexate
[a]When used in conjunction with IFX or ADA
[b]When used in conjunction with IFX or ADA

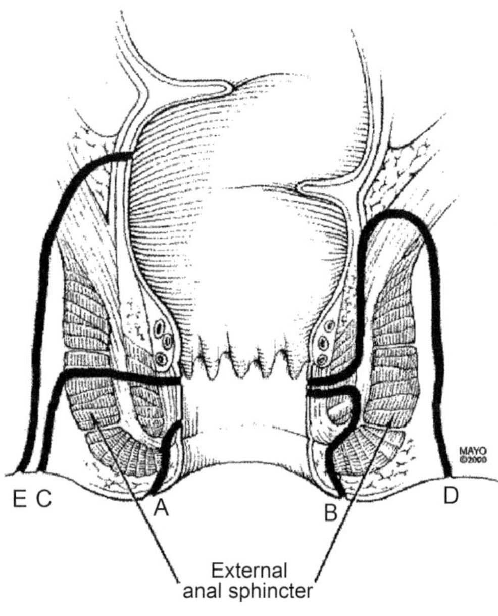

Fig. 37.1 The Parks classification. (**a**) A superficial fistula tracks below both the internal anal sphincter and external anal sphincter complexes. (**b**) An intersphincteric fistula tracks between the internal anal sphincter and the external anal sphincter in the intersphincteric space. (**c**) A transsphincteric fistula tracks from the intersphincteric space through the external anal sphincter. (**d**) A suprasphincteric fistula leaves the intersphincteric space over the top of the puborectalis and penetrates the levator muscle before tracking down to the skin. (**e**) An extrasphincteric fistula tracks outside of the external anal sphincter and penetrates the levator muscle into the rectum. Reprinted with permission from Parks et al., A classification of fistula-in-ano, The British Journal of Surgery, 1976, page 5 and Sandborn et al., AGA Technical Review on Perianal Crohn's Disease, Gastroenterology, 2003, page 1510. [3, 4] © British Journal of Surgery Society Ltd. Reproduced with permission granted by John Wiley & Sons Ltd on behalf of the BJSS Ltd and Elsevier on behalf of Gastroenterology

In a 2003 review on perianal CD published by the American Gastroenterological Association, perianal fistulas were classified clinically as "simple" or "complex" [4]. A simple fistula is low, has a single external opening and lacks findings consistent with a perianal abscess, rectovaginal fistula, anorectal stricture, or proctitis. Conversely, a complex fistula is high, may have multiple external openings and may have findings consistent with a perianal abscess, rectovaginal fistula, anorectal stricture or proctitis. While symptomatic simple perianal fistulas can be treated with either non-cutting seton placement or fistulotomy when used in conjunction with medical therapy, complex perianal fistulas usually require a combination of medical and surgical management in addition to non-cutting seton placement.

Investigation of Suspected Fistulizing Disease: Clinical Evaluation, Radiological Imaging, and Endoscopic Assessment

In the past, clinical evaluation and examination under anesthesia (EUA) were the primary methods of fistula evaluation. Antiquated imaging modalities including fistulography and computed tomography (CT) have been replaced by magnetic resonance imaging (MRI) and endoscopic ultrasound (EUS), which provide better resolution of perianal anatomy and avoid the risks of radiation. MRI and EUS are increasingly being used as tools that aid in diagnosis, monitor therapeutic efficacy, rule out complications (i.e., perianal abscess), and assist in surgical planning. Not only can MRI better delineate perianal anatomy preoperatively, but it is also a better predictor of surgical outcomes when compared to EUA, having a positive predictive value of 73 % and negative predictive value of 87 % [5].

A prospective triple-blinded study by Schwartz et al. demonstrated that EUS, EUA, and MRI have similar accuracy (87–91 %) in determining perianal fistula anatomy [6]. It is recommended that any two of the tests be combined to evaluate pFCD as the accuracy approaches 100 %. When comparing EUS to pelvic MRI, EUS is an operator dependent technique and is more likely to miss ischioanal fossa or supralevator abscesses whereas pelvic MRI may have a tendency to miss superficial fistula tracts. Ultimately, the exact imaging modality used in combination with EUA depends on local expertise and availability.

In addition to EUA and imaging, endoscopy should always be performed prior to the surgical treatment of pFCD as the presence of proctitis precludes definitive surgical management prior to medical therapy. Furthermore, if an anal stricture is present and malignancy has been excluded, endoscopic dilation should be attempted.

Definitions of Perianal Fistula Healing

Various symptom indices and imaging criteria have been used to define fistula healing and therefore the definition of "response to therapy" varies among studies. The perianal disease activity index (PDAI) was first described in 1995 and consists of five domains: discharge, pain/restriction of activities, restriction of sexual activity, type of perianal disease, and degree of induration [7]. The difficulty with using the PDAI is that there is no validated cutoff for fistula healing. The finger-compression technique has also been used to assess fistula drainage and was first used in a randomized controlled trial with infliximab (IFX) [8]. It is becoming increasingly apparent that radiological healing of fistulous tracts lags behind clinical remission by a median of 1 year [9]. Therefore, repeated imaging in the form of either MRI or EUS should be strongly considered within 6–12 months after initiating therapy.

Medical Treatments for Perianal Fistulizing Crohn's Disease

Antibiotics

Antibiotics such as ciprofloxacin and metronidazole are the most commonly prescribed treatment for pFCD in spite of the lack of evidence from placebo-controlled trials. They are prescribed as both a primary treatment and as a secondary treatment for complications such as abscesses that arise from fistulas. In one of the earliest published case series by Bernstein et al., 10 of 18 Crohn's patients (56 %) with perineal disease demonstrated complete healing with a 10-week course of metronidazole [10]. Topical 10 % metronidazole ointment has also been studied in 74 patients in a randomized placebo-controlled study, suggesting a beneficial effect on perianal discharge and pain [11]. Nevertheless, the majority of patients experience a recurrence of perineal disease months after metronidazole cessation. In the only randomized, double-blind, placebo-controlled trial involving antibiotics, there was a trend towards clinical remission and response occurring more frequently in the group treated with ciprofloxacin compared to patients treated with either metronidazole or placebo [12]. However, this trial was underpowered ($n=25$) and the majority of patients assigned to the metronidazole arm did not complete the prescribed 10-week course.

Evidence suggests that combination antibiotic therapy with anti-tumor necrosis factor α (anti-TNF α) therapy provides additional symptomatic benefit. In a double-blind, placebo-controlled trial, 76 CD patients with active perianal fistulizing disease were randomized to either adalimumab (ADA) monotherapy or ADA and ciprofloxacin for 12 weeks after ADA induction [13]. A significantly higher number of patients demonstrated both a partial (71 % vs. 47 %, $p=0.047$) and complete (65 % vs. 33 %, $p=0.009$) clinical response of fistula closure at 12 weeks in the combination therapy group. While the difference in fistula closure rates was not maintained at 24 weeks, the trend in favor of combination therapy remained. In a similarly designed study with IFX and ciprofloxacin, patients treated with combination therapy tended to have a better clinical response at week 18 (OR = 2.37 [0.94–5.98], $p=0.07$) [14]. Accordingly, antibiotics should be used as a co-induction agent in pFCD with ciprofloxacin being better-tolerated than metronidazole.

6-Mercaptopurine/Azathioprine

Although historically the daily recommended doses for 6-mercaptopurine (6-MP) and azathioprine (AZA) have been 1.5 and 2.5 mg/kg respectively, the ideal dosing regimen or optimal thiopurine metabolite levels are unknown in the setting of pFCD. In one of the first randomized, double-blinded studies of thiopurines, there was a trend towards fistula closure in the 6-MP group (31 % vs. 6 %) [15]. Subsequently, a meta-analysis of 6-MP and AZA use in CD demonstrated that fistulae improved with therapy (OR 4.44 [1.50–13.20]) [16]. While data exists for the use of thiopurines as maintenance treatment for pFCD, they are second-line therapies when compared to anti-TNF α drugs and are best used as concomitant therapy.

Tacrolimus/Cyclosporine

Calcineurin inhibitors have been used with modest benefit in cases of medically refractory pFCD. In both a randomized placebo-controlled trial and small pilot study of oral tacrolimus, tacrolimus-treated patients were significantly more likely to experience fistula closure that was documented clinically in the former study and radiologically by MRI in the latter [17, 18]. Topical tacrolimus was also explored in a small randomized, placebo-controlled study of 12 patients with pFCD [19]. Only one of six patients in the active treatment group had a complete response defined as cessation of drainage of all fistulas after 12 weeks. Evidence for the use of cyclosporine is equally sparse. In a case series of nine patients with fistulizing CD, the majority initially responded to IV cyclosporine, but after transitioning to oral cyclosporine and subsequent discontinuation, only two patients remained in prolonged remission [20]. The authors postulated that this outcome related to the inadequate overlap of concomitant therapy with either 6-MP or AZA prior to the withdrawal of cyclosporine.

Infliximab

Two large randomized placebo-controlled trials have demonstrated the efficacy of IFX for inducing and maintaining fistula closure in CD. The first trial in fistulizing CD was carried out by Present et al. and included 94 Crohn's patients randomized to placebo, IFX 5 mg/kg or IFX 10 mg/kg [8]. A reduction in 50 % or more from baseline in the number of draining fistula openings was noted in 62 % of the IFX group compared to 26 % of the placebo group ($p=0.002$). Moreover, complete fistula closure was demonstrated in 46 % of the IFX group compared to 13 % of the placebo group ($p=0.001$). The beneficial effect of IFX in this study was not dose-related.

In the ACCENT II trial, time to loss of response was significantly longer in patients receiving IFX 5 mg/kg maintenance every 8 weeks compared to placebo (>40 weeks vs. 14 weeks, $p<0.001$) [21]. Furthermore, at week 54, a greater number of patients in the IFX arm had a complete absence of draining fistulas (36 % vs. 19 %, $p=0.009$). Lichtenstein et al. have also shown that IFX 5 mg/kg maintenance therapy every 8 weeks significantly reduces hospitalizations, surgeries and procedures in CD patients with fistulizing disease [22].

Adalimumab

Although ADA has been used in the setting of IFX failures for the treatment of pFCD, recent evidence supports using ADA in anti-TNF naïve patients. The initial CLASSIC-1 and GAIN trials did not show any benefit of ADA compared to placebo with respect to clinically documented fistula closure; however, this could have occurred as the comparison was made too early at week 4 [23, 24]. In an open-label extension of the CHARM trial, not only was ADA more effective than placebo for inducing fistula healing, but also 28/31 patients (90 %) with healed fistulas at week 56 maintained healing after 1 year of open label ADA [25]. Moreover, in a retrospective multicenter Spanish study, 39 anti-TNF naïve CD patients were followed for 1 year after the initiation of ADA for pFCD [26]. The majority of patients received induction doses of 160 and 80 mg of ADA at week 0 and 2 respectively followed by 40 mg every other week. While 41 % of patients were maintained in clinical remission, 8 % exhibited partial clinical response. A smaller subset of 14 patients was also followed radiologically with MRI revealing fistula tract healing in 43 % at 1 year.

Certolizumab

Among the anti-TNF α antagonists, the least evidence for pFCD exists for certolizumab pegol (CZP). The PRECISE-I and PRECISE-II trials were not powered to examine the efficacy of CZP on fistula closure [27, 28]. Post hoc analyses were performed on a subgroup of patients (55/58 patients with fistulas had pFCD) from the PRECISE II placebo-controlled study, looking at the outcome of fistula closure at week 26 [29]. Although there was no statistical difference in the primary endpoint of prespecified definition of fistula closure (≥50 % closure at two consecutive post-baseline visits ≥3 weeks apart) between the CZP and placebo groups, a significantly greater number of patients randomized to CZP demonstrated complete clinical fistula closure at week 26 compared to placebo (36 % vs. 17 %, $p=0.038$).

Surgery

EUA allows for complete clinical assessment, incision and drainage of an abscess, and seton placement prior to the initiation of biologics for pFCD. In a retrospective case series, Regueiro and Mardini determined that patients with pFCD treated with IFX are more likely to maintain fistula closure if treatment is preceded by EUA and seton placement, especially in the setting of complex fistulas [30]. Nevertheless, the optimal timing of seton removal is unknown.

Surgical management varies based on the type of fistula ("simple" vs. "complex") as well as the presence or absence of anal stenosis or proctitis. One of the primary surgical concerns is postoperative anal incontinence secondary to sphincter injury. Several surgical techniques are available to treat pFCD including laying open a fistula tract (fistulotomy), conducting a ligation of the intersphincteric fistula tract (LIFT procedure), injecting bioprosthetic plug or fibrin glue, creating an advancement flap (AF) or diverting stoma, and as a last resort, performing a proctectomy. Unfortunately, many patients develop issues with perineal wound healing and subsequent chronic perineal sinuses after proctectomy.

Conclusion

While the optimal medical management of pFCD includes antibiotics with either IFX or ADA with or without a concomitant thiopurine for induction therapy, surgical therapy should be considered simultaneously to achieve the best outcomes (Figs. 37.2 and 37.3). Even in the era of biologics and advanced surgical techniques, perianal disease can be refractory. Clinicians should be alert to the rare but devastating possibility that malignancy may contribute to the refractoriness of pFCD. Given that fistula response rates for IFX and

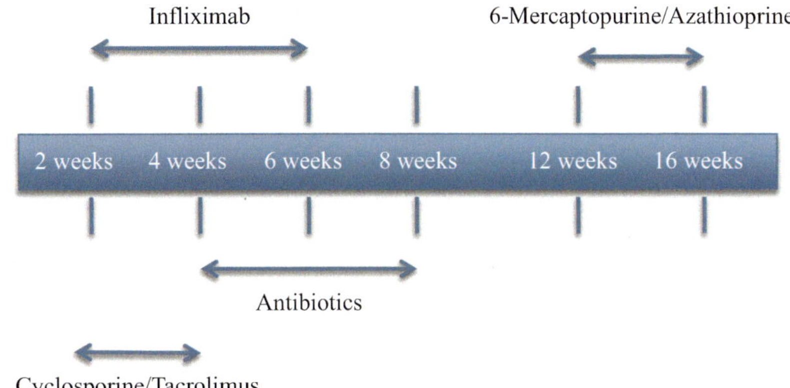

Fig. 37.2 Expected time to clinical response for perianal fistulas

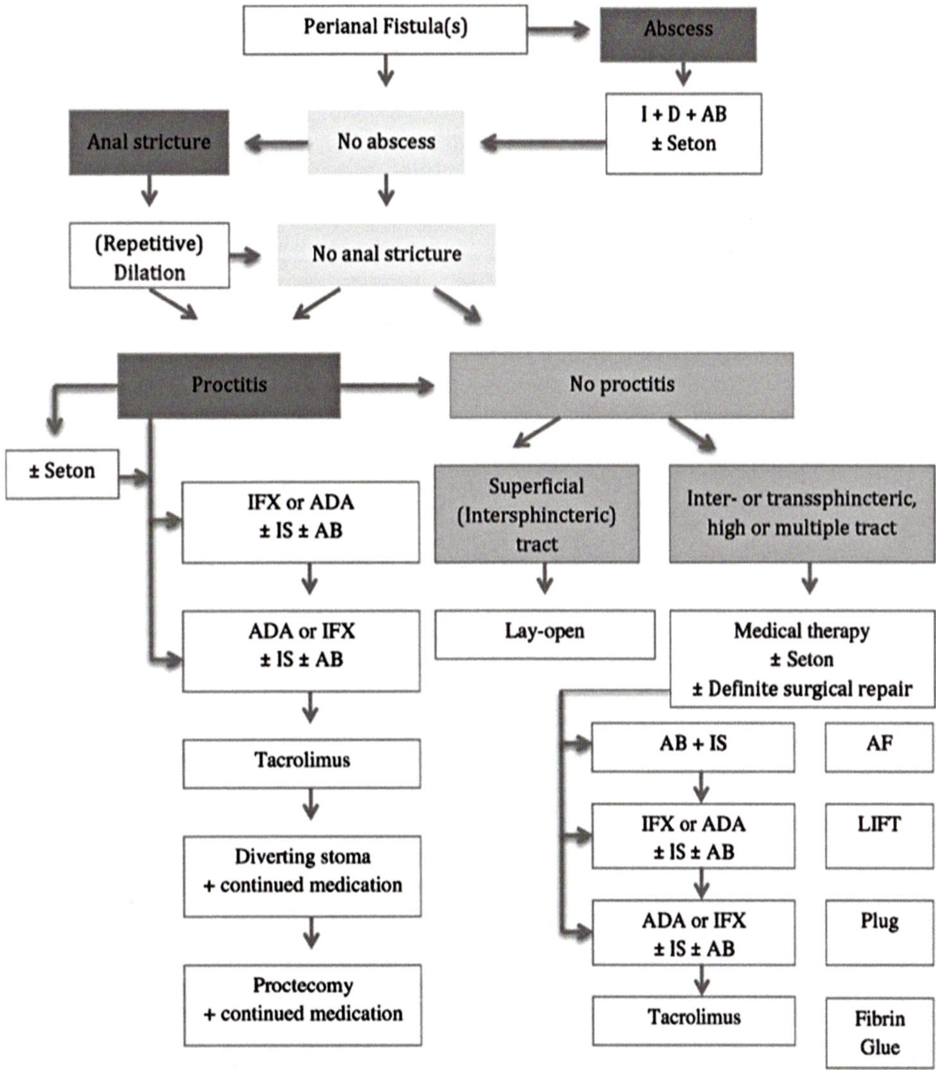

Fig. 37.3 Treatment algorithm for perianal fistulizing Crohn's disease. *AB* antibiotics, *ADA* adalimumab, *AF* advancement flap, *D* drainage, *I* incision, *IFX* infliximab, *IS* immunosuppressants, *LIFT* ligation of the intersphincteric fistula tract. Reprinted and reproduced from [A global consensus on the classification, diagnosis and multidisciplinary treatment of perianal fistulising Crohn's disease, Gecse et al., Volume 63, page 1389, © 2014] [31] with permission from BMJ Publishing Group Ltd

ADA are approximately 50 %, CD patients and clinicians eagerly await the development of more efficacious therapies for this disabling Crohn's phenotype.

References

1. Yarur AJ, Strobel SG, Deshpande AR, Abreu MT. Predictors of aggressive inflammatory bowel disease. Gastroenterol Hepatol. 2011;7:652–9.
2. Schwartz DA, Loftus Jr EV, Tremaine WJ, Panaccione R, Harmsen WS, Zinsmeister AR, et al. The natural history of fistulizing Crohn's disease in Olmsted County, Minnesota. Gastroenterology. 2002;122:875–80.
3. Parks AG, Gordon PH, Hardcastle JD. A classification of fistula-in-ano. Br J Surg. 1976;63:1–12.
4. Sandborn WJ, Fazio VW, Feagan BG, Hanauer SB. AGA technical review on perianal Crohn's disease. Gastroenterology. 2003;125: 1508–30.
5. Spencer JA, Chapple K, Wilson D, Ward J, Windsor ACJ, Ambrose NS. Outcome after surgery for perianal fistula: predictive value of MR imaging. AJR Am J Roentgenol. 1998;171:403–9.
6. Schwartz DA, Wiersema MJ, Dudiak KM, Fletcher JG, Clain JE, Tremaine WJ, et al. A comparison of endoscopic ultrasound, magnetic resonance imaging, and exam under anesthesia for evaluation of Crohn's perianal fistulas. Gastroenterology. 2001;121:1064–72.
7. Irvine EJ. Usual therapy improves perianal Crohn's disease as measured by a new disease activity index. J Clin Gastroenterol. 1995;20:27–32.
8. Present DH, Rutgeerts P, Targan S, Hanauer SB, Mayer L, van Hogezand RA, et al. Infliximab for the treatment of fistulas in patients with Crohn's disease. N Engl J Med. 1999;340:1398–405.
9. Tozer P, Ng SC, Siddiqui MR, Plamondon S, Burling D, Gupta A, et al. Long-term MRI-guided combined anti-TNF-α and thiopurine therapy for Crohn's perianal fistulas. Inflamm Bowel Dis. 2012;18:1825–34.
10. Bernstein LH, Frank MS, Brandt LJ, Boley SJ. Healing of perineal Crohn's disease with metronidazole. Gastroenterology. 1980;79: 357–65.
11. Maeda Y, Ng SC, Durdey P, Burt C, Torkington J, Rao PKD, et al. Randomized clinical trial of metronidazole ointment versus placebo in perianal Crohn's disease. Br J Surg. 2010;97:1340–7.
12. Thia KT, Mahadevan U, Feagan BG, Wong C, Cockeram A, Bitton A, et al. Ciprofloxacin or metronidazole for the treatment of perianal fistulas in patients with Crohn's disease: a randomized, double-blind, placebo-controlled pilot study. Inflamm Bowel Dis. 2009;15:17–24.
13. Dewint P, Hansen BE, Verhey E, Oldenburg B, Hommes DW, Pierik M, et al. Adalimumab combined with ciprofloxacin is superior to adalimumab monotherapy in perianal fistula closure in Crohn's disease: a randomised, double-blind, placebo controlled trial (ADAFI). Gut. 2014;63:292–9.
14. West RL, Woude CJ, Hansen BE, Felt-Bersma RJF, Tilburg AJP, Drapers JAG, et al. Clinical and endosonographic effect of ciprofloxacin on the treatment of perianal fistulae in Crohn's disease with infliximab: a double-blind placebo-controlled study. Aliment Pharmacol Ther. 2004;20:1329–36.
15. Present DH, Korelitz BI, Wisch N, Glass JL, Sachar DB, Pasternack BS. Treatment of Crohn's disease with 6-mercaptopurine. N Engl J Med. 1980;302:981–7.
16. Pearson DC, May GR, Fick GH, Sutherland LR. Azathioprine and 6-mercaptopurine in Crohn disease. Ann Intern Med. 1995;122: 132–42.
17. Sandborn WJ, Present DH, Isaacs KL, Wolf DC, Greenberg E, Hanauer SB, et al. Tacrolimus for the treatment of fistulas in patients with Crohn's disease: a randomized, placebo-controlled trial. Gastroenterology. 2003;125:380–8.
18. Gonzalez-Lama Y, Abreu L, Vera MI, Pastrana M, Tabernero S, Revilla J, et al. Long-term oral tacrolimus therapy in refractory to infliximab fistulizing Crohn's disease. Inflamm Bowel Dis. 2005;11:8–15.
19. Hart AL, Plamondon S, Kamm MA. Topical tacrolimus in the treatment of perianal Crohn's disease. Inflamm Bowel Dis. 2007;13: 245–53.
20. Egan LJ, Sandborn WJ, Tremaine WJ. Clinical outcome following treatment of refractory inflammatory and fistulizing Crohn's disease with intravenous cyclosporine. Am J Gastroenterol. 1998;93:442–8.
21. Sands BE, Anderson FH, Bernstein CN, Chey WY, Feagan BG, Fedorak RN, et al. Infliximab maintenance therapy for fistulizing Crohn's disease. N Engl J Med. 2004;350:876–85.
22. Lichtenstein GR, Yan S, Bala M, Blank M, Sands BE. Infliximab maintenance treatment reduces hospitalizations, surgeries, and procedures in fistulizing Crohn's disease. Gastroenterology. 2005;128:862–9.
23. Hanauer SB, Sandborn WJ, Rutgeerts P, Fedorak RN, Lukas M, MacIntosh D, et al. Human anti-tumor necrosis factor monoclonal antibody (adalimumab) in Crohn's disease: the CLASSIC-I trial. Gastroenterology. 2006;130:323–33.
24. Sandborn WJ, Rutgeerts P, Enns R, Hanauer SB, Colombel J-F, Panaccione R, et al. Adalimumab induction therapy for Crohn disease previously treated with infliximab. Ann Intern Med. 2007;146:829–38.
25. Colombel JF, Schwartz DA, Sandborn WJ, Kamm MA, D'Haens G, Rutgeerts P, et al. Adalimumab for the treatment of fistulas in patients with Crohn's disease. Gut. 2009;58:940–8.
26. Castaño-Milla C, Chaparro M, Saro C, Barreiro-de Acosta M, García-Albert AM, Bujanda L, et al. Effectiveness of adalimumab in perianal fistulas in Crohn's disease patients naive to anti-TNF therapy. J Clin Gastroenterol. 2015;49:34–40.
27. Schreiber S, Khaliq-Kareemi M, Lawrance IC, Thomsen OØ, Hanauer SB, McColm J, et al. Maintenance therapy with certolizumab pegol for Crohn's disease. N Engl J Med. 2007;357:239–50.
28. Sandborn WJ, Feagan BG, Stoinov S, Honiball PJ, Rutgeerts P, Mason D, et al. Certolizumab pegol for the treatment of Crohn's disease. N Engl J Med. 2007;357:228–38.
29. Schreiber S, Lawrance IC, Thomsen OØ, Hanauer SB, Bloomfield R, Sandborn WJ. Randomised clinical trial: certolizumab pegol for fistulas in Crohn's disease—subgroup results from a placebo-controlled study. Aliment Pharmacol Ther. 2011;33:185–93.
30. Regueiro M, Mardini H. Treatment of perianal fistulizing Crohn's disease with infliximab alone or as an adjunct to exam under anesthesia with Seton placement. Inflamm Bowel Dis. 2003;9:98–103.
31. Gecse KB, Bemelman W, Kamm MA, Stoker J, Khanna R, Ng SC, et al. A global consensus on the classification, diagnosis and multidisciplinary treatment of perianal fistulising Crohn's disease. Gut. 2014;63:1381–92.

Part V

Therapy: Ulcerative Colitis

Sulfasalazine and 5-Aminosalicylates for Ulcerative Colitis

38

Reena Khanna and John K. Marshall

Chemical Structure and Pharmacokinetics

Sulfasalazine consists of 5-ASA linked to a sulfa moiety by a di-azo bond. After oral administration, a portion of the dose is absorbed in the small bowel. Of this fraction, the majority enters enterohepatic circulation and returns to the small intestine via bile, while a minute amount is excreted in the urine [2]. Most of the ingested sulfasalazine reaches the colon where bacterial diazoreductase cleaves 5-ASA from sulfapyridine. Sulfapyridine is absorbed and undergoes hepatic acetylation and hydroxylation, with subsequent urinary excretion. Most 5-ASA is eliminated in the feces, but a small fraction is absorbed and inactivated by acetylation in intestinal epithelial cells and in the liver [3]. Acetyl-5-ASA enters the systemic circulation and undergoes urinary excretion [4].

5-ASA is the major active therapeutic component of sulfasalazine [5]. Although sulfapyridine has been suggested to exert independent therapeutic effects through induction of T cell apoptosis [6], it also contributes to the poor oral tolerability and adverse effect profile of sulfasalazine [3]. Alternate 5-ASA formulations were developed to improve tolerability while optimizing delivery to specific segments of the gastrointestinal tract. Despite such chemical modifications, newer formulations of 5-ASA appear to retain pharmacokinetic profiles similar to sulfasalazine.

Balsalazide consists of a 5-ASA molecule linked to an inert carrier, 4-aminobenzoyl-B-alanine, by a di-azo bond [3]. Similarly, olsalazine joins two 5-ASA molecules with a di-azo bond. Like sulfasalazine, olsalazine and balsalazide have low bioavailability with almost complete delivery to the colon where the di-azo bond is cleaved by bacterial azoreductase. Per weight, olsalazine delivers more 5-ASA to the colon than sulfasalazine [3].

Mesalamine refers to 5-ASA monomers that are delivered to various segments of the gastrointestinal tract using pH-mediated or time-based coatings and release mechanisms. One formulation uses ethylcellulose-coated granules to release 5-ASA throughout the small intestine and colon. Others use the acrylic resin Eudragit as a coating to release drug in the distal small bowel and colon as pH rises. A more recent formulation uses a multimatrix structure to encapsulate 5-ASA in an inner lipophilic matrix, a hydrophobic matrix, and an outer polymethacrylate coating. The result is a time- and pH-based release of 5-ASA in the terminal ileum and throughout the colon (Fig. 38.1) [2, 7].

Mechanism of Action

Sulfasalazine has been suggested to exert its clinical effects through anti-inflammatory, immunosuppressive, and bacteriostatic mechanisms. Downregulation of the inflammatory response by sulfasalazine is mediated by inhibition of granulocyte functions including degranulation, chemotaxis, migration [2, 8], and superoxide production [9]. It also acts on several arachidonic acid metabolism pathways resulting in a net increase in prostaglandins which possess both anti-inflammatory and immunosuppressive effects, and a decrease in pro-inflammatory lipoxygenase [9] titers. Immunologically, sulfasalazine inhibits the activity of natural killer cells and T-cells [6, 8]. The sulfapyridine moiety has in vitro bactericidal activity in human blood [1, 10].

5-ASA has been shown to decrease leukotriene production, remove free radicals, and inhibit leukocyte chemotaxis in vitro and in vivo models. 5-ASA has also been postulated to inhibit the nuclear factor-kappa B pathway, decrease oxidative stress induced cell injury and apoptosis, increase heat

R. Khanna, M.D., F.R.C.P.C.
Department of Medicine, University of Western Ontario, London, ON, Canada

J.K. Marshall, M.D., M.Sc., F.R.C.P.C. (✉)
Department of Medicine, Farncombe Family Digestive Health Research Institute, McMaster University, Hamilton, ON, Canada

Division of Gastroenterology (2F59), McMaster University Medical Centre, 1280 Main Street West, Hamilton, ON L8S 4K1, Canada
e-mail: marshllj@mcmaster.ca

D.C. Baumgart (ed.), *Crohn's Disease and Ulcerative Colitis*, DOI 10.1007/978-3-319-33703-6_38

Sulfasalazine

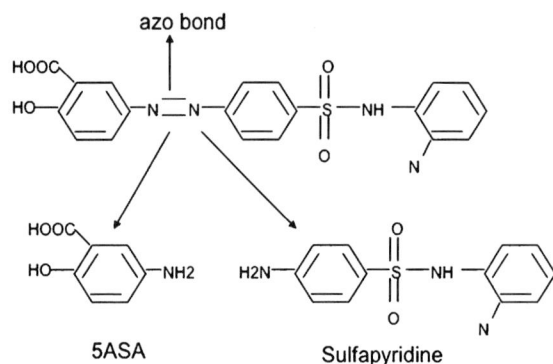

azo bond

HOOC
HO
N=N
O
S
NH
O
N

HOOC
HO
NH2
H2N
O
S
NH
O
N

5ASA
Sulfapyridine

Olsalazine

HOOC
HO
N=N
COOH
OH

5ASA
5ASA

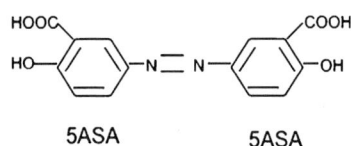

Mesalamine

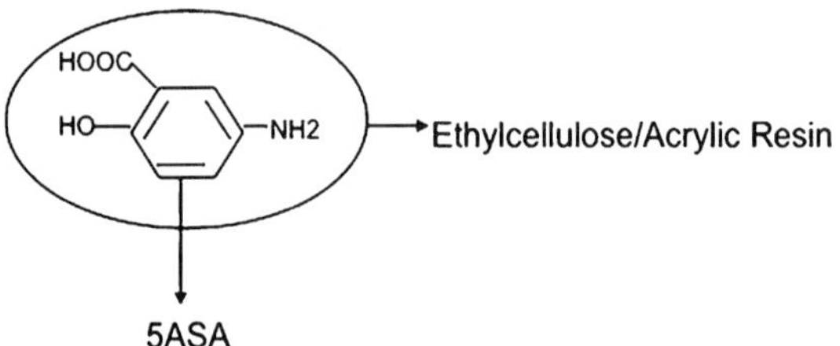

Balsalazide

HOOC
HO
N=N
O
C
NH
CH2
CH2
COOH

5ASA
4-aminobenzoyl-B-alanine

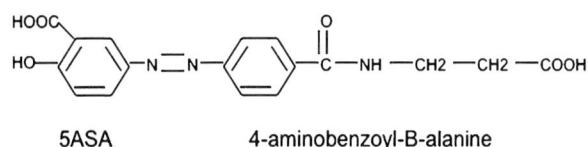

Fig. 38.1 Chemical structures of sulfasalazine and 5-ASA derivatives [2, 3]

shock protein response, decrease leukotriene production, and alter prostaglandin metabolism in colonic epithelial cells [3]. Patients with ulcerative colitis who are treated with 5-ASA have lower fecal concentrations of prostaglandin E2 [11].

The primary mechanism of action of 5-ASA may be activation of gamma-form peroxisome proliferator-activated receptors (PPAR-gamma) in colonic epithelial cells. These receptors play a role in inducing transcription in response to environmental cues, and are activated in vivo primarily by colonic bacteria. Evidence for PPAR-gamma involvement in ulcerative colitis is derived from the observation that heterozygote knock-out mice develop colonic inflammation. Interestingly, PPAR-gamma is known to have antiproliferative effects, while influencing differentiation and apoptosis. Cumulatively, these may protect against the development of colonic dysplasia and neoplasia in ulcerative colitis [3].

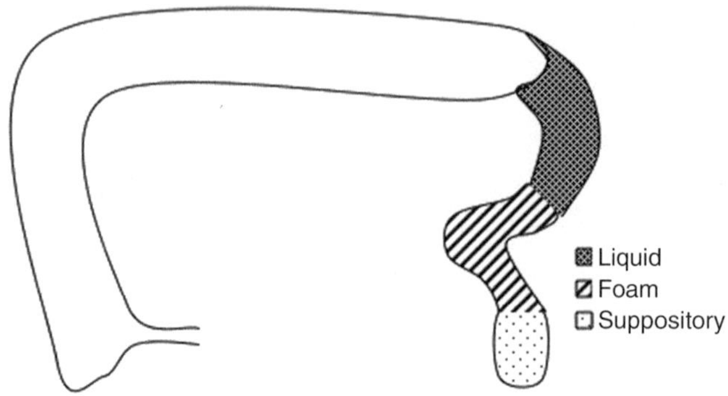

Fig. 38.2 Proximal distribution of rectal 5-ASA therapy [12]

Formulations

5-ASA is believed to act topically, in that direct mucosal contact is required for its therapeutic effect. Accordingly, 5-ASA is available in both oral and rectal preparations. Although oral therapy is more commonly used in clinical practice [12], rectal therapy is effective in treating left-sided disease [13]. As rectal administration cannot deliver drug reliably beyond the splenic flexure, this defines the proximal margin for primary rectal therapy [12]. However, rectal therapy may still augment the efficacy of oral 5-ASA in patients with more extensive disease [14]. Rectal therapy also delivers medication to the site of maximal inflammation, while limiting systemic absorption and associated side effects. However, uptake of rectal therapy may be limited by poor patient acceptance [12].

The proximal distribution of 5-ASA differs among suppositories, foams, and liquid enemas [12]. Suppositories deliver drug only to the rectum, as evidenced by scintigraphic studies [15, 16]. Foam preparations reach the sigmoid colon [16, 17], while enemas deliver medication up to the splenic flexure [12, 16, 18]. The proximal spread of an enema is dependent upon its volume [12] and viscosity [19]. All formulations of 5-ASA are equally effective in inducing remission [20], but foam based products offer more uniform colonic coating [21] and greater patient comfort [22] than liquid enema. Enema retention optimizes efficacy and is improved with greater viscosity [19] but reduced by disease severity (Fig. 38.2) [23].

Efficacy

Oral Formulations

Controlled trials report symptomatic remission in up to 61 % of patients taking oral 5-ASA [24–26], and a meta-analysis reported a significant relative risk of 0.86 (95 % CI 0.81–0.91) versus placebo for failure of 5-ASA to induce remission [27]. For the induction of remission with 5-ASA the number need to treat has been estimated to be 10, while the number needed to treat to maintain remission is 6 [28].

Both sulfasalazine and 5-ASA are used to induce and maintain remission of ulcerative colitis and have roughly similar efficacy for both indications [29]. However, 5-ASA may induce clinical and endoscopic improvement more quickly and is better tolerated [26]. In a recent meta-analysis the relative risk of relapse was 0.69 (95 % CI 0.62–0.77) for oral 5-ASA versus placebo [30]. For maintenance of remission, sulfasalazine was superior to 5-ASA, but individual trials have been criticized for enrolling patients known to be tolerant of this medication.

Rectal Formulations

Rectal 5-ASA is a first line therapy for both induction and maintenance of remission in patients with mild to moderately active distal ulcerative colitis [12]. A meta-analysis of five trials found topical 5-ASA to be superior to placebo, with pooled odds ratio 7.36 (95 % CI 4.72–11.47) for symptomatic improvement and 10.37 (95 % CI 5.72–18.8) for symptomatic remission. Rectal 5-ASA also induced mucosal healing, with odds ratios for endoscopic and histologic remission of 8.23 (95 % CI 4.08–16.58) and 12.47 (95 % CI 3.75–41.43), respectively [13, 31]. No dose-response relationship has been defined for rectal 5-ASA, and efficacy does not appear to differ among suppository, foam and enema preparations.

Rectal 5-ASA is more effective than rectal corticosteroids, with pooled odds ratios for symptomatic, endoscopic and histologic remission of 2.42 (95 % CI 1.72–3.41), 1.89 (95 % CI 1.29–2.76) and 2.03 (95 % CI 1.28–3.2), respectively [31, 32]. When compared to oral 5-ASA therapy, rectal treatment is as least as effective in inducing remission, and may be superior as indicated by physician and patient global improvement scores [12, 31, 33].

Rectal 5-ASA is more effective than placebo for maintaining remission of distal ulcerative colitis [33]. A meta-analysis pooling data from four placebo-controlled trials found that rectal 5-ASA had a pooled odds ratio of 5.6 (95 % CI 3.0–10.5) for maintaining symptomatic remission [12] and was superior to oral 5-ASA in three trials with a pooled a pooled odds ratio of 2.3 (95 % CI 3.0–10.5) [12].

Combination Therapy

The combination of oral and rectal 5-ASA is superior to either monotherapy [14, 34, 35], even among patients with extensive or pan-colitis. This may reflect either increased local concentrations of active drug or improved distribution of drug through the affected segments. Combination therapy is superior in patients at high risk for relapse, as the addition of rectal 5-ASA to oral therapy results in significantly fewer recurrences [34, 35], clinic visits, hospitalizations, and endoscopic evaluations [35]. Combination 5-ASA therapy also decreases steroid usage [35], making dual therapy an effective alternative for patients judged to be at high risk of disease exacerbation. The combination of rectal 5-ASA and topical steroids also achieves higher remission rates than either agent as monotherapy [36]. Combination strategies should be considered in patients who fail 5-ASA monotherapy as an alternative to systemic corticosteroids to avoid steroid-related adverse effects.

Dose Response

The optimal dosing of 5-ASA for both induction and maintenance of remission remains controversial. Doses less than 2.0 g daily are not recommended for induction therapy [37]. For mild to moderately active disease, lower daily doses (2.0–2.4 g) and higher daily doses (4.0–4.8 g) have demonstrated similar efficacy in clinical trials [38, 39]. However, the 4.8 g dosage may be more effective in some subgroups, such as patients with moderately active versus mild disease [40]. The gain in efficacy achieved by adding rectal to oral 5-ASA therapy does provide corollary evidence that increased luminal drug levels improve efficacy, although this may also reflect an improved distribution of drug throughout the colon. Once daily dosing of oral 5-ASA for induction therapy appears to be no less effective than split dosing [27].

Following induction, 5-ASA is efficacious as maintenance therapy [29, 41], when administered at daily doses of 1.5–4.8 g [40]. A weak dose response was observed in a recent meta-analysis [30]. Although there appears to be a dose dependent effect for sulfasalazine, 2 g daily is often prescribed due to the limited tolerability of higher doses [42]. Once daily dosing of 5-ASA for maintenance of remission appears to be at least as effective as split dosing and may help long-term compliance [30, 43].

No dose response has been observed for the induction or maintenance of remission with rectal 5-ASA formulations [13].

Duration

The optimal duration of induction therapy has not been defined, and may vary among formulations of 5-ASA [24]. Most efficacy trials have evaluated 8 weeks of therapy [24–26], but response is often observed sooner [24]. Improvement in stool frequency has been reported 4 weeks after initiating sulfasalazine, with resolution of bleeding after 8 weeks [26]. Improvements in bowel frequency [24, 26], rectal bleeding [24, 25], endoscopic appearance, and physician global assessment [24] have been observed as early as 2 weeks after starting oral 5-ASA.

Similarly, the optimal duration of maintenance therapy with 5-ASA remains unknown, as no controlled trials have addressed this question. Lifelong 5-ASA therapy has been advocated both to decrease the frequency of disease flares and to reduce the risk of colorectal cancer. However, nonadherence can be problematic. Noncompliance is highest among single males, patients with left-sided colitis, and those on more complicated dosing regimens [44]. Once-daily dosing of oral 5-ASA can enhance compliance [43]. Decisions to continue long-term maintenance therapy should consider patient preferences, and patient education [1].

Safety

The frequency of adverse events attributed to sulfasalazine and 5-ASA is highly variable in the literature, in part because of variations in dose, formulation, and event definition [7]. Adverse events are less common with 5-ASA than with sulfasalazine [7], likely from loss of the sulfapyridine moiety [3]. One review found no significant difference in the rate of adverse events between 5-ASA and placebo. A study that followed patients for 8 years reported drug-related adverse events in 20 % of patients treated with sulfasalazine versus 6.5 % of those treated with 5-ASA [45]. The most common adverse effects of sulfasalazine were dyspepsia, rash, and headache, in 62 %, 35 %, and 27 % of patients respectively [45]. Of note, 40 % of patients that were initially intolerant of sulfasalazine successfully underwent desensitization through a protocol of gradual dose escalation [45]. The overall rate of adverse effects with 5-ASA is 1.5 % in patients never exposed to sulfasalazine, 4 % in patients with prior sulfasalazine exposure, and 22 % in patients with prior sulfasalazine intolerance [45]. This overlap suggests that some intolerance to sulfasalazine can be attributed to 5-ASA [46]. Common adverse effects of 5-ASA include rash, diarrhea, headache, and fever, which occur in 37 %, 25 %, 17 % and 17 % of patients, respectively [45]. Other organ-specific adverse effects are summarized in Table 38.1.

Table 38.1 Summary of the adverse events reported with sulfasalazine and 5-ASA

Renal:	Gastrointestinal:
– Asymptomatic elevation in creatinine	– Dyspepsia
– Asymptomatic decline in creatinine clearance	– Diarrhea
– Nephrotic syndrome	– Pancreatitis
– Tubulointerstitial nephritis	
– Sulfapyridine stones	Respiratory:
	– Pulmonary eosinophilia
Hematologic:	
– Leucopenia	Neurological:
– Anemia	– Benign headaches
– Heinz body anemia	– Intracranial hypertension
– Hemolysis	– Sensorimotor neuropathy
– Immune complex hemolytic anemia	
– Folate deficiency anemia	Immune:
	– Lupus-like syndrome
Cardiac:	– Erythroderma
– Pericarditis	– Toxic epidermal necrolysis
– Myocarditis	– Hypersensitivity reactions
	– Hepatoxicity
Reproduction:	– Jaundice
– Spermatic abnormalities	– Thrombocytopenia
– Motility	– Peripheral eosinophilia
– Form	
– Concentration	Topical:
– Folate deficiency	– Discomfort
– Diarrhea in the infant	– Inconvenient drug administration

Renal

A variety of renal complications of 5-ASA therapy have been reported. However, it is important to note that renal disease may also be a primary complication of inflammatory bowel disease itself. Known renal manifestations of inflammatory bowel disease include nephrolithiasis, urinary obstruction, fistulization, glomerular disease, protein-losing nephropathy, secondary amyloidosis, and renal failure [47].

Long-term 5-ASA and sulfasalazine have been associated with a gradual increase in serum creatinine levels and a decline in creatinine clearance. These changes have been correlated with both the duration of therapy and the total daily dosage. One study reported a decline in creatinine clearance from 104.6 to 93.1 ml/min, and suggested that baseline renal dysfunction was predictive of subsequent renal decline [48]. However, the clinical significance of such small changes and their causal relationship to 5-ASA exposure have yet to be established. Still, patients on long-term 5-ASA therapy have been advised to have annual testing for renal function.

Sulfasalazine-induced nephrotic syndrome is an unusual complication of 5-ASA therapy that is believed to be mediated via podocyte toxicity and may be reversible with systemic corticosteroids [49]. Sulfapyridine stones have also been reported [50] following acetylation and renal excretion. Tubulointerstitial nephritis has been reported in patients receiving 5-ASA therapy, but its pathogenesis is unclear and it may be an extra-intestinal manifestation of inflammatory bowel disease [45, 48].

Hematologic

Hematologic toxicities have been attributed more to sulfasalazine than to 5-ASA. A reversible leucopenia has been associated with serum sulfapyridine concentrations greater than 50 mcg/ml. Sulfapyridine is acetylated to form N-acetylsulfapyridine by N-acetyltransferase 2 (NAT2). Case reports suggest that a NAT2 variant results in slow acetylation which subsequently increases serum sulfapyridine levels and predisposes to drug toxicity [51]. Sulfasalazine is known to induce Heinz body anemia in patients with hemoglobinopathies, as well as hemolysis in patients with glucose-6-phosphate dehydrogenase deficiency. Rare idiosyncratic immune complex hemolytic anemia in patients without an underlying disease process has also been described [52]. Sulfasalazine can also induce folate deficiency (see below), although inadequate folate intake is uncommon in patients consuming unrestricted diets [53].

Cardiac

Both sulfasalazine and 5-ASA have also been associated with isolated pericarditis as a hypersensitivity reaction within 2 weeks of medication initiation or following dose escalation. Sulfasalazine has also been associated with pericarditis in the context of a systemic lupus-like reaction. There is variable experience with recurrence of sulfasalazine-induced pericarditis when patients are rechallenged with 5-ASA. Sulfasalazine and 5-ASA-induced pericarditis appear to resolve with medication discontinuation [54].

Myocarditis is a rare but life-threatening extra-intestinal manifestation of inflammatory bowel disease, but has also been reported after 5-ASA therapy. A case report describes eosinophilic cardiac infiltrates consistent with a hypersensitivity reaction, improvement of cardiac function with withdrawal of 5-ASA, and recurrence of myocarditis with 5-ASA rechallenge. 5-ASA-induced myocarditis has been successfully treated with steroids and azathioprine [55].

Reproductive

Fertility is affected in all male patients treated with sulfasalazine as determined by seminal fluid analysis. Abnormalities in sperm motility, form, and concentration occur in 92 %, 42 %, and 40 %, respectively. There is no known correlation with sulfasalazine dose [56], but form and concentration have been observed to improve when patients are switched to 5-ASA [45, 56]. Motility improves to a lesser degree. Men have been encouraged to discontinue sulfasalazine or switch to 5-ASA three months prior to conception as the life span of sperm is 120 days [57].

Sulfasalazine and most 5-ASA products carry an FDA class B designation for use in pregnancy, meaning that there is no evidence of fetal risk but randomized controlled data are lacking. Olsalazine, in contrast, is a class C medication. Although there is no evidence to suggest an increase in congenital abnormalities with sulfasalazine therapy, the potential for medication induced folate deficiency exists. This has prompted the recommendation for women on sulfasalazine to take oral folate supplements prior to conception and throughout pregnancy [57]. Unlike other sulfa-based medications, sulfasalazine does not lead to the displacement of bilirubin or kernicterus in the infant. Thus breast-feeding is considered low-risk [57].

A meta-analysis of pregnancy outcomes in women with inflammatory bowel disease exposed to 5-ASA during gestation, showed nonsignificant trends towards higher rates of congenital abnormalities, stillbirths, spontaneous abortions, preterm deliveries, and low birth weight, when compared with those who had not received medications [58]. Although 5-ASA from breast-milk can lead to diarrhea in the infant, this is not a contraindication to continuing treatment during lactation, provided that attention is given to stool changes and infant hydration [57]. Overall, the evidence supports the safety of sulfasalazine and 5-ASA during pregnancy and lactation. The risks of these medications are thought to be less than the harm associated with severe disease exacerbations during pregnancy [57].

Gastrointestinal

Gastrointestinal symptoms are the most common adverse effect associated with sulfasalazine and 5-ASA. Up to 62 % of patients on sulfasalazine experience dyspepsia, while up to 25 % of those on 5-ASA develop paradoxical diarrhea [45]. 5-ASA-induced diarrhea is idiosyncratic and can occur at any dosage, and even after a single administration [59–61]. A possible risk factor for this is extensive or pan-colitis [59]. Several mechanisms for this effect have been invoked, including accelerated orocecal transit [59] and increased small intestinal fluid secretion [59, 62]. The observation that an individual may develop diarrhea with one 5-ASA formulation, while remaining tolerant to another [59, 60] suggests intestinal sensitivity to an inert compound within the medication [60] as the causative mechanism in a subgroup of patients. It is challenging to distinguish disease activity from adverse effect, except that drug-induced diarrhea is generally mild and responds to medication withdrawal [45, 60, 61].

Case reports have associated acute pancreatitis with wide range of 5-ASA and sulfasalazine doses [63] (0.8–5 g daily) [64] and treatment durations [63, 65] (2 days to 2 years) [64], suggesting an idiosyncratic reaction [63, 64]. Although cases are generally mild, fatal necrotizing pancreatitis has also been described with sulfasalazine [64]. An analysis of population-based hospital discharges, however, found no attributable risk of acute pancreatitis for either sulfasalazine or 5-ASA. This study suggested that the underlying inflammatory bowel disease may be causative [66]. Disease related pancreatitis is thought to be mediated by cholesterol and pigment stones due to ileal disease, structural abnormalities of the duodenum, and immunological derangements [64].

Respiratory

Although sulfasalazine-induced pulmonary toxicity is rare, its most commonly described manifestation is pulmonary eosinophilia attributed to the sulfapyridine moiety. This appears to resolve with discontinuation of sulfasalazine [67] and relapses on rechallenge with sulfasalazine but not 5-ASA [68]. However a similar clinical presentation, including biopsy proven interstitial pulmonary fibrosis has been reported with 5-ASA [69].

Neurological

Benign headaches are common with sulfasalazine therapy [45], but rare reports have associated intracranial hypertension with both sulfasalazine and 5-ASA [70]. A sensorimotor neuropathy mediated by sulfasalazine and, much less frequently, 5-ASA has been reported. A case report temporally associated lower limb dysesthesia and gait abnormality with 5-ASA [71]. The mechanisms for such neurological toxicities remain unknown, but there is reported improvement with drug withdrawal [70, 71].

Immunological

Sulfasalazine and 5-ASA have been associated with the development of lupus-like syndromes, including lupus nephritis [72]. Both agents have also been associated with erythroderma and toxic epidermal necrolysis. Caution should be exercised in using 5-ASA products in patients with severe reactions to sulfasalazine, even when topical therapy has previously been tolerated [73]. Other hypersensitivity reactions have manifested as hepatoxicity, thrombocytopenia, and peripheral eosinophilia, even after several years of drug exposure [74].

Rectal Therapy

The extent of systemic absorption from rectally administered 5-ASA is dependent upon the acidity of the topical preparation, and is lower in active disease states. Despite this variability, topical 5-ASA results in substantially lower systemic drug distribution than oral formulations as determined by urinary excretion and serum metabolite analysis. Thus, rectal formulations result in significantly fewer systemic adverse effects than oral therapy. In fact, the majority of adverse events attributed to topical 5-ASA is due to discomfort and inconvenience from drug administration [12].

Cancer Prevention

The risk of colorectal cancer in patients with ulcerative colitis increases with duration of disease and the extent of inflammation. Additional risk factors in this population include concomitant primary sclerosing cholangitis, folate deficiency, and a family history of colorectal cancer [75, 76]. Currently, management of this risk involves colonoscopic surveillance and colectomy for dysplasia [77, 78]. This has prompted the search for more cost effective, less invasive methods for primary prevention [77].

In ulcerative colitis, the development of dysplasia is believed to be secondary to the increased cellular turnover associated with chronic inflammation [79, 80] and altered prostaglandin metabolism [81]. Despite this, corticosteroids have not been shown to decrease cancer risk [75]. 5-ASA has been postulated to exert primary chemoprotective effects via mechanisms other than its control of disease activity [79]. Nonsteroidal anti-inflammatory drugs (NSAIDs) are associated with a decreased rate of colon cancer in the general population, in patients with familial adenomatous polyposis [76], and in animal models [76, 79]. Mesalamine instilled as an enema in patients with sporadic colon cancer induces apoptosis in tumor cells [82], which may be mediated by inhibition of nuclear factor kappa B [79]. Additionally, NSAIDs and 5-ASA activate peroxisome proliferator-activator receptor gamma which leads to anti-inflammatory and antiproliferative effects in colonic epithelium [79, 80]. These agents also display antioxidant properties [79]. Cumulatively, this evidence has prompted investigation of 5-ASA as a means of chemoprevention in ulcerative colitis.

Of note, an increase in colorectal cancer among patients with ulcerative colitis is not seen in Denmark, which has been attributed to widespread and longstanding use of 5-ASA maintenance therapy [76]. Observational data have associated 5-ASA therapy with a 70 % reduction in colorectal carcinoma [75, 78, 83]. This protective effect is greatest when mesalamine is taken at doses greater than 1.2 g daily [75, 83]. One study suggested that the risk of colorectal carcinoma or dysplasia in these patients decreases by 16 % for each 1000 g increase in the cumulative dosage of 5-ASA and by 56 % for each 1 g incremental increase in daily dose [83]. Although protective effects are seen with daily sulfasalazine doses greater than 2 g, its protective effect seems less robust [75]. This may be secondary to alterations in folate metabolism, as folate deficiency is an independent risk for colon cancer [79].

Two recent cohort studies have questioned the role of 5-ASA in primary chemoprevention. In a nested case–control analysis of patients enrolled in a rigorous surveillance program at St. Mark's Hospital in the UK, histological inflammation was the only significant factor in the development of colorectal cancer [81]. A similar study of a cohort of patients followed in the USA reached a similar conclusion [84]. Neither analysis identified 5-ASA or sulfasalazine as an independent risk factor, suggesting that the chemopreventive benefit of these agents lies primarily in their ability to control disease activity.

Cost-Effectiveness

The cost-effectiveness of 5-ASA therapy for ulcerative colitis has been evaluated in several economic analyses. A cost-utility decision analysis concluded that a daily 5-ASA dose of 4.8 g was less costly and more effective than a daily 5-ASA dose of 2.4 g over a limited time horizon of 12 weeks in patients with moderately active disease, with fewer hospitalizations and surgeries [85]. Maintenance 5-ASA therapy has also been estimated to cost approximately $8810 (US) for each flare that is prevented [86], although this estimate was highly sensitive to variations in 5-ASA cost, rates of flare, rates of colectomy and health state utility. In a Markov simulation model, 5-ASA therapy allowed cost-effective extension of colonoscopic surveillance intervals from 1 to 3 years [87].

Conclusions

Despite new developments in the management of inflammatory bowel disease, sulfasalazine and 5-ASA have maintained a prominent role in the treatment of ulcerative colitis, and this role is emphasized in recent clinical practice guidelines [88]. Over time, both oral and topical formulations have proven their efficacy as induction and maintenance therapies [12, 27, 30] and possibly in chemoprevention of colorectal cancer [75, 83]. As these agents are well-tolerated [45] and cost-effective [34], sulfasalazine and 5-ASA are advocated as first line therapy for mild to moderate disease activity, and will likely maintain their key role in management algorithms.

References

1. Moshkovska T, Mayberry JF. Duration of treatment with 5-aminosalicylic acid compounds. World J Gastroenterol. 2007;13:4310–5.
2. Cohen H, Das K. The metabolism of mesalamine and its possible use in colonic diverticulitis as an anti-inflammatory agent. J Clin Gastroenterol. 2006;40 Suppl 3:150–4.
3. Desreumaux P, Ghosh S. Mode of action and delivery of 5-aminosalicylic acid—new evidence. Aliment Pharmacol Ther. 2006;24 Suppl 1:2–9.
4. Bondesen S, Nielsen OH, Schou JB, Jensen PH, Lassen LB, Binder V, et al. Steady-state kinetics of 5-aminosalicylic acid and sulfapyridine during sulfasalazine prophylaxis in ulcerative colitis. Scand J Gastroenterol. 1986;21:693–700.
5. Van Hees PA, Bakker JH, van Tongeren JH. Effect of sulphapyridine, 5-aminosalicylic acid, and placebo in patients with idiopathic proctitis: a study to determine the active therapeutic moiety of sulfasalazine. Gut. 1980;21:632.
6. Doering J, Begue B, Lentze MJ, et al. Induction of T lymphocyte apoptosis by sulfasalazine in patients with Crohn's disease. Gut. 2004;53:1632–8.
7. Loftus EV, Kane SV, Bjorkman D. Systematic review: short-term adverse effects of 5-aminosalicylic acid agents in the treatment of ulcerative colitis. Aliment Pharmacol Ther. 2004;19:179.
8. MacDermott RP. Progress in understanding the mechanisms of action of 5-aminosalicylic acid. Am J Gastroenterol. 2000;95: 3343–5.
9. Simmonds NJ, Millar AD, Blake DR, Rampton DS. Antioxidant effects of aminosalicylates and potential new drugs for inflammatory bowel disease: assessment in cell-free systems and inflamed human colorectal biopsies. Aliment Pharmacol Ther. 1999;13:363–72.
10. Lowell F, Spring W, Finland M. Bactericidal action of sodium sulfapyridine and of a glucose-sulfapyridine solution in human blood. J Clin Invest. 1940;19:215–8.
11. Lauritsen K, Staerk Laursen L, Bukhave K, Rask-Madsen J. Longterm olsalazine treatment: pharmacokinetics, tolerance and effects on local eicosanoid formation in ulcerative colitis and Crohn's colitis. Gut. 1988;29:974–82.

12. Marshall JK, Irvine EJ. Putting rectal 5-aminosalicylic acid in its place: the role in distal ulcerative colitis. Am J Gastroenterol. 2000;95:1628–36.
13. Marshall JK, Irvine EJ. Rectal aminosalicylate therapy for distal ulcerative colitis: a meta-analysis. Aliment Pharmacol Ther. 1995; 9:293.
14. Marteau P, Probert CS, Lindgren S, Gassul M, Tan TG, Dignass A, et al. Combined oral and enema treatment with Pentasa (mesalazine) is superior to oral therapy alone in patients with extensive mild/moderate active ulcerative colitis: a randomised, double blind, placebo controlled study. Gut. 2005;54:960–5.
15. Williams CN, Haber G, Aquino JA. Double-blind, placebo-controlled evaluation of 5-ASA suppositories in active distal proctitis and measurement of extent of spread using 99mTc-labeled 5-ASA suppositories. Dig Dis Sci. 1987;32:71S–5.
16. Brown J, Haines S, Wilding IR. Colonic spread of three rectally administered mesalazine (Pentasa) dosage forms in healthy volunteers as assessed by gamma scintigraphy. Aliment Pharmacol Ther. 1997;11:685–91.
17. Wilding IR, Kenyon CJ, Chauhan S, Hooper G, Marshall S, McCracken JS, et al. Colonic spreading of a non-chlorofluorocarbon mesalazine rectal foam enema in patients with quiescent ulcerative colitis. Aliment Pharmacol Ther. 1995;9:161–6.
18. Kruis W, Büll U, Eisenburg J, Paumgartner G. Retrograde colonic spread of sulphasalazine enemas. Scand J Gastroenterol. 1982;17:933–8.
19. Otten MH, De Haas G, Van den Ende R. Colonic spread of 5-ASA enemas in healthy individuals, with a comparison of their physical and chemical characteristics. Aliment Pharmacol Ther. 1997;11: 693–7.
20. Cortot A, Maetz D, Degoutte E, Delette O, Meunier P, Tan G, et al. Mesalamine foam enema versus mesalamine liquid enema in active left-sided ulcerative colitis. Am J Gastroenterol. 2008;103:3106–14.
21. Campieri M, Paoluzi P, D'Albasio G, Brunetti G, Pera A, Barbara L, et al. Better quality of therapy with 5-ASA colonic foam in active ulcerative colitis: A multicenter comparative trial with 5-ASA enema. Dig Dis Sci. 1993;38:1843.
22. Campieri M, Corbelli C, Gionchetti P, Brignola C, Belluzzi A, Di Febo G, et al. Spread and distribution of 5-ASA colonic foam and 5-ASA enema in patients with ulcerative colitis. Dig Dis Sci. 1992;37:1890–7.
23. Gionchetti P, Venturi A, Rizzello F, Corbelli C, Fanti S, Ferretti M, et al. Retrograde colonic spread of a new mesalazine rectal enema in patients with distal ulcerative colitis. Aliment Pharmacol Ther. 1997;11:679–84.
24. Pruitt R, Hanson J, Safdi M, et al. Balsalazide is superior to mesalamine in the time to improvement of signs and symptoms of acute mild-to-moderate ulcerative colitis. Am J Gastroenterol. 2002;97:3078.
25. Lichtenstein GR, Kamm MA, Boddu P, et al. Effect of once- or twice-daily MMX mesalamine (SPD476) for the induction of remission of mild to moderately active ulcerative colitis. Clin Gastroenterol Hepatol. 2007;5:95.
26. Mansfield JC, Giaffer MH, Cann PA, et al. A double-blind comparison of balsalazide, 675 g, and sulfasalazine, 3 g, as sole therapy in the management of ulcerative colitis. Aliment Pharmacol Ther. 2002;16:69.
27. Feagan BG, MacDonald JK. Oral 5-aminosalicylic acid for induction of remission in ulcerative colitis. Cochrane Database Syst Rev. 2012;10:CD000543.
28. Bebb JR, Scott BB. How effective are the usual treatments for ulcerative colitis? Aliment Pharmacol Ther. 2004;20:143–9.
29. Nikfar S, Rahimi R, Rezaie A, Abdollahi M. A meta-analysis of the efficacy of sulfasalazine in comparison with 5-aminosalicylates in the induction of improvement and maintenance of remission in patients with ulcerative colitis. Dig Dis Sci. 2009;54:1157–70.
30. Feagan BG, Macdonald JK. Oral 5-aminosalicylic acid for maintenance of remission in ulcerative colitis. Cochrane Database Syst Rev. 2012;10:CD000544.
31. Marshall JK, Thabane M, Steinhart AH, Newman JR, Anand A, Irvine EJ. Rectal 5-aminosalicylic acid for induction of remission in ulcerative colitis. Cochrane Database Syst Rev. 2010;1:CD004115.
32. Marshall JK, Irvine EJ. Rectal corticosteroids versus alternative treatments in ulcerative colitis: a meta-analysis. Gut. 1997;40: 775–81.
33. Cohen RD, Woseth DM, Thisted RA, et al. A meta-analysis and overview of the literature on treatment options for left-sided ulcerative colitis and ulcerative proctitis. Am J Gastroenterol. 2000;95:1263.
34. Piodi LP, Ulivieri FM, Cermesoni L, Cesana BM. Long-term intermittent treatment with low-dose 5-aminosalicylic enemas is efficacious for remission maintenance in ulcerative colitis. Scand J Gastroenterol. 2004;39:154–7.
35. Frieri G, Pimpo M, Galletti B, Palumbo G, Corrao G, Latella G, et al. Long-term oral plus topical mesalazine in frequently relapsing ulcerative colitis. Dig Liver Dis. 2005;37:92–6.
36. Mulder CJJ, Fockens P, Meijer LWR, et al. Beclomethasone dipropionate (3 mg) versus 5-aminosalicylic acid (2 g) versus the combination (3 mg/2 g) as retention enemas in active ulcerative proctitis. Eur J Gastroenterol Hepatol. 1996;8:549–53.
37. Ford AC, Achkar JP, Khan KJ, Kane SV, Talley NJ, Marshall JK, et al. Efficacy of 5-aminosalicylates in ulcerative colitis: systematic review and meta-analysis. Am J Gastroenterol. 2011;106:601–16.
38. Hanauer SB, Sandborn WJ, Kornbluth A, et al. Delayed-release oral mesalamine at 4.8 g/day (800 mg tablet) for the treatment of moderately active ulcerative colitis: the ASCEND II trial. Am J Gastroenterol. 2005;100:2478.
39. Kamm MA, Sandborn WJ, Gassull M, et al. Once-daily, high-concentration MMX mesalamine in active ulcerative colitis. Gastroenterology. 2007;132:66–75.
40. Hanauer SB, Sandborn WJ, Dallaire C, Archambault A, Yacyshyn B, Yeh C, et al. Delayed-release oral mesalamine 4.8 g/day (800 mg tablets) compared to 2.4 g/day (400 mg tablets) for the treatment of mildly to moderately active ulcerative colitis: the ASCEND I trial. Can J Gastroenterol. 2007;21:827–34.
41. Kruis W, Bar-Meir S, Feher J, Mickisch O, Mlitz H, Faszczyk M, et al. The optimal dose of 5-aminosalicylic acid in active ulcerative colitis: a dose-finding study with newly developed mesalamine. Clin Gastroenterol Hepatol. 2003;1:36–43.
42. Azad Khan AK, Howes DT, Piris J, et al. Optimum dose of sulphasalazine for maintenance treatment in ulcerative colitis. Gut. 1980;21:232.
43. Ford AC, Khan KJ, Sandborn WJ, Kane SV, Moayyedi P. Once-daily dosing vs. conventional dosing schedule of mesalamine and relapse of quiescent ulcerative colitis: a systematic review and meta-analysis. Am J Gastroenterol. 2011;106:2070–7.
44. Kane SV, Cohen RD, Aikens JE, Hanauer SB. Prevalence of nonadherence with maintenance mesalamine in quiescent ulcerative colitis. Am J Gastroenterol. 2001;96:2929–33.
45. Di Paolo MC, Paoluzi OA, Pica R, Iacopini F, Crispino P, Rivera M, et al. Sulphasalazine and 5-aminosalicylic acid in long-term treatment of ulcerative colitis: report on tolerance and side-effects. Dig Liver Dis. 2001;33:563–9.
46. Fardy JM, Lloyd DA, Reynolds RP. Adverse effects with oral 5-aminosalicyclic acid. J Clin Gastroenterol. 1988;10:635–7.
47. Uslu N, Demir H, Saltik-Temizel IN, Topaloğlu R, Gürakan F, Yüce A. Acute tubular injury associated with mesalazine therapy in an adolescent girl with inflammatory bowel disease. Dig Dis Sci. 2007;52:2926–9.
48. Patel H, Barr A, Jeejeebhoy KN. Renal effects of long-term treatment with 5-aminosalicylic acid. Can J Gastroenterol. 2009;23: 170–6.

49. Molnár T, Farkas K, Nagy F, Iványi B, Wittmann T. Sulfasalazine-induced nephrotic syndrome in a patient with ulcerative colitis. Inflamm Bowel Dis. 2010;16:552–3.
50. Russinko PJ, Agarwal S, Choi MJ, Kelty PJ. Obstructive nephropathy secondary to sulfasalazine calculi. Urology. 2003;62:748.
51. Teshima D, Hino B, Makino K, Yano T, Itoh Y, Joh Y, et al. Sulphasalazine-induced leucopenia in a patient with renal dysfunction. J Clin Pharm Ther. 2003;28:239–42.
52. Teplitsky V, Virag I, Halabe A. Immune complex haemolytic anaemia associated with sulfasalazine. BMJ. 2000;320:1113.
53. Spindel E. Sulfasalazine and folate deficiency. JAMA. 1983; 250:900.
54. Perrot S, Aslangul E, Szwebel T, Gadhoum H, Romnicianu S, Le Jeunne C. Sulfasalazine-induced pericarditis in a patient with ulcerative colitis without recurrence when switching to mesalazine. Int J Colorectal Dis. 2007;22:1119–21.
55. Stelts S, Taylor MH, Nappi J, Van Bakel AB. Mesalamine-associated hypersensitivity myocarditis in ulcerative colitis. Ann Pharmacother. 2008;42:904–5.
56. Riley SA, Lecarpentier J, Mani V, Goodman MJ, Mandal BK, Turnberg LA. Sulphasalazine induced seminal abnormalities in ulcerative colitis: results of mesalazine substitution. Gut. 1987;28: 1008–12.
57. Mahadevan U, Kane S. American Gastroenterological Association Institute technical review on the use of gastrointestinal medications in pregnancy. Gastroenterology. 2006;131:283–311.
58. Rahimi R, Nikfar S, Rezaie A, Abdollahi M. Pregnancy outcome in women with inflammatory bowel disease following exposure to 5-aminosalicylic acid drugs: a meta-analysis. Reprod Toxicol. 2008;25:271–5.
59. Giaffer MA, O'Brien CJ, Holdsworth CD. Clinical tolerance to three 5-aminosalicylic acid releasing preparations in patients with inflammatory bowel disease intolerant or allergic to sulfasalazine. Aliment Pharmacol Ther. 1992;6:51–9.
60. Rao SS, Cann PA, Holdsworth CD. Clinical experience of the tolerance of mesalazine and olsalazine in patients intolerant of sulphasalazine. Scand J Gastroenterol. 1987;22:332–6.
61. Turunen U, Elomaa I, Anttila K, Seppala K. Mesalazine tolerance in patients with inflammatory bowel disease and previous intolerance or allergy to sulphasalazine or sulphonamides. Scand J Gastroenterol. 1987;22:798–802.
62. Kles KA, Vavricka SR, Turner JR, Musch MW, Hanauer SB, Chang EB. Comparative analysis of the in vitro prosecretory effects of balsalazide, sulfasalazine, olsalazine, and mesalamine in rabbit distal ileum. Inflamm Bowel Dis. 2005;11:253–7.
63. Fiorentini MT, Fracchia M, Galatola G, Barlotta A, De la Pierre M. Acute pancreatitis during oral 5-aminosalicylic acid therapy. Dig Dis Sci. 1990;35:1180–2.
64. Pitchumoni CS, Rubin A, Das K. Pancreatitis in inflammatory bowel diseases. J Clin Gastroenterol. 2010;44:246–53.
65. Fernandez J, Sala M, Panes J, Feu F, Navarro S, Teres J. Acute pancreatitis after long-term 5-aminosalicylic acid therapy. Am J Gastroenterol. 1997;92:2302–3.
66. Munk EM, Pedersen L, Floyd A, Nørgård B, Rasmussen HH, Sørensen HT. Inflammatory bowel diseases, 5-aminosalicylic acid and sulfasalazine treatment and risk of acute pancreatitis: a population-based case-control study. Am J Gastroenterol. 2004;99: 884–8.
67. Sullivan SN. Sulfasalazine lung. Desensitization to sulfasalazine and treatment with acrylic coated 5-ASA and azodisalicylate. J Clin Gastroenterol. 1987;9:461–3.
68. Scherpenisse J, van der Valk PD, van den Bosch JM, van Hees PA, Nadorp JH. Olsalazine as an alternative therapy in a patient with sulfasalazine-induced eosinophilic pneumonia. J Clin Gastroenterol. 1988;10:218–20.
69. Lázaro MT, García-Tejero MT, Díaz-Lobato S. Mesalamine-induced lung disease. Arch Intern Med. 1997;157:462.
70. Sevgi E, Yalcin G, Kansu T, Varli K. Drug induced intracranial hypertension associated with sulphasalazine treatment. Headache. 2008;48:296–8.
71. Ono K, Iwasa K, Shirasaki H, Takamori M. Sensorimotor polyneuropathy with 5-aminosalicylic acid: a case report. J Clin Neurosci. 2003;10:386–9.
72. Gunnarsson I, Pettersson E, Lindblad S, Ringertz B. Olsalazine-induced lupus syndrome. Scand J Rheumatol. 1997;26:65–6.
73. Iemoli E, Piconi S, Ardizzone S, Bianchi Porro G, Raimond F. Erythroderma and toxic epidermal necrolysis caused by to 5-aminosalicylic acid. Inflamm Bowel Dis. 2006;12:1007–8.
74. Nayar M, Cunliffe W, Cross P, Oppong K. Mesalazine-induced jaundice, eosonophilia, and thrombocytopenia. Inflamm Bowel Dis. 2008;14:1320–1.
75. Eaden J, Abrams K, Ekbom A, Jackson E, Mayberry J. Colorectal cancer prevention in ulcerative colitis: a case-control study. Aliment Pharmacol Ther. 2000;14:145–53.
76. Eaden J. Review article: the data supporting a role for aminosalicylates in the chemoprevention of colorectal cancer in patients with inflammatory bowel disease. Aliment Pharmacol Ther. 2003;18 Suppl 2:15–21.
77. Rubin DT, Lashner BA. Will a 5-ASA a day keep the cancer (and dysplasia) away? Am J Gastroenterol. 2005;100:1354–6.
78. Velayos FS, Terdiman JP, Walsh JM. Effect of 5-aminosalicylate use on colorectal cancer and dysplasia risk: a systematic review and metaanalysis of observational studies. Am J Gastroenterol. 2005; 100:1345–53.
79. Ryan BM, Russel MG, Langholz E, Stockbrugger RW. Aminosalicylates and colorectal cancer in IBD: a not-so bitter pill to swallow. Am J Gastroenterol. 2003;98:1682–7.
80. Stolfi C, Pellegrini R, Franze E, Pallone F, Monteleone G. Molecular basis of the potential of mesalazine to prevent colorectal cancer. World J Gastroenterol. 2008;14:4434–9.
81. Rutter M, Saunders B, Wilkinson K, et al. Severity of inflammation is a risk factor for colorectal neoplasia in ulcerative colitis. Gastroenterology. 2004;126:451–9.
82. Bus PJ, Nagtegaal ID, Verspaget HW, et al. Mesalazine induced apoptosis of colorectal cancer: on the verge of a new chemopreventive era? Aliment Pharmacol Ther. 1999;13:1397–402.
83. Rubin DT, LoSavio A, Yadron N, Huo D, Hanauer SB. Aminosalicylate therapy in the prevention of dysplasia and colorectal cancer in ulcerative colitis. Clin Gastroenterol Hepatol. 2006;4: 1346–50.
84. Gupta RB, Harpaz N, Itzkowitz S, et al. Histologic inflammation is a risk factor for progression to colorectal neoplasia in ulcerative colitis: a cohort study. Gastroenterology. 2007;133:1099–105.
85. Buckland A, Bodger K. The cost-utility of high dose oral mesalazine for moderately active ulcerative colitis. Aliment Pharmacol Ther. 2008;28:1287–96.
86. Yen EF, Kane SV, Ladabaum U. Cost-effectiveness of 5-aminosalicylic acid therapy for maintenance of remission in ulcerative colitis. Am J Gastroenterol. 2008;103:3094–105.
87. Rubenstein JH, Waljee AK, Jeter JM, Velayos FS, Ladabaum U, Higgins PD. Cost effectiveness of ulcerative colitis surveillance in the setting of 5-aminosalicylates. Am J Gastroenterol. 2009;104: 2222–32.
88. Bressler B, Marshall JK, Bernstein CN, Bitton A, Jones J, Leontiadis GL, et al. Toronto Ulcerative Colitis Consensus Group. Clinical practice guidelines for the medical management of ulcerative colitis: the Toronto Consensus. Gastroenterology. 2015;148:1035–58.
89. Nielsen ST, Beninati L, Buonato CB. Sulfasalazine and 5-aminosalicylic acid inhibit contractile leukotriene formation. Scand J Gastroenterol. 1988;23:272–6.

Conventional Therapy of Ulcerative Colitis: Corticosteroids

39

Kirstin Taylor and Peter R. Gibson

Corticosteroids are long established as effective agents for the induction of remission of ulcerative colitis. This was initially proven by Truelove and Witts in 1955 [1], and had significant impact on a disease with a once high mortality (61 %) [2]. Concern regarding the safety profile of corticosteroids has made them less desirable, albeit sometimes necessary, and has led to the development of formulations to reduce systemic bioavailability, along with steroid-sparing therapeutic strategies.

Corticosteroids exert their anti-inflammatory effects through influencing multiple signal transduction pathways via the glucocorticoid receptor. Most importantly, they downregulate inflammatory genes and upregulate anti-inflammatory genes through interaction with the transcription factors, activator protein 1 (AP-1) and nuclear factor-kB (NFkB) [3]. Corticosteroids have additional posttranscriptional effects on inflammatory protein synthesis through reduction in stability of mRNA [4]. Furthermore, they have direct effects on both sodium and water absorption from the left colon, improving diarrhea through reduction in stool volume [5].

Efficacy According to Route of Administration and Dosage

Corticosteroids for ulcerative colitis may be administered intravenously (methylprednisolone, hydrocortisone, dexamethasone), orally (prednisone, prednisolone, budesonide MMX, beclomethasone dipropionate), and rectally as enemas or suppositories (prednisolone metasulfobenzoate, beclomethasone, hydrocortisone, budesonide). The results of randomized controlled trials of corticosteroids in ulcerative colitis are shown in Tables 39.1 and 39.2.

Oral Therapy for Moderate to Severe Ulcerative Colitis

Oral corticosteroids are effective for the induction of remission in patients with moderate to severe ulcerative colitis [38], in milder disease that is refractory to sulfasalazine or mesalazine, and in patients who have responded to initial treatment with intravenous corticosteroids following hospitalization for acute severe disease. Prednisone and prednisolone are well absorbed after oral administration, with a high bioavailability (over 70 %). Absorption may be delayed, however, in patients with severe ulcerative colitis [39]. Although a daily dose of 40 mg prednisolone is more effective than 20 mg, doses above this threshold have not demonstrated incremental benefit, but are associated with increased adverse effects [40]. Single daily dosing is as effective as split-dosing and causes less adrenal suppression [41]. Both clinical and endoscopic response can be seen following 2 weeks of treatment with oral prednisolone [12, 20]. Those who have not responded by then are considered to have corticosteroid-refractory disease and should be treated with anti-tumor necrosis factor (anti-TNF) therapy, tacrolimus or intravenous corticosteroid therapy [42]. The optimal tapering regimen has not been determined but the dose is usually reduced over 8–12 weeks.

Oral Therapy with Low Systemic Bioavailability

Budesonide-MMX

Budesonide has an intrinsic potency, as measured by affinity to the glucocorticoid receptor, about 15 times higher than that of prednisolone [43]. It has been shown to be effective for ileocecal Crohn's disease, with fewer side effects than prednisolone due to extensive first-pass metabolism in the

K. Taylor, M.B.B.S., M.R.C.P.(UK)
P.R. Gibson, M.D., F.R.A.C.P. (✉)
Department of Gastroenterology, The Alfred Hospital and Monash University, Melbourne, VIC, Australia
e-mail: kirstin.taylor@alfred.org.au; peter.gibson@monash.edu

D.C. Baumgart (ed.), *Crohn's Disease and Ulcerative Colitis*, DOI 10.1007/978-3-319-33703-6_39

Table 39.1 Randomized controlled trials of intravenous or oral corticosteroids in patients with ulcerative colitis

Study	Corticosteroid (starting dose)	Comparator	No. of patients	Disease extent	Duration (weeks)	End-points	Remission	NNT (95 % CI)
Intravenous								
Meyers [6] 1983	Hydrocortisone (300 mg daily)	Corticotropin (ACTH) 120 U/day	66	26 % sigmoid 48 % left sided 26 % pan	10 days	Clinical remission according to prior oral steroids	Prior steroids: 53 % hydrocortisone 25 % corticotropin ($p<0.05$) No prior steroids: 27 % hydrocortisone 63 % corticotropin (p=NS)	n/a
Oral—moderate–severe								
Truelove and Witts [7] 1954	Cortisone (100 mg OD in majority)	Placebo	210	Not reported	6	Clinical and hematological remission	16 % placebo 41 % cortisone ($p<0.001$)	4 (2.7–7.3)
Hawthorne [8] 1993	Fluticasone propionate (5 mg QD)	Prednisolone (40 mg OD)	205[a]	Left sided or pan—numbers not stated	4	Investigators overall assessment of remission	28 % prednisolone 25 % fluticasone (p=NS)	n/a
Oral—mild to moderate								
Lennard-Jones [9] 1960	Prednisone (40–60 mg OD, dose tapered)	Placebo	37	All distal	3–4	Clinical and endoscopic remission	17 % placebo 68 % prednisone ($p<0.01$)	2 (1.3–4.1)
Danish 5ASA Group [10] 1987	Prednisolone (25 mg OD)	Mesalazine enema (1 g OD)	123	All distal	2–4	Clinical and endoscopic response	77 % mesalazine 72 % prednisolone (p=NS)	n/a
Angus [11] 1992	Fluticasone propionate (5 mg QID)	Placebo	59[b]	44 % proctitis, 20 % sigmoid 36 % distal	4	Clinical and endoscopic remission	17 % placebo 13 % fluticasone propionate (p=NS)	n/a
Lofberg [12] 1996	Budesonide CR capsule (10 mg OD)	Prednisolone (40 mg OD)	72	40 % left-sided 60 % extensive	9	Endoscopic remission	12 % prednisolone 16 % budesonide (p=NS)	n/a
Gross [13] 2011	Budesonide CR capsule (9 mg OD)	Mesalazine (1 g TDS)	343	55 % sigmoid 25 % left-sided 20 % pan	8	Clinical remission	54.8 % mesalazine 39.5 % budesonide ($p=0.52$ for noninferiority)	n/a
D'Haens [14] 2010	Budesonide MMX (9 mg OD)	Placebo	36	All left-sided	4	Clinical and endoscopic remission and/or reduction in CAI by $\geq$50 %	33.3 % placebo 47.1 % budesonide (p=NS)	n/a

Sandborn [15] 2012	Budesonide MMX (9 mg or 6 mg OD)	Mesalazine (2.4 g OD) or Placebo	509	28 % sigmoid 29 % left sided 41 % extensive 2 % unknown	8	Clinical and endoscopic remission	7 % placebo 12 % mesalazine (p=NS) 13 % budesonide MMX 6 mg (p=NS) 18 % budesonide MMX 9 mg (p=0.01)	budesonide MMX 9 mg 10 (5.5–45.3)
Travis [16] 2014	Budesonide MMX (9 or 6 mg OD)	Ileal-release (IR) budesonide (9 mg OD) or Placebo	509	41 % sigmoid 39 % left sided 20 % extensive	8	Clinical and endoscopic remission	3 % placebo 10 % IR 7 % MMX 6 mg 15 % MMX 9 mg (p=0.0008)	budesonide MMX 9 mg 9 (5.3–20.2)
Bossa [17] 2008	Prednisolone (0.5 mg/kg daily dose)	DEE[c] (two *intravenous infusions*, 2 weeks apart) or Placebo	40	65 % distal 25 % left-sided 10 % pan	8	Endoscopic remission	10 % placebo 80 % prednisolone 75 % DEE (p<0.001)	Prednisolone: 2 (1–2.6) DEE: 2 (1.1–2.6)
Rizzello [18] 2002	Beclomethasone dipropionate (5 mg OD)+mesalazine (3.2 g OD)	Placebo+mesalazine (3.2 g OD)	119	71 % left-sided 29 % pancolitis	4	Clinical remission	34 % placebo 59 % beclomethasone (p=0.008)	5 (2.4–14.7)
Van Assche [19] 2015	Beclomethasone dipropionate (5 mg OD)	Prednisone (40 mg OD)	282	3 % proctitis, 43 % sigmoid 36 % left-sided 18 % pancolitis	4	Clinical and endoscopic response	66 % prednisone 65 % beclomethasone (p=NS)	n/a
Rhodes [20] 2008	Prednisolone metasulfobenzoate [PM] (20 mg or 30 mg BD)	Prednisolone (40 mg, in two divided doses)	181	2 % proctitis 36 % sigmoid 30 % left-sided 25 % extensive 6 % unknown	24	Visual analog scale for assessment of symptoms at 2 and 6 months	Symptoms at 2 months: 6.9 cm prednisolone 7.4 cm PM 40 mg 6.3 cm PM 60 mg PM (p=NS)	n/a

[a]Included mild severity [b]severity not stated [c]DEE=dexamethasone 21-P-encapsulated erythrocytes
Abbreviations: n/a not applicable, *NS* not significant, *OD* once daily, *BD* twice daily, *TDS* three times daily, *QID* four times daily

Table 39.2 Randomized controlled trials of rectally delivered corticosteroids in patients with mild–moderate ulcerative colitis

Study	Corticosteroid (starting dose)	Comparator	No. of patients	Disease extent	Duration (weeks)	Criteria to define remission	Remission	NNT (95 % CI)
Hanauer [21] 1998	Budesonide (0.5 mg, 2 mg or 8 mg OD)	Placebo	233	All distal	6	Clinical and endoscopic remission	8 % placebo 12 % 0.5 mg (p=NS) 27 % 2 mg ($p \leq 0.05$) 35 % 8 mg ($p \leq 0.001$)	2 mg: 6 (3.1–20.4)
Lindgren [22] 2002	Budesonide (2 mg OD)	Budesonide (2 mg BD)	149	Proctitis and distal (not stated)	8	Clinical and endoscopic remission	54 % BD 51 % OD (p=NS)	n/a
Sandborn [23] 2015	Budesonide[a] (2 mg BD)	Placebo[a]	546 (2 studies)	28 % proctitis, 71 % distal 1 % unknown	6	Clinical and endoscopic remission	24 % placebo 41 % budesonide ($p<0.0001$)	6 (4–10.6)
Bansky [24] 1987	Beclomethasone dipropionate (0.5 mg OD)	Betamethasone phosphate (5 mg OD)	16 (18 flares of colitis)	22 % rectum 56 % sigmoid 17 % descending 5 % transverse	20 days	Clinical, endoscopic, and histologic remission considered separately	Endoscopic remission: 33 % betamethasone 44 % beclomethasone (p=NS)	n/a
Van der Heide [25] 1988	Beclomethasone dipropionate (1 mg OD)	Prednisolone disodium phosphate (30 mg OD)	18	All distal	4	Clinical, endoscopic, histologic response considered separately	Clinical and endoscopic response: 100 % prednisolone 40 % beclomethasone (p=0.01)	n/a
Halpern [26] 1991	Beclomethasone dipropionate (0.5 mg OD)	Betamethasone phosphate (5 mg OD)	32 (40 flares of colitis)	All distal	4	Clinical, endoscopic, and histologic response considered separately	Clinical remission: 45 % betamethasone 60 % beclomethasone (p=NS)	n/a
Mulder [27] 1996	Beclomethasone dipropionate (3 mg OD) ± mesalazine (2 g OD)	Mesalazine (2 g OD)	60	All distal	4	Clinical, endoscopic, and histologic response considered separately	Clinical response: 76 % mesalazine 70 % beclomethasone 100 % beclomethasone plus mesalazine ($p<0.01$ vs either agent alone)	4 (2–10.1)
Campieri [28] 1998	Beclomethasone dipropionate (3 mg OD)	Prednisolone Na phosphate (30 mg OD)	157	3 % proctitis 4 % sigmoid 93 % distal	4	Clinical, endoscopic, and histologic response considered separately	Clinical and endoscopic remission: 25 % prednisolone Na phosphate 29 % beclomethasone dipropionate (p=NS)	n/a
Biancone [29] 2007	Beclomethasone dipropionate[b] (3 mg od)	Mesalazine[b] (2 g OD)	99	All distal colitis	8	Clinical and endoscopic remission at week 4	28 % mesalazine 24 % beclomethasone dipropionate (p=NS)	n/a

McIntyre [30] 1985	Prednisolone metasulfobenzoate (20 mg OD)	Prednisolone-21-phosphate (20 mg OD)	40	50 % proctitis 50 % sigmoid	2	Clinical, endoscopic, and histologic response considered separately	Clinical response: 70 % prednisolone -21-phosphate 75 % prednisolone metasulphobenzoate	n/a
Riley [31] 1989	Prednisolone metasulfobenzoate (20 mg OD)	Sucralfate enema (4 g OD)	44	34 % proctitis 50 % sigmoid 16 % left-sided	4	Clinical, endoscopic, and histologic response considered separately	Resolution of rectal bleeding: 68 % vs 27 % ($p<0.02$) Endoscopic remission: 36 % vs 32 % (p=NS)	n/a
Cobden [32] 1991	Prednisolone metabenzoate (20 mg BD)	Mesalazine (800 mg orally QD)	37	38 % proctitis 51 % sigomoid 11 % left-sided	4	Clinical, endoscopic, and histologic response considered separately	Clinical, endoscopic, and histologic responses similar (p=NS)	n/a
Mulder [33] 1988	Prednisolone Na phosphate (30 mg OD)	Mesalazine (3 g OD)	29	All distal colitis	4	Clinical, endoscopic, and histologic response considered separately	Clinical response: 74 % mesalazine 79 % prednisolone (p=NS)	n/a
O'Donnell [34] 1992	Prednisolone Na phosphate (20 g OD)	PAS[c] (2 g OD)	53	All distal colitis	6	Clinical, endoscopic, and histologic response considered separately	Clinical remission: 23.8 % PAS 37.5 % prednisolone (p=NS)	n/a
Sharma [35] 1992	Prednisolone Na phosphate (20 g OD)	PAS (2 g OD)	40	11 % proctitis 89 % sigmoid	4	Clinical, endoscopic, and histologic response considered separately	Similar clinical response (p=NS) Endoscopic remission: 90 % PAS 40 % prednisolone ($p<0.01$)	n/a
Campieri [36] 1987	Hydrocortisone (100 mg OD)	Mesalazine (4 g OD)	86	All left-sided colitis	2	Clinical, endoscopic, and histologic response considered separately	Greater improvement in clinical, endoscopic, and histologic response for mesalazine ($p<0.0005$)	n/a
Bianchi Porro [37] 1995	Hydrocortisone (100 mg OD)	Mesalazine (1 g OD)	52	All distal colitis	3	Clinical and endoscopic response considered separately	Similar clinical and endoscopic response between groups (p=NS)	n/a

[a]Foam enema [b]liquid or foam enema [c]para-amino salicylic acid

liver [44]. Budesonide-MMX is a novel formulation that utilizes multimatrix technology to release the drug in the colon. It contains a gastro-resistant polymer coating that dissolves at a pH greater than 7, thereby delaying release during transit through the stomach and duodenum until the ileum is reached. A budesonide-containing lipophilic matrix then allows release of budesonide at a controlled rate throughout the colon [45]. In two trials, budesonide-MMX at a dose of 9 mg a day was shown to be well-tolerated and more effective than placebo for inducing remission in patients with mild–moderate ulcerative colitis [15, 16]. A small study of budesonide-MMX 10 mg in active extensive and left-sided ulcerative colitis showed similar efficacy to 40 mg of prednisolone with regard to endoscopic improvement. It may have a role in patients with disease that does not respond to mesalazine, before initiation of systemically acting corticosteroids.

Beclomethasone Dipropionate

The oral, prolonged-release formulation of beclomethasone dipropionate (Clipper) has an acid-resistant methacrylate film coating (Eudragit L100/55) that prevents the tablets from dissolving in the stomach, and a modified release core of hydroxypropyl methylcellulose (Methocel K4M) that dissolves at pH values below 6, allowing for release of the drug in the mid-distal ileum and colon [46]. Beclomethasone dipropionate is a prodrug with weak glucocorticoid receptor binding affinity, but it is hydrolyzed to its active metabolite, beclomethasone 17-monopropionate following contact with the gut mucosa. Beclomethasone 17-monopropionate is highly potent, with glucocorticoid receptor binding affinity approximately 80 times that of prednisolone [47]. As with budesonide, there is extensive first-pass metabolism. Its efficacy has been shown to be similar to that of mesalazine [48], and a recent trial has shown noninferiority with regard to clinical efficacy and safety of beclomethasone dipropionate 5 mg daily for 4 weeks followed by 5 mg on alternate days for 4 weeks, compared to oral prednisolone at an initial dose of 40 mg daily for 2 weeks then tapered by 10 mg a fortnight [19].

Prednisolone Metasulfobenzoate

Oral prednisolone metasulfobenzoate (Predocol) has an acid-resistant coating (Eudragit L) that dissolves at a pH of 6 (corresponding to the mid-ileum) to release around 200 pellets. These pellets contain active drug in a controlled-release matrix, and spread throughout the colon [49]. Mucosal levels of prednisolone within the colon are similar to those achieved with conventional prednisolone, with minimal systemic absorption [50]. A randomized controlled trial of Predocol 40 mg daily for 6 months versus prednisolone at an initial dose of 40 mg daily for 2 weeks, tapering to stop at 8 weeks, showed similar efficacy between the groups, with fewer perceived steroid-related side effects in the Predocol group [20].

Topical Therapy

Topical corticosteroids are effective therapy for left-sided ulcerative colitis, with second-generation formulations (budesonide and beclomethasone dipropionate enemas) showing similar efficacies to topical mesalazine [51, 52]. Corticosteroids absorbed from the rectum (as opposed to the proximal gastrointestinal tract) do not undergo first-pass metabolism in the liver, and can result in adrenal suppression [53]. Studies of systemic bioavailability of topical corticosteroids in healthy subjects show high variability: from 2 % to 90 % of hydrocortisone administered as an enema was available systemically [54, 55]. The presence of rectal inflammation may reduce systemic absorption [56].

In active left-sided ulcerative colitis, budesonide enemas (2 mg, once a day) have shown similar endoscopic, histological and clinical response rates compared to both hydrocortisone foam (125 mg, once a day) and prednisolone (31.25 mg, once a day) enemas, but without the significant reduction in plasma cortisol levels seen with hydrocortisone [57] and prednisolone [58]. Beclomethasone dipropionate enemas (3 mg, once a day) also had a similar response compared with prednisolone enemas, again without the reduction in cortisol levels seen with prednisolone [28]. Budesonide foam enemas are better tolerated than budesonide liquid enemas and are just as effective [59].

Intravenous Therapy for Acute Severe Ulcerative Colitis

The optimum dose of corticosteroid for acute severe ulcerative colitis has not been established. However, hydrocortisone 300–400 mg intravenously every 24 h (or equivalent) is recommended based on clinical trial data, with an overall response rate of 67 % [60]. Again, higher doses are no more effective and lower doses are less effective. Therapy extending beyond 7–10 days provides no additional benefit [60]. The response to intravenous corticosteroids should be assessed objectively at day 3 to determine those who might need salvage therapy with ciclosporin or infliximab [61]. Predictors of poor response to medical therapy, with the need for early colectomy, include clinical markers (stool frequency), biochemical markers (elevated CRP, low albumin), radiological signs (colonic dilatation or mucosal islands on plain X-ray), and endoscopic appearance (severe ulceration) [62].

How to Manage Corticosteroid Withdrawal

Although they are effective agents for induction of remission of active ulcerative colitis, corticosteroids are not beneficial in maintaining remission [63–65]. Short courses (<3 weeks) and low starting doses (<15 mg prednisolone) of oral corticosteroids are associated with early relapse [40]. It is recommended that corticosteroids are tapered over several weeks, first to avoid rapid relapse, secondly, to allow the introduction or optimization of mesalazine, immunomodulators (thiopurines or methotrexate), and biological therapy, and thirdly, to allow resumption of usual function of the hypothalamic–pituitary–adrenal axis. The most favorable regimen for corticosteroid tapering has not been determined, but a standardized taper can identify early those who are corticosteroid-dependent [66]. Arthralgia and myalgia can occur as corticosteroids are tapered. This usually responds to paracetamol and reassurance, but improvement can take several months and some patients need reintroduction of corticosteroids with a slower taper [67].

Corticosteroid Resistance

Up to one-third of patients with ulcerative colitis fail to respond to standard courses of corticosteroid therapy and have corticosteroid-resistant disease [61, 68]. This may be due to a superimposed pathogen, such as cytomegalovirus infection or *Clostridium difficile* toxin, which should be excluded. An association between glucocorticoid receptor polymorphisms and corticosteroid resistance in IBD has been postulated, but a meta-analysis of five studies involving 942 cases was underpowered to detect this [69].

Corticosteroid resistance may occur downstream in the glucocorticoid receptor-signaling pathway via inflammatory cytokines. Tumor necrosis factor α (TNF-α) decreases corticosteroid sensitivity in monocytes by downregulation of the glucocorticoid receptor [70], and in patients with ulcerative colitis, mucosal levels of this inflammatory cytokine, along with IL-6 and IL-8, are higher in corticosteroid-resistant patients [71]. Infliximab, a TNF-α blocker, is effective for corticosteroid-resistant disease [72], as too are the calcineurin inhibitors, ciclosporin and tacrolimus [73, 74]. Calcineurin participates in the synthesis of interleukin-2 (IL-2), which has been implicated in the development of corticosteroid-resistant T lymphocytes. However, a trial of basiliximab, a monoclonal antibody that binds to and blocks CD25 on activated T lymphocytes, inhibiting IL-2 binding and IL-2 mediated proliferation, did not show an increased effectiveness of corticosteroids for induction of remission in outpatients with moderate to severe, steroid-resistant ulcerative colitis [75].

Corticosteroids in Pediatric Patients

Oral corticosteroids are effective treatment for induction of remission of ulcerative colitis in children, with a response rate of up to 90 % [76]. Dose-finding and optimal tapering studies have not been performed in pediatric disease but expert consensus recommends a dose of oral prednisolone 1 mg/kg (up to 40 mg a day), taken as a single dose, and tapered over 11 weeks [77]. Compared with adult-onset disease, corticosteroid dependency following corticosteroid treatment at diagnosis is higher in children (45 % of children compared with 9 % of adults over 1 year follow-up) [78].

Growth failure and malnutrition are less common in children with ulcerative colitis than those with Crohn's disease [79]. However, corticosteroids can suppress growth through effects on insulin-like growth factor (IGF)-1 [80], and the chondrocytes of the growth plates of the long bones [81]. Additionally, other corticosteroid-induced complications, including glaucoma, cataracts, and osteoporosis, are seen at a higher rate of in children than in adults [82], making corticosteroid-sparing strategies of paramount importance.

Side Effects of Corticosteroids

Corticosteroid side effects are manifold and involve multiple organ systems. This list is by no means exhaustive but considers those complications most pertinent to ulcerative colitis.

Metabolic Derangement

Hyperglycemia is one of the commonest metabolic derangements associated with corticosteroid use, and the development of diabetes mellitus is related to corticosteroid dose and duration [83]. Even short-term elevation of blood glucose is associated with adverse outcomes, and, therefore, this complication should be proactively sought and managed [84]. Sodium retention (leading on to fluid retention and hypertension) and hypokalemia are seen with corticosteroids with strong mineralocorticoid effects (e.g., hydrocortisone) [85], and tends to be a lesser issue in those with minimal mineralocorticoid activity (e.g., dexamethasone) [86]. Hypercholesterolemia, hypertriglyceridemia, atherogenesis and hepatic steatosis can complicate prolonged corticosteroid therapy [87, 88].

Neuropsychiatric Effects

Mood disorders can occur in up to 60 % of patients treated with corticosteroids [89], with severe psychiatric reactions (psychotic and affective symptoms) in approximately 5 % [90]. Effects are usually seen within 2 weeks of commencing therapy, and are associated with doses of prednisolone greater than 40 mg a day (or equivalent), hypoalbuminaemia, and defects in the blood–brain barrier [91]. Patients who display symptoms of psychosis or mania should undergo urgent psychiatric assessment. Symptoms usually resolve within 6 weeks of stopping therapy, and prophylaxis with olanzapine or lithium should be considered in those in whom further corticosteroid therapy cannot be avoided [91].

Infection

The risk of common-or-garden [92], opportunistic [93], and postoperative [94] infection is increased in IBD patients taking corticosteroids. Pooled data from 71 controlled trials of corticosteroid therapy for all indications showed that patients taking more than 40 mg a day of prednisone were at greatest risk for infection, with no increased risk at doses of less than 10 mg a day, or a cumulative dose of less than 700 mg of prednisone (with a specific relative risk for infection in patients receiving corticosteroids for intestinal disease of 1.4) [95]. Advanced age and diabetes both independently predispose patients with IBD to infections [93], and this risk is augmented further with corticosteroid use [96, 97].

Infections of specific relevance to patients with ulcerative colitis treated with corticosteroids include:

- *Clostridium difficile*: IBD, colitis in particular, is an independent risk factor for *C. difficile* infection, and corticosteroid therapy, regardless of dose and duration, is associated with a threefold increase in risk compared with other immunomodulators or biological agents (perhaps in part due to their use in more severe or active disease, and their lower rates of mucosal healing) [98].
- *Pneumocystis jirovecii*: Pneumonia due to this organism is associated with corticosteroid use, both alone and in combination with other immunomodulators in IBD [99]. Current European Crohn's and Colitis Organization guidelines recommend prophylaxis with cotrimoxazole for patients on three immunomodulators, where one is a biological agent or calcineurin inhibitor [100].
- *Cytomegalovirus (CMV)*: CMV infection is frequently reactivated in patients with ulcerative colitis treated with corticosteroids, but in most circumstances this is not clinically relevant and does not require cessation of immunomodulators [101]. CMV colitis, however, is associated with severity of the underlying disease, with a reported prevalence of 4.5–16.6 % of patients with severe colitis, and as high as 25 % in patients requiring colectomy for severe, corticosteroid-refractory disease [102]. To make the diagnosis, CMV must be found in colonic tissue: CMV inclusion bodies on hematoxylin and eosin staining, positive immunohistochemistry, and/or colonic tissue CMV polymerase chain resistance (PCR) positivity with >250 copies of CMV DNA/mg of tissue [103].
- Whether CMV contributes to the pathogenesis of severe colitis, or is simply a bystander in severe disease, has not been established. Evidence for causation includes the remission rates for colitis after antiviral therapy (usually intravenous ganciclovir 5 mg/kg for 2 weeks) in IBD patients with CMV infection, of 67–100 % [102], with restoration of efficacy of immunomodulators after treatment [103]. The use of infliximab in CMV infection in ulcerative colitis has been investigated in small case series, with no worsening of the colitis or the infection [104], and in some instances it has shown improvement in both clinical response of the ulcerative colitis, and loss of CMV PCR positivity from colonic tissue [105]. TNFα plays a major role in reactivation of CMV [106] and thus its blockade with anti-TNFα therapy might prevent its reactivation, alongside the benefits in treating the underlying ulcerative colitis. Thus, infliximab could be considered alongside antiviral therapy in patients with corticosteroid-refractory ulcerative colitis and superimposed CMV colitis. Such an approach requires further study.
- *Tuberculosis (TB)*: Biological agents have garnered much attention with respect to the risk of TB [107]. However, corticosteroids can also lead to reactivation of TB, and may cause false negative results when testing for latent disease [108]. It is well established that patients are screened for TB prior to initiation of immunomodulators such as thiopurines, methotrexate, or biological agents, but testing prior to commencement of corticosteroid therapy is often overlooked.
- *Hepatitis B virus*: The hepatitis B virus (HBV) genome contains a corticosteroid-response receptor on the hepatitis B core protein which upregulates HBV replication [109]. Prolonged courses of corticosteroids (over 3 months) are associated with deranged liver function tests in IBD patients with HBV infection (surface antigen positive, regardless of HBV DNA level) [110] and these patients should receive prophylactic antiviral therapy with tenofovir or entecavir (nucleotide/nucleoside analogs), which should be continued for 12 months following the cessation of immunosuppressant therapy [111]. Reactivation of prior HBV infection (surface antigen negative, core antibody positive) rarely occurs in IBD [112] and, therefore, routine prophylaxis is not required, unless the HBV DNA is detectable. If this is the case,

management is the same as for those with HBV surface antigen positivity. Those patients who are HBV surface antigen negative, core antibody positive, and HBV DNA negative should have HBV DNA levels and liver function tests monitored every 1–3 months, and should be treated with a nucleotide/nucleoside analog if the HBV DNA becomes detectable, before derangement in the liver function tests [111].

Live vaccinations should not be given within 4 weeks prior to initiation of therapy, during therapy, or within 3 months of cessation of therapy with high-dose corticosteroids (equivalent to a daily dose of ≥20 mg prednisolone for ≥14 days) [113]. Although the evidence for this recommendation is weak specifically for corticosteroids in IBD, the evidence of harm of live vaccinations in other similarly immunosuppressed patient groups has led to numerous guidelines strongly advising against their use in patients with chronic inflammatory diseases on high level immunosuppression [100, 114, 115].

Bone Disease

The prevalence of osteoporosis in patients with IBD is reported at 17–41 %, and osteopenia at 22–67 % [116]. The variation in prevalence estimates results from differences in population characteristics, age, disease extent and duration, dual energy X-ray absorptiometry methodology, and study design. Low bone mineral density in IBD is often attributed to corticosteroid use, but can be detected prior to initiation of therapy [117]. Factors pertinent to IBD, such as poor intake of calcium, vitamin D, and vitamin K, the effect of inflammatory cytokines, and hypogonadism [116], along with more general factors (e.g., smoking), are important modifiable risks to consider in low bone mineral density.

Corticosteroids cause bone mineral loss through several mechanisms, including increased apoptosis of osteoblasts and osteocytes, impaired differentiation of osteoblasts, and increased longevity of osteoclasts [118]. Bone loss is dose-dependent, occurring at doses of over 5 mg of prednisolone a day [119]. Following cessation of corticosteroids, new bone formation recurs although bone mass rarely recovers completely [120]. Rapid bone loss occurs on commencing corticosteroids and co-prescription of calcium and vitamin D3 supplements has been shown to partially ameliorate this [121].

Osteonecrosis is a serious complication of corticosteroid therapy, occurring in 0.5–4.3 % [122, 123] of IBD patients and usually involving the hips. However, multiple joints in the same patient may be affected without symptoms, most likely the shoulders and knees, and these should therefore be investigated [123]. There is some evidence that IBD lowers the cumulative dose threshold of corticosteroids needed to induce osteonecrosis, compared with other conditions [124].

Should Steroids Still Be Part of the Therapeutic Arsenal in Ulcerative Colitis?

The efficacy of corticosteroids for induction of remission of moderate–severely active ulcerative colitis is not in dispute, but in order to minimize their side effects, they should be used at the lowest effective dose for the shortest possible duration, with early consideration of initiating corticosteroid-sparing therapies. Early clinical review should take place to detect those who are corticosteroid-dependent or -refractory, and to monitor for complications, with rapid access to alternative agents when needed. In such circumstances, therapy with a swift onset of action is necessary but is usually expensive. Infliximab has clear evidence of efficacy in these patients [125], and the combination with azathioprine appears to be more effective than either drug alone [126]. Granulocyte apheresis is another potential option, albeit less accessible, with evidence largely from uncontrolled studies. In one such study of corticosteroid-refractory or corticosteroid-dependent UC, 5 weeks of granulocyte apheresis, one session a week, led to clinical remission in 71 % of patients by the end of treatment, with 48 % in remission at 1 year [127].

Corticosteroids still have a place in the management of ambulatory patients with active ulcerative colitis as induction agents. However, there are multiple aspects to optimally applying them in order to maximize efficacy of corticosteroids while minimizing the risk, as detailed in Table 39.3.

Conclusion

An awareness of the appropriate use and risks of corticosteroids, and early initiation of corticosteroid-sparing therapy are important in reducing complications associated with prolonged use. Unfortunately, they remain a tempting option: conventional corticosteroids are cheap, easy to prescribe and use, rapidly acting, and readily available. Extensively metabolized or poorly absorbed second-generation corticosteroids provide more acceptable safety profiles but are not a panacea. Testing to predict steroid responsiveness [69], the use of steroid-sensitizing drugs [75], or novel therapies to enhance the desirable effects of corticosteroid therapy whilst minimizing the adverse effects [128] had shown initial promise, but later studies were less encouraging. Timely decisions regarding colectomy for patients failing medical therapy in the acute setting, and those who are corticosteroid-dependent despite appropriate escalation of therapy, remain essential.

Table 39.3 Corticosteroid therapy for induction of remission of ulcerative colitis in the outpatient setting—maximizing efficacy and minimizing risk

Who should be treated with oral or topical corticosteroids?	• Those with moderate—severely active UC, not requiring hospitalization • Those with milder disease that fails to respond to oral and topical mesalazine
What should be considered before starting therapy?	• Prior corticosteroid use and cumulative dose • Careful history and infection screen (to include tuberculosis, hepatitis B and C, HIV, varicella) • Timing of administration of live vaccines (>4 weeks before starting if can be safely delayed) • Previous side effects, particularly neuropsychiatric effects • Concurrent medical problems, e.g., diabetes mellitus, osteoporosis, infection, glaucoma • Pregnancy • Drug interactions: antibiotics, antifungals, antivirals, anticonvulsants, anticoagulants, diuretics, nonsteroidal anti-inflammatory drugs • Warn patient of potential side effects and to seek prompt medical advice if concerned
Which corticosteroid should be used?	• Prednisolone 40 mg once daily (ideally in the morning) in those with moderate–severely active UC • Consider an oral or topical (for distal disease) second-generation corticosteroid in those with milder disease failing to respond to mesalazine (e.g., oral budesonide MMX 9 mg/day or oral beclomethasone dipropionate 5 mg/day). Systemic toxicity can still manifest with these drugs and so they are not suitable for long-term maintenance therapy
What co-prescriptions should be considered?	• Calcium and vitamin D supplementation during corticosteroid course • Proton-pump inhibitors in those with increased risk of gastrointestinal bleeding, e.g., previous peptic ulcer disease, concurrent nonsteroidal anti-inflammatory drugs
When and how should response be assessed?	• Clinical and biomarker response should be assessed at 2 weeks
How should corticosteroid-refractory disease be managed?	• If no response by 2 weeks with oral therapy, or an earlier deterioration, consider intravenous corticosteroids, infliximab, vedolizumab, or tacrolimus • If partial response only, consider thiopurine or methotrexate if slow onset of action will be tolerated • Repeat stool cultures and testing for *Clostridium difficile* toxin • Consider colonic biopsy for cytomegalovirus infection
How long should therapy be given and how should it be withdrawn?	• In those responding to oral corticosteroids at 2 weeks, taper over the following 6–10 weeks • Use a standard tapering regimen to detect those with early relapse or corticosteroid dependence • In those who relapse early or who develop myalgia and arthralgia on withdrawal, reintroduce the lowest efficacious dose of corticosteroid and then taper more slowly; if early relapse again, repeat action and add thiopurine or methotrexate • Topical second-generation corticosteroids may be given for up to 8 weeks in those with distal disease who have responded but are not yet in remission
How should remission be maintained?	• Optimize oral and topical mesalazine • Consider early introduction of a thiopurine and/or biological therapy in those who show signs of relapse, corticosteroid dependence or who have required >1 course of corticosteroids in the previous year

References

1. Truelove SC, Witts LJ. Cortisone in ulcerative colitis. Br Med J. 1955;2:1041–8.
2. Edwards FC, Truelove SC. The course and prognosis of ulcerative colitis. Gut. 1963;4:299–315.
3. McKay LI, Cidlowski JA. Cross-talk between nuclear factor-kappa B and the steroid hormone receptors: mechanisms of mutual antagonism. Mol Endocrinol. 1998;12:45–56.
4. Barnes PJ. How corticosteroids control inflammation: Quintiles Prize Lecture 2005. Br J Pharmacol. 2006;148(3):245–54.
5. Sandle GI, Hayslett JP, Binder HJ. Effect of glucocorticoids on rectal transport in normal subjects and patients with ulcerative colitis. Gut. 1986;27(3):309–16.
6. Meyers S, Sachar DB, Goldberg JD, Janowitz HD. Corticotropin versus hydrocortisone in the intravenous treatment of ulcerative colitis. A prospective, randomized, double-blind clinical trial. Gastroenterology. 1983;85(2):351–7.
7. Truelove SC, Witts LJ. Cortisone in ulcerative colitis; preliminary report on a therapeutic trial. Br Med J. 1954;2(4884):375–8.
8. Hawthorne AB, Record CO, Holdsworth CD, Giaffer MH, Burke DA, Keech ML, et al. Double blind trial of oral fluticasone propionate v prednisolone in the treatment of active ulcerative colitis. Gut. 1993;34(1):125–8.

9. Lennard-Jones JE, Longmore AJ, Newell AC, Wilson CW, Jones FA. An assessment of prednisone, salazopyrin, and topical hydrocortisone hemisuccinate used as out-patient treatment for ulcerative colitis. Gut. 1960;1:217–22.
10. Topical 5-aminosalicylic acid versus prednisolone in ulcerative proctosigmoiditis. A randomized, double-blind multicenter trial. Danish 5-ASA Group. Digest Dis Sci. 1987;32(6):598–602.
11. Angus P, Snook JA, Reid M, Jewell DP. Oral fluticasone propionate in active distal ulcerative colitis. Gut. 1992;33(5):711–4.
12. Lofberg R, Danielsson A, Suhr O, Nilsson A, Schioler R, Nyberg A, et al. Oral budesonide versus prednisolone in patients with active extensive and left-sided ulcerative colitis. Gastroenterology. 1996;110(6):1713–8.
13. Gross V, Bunganic I, Belousova EA, Mikhailova TL, Kupcinskas L, Kiudelis G, et al. 3 g mesalazine granules are superior to 9 mg budesonide for achieving remission in active ulcerative colitis: a double-blind, double-dummy, randomised trial. J Crohns Colitis. 2011;5(2):129–38.
14. D'Haens GR, Kovacs A, Vergauwe P, Nagy F, Molnar T, Bouhnik Y, et al. Clinical trial: preliminary efficacy and safety study of a new Budesonide-MMX(R) 9 mg extended-release tablets in patients with active left-sided ulcerative colitis. J Crohns Colitis. 2010;4(2):153–60.
15. Sandborn WJ, Travis S, Moro L, Jones R, Gautille T, Bagin R, et al. Once-daily budesonide MMX(R) extended-release tablets induce remission in patients with mild to moderate ulcerative colitis: results from the CORE I study. Gastroenterology. 2012;143(5):1218–26.e1–2.
16. Travis SP, Danese S, Kupcinskas L, Alexeeva O, D'Haens G, Gibson PR, et al. Once-daily budesonide MMX in active, mild-to-moderate ulcerative colitis: results from the randomised CORE II study. Gut. 2014;63(3):433–41.
17. Bossa F, Latiano A, Rossi L, Magnani M, Palmieri O, Dallapiccola B, et al. Erythrocyte-mediated delivery of dexamethasone in patients with mild-to-moderate ulcerative colitis, refractory to mesalamine: a randomized, controlled study. Am J Gastroenterol. 2008;103(10):2509–16.
18. Rizzello F, Gionchetti P, D'Arienzo A, Manguso F, Di Matteo G, Annese V, et al. Oral beclometasone dipropionate in the treatment of active ulcerative colitis: a double-blind placebo-controlled study. Aliment Pharmacol Ther. 2002;16(6):1109–16.
19. Van Assche G, Manguso F, Zibellini M, Cabriada Nuno JL, Goldis A, Tkachenko E, et al. Oral prolonged release beclomethasone dipropionate and prednisone in the treatment of active ulcerative colitis: results from a double-blind, randomized, parallel group study. Am J Gastroenterol. 2015;110(5):708–15.
20. Rhodes JM, Robinson R, Beales I, Pugh S, Dickinson R, Dronfield M, et al. Clinical trial: oral prednisolone metasulfobenzoate (Predocol) vs. oral prednisolone for active ulcerative colitis. Aliment Pharmacol Ther. 2008;27(3):228–40.
21. Hanauer SB, Robinson M, Pruitt R, Lazenby AJ, Persson T, Nilsson LG, et al. Budesonide enema for the treatment of active, distal ulcerative colitis and proctitis: a dose-ranging study. U.S. Budesonide enema study group. Gastroenterology. 1998;115(3): 525–32.
22. Lindgren S, Lofberg R, Bergholm L, Hellblom M, Carling L, Ung KA, et al. Effect of budesonide enema on remission and relapse rate in distal ulcerative colitis and proctitis. Scand J Gastroenterol. 2002;37(6):705–10.
23. Sandborn WJ, Bosworth B, Zakko S, Gordon GL, Clemmons DR, Golden PL, et al. Budesonide foam induces remission in patients with mild to moderate ulcerative proctitis and ulcerative proctosigmoiditis. Gastroenterology. 2015;148(4):740–50.e2.
24. Bansky G, Buhler H, Stamm B, Hacki WH, Buchmann P, Muller J. Treatment of distal ulcerative colitis with beclomethasone enemas: high therapeutic efficacy without endocrine side effects. A prospective, randomized, double-blind trial. Dis Colon Rectum. 1987;30(4):288–92.
25. van der Heide H, van den Brandt-Gradel V, Tytgat GN, Endert E, Wiltink EH, Schipper ME, et al. Comparison of beclomethasone dipropionate and prednisolone 21-phosphate enemas in the treatment of ulcerative proctitis. J Clin Gastroenterol. 1988;10(2): 169–72.
26. Halpern Z, Sold O, Baratz M, Konikoff F, Halak A, Gilat T. A controlled trial of beclomethasone versus betamethasone enemas in distal ulcerative colitis. J Clin Gastroenterol. 1991;13(1): 38–41.
27. Mulder CJ, Fockens P, Meijer JW, van der Heide H, Wiltink EH, Tytgat GN. Beclomethasone dipropionate (3 mg) versus 5-aminosalicylic acid (2 g) versus the combination of both (3 mg/2 g) as retention enemas in active ulcerative proctitis. Eur J Gastroenterol Hepatol. 1996;8(6):549–53.
28. Campieri M, Cottone M, Miglio F, Manenti F, Astegiano M, D'Arienzo A, et al. Beclomethasone dipropionate enemas versus prednisolone sodium phosphate enemas in the treatment of distal ulcerative colitis. Aliment Pharmacol Ther. 1998;12(4):361–6.
29. Biancone L, Gionchetti P, Blanco Gdel V, Orlando A, Annese V, Papi C, et al. Beclomethasone dipropionate versus mesalazine in distal ulcerative colitis: a multicenter, randomized, double-blind study. Dig Liver Dis. 2007;39(4):329–37.
30. McIntyre PB, Macrae FA, Berghouse L, English J, Lennard-Jones JE. Therapeutic benefits from a poorly absorbed prednisolone enema in distal colitis. Gut. 1985;26(8):822–4.
31. Riley SA, Gupta I, Mani V. A comparison of sucralfate and prednisolone enemas in the treatment of active distal ulcerative colitis. Scand J Gastroenterol. 1989;24(8):1014–8.
32. Cobden I, al-Mardini H, Zaitoun A, Record CO. Is topical therapy necessary in acute distal colitis? Double-blind comparison of high-dose oral mesalazine versus steroid enemas in the treatment of active distal ulcerative colitis. Aliment Pharmacol Ther. 1991;5(5):513–22.
33. Mulder CJ, Tytgat GN, Wiltink EH, Houthoff HJ. Comparison of 5-aminosalicylic acid (3 g) and prednisolone phosphate sodium enemas (30 mg) in the treatment of distal ulcerative colitis. A prospective, randomized, double-blind trial. Scand J Gastroenterol. 1988;23(8):1005–8.
34. O'Donnell LJ, Arvind AS, Hoang P, Cameron D, Talbot IC, Jewell DP, et al. Double blind, controlled trial of 4-aminosalicylic acid and prednisolone enemas in distal ulcerative colitis. Gut. 1992;33(7):947–9.
35. Sharma MP, Duphare HV, Dasarathy S. A prospective randomized double blind trial comparing prednisolone and 4-aminosalicylic acid enemas in acute distal ulcerative colitis. J Gastroenterol Hepatol. 1992;7(2):173–7.
36. Campieri M, Gionchetti P, Belluzzi A, Brignola C, Migaldi M, Tabanelli GM, et al. Efficacy of 5-aminosalicylic acid enemas versus hydrocortisone enemas in ulcerative colitis. Dig Dis Sci. 1987;32(12 Suppl):67s–70s.
37. Bianchi Porro G, Ardizzone S, Petrillo M, Fasoli A, Molteni P, Imbesi V. Low Pentasa dosage versus hydrocortisone in the topical treatment of active ulcerative colitis: a randomized, double-blind study. Am J Gastroenterol. 1995;90(5):736–9.
38. Ford AC, Bernstein CN, Khan KJ, Abreu MT, Marshall JK, Talley NJ, et al. Glucocorticosteroid therapy in inflammatory bowel disease: systematic review and meta-analysis. Am J Gastroenterol. 2011;106(4):590–9.
39. Elliott PR, Powell-Tuck J, Gillespie PE, Laidlow JM, Lennard-Jones JE, English J, et al. Prednisolone absorption in acute colitis. Gut. 1980;21(1):49–51.
40. Baron JH, Connell AM, Kanaghinis TG, Lennard-Jones JE, Jones AF. Out-patient treatment of ulcerative colitis. Comparison between three doses of oral prednisone. Br Med J. 1962;2(5302): 441–3.

41. Powell-Tuck J, Bown RL, Lennard-Jones JE. A comparison of oral prednisolone given as single or multiple daily doses for active proctocolitis. Scand J Gastroenterol. 1978;13(7):833–7.
42. Dignass A, Lindsay JO, Sturm A, Windsor A, Colombel JF, Allez M, et al. Second European evidence-based consensus on the diagnosis and management of ulcerative colitis. Part 2: Current management. J Crohns Colitis. 2012;6(10):991–1030.
43. Centre for Drug Evaluation and Research. Pharmacology review. Budesonide modified release capsules. 2001. Available from: http://www.accessdata.fda.gov/drugsatfda_docs/nda/2001/21-324_Entocort_pharmr.pdf. Accessed 20 July 2015.
44. Seow CH, Benchimol EI, Griffiths AM, Otley AR, Steinhart AH. Budesonide for induction of remission in Crohn's disease. Cochrane Database Syst Rev. 2008;(3):Cd000296.
45. Ferring Pharmaceuticals Ltd. Cortiment 9 mg, prolonged release tablets: summary of product characteristics 2014. Available from: http://www.mhra.gov.uk/home/groups/spcpil/documents/spcpil/con1437715186489.pdf. Accessed 20 July 2015.
46. Steed KP, Hooper G, Ventura P, Musa R, Wilding IR. The in vivo behaviour of a colonic delivery system: a pilot study in man. Int J Pharm. 1994;112(3):199–206.
47. Fasci Spurio F, Aratari A, Margagnoni G, Doddato MT, Chiesara F, Papi C. Oral beclomethasone dipropionate: a critical review of its use in the management of ulcerative colitis and Crohn's disease. Curr Clin Pharmacol. 2012;7(2):131–6.
48. Campieri M, Adamo S, Valpiani D, D'Arienzo A, D'Albasio G, Pitzalis M, et al. Oral beclometasone dipropionate in the treatment of extensive and left-sided active ulcerative colitis: a multicentre randomised study. Aliment Pharmacol Ther. 2003;17(12):1471–80.
49. Ford GA, Oliver PS, Shepherd NA, Wilkinson SP. An Eudragit-coated prednisolone preparation for ulcerative colitis: pharmacokinetics and preliminary therapeutic use. Aliment Pharmacol Ther. 1992;6(1):31–40.
50. Bell GD EJ, Spiers C, Nylander D, Hancock JM, Rowland RS. Colonic mucosal concentrations of prednisolone following oral administration of a novel formulation of prednisolone metasulphobenzoate (Predocol) [Abstract]. Gut. 2000;(Suppl 46):T29.
51. Manguso F, Balzano A. Meta-analysis: the efficacy of rectal beclomethasone dipropionate vs. 5-aminosalicylic acid in mild to moderate distal ulcerative colitis. Aliment Pharmacol Ther. 2007;26(1):21–9.
52. Lemann M, Galian A, Rutgeerts P, Van Heuverzwijn R, Cortot A, Viteau JM, et al. Comparison of budesonide and 5-aminosalicylic acid enemas in active distal ulcerative colitis. Aliment Pharmacol Ther. 1995;9(5):557–62.
53. Farmer RG, Schumacher OP. Treatment of ulcerative colitis with hydrocortisone enemas. Comparison of absorption and clinical response with hydrocortisone alcohol and hydrocortisone acetate. Am J Gastroenterol. 1970;54(3):229–36.
54. Mollmann H, Barth J, Mollmann C, Tunn S, Krieg M, Derendorf H. Pharmacokinetics and rectal bioavailability of hydrocortisone acetate. J Pharm Sci. 1991;80(9):835–6.
55. Lima JJ, Giller J, Mackichan JJ, Jusko WJ. Bioavailability of hydrocortisone retention enemas in normal subjects. Am J Gastroenterol. 1980;73(3):232–7.
56. Petitjean O, Wendling JL, Tod M, Louchahi K, Nicolas P, Perret G, et al. Pharmacokinetics and absolute rectal bioavailability of hydrocortisone acetate in distal colitis. Aliment Pharmacol Ther. 1992;6(3):351–7.
57. Tarpila S, Turunen U, Seppala K, Aukee S, Pikkarainen P, Elomaa I, et al. Budesonide enema in active haemorrhagic proctitis—a controlled trial against hydrocortisone foam enema. Aliment Pharmacol Ther. 1994;8(6):591–5.
58. Lofberg R, Ostergaard Thomsen O, Langholz E, Schioler R, Danielsson A, Suhr O, et al. Budesonide versus prednisolone retention enemas in active distal ulcerative colitis. Aliment Pharmacol Ther. 1994;8(6):623–9.
59. Gross V, Bar-Meir S, Lavy A, Mickisch O, Tulassay Z, Pronai L, et al. Budesonide foam versus budesonide enema in active ulcerative proctitis and proctosigmoiditis. Aliment Pharmacol Ther. 2006;23(2):303–12.
60. Turner D, Walsh CM, Steinhart AH, Griffiths AM. Response to corticosteroids in severe ulcerative colitis: a systematic review of the literature and a meta-regression. Clin Gastroenterol Hepatol. 2007;5(1):103–10.
61. Travis SP, Farrant JM, Ricketts C, Nolan DJ, Mortensen NM, Kettlewell MG, et al. Predicting outcome in severe ulcerative colitis. Gut. 1996;38(6):905–10.
62. Travis S, Satsangi J, Lémann M. Predicting the need for colectomy in severe ulcerative colitis: a critical appraisal of clinical parameters and currently available biomarkers. Gut. 2011;60(1):3–9.
63. Truelove SC, Witts LJ. Cortisone and corticotrophin in ulcerative colitis. Br Med J. 1959;1(5119):387–94.
64. Lennard-Jones JE, Misiewicz JJ, Connell AM, Baron JH, Jones FA. Prednisone as maintenance treatment for ulcerative colitis in remission. Lancet. 1965;1(7378):188–9.
65. Powell-Tuck J, Bown RL, Chambers TJ, Lennard-Jones JE. A controlled trial of alternate day prednisolone as a maintenance treatment for ulcerative colitis in remission. Digestion. 1981;22(5):263–70.
66. Lichtenstein GR, Abreu MT, Cohen R, Tremaine W. American Gastroenterological Association Institute technical review on corticosteroids, immunomodulators, and infliximab in inflammatory bowel disease. Gastroenterology. 2006;130(3):940–87.
67. Keenan GF. Management of complications of glucocorticoid therapy. Clin Chest Med. 1997;18(3):507–20.
68. Faubion Jr WA, Loftus Jr EV, Harmsen WS, Zinsmeister AR, Sandborn WJ. The natural history of corticosteroid therapy for inflammatory bowel disease: a population-based study. Gastroenterology. 2001;121(2):255–60.
69. Chen HL, Li LR. Glucocorticoid receptor gene polymorphisms and glucocorticoid resistance in inflammatory bowel disease: a meta-analysis. Dig Dis Sci. 2012;57(12):3065–75.
70. Franchimont D, Martens H, Hagelstein MT, Louis E, Dewe W, Chrousos GP, et al. Tumor necrosis factor alpha decreases, and interleukin-10 increases, the sensitivity of human monocytes to dexamethasone: potential regulation of the glucocorticoid receptor. J Clin Endocr Metab. 1999;84(8):2834–9.
71. Ishiguro Y. Mucosal proinflammatory cytokine production correlates with endoscopic activity of ulcerative colitis. J Gastroenterol. 1999;34(1):66–74.
72. Jarnerot G, Hertervig E, Friis-Liby I, Blomquist L, Karlen P, Granno C, et al. Infliximab as rescue therapy in severe to moderately severe ulcerative colitis: a randomized, placebo-controlled study. Gastroenterology. 2005;128(7):1805–11.
73. Lichtiger S, Present DH, Kornbluth A, Gelernt I, Bauer J, Galler G, et al. Cyclosporine in severe ulcerative colitis refractory to steroid therapy. N Engl J Med. 1994;330(26):1841–5.
74. Chow DK, Leong RW. The use of tacrolimus in the treatment of inflammatory bowel disease. Expert Opin Drug Saf. 2007;6(5):479–85.
75. Sands BE, Sandborn WJ, Creed TJ, Dayan CM, Dhanda AD, Van Assche GA, et al. Basiliximab does not increase efficacy of corticosteroids in patients with steroid-refractory ulcerative colitis. Gastroenterology. 2012;143(2):356–64.e1.
76. Beattie RM, Nicholls SW, Domizio P, Williams CB, Walker-Smith JA. Endoscopic assessment of the colonic response to corticosteroids in children with ulcerative colitis. J Pediatr Gastroenterol Nutr. 1996;22(4):373–9.

77. Turner D, Levine A, Escher JC, Griffiths AM, Russell RK, Dignass A, et al. Management of pediatric ulcerative colitis: joint ECCO and ESPGHAN evidence-based consensus guidelines. J Pediatr Gastroenterol Nutr. 2012;55(3):340–61.
78. Jakobsen C, Bartek Jr J, Wewer V, Vind I, Munkholm P, Groen R, et al. Differences in phenotype and disease course in adult and pediatric inflammatory bowel disease—a population-based study. Aliment Pharmacol Ther. 2011;34(10):1217–24.
79. Rocha R, Santana GO, Almeida N, Lyra AC. Analysis of fat and muscle mass in patients with inflammatory bowel disease during remission and active phase. Br J Nutr. 2009;101(5):676–9.
80. Hokken-Koelega AC, Stijnen T, de Muinck Keizer-Schrama SM, Blum WF, Drop SL. Levels of growth hormone, insulin-like growth factor-I (IGF-I) and -II, IGF-binding protein-1 and -3, and cortisol in prednisone-treated children with growth retardation after renal transplantation. J Clin Endocr Metab. 1993;77(4): 932–8.
81. Mushtaq T, Farquharson C, Seawright E, Ahmed SF. Glucocorticoid effects on chondrogenesis, differentiation and apoptosis in the murine ATDC5 chondrocyte cell line. J Endocrinol. 2002;175(3): 705–13.
82. Uchida K, Araki T, Toiyama Y, Yoshiyama S, Inoue M, Ikeuchi H, et al. Preoperative steroid-related complications in Japanese pediatric patients with ulcerative colitis. Dis Colon Rectum. 2006; 49(1):74–9.
83. Gurwitz JH, Bohn RL, Glynn RJ, Monane M, Mogun H, Avorn J. Glucocorticoids and the risk for initiation of hypoglycemic therapy. Arch Intern Med. 1994;154(1):97–101.
84. Clore JN, Thurby-Hay L. Glucocorticoid-induced hyperglycemia. Endocr Pract. 2009;15(5):469–74.
85. Clyburn EB, DiPette DJ. Hypertension induced by drugs and other substances. Semin Nephrol. 1995;15(2):72–86.
86. Hulter HN, Licht JH, Bonner Jr EL, Glynn RD, Sebastian A. Effects of glucocorticoid steroids on renal and systemic acid-base metabolism. Am J Physiol. 1980;239(1):F30–43.
87. Nashel DJ. Is atherosclerosis a complication of long-term corticosteroid treatment? Am J Med. 1986;80(5):925–9.
88. Peckett AJ, Wright DC, Riddell MC. The effects of glucocorticoids on adipose tissue lipid metabolism. Metabolism. 2011; 60(11):1500–10.
89. Bolanos SH, Khan DA, Hanczyc M, Bauer MS, Dhanani N, Brown ES. Assessment of mood states in patients receiving long-term corticosteroid therapy and in controls with patient-rated and clinician-rated scales. Ann Allerg Asthma Immunol. 2004; 92(5):500–5.
90. Lewis DA, Smith RE. Steroid-induced psychiatric syndromes. A report of 14 cases and a review of the literature. J Affect Disorder. 1983;5(4):319–32.
91. West S, Kenedi C. Strategies to prevent the neuropsychiatric side-effects of corticosteroids: a case report and review of the literature. Curr Opin Organ Transplant. 2014;19(2):201–8.
92. Lichtenstein GR, Feagan BG, Cohen RD, Salzberg BA, Diamond RH, Price S, et al. Serious infection and mortality in patients with Crohn's disease: more than 5 years of follow-up in the TREAT registry. Am J Gastroenterol. 2012;107(9):1409–22.
93. Toruner M, Loftus Jr EV, Harmsen WS, Zinsmeister AR, Orenstein R, Sandborn WJ, et al. Risk factors for opportunistic infections in patients with inflammatory bowel disease. Gastroenterology. 2008;134(4):929–36.
94. Subramanian V, Saxena S, Kang JY, Pollok RC. Preoperative steroid use and risk of postoperative complications in patients with inflammatory bowel disease undergoing abdominal surgery. Am J Gastroenterol. 2008;103(9):2373–81.
95. Stuck AE, Minder CE, Frey FJ. Risk of infectious complications in patients taking glucocorticosteroids. Rev Infect Dis. 1989; 11(6):954–63.
96. Brassard P, Bitton A, Suissa A, Sinyavskaya L, Patenaude V, Suissa S. Oral corticosteroids and the risk of serious infections in patients with elderly-onset inflammatory bowel diseases. Am J Gastroenterol. 2014;109(11):1795–802. quiz 803.
97. Ananthakrishnan AN, Cagan A, Cai T, Gainer VS, Shaw SY, Churchill S, et al. Diabetes and the risk of infections with immunomodulator therapy in inflammatory bowel diseases. Aliment Pharmacol Ther. 2015;41(11):1141–8.
98. Schneeweiss S, Korzenik J, Solomon DH, Canning C, Lee J, Bressler B. Infliximab and other immunomodulating drugs in patients with inflammatory bowel disease and the risk of serious bacterial infections. Aliment Pharmacol Ther. 2009;30(3): 253–64.
99. Long MD, Farraye FA, Okafor PN, Martin C, Sandler RS, Kappelman MD. Increased risk of Pneumocystis jirovecii pneumonia among patients with inflammatory bowel disease. Inflamm Bowel Dis. 2013;19(5):1018–24.
100. Rahier JF, Magro F, Abreu C, Armuzzi A, Ben-Horin S, Chowers Y, et al. Second European evidence-based consensus on the prevention, diagnosis and management of opportunistic infections in inflammatory bowel disease. J Crohns Colitis. 2014;8(6):443–68.
101. Matsuoka K, Iwao Y, Mori T, Sakuraba A, Yajima T, Hisamatsu T, et al. Cytomegalovirus is frequently reactivated and disappears without antiviral agents in ulcerative colitis patients. Am J Gastroenterol. 2007;102(2):331–7.
102. Sager K, Alam S, Bond A, Chinnappan L, Probert CS. Review article: cytomegalovirus and inflammatory bowel disease. Aliment Pharmacol Ther. 2015;41(8):725–33.
103. Roblin X, Pillet S, Oussalah A, Berthelot P, Del Tedesco E, Phelip JM, et al. Cytomegalovirus load in inflamed intestinal tissue is predictive of resistance to immunosuppressive therapy in ulcerative colitis. Am J Gastroenterol. 2011;106(11):2001–8.
104. D'Ovidio V, Vernia P, Gentile G, Capobianchi A, Marcheggiano A, Viscido A, et al. Cytomegalovirus infection in inflammatory bowel disease patients undergoing anti-TNFalpha therapy. J Clin Virol. 2008;43(2):180–3.
105. Criscuoli V, Mocciaro F, Orlando A, Rizzuto MR, Renda MC, Cottone M. Cytomegalovirus disappearance after treatment for refractory ulcerative colitis in 2 patients treated with infliximab and 1 patient with leukapheresis. Inflamm Bowel Dis. 2009; 15(6):810–1.
106. Nakase H, Honzawa Y, Toyonaga T, Yamada S, Minami N, Yoshino T, et al. Diagnosis and treatment of ulcerative colitis with cytomegalovirus infection: importance of controlling mucosal inflammation to prevent cytomegalovirus reactivation. Intest Res. 2014;12(1):5–11.
107. Keane J, Gershon S, Wise RP, Mirabile-Levens E, Kasznica J, Schwieterman WD, et al. Tuberculosis associated with infliximab, a tumor necrosis factor alpha-neutralizing agent. N Engl J Med. 2001;345(15):1098–104.
108. Belard E, Semb S, Ruhwald M, Werlinrud AM, Soborg B, Jensen FK, et al. Prednisolone treatment affects the performance of the QuantiFERON gold in-tube test and the tuberculin skin test in patients with autoimmune disorders screened for latent tuberculosis infection. Inflamm Bowel Dis. 2011;17(11):2340–9.
109. Tur-Kaspa R, Burk RD, Shaul Y, Shafritz DA. Hepatitis B virus DNA contains a glucocorticoid-responsive element. Proc Natl Acad Sci U S A. 1986;83(6):1627–31.
110. Park SH, Yang SK, Lim YS, Shim JH, Yang DH, Jung KW, et al. Clinical courses of chronic hepatitis B virus infection and inflammatory bowel disease in patients with both diseases. Inflamm Bowel Dis. 2012;18(11):2004–10.
111. EASL clinical practice guidelines: management of chronic hepatitis B virus infection. J Hepatol. 2012;57(1):167–85.
112. Loras C, Gisbert JP, Minguez M, Merino O, Bujanda L, Saro C, et al. Liver dysfunction related to hepatitis B and C in patients

with inflammatory bowel disease treated with immunosuppressive therapy. Gut. 2010;59(10):1340–6.
113. General recommendations on immunization—recommendations of the Advisory Committee on Immunization Practices (ACIP). MMWR Recommendations and reports: morbidity and mortality weekly report. Centers for Disease Control. 2011;60(2):1–64. http://www.cdc.gov/mmwr/preview/mmwrhtml/rr6002a1.htm?s_cid=rr6002a1_w. Accessed 20 July 2015.
114. Rubin LG, Levin MJ, Ljungman P, Davies EG, Avery R, Tomblyn M, et al. 2013 IDSA clinical practice guideline for vaccination of the immunocompromised host. Clin Infect Dis. 2014;58(3):309–18.
115. Heijstek MW, Ott de Bruin LM, Bijl M, Borrow R, van der Klis F, Kone-Paut I, et al. EULAR recommendations for vaccination in pediatric patients with rheumatic diseases. Ann Rheum Dis. 2011;70(10):1704–12.
116. Tigas S, Tsatsoulis A. Endocrine and metabolic manifestations in inflammatory bowel disease. Ann Gastroenterol. 2012;25(1): 37–44.
117. Sylvester FA, Wyzga N, Hyams JS, Davis PM, Lerer T, Vance K, et al. Natural history of bone metabolism and bone mineral density in children with inflammatory bowel disease. Inflamm Bowel Dis. 2007;13(1):42–50.
118. den Uyl D, Bultink IEM, Lems WF. Advances in glucocorticoid-induced osteoporosis. Curr Rheumatol Rep. 2011;13(3):233–40.
119. Tannirandorn P, Epstein S. Drug-induced bone loss. Osteoporosis Int. 2000;11(8):637–59.
120. Adachi JD, Rostom A. Metabolic bone disease in adults with inflammatory bowel disease. Inflamm Bowel Dis. 1999;5(3): 200–11.
121. Homik J, Suarez-Almazor ME, Shea B, Cranney A, Wells G, Tugwell P. Calcium and vitamin D for corticosteroid-induced osteoporosis. Cochrane Database Syst Rev. 2000;(2):Cd000952.
122. Freeman HJ, Freeman KJ. Prevalence rates and an evaluation of reported risk factors for osteonecrosis (avascular necrosis) in Crohn's disease. Can J Gastroenterol. 2000;14(2):138–43.
123. Vakil N, Sparberg M. Steroid-related osteonecrosis in inflammatory bowel disease. Gastroenterology. 1989;96(1):62–7.
124. Klingenstein G, Levy RN, Kornbluth A, Shah AK, Present DH. Inflammatory bowel disease related osteonecrosis: report of a large series with a review of the literature. Aliment Pharmacol Ther. 2005;21(3):243–9.
125. Rutgeerts P, Sandborn WJ, Feagan BG, Reinisch W, Olson A, Johanns J, et al. Infliximab for induction and maintenance therapy for ulcerative colitis. N Engl J Med. 2005;353(23):2462–76.
126. Panaccione R, Ghosh S, Middleton S, Marquez JR, Scott BB, Flint L, et al. Combination therapy with infliximab and azathioprine is superior to monotherapy with either agent in ulcerative colitis. Gastroenterology. 2014;146(2):392–400.e3.
127. Sacco R, Romano A, Mazzoni A, Bertini M, Federici G, Metrangolo S, et al. Granulocytapheresis in steroid-dependent and steroid-resistant patients with inflammatory bowel disease: a prospective observational study. J Crohns Colitis. 2013;7(12): e692–7.
128. Bossa F, Annese V, Valvano MR, Latiano A, Martino G, Rossi L, et al. Erythrocytes-mediated delivery of dexamethasone 21-phosphate in steroid-dependent ulcerative colitis: a randomized, double-blind Sham-controlled study. Inflamm Bowel Dis. 2013;19(9):1872–9.

Medical Management of Ulcerative Colitis: Conventional Therapy—Azathioprine

40

Barrett G. Levesque and Edward V. Loftus Jr.

Introduction

Induction therapy with cortisone for ulcerative colitis was first described by Dearing and Brown of Mayo Clinic in 1950 [1], and the final results of a randomized clinical trial by Truelove and Witts of Oxford were published in 1955 [2]. By 1965, Lennard-Jones and colleagues had definitively shown that prednisone was not effective in maintaining remission in ulcerative colitis [3]. Alternative immunosuppressive agents which would maintain clinical remission and spare the side effects of long-term corticosteroids were sought. Azathioprine (AZA) was originally demonstrated as a therapy for ulcerative colitis in 1966 by Bowen and colleagues at the University of Chicago [4]. In an open-label case series, ten hospitalized patients were treated with relatively high doses of AZA (4-6 mg/kg/day) which was then continued in the outpatient setting. Most patients improved; however, the results were confounded by other medications and lacked a control group [4]. In the subsequent four decades, controlled trials of AZA have revealed mixed results in induction and maintenance for ulcerative colitis [5–8]. The role of AZA in the treatment of ulcerative colitis has continued to be debated due its evidence base of predominantly heterogenous small clinical trials and the advent of biologic therapy. The following chapter on AZA in the treatment of ulcerative colitis emphasizes practical implications of pharmacology and metabolism, efficacy estimates from clinical trials, safety, and practical dosing and toxicity monitoring methods for clinical practice.

B.G. Levesque, M.D., M.S.
Division of Gastroenterology, University of California San Diego, La Jolla, CA, USA

E.V. Loftus Jr., M.D. (✉)
Division of Gastroenterology & Hepatology, Mayo Clinic, 200 First Street, S.W., Rochester, MN 55905, USA
e-mail: loftus.edward@mayo.edu

Pharmacology and Metabolism

AZA is a prodrug which undergoes approximately 88 % conversion to mercaptopurine (6MP) by nonenzymatic nucleophilic attack in red blood cells and other tissues [9, 10] (Fig. 40.1). AZA is 55 % 6MP by molecular weight, and a conversion factor of 2.07 is used to convert a dose of 6MP to AZA dose [11]. Xanthine oxidase, thiopurine methyltransferase (TPMT), and hypoxanthine phosphoribosyl transferase are the three enzyme systems that break down 6MP to 6-thiouric acid, 6 methylmercaptopurine (6MMP), and precursors of the active 6-thioguanine nucleotides (6-TGN) [12], respectively. The mechanism of action of AZA and 6MP has not been fully elucidated. 6-TGN are incorporated into nucleic acid and subsequently inhibit synthesis of protein, ribonucleic acid (RNA), and deoxyribonucleic acid (DNA) [12]. The conversion of 6MP to 6MMP by TPMT is subject to different rates due to genetic variation in TPMT activity. Approximately 0.3 % of the population is homozygous for the mutant inactive form of TPMT, 11 % are heterozygous with intermediate activity, and 89 % have normal activity [13]. The half-life of 6-TGN in red blood cells is 3–13 days, and may take 4 days to 3 years to reach a steady state [14]. While intravenous loading doses of AZA have been shown to be feasible, and initial reports seemed promising [15, 16], a randomized placebo-controlled trial of intravenous loading in Crohn's disease showed no difference in time to clinical response [17]. Interestingly, steady state levels of 6-TGN occurred by week 2 in both groups. In general, a therapeutic clinical response may take 2–4 months for most patients [17, 18].

Several aspects of AZA metabolism have clinical implications. An inverse association between TPMT enzyme activity and 6TGN concentration has been suggested [15], which supports the clinical experience that patients with intermediate TPMT activity levels are more likely to respond to lower doses of AZA therapy than patients with normal TPMT activity level. Due to the risk of life-threatening

D.C. Baumgart (ed.), *Crohn's Disease and Ulcerative Colitis*, DOI 10.1007/978-3-319-33703-6_40

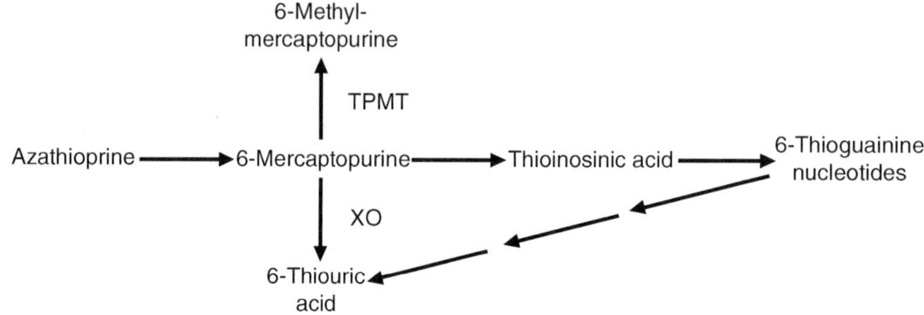

Fig. 40.1 Metabolism of azathioprine. *TMPT* thiopurine methyltransferase, *HPRT* hypoxanthine phosphoribosyl transferase, *XO* xanthine oxidase. Reproduced from Chan GL, Erdmann GR, Gruber SA, et al. Azathioprine metabolism: Pharmacokinetics of 6MP, 6-thiouric acid and 6-thioguanine nucleotides in renal transplant patients. J Clin Pharmacol 1990;30:358–63. (Copyright 1960 by SAGE Publications, Reprinted with Permission by SAGE Publications)

myelosuppression in patients who completely lack TPMT activity, it is prudent to check a TPMT genotype or phenotype (i.e., activity level) prior to beginning AZA or 6MP. For patients with normal genotype or activity level, it is reasonable to start 2–2.5 mg/kg body weight daily of AZA or 1.0–1.25 mg/kg daily of 6MP. For patients with heterozygous genotype or intermediate activity level, the recommended starting dose is 1–1.25 mg/kg daily for AZA and 0.5 mg/kg daily for 6MP. Beginning patients on low doses (e.g., 50 mg daily) of AZA to reduce toxicity, and then slowly increasing this dose over several weeks, is not consistent with the pharmacology, in that dose-dependent toxicity (such as bone marrow suppression) will be delayed, but not prevented, and idiosyncratic reactions (e.g., drug fever, pancreatitis, arthralgia, rash) will not be prevented [11].

Assays for 6-TGN and 6-MMP metabolites are commercially available. 6-TGN levels greater than 235–250 pmol/8 × 10 (8) erythrocytes and 6-MMP levels greater than 5700 pmol/8 × 10(8) erythrocytes have been correlated with therapeutic response and hepatotoxicity, respectively [19, 20]. Routine measurement of TPMT activity level or genotype often helps determine the correct starting dose of AZA or 6MP, and likely limits the utility of universal measurement of 6-TGN metabolites. Nonresponders may have high or low 6-TGN levels [19] and there is scant safety data above 2.5 mg/kg/day of thiopurine in inflammatory bowel disease (IBD). A meta-analysis of 12 studies examining the use of 6-TGN metabolite levels in IBD showed that median 6-TGN levels were 66 pmol/8 × 10(8) red blood cells higher among responders than nonresponders, but there was significant heterogeneity [21]. Patients with levels above a threshold of 230–260 pmol/8 × 10(8) erythrocytes had a remission rate of 62 %, while those with levels below the threshold had a remission rate of 36 %. However, a prospective randomized controlled trial was unable to show that a strategy of adjusting AZA dose according to 6-TGN concentrations was superior to standard weight-based AZA dosing among patients with Crohn's disease who had normal TPMT levels [22]. Patients with and without hepatoxicity may have high 6-MMP levels; however, elevation in alanine aminotransferase (ALT) in patients without other liver disease on AZA often warrants decreasing the dose of AZA and following the ALT level. The 6-TGN and 6-MMP levels may have the most clinical utility in assessing patients with no or incomplete response, when patient noncompliance is suspected, and in the 10 % of patients who are TPMT heterozygotes.

Allopurinol competes with xanthine oxidase, increases levels of 6TGN, and shunts metabolism away from the production of 6MMP, which is a metabolite associated with hepatoxicity [23]. The addition of allopurinol may correct an unfavorable ratio of 6-TGN to 6MMP by reducing 6MMP concentrations while raising 6-TGN concentrations [24]. The addition of allopurinol to AZA, and subsequent substantial dose reduction of AZA, has been suggested in patients with hepatoxicity [23, 25], arthralgias, or nausea [26]. However, this strategy is controversial, and in some experiences has been associated with high rates of opportunistic infections [27] despite small prospective studies showing the safety of long-term use [25, 28]. Selected use of thioguanine as a therapy has been shown to be associated with early hepatic nodular hyperplasia disease of the liver [29], and is not used in our clinical practice.

Efficacy Estimates for Induction and Maintenance Therapy

The efficacy of AZA has been shown to depend on the state of ulcerative colitis activity (i.e., whether the disease is active or in remission), and the relatively small clinical trials have examined the separate issues of its use as an adjunct or alternative to steroids and/or 5-ASA therapy in these disease states. Two systematic reviews of the efficacy of AZA in ulcerative colitis concluded that the use of AZA was of modest benefit in ulcerative colitis, with pooled odds ratios ranging from 1.4 to 2.6 depending on the particular outcome studied [30, 31].

However, one could argue that the individual studies upon which these pooled analyses have been based have been heterogeneous with respect to disease activity, outcome measures, blinding of patients and investigators, controls (placebo vs. 5-ASA), and lengths of follow-up, precluding our ability to synthesize an average result across all of the trials and make an overall conclusion in either direction [32].

Overall, AZA has had mixed results in trials examining its efficacy as an induction agent in active ulcerative colitis. Controlled trials by Jewell and colleagues and Caprilli et al. in the 1970s were among the first to show that AZA was not superior to placebo as an adjunct to corticosteroids or an alternative to sulfasalazine in the treatment of active ulcerative colitis over 1–3 months [5, 6]. In 2000, Sood and colleagues examined AZA as an adjunct to starting sulfasalazine and steroids in severe relapsing ulcerative colitis. There was not a significant difference in achieving remission among the two groups over a year [33]. In 2006, Ardizzone and colleagues showed AZA to be more effective than 5-aminosalicylic acid (3200 mg daily) in attaining steroid-free remission in steroid-dependent ulcerative colitis (53 % vs. 21 %, $p=.006$); however, the patients were not blinded to the type of therapy [34]. Nonetheless, remission was defined both on clinical and endoscopic disease activity, and AZA was superior to placebo in both per-protocol and intention-to-treat analyses [34].

Controlled trials of AZA for the maintenance of remission in steroid-dependent ulcerative colitis have been more promising, but have still shown mixed results. Jewell and colleagues showed no significant difference in remission rates between AZA (1.5–2.5 mg/kg/day) and placebo (40 % and 23 %, respectively ($p=.18$)) among 80 patients over 11 months, where relapse was defined as recurrent blood in the stool and endoscopic evidence of inflammation [5]. A controlled withdrawal trial by Hawthorne et al. in 1992 again showed no significant difference between AZA and placebo as an adjunctive therapy for chronically active ulcerative colitis over 12 months [35]. However, the relapse rates among patients in remission after a year of AZA or placebo were 36 % and 59 %, respectively, and this small trial of 79 patients may have been under-powered [35]. In 2002, Sood and colleagues showed that the addition of AZA to steroids and sulfasalazine in 35 newly diagnosed patients with severe CUC was superior to the addition of placebo in maintaining remission over a year [36]. Rates of relapse were 24 % and 56 % with adjunct AZA and placebo, respectively [36]. In a small open-label study ($n=25$), Sood et al. did not show a difference in remission rates with severe ulcerative colitis [37]. The discontinuation of AZA in patients in steroid-free remission has been associated with high rates of relapse in a long-term retrospective analysis [38]. The proportion of relapsing patients at 1 year, 2 years and 5 years was one third, one half, and two thirds, respectively [38]. A 2012 Cochrane meta-analysis of the effectiveness of thiopurines for maintaining remission in ulcerative colitis examined 6 studies including 286 patients with ulcerative colitis suggested 32 % and 47 % risk reductions in failure to maintain remission with AZA and 6MP, respectively [39].

Safety and Monitoring

Thiopurine therapies in inflammatory bowel disease (IBD) have the potential for significant adverse reactions. Thorough patient education prior to initiating therapy is advised for clinicians initiating or continuing these medications. There are several classes of adverse reactions: dose-dependent, dose-independent, infection risk, and malignancy risk.

Myelosuppression is a dose-dependent adverse reaction that may occur both early and late in AZA therapy [40, 41]. By testing for TPMT activity level or genotype, the 0.3 % of patients without any TPMT activity should be prevented from receiving AZA or 6MP, which for them could cause rapid development of life-threatening cytopenia. For patients with normal and intermediate TPMT activity, frequent monitoring of complete blood counts (CBC) and liver transaminase and alkaline phosphatase is recommended. A genetic analysis of patients with myelosuppression on AZA therapy showed that only 27 % carried mutant alleles [42]. Mesalamine-containing medications may potentiate myelosuppression [43]; however, dose reductions or changes in monitoring are not typically needed. A recent large retrospective cohort study showed that severe neutropenia and thrombocytopenia occur most often in the first 8 weeks of therapy [41]; however, myelosuppression has been shown to occur even a decade after starting therapy [40]. An example of monitoring would be to check a complete blood count at baseline, then weekly for a month, biweekly for 2 months, and then monthly for the first year of therapy. Provided that cell counts have been stable, one could consider decreasing the frequency of CBC monitoring to once every 3 months after the first year. Alanine aminotransferase and alkaline phosphatase may be checked at baseline, 4 weeks, and then every 3 months if normal. Increasing mean corpuscular volume is correlated with increasing 6-TGN concentration and may be an inexpensive alternative to metabolite monitoring [44]. Leukopenia warrants stopping the medication for 2 weeks and restarting at a lower dose once leukopenia has resolved, whereas borderline leukopenia may be an indication of more frequent monitoring. Even mild elevations in hepatic enzymes are concerning, and if other etiologies are excluded, warrant discontinuing the medication due to risks in the long term of progressive liver disease such fibrosis and nodular hyperplasia. Approximately 25 % of patients may have resolution of mild elevations of transaminases after changing from AZA to 6MP [45].

Dose-independent adverse reactions to AZA include drug fever, pancreatitis, hair loss, arthralgias, and nausea and rash [11]. Drug fever typically presents within 2 weeks of starting therapy, and requires immediate cessation of the thiopurine. The risk of pancreatitis in AZA therapy is approximately 3 %, and also typically occurs within the first 2 weeks of therapy and requires cessation of therapy as well [46, 47]. AZA-associated pancreatitis is most often mild, but can be severe [47]. After either high drug fever or pancreatitis, it is not recommended to change from AZA to 6MP or 6MP to AZA. However, 6MP may be tolerated in 60 % of patients who develop other intolerances such as flu-like illness, nausea, vomiting, and rash while on AZA [45].

Infection is of significant concern in patients with ulcerative colitis taking AZA or 6MP. Patients taking AZA for ulcerative colitis are at an increased risk of opportunistic infections [48]. Increased risk of tuberculosis is not limited to biologic therapy—a large retrospective cohort study of patients in the UK General Practice Research Database treated prior to the era of biologic therapy showed a greater than twofold unadjusted relative risk of active tuberculosis in patients with IBD compared to the general population, although this may have been confounded by cigarette smoking and corticosteroid use [49]. The potential risks of AZA or 6MP must be balanced against the risks of either long-term corticosteroid use, which has been associated with infection and increased mortality risk [50], or severe disease activity with its risk of toxic mega-colon and septicemia. Although often overlooked in clinical practice, vaccination for influenza virus and *Streptococcus pneumoniae* are recommended for IBD patients considering or taking AZA or 6MP [51]. Live vaccines in immunosuppressed patients are generally contraindicated; however, varicella zoster vaccination may be considered in patients taking less than 3 mg/kg body weight daily of AZA [52]. Reactivation of latent hepatitis B virus is a risk for patients treated with AZA, and hepatitis B surface antigen should be checked prior to initiating therapy for patients with any risk factors for the disease [52].

Thiopurine therapy in IBD carries an increased risk of lymphoma. A meta-analysis by Kandiel et al. in 2005 of five single-center studies and one population-based study, totaling 3891 patients, showed a relative risk of 4.18 for lymphoma with patients treated with thiopurines for IBD compared to the general population [53]. Of note, the "number-needed-to harm" varied from 4357 in 20–29-year-olds to 355 in 70–79-year-olds [53]. A meta-analysis of patients taking anti-tumor necrosis factor (TNF) therapy and AZA showed 13 cases of non-Hodgkin's lymphoma among 8905 patients with 21,178 years of follow-up (6.1 cases per 10,000 patient-years, median follow-up of 48–201 weeks) where most patients had previous immunomodulator exposure [54]. The recent results from the CESAME study group in France followed 19,486 patients with a median follow-up of 35 months (IQR, 29–40 months) [55]. The adjusted hazard ratio for lymphoma in patients treated with thiopurines for IBD compared to those without was 5.28 (95 % CI, 2.01–13.9). Incidence rates of lymphoma in patients continuing thiopurine varied from 0.37 cases per 1000 person-years in patients less than 50 years old, 2.58 per 1000 in those 50–65 years, and 5.4 per 1000 in patients greater than 65 years old [55]. The most recently published meta-analysis of lymphoma risk in IBD patients treated with thiopurines estimated an almost threefold elevation in lymphoma risk in population-based studies; current use but not previous use was associated with elevated risk [56].

There are conflicting data as to whether there is a constant or cumulative risk of lymphoma with AZA therapy; in study of 4734 US military veterans with ulcerative colitis who were treated with a thiopurine, the risk of lymphoma rose considerably during the fourth year of thiopurine therapy, but decreased rapidly after cessation of thiopurines [57]. However, in the French study there were the same number of lymphomas reported in the first and third year of the study, and in the post-transplant setting the risk of post-transplant lymphoma has been shown to be constant given a constant dose of immunosuppression [55]. Most lymphomas associated with immunosuppression are Epstein–Barr virus (EBV)-positive, as was shown in a referral-based study from Mayo Clinic [58]. Of note, there were two cases of fatal post-mononucleosis lymphoproliferative disorder in EBV-negative patients in the CESAME cohort [55], and further research is merited into whether AZA should be avoided in these patients. There have been scattered cases of fatal hepatosplenic T-cell lymphoma in almost exclusively young male patients taking the combination of AZA/6MP and anti-TNF therapy for IBD [59]. The absolute risk of hepatosplenic T cell lymphoma in young men on combination therapy has been estimated to be approximately 1 in 3500 [60] There is an increased risk of non-melanoma skin cancers in patients on AZA therapy [61, 62], with an absolute risk increase of 14 % (adjusted OR 4.27; 95 % CI 2.08–5.29) among patients taking thiopurines for greater than 1 year [61]. Sunscreen and regular skin exams are recommended for patients on AZA therapy.

The uncertainty of risks of AZA for ulcerative colitis during pregnancy is a challenge for clinicians and patients. Women with ulcerative colitis who plan to become pregnant seek medical care to help them reach their goals of healthy pregnancies and healthy children. Active ulcerative colitis during conception and pregnancy has been associated with an increased risk of adverse perinatal outcomes [63, 64]. A recent study group described the pregnancy outcomes of a cohort of 204 women with IBD followed prospectively in France who were treated with and without thiopurines [65]. Approximately 40 % of the patients were treated with thiopurines as part of their medical regimen, and their pregnancy outcomes were compared to patients who were not receiving them to assess primarily for differences in live births, prematurity, birth weight and congenital abnormalities. All groups had rates of live births in the range of the general population. Furthermore, the overall rates of congenital malformations in patients receiving medication (3.5 %) were not significantly greater than the general population in France. The study was limited by its power to detect only a relatively large (five-fold) relative increase in malformations in the treatment groups. Although there were higher rates of prematurity and low birth weight among all of the patients that are concerning, the severity and impact of these differences on neonatal outcomes is not clear. For example, although many studies have reported preterm deliveries in IBD, most occur after 35 weeks gestation [66, 67]. Larger prospective studies are needed to detect small incremental increase in risks of AZA during pregnancy, such as the ongoing the Pregnancy in Inflammatory Bowel Disease and Neonatal Outcomes (PIANO) registry in the USA [68]. Currently, it is recommended that risks and benefits of AZA be discussed in order to enable patients to make an informed decision regarding its use during pregnancy; however, there is not sufficient evidence to recommend discontinuing AZA for patients in whom it is indicated.

Summary and Future Directions

Thiopurines are effective medications for many patients with ulcerative colitis. Genetic variation in the population leading to variable metabolism of AZA or 6MP warrants initial and ongoing laboratory monitoring throughout the course of treatment for dose-dependent toxicities. Dose-independent toxicity often occurs in the first few weeks of therapy, and some reactions may be avoided by switching from AZA to 6MP. Infections are a primary risk of therapy which merit vaccination prior to therapy, checking for latent disease, and close monitoring for signs of infection. There is an elevated relative risk of lymphoma during therapy; however, the absolute risk is relatively low. Ongoing clinical trials may show if the combination of AZA and biologic therapy is more effective in ulcerative colitis than either therapy alone, as has been shown in the case of Crohn's disease [69].

References

1. Dearing WH, Brown PW. Experiences with cortisone and ACTH in chronic ulcerative colitis. Proc Staff Meet Mayo Clin. 1950;25: 486–8.
2. Truelove SC, Witts LJ. Cortisone in ulcerative colitis; final report on a therapeutic trial. Br Med J. 1955;2:1041–8.
3. Lennard-Jones JE, Misiewicz JJ, Connell AM, Baron JH, Jones FA. Prednisone as maintenance treatment for ulcerative colitis in remission. Lancet. 1965;1:188–9.
4. Bowen GE, Irons Jr GV, Rhodes JB, Kirsner JB. Early experiences with azathioprine in ulcerative colitis; a note of caution. JAMA. 1966;195:460–4.
5. Jewell DP, Truelove SC. Azathioprine in ulcerative colitis: final report on controlled therapeutic trial. Br Med J. 1974;4:627–30.
6. Caprilli R, Carratu R, Babbini M. Double-blind comparison of the effectiveness of azathioprine and sulfasalazine in idiopathic proctocolitis. Preliminary report Am J Dig Dis. 1975;20:115–20.
7. Kirk AP, Lennard-Jones JE. Controlled trial of azathioprine in chronic ulcerative colitis. Br Med J (Clin Res Ed). 1982;284: 1291–2.
8. Rosenberg JL, Wall AJ, Levin B, Binder HJ, Kirsner JB. A controlled trial of azathioprine in the management of chronic ulcerative colitis. Gastroenterology. 1975;69:96–9.
9. Elion G. The comparative metabolism of Imuran and 6-mercaptopurine in man. Proc Am Assoc Cancer Res. 1969;10:21.
10. De Miranda P, Beacham 3rd LM, Creagh TH, Elion GB. The metabolic fate of the methylnitroimidazole moiety of azathioprine in the rat. J Pharmacol Exp Ther. 1973;187:588–601.
11. Sandborn WJ. A review of immune modifier therapy for inflammatory bowel disease: azathioprine, 6-mercaptopurine, cyclosporine, and methotrexate. Am J Gastroenterol. 1996;91:423–33.
12. Lennard L. The clinical pharmacology of 6-mercaptopurine. Eur J Clin Pharmacol. 1992;43:329–39.
13. Weinshilboum RM, Sladek SL. Mercaptopurine pharmacogenetics: monogenic inheritance of erythrocyte thiopurine methyltransferase activity. Am J Hum Genet. 1980;32:651–62.
14. Lennard L, Harrington CI, Wood M, Maddocks JL. Metabolism of azathioprine to 6-thioguanine nucleotides in patients with pemphigus vulgaris. Br J Clin Pharmacol. 1987;23:229–33.
15. Sandborn WJ, Van OEC, Zins BJ, Tremaine WJ, Mays DC, Lipsky JJ. An intravenous loading dose of azathioprine decreases the time to response in patients with Crohn's disease. Gastroenterology. 1995;109:1808–17.
16. Mahadevan U, Tremaine WJ, Johnson T, Pike MG, Mays DC, Lipsky JJ, et al. Intravenous azathioprine in severe ulcerative colitis: a pilot study. Am J Gastroenterol. 2000;95:3463–8.
17. Sandborn WJ, Tremaine WJ, Wolf DC, Targan SR, Sninsky CA, Sutherland LR, et al. Lack of effect of intravenous administration on time to respond to azathioprine for steroid-treated Crohn's disease. North American Azathioprine Study Group. Gastroenterology. 1999;117:527–35.
18. Pearson DC, May GR, Fick GH, Sutherland LR. Azathioprine and 6-mercaptopurine in Crohn disease. A meta-analysis. Ann Intern Med. 1995;123:132–42.
19. Dubinsky MC, Lamothe S, Yang HY, Targan SR, Sinnett D, Theoret Y, et al. Pharmacogenomics and metabolite measurement for 6-mercaptopurine therapy in inflammatory bowel disease. Gastroenterology. 2000;118:705–13.
20. Cuffari C, Hunt S, Bayless T. Utilisation of erythrocyte 6-thioguanine metabolite levels to optimise azathioprine therapy in patients with inflammatory bowel disease. Gut. 2001;48:642–6.
21. Osterman MT, Kundu R, Lichtenstein GR, Lewis JD. Association of 6-thioguanine nucleotide levels and inflammatory bowel disease activity: a meta-analysis. Gastroenterology. 2006;130:1047–53.
22. Reinshagen M, Schutz E, Armstrong VW, Behrens C, von Tirpitz C, Stallmach A, et al. 6-Thioguanine nucleotide-adapted azathioprine therapy does not lead to higher remission rates than standard therapy in chronic active Crohn disease: results from a randomized, controlled, open trial. Clin Chem. 2007;53:1306–14.
23. Sparrow MP, Hande SA, Friedman S, Cao D, Hanauer SB. Effect of allopurinol on clinical outcomes in inflammatory bowel disease nonresponders to azathioprine or 6-mercaptopurine. Clin Gastroenterol Hepatol. 2007;5:209–14.
24. Gardiner SJ, Gearry RB, Burt MJ, Chalmers-Watson T, Chapman BA, Ross AG, et al. Allopurinol might improve response

to azathioprine and 6-mercaptopurine by correcting an unfavorable metabolite ratio. J Gastroenterol Hepatol. 2011;26:49–54.

25. Ansari A, Elliott T, Baburajan B, Mayhead P, O'Donoghue J, Chocair P, et al. Long-term outcome of using allopurinol co-therapy as a strategy for overcoming thiopurine hepatotoxicity in treating inflammatory bowel disease. Aliment Pharmacol Ther. 2008;28: 734–41.
26. Ansari A, Patel N, Sanderson J, O'Donoghue J, Duley JA, Florin TH. Low-dose azathioprine or mercaptopurine in combination with allopurinol can bypass many adverse drug reactions in patients with inflammatory bowel disease. Aliment Pharmacol Ther. 2010;31:640–7.
27. Govani SM, Higgins PD. Combination of thiopurines and allopurinol: adverse events and clinical benefit in IBD. J Crohns Colitis. 2010;4:444–9.
28. Leung Y, Sparrow MP, Schwartz M, Hanauer SB. Long term efficacy and safety of allopurinol and azathioprine or 6-mercaptopurine in patients with inflammatory bowel disease. J Crohns Colitis. 2009;3:162–7.
29. Geller SA, Dubinsky MC, Poordad FF, Vasiliauskas EA, Cohen AH, Abreu MT, et al. Early hepatic nodular hyperplasia and submicroscopic fibrosis associated with 6-thioguanine therapy in inflammatory bowel disease. Am J Surg Pathol. 2004;28:1204–11.
30. Leung Y, Panaccione R, Hemmelgarn B, Jones J. Exposing the weaknesses: a systematic review of azathioprine efficacy in ulcerative colitis. Dig Dis Sci. 2008;53:1455–61.
31. Gisbert JP, Linares PM, McNicholl AG, Mate J, Gomollon F. Meta-analysis: the efficacy of azathioprine and mercaptopurine in ulcerative colitis. Aliment Pharmacol Ther. 2009;30:126–37.
32. Levesque BG, Olkin I. Azathioprine and ulcerative colitis: a "second-look" meta-analysis. Dig Dis Sci. 2010;55:1186–8.
33. Sood A, Midha V, Sood N, Kaushal V. Role of azathioprine in severe ulcerative colitis: one-year, placebo-controlled, randomized trial. Indian J Gastroenterol. 2000;19:14–6.
34. Ardizzone S, Maconi G, Russo A, et al. Randomised controlled trial of azathioprine and 5-aminosalicylic acid for treatment of steroid dependent ulcerative colitis. Gut. 2006;55:47–53.
35. Hawthorne AB, Logan RF, Hawkey CJ, et al. Randomised controlled trial of azathioprine withdrawal in ulcerative colitis. BMJ. 1992;305:20–2.
36. Sood A, Kaushal V, Midha V, Bhatia KL, Sood N, Malhotra V. The beneficial effect of azathioprine on maintenance of remission in severe ulcerative colitis. J Gastroenterol. 2002;37:270–4.
37. Sood A, Midha V, Sood N, Avasthi G. Azathioprine versus sulfasalazine in maintenance of remission in severe ulcerative colitis. Indian J Gastroenterol. 2003;22:79–81.
38. Cassinotti A, Actis GC, Duca P, Massari A, Colombo E, Gai E, et al. Maintenance treatment with azathioprine in ulcerative colitis: outcome and predictive factors after drug withdrawal. Am J Gastroenterol. 2009;104:2760–7.
39. Timmer A, McDonald JW, Tsoulis DJ, Macdonald JK, et al. Azathioprine and 6-mercaptopurine for maintenance of remission in ulcerative colitis. Cochrane Database Syst Rev. 2012;9:CD000478.
40. Connell WR, Kamm MA, Ritchie JK, Lennard-Jones JE. Bone marrow toxicity caused by azathioprine in inflammatory bowel disease: 27 years of experience. Gut. 1993;34:1081–5.
41. Lewis JD, Abramson O, Pascua M, Liu L, Asakura LM, Velayos FS, et al. Timing of myelosuppression during thiopurine therapy for inflammatory bowel disease: implications for monitoring recommendations. Clin Gastroenterol Hepatol. 2009;7:1195–201. quiz 1141–2.
42. Colombel JF, Ferrari N, Debuysere H, Marteau P, Gendre JP, Bonaz B, et al. Genotypic analysis of thiopurine S-methyltransferase in patients with Crohn's disease and severe myelosuppression during azathioprine therapy. Gastroenterology. 2000;118:1025–30.
43. Hande S, Wilson-Rich N, Bousvaros A, Zholudev A, Maurer R, Banks P, et al. 5-Aminosalicylate therapy is associated with higher 6-thioguanine levels in adults and children with inflammatory bowel disease in remission on 6-mercaptopurine or azathioprine. Inflamm Bowel Dis. 2006;12:251–7.
44. Thomas Jr CW, Lowry PW, Franklin CL, Weaver AL, Myhre GM, Mays DC, et al. Erythrocyte mean corpuscular volume as a surrogate marker for 6-thioguanine nucleotide concentration monitoring in patients with inflammatory bowel disease treated with azathioprine or 6-mercaptopurine. Inflamm Bowel Dis. 2003;9:237–45.
45. Lees CW, Maan AK, Hansoti B, Satsangi J, Arnott ID. Tolerability and safety of mercaptopurine in azathioprine-intolerant patients with inflammatory bowel disease. Aliment Pharmacol Ther. 2008;27:220–7.
46. Weersma RK, Peters FT, Oostenbrug LE, van den Berg AP, van Haastert M, Ploeg RJ, et al. Increased incidence of azathioprine-induced pancreatitis in Crohn's disease compared with other diseases. Aliment Pharmacol Ther. 2004;20:843–50.
47. Bermejo F, Lopez-Sanroman A, Taxonera C, Gisbert JP, Perez-Calle JL, Vera I, et al. Acute pancreatitis in inflammatory bowel disease, with special reference to azathioprine-induced pancreatitis. Aliment Pharmacol Ther. 2008;28:623–8.
48. Toruner M, Loftus Jr EV, Harmsen WS, Zinsmeister AR, Orenstein R, Sandborn WJ, et al. Risk factors for opportunistic infections in patients with inflammatory bowel disease. Gastroenterology. 2008;134:929–36.
49. Aberra FN, Stettler N, Brensinger C, Lichtenstein GR, Lewis JD. Risk for active tuberculosis in inflammatory bowel disease patients. Clin Gastroenterol Hepatol. 2007;5:1070–5.
50. Lichtenstein GR, Feagan BG, Cohen RD, Salzberg BA, Diamond RH, Chen DM, et al. Serious infections and mortality in association with therapies for Crohn's disease: TREAT registry. Clin Gastroenterol Hepatol. 2006;4:621–30.
51. Melmed GY, Ippoliti AF, Papadakis KA, Tran TT, Birt JL, Lee SK, et al. Patients with inflammatory bowel disease are at risk for vaccine-preventable illnesses. Am J Gastroenterol. 2006;101: 1834–40.
52. Wasan SK, Baker SE, Skolnik PR, Farraye FA. A practical guide to vaccinating the inflammatory bowel disease patient. Am J Gastroenterol. 2010;105:1231–8.
53. Kandiel A, Fraser AG, Korelitz BI, Brensinger C, Lewis JD. Increased risk of lymphoma among inflammatory bowel disease patients treated with azathioprine and 6-mercaptopurine. Gut. 2005;54:1121–5.
54. Siegel CA, Marden SM, Persing SM, Larson RJ, Sands BE. Risk of lymphoma associated with combination anti-tumor necrosis factor and immunomodulator therapy for the treatment of Crohn's disease: a meta-analysis. Clin Gastroenterol Hepatol. 2009;7:874–81.
55. Beaugerie L, Brousse N, Bouvier AM, Colombel JF, Lemann M, Cosnes J, et al. Lymphoproliferative disorders in patients receiving thiopurines for inflammatory bowel disease: a prospective observational cohort study. Lancet. 2009;374:1617–25.
56. Kotlyar DS, Lewis JD, Beaugerie L, Tierney A, Brensinger CM, Gisbert JP, et al. Risk of lymphoma in patients with inflammatory bowel disease treated with azathioprine and 6-mercaptopurine: a meta-analysis. Clin Gastroenterol Hepatol. 2015;13:847–58.e4. quiz e48–50.
57. Khan N, Abbas AM, Lichtenstein GR, Loftus Jr EV, Bazzano LA. Risk of lymphoma in patients with ulcerative colitis treated with thiopurines: a nationwide retrospective cohort study. Gastroenterology. 2013;145:1007–15.e3.
58. Dayharsh GA, Loftus Jr EV, Sandborn WJ, Tremaine WJ, Zinsmeister AR, Witzig TE, et al. Epstein-Barr virus-positive lymphoma in patients with inflammatory bowel disease treated with azathioprine or 6-mercaptopurine. Gastroenterology. 2002;122:72–7.

59. Mackey AC, Green L, Liang LC, Dinndorf P, Avigan M. Hepatosplenic T cell lymphoma associated with infliximab use in young patients treated for inflammatory bowel disease. J Pediatr Gastroenterol Nutr. 2007;44:265–7.
60. Kotlyar DS, Osterman MT, Diamond RH, Porter D, Blonski WC, Wasik M, et al. A systematic review of factors that contribute to hepatosplenic T-cell lymphoma in patients with inflammatory bowel disease. Clin Gastroenterol Hepatol. 2011;9:36–41.e1.
61. Long MD, Herfarth HH, Pipkin CA, Porter CQ, Sandler RS, Kappelman MD. Increased risk for non-melanoma skin cancer in patients with inflammatory bowel disease. Clin Gastroenterol Hepatol. 2010;8:268–74.
62. Long MD, Kappelman MD, Pipkin CA. Nonmelanoma skin cancer in inflammatory bowel disease: a review. Inflamm Bowel Dis. 2011;17(6):1423–7.
63. Baiocco PJ, Korelitz BI. The influence of inflammatory bowel disease and its treatment on pregnancy and fetal outcome. J Clin Gastroenterol. 1984;6:211–6.
64. Bush MC, Patel S, Lapinski RH, Stone JL. Perinatal outcomes in inflammatory bowel disease. J Matern Fetal Neonatal Med. 2004;15:237–41.
65. Coelho J, Beaugerie L, Colombel JF, Hebuterne X, Lerebours E, Lemann M, et al. Pregnancy outcome in patients with inflammatory bowel disease treated with thiopurines: cohort from the CESAME Study. Gut. 2011;60:198–203.
66. Dominitz JA, Young JC, Boyko EJ. Outcomes of infants born to mothers with inflammatory bowel disease: a population-based cohort study. Am J Gastroenterol. 2002;97:641–8.
67. Nguyen GC, Boudreau H, Harris ML, Maxwell CV. Outcomes of obstetric hospitalizations among women with inflammatory bowel disease in the United States. Clin Gastroenterol Hepatol. 2009;7:329–34.
68. Mahadevan U, Martin CF, Sandler RS, Kane SV, Dubinsky M, Lewis JD, et al. A multi-center national prospective study of pregnancy and neonatal outcomes in women with inflammatory bowel disease exposed to immunomodulators and biologic therapy. Gastroenterology. 2009;136:A-88.
69. Colombel JF, Sandborn WJ, Reinisch W, Mantzaris GJ, Kornbluth A, Rachmilewitz D, et al. Infliximab, azathioprine, or combination therapy for Crohn's disease. N Engl J Med. 2010;362:1383–95.

Calcineurin Inhibitors in Ulcerative Colitis

41

Andreas Fischer and Daniel C. Baumgart

Cyclosporine for the Induction of Remission in Ulcerative Colitis

When Cyclosporine A (CsA) was introduced in the early 1980s, it marked a turning point in transplantation medicine. For the first time, a potent T-cell selective agent was available that lacked myelotoxic effects (a major limitation of azathioprine in the pre-CsA era), thereby not just improving survival of renal allografts,but also allowing for the successful establishment of immunosuppressive protocols in heart, lung, and liver transplantation [1]. Originally isolated in the Sandoz-Labs in Basel in the early 1970s from soil samples containing the fungus *Tolypocladium inflatum*, CsA acts by binding to the peptidyl-prolyl cis–trans isomerase cyclophilin A (CpA). The CpA-CsA complex then inhibits calcineurin, a serine/threonine phosphatase that dephosphorylates transcription factors of the NFAT (nuclear factor of activated T cells) family, thereby enabling their translocation to the nucleus [2]. As NFATs control the production of interleukin-2 and other cytokines and co-stimulatory molecules necessary for the growth and differentiation of T-cells [3, 4], calcineurin inhibition results in a profound suppression of T-cell activation.

A first report on the successful use of CsA in a patient with ulcerative colitis was published as early as 1984 [5]. Six years later, Lichtiger and Present published the results of a prospective uncontrolled trial investigating the efficacy of intravenous CsA in 15 patients with severe ulcerative colitis refractory to corticosteroids, which led to clinical response in 73 % of patients, thus enabling them to avoid imminent colectomy [6]. Based on these results, a prospective randomized double-blind controlled trial comparing intravenous CsA to placebo in severe ulcerative colitis refractory to corticosteroids was initiated at the Mt. Sinai Hospital in New York and the University of Chicago Hospital, that resulted in the seminal publication of Lichtiger et al. in 1994. In this report, 9 out of 11 patients (82 %) receiving CsA displayed a clinical response to therapy within a mean of 7 days as compared to 0 out of 9 patients receiving placebo, 5 of which later received open-label CsA and reached clinical response [7].

Given these impressive results that were later confirmed in a number of open-label observational studies [8–11], the trial was terminated early and CsA became the first pharmaceutical agent with proven efficacy in acute severe steroid-refractory colitis. Of note, a randomized double-blind placebo controlled trial investigated the efficacy of intravenous CsA as a "stand-alone" agent for severe ulcerative colitis as compared with traditional corticosteroid therapy and found response rates of 64 % in the CsA arm as compared to 53 % in the methylprednisolone arm ($p=0.4$) [12]. Thus, monotherapy with CsA might pose a rescue option for those patients with acute severe ulcerative colitis, in which intravenous corticosteroid treatment is precluded by factors such as susceptibility to steroid psychosis or uncontrolled hypertension.

Whereas early studies employed an initial daily CsA dose of 4 mg/kg, a subsequent double-blind placebo controlled randomized trial compared the efficacy of "high dose" CsA with a lower dosing schedule starting with 2 mg/kg and aiming for stable blood concentrations between 150 and 250 ng/ml. No differences were found between both arms with response rates of 84 % vs. 85 % after 8 days of treatment [13], suggesting that lower doses of CsA are equally effective and consequently, a starting dose of 2 mg/kg has become the standard of care. However, even with low dose CsA, adverse events are common, with impaired renal function, hypertension, headache, paresthesia, myalgia, tremor, and gingival hyperplasia being the most frequently reported side effects affecting up to a third of patients [7–10, 12, 13]. It is

A. Fischer (✉) • D.C. Baumgart
Department of Gastroenterology and Hepatology, Inflammatory Bowel Disease Center, Charité Medical Center—Virchow Hospital, Medical School of the Humboldt University of Berlin, 13344 Berlin, Germany
e-mail: andi.fischer@charite.de

D.C. Baumgart (ed.), *Crohn's Disease and Ulcerative Colitis*, DOI 10.1007/978-3-319-33703-6_41

important to correct low blood magnesium levels before initiation of intravenous CsA therapy as the risk of neurotoxicity and nephrotoxicity is increased when hypomagnesaemia is present [14, 15]. As CsA itself can lead to reduced magnesium reabsorption, frequent monitoring of blood magnesium levels is advised during CsA therapy [15]. In addition, caution should be exercised in patients with serum cholesterol levels <100 mg/dl as neurotoxicity is increased under these conditions [16].

Role of Cyclosporine in the Maintenance of Remission

Generally, patients responding to intravenous CsA will be switched to an oral formulation of the drug (typically 5–8 mg/kg divided in two doses, aiming at whole blood trough levels between 100 and 200 ng/ml) for about 3 months, after which therapy should be discontinued due to the risk of irreversible nephrotoxicity [17]. Long-term follow-up studies have made it clear, however, that the majority of patients who initially avoided colectomy will eventually require surgery when treated with CsA alone. For example, Cheifetz et al. reported on the outcome of 60 patients, who initially responded to intravenous CsA and were then switched to oral CsA for 6 months. Within a mean follow-up of 3 years, 76 % of patients receiving no concomitant immunosuppression had to undergo colectomy, whereas only 1 out of 24 patients (4 %) in which 6-mercaptopurine (6-MP) was started shortly after hospital discharge required colectomy [18].

Similarly, in a retrospective cohort study from the University of Chicago, 80 % of initial CsA responders who went on to receive 6-MP or azathioprine avoided colectomy during a 5-year follow-up period whereas 45 % of patients not receiving thiopurine-based immunosuppression ultimately required surgery [9]. The positive impact of a maintenance therapy with purine analogues was furthermore confirmed in a recent observational trial, in which azathioprine use displayed a highly significant association with long term remission and the avoidance of colectomy in CsA responders followed for at least 5 years [19].

Based on these data, treatment with an oral formulation of the drug in responders to intravenous CsA is regarded as a bridging therapy until thiopurine immunosuppressants become effective. Consequently, rescue therapy with CsA appears to be of little use when there are contraindications against maintenance therapy with azathioprine or 6-MP. In line with this, rescue therapy with CsA was demonstrated to be less effective in the long term when previous maintenance therapy with 6-MP or azathioprine had failed, which was illustrated in an observational cohort study that reported a colectomy rate of 88 % within 1 year for patients in which CsA was started after failure of maintenance therapy with purine analogues as compared to 52 % of patients receiving de novo azathioprine with CsA [10]. As a significant proportion of patients treated with cyclosporine will thus require a colectomy later on, the potential impact of this therapy on postoperative complications is an important issue. In this respect, two retrospective cohort studies did not find a significant increase in infectious or noninfectious postoperative complications [20, 21].

When initiating thiopurine maintenance treatment, great caution has to be paid during the time when patients are on a triple immunosuppressive therapy consisting of steroids, CsA, and azathioprine/6-MP as the risk for serious infection is severely increased. This is highlighted by the data published by Arts et al., reporting three deaths from opportunistic infections (one from *Pneumocystis jirovecii* pneumonia, two from *Aspergillus fumigatus* pneumonia) among patients receiving triple combined immunosuppressive treatment [22] as well as a Belgian cohort study, in which 3 out of 118 patients receiving CsA died, again from *Pneumocystis* pneumonia and systemic aspergillosis [10]. Consequently, it is advised that patients treated with combined immunosuppression should receive prophylaxis against *pneumocystis jirovecii* pneumonia with co-trimoxazole [23]. Whether novel agents like the $\alpha_4\beta_7$-antagonist vedolizumab will expand the therapeutic options for the maintenance of remission after induction with CsA remains to be established in clinical trials.

Tacrolimus for the Induction of Remission in Ulcerative Colitis

As a consequence of the various toxicities associated with the use of cyclosporine, an intense search for novel immunosuppressants began which in 1984 led to the discovery of a macrolide produced by *Streptomyces tsukubaensis* that was initially termed FK-506 and later renamed into tacrolimus (for tsukuba macrolide immunosuppressant; Fig. 41.1) [24]. Similar to cyclosporine, tacrolimus acts by inhibiting calcineurin, although it does not bind to cyclophilin A, but a protein termed FKBP (for FK binding protein) [25]. In addition, tacrolimus was demonstrated to suppress the production of proinflammatory cytokines in activated macrophages and promote their apoptosis [26]. The immunosuppressive potency of tacrolimus vastly exceeds that of cyclosporine [24, 27] and the compound has been approved for the prevention of allograft rejection in patients undergoing kidney or liver transplantation.

First evidence for a potential role of tacrolimus in the treatment of ulcerative colitis came from animal models of IBD, where the drug not just attenuated inflammation but also extraintestinal manifestations [28–31]. As a result, its use in ulcerative colitis was investigated in a number of uncontrolled case series employing 7–40 patients and

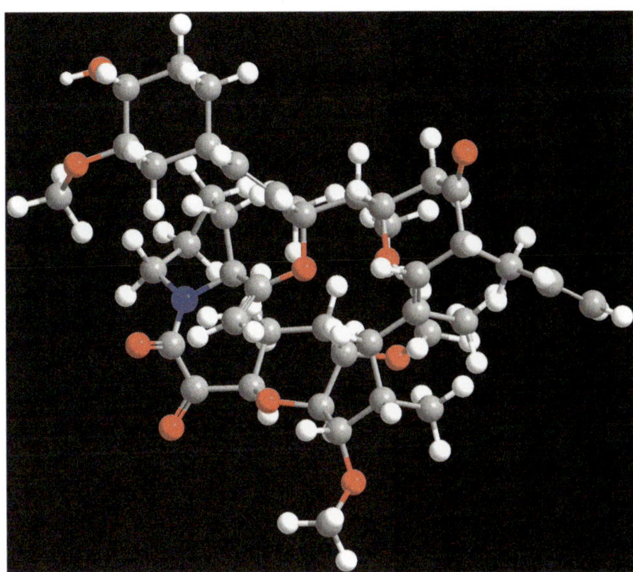

Fig. 41.1 Structure of tacrolimus

reporting response rates between 60 % and 96 % and remission rates between 34 % and 74 % [32–36]. In 2006, a first double-blind randomized controlled trial comparing two arms with low (5–10 ng/ml) and high (10–15 ng/ml) tacrolimus trough levels to placebo in a total of 60 patients with moderately or severely active ulcerative colitis was published [37]. As opposed to the pivotal initial trials with cyclosporine, the majority of patients in this study was not refractory to corticosteroid treatment, but mostly had a steroid-dependent course of disease. Clinical response was observed in 68 % and 38 % of patients in the high and low dose group, respectively, as compared to 10 % in the placebo group within 2 weeks of therapy. Although statistical significance was not attained in the low trough level group and the study has been criticized for the inclusion of patients with less severe disease [38], this trial provided the first data on the short-term efficacy of tacrolimus in a double-blind randomized design.

Following up on these results, the same group later on conducted a second double-blind placebo-controlled trial in 62 patients with steroid-dependent or -refractory ulcerative colitis aiming for tacrolimus trough levels between 10 and 15 ng/ml. Clinical response was seen 50 % in the tacrolimus group as compared to 13 % in the placebo group ($p=0.003$) [39]. Importantly, this trial also reported rates for mucosal healing, demonstrating superiority of tacrolimus (44 %) over placebo (13 %). Again, patients investigated clearly suffered from less severe disease as compared to those in the earlier cyclosporine trials which is also evidenced by the fact that none of the patients in either the tacrolimus or placebo group underwent colectomy during a 12 week open label extension. There are, however, observational trials that selectively addressed the impact of tacrolimus as a rescue therapy in truly steroid-refractory patients yielding response rates broadly comparable to those seen with CsA [33–35], suggesting tacrolimus as a viable alternative to CsA in these situations.

Taken together, evidence from randomized controlled trials as well as numerous case series summarized in Table 41.1 suggests that tacrolimus is effective in the induction of remission in both moderate and severe ulcerative colitis. Initiating therapy with oral administration of the drug (0.1 mg/kg/day divided in two doses) appears to be equally effective as compared to continuous infusion at least in patients with less severe disease and whereas target trough levels between 10 and 15 ng/ml are supported by both randomized controlled trials, various case series suggest that aiming for lower serum concentrations (5–10 ng/ml) might be sufficient, especially once remission has been reached. Target levels with oral administration of tacrolimus will be met more rapidly when patients are fasting as the rate and extent of tacrolimus absorption is significantly decreased in the presence of food [44, 45].

As tacrolimus is metabolized via the cytochrome P-450 (CYP) enzymes 3A4 and 3A5, polymorphisms in the genes encoding for these proteins might have an additional impact on whole blood trough levels and therapeutic efficacy of the drug. A Japanese cohort study found that CYP3A5 non-expressers were significantly more likely to reach optimal trough levels on days 2–5 of therapy and displayed significantly higher remission rates as compared to patients expressing CYP3A5 [46]. Of note, the frequency of CYP3A5 non-expressers is much higher in Caucasians as compared to Asians [47] and an impact of CYP3A5 polymorphisms on tacrolimus response could not be replicated in a cohort of German patients [43]. The latter report, however, identified three alleles of the ABCB1 gene encoding for the drug efflux pump P-glycoprotein that were associated with significantly higher short-term remission rates [43].

Adverse effects in studies investigating tacrolimus for the induction of remission affected up to 50 % of patients and most frequently included an increase in serum creatinine, tremor, paraesthesia, and hypertension, but were generally mild and seldom required cessation of therapy [34, 37, 40, 48]. Special caution, however, is advised with respect to potential drug interactions, e.g., with macrolide antibiotics, antiepileptic and antifungal drugs as well as antiretroviral medication [49].

Role of Tacrolimus in the Maintenance of Remission

In contrast to CsA, long-term treatment with tacrolimus appears to be justifiable under safety considerations. Data assessing a potential role of tacrolimus in the maintenance of remission are, however, sparse and no randomized controlled

Table 41.1 Studies investigating the role of tacrolimus in the induction of remission in adult patients with ulcerative colitis

Reference	Year	Trial design	*n*	Disease severity	Route	Starting dose (mg/kg/day)	Trough level (ng/ml)	Response rate (%)	Remission rate (%)	Colectomy rate (%)
Fellermann et al. [40]	1998	Retrospective	7	Severe	i.v.	0.01–0.02	8.7–16	83	67	17
Fellermann et al. [33]	2002	Retrospective	38	Severe	i.v. or p.o.	0.01–0.02 (i.v.) 0.1–0.2 (p.o.)	9–13	60	34	8
Högenauer et al. [35]	2003	Retrospective	9	Moderate to severe	p.o.	0.15	13	89	67	11
Baumgart et al. [34]	2003	Retrospective	23	Severe	p.o.	0.1	4–6	96	74	4
Ogata et al. [37]	2006	RCT	19	Moderate to severe	p.o.	0.1	10–15	68.4	20	0
Ogata et al. [37]	2006	RCT	21	Moderate to severe	p.o.	0.1	5–10	38.1	11	0
Baumgart et al. [36]	2006	Retrospective	40	Severe	p.o.	0.1	4–8	78	45	NR
Ng et al. [41]	2007	Retrospective	6	Moderate to severe	p.o.	0.1	5–10	67	50	0
Yamamoto et al. [42]	2008	Retrospective	27	NR	p.o.	0.1	10–15	78	70	0
Herrlinger et al. [43]	2011	Retrospective	84	NR	i.v. or p.o.	0.1–0.2	10	75	61	25
Ogata et al.	2012	RCT	32	Moderate to severe	p.o.	2–5 mg/day	10–15	50	9	0
Schmidt et al.	2013	Retrospective	130	Moderate to severe	p.o.	0.1	NR	NR	72	14
Thin et al.	2013	Retrospective	24	Moderate to severe	p.o.	0.1	8–12	50	33	NR
Mizoshita et al.	2013	Retrospective	30	Moderate to severe	p.o.	NR	10–15	46	13	3
Inoue et al.	2013	Retrospective	11	Moderate to severe	p.o.	0.1	10–15	100	73	0
Hirai et al.	2014	Retrospective	40	Moderate to severe	p.o.	0.1	10–15	NR	31	9
Kawakami et al.	2015	Prospective observational	49	Moderate to severe	p.o.	0.1	10–15	90	76	6
Ikeya et al.	2015	Retrospective	44	Moderate to severe	p.o.	0.1	10–15	86	66	16

For studies reporting data on short- and long-term outcome, only results with respect to the induction of remission are given

trials investigating its long-term use have been conducted up to now. Retrospective cohort series reported colectomy-free survival rates between 66 % and 78 % within up to 39 months [33, 36, 42], suggesting that surgery can be avoided or at least delayed in a substantial percentage of patients who achieve remission upon treatment with tacrolimus. However, the majority of patients in these studies received concomitant or subsequent therapy with thiopurines or biologics so that the impact of tacrolimus on the maintenance of remission cannot be directly assessed from these data.

In contrast, a recent retrospective French cohort study reported on the outcome of 21 patients, who were maintained on a tacrolimus monotherapy after induction with this drug. In this challenging group of patients, all of which had failed previous therapies with corticosteroids, immunomodulators, and TNF antagonists, clinical remission was maintained at 52 weeks in 38 %, whereas 29 % displayed clinical failure and 33 % experienced adverse events resulting in cessation of therapy [50]. Remission rates, however, declined to 14 % after 3 years, suggesting that long-term therapy with tacrolimus is unlikely to change the course of disease in patients resistant to other conventional and biological therapies.

Another case series compared the outcome of maintenance treatment with tacrolimus to a cohort receiving purine analogues and found remission rates of 51 % and 59 % after 52 weeks [51]. Again, however, these rates declined to 19 % in the tacrolimus group and 36 % in the thiopurine group after 3 years with even lower rates in patients who previously failed therapy with purine analogues (25 % and 0 % after 1 and 3 years, respectively). Thus, these data suggest that similar to

CsA, tacrolimus is most effective in inducing remission in ulcerative colitis when treatment with corticosteroids has failed, whereas it appears to have limited value in the maintenance of remission. Adverse events were common in studies investigating the long-term use of tacrolimus and tend to affect 40–50 % of patients. Paraesthesia, tremor, infections, headache, and renal impairment, as well as hypertension, leucopenia, and arthralgia, were most frequently reported, leading to cessation of therapy in about 20 % of patients [42, 50–52].

Topical Application of Calcineurin Inhibitors in Ulcerative Colitis

Given the risks associated with systemic immunosuppression in general and the specific toxicities of both CsA and tacrolimus, topical application of these compounds to areas of active inflammation seems to be an appealing approach. A first small open-label case series, in which CsA was administered topically as retention enemas in ulcerative proctitis, reported clinical and sigmoidoscopic improvement in six out of eight patients as early as 1989 [53]. Subsequent uncontrolled studies found response rates between 50 % and 60 % with topical application of CsA in patients with acute severe proctitis, pouchitis, or left-sided colitis [54–56], so that a first randomized double-blind placebo-controlled trial comparing CsA to placebo enemas in a total of 40 patients suffering from mild to moderately active left-sided colitis was initiated. This trial, however, failed to show a significant effect of topically administered cyclosporine within 4 weeks as 40 % in the CsA group improved clinically as opposed to 45 % of patients in the placebo group [57]. Although it has been suggested that more frequent dosing schedules, alternative enema vehicles, or the restriction of topical CsA administration to patients suffering from ulcerative proctitis might be worthwhile to be investigated in future studies, no such trials have been reported up to now, and thus, topical therapy with CsA is currently not supported by prospective evidence.

As for tacrolimus, no randomized controlled trials investigating its topical application have been published up to now. There are, however, data from two small case series suggesting that rectal administration of tacrolimus might have a place in the treatment of ulcerative proctitis. In a first report, six out of eight patients suffering from ulcerative proctitis resistant to oral and topical aminosalicylates, steroids and immunomodulators achieved remission upon 8 weeks of therapy with rectal tacrolimus given at doses between 0.9 and 3 mg twice daily, which produced trough serum levels between undetectable and 7 ng/ml [58]. A second case series described 12 patients with ulcerative proctitis that had failed to respond to local corticosteroids either alone or in combination with topical 5-ASA and were treated with rectal tacrolimus given either as suppositories or enemas at 2–4 mg per day. Ten out of 12 patients (83 %) displayed clinical response to therapy with four patients achieving mucosal healing [59]. Response rates were lower for patients with ulcerative colitis extending beyond 15 cm from the anal verge (three out of five patients equalling 60 %) and no systemic side effects were reported. Interestingly, this study not only included whole blood trough levels (2.5 ng/ml and 0.7 ng/ml in patients receiving enemas or suppositories, respectively), but also assessed tacrolimus concentrations found in mucosal biopsies, which exceeded 100 ng/mg on average.

Another case series furthermore suggested that topical tacrolimus might be an effective treatment option for patients suffering from pouchitis unresponsive to a therapy with ciprofloxacin or metronidazole as all of ten patients treated with tacrolimus retention enemas (4–5 mg per day, given as a single enema) displayed a reduction in their Pouchitis Disease Activity Index (PDAI; mean reduction from 15.9 ± 0.8 to 7.8 ± 0.8 points; $p < 0.01$) with seven out of ten patients achieving clinical remission [60]. Similar to other studies, trough levels between 2.6 and 3.8 ng/ml were reported in this case series resulting from colonic absorption as demonstrated in a study with healthy volunteers [61]. Topical administration appears therefore not a suitable way to prevent systemic tacrolimus exposure.

Other strategies aiming at selectively targeting tacrolimus administration to areas of inflamed mucosa such as entrapment of the drug into nanoparticles or coupling it to pH-sensitive spheres have yielded promising results in animal models, but no data on their clinical use have been published up to now [62–64].

Positioning of Calcineurin Inhibitors in Acute Severe Steroid Refractory Ulcerative Colitis

With the advent of biological therapies, alternative options for the medical management of acute severe ulcerative colitis resistant to corticosteroids emerged. Following a number of uncontrolled case series [65–67], a randomized placebo-controlled trial found that 71 % of patients with severe to moderately severe ulcerative colitis not responding to conventional treatment avoided colectomy within a 90 day period after a single infusion of infliximab (IFX) vs. 33 % in the placebo group, thus establishing efficacy of IFX for the induction of remission in this setting [68].

In a seminal randomized controlled multicenter trial, Laharie et al. compared the ability of IFX and CsA to elicit a treatment response in 115 patients suffering from an acute severe flare of ulcerative colitis that had previously failed a course of high-dose intravenous steroids. Patients were assigned to receive either induction therapy with intravenous CsA followed by oral CsA for 3 months or three infusions of IFX at weeks 0, 2, and 6 and maintenance therapy with azathioprine was started in all patients demonstrating clinical response at day 7. Treatment failure as defined by absence of a clinical response at day 7, a relapse between day 7 and day 98, absence of steroid-free remission at day 98, a severe adverse event leading to treatment interruption, colectomy, or death occurred in 60 % of patient assigned to CsA vs. 54 % treated with IFX, suggesting that both compounds are equally effective in this setting [69]. This notion was later corroborated in a long-term follow-up recently presented in abstract form: In the CsA group, 30 %, 35 %, and 39 % of patients had to undergo colectomy within 1, 2, and 5 years, respectively, whereas 30 %, 32 %, and 35 % of patients initially treated with IFX required surgery within this time frame [70]. A meta-analysis of 6 retrospective cohort studies describing 321 patients receiving infliximab or cyclosporine as rescue therapy in acute severe steroid-refractory similarly concluded that both of these options are comparable in terms of efficacy and the incidence of adverse events [71].

Data directly comparing tacrolimus to IFX have not been published up to now, but considering the efficacy data outlined above, it appears reasonable to assume equivalence of tacrolimus and CsA. Thus, salvage therapies with calcineurin antagonists and infliximab can be regarded as equally effective options in the setting of acute severe steroid resistant ulcerative colitis. Choice of treatment should therefore be guided by physician and center experience and consider patient characteristics and different adverse event profiles associated with both classes of compounds. However, in patients who failed maintenance therapy with purine analogues or are thiopurine intolerant, infliximab should be preferred over calcineurin antagonists for reasons of the marginal long-term remission rates in this group of patients when treated with tacrolimus.

Given the risks and toxicities associated with long-term immunosuppressive treatment as well as the increasing risk of colorectal cancer with the need for regular surveillance colonoscopies in long-standing ulcerative colitis, surgery should also be discussed with every patient presenting with acute severe steroid resistant ulcerative colitis. This is all the more important when previous therapies with both thiopurines and anti-TNF antibodies have failed, as these patients lack a reasonable option for maintenance therapy if remission can be induced by CsA or tacrolimus. Similarly, although sequential salvage therapies with infliximab and calcineurin antagonists in patients who have failed rescue therapy with either of these agents were demonstrated to be successful in the short term in 25–40 % of patients [72–74], these strategies have been associated with considerable morbidity and even mortality as well as uncertain long-term prospects, so that surgery should be strongly considered in this group of patients.

References

1. Kahan BD. Cyclosporine. N Engl J Med. 1989;321(25):1725–38.
2. Bram RJ, Hung DT, Martin PK, Schreiber SL, Crabtree GR. Identification of the immunophilins capable of mediating inhibition of signal transduction by cyclosporin A and FK506: roles of calcineurin binding and cellular location. Mol Cell Biol. 1993;13(8):4760–9.
3. Rao A, Luo C, Hogan PG. Transcription factors of the NFAT family: regulation and function. Annu Rev Immunol. 1997;15:707–47.
4. Shibasaki F, Price ER, Milan D, McKeon F. Role of kinases and the phosphatase calcineurin in the nuclear shuttling of transcription factor NF-AT4. Nature. 1996;382(6589):370–3.
5. Gupta S, Keshavarzian A, Hodgson HJ. Cyclosporin in ulcerative colitis. Lancet. 1984;2(8414):1277–8.
6. Lichtiger S, Present DH. Preliminary report: cyclosporin in treatment of severe active ulcerative colitis. Lancet. 1990;336(8706):16–9.
7. Lichtiger S, Present DH, Kornbluth A, Gelernt I, Bauer J, Galler G, et al. Cyclosporine in severe ulcerative colitis refractory to steroid therapy. N Engl J Med. 1994;330(26):1841–5.
8. Stack WA, Long RG, Hawkey CJ. Short- and long-term outcome of patients treated with cyclosporin for severe acute ulcerative colitis. Aliment Pharmacol Ther. 1998;12(10):973–8.
9. Cohen RD, Stein R, Hanauer SB. Intravenous cyclosporin in ulcerative colitis: a five-year experience. Am J Gastroenterol. 1999;94(6): 1587–92.
10. Moskovitz DN, Van Assche G, Maenhout B, Arts J, Ferrante M, Vermeire S, et al. Incidence of colectomy during long-term follow-up after cyclosporine-induced remission of severe ulcerative colitis. Clin Gastroenterol Hepatol. 2006;4(6):760–5.
11. Kobayashi T, Naganuma M, Okamoto S, Hisamatsu T, Inoue N, Ichikawa H, et al. Rapid endoscopic improvement is important for 1-year avoidance of colectomy but not for the long-term prognosis in cyclosporine A treatment for ulcerative colitis. J Gastroenterol. 2010;45(11):1129–37.
12. D'Haens G, Lemmens L, Geboes K, Vandeputte L, Van Acker F, Mortelmans L, et al. Intravenous cyclosporine versus intravenous corticosteroids as single therapy for severe attacks of ulcerative colitis. Gastroenterology. 2001;120(6):1323–9.
13. Van Assche G, D'Haens G, Noman M, Vermeire S, Hiele M, Asnong K, et al. Randomized, double-blind comparison of 4 mg/kg versus 2 mg/kg intravenous cyclosporine in severe ulcerative colitis. Gastroenterology. 2003;125(4):1025–31.
14. Thompson CB, June CH, Sullivan KM, Thomas ED. Association between cyclosporin neurotoxicity and hypomagnesaemia. Lancet. 1984;2(8412):1116–20.
15. Miura K, Nakatani T, Asai T, Yamanaka S, Tamada S, Tashiro K, et al. Role of hypomagnesemia in chronic cyclosporine nephropathy. Transplantation. 2002;73(3):340–7.
16. de Groen PC, Aksamit AJ, Rakela J, Forbes GS, Krom RA. Central nervous system toxicity after liver transplantation. The role of cyclosporine and cholesterol. N Engl J Med. 1987;317(14):861–6.
17. Durai D, Hawthorne AB. Review article: how and when to use ciclosporin in ulcerative colitis. Aliment Pharmacol Ther. 2005;22(10):907–16.
18. Cheifetz AS, Stern J, Garud S, Goldstein E, Malter L, Moss AC, et al. Cyclosporine is safe and effective in patients with severe ulcerative colitis. J Clin Gastroenterol. 2011;45(2):107–12.
19. Miyake N, Ando T, Ishiguro K, Maeda O, Watanabe O, Hirayama Y, et al. Azathioprine is essential following cyclosporine for patients with steroid-refractory ulcerative colitis. World J Gastroenterol. 2015;21(1):254–61.
20. Nelson R, Liao C, Fichera A, Rubin DT, Pekow J. Rescue therapy with cyclosporine or infliximab is not associated with an increased risk for postoperative complications in patients hospitalized for severe steroid-refractory ulcerative colitis. Inflamm Bowel Dis. 2014;20(1):14–20.

21. Hyde GM, Jewell DP, Kettlewell MG, Mortensen NJ. Cyclosporin for severe ulcerative colitis does not increase the rate of perioperative complications. Dis Colon Rectum. 2001;44(10):1436–40.
22. Arts J, D'Haens G, Zeegers M, Van Assche G, Hiele M, D'Hoore A, et al. Long-term outcome of treatment with intravenous cyclosporin in patients with severe ulcerative colitis. Inflamm Bowel Dis. 2004;10(2):73–8.
23. Rahier JF, Ben-Horin S, Chowers Y, Conlon C, De Munter P, D'Haens G, et al. European evidence-based Consensus on the prevention, diagnosis and management of opportunistic infections in inflammatory bowel disease. J Crohns Colitis. 2009;3(2):47–91.
24. Kino T, Hatanaka H, Hashimoto M, Nishiyama M, Goto T, Okuhara M, et al. FK-506, a novel immunosuppressant isolated from a Streptomyces. I. Fermentation, isolation, and physico-chemical and biological characteristics. J Antibiot (Tokyo). 1987;40(9):1249–55.
25. Sigal NH, Dumont FJ. Cyclosporin A, FK-506, and rapamycin: pharmacologic probes of lymphocyte signal transduction. Annu Rev Immunol. 1992;10:519–60.
26. Yoshino T, Nakase H, Honzawa Y, Matsumura K, Yamamoto S, Takeda Y, et al. Immunosuppressive effects of tacrolimus on macrophages ameliorate experimental colitis. Inflamm Bowel Dis. 2010;16(12):2022–33.
27. Thomson AW, Carroll PB, McCauley J, Woo J, Abu-Elmagd K, Starzl TE, et al. FK 506: a novel immunosuppressant for treatment of autoimmune disease. Rationale and preliminary clinical experience at the University of Pittsburgh. Springer Semin Immunopathol. 1993;14(4):323–44.
28. Aiko S, Conner EM, Fuseler JA, Grisham MB. Effects of cyclosporine or FK506 in chronic colitis. J Pharmacol Exp Ther. 1997;280(2):1075–84.
29. Hoshino H, Goto H, Sugiyama S, Hayakawa T, Ozawa T. Effects of FK506 on an experimental model of colitis in rats. Aliment Pharmacol Ther. 1995;9(3):301–7.
30. Higa A, McKnight GW, Wallace JL. Attenuation of epithelial injury in acute experimental colitis by immunomodulators. Eur J Pharmacol. 1993;239(1–3):171–6.
31. Takizawa H, Shintani N, Natsui M, Sasakawa T, Nakakubo H, Nakajima T, et al. Activated immunocompetent cells in rat colitis mucosa induced by dextran sulfate sodium and not complete but partial suppression of colitis by FK506. Digestion. 1995;56(3):259–64.
32. Bousvaros A, Kirschner BS, Werlin SL, Parker-Hartigan L, Daum F, Freeman KB, et al. Oral tacrolimus treatment of severe colitis in children. J Pediatr. 2000;137(6):794–9.
33. Fellermann K, Tanko Z, Herrlinger KR, Witthoeft T, Homann N, Bruening A, et al. Response of refractory colitis to intravenous or oral tacrolimus (FK506). Inflamm Bowel Dis. 2002;8(5):317–24.
34. Baumgart DC, Wiedenmann B, Dignass AU. Rescue therapy with tacrolimus is effective in patients with severe and refractory inflammatory bowel disease. Aliment Pharmacol Ther. 2003;17(10):1273–81.
35. Högenauer C, Wenzl HH, Hinterleitner TA, Petritsch W. Effect of oral tacrolimus (FK 506) on steroid-refractory moderate/severe ulcerative colitis. Aliment Pharmacol Ther. 2003;18(4):415–23.
36. Baumgart DC, Pintoffl JP, Sturm A, Wiedenmann B, Dignass AU. Tacrolimus is safe and effective in patients with severe steroid-refractory or steroid-dependent inflammatory bowel disease—a long-term follow-up. Am J Gastroenterol. 2006;101(5):1048–56.
37. Ogata H, Matsui T, Nakamura M, Iida M, Takazoe M, Suzuki Y, et al. A randomised dose finding study of oral tacrolimus (FK506) therapy in refractory ulcerative colitis. Gut. 2006;55(9):1255–62.
38. Baumgart DC, Macdonald JK, Feagan B. Tacrolimus (FK506) for induction of remission in refractory ulcerative colitis. Cochrane Database Syst Rev. 2008;3:CD007216.
39. Ogata H, Kato J, Hirai F, Hida N, Matsui T, Matsumoto T, et al. Double-blind, placebo-controlled trial of oral tacrolimus (FK506) in the management of hospitalized patients with steroid-refractory ulcerative colitis. Inflamm Bowel Dis. 2012;18(5):803–8.
40. Fellermann K, Ludwig D, Stahl M, David-Walek T, Stange EF. Steroid-unresponsive acute attacks of inflammatory bowel disease: immunomodulation by tacrolimus (FK506). Am J Gastroenterol. 1998;93(10):1860–6.
41. Ng SC, Arebi N, Kamm MA. Medium-term results of oral tacrolimus treatment in refractory inflammatory bowel disease. Inflamm Bowel Dis. 2007;13(2):129–34.
42. Yamamoto S, Nakase H, Mikami S, Inoue S, Yoshino T, Takeda Y, et al. Long-term effect of tacrolimus therapy in patients with refractory ulcerative colitis. Aliment Pharmacol Ther. 2008;28(5):589–97.
43. Herrlinger KR, Koc H, Winter S, Teml A, Stange EF, Fellermann K, et al. ABCB1 single-nucleotide polymorphisms determine tacrolimus response in patients with ulcerative colitis. Clin Pharmacol Ther. 2011;89(3):422–8.
44. Bekersky I, Dressler D, Mekki QA. Effect of low- and high-fat meals on tacrolimus absorption following 5 mg single oral doses to healthy human subjects. J Clin Pharmacol. 2001;41(2):176–82.
45. Naganuma M, Fujii T, Watanabe M. The use of traditional and newer calcineurin inhibitors in inflammatory bowel disease. J Gastroenterol. 2011;46(2):129–37.
46. Hirai F, Takatsu N, Yano Y, Satou Y, Takahashi H, Ishikawa S, et al. Impact of CYP3A5 genetic polymorphisms on the pharmacokinetics and short-term remission in patients with ulcerative colitis treated with tacrolimus. J Gastroenterol Hepatol. 2014;29(1):60–6.
47. Kuehl P, Zhang J, Lin Y, Lamba J, Assem M, Schuetz J, et al. Sequence diversity in CYP3A promoters and characterization of the genetic basis of polymorphic CYP3A5 expression. Nat Genet. 2001;27(4):383–91.
48. Schmidt KJ, Herrlinger KR, Emmrich J, Barthel D, Koc H, Lehnert H, et al. Short-term efficacy of tacrolimus in steroid-refractory ulcerative colitis—experience in 130 patients. Aliment Pharmacol Ther. 2013;37(1):129–36.
49. Chow DK, Leong RW. The use of tacrolimus in the treatment of inflammatory bowel disease. Expert Opin Drug Saf. 2007;6(5):479–85.
50. Boschetti G, Nancey S, Moussata D, Stefanescu C, Roblin X, Chauvenet M, et al. Tacrolimus induction followed by maintenance monotherapy is useful in selected patients with moderate-to-severe ulcerative colitis refractory to prior treatment. Dig Liver Dis. 2014;46(10):875–80.
51. Yamamoto S, Nakase H, Matsuura M, Masuda S, Inui K, Chiba T. Tacrolimus therapy as an alternative to thiopurines for maintaining remission in patients with refractory ulcerative colitis. J Clin Gastroenterol. 2011;45(6):526–30.
52. Landy J, Wahed M, Peake ST, Hussein M, Ng SC, Lindsay JO, et al. Oral tacrolimus as maintenance therapy for refractory ulcerative colitis—an analysis of outcomes in two London tertiary centres. J Crohns Colitis. 2013;7(11):e516–21.
53. Brynskov J, Freund L, Thomsen OO, Andersen CB, Rasmussen SN, Binder V. Treatment of refractory ulcerative colitis with cyclosporin enemas. Lancet. 1989;1(8640):721–2.
54. Sandborn WJ, Tremaine WJ, Schroeder KW, Steiner BL, Batts KP, Lawson GM. Cyclosporine enemas for treatment-resistant, mildly to moderately active, left-sided ulcerative colitis. Am J Gastroenterol. 1993;88(5):640–5.
55. Winter TA, Dalton HR, Merrett MN, Campbell A, Jewell DP. Cyclosporin A retention enemas in refractory distal ulcerative colitis and 'pouchitis'. Scand J Gastroenterol. 1993;28(8):701–4.
56. Ranzi T, Campanini MC, Velio P, Quarto di Palo F, Bianchi P. Treatment of chronic proctosigmoiditis with cyclosporin enemas. Lancet. 1989;2(8654):97.
57. Sandborn WJ, Tremaine WJ, Schroeder KW, Batts KP, Lawson GM, Steiner BL, et al. A placebo-controlled trial of cyclosporine enemas for mildly to moderately active left-sided ulcerative colitis. Gastroenterology. 1994;106(6):1429–35.

58. Lawrance IC, Copeland TS. Rectal tacrolimus in the treatment of resistant ulcerative proctitis. Aliment Pharmacol Ther. 2008;28(10):1214–20.
59. van Dieren JM, van Bodegraven AA, Kuipers EJ, Bakker EN, Poen AC, van DH, et al. Local application of tacrolimus in distal colitis: feasible and safe. Inflamm Bowel Dis. 2009;15(2):193–8.
60. Uchino M, Ikeuchi H, Matsuoka H, Bando T, Hida N, Nakamura S, et al. Topical tacrolimus therapy for antibiotic-refractory pouchitis. Dis Colon Rectum. 2013;56(10):1166–73.
61. Tsunashima D, Kawamura A, Murakami M, Sawamoto T, Undre N, Brown M, et al. Assessment of tacrolimus absorption from the human intestinal tract: open-label, randomized, 4-way crossover study. Clin Ther. 2014;36(5):748–59.
62. Lamprecht A, Yamamoto H, Takeuchi H, Kawashima Y. Nanoparticles enhance therapeutic efficiency by selectively increased local drug dose in experimental colitis in rats. J Pharmacol Exp Ther. 2005;315(1):196–202.
63. Lamprecht A, Yamamoto H, Takeuchi H, Kawashima Y. A pH-sensitive microsphere system for the colon delivery of tacrolimus containing nanoparticles. J Control Release. 2005;104(2):337–46.
64. Lamprecht A, Yamamoto H, Ubrich N, Takeuchi H, Maincent P, Kawashima Y. FK506 microparticles mitigate experimental colitis with minor renal calcineurin suppression. Pharm Res. 2005;22(2): 193–9.
65. Kaser A, Mairinger T, Vogel W, Tilg H. Infliximab in severe steroid-refractory ulcerative colitis: a pilot study. Wien Klin Wochenschr. 2001;113(23-24):930–3.
66. Gornet JM, Couve S, Hassani Z, Delchier JC, Marteau P, Cosnes J, et al. Infliximab for refractory ulcerative colitis or indeterminate colitis: an open-label multicentre study. Aliment Pharmacol Ther. 2003;18(2):175–81.
67. Kohn A, Prantera C, Pera A, Cosintino R, Sostegni R, Daperno M. Infliximab in the treatment of severe ulcerative colitis: a follow-up study. Eur Rev Med Pharmacol Sci. 2004;8(5):235–7.
68. Järnerot G, Hertervig E, Friis-Liby I, Blomquist L, Karlen P, Grännö C, et al. Infliximab as rescue therapy in severe to moderately severe ulcerative colitis: a randomized, placebo-controlled study. Gastroenterology. 2005;128(7):1805–11.
69. Laharie D, Bourreille A, Branche J, Allez M, Bouhnik Y, Filippi J, et al. Ciclosporin versus infliximab in patients with severe ulcerative colitis refractory to intravenous steroids: a parallel, open-label randomised controlled trial. Lancet. 2012;380(9857):1909–15.
70. Laharie D, Bourreille A, Branche J, Allez M, Bouhnik Y, Filippi J, et al., editors. OP017 Long-term outcomes in a cohort of patients with acute severe ulcerative colitis refractory to intravenous steroids treated with cyclosporine or infliximab. Inflammatory Bowel Diseases— 10th Congress of ECCO; 2015; Barcelona.
71. Chang KH, Burke JP, Coffey JC. Infliximab versus cyclosporine as rescue therapy in acute severe steroid-refractory ulcerative colitis: a systematic review and meta-analysis. Int J Colorectal Dis. 2013;28(3):287–93.
72. Maser EA, Deconda D, Lichtiger S, Ullman T, Present DH, Kornbluth A. Cyclosporine and infliximab as rescue therapy for each other in patients with steroid-refractory ulcerative colitis. Clin Gastroenterol Hepatol. 2008;6(10):1112–6.
73. Herrlinger KR, Barthel DN, Schmidt KJ, Buning J, Barthel CS, Wehkamp J, et al. Infliximab as rescue medication for patients with severe ulcerative/indeterminate colitis refractory to tacrolimus. Aliment Pharmacol Ther. 2010;31(9):1036–41.
74. Leblanc S, Allez M, Seksik P, Flourie B, Peeters H, Dupas JL, et al. Successive treatment with cyclosporine and infliximab in steroid-refractory ulcerative colitis. Am J Gastroenterol. 2011;106(4):771–7.

Biologic Therapy in Moderate-to-Severe Ulcerative Colitis: Infliximab

42

Mindy Lam and Brian Bressler

Tumor Necrosis Factor and Ulcerative Colitis

The role of tumor necrosis factor α (TNF-α) proinflammatory cytokine in the pathogenesis of ulcerative colitis (UC) has been debated [1–5]. Inflammatory cascade involves activation of CD4+ T-lymphocytes into T helper (Th)-1 and Th-2 cells. Activation of Th-1 cells leads to secretion of interferon gamma (IFNγ), and interleukin (IL)-2, IL-12, and IL-18. In contrast, activation of Th-2 cells leads to secretion of IL-4, IL-5, IL-6, IL-10, and IL-13. TNF-α expression from macrophages and monocytes is stimulated by Th-1 response by the release of IFNγ.

The cytokine profile of UC has an atypical Th-2 pattern and reduced Th-1 response. CD4 natural-killing T cell in UC expresses intracellular IL-13; this is unique in UC and not found in Crohn's disease [6]. While intestinal cytokine messenger ribonucleic acid (mRNA) analysis show increased levels of IL-1β, IL-4, IL-5, IL-8, IL-12p40, IFNγ, and TNF-α [7]. Despite this atypical pattern, elevated levels of TNF-α likely contributes to the effectiveness of anti-TNF-α therapy in UC.

TNF-α is produced as a 212-amino acid type II transmembrane protein in stable homotrimers or secreted 17-kDa form. The circulating soluble TNF-α is formed from cleavage of the transmembrane form by TNF-α converting enzyme (TACE). The circulating soluble TNF-α binds to two different TNF-α receptors, TNF receptor 1 (TNFR1) and TNF receptor 2 (TNFR2) expressed in most tissues, leading to activation of other macrophages and augmenting T cell response with increased recruitment of neutrophils and induction of granuloma formation [8, 9].

M. Lam • B. Bressler (✉)
Division of Gastroenterology, University of British Columbia, Vancouver, BC, Canada
e-mail: brian_bressler@hotmail.com

Molecular Structure of Infliximab

Infliximab is a chimeric IgG1 monoclonal antibody of 149 kDa that binds and neutralizes TNF-α specifically. Binding of infliximab to the transmembrane TNF-α induces apoptosis of those cells in vitro. The binding of infliximab to soluble TNF-α prevents binding of TNF-α to TNFR. The Food and Drug Administration (FDA) approved infliximab in September 16, 2005 for use in moderate-to-severe UC that failed conventional therapy. The European Medicines Agency approved infliximab for ulcerative colitis, in 2006.

Pharmacokinetics of Infliximab

Infliximab showed a linear relationship between the dose administered and maximum serum concentration; it has an association constant of 10^{10} M^{-1} to TNF-α. The volume of distribution at steady state was independent of dose and indicated that infliximab was distributed primarily within the vascular compartment. The median half-life of infliximab is 7.7–9.5 days [10].

Efficacy of Infliximab in Ulcerative Colitis

The definition of efficacy of medical therapy in UC may be subject to varying interpretations. Efficacy may mean steroid-free clinical remission for some, or it may mean mucosal healing for others; both of these definitions are academic and may not have much relevance to patients as they do for their clinicians. Efficacy, for most patients, means maintaining a good quality of life, avoiding colectomy, and reducing risk of complications related to UC such as colorectal cancer. Prior to the biologics era, the probability of colectomy within the first 5 years of diagnosis ranges from 9 % in distal colitis to 35 % in pancolitis [11]. Several clinical trials have shown that infliximab is efficacious in

D.C. Baumgart (ed.), *Crohn's Disease and Ulcerative Colitis*, DOI 10.1007/978-3-319-33703-6_42

induction and maintenance of remission and reduces colectomy rates in UC.

Initial small clinical trials showed conflicting results for infliximab for UC [12–16]. Rutgeerts et al. set forth to perform the much-needed multicenter randomized double blind, placebo-controlled efficacy trial for the use of infliximab in induction and maintenance of remission in UC [17]. Moderately to severely active UC patients (defined as full Mayo score of 6–12) despite the use of conventional therapy were enrolled and randomized to receive placebo, or infliximab 5 or 10 mg/kg at 0, 2, 6 weeks, and then every 8 weeks thereafter [18]. ACT 1 patients received treatment up to week 46 and were observed to week 54, and ACT 2 patients received treatment up to week 22 and were observed to week 30. The primary outcome was clinical response at week 8, defined by decrease from baseline total Mayo score of at least 3 points and at least 30 %, with an accompanying decrease in the rectal bleeding subscore of at least 1 point or absolute subscore of 0 or 1. The ACT trials demonstrated that significantly higher proportion of patients achieved induction and maintenance of clinical response or remission at weeks 8, 30 and week 54 (in ACT 1) at either 5 or 10 mg/kg dosing, compared to placebo.

To further assess if treatment with infliximab reduces colectomy rates, Sandborn et al. carried out an analysis of ACT data on the colectomy-sparing effect of infliximab therapy in UC [19]. Six hundred and thirty of 728 (87 %) randomized patients had complete colectomy follow-up data through 54 weeks. Eighty-two patients (36 from placebo, 28 and 18 from infliximab 5 and 10 mg/kg respectively) had colectomy within 54 weeks. The cumulative incidence of colectomy was significantly higher in placebo group than infliximab groups, with an absolute risk reduction of 7 % (95 % confidence interval of 0.01–0.12) and 41 % reduction in risk of colectomy for infliximab groups compared to placebo.

These studies demonstrate that infliximab is efficacious in the management of moderately to severely active UC.

Clinical Practice

Many questions remained regarding the optimal use of infliximab for the management of UC. The requirement of a concomitant immunosuppressant with infliximab was one of the most pressing issues.

Panaccione et al. set out to address this question by comparing efficacies of infliximab, purine antimetabolites, or combination of infliximab and purine antimetabolites. UC SUCCESS was a randomized, double blinded, double dummy efficacy trial, the primary outcome was proportion of patients in corticosteroid-free remission defined as total Mayo score of 2 points or less with no individual subscore greater than 1 point, and without use of corticosteroids at week 16 [20]. There was significantly higher proportion of patients in combination therapy (infliximab and azathioprine) achieving corticosteroid-free remission than azathioprine or infliximab alone at week 16, the difference was twofold. In light of these new evidence, the Toronto Consensus formulized guidelines for management of non-hospitalized UC addressing this specific issue by stating that combination therapy with thiopurine when initiating infliximab therapy is preferred [21]. Concomitant use of immunosuppression therapy has been shown to reduce the likelihood of anti-infliximab antibody formation. UC SUCCESS showed that less percentage of patients developed antibodies to infliximab at week 16 from the combination therapy group (infliximab and azathioprine) at 3 %, compared to infliximab monotherapy at 19% [20]. Armuzzi et al. demonstrated in a prospective observational trial that predictor for steroid-free clinical remission at 6 and 12 months were thiopurine-naïve status (hazard ratio (HR) of 2.5 and 2.8 respectively), and combination therapy (HR 2.1 and 2.2 respectively) [22]. Furthermore, a systematic review and meta-analysis of four controlled trials showed that clinical remission rate was significantly lower for infliximab monotherapy group than combination of infliximab and immunosuppressant therapy, with an odds ratio (OR) of 0.5 (95 % confidence interval of 0.34–0.73) [23].

The evidence for combination with methotrexate and infliximab is not as clear as that for thiopurine in the induction and maintenance of active UC. This may stem from the fact that the evidence for methotrexate in UC treatment has not been convincing [24–26]. The Cochrane systematic review included two randomized controlled trials comparing methotrexate with placebo in active UC [27]. The review included 101 patients and there was no statistical significant difference in clinical remission rate and complete withdrawal from steroid therapy, with a risk ratio of 0.96 (95 % confidence interval of 0.58–1.59). However, methotrexate used in combination with infliximab have been shown to reduced immunogenicity and increase infliximab trough levels in other conditions, such as Crohn's disease, rheumatoid arthritis, and psoriasis. COMMIT is a trial to compare infliximab monotherapy to infliximab with methotrexate combination therapy in steroid-dependent Crohn's disease [28]. The anti-infliximab antibody formation was 4 % in combination therapy compared to 20 % infliximab monotherapy, correlating to a higher trough level of 6.35 μg/mL in the combination group compared to 3.75 μg/mL in infliximab monotherapy group.

In patients with UC refractory to thiopurines or corticosteroids, TNF-α antagonist should be used for induction to complete corticosteroid-free remission. This has been shown in meta-analysis of randomized controlled trials to be efficacious in those who failed to respond to corticosteroids. Five trials showed that infliximab was superior to placebo in inducing endoscopic remission (Relative risk for no remission is 0.72 with 95 % confidence interval of 0.57–0.91).

For patients who responded to TNF-α antagonist therapy, it should be continued on as maintenance therapy.

Inpatient

There is much less literature in evaluating optimal management of hospitalized UC patients, however recently clinical practice guidelines has been published to help clinicians manage this challenging group of patients [29]. Infliximab is the only approved biologic to date to be studied in a randomized control trial for efficacy in hospitalized UC patients [12, 13]. Jarnerot et al. performed a randomized double-blind trial of infliximab or placebo in hospitalized ulcerative colitis patients not responding to conventional treatment; patients were randomized to infliximab or placebo on day 4 or day 6–8 after starting corticosteroid treatment [15]. The primary outcome was colectomy or death within 90 days after infliximab infusion. The odds of needing colectomy in the placebo group were 4.9 times the odds of colectomy in the infliximab group (95 % confidence interval 1.4–17). A meta-analysis of randomized controlled trials of both moderate-to-severe UC in ambulatory and hospitalized settings showed that induction of clinical and endoscopic remission was superior in infliximab group compared to placebo. The relative risk was 3.22 (95 % confidence interval of 2.18–4.76, number needed to treat (NNT) of 5) and 1.88 (95 % confidence interval of 1.54–2.28, NNT of 4) respectively [30].

Assessment for response to second-line medical therapy should be made within day 5–7 after initiation, as not to delay surgical therapy if needed. The Jarnerot study did not define mean time to response; however, mean time to colectomy was 8 days after initiation of infliximab therapy [15]. Those who responded to first dose of infliximab should complete induction regimen at weeks 2 and 6, followed by maintenance therapy.

Optimization

Trough serum infliximab level is a predictor of clinical outcome for treatment in UC. A prospective observational trial by Seow et al. showed that detectable trough serum infliximab level after three induction doses followed by maintenance scheduled doses predicts clinical remission, endoscopic improvement, and lower risk of colectomy [31]. Adedokun et al. also showed that infliximab concentration and the infliximab antibodies influence response [32]. Infliximab concentration of approximately 41 μg/mL 2 weeks after induction is complete and an infliximab concentration of approximately 4 μg/mL during maintenance are desirable levels to achieve optimal outcomes.

Although infliximab is an effective therapy in UC, clinician should recognize if there is inadequate response, as optimizing the exposure of infliximab with the guidance of therapeutic drug monitoring is important.

Adverse Events

There is much more safety data for infliximab and Crohn's disease compared to UC, but it is assumed that the risks are similar in both [33].

Opportunistic infection has been reported, including a variety of infectious such as herpes zoster, various fungal infection, herpes simplex, candida, tuberculosis (TB), aspergillosis, and cryptococcosis. Many cases involve disseminated or military TB. Hepatitis B reactivation has been associated with infliximab in chronic carriers. Patient should be tested for HBV infection before initiation of therapy, expert treatment of hepatitis B is recommended prior to infliximab initiation.

A case report of infant death from disseminated Bacillus Calmette–Guérin (BCG) after administration of the BCG vaccine to a 4.5-month-old infant born to a mother who had received infliximab therapy for CD during pregnancy has brought attention to the potential dangers of these medications, not only on the immediate neonatal outcome but also on the lasting effects on infants [34]. As such, live vaccines or therapeutic infectious agents should not be given while on infliximab.

Lymphoproliferative disorders, especially non-Hodgkin's lymphoma, have been reported, mostly in patients on concomitant immunosuppressants. Despite these case reports, the safety of infliximab is best summarized from the on-going prospective study, Crohn's Therapy, Resource, Evaluation, and Assessment Tool (TREAT™) Registry, examining the long-term outcomes of Crohn's disease treatment, including infliximab [35]. As of February 23, 2010, 3764 Crohn's disease patients exposed to infliximab therapy was analyzed. The cancer incidences were similar between those exposed to infliximab compared to those exposed to other treatments. Multivariate Cox regression analysis shows that baseline age (hazard ratio (HR) 1.59/10 years, $P<0.001$), disease duration (HR 1.64/10 years, $P=0.012$), and smoking (HR 1.38, $P=0.045$) were associated with risk of malignancy, while immunosuppressive therapy (HR 1.43; $P=0.11$), infliximab therapy (HR 0.59, $P=0.16$), or a combination (HR 1.22, $P=0.34$) was not associated with risk of malignancy.

Furthermore, a meta-analysis of efficacy and safety of TNF-antagonists in Crohn's disease included 5356 patients, and found that anti-TNF therapy did not increase risk of death, malignancy, or serious infections [36].

Other rare case-reports but significant concerns with infliximab therapy have emerged include demyelinating disease, lupus-like syndrome, and psoriaform skin disease.

Increase antinuclear antibody (ANA) autoantibodies and lupus-like syndrome were noted in clinical trials of infliximab. Between January 2000 and December 2012, there has been 39 reports of lupus-like syndrome involving TNF-antagonist; 25 of these were associated with infliximab [37]. The most common was cutaneous and rheumatologic manifestation and ANA autoantibodies were present in all cases, with anti-DNA in 77.8 % of the cases. Symptoms often improve with discontinuation of TNF-antagonist therapy. The reporting odds ratio of infliximab and lupus is 10.97 (95 % confidence interval of 7.27–16.56).

Since March 30, 2012, there have been 81 cases of infliximab-induced psoriasis, with symptoms occurring between 2 weeks and 6.5 years of infliximab therapy; only four of these cases were in the setting of UC and 30 in Crohn's disease. Majority developed palmoplantar pustular psoriasis (20 cases) or pustular psoriasis (12 cases) [38].

Other safety concerns include use in congestive heart failure and rare risk of hepatotoxicity and pancytopenia. Infliximab is contraindicated in NYHA Class III/IV congestive heart failure. Hepatotoxicity with acute liver failure, jaundice, hepatitis, and cholestasis has been reported rarely in those receiving infliximab. Pancytopenia in infliximab therapy has been reported in post-marketing use; however, many of these cases are on concomitant medications.

Conclusion

Infliximab is a safe and effective agent for induction and maintenance of ulcerative colitis. The use of this medication in both hospitalized and ambulatory settings has been a major advancement in the care of patients with ulcerative colitis. In current practice it is our expectation when starting a patient with UC on infliximab, we will improve the chance of this particular patient to live a normal life with UC, with a reduced risk of requiring steroids and ultimately a reduced risk of colectomy.

References

1. Mizoguchi E, Mizoguchi A, Takedatsu H, Cario E, de Jong YP, Ooi CJ, et al. Role of tumor necrosis factor receptor 2 (TNFR2) in colonic epithelial hyperplasia and chronic intestinal inflammation in mice. Gastroenterology. 2002;122(1):134–44.
2. Melgar S, Yeung MM, Bas A, Forsberg G, Suhr O, Oberg A, et al. Over-expression of interleukin 10 in mucosal T cells of patients with active ulcerative colitis. Clin Exp Immunol. 2003;134(1):127–37.
3. Leeb SN, Vogl D, Gunckel M, Kiessling S, Falk W, Goke M, et al. Reduced migration of fibroblasts in inflammatory bowel disease: role of inflammatory mediators and focal adhesion kinase. Gastroenterology. 2003;125(5):1341–54.
4. Ten Hove T, The Olle F, Berkhout M, Bruggeman JP, Vyth-Dreese FA, Slors JF, et al. Expression of CD45RB functionally distinguishes intestinal T lymphocytes in inflammatory bowel disease. J Leukoc Biol. 2004;75(6):1010–5.
5. Amasheh S, Barmeyer C, Koch CS, Tavalali S, Mankertz J, Epple HJ, et al. Cytokine-dependent transcriptional down-regulation of epithelial sodium channel in ulcerative colitis. Gastroenterology. 2004;126(7):1711–20.
6. Fuss IJ, Heller F, Boirivant M, Leon F, Yoshida M, Fichtner-Feigl S, et al. Nonclassical CD1d-restricted NK T cells that produce IL-13 characterize an atypical Th2 response in ulcerative colitis. J Clin Invest. 2004;113(10):1490–7.
7. Sawa Y, Oshitani N, Adachi K, Higuchi K, Matsumoto T, Arakawa T. Comprehensive analysis of intestinal cytokine messenger RNA profile by real-time quantitative polymerase chain reaction in patients with inflammatory bowel disease. Int J Mol Med. 2003;11(2):175–9.
8. Sands BE, Kaplan GG. The role of TNFa in ulcerative colitis. J Clin Pharmacol. 2007;47(8):930–41.
9. Theiss AL, Simmons JG, Jobin C, Lund PK. Tumor necrosis factor (TNF)a increases collagen accumulation and proliferation in intestinal myofibroblasts via TNF receptor 2. J Biol Chem. 2005;280:36099–109.
10. Remicade. Janssen. 2015.
11. Langholz E, Munkholm P, Davidsen M, Binder V. Colorectal cancer risk and mortality in patients with ulcerative colitis. Gastroenterology. 1992;103:1444–51.
12. Sands BE, Tremaine WJ, Sandborn WJ, Rutgeerts PJ, Hanauer SB, Mayer L, et al. Infliximab in the treatment of severe, steroid-refractory ulcerative colitis: a pilot study. Inflamm Bowel Dis. 2001;7(2):83–8.
13. Probert CS, Hearing SD, Schreiber S, Kuhbacher T, Ghosh S, Arnott ID, et al. Infliximab in moderately severe glucocorticoid resistant ulcerative colitis: a randomised controlled trial. Gut. 2003;52(7):998–1002.
14. Ochsenkuhn T, Sackmann M, Goke B. Infliximab for acute, not steroid-refractory ulcerative colitis: a randomized pilot study. Eur J Gastroenterol Hepatol. 2004;16(11):1167–71.
15. Jamerot G, Hertervig E, Frils-Liby K, Blomquist L, Karlen P, Granno C, et al. Infliximab as rescue therapy in severe to moderately severe ulcerative colitis: a randomized, placebo-controlled study. Gastroenterology. 2005;128(7):1805–11.
16. Chey WY. Infliximab for patients with refractory ulcerative colitis. Inflamm Bowel Dis. 2001;7 Suppl 1:S30–3.
17. Rutgeerts P, Sandborn WJ, Feagan BG, Reinisch W, Olson A, Johanns J, et al. Infliximab for induction and maintenance therapy for ulcerative colitis. N Engl J Med. 2005;353:2462–76.
18. Schroeder KW, Tremaine WJ, Ilstrup DM. Coated oral 5-aminosalicylic acid therapy for mildly to moderately active ulcerative colitis. A randomized study. N Engl J Med. 1987;317(26):1625–9.
19. Sandborn WJ, Rutgeerts P, Feagan BG, Reinisch W, Olson A, Johanns J, et al. Colectomy rate comparison after treatment of ulcerative colitis with placebo or infliximab. Gastroenterology. 2009;137(4):1250–60.
20. Panaccione R, Ghosh S, Middleton S, Marquez JR, Scott BB, Flint L, et al. Combination therapy with infliximab and azathioprine is superior to monotherapy with either agent in ulcerative colitis. Gastroenterology. 2014;146(2):392–400.
21. Bressler B, Marshall JK, Bernstein CN, Bitton A, Johnes J, Leontiadis GI, et al. Clinical practice guidelines for the medical management of nonhospitalized ulcerative colitis: the Toronto consensus. Gastroenterology. 2015;148(5):1035–58.
22. Armuzzi A, Pugliese D, Danese S, Rizzo G, Felice C, Marzo M, et al. Infliximab in steroid-dependent ulcerative colitis: effectiveness and predictors of clinical and endoscopoic remission. Inflamm Bowel Dis. 2013;19(5):1065–72.
23. Christophorou D, Funakoshi N, Duny Y, Valats JC, Bismuth M, Pineton De Chambrun G, et al. Systematic review with

meta-analysis: infliximab and immunosuppressant therapy vs. infliximab alone for active ulcerative colitis. Aliment Pharmacol Ther. 2015;41(7):603–12.

24. Baron TH, Truss CD, Elson CO. Low-dose oral methotrexate in refractory inflammatory bowel disease. Dig Dis Sci. 1993;38(10):1851–6.
25. Cummings JR, Herrlinger KR, Travis SP, Gorard DA, McIntyre AS, Jewell DP. Oral methotrexate in ulcerative colitis. Aliment Pharmacol Ther. 2005;21(4):385–9.
26. Khan N, Abbas AM, Moehlen M, Balart L. Methotrexate in ulcerative colitis: a nationwide retrospective cohort from the Veterans Affairs Health Care System. Inflamm Bowel Dis. 2013;19(7):1379–83.
27. Chande N, Wang Y, MacDonald JK, McDonald JW. Methotrexate for induction of remission in ulcerative colitis. Cochrane Database Syst Rev. 2014;8:CD006618.
28. Feagan BG, McDonald JW, Panaccione R, Enns RA, Bernstein CN, Ponich TP, et al. Methotrexate in combination with infliximab is no more effective than infliximab alone in patients with Crohn's disease. Gastroenterology. 2014;146(3):681–8.
29. Bitton A, Buie D, Enns R, Feagan BG, Jones JL, Marshall JK, et al. Treatment of hospitalized adult patients with severe ulcerative colitis: Toronto consensus statements. Am J Gastroenterol. 2012;107(2):179–94.
30. Lawson MM, Thomas AG, Akobeng AK. Tumour necrosis factor alpha blocking agents for induction of remission in ulcerative colitis. Cochrane Database Syst Rev. 2006;19(3):CD005112.
31. Seow CH, Newman A, Irwin SP, Steinhart AH, Silverberg MS, Greenberg GR. Trough serum infliximab: a predictive factor of clinical outcome for infliximab treatment in acute ulcerative colitis. Gut. 2010;59(1):49–54.
32. Adedokun OJ, Sandborn WJ, Feagan BG, Rutgeerts P, Xu Z, Marano CW, et al. Association between serum concentration of infliximab and efficacy in adult patients with ulcerative colitis. Gastroenterology. 2014;147(6):1296–307.
33. Safety update on TNF-a antagonists: infliximab and etanercept. 2015. http://www.fda.gov/ohrms/dockets/ac/01/briefing/3779b2_01_cber_safety%20_revision2.pdf. Accessed Aug 2015.
34. Cheent K, Nolan J, Shariq S, Kiho L, Pal A, Arnold J. Case Report: Fatal case of disseminated BCG infection in an infant born to a mother taking infliximab for Crohn's disease. J Crohns Colitis. 2010;4(5):603–5.
35. Lichtenstein GR, Feagan BG, Cohen RD, Salzberg BA, Diamond RH, Langholff W, et al. Drug therapies and the risk of malignancy in Crohn's disease: results from the TREAT™ Registry. Am J Gastroenterol. 2014;109(2):212–23.
36. Peyrin-Biroulet L, Deltenre P, de Suray N, Branche J, Sandborn WJ, Colombel JF. Efficacy and safety of tumor necrosis factor antagonists in Crohn's disease: meta-analysis of placebo-controlled trials. Clin Gastroenterol Hepatol. 2008;6(6):644–53.
37. Moulis G, Sommet A, Lapeyre-Mestre M, Montastruc JL. Association Francaise des Centres Regionaux de PharmacoVigilance. Rheumatology (Oxford). 2014;54(10):1864–71.
38. Famenini S, Wu JJ. Infliximab-induced psoriasis in treatment of Crohn's disease-associated ankylosing spondylitis: case report and review of 142 cases. J Drugs Dematol. 2013;12(8):939–43.

43 Biologic Therapy of Ulcerative Colitis: Adalimumab

Walter Reinisch

Introduction

Ulcerative colitis is a chronic inflammatory condition which can progress over time towards extensive colonic involvement and/or severe activity which renders colectomy inevitable in up to 10 % of all cases [1]. Elevated levels of TNF-α have been detected in samples of colon tissue, blood, stool, and urine of pediatric and adult patients with ulcerative colitis, suggesting a substantial pathophysiological role of this proinflammatory cytokine [2–5].

Actually, many features of an excessive production of TNF-α have been described in ulcerative colitis, including activation of macrophages and T cells, expression of adhesion molecules on vascular endothelium or increased migration of neutrophils into the colonic mucosa [6]. Targeting TNF-α has been shown to provide a successful mechanism of action in ulcerative colitis and meanwhile three originator anti-TNF agents, infliximab, adalimumab, and golimumab, have been approved by the US Food and Drug Administration (FDA) and the European Medicines Agency (EMA) for use in treating adult patients with moderate to severely active ulcerative colitis. The focus of this article is to highlight the scientific evidence of adalimumab in the management of patients with ulcerative colitis.

Adalimumab is a recombinant, fully human recombinant monoclonal IgG1 antibody which binds specifically and with high affinity to the soluble and transmembrane forms of TNF-α and inhibits the binding of TNF-α with its receptor. Adalimumab is approved in the USA and Europe for the treatment of a diversity of immune mediated inflammatory diseases including rheumatoid arthritis, juvenile idiopathic arthritis, psoriatic arthritis, ankylosing spondylitis, psoriasis, as well as adult and pediatric Crohn's disease. Adalimumab is administered subcutaneously every other week with the option to reduce the dosing interval to weekly injections.

W. Reinisch (✉)
Division of Gastroenterology, Department of Medicine, McMaster University, 1280 Main Street West, Hamilton, ON L8N 3Z5, Canada
e-mail: reinisw@mcmaster.ca

Adalimumab

The Early Non-controlled Experience with Adalimumab

Several small open-label trials and case reports suggested that adalimumab can induce remission in patients with UC even in those failing previous treatment with infliximab [7–12]. In the largest of those series 30 patients with active ulcerative colitis having previously failed standard medications including infliximab were treated with adalimumab 160 mg at week 0 and 80 mg at week 2 and subsequently with 40 mg every other week. In case of non-response maintenance dose could be increased to adalimumab 40 mg weekly. After a mean follow-up of 48 weeks 15 patients (50 %) continued on adalimumab. Patients who achieved short-term clinical response at week 12 were less likely to undergo colectomy during follow-up [12].

Randomized Controlled Trials with Adalimumab

The safety and efficacy of adalimumab in ulcerative colitis were evaluated in two pivotal randomized, placebo-controlled, double-blind, phase III clinical studies named ULTRA 1 and ULTRA 2, where ULTRA stands for Ulcerative Colitis Long-Term Remission and Maintenance with Adalimumab. Eligible were patients who had moderately to severely active ulcerative colitis with a Mayo score of ≥6 points and an endoscopic subscore of ≥2 points despite having previously received or being on concurrent treatment with corticosteroids and/or immunosuppressants such as azathioprine or 6-MP. Whereas ULTRA 1 only enrolled

D.C. Baumgart (ed.), *Crohn's Disease and Ulcerative Colitis*, DOI 10.1007/978-3-319-33703-6_43

patients naïve to anti-TNF-α agents, 40 % of subjects in ULTRA 2 had previously been exposed to infliximab but no longer than 8 weeks before baseline [13, 14]. In 2012, the results from the ULTRA program which included 1.094 patients led to the approval by FDA and EMA of adalimumab for use in adult patients with moderately to severely active ulcerative colitis who were nonresponders or intolerant to conventional therapy (in the EU including corticosteroids and the thiopurines, 6-mercaptopurine or azathioprine).

ULTRA 1 was the induction study of the ULTRA program. The primary endpoint, remission defined by a Mayo score ≤2 with no individual subscore >1, was set at week 8. Three hundred and ninety patients were randomized (1:1:1) to adalimumab 160/80 or adalimumab 80/40 at weeks 0 and 2 followed by adalimumab 40 mg at weeks 4 and 6, or placebo. At week 8, 18.5 % of patients in the adalimumab 160/80 group ($p=0.031$ vs. placebo) and 10.0 % in the adalimumab 80/40 group ($p=0.833$ vs. placebo) were in remission, compared with 9.2 % in the placebo group. Clinical response and mucosal healing as secondary endpoints were not significantly different among the three groups. Baseline clinical variables, such as extensive disease, high disease activity (Mayo score ≥ 10), and high levels of systemic inflammation (C-reactive protein ≥ 10 mg/L), were associated with a lower proportion of patients in clinical remission in a post hoc analysis. The authors also suggested the possibility that a substantial proportion of patients with ulcerative colitis may have required a higher dose of adalimumab to induce remission as remission rates in patients with a body weight less than 82 kg were more than twice for patients above 82 kg in the 160/80 mg dose group [13].

After the 8 week induction period patients could enter an open-label extension study while being maintained on adalimumab 40 mg EOW dosing regimen for 52 weeks. In case of loss-of-response an option to escalate the dose to 40 mg weekly was provided. At week 52 25.6 % of patients without dose escalation were in remission, whereas including subjects with dose escalation the corresponding number was 29.5 % [15].

The ULTRA 2 trial was the induction and maintenance study of the program with the proportion of patients achieving remission at week 8 and week 52 as co-primary endpoints. Four hundred and ninety-four patients were randomized to receive adalimumab 160 mg at week 0, 80 mg at week 2, and 40 mg EOW, or placebo, through to 52 weeks. Clinical remission at week 8 and week 52 were achieved in 16.5 % of patients in the adalimumab arm versus 9.3 % of patients in the placebo arm ($P=0.019$) and in corresponding 17.3 % versus 8.5 % ($P=0.004$), respectively. Also the secondary endpoints response and endoscopic remission were achieved after induction and maintenance (endoscopic remission defined as endoscopic Mayo subscore of 0 or 1 at week 8: 41.1 %, adalimumab vs 31.7 %, placebo, $P=0.032$; at week 52: 25 % vs 15.4 %, $P=0.009$). Stratifying patients based on prior exposure to anti-TNF-α agents revealed significant differences in clinical remission in favor of adalimumab among naïve patients both at week 8 and 52, whereas among anti-TNF-α-exposed patients this could be shown only at week 52 (10.2 %, adalimumab and 3 %, placebo, $P=0.039$) [14].

As the treat-through design applied in ULTRA 2 does not necessarily reflect clinical practice a post hoc intention-to-treat analysis addressed the question of week 52 clinical outcomes among the 123 patients who were randomized to adalimumab and achieved a clinical response, as per their partial Mayo score at week 8. Of these, 30.9 %, 49.6 %, and 43.1 % achieved clinical remission, clinical response, and mucosal healing at week 52, respectively. Of the adalimumab-treated patients taking corticosteroids at baseline and responded at week 8, 21.1 % achieved corticosteroid-free remission and 37.8 % were corticosteroid-free at week 52, without significant differences among the anti-TNFα-naïve and exposed patients [16].

The safety profile of adalimumab in ULTRA 1 and ULTRA 2 was comparable to that of placebo with rates of adverse events similar to those reported from studies of other approved indications. The presence of human anti-adalimumab antibodies (AAA) and low trough serum adalimumab levels have been reported to be associated with unfavorable long-term outcomes in patients with Crohn's disease, whereas corresponding data from ulcerative colitis are scarce and don't allow robust conclusions yet. Body weight, occurrence of AAA, and plasma albumin were significant covariates on estimated apparent clearance. Pharmacokinetic modeling lead to the justification of an alternative and higher dosing of adalimumab during the induction phase. A corresponding high-dose induction study with adalimumab in ulcerative colitis is currently recruiting.

A combined analysis of patients that received 160 mg/80 mg induction therapy of adalimumab or placebo in ULTRA 1 and ULTRA 2 ($n=963$) revealed significant reductions in risk of all-cause, UC-related, and UC- or drug-related hospitalizations (by 40 %, 50 %, and 47 %, respectively; $P<0.05$ for all comparisons) within the first 8 weeks in favor of adalimumab. This benefit of adalimumab over placebo was further observed during 52 weeks. Facing an overall low colectomy rate in the ULTRA program, the number of colectomies did not differ significantly between patients given adalimumab versus placebo [17].

A registration trial in 273 anti-TNF-α naive Japanese patients with ulcerative colitis who were refractory to corticosteroids, immunomodulators, or both and who were randomized to placebo, adalimumab 80 mg/40 mg at weeks 0/2 and then 40 mg every other week, or adalimumab 160 mg/80 mg at weeks 0/2 and then 40 mg every other week confirmed in general the safety and efficacy of adalimumab in an Asian patient population. Whereas at week 8, remission rates were similar among treatment arms, but more patients treated with adalimumab 160/80 achieved response and mucosal healing compared with placebo, all those endpoints were achieved significantly more often with adalimumab at week 52 [18].

Open Label Long-Term Study with Adalimumab

All patients who completed ULTRA 1 or ULTRA 2 could enter the open-label extension, ULTRA 3. Patients who completed ULTRA 2 on blinded therapy (either adalimumab or placebo) received open-label adalimumab 40 mg every other week in ULTRA 3. Patients who completed the lead-in study (ULTRA 1 or ULTRA 2) on open-label adalimumab 40 mg every other week or weekly continued their same dosing regimens in ULTRA 3. Escalation to 40 mg weekly dosing was allowed after week 12 of ULTRA 3 for inadequate response or disease flare. Corticosteroid tapering was allowed after week 12 of ULTRA 3 for patients with a clinical response, but if corticosteroid tapering was begun in ULTRA 1 or ULTRA 2, patients could continue their corticosteroid taper upon entry into ULTRA 3. A total of 600/1094 patients enrolled in ULTRA 1 or 2 were randomized to receive adalimumab and 199 of these remained on adalimumab after 4 years of follow-up. Rates of remission per partial Mayo score, mucosal healing, and corticosteroid discontinuation at week 208 were 24.7 %, 27.7 % (non-responder imputation), and 59.2 % (observed), respectively. Of the patients who were followed up in ULTRA 3 remission per partial Mayo score and mucosal healing were maintained by 63.6 % and 59.9 % of patients, respectively (non-responder imputation). The adverse event rates were stable over time [19].

Meta-Analysis Assessing Adalimumab in Ulcerative Colitis

A number of meta-analysis assessed the efficacy of adalimumab in moderately to severely active ulcerative colitis. From the results of a network meta-analysis of seven double-blind, placebo-controlled trials the authors suggested that among anti-TNF-α agents infliximab is more effective to induce clinical response (odds ratio, 2.36 [95 % credible interval, 1.22–4.63]) and mucosal healing (odds ratio, 2.02 [95 % credible interval, 1.13–3.59]) than adalimumab. No other significant differences in the induction performance between adalimumab, infliximab, golimumab, and vedolizumab were noted. For maintenance studies the risk of bias was deemed too high to allow robust conclusions. However, results from indirect comparisons, as such by network-meta-analysis need to be interpreted with cautions as no direct comparison from head-to-head studies between any biologics is yet available [20].

Recent Real-Life Experience

Since the publication of the ULTRA trials some real-life experiences with adalimumab in ulcerative colitis have been published. From a single center experience on 73 patients with ulcerative colitis, all previously exposed to infliximab, response rates to adalimumab at weeks 12 and 52 of 75 % and 52 %, respectively, were reported. However, 22 patients needed a dose escalation and 35 discontinued treatment within the first year. Primary response to infliximab and serum adalimumab concentrations were independent predictors for induction and maintenance response. The thresholds of serum adalimumab concentrations for response at week 12 and 52 were 4.58 μg/mL and 7.0 μg/mL, respectively [21].

An Italian multicenter study on 88 patients represents the largest real-life series of patients with ulcerative colitis treated with adalimumab so far. The majority of patients received an induction dose of 160 mg/80 mg adalimumab followed by 40 mg biweekly, had been previously treated with infliximab and/or immunosuppressants, and were either steroid-dependent or -refractory. Sustained clinical remission, defined as a partial Mayo score of ≤1 week from 12 up to week 24 and 54 was achieved by 17 % of patients. Among the 60 patients who were taking steroids at baseline, steroid-free remission was achieved in 40.0 % at week 54. Among the 57 patients in whom baseline and follow-up endoscopy after a median of 11 months was available 49.1 % achieved mucosal healing. The fact that 25 % of the patients required colectomy within a median of 5.5 months mirrors the disease severity of the treated patients. The rate of colectomy was higher in the infliximab-exposed group than in the infliximab-naïve group (28.9 % vs 10.5 %) [22].

Consensus

A consensus panel installed by the Canadian Association of Gastroenterology published guideline recommendations for the use of anti-TNF-α agents in patients with ulcerative colitis. Interestingly, a differentiation of the clinical efficacy between infliximab, adalimumab, and golimumab was not performed and statements are considered class-related without prioritizing the use of one anti-TNF-α agent over another. As such, anti-TNF-α agents are recommended in patients with ulcerative colitis who failed corticosteroids or thiopurines or who are steroid-dependent in order to induce and maintain steroid-free complete remission, which is defined as both symptomatic and endoscopic remission. When starting anti-TNF-α therapy a combination with a thiopurine or methotrexate rather than the use as monotherapy is recommended. Symptomatic response should be evaluated in 8–12 weeks. In patients who respond to anti-TNF-α induction therapy, treatment should be continued, whereas in those who have experienced a suboptimal response dose intensification is recommended. The latter applies also to subjects who lose response to anti-TNF-α maintenance therapy [23].

Conclusion

Anti-TNF alpha agents have hugely expanded our therapeutic armamentarium against ulcerative colitis. For a long time infliximab was the sole representative of this class of agents approved for use in ulcerative colitis. Now, adalimumab and golimumab are posing therapeutic in-class alternatives. Adalimumab is effective to induce and maintain remission in patients with ulcerative colitis; however, the right timing of treatment initiation is substantial to realize its full therapeutic potential. Post hoc analyses suggest that with increasing disease severity and inflammatory burden the likelihood of a response diminishes. Furthermore, adalimumab is apparently less effective in patients who have failed a previous exposure to infliximab. This and the fact of self-administration of the drug would favor its use in a more moderately active patient population than applying it in the severely active disease arena. Some early pharmacokinetic data of adalimumab in ulcerative colitis point to underdosing with the conventional 160 mg/80 mg induction scheme and have subsequently incited the initiation of high-dose induction studies (SERENE) in both ulcerative colitis and Crohn's disease. As a consequence, individualized induction treatment with adalimumab could become a not too far-fetched reality soon. Al Jolson's quote "you ain't heard nothing yet" from the first talking movie the Jazz Singer when evoking the transition of silent movies into a new age of cinema might also apply to forecasting the true potential of adalimumab in ulcerative colitis. In any case, Al Jolson was right then.

References

1. Solberg IC, Lygren I, Jahnsen J, Aadland E, Høie O, Cvancarova M, et al. Clinical course during the first 10 years of ulcerative colitis: results from a population-based inception cohort (IBSEN Study). Scand J Gastroenterol. 2009;44:431–40.
2. Murch SH, Lamkin VA, Savage MO, Walker-Smith JA, MacDonald TT. Serum concentrations of tumor necrosis factor alpha in childhood chronic inflammatory bowel disease. Gut. 1991;32:913–7.
3. Masuda H, Iwai S, Tanaka T, Hayakawa S. Expression of IL-8, TNF-alpha and IFN-gamma m-RNA in ulcerative colitis, particularly in patients with inactive phase. J Clin Lab Immunol. 1995;46:111–23.
4. Nielsen OH, Gionchetti P, Ainsworth M, Vainer B, Campieri M, Borregaard N, et al. Rectal dialysate and fecal concentrations of neutrophil gelatinase-associated lipocalin, interleukin-8, and tumor necrosis factor-alpha in ulcerative colitis. Am J Gastroenterol. 1999;94:2923–8.
5. Breese EJ, Michie CA, Nicholls SW, Murch SH, Williams CB, Domizio P, et al. Tumor necrosis factor alpha-producing cells in the intestinal mucosa of children with inflammatory bowel disease. Gastroenterology. 1994;106:1455–66.
6. Sands BE, Kaplan GG. The role of TNF alpha in ulcerative colitis. J Clin Pharmacol. 2007;47:930–41.
7. Peyrin-Biroulet L, Laclotte C, Roblin X, Bigard MA. Adalimumab induction therapy for ulcerative colitis with intolerance or lost response to infliximab: an open-label study. World J Gastroenterol. 2007;13:2328–32.
8. Oussalah A, Laclotte C, Chevaux JB, Bensenane M, Babouri A, Serre AA, et al. Long-term outcome of adalimumab therapy for ulcerative colitis with intolerance or lost response to infliximab: a single-centre experience. Aliment Pharmacol Ther. 2008 Oct 15;28:966–72.
9. Afif W, Leighton JA, Hanauer SB, Loftus Jr EV, Faubion WA, Pardi DS, et al. Open-label study of adalimumab in patients with ulcerative colitis including those with prior loss of response or intolerance to infliximab. Inflamm Bowel Dis. 2009;15:1302–7.
10. Barreiro-de Acosta M, Lorenzo A, Dominguez-Munoz JE. Adalimumab in ulcerative colitis: two cases of mucosal healing and clinical response at two years. World J Gastroenterol. 2009;15:3814–6.
11. Gies N, Kroeker KI, Wong K, Fedorak RN. Treatment of ulcerative colitis with adalimumab or infliximab: long-term follow-up of a single-centre cohort. Aliment Pharmacol Ther. 2010;32:522–8.
12. Taxonera C, Estellés J, Fernández-Blanco I, Merino O, Marín-Jiménez I, Barreiro-de Acosta M, et al. Adalimumab induction and maintenance therapy for patients with ulcerative colitis previously treated with infliximab. Aliment Pharmacol Ther. 2011;33:340–8.
13. Reinisch W, Sandborn WJ, Hommes DW, D'Haens G, Hanauer S, Schreiber S, et al. Adalimumab for induction of clinical remission in moderately to severely active ulcerative colitis: results of a randomised controlled trial. Gut. 2011;60:780–7.
14. Sandborn WJ, van Assche G, Reinisch W, Colombel JF, D'Haens G, Wolf DC, et al. Adalimumab induces and maintains clinical remission in patients with moderate-to-severe ulcerative colitis. Gastroenterology. 2012;142:257–65.
15. Reinisch W, Sandborn WJ, Panaccione R, Huang B, Pollack PF, Lazar A, et al. 52-week efficacy of adalimumab in patients with moderately to severely active ulcerative colitis who failed corticosteroids and/or immunosuppressants. Inflamm Bowel Dis. 2013;19:1700–9.
16. Sandborn WJ, Colombel JF, D'Haens G, Van Assche G, Wolf D, Kron M, et al. One-year maintenance outcomes among patients with moderately-to-severely active ulcerative colitis who responded to induction therapy with adalimumab: subgroup analyses from ULTRA 2. Aliment Pharmacol Ther. 2013;37:204–13.
17. Feagan BG, Sandborn WJ, Lazar A, Thakkar RB, Huang B, Reilly N, et al. Adalimumab therapy is associated with reduced risk of hospitalization in patients with ulcerative colitis. Gastroenterology. 2014;146:110–8.
18. Suzuki Y, Motoya S, Hanai H, Matsumoto T, Hibi T, Robinson AM, et al. Efficacy and safety of adalimumab in Japanese patients with moderately to severely active ulcerative colitis. J Gastroenterol. 2014;49:283–94.

19. Colombel JF, Sandborn WJ, Ghosh S, Wolf DC, Panaccione R, Feagan B, et al. Four-year maintenance treatment with adalimumab in patients with moderately to severely active ulcerative colitis: Data from ULTRA 1, 2, and 3. Am J Gastroenterol. 2014;109:1771–80.
20. Danese S, Fiorino G, Peyrin-Biroulet L, et al. Biological agents for moderately to severely active ulcerative colitis: a systematic review and network meta-analysis. Ann Intern Med. 2014;160:704–11.
21. Baert F, Vande Casteele N, Tops S, et al. Prior response to infliximab and early serum drug concentrations predict effects of adalimumab in ulcerative colitis. Aliment Pharmacol Ther. 2014;40:1324–32.
22. Italian Group for the Study of Inflammatory Bowel Disease, Armuzzi A, Biancone L, Daperno M, et al. Adalimumab in active ulcerative colitis: a "real-life" observational study. Dig Liver Dis. 2013;45:738-43.
23. Bressler B, Marshall JK, Bernstein CN, et al. Clinical practice guidelines for the medical management of nonhospitalized ulcerative colitis: the Toronto consensus. Gastroenterology. 2015;148:1035–58.

Biologic Therapy of Ulcerative Colitis: Golimumab

44

Mark A. Samaan and Peter M. Irving

Abbreviations

UC	Ulcerative colitis
QoL	Quality of fife
TNF	Tumor necrosis factor
MH	Mucosal healing
CRP	C-reactive protein
PURSUIT	Program of Ulcerative colitis Research Studies Utilizing an Investigational Treatment
ACT	Active ulcerative colitis trials
ULTRA	Ulcerative colitis long-term remission and maintenance with adalimumab

Introduction and Preclinical Studies

Golimumab (Simponi®, Janssen Biotech, Inc., Horsham, PA, USA) is the most recent anti-TNF agent to be approved for the treatment of moderately to severely active ulcerative colitis (UC), infliximab and adalimumab already being available for this indication. Although it was approved for use in rheumatoid arthritis, psoriatic arthritis, and ankylosing spondylitis in 2009, it was not until 2013 that the US Food and Drug Administration (FDA) and the European Medicines Agency (EMA) granted approval for UC. Golimumab is a transgenic, fully human monoclonal immunoglobulin G1 antibody that is synthesized from TNF-immunized transgenic mice expressing human immunoglobulin G [1, 2]. It differs from earlier anti-TNF agents in both its TNF binding affinity and protein stability [3]. In vitro studies have demonstrated that golimumab binds to both bioactive forms of TNF (membrane-bound and soluble TNF) more avidly than infliximab or adalimumab [4]. This superior affinity has been shown to result in more potent neutralization of TNF-induced cytotoxicity and endothelial cell activity. Subsequent in vivo studies (carried out in a murine model of TNF-mediated arthritis) have also suggested golimumab is more potent than infliximab with doses of 1 and 10 mg/kg significantly delaying disease progression, whereas infliximab was only effective at 10 mg/kg [4]. The excellent protein stability profile of golimumab is also relevant. This property means it can be prepared as a high concentration liquid formulation, making subcutaneous administration possible. This contrasts with infliximab which, owing to its inferior conformational stability, must be stored as a powder and reconstituted before being administered intravenously [4].

Golimumab as Induction Treatment

Data to support golimumab's approval for induction of remission in UC was generated by the PURSUIT-SC trial program. This trial was a randomized, double-blind, placebo-controlled integrated phase 2 and 3 study designed to evaluate the safety and efficacy of subcutaneous golimumab for the induction of remission in moderate-to-severe UC [5]. In conjunction with this, an equivalent IV trial program was commenced (PURSUIT-IV) assessing 2 and 4 mg/kg doses. However, as interim analysis suggested that induction regimens in the SC trial resulted in better clinical efficacy and pharmacokinetic profiles than in the IV trial, only the SC trial was taken forward.

Subjects enrolled to PURSUIT-SC were required to have failed or responded inadequately to standard therapy including oral 5-aminosalicylates, thiopurines, or oral corticosteroids. Patients who had previously been treated with

M.A. Samaan • P.M. Irving (✉)
Department of Gastroenterology, Guy's and St Thomas' Hospital, First Floor College House, North Wing, St Thomas' Hospital, Westminster Bridge Road, London SE1 7EH, UK
e-mail: Peter.Irving@gstt.nhs.uk

D.C. Baumgart (ed.), *Crohn's Disease and Ulcerative Colitis*, DOI 10.1007/978-3-319-33703-6_44

anti-TNF therapy were excluded from taking part in the study. At least moderate disease activity was required, defined as a Mayo score of 6–12 with an endoscopic subscore of 2 or more. Endoscopies were scored by the local investigator rather than being centrally read [6].

The initial phase 2 portion of the study was conducted to determine the dose–response relationship of subcutaneous golimumab. The data generated from this part of the study was then used to inform the design of the phase 3 portion of the trial, designed to evaluate efficacy. In the phase 2 study 169 patients were randomized to receive either placebo or one of three induction regimens: subcutaneous golimumab administered at weeks 0 and 2 in doses of 100/50, 200/100, or 400/200 mg. After safety, pharmacokinetic and efficacy analyses, the 200/100 and 400/200 mg doses were selected for continuation in the phase 3 study.

Seven hundred and seventy-four patients were enrolled into the phase 3 portion of PURSUIT. The study's primary endpoint was clinical response at week 6 defined as a decrease in the Mayo score by at least three points and by 30 % or more, with a bleeding subscore of 0 or 1, or decrease ≥1. Clinical remission was a secondary endpoint and was defined as a Mayo score ≤2 (with no sub-score greater than 1). Additional secondary endpoints included rates of mucosal healing (MH) and impact on Quality of life (QoL). MH was defined as a Mayo endoscopic sub-score of 0 or 1 and QoL was quantified using the Inflammatory Bowel Disease Questionnaire (IBDQ).

The study demonstrated positive findings for the primary and all secondary endpoints. A significantly larger proportion of subjects in the golimumab treated groups had achieved clinical response, clinical remission (Fig. 44.1), MH and had greater IBDQ scores when compared with placebo. Clinical response at week 6, the primary endpoint, was significantly greater in the 400/200 mg (55 %) and 200/100 mg (51 %) groups compared with placebo (30 %, $p<0.0001$ for both treatment groups) as were MH rates (400/200 mg—45 %, 200/100 mg 42 %, placebo—29 %; $p<0.0001$ and <0.0014 respectively). In addition, although a Mayo score of 0 or 1 has been shown to be a clinically meaningful endpoint [7], as part of the endoscopic evaluation a more stringent endoscopic endpoint, Mayo 0 (normal mucosa or inactive disease) was also investigated (Fig. 44.2). Whilst this endpoint was uncommon in participants at week 6, it occurred more commonly in golimumab-treated patients than those receiving placebo (12 %—400/200 mg regimen vs 4 %—placebo, $p<0.0001$). Clinical remission was also more common in golimumab treated patients approximately 18 % of whom entered remission compared with only 6 % of the placebo group ($p<0.0001$) resulting in a number needed to treat of approximately eight patients [8].

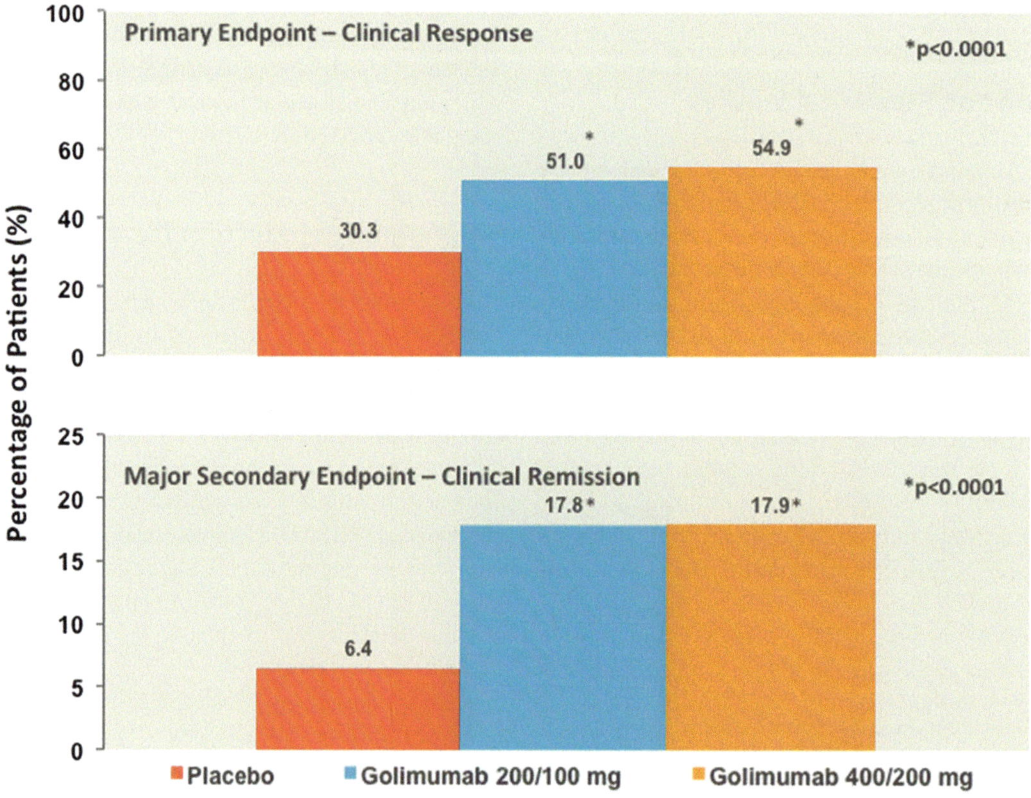

Fig. 44.1 Clinical response (*above*) and remission (*below*) rates for golimumab induction therapy in PURSUIT-SC

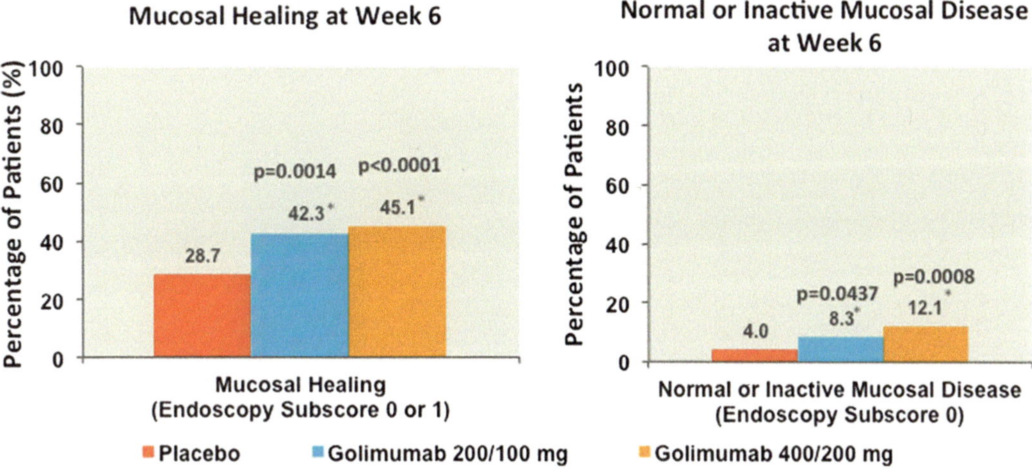

Fig. 44.2 Rates of mucosal healing (Mayo 1 or 0, *left panel*) and inactive mucosal disease (Mayo 0 only, *right panel*) at week 6 in PURSUIT-SC

Biochemical evidence of improvement was also demonstrated with the mean C-reactive protein (CRP) concentration declining to a greater extent in the 400/200 and 200/100 mg groups compared with placebo; fecal calprotectin was not measured.

The authors of the PURSUIT-SC study concluded that subcutaneous golimumab induces clinical response, remission and mucosal healing and improves quality of life in patients with active UC. Based on these results both the EMA and FDA approved the same induction regimen: 200 mg at week 0 and 100 mg at week 2, independent of weight.

However, subsequent comment on the trial outcome has suggested that although these endpoints are conventional (they parallel those used in trials of infliximab [9] and adalimumab [10]) and were achieved, they may not tell clinicians all they need to know about the drug. For example, although golimumab is superior to placebo, it remains true that the vast majority of patients who respond to the drug are still symptomatic, on concomitant steroids, and without a "normal or inactive" mucosal appearance [8].

Golimumab as Maintenance Treatment

All subjects from the PURSUIT-SC trial program were eligible for enrollment into the PURSUIT-Maintenance (PURSUIT-M) study (Fig. 44.3) [11]. The 464 patients who achieved a clinical response with golimumab induction therapy were subsequently randomized to either placebo or treatment with 50 or 100 mg of golimumab administered every 4 weeks. A further 129 patients who had responded to placebo continued on placebo maintenance therapy, and 635 patients who did not respond (to either placebo or golimumab) received open-label golimumab 100 mg every 4 weeks (Fig. 44.4). The primary end point was clinical response maintained through to week 54. To demonstrate maintained response patients were assessed using the partial Mayo score at 4 weekly intervals with the addition of the endoscopic component (to generate the full Mayo score) at weeks 30 and week 54. Patients who met predefined criteria for a clinical flare at any time point underwent an endoscopy to confirm loss of response.

Golimumab was shown to maintain response in 47 % and 50 % of patients who received 50 or 100 mg golimumab every 4 weeks, respectively, versus 31 % in the placebo group ($p=0.010$ and $p<0.001$, respectively), thus meeting the trial's primary endpoint (Fig. 44.5).

The secondary endpoint of clinical remission at both weeks 30 and 54 was achieved by 16 %, 23 %, and 28 % in the placebo, golimumab 50 mg, and golimumab 100 mg groups, respectively (Fig. 44.5). This difference reached statistical significance in the 100 mg group but not in the 50 mg group, despite a numerical advantage being seen ($p=0.122$ and $p=0.004$ for 50 mg and 100 mg golimumab-treated patients versus placebo). Additional secondary endpoints of MH, and corticosteroid-free remission by week 54 were also significantly more likely to occur in patients treated with golimumab compared with placebo.

Based on the results of PURSUIT-M, golimumab was approved by both the EMA and FDA. However, the dosing regimen approved by each differs slightly. In the USA, all patients receive 100 mg every 4 weeks, whilst in Europe patients below 80 kg receive 50 mg every 4 weeks and only those over 80 kg receive 100 mg every 4 weeks.

The design of PURSUIT-M was novel in several ways. Firstly, its definition of maintained response was more stringent than any previously seen in a UC trial. Long-term continuous efficacy was evaluated over the course of 15 prospective assessments without loss of response permitted at

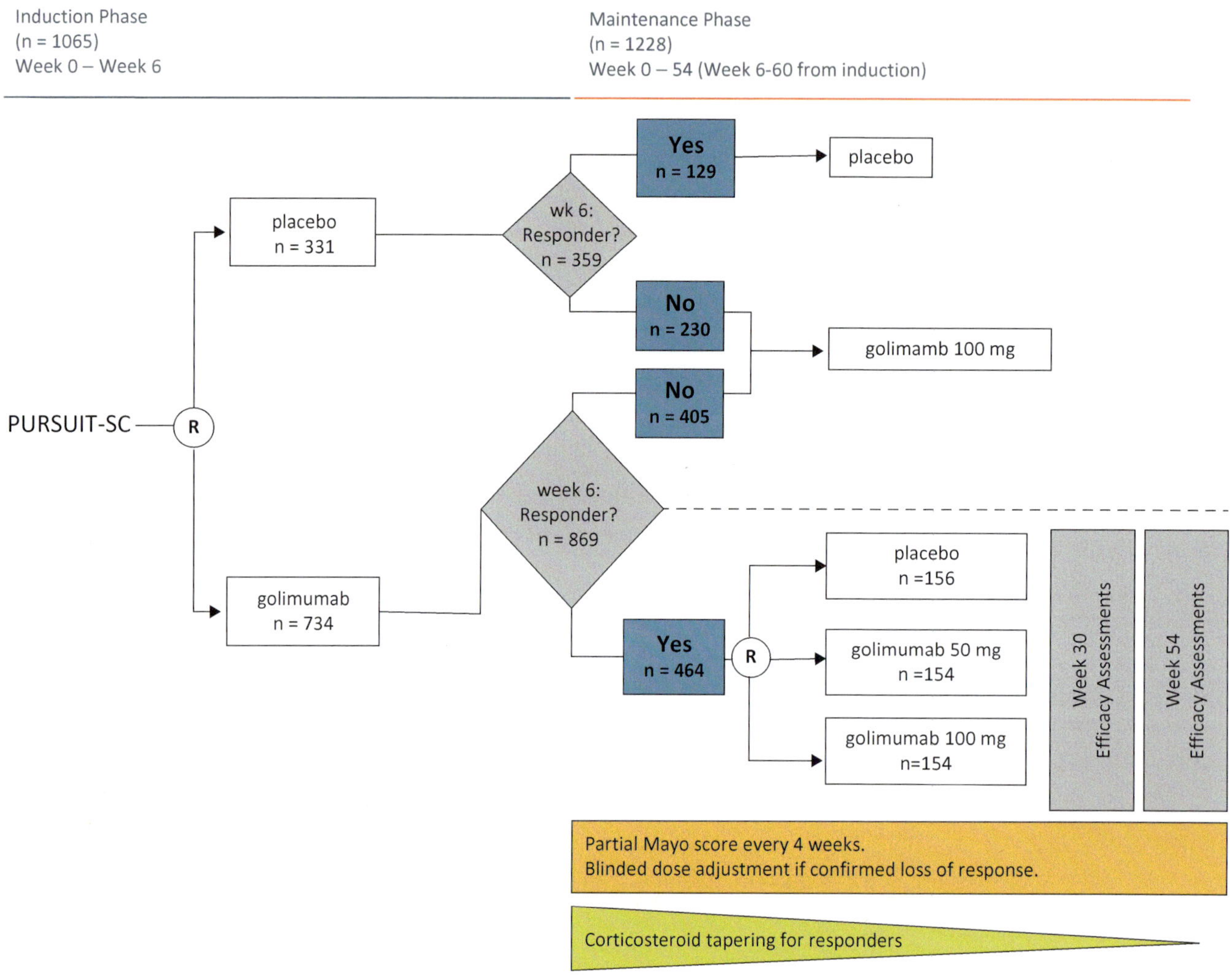

Fig. 44.3 Overview of the study design of the PURSUIT program

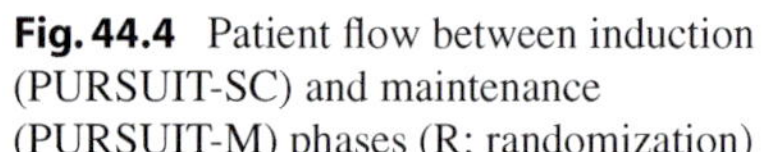

Fig. 44.4 Patient flow between induction (PURSUIT-SC) and maintenance (PURSUIT-M) phases (R; randomization)

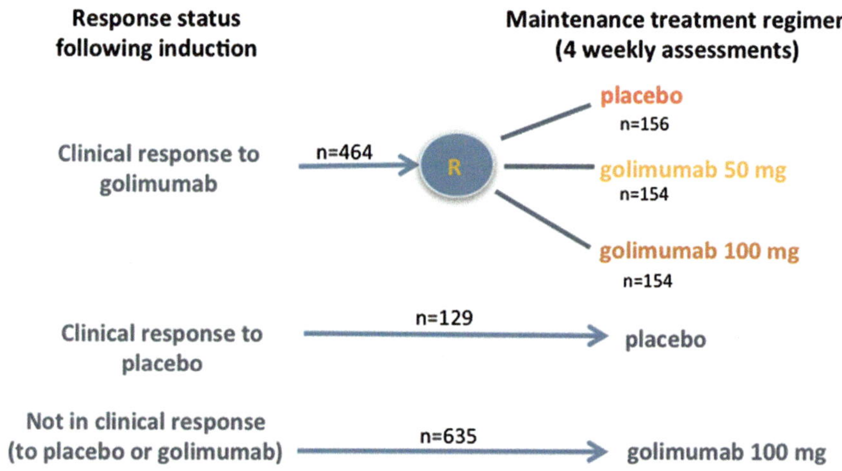

any time-point (Fig. 44.6). This compares with three assessments undertaken as part of the ACT-1 [9] maintenance trial or the two seen in the ACT-2 [9] and ULTRA [10] maintenance trials. Second, PURSUIT-M was the first randomized withdrawal study of an anti-TNF in UC, thus clarifying that induction only is insufficient to maintain a long-term response.

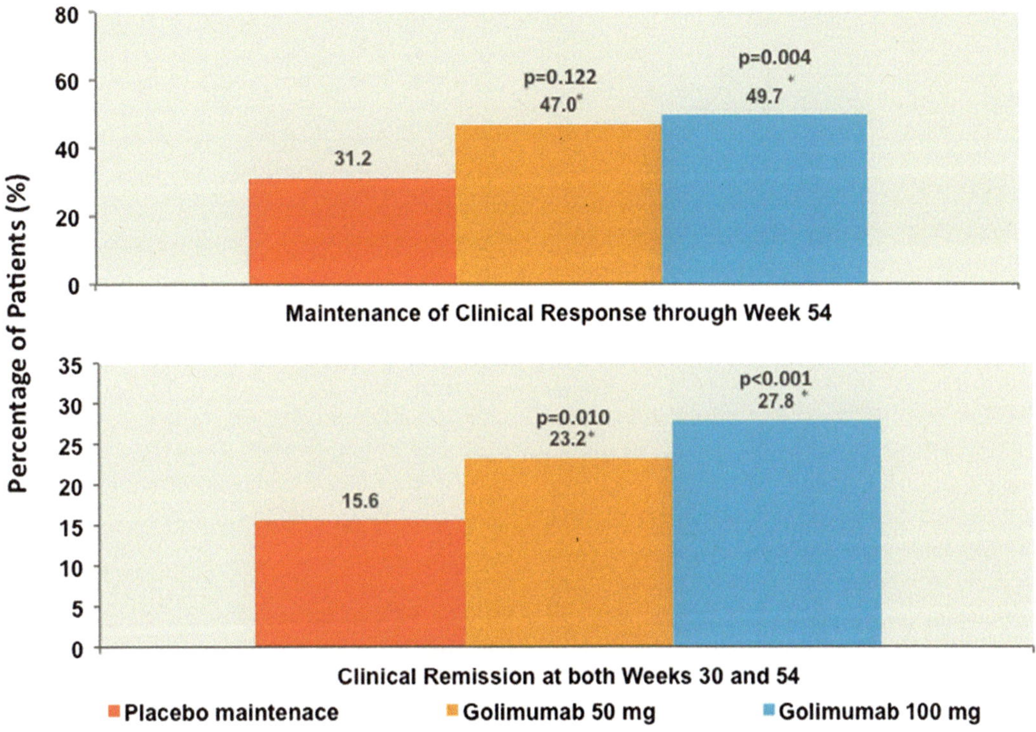

Fig. 44.5 Proportion of golimumab induction responders who maintained clinical response through week 54 (*above*) achieved clinical remission at both weeks 30 and 54 (*below*)

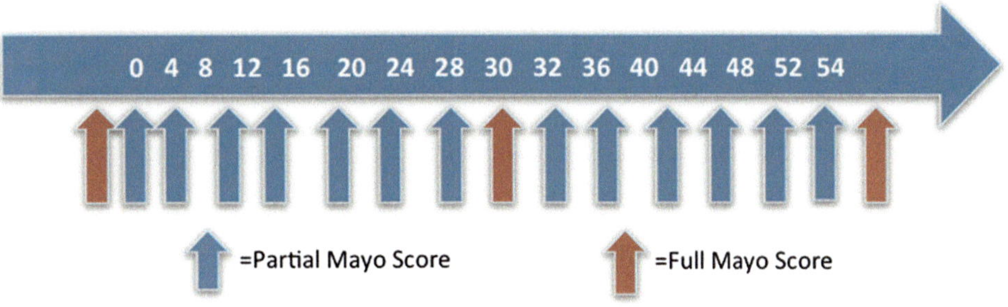

Fig. 44.6 Diagram demonstrating distribution of the fifteen clinical assessments (two of which included endoscopy) made as part of PURSUIT-M

Safety

It remains too early for any safety registry data for golimumab in inflammatory bowel disease to mirror the results from the infliximab (TREAT [12]) and adalimumab (PYRAMID [13]) registries. However, safety analyses from the PURSUIT trials and results as well as long-term extensions of randomized controlled trials carried out in rheumatoid diseases help to inform this area [14]. During the PURSUIT trial program the observed safety signals were reassuring and consistent with experience gained from use in rheumatoid arthritis as well as with the safety profile of the other anti-TNF agents. Four cases of tuberculosis were seen, all in golimumab-treated patients (who were also receiving corticosteroids) living in endemic regions, with one resulting death. This finding should serve to underscore the importance of robust pretreatment screening for tuberculosis in clinical practice. Overall, the percentage of patients with adverse events were similar across the golimumab treatment groups but were somewhat higher compared with the placebo group. However, when the safety data were normalized to 100 years of patient follow-up, the incidence of adverse events was comparable across each of the treatment groups (Table 44.1). The most commonly observed adverse events (other than UC flare) were nasopharyngitis, headache, and arthralgia. Injection site reactions were more common in golimumab treated patients and occurred in 7.1 % of patients receiving 100 mg golimumab, 1.9 % receiving 50 mg golimumab and 1.9 % receiving placebo. Other than this finding, no significant dose-dependent accumulation of adverse events was seen.

Table 44.1 Key safety findings, normalized to 100 patient-years of follow-up through to week 54

		Golimumab	
	Placebo ($n=156$)	50 mg ($n=154$)	100 mg ($n=154$)
	Number of specified events per 100-PYs of FU		
Adverse event	211	187	173
Serious adverse events	13	10	17
Infections	55	61	60
Serious infections	3	4	4
Adverse events leading to discontinuation of study agent	10	6	10

In a 3-year follow-up of 2226 patients with rheumatological conditions (rheumatoid arthritis, psoriatic arthritis, or ankylosing spondylitis) treated with golimumab in clinical trials, it was observed that golimumab 100 mg showed numerically higher incidences of serious infections, demyelinating events, and lymphoma than 50 mg [14]. Although none of these differences reached statistical significance, further longitudinal safety data is yet to be reported at 5 years to clarify further the relationship with these potential long-term adverse effects.

Pharmacokinetic Data and Exposure–Response Relationship

Analysis of serum golimumab concentrations during PURSUIT was carried out using a validated assay and revealed that serum concentrations were dose-proportional. Furthermore, there was an exposure–response relationship in that those with higher serum concentrations of golimumab had higher rates of response and remission as well as greater improvement in median composite Mayo scores. The median trough level serum concentration (measured prior to administrations at weeks 8, 12, 20, 28, 36, and 44) was 0.69–0.83 μg/mL in the golimumab 50 mg group and 1.33–1.58 μg/mL in the golimumab 100 mg group. Steady-state pharmacokinetics was achieved after approximately 8 weeks of maintenance treatment with no carry-over effect observed from the induction dose regimen received. Further pharmacokinetic analysis demonstrated that the bioavailability of golimumab is approximately 52 % and that its half-life is approximately 10.5 days. These values compare with 64 % and approximately 14 days for adalimumab [15].

In PURSUIT-SC the change from baseline Mayo score and rates of clinical response and clinical remission at week 6 increased with increasing quartiles of serum golimumab concentration (Fig. 44.7). In the subsequent maintenance trial, a combined analysis of patients randomized to golimumab 50 and 100 mg groups showed that more patients in the higher serum golimumab concentration quartiles achieved clinical response through to week 54, or clinical remission at both weeks 30 and 54, when compared with those in the lower serum concentration quartiles (Fig. 44.8). This raises the possibility that dose escalation could be an effective strategy for patients with lower drug levels although, it should be noted that there was no difference in the rate of clinical response in secondary nonresponders who received dose escalation, compared to those who maintained the 50 mg dose albeit only in a small number of patients [8].

Despite demonstrating an exposure–response relationship, quartile data does not allow identification of a therapeutic range and, in particular, a minimum threshold and further dedicated, prospective trials are warranted for this purpose in UC. Initial studies have been carried out to investigate golimumab serum drug levels and antidrug antibodies in rheumatoid arthritis [16]. In a prospective, observational cohort study consisting of 37 patients a similar correlation between trough level quartile and response was observed as described above. The lowest quartile (golimumab < 0.25 mg/L) comprised 32 % of all nonresponders, whilst the highest (golimumab > 1.4 mg/L) comprised 47 % of all responders. Data such as these could be used to optimize the use of golimumab in clinical practice and possibly also inform prospective therapeutic drug monitoring trials employing trough levels to drive dosing. Amongst the patients with rheumatoid arthritis treated with golimumab, three patients were found to have high antidrug antibody titers. These resulted in undetectable golimumab levels and poor clinical outcome. Antidrug antibodies were also detected in a small minority of patients (2.9 %) in the PURSUIT trials and the majority of these (67.7 %) were found to be neutralizing. Their occurrence was significantly less common in patients who were receiving concomitant immunomodulators (1.1 %) compared with patients who were not (3.8 %). These findings argue for the use of golimumab in combination with an immunomodulatory drug to optimize its efficacy, although future research comparing combination to monotherapy is necessary to establish whether combination therapy is associated with clinical benefit and to understand the risk benefit ratio.

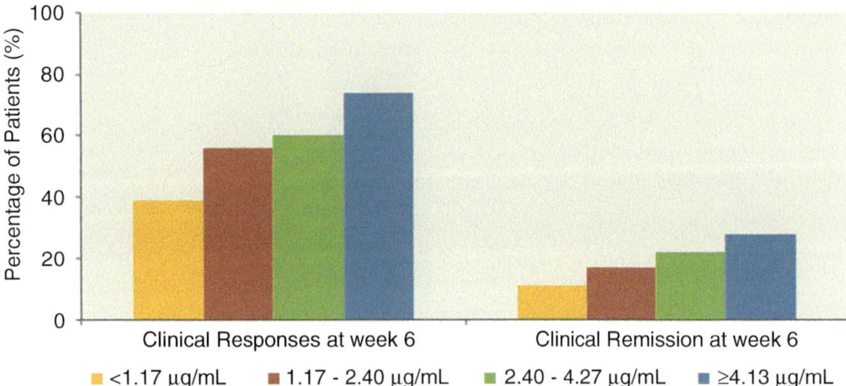

Fig. 44.7 Proportion of patients achieving clinical response (*left*) and remission (*right*) by serum golimumab concentration at week 6 in PURSUIT-SC

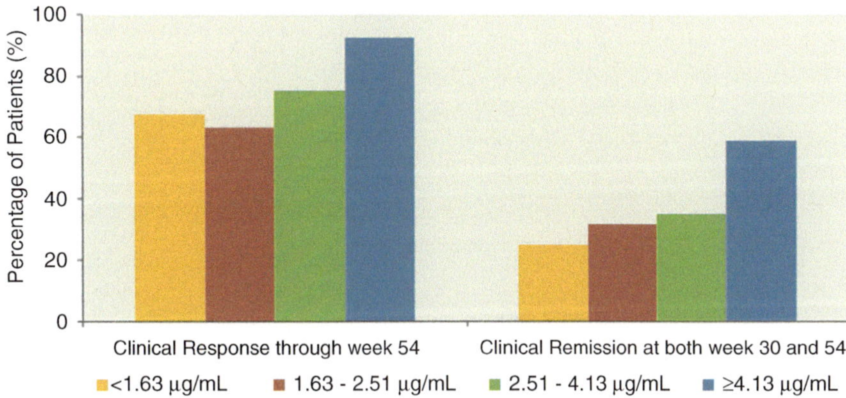

Fig. 44.8 Proportion of patients with clinical response through to week 54 (*left*) or in clinical remission at both weeks 30 and 54 (*right*) by serum golimumab concentration quartiles at week 54 in PURSUIT-M

The Position of Golimumab in the UC Therapeutic Algorithm

Where golimumab is positioned in the treatment of moderate to severe UC will depend on a number of factors some of which will vary across individual healthcare systems, centers, clinicians and patients. Its pattern and frequency of use will, therefore, likely vary. No head-to-head trials have been performed comparing different anti-TNF agents in UC; however, a network meta-analysis, comprising 2282 patients receiving anti-TNF (infliximab, adalimumab or golimumab) or vedolizumab for UC [17] has been published. This identified a trend suggesting that infliximab may be slightly more effective than the other biologic agents although the only statistically significant difference was seen when comparing the ability of infliximab and adalimumab in inducing clinical response (odds ratio 2.36; confidence interval 1.22–4.63) and mucosal healing (odds ratio 2.0; confidence interval 1.13–3.59). It is important to remember the weaknesses of comparing results from different trials; however, golimumab and adalimumab seem to be approximately equivalent in terms of efficacy and safety. From the perspective of patient comfort, golimumab would seem favorable owing to its 4 weekly administration schedule compared with every other week (or every week in the case of dose intensification) for adalimumab.

The use of golimumab as a rescue therapy in acute severe hospitalized patients with UC has not been studied and infliximab will remain the anti-TNF agent of choice for these patients. Golimumab has also not been evaluated formally in patients who have failed other anti-TNF agents. As both primary non-response and secondary loss of response to anti-TNF therapy are common, the effectiveness of golimumab as a second line anti-TNF agent needs to be determined. Finally, whether vedolizumab will eventually become the preferred biologic for UC currently remains unclear. The positioning of anti-TNF and anti-adhesion molecule therapy will become apparent as experience of use of the latter increases.

Summary and Conclusion

Golimumab is licensed for use in moderate-to-severe UC based on proven efficacy in the induction and maintenance of clinical response and remission. This evidence was generated in high-quality, well-designed, and large-scale randomized controlled trials, which also demonstrated its safety. Although long-term safety data from a prospectively maintained registry in IBD is not yet available, results from such cohorts in rheumatology are reassuring and in keeping with other the anti-TNF agents.

Its dosing schedule and route of administration are factors that may lead clinicians and patients to favor it over alternative anti-TNF agents in certain scenarios and its use is therefore likely to increase. However, many questions regarding its optimal use and comparative effectiveness remain to be answered, these include; does dose escalation improve efficacy amongst nonresponders? Does trough level target driven dosing yield better results? Is combination therapy favorable to monotherapy? What role do antidrug antibodies play, and can they be overcome by dose escalation or immunomodulation? How effective is golimumab in the setting of previous anti-TNF failure? How would golimumab compare to other anti-TNF agents and vedolizumab in head-to-head trials?

These questions will require dedicated trials to generate the necessary evidence to allow clinicians and patients to get the most out of this new agent in the treatment of UC.

Disclosures Mark A. Samaan—Hospira: Advisory board and training, Takeda: Lecturing.

Peter M. Irving—Honoraria for acting in an advisory capacity or speaking on behalf of MSD, Abbvie, Takeda, Shire, Ferring, Tillott's Pharma, Warner Chilcott, Genentech, Pharmacosmos. Research support: MSD.

References

1. Hutas G. Golimumab, a fully human monoclonal antibody against TNFalpha. Curr Opin Mol Ther. 2008;10(4):393–406.
2. Lonberg N. Human antibodies from transgenic animals. Nat Biotechnol. 2005;23(9):1117–25.
3. Lowenberg M, de Boer N, Hoentjen F. Golimumab for the treatment of ulcerative colitis. Clin Exp Gastroenterol. 2014;7:53–9. Pubmed Central PMCID: 3958527.
4. Shealy DJ, Cai A, Staquet K, Baker A, Lacy ER, Johns L, et al. Characterization of golimumab, a human monoclonal antibody specific for human tumor necrosis factor alpha. mAbs. 2010;2(4):428–39. Pubmed Central PMCID: 3180089.
5. Sandborn WJ, Feagan BG, Marano C, Zhang H, Strauss R, Johanns J, et al. Subcutaneous golimumab induces clinical response and remission in patients with moderate-to-severe ulcerative colitis. Gastroenterology. 2014;146(1):85–95.
6. Feagan BG, Sandborn WJ, D'Haens G, Pola S, McDonald JW, Rutgeerts P, et al. The role of centralized reading of endoscopy in a randomized controlled trial of mesalamine for ulcerative colitis. Gastroenterology. 2013;145(1):149–57.e2.
7. Sandborn WJ, Rutgeerts P, Feagan BG, Reinisch W, Olson A, Johanns J, et al. Colectomy rate comparison after treatment of ulcerative colitis with placebo or infliximab. Gastroenterology. 2009;137(4):1250–60. quiz 520.
8. Hanauer SB. Still in pursuit. Gastroenterology. 2014;146(1):13–5.
9. Rutgeerts P, Sandborn WJ, Feagan BG, Reinisch W, Olson A, Johanns J, et al. Infliximab for induction and maintenance therapy for ulcerative colitis. N Engl J Med. 2005;353(23):2462–76.
10. Sandborn WJ, van Assche G, Reinisch W, Colombel JF, D'Haens G, Wolf DC, et al. Adalimumab induces and maintains clinical remission in patients with moderate-to-severe ulcerative colitis. Gastroenterology. 2012;142(2):257–65.e1–3.
11. Sandborn WJ, Feagan BG, Marano C, Zhang H, Strauss R, Johanns J, et al. Subcutaneous golimumab maintains clinical response in patients with moderate-to-severe ulcerative colitis. Gastroenterology. 2014;146(1):96–109.e1.
12. Lichtenstein GR, Feagan BG, Cohen RD, Salzberg BA, Diamond RH, Price S, et al. Serious infection and mortality in patients with Crohn's disease: more than 5 years of follow-up in the TREAT registry. Am J Gastroenterol. 2012;107(9):1409–22. Pubmed Central PMCID: 3438468.
13. D'Haens G, Reinisch W, Satsangi J, Loftus E, Panaccione R, Tokimoto D, et al. PYRAMID registry: an observational study of adalimumab in Crohn's disease: results at year 3. Inflamm Bowel Dis. 2011;17:S21.
14. Kay J, Fleischmann R, Keystone E, Hsia EC, Hsu B, Mack M, et al. Golimumab 3-year safety update: an analysis of pooled data from the long-term extensions of randomized, double-blind, placebo-controlled trials conducted in patients with rheumatoid arthritis, psoriatic arthritis or ankylosing spondylitis. Ann Rheum Dis. 2015;74(3):538–46. Pubmed Central PMCID: 4345908.
15. Mease PJ. Adalimumab in the treatment of arthritis. Ther Clin Risk Manag. 2007;3(1):133–48. Pubmed Central PMCID: 1936294.
16. Kneepkens EL, Plasencia C, Krieckaert CL, Pascual-Salcedo D, van der Kleij D, Nurmohamed MT, et al. Golimumab trough levels, antidrug antibodies and clinical response in patients with rheumatoid arthritis treated in daily clinical practice. Ann Rheum Dis. 2014;73(12):2217–9.
17. Danese S, Fiorino G, Peyrin-Biroulet L, Lucenteforte E, Virgili G, Moja L, et al. Biological agents for moderately to severely active ulcerative colitis: a systematic review and network meta-analysis. Ann Intern Med. 2014;160(10):704–11.

Biologic Therapy of Ulcerative Colitis: Natalizumab, Vedolizumab, Etrolizumab (rHUMab Beta 7), Anti-MAdCAM

45

Severine Vermeire

Treatment Goal in Ulcerative Colitis (UC)

Following the introduction of biologic agents, of which the anti-tumor necrosis factor (TNF) antibodies have occupied the scene in the last decade, the treatment goal for patients with UC has shifted from symptom control towards steroid-free remission and healing of the mucosa. How endoscopic healing is achieved is less important, as long as it is done in a timely manner and chronic use of steroids is avoided. The degree of mucosal healing is still a matter of debate. Whereas disappearance of frank ulcers and overt bleeding is unanimously accepted, it is less clear if some persistence of friability and decreased vascular pattern can be left alone. Furthermore, presence of basal plasmacytosis in the lamina propria seen on histology has been confirmed by several groups as a marker of relapse, therefore even suggesting that histologic healing should be studied in the future [1].

Anti-Cell Adhesion Strategies as a Novel Therapeutic Class in IBD

The relatively high treatment failure rate of anti-TNF therapy (both primary or secondary loss of response), especially in UC, urged the need for new agents targeting other pathways involved in the disease pathogenesis. A promising idea is to dampen the influx of immune cells towards the inflamed sites in the intestinal mucosa, rather than targeting inflammatory cells and mediators that are already present: the so-called anti-cell adhesion molecules. T cells originate in the bone marrow and mature in the lymph nodes by differentiating into regulatory or effector cells. This occurs thanks to the activation by dendritic cells after they have recognized the antigen (Ag). The effector T cells have receptors that enable them to migrate to the inflamed tissue, mainly through the post-capillary venules. One of the crucial points of the increased immune response in inflammatory bowel disease (IBD) is the increased migration of T cells to the intestinal tract. Leucocytes travel at high speed through the vasculature, and in order to migrate to tissues such as the intestinal tract, there is a sequential adhesion system consisting of the capture, tethering, rolling, activation, adhesion and migration through the vascular wall [2, 3]. The capture of the T cells to the endothelium is mediated through the interaction between selectins (L-selectins expressed by leucocytes and P- and E-selectins that are found on the endothelium) and oligosaccharide moieties that act as ligands. This weak and transient interaction allows leucocytes first to slow their speed in the vascular flow and then to roll through the vascular wall by going from one selectin to another. There are several arguments favoring the development of anti-leukocyte migration strategies in UC. First, UC is characterized by a strong adhesion molecule-mediated mucosal infiltration of leukocytes [4] (Fig. 45.1). Next, VCAM-1, the ligand for integrin $\alpha4\beta1$, is upregulated in the vascular endothelium of the inflamed gut [5]. Furthermore, MADCAM, ligand for integrin $\alpha4\beta7$ ligand which is responsible for the trafficking of lymphocytes to the gut, is also upregulated in IBD mucosa.

Attempts to suppress inflammation in a gut-selective way have been successful with antibodies targeting alpha4 beta7+ T-lymphocytes, which have a phenotype of intestinal homing lymphocytes. This class of drugs is certainly anticipated to be superior from a safety perspective. Preclinical studies showed efficacy of blocking integrin $\alpha4(\beta7)$ in the spontaneous cotton-top tamarin colitis model [6, 7]. More recently, the genetic association between IBD and integrins (ITGAL = integrin alpha–L), chemokines and chemokine receptors has been uncovered. The main

S. Vermeire, M.D., Ph.D. (✉)
Department of Gastroenterology, University Hospitals Leuven, Leuven, Belgium
e-mail: Severine.Vermeire@uzleuven.be

D.C. Baumgart (ed.), *Crohn's Disease and Ulcerative Colitis*, DOI 10.1007/978-3-319-33703-6_45

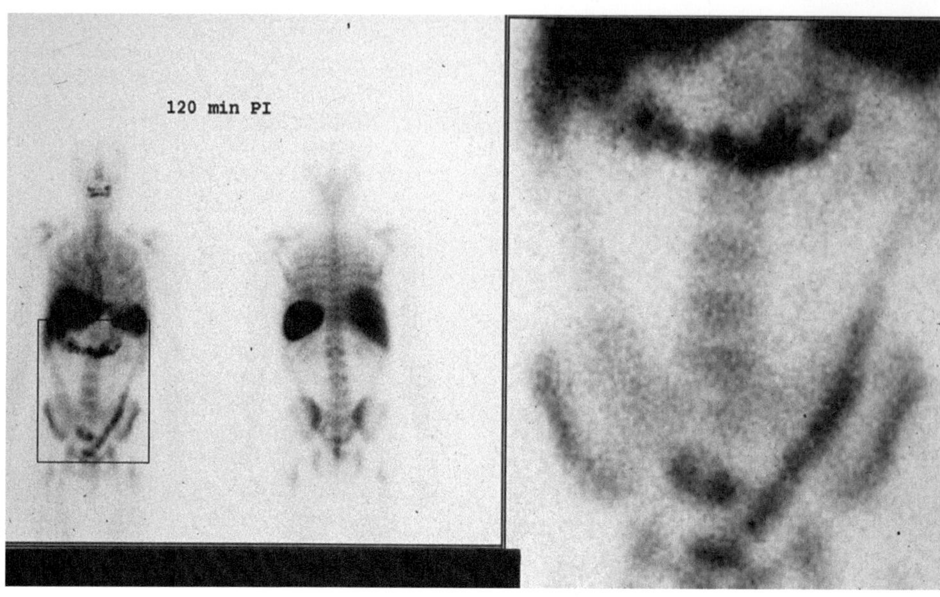

Fig. 45.1 Tc-99 m HMPAO WBC scintigraphy in a patient with ulcerative colitis (*left*) whole-body image and (*right*) a detail of the abdomen. Rapid migration of lymphocytes from the peripheral circulation to the colon is seen

cell populations responsible for the adaptive immune response in the gut are antigen-presenting cells, which can be professional (dendritic cells) or not professional (epithelial cells), effector cells (effector T cells, granulocytes, natural killer, macrophages, etc.), regulatory T cells, and mucosal B cells. Secondary adhesion molecules are members of the family of integrins. These allow leucocytes to stop rolling and start migration and extravasation through the vascular wall. The expression of integrins is activated by chemokines, which are released by T cells. Integrins involved in the T-cell migration are as follows: leucocyte function-associated antigen 1 (LFA-1 or $\alpha 2\beta 2$) and the two $\alpha 4$-integrins ($\alpha 4\beta 7$ and $\alpha 1\beta 7$). The subunit α is implied in the specificity and the subunit β in signal pathways. For the migration of the leucocytes, these integrins bind to specific ligands at the endothelium called addressins or adhesion molecules. The $\alpha 2\beta 2$ integrin, expressed on neutrophils, interacts with intercellular adhesion molecule-1 (ICAM-1) that is expressed on leucocytes, dendritic cells, fibroblasts, epithelial cells, and endothelial cells. The $\alpha 4\beta 1$ integrin is composed of one $\beta 1$ chain and one $\alpha 4$ chain and is expressed on most leucocytes, but not on neutrophils. The $\alpha 4\beta 1$ integrin binds to vascular cell adhesion molecule-1 (VCAM-1) and to components of the extracellular matrix such as fibronectin and thrombospondin. The third family is the $\alpha 4\beta 7$ integrin, which is expressed on the lymphocytes that colonize the gut and gut-associated lymphoid tissues and interacts with the mucosal addressin-cell adhesion molecule 1 (MAdCAM-1). The MAdCAM-1 ligand is expressed in the endothelial venules in the small intestine, in the Peyer's patches and the colon, and the interaction with integrin $\alpha 4\beta 7$ activates the migration of lymphocytes to Peyer's patches. Therefore, the interaction between $\alpha 4\beta 7$ and MAdCAM-1 is gut-specific.

Natalizumab (Tysabri)

Anti-integrin strategies have been developed and two compounds have received FDA/EMA approval so far. Natalizumab, a human anti-alpha4 integrin antibody, was developed first and the clinical development with the ENCORE & ENACT trials met their primary endpoint [8, 9]. The drug received a FDA-fast track approval for treatment of moderate-to-severe Crohn's disease, not responding to standard drugs. However, following a number of fatal case reports of patients treated with natalizumab who developed progressive multifocal leukoencephalopathy (PML), a neurological disorder caused by reactivation of JC virus in the brain, further drug development was stopped [10, 11] (Fig. 45.2). In 2008, the US Food and Drug Administration (FDA) approved natalizumab (Tysabri) for the treatment of moderate-to-severe Crohn's disease. Crohn's disease patients who are started on Tysabri must be enrolled in a special restricted distribution program called CD TOUCH (Crohn's Disease-Tysabri Outreach Unified Commitment to Health). Under CD-TOUCH, physicians evaluate CD patients after 3 months of Tysabri treatment to determine if they have improved on Tysabri and if not, patients should discontinue further treatment. Previously, in 2006, Tysabri was approved by FDA to treat relapsing forms of multiple sclerosis.

Vedolizumab (Entyvio)

The necessity to develop a gut-selective drug became clear after reports of PML with the non-gut specific anti-alpha4 integrin natalizumab. Vedolizumab was developed soon after and inhibits the binding of alpha4beta 7 integrin to its receptor MadCam, hence selectively inhibiting homing of T-lymphocytes

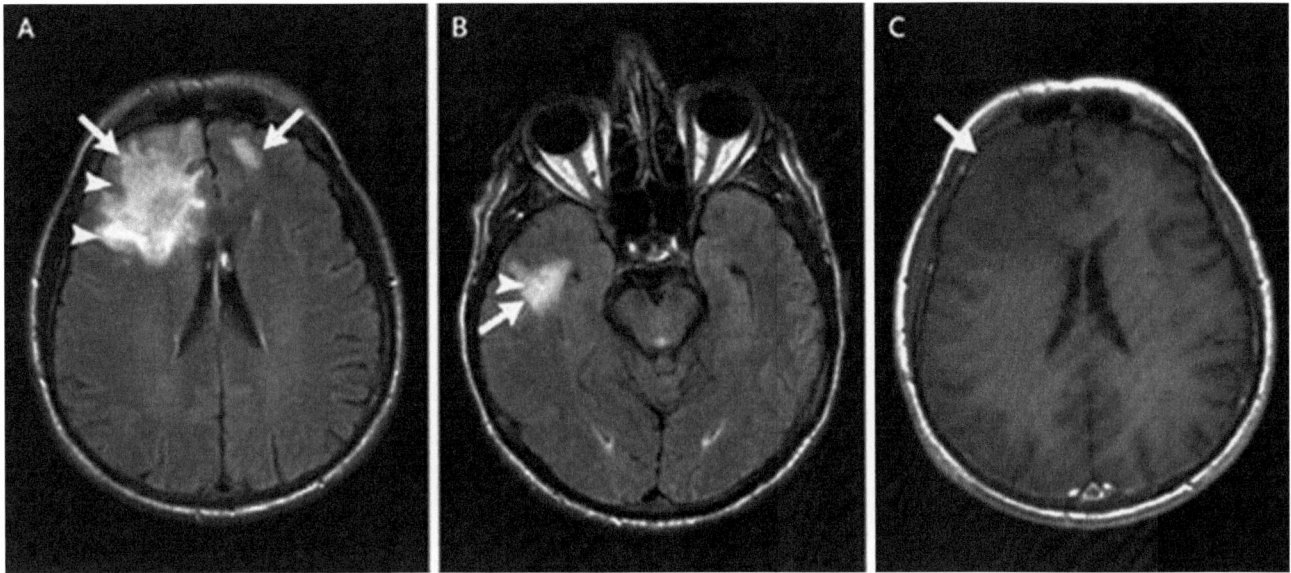

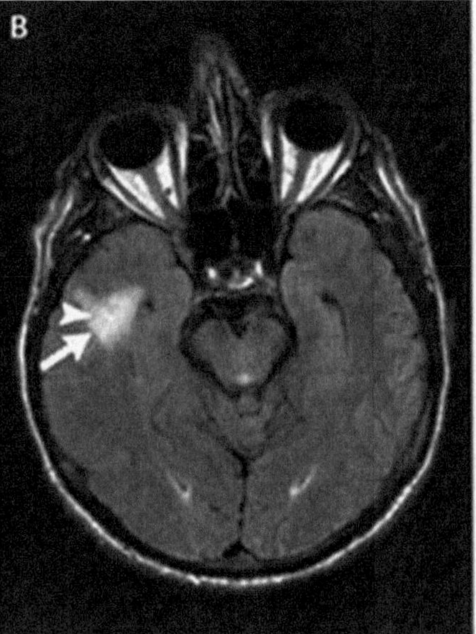

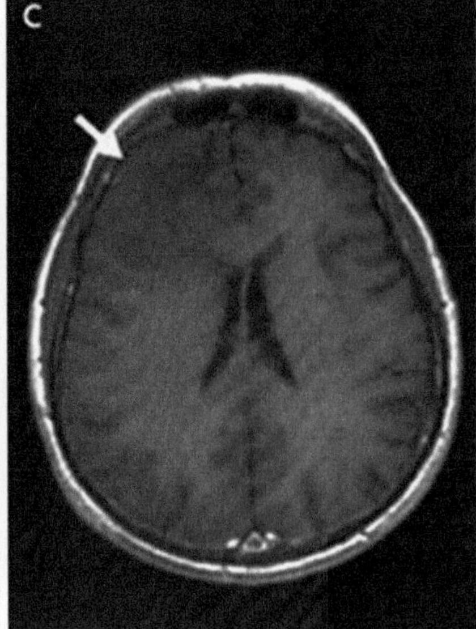

Fig. 45.2 Brain MRI in a IBD patient treated with natalizumab shows progressive multifocal leucoencephalopathy (Van Assche G et al. N Engl J Med 2005;353:362–36)

to the gut. Feagan et al. studied vedolizumab, in a randomized, double-blind trial of 29 patients with moderately severe UC [12]. Three single doses of vedolizumab 0.15, 0.5, and 2.0 mg/kg or placebo were studied. Follow-up studies looked at repeated doses: in the study by Feagan et al., 181 patients with active UC were randomized to receive vedolizumab 0.5, 2 mg/kg or matched placebo on days 1 and 29 [13]. The study by Parikh et al. included 47 patients and doses of 2, 6, 10 mg/kg or placebo, administered on days 1, 15, 29, and 85 [14]. The large GEMINI I phase III trial in UC was an integrated induction and maintenance study and met the primary endpoint of clinical response at week 6 [15]. In the trial of induction therapy, 374 patients (cohort 1) received vedolizumab at a dose of 300 mg or placebo intravenously at weeks 0 and 2, and 521 patients (cohort 2) received open-label vedolizumab at weeks 0 and 2. In the trial of maintenance therapy, patients who had a response to vedolizumab at week 6 were randomly assigned to continue receiving vedolizumab every 8 or 4 weeks or to switch to placebo for up to 52 weeks. At week 6, 47 % of UC patients treated with vedolizumab responded and 41 % showed healing (in contrast to 25 % for both endpoints in the placebo group). The long-term results were even more impressive as 45 % of patients treated with vedolizumab q4 weeks were in corticosteroid free remission at week 52 (14 % in the placebo arm) and 56 % had mucosal healing (20 % in the placebo arm). The GEMINI programs demonstrated superior efficacy in induction and maintenance of remission and in May 2014, vedolizumab was approved by FDA and also by the European Medicines Agency (EMA) for treatment of CD and UC [15, 16] (Fig. 45.3). An open-label GEMINI-long term safety (LTS) trial, is currently running and will be completed in March 2016 (NCT00790933).

Etrolizumab

Etrolizumab is a humanized IgG1 monoclonal antibody to β7 integrin expressed on lymphocytes. Etrolizumab inhibits therefore trafficking of T-lymphocytes into the gastrointestinal mucosa through interaction between alpha4 beta7 with MadCam but also blocks retention of lymphocytes in the gut epithelium by blocking interaction of alphaE beta7 and its ligand E-Cadherin. As such, etrolizumab is also gut-selective and does not interfere with leukocyte trafficking to the central nervous system or to other non-mucosal tissues and PML is also not expected to occur with this compound. The exact role of Alpha-E positive lymphocytes in human IBD is unknown and this cell population accounts for less than 1 % of all circulating lymphocytes in the peripheral blood.

A phase 1 study with etrolizumab showed a good safety profile [17]. The phase 2 study conducted in UC included 124 patients who were randomized to placebo or a low (100 mg) or high (300 mg + loading dose) of SC dosed etrolizumab q 4 weekly [18]. The primary endpoint was clinical remission at week 10. A significantly higher proportion of patients treated with etrolizumab low dose (21 %) or high dose + loading dose (10 %) met the primary endpoint of clinical remission compared to placebo (0 %). The effect was entirely driven by the anti-TNF naïve patient population, although the low sample size of this phase 2 study precludes from making strong statements about this observation. Interestingly, patients with high alpha-E (ITGAE) gene expression in their baseline colon biopsies had a higher likelihood of achieving clinical remission that patients with low alphaE gene expression (using a median cutoff value to define high and low expression). In addition a high numbers

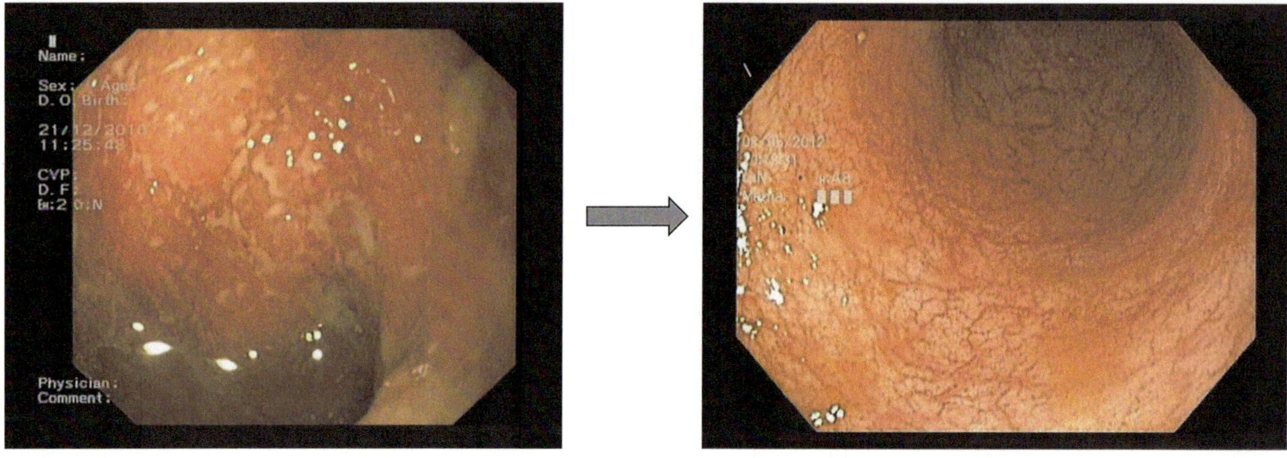

Fig. 45.3 Endoscopic picture of patient with left-sided ulcerative colitis (*left*) shows endoscopic healing after treatment with vedolizumab (*right*)

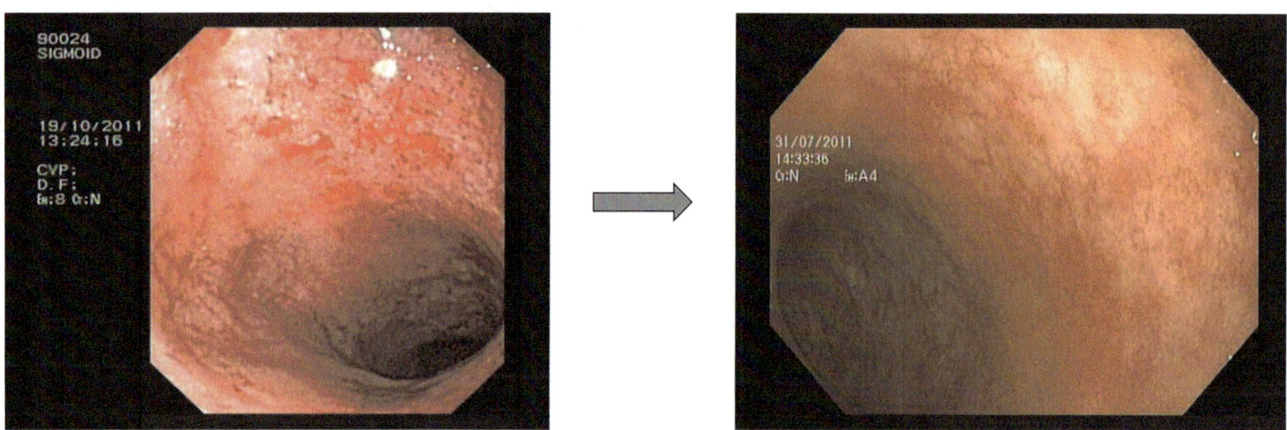

Fig. 45.4 Endoscopic picture of patient with ulcerative colitis before (*left*) and after (*right*) treatment with etrolizumab

of αE+ cells predicted a higher remission rate. Based on these encouraging results, a large phase 3 program with etrolizumab is ongoing in anti-TNF naïve and experienced patients and includes besides placebo-controlled studies also a number of trial designs with active comparator arm against anti-TNF agents (e.g., NCT02136069, NCT02163759) (Fig. 45.4). Results are expected in 2017. The alpha-E positivity in the colonic biopsies will be checked to validate the findings of the phase 2 study on the role of alphaE as predictor of response.

Anti-MadCam

Similar to inhibition of integrins expressed on gut lymphocytes, their respective ligands on the endothelial wall can also be the target. An anti-MadCam monoclonal antibody has been developed by Pfizer and a first-in-human study explored the safety and preliminary efficacy of this compound in ulcerative colitis (trial Register No. NCT00928681). A total of 80 patients with active UC received single or multiple (three doses, 4-week intervals) doses of anti-MadCam 0.03–10 mg/kg IV/SC, or placebo [19]. The overall responder/remission rates at 4 and 12 weeks were 52 %/13 % and 42 %/22 %, respectively with combined anti-MadCam doses compared with 32 %/11 % and 21 %/0 %, respectively with placebo. Clinical results were paralleled by a decrease in fecal calprotectin levels in patients treated with active drug compared to placebo. This led to the larger phase 2 study assessing different doses (7.5, 22.5, 75, or 225 mg) of anti-MadCam or placebo [20]. Primary endpoint was clinical remission at week 12 and was met for the 7.5, 22.5, and 75 mg doses, as compared to placebo. Interestingly, a bell-shaped dose-response curve was again seen with highest efficacy observed in patients receiving the 22.5 mg dose. This bell-shaped response curve was also observed in the etrolizumab phase 2 study where the low 100 mg dose showed superior results than the high 300 mg+loading dose group, and also in an early vedolizumab phase 2 study, the same observation was made. This poses the question if higher doses of drugs belonging to this mode of action, may also interfere with migration or activity of other cells such as regulatory T-cells? Another intriguing finding was the fact that the effect of anti-Madcam was observed almost exclusively in TNF-naïve patients, similar to what was seen with etrolizumab, and to a lesser extent with vedolizumab. If this represents a more refractory patient population is unclear at present.

Ideal Time Point for Assessment of Response with Anti-CAM

Compared to the anti-TNF drugs, and following their mechanism of action, anti-leukocyte trafficking drugs have a slower onset of action. The GEMINI I study with vedolizumab assessed response and remission in UC at week 6 and met its primary endpoint [15]. Etrolizumab in the phase 2 study met its primary endpoint of clinical remission at week 10 [18] and the recently completed phase 2 study with anti-Madcam in UC assessed response and remission no earlier than week 12 [20]. It therefore seems that the optimum time point for assessment of response or remission will most likely be situated 10 weeks or more following the first administration. Real-life cohort studies in the coming years will undoubtedly learn when physicians should reassess before determining primary non-response. This also implies that bridging strategies will need to be adopted to enhance symptom control in the first weeks. What the most optimal bridging strategy for induction of remission will be, is unknown at this moment but fast-induction agents such as corticosteroids, anti-TNF and even cyclosporine have already been proposed. While efficacy is important, the safety profile of combining 2 or more immunosuppressive agents however also needs to be considered, as will be the economic cost.

Maintenance of Response and Remission

The true benefit of the class of anti-trafficking agents lies in their ability to maintain remission and mucosal healing. Long-term maintenance results of vedolizumab q8 weeks in GEMINI I showed remission rates at week 52 of 45 %, corticosteroid-free remission rates of 45 % and mucosal healing of 56 %. The GEMINI Long Term Safety (LTS) study released results from 3 year maintenance therapy with sustained remission rates in >90 % of patients, suggesting only minor loss of response. Although data on immunogenicity and drug exposure are limited thus far, only 4 % of patients developed antidrug antibodies in GEMINI I and II [15, 16].

Biologic-Naïve Patients: Anti-TNF or Anti-Leucocyte Trafficking?

The most challenging question at present probably in a patient with moderate to severe UC failing 5-ASA, steroids and/or azathioprine, is which biologic therapy to start? Until 1 year ago only anti-TNF was available and physicians used parameters such as disease severity and patient preferences to guide the therapeutic decision to infliximab, adalimumab, or golimumab. With the advent of vedolizumab, the choice of treatment expands and with this, also the need for predictive biomarkers or mucosal signatures of response. A personalized therapeutic approach is very well known and applied already in other disease areas. In oncology, gene expression profiling has been successfully used to identify transcriptional signatures that predict several aspects of disease behavior, including risk of metastasis and response to chemotherapy [21, 22]. These gene expression-based biomarkers have also been translated into clinical practice and have received FDA-approval [23]. In contrast, in autoimmune and inflammatory disorders, such techniques have generally not detected signatures with equivalent prognostic utility. Typically, the tissues examined (peripheral blood mononuclear cells (PBMCs), mucosal biopsies, …) are heterogeneous, and hence any transcriptional variation detected will predominantly reflect differences in the cellular composition between samples. We previously identified a mucosal gene signature to predict response to infliximab in IBD [24]. The most exciting data in this respect, as addressed above, have been generated for etrolizumab. In the phase 2 study, response and remission rates were enriched in patients expressing high alphaE+ cells (defined as below or above the median) [18] and in a follow-up study, it was shown that levels of Granzyme A and Integrin alphaE mRNAs in colon tissues can identify patients with UC who are most likely to benefit from etrolizumab [25]. If this finding is confirmed in the large phase 3 studies, then this may well become the first clinically useful biomarker for predicting response to this drug.

Safety

Whereas the first molecule in the class of anti-cell adhesion molecules, natalizumab, was non-gut selective, the compounds which followed have a gut-selective mode of action. This renders a possible safety advantage over anti-TNF agents, that have been associated with serious opportunistic infections, rare malignancies such as hepato-splenic T-cell lymphomas and melanomas, and with psoriasiform skin eruptions or alopecia.

The gut-selectivity of vedolizumab and the other agents etrolizumab and anti-MadCam has been further demonstrated by lack of MadCam expression in human brain (in contrast to expression of VCAM-1 in the brain). The effect of vedolizumab on cerebrospinal fluid was also studied in healthy volunteers receiving a single dose of vedolizumab and who underwent a lumbar punction pretreatment and at week 5 post-treatment. No changes in CD4/CD8 ratio was observed. Similarly, the effects of anti-MadCam on CSF were studied in Crohn's patients in the TOSCA study and no changes in CSGF composition following anti-MadCam treatment were observed. Wyant et al. studied the seroconversion of IM Hepatitis B vaccination or oral cholera vaccine following treatment with vedolizumab in healthy volunteers. Whereas the anti-HBs titers were similar between placebo or vedolizumab, the mean anti cholera toxin IgG levels were significantly higher in placebo-treated individuals as compared to vedo-exposed individuals, demonstrating the gut-selective mode of action of the latter. Of course long-term safety registries are ongoing with all agents in this class, although at this moment, no cases of PML have been reported. Patients in the GEMINI programs with vedolizumab were actively monitored for PML with very frequent screenings. Any unexplained neurological symptom also needed further evaluation.

With regard to overall safety of vedolizumab, no statistically significant difference has been observed in the proportion of patients who experienced any adverse event (AE) or serious adverse events. Commonly reported AEs in the studies included worsening of UC, headache, nasopharyngitis, upper respiratory tract infection, nausea, and abdominal pain.

References

1. Peyrin-Biroulet L, Bressenot A, Kampman W. Histologic remission: the ultimate therapeutic goal in ulcerative colitis? Clin Gastroenterol Hepatol. 2014;12:929–34.
2. Koizumi M, King N, Lobb R, Benjamin C, Podolsky DK. Expression of vascular adhesion molecules in inflammatory bowel disease. Gastroenterology. 1992;103(3):840–7.
3. Briskin M, Winsor-Hines D, Shyjan A, Cochran N, Bloom S, Wilson J, et al. Human mucosal addressin cell adhesion molecule-1 is preferentially expressed in intestinal tract and associated lymphoid tissue. Am J Pathol. 1997;151(1):97–110.
4. Bennink R, Peeters M, D'Haens G, Rutgeerts P, Mortelmans L. Tc-99m HMPAO white blood cell scintigraphy in the assessment of the extent and severity of an acute exacerbation of ulcerative colitis. Clin Nucl Med. 2001;26:99–104.
5. Souza HS, Elia CC, Spencer J, MacDonald TT. Expression of lymphocyte-endothelial receptor-ligand pairs, alpha4beta7/MAdCAM-1 and OX40/OX40 ligand in the colon and jejunum of patients with inflammatory bowel disease. Gut. 1999;45(6):856–63.
6. Podolsky DK, Lobb R, King N, Benjamin CD, Pepinsky B, Sehgal P, et al. Attenuation of colitis in the cotton-top tamarin by anti-alpha 4 integrin monoclonal antibody. J Clin Invest. 1993;92(1):372–80.
7. Hesterberg PE, Winsor-Hines D, Briskin MJ, Soler-Ferran D, Merrill C, Mackay CR, et al. Rapid resolution of chronic colitis in the cotton-top tamarin with an antibody to a gut-homing integrin alpha 4 beta 7. Gastroenterology. 1996;111(5):1373–80.
8. Sandborn WJ, Colombel JF, Enns R, Feagan BG, Hanauer SB, Lawrance IC, et al. Natalizumab induction and maintenance therapy for Crohn's disease. N Engl J Med. 2005;353(18):1912–25.
9. Targan SR, Feagan BG, Fedorak RN, Lashner BA, Panaccione R, Present DH, et al. Natalizumab for the treatment of active Crohn's disease: results of the ENCORE Trial. Gastroenterology. 2007;132(5):1672–83.
10. Van Assche G, Van Ranst M, Sciot R, Dubois B, Vermeire S, Noman M, et al. Progressive multifocal leukoencephalopathy after natalizumab therapy for Crohn's disease. N Engl J Med. 2005;353(4):362–8.
11. Bloomgren G, Richman S, Hotermans C, Subramanyam M, Goelz S, Natarajan A, et al. Risk of natalizumab-associated progressive multifocal leukoencephalopathy. N Engl J Med. 2012;366(20):1870–80.
12. Feagan BG, McDonald J, Greenberg G, Wild G, Pare P, Fedorak RN, et al. An ascending dose trial of a humanized A4B7 antibody in ulcerative colitis (UC). Gastroenterology. 2000;118(4, Part 1):A874.
13. Feagan BG, Greenberg GR, Wild G, Fedorak RN, Pare P, McDonald JW, et al. Treatment of ulcerative colitis with a humanized antibody to the alpha4beta7 integrin. N Engl J Med. 2005; 352:2499–507.
14. Parikh A, Leach T, Wyant T, Scholz C, Sankoh S, Mould DR, et al. Vedolizumab for the treatment of active ulcerative colitis: a randomized controlled phase 2 dose-ranging study. Inflamm Bowel Dis. 2012;18:1470–9.
15. Feagan BG, Rutgeerts P, Sands BE, Hanauer S, Colombel JF, Sandborn WJ, et al. Vedolizumab as induction and maintenance therapy for ulcerative colitis. N Engl J Med. 2013;369:699–710.
16. Sandborn WJ, Feagan BG, Rutgeerts P, Hanauer S, Colombel JF, Sands BE, et al. Vedolizumab as induction and maintenance therapy for Crohn's disease. N Engl J Med. 2013;369:711–21.
17. Rutgeerts PJ, Fedorak RN, Hommes DW, et al. A randomised phase I study of etrolizumab (rhuMAb beta7) in moderate to severe ulcerative colitis. Gut. 2013;62:1122–30.
18. Vermeire S, O'Byrne S, Keir M, Williams M, Lu TT, Mansfield JC, et al. Etrolizumab as induction therapy for ulcerative colitis: a randomised, controlled, phase 2 trial. Lancet. 2014;384:309–18.
19. Vermeire S, Ghosh S, Panes J, Dahlerup JF, Luegering A, Sirotiakova J, et al. The mucosal addressin cell adhesion molecule antibody PF-00547,659 in ulcerative colitis: a randomised study. Gut. 2011;60:1068–75.
20. Vermeire S, Sandborn W, Danese S, et al. OP021. TURANDOT: a randomized, multicenter double-blind, placebo-controlled study of the safety and efficacy of Anti-MAdCAM Antibody PF-00547659 (PF) in patients with moderate to severe Ulcerative Colitis (UC). J Crohns Colitis. 2015;9:S13.
21. Chang JC et al. Gene expression profiling for the prediction of therapeutic response to docetaxel in patients with breast cancer. Lancet. 2003;362:362–9.
22. Watanabe T et al. Gene expression signature for recurrence in stage III colorectal cancers. Cancer. 2009;115:283–92.
23. De Roock W et al. Effects of KRAS, BRAF, NRAS, and PIK3CA mutations on the efficacy of cetuximab plus chemotherapy in chemotherapy-refractory metastatic colorectal cancer: a retrospective consortium analysis. Lancet Oncol. 2010;11:753–62.
24. Arijs I et al. Mucosal gene signatures to predict response to infliximab in patients with ulcerative colitis. Gut. 2009;58:1612–9.
25. Tew GW, Hackney JA, Gibbons D, Lamb CA, Luca D, Egen JG, et al. Association between response to etrolizumab and expression of integrin αE and granzyme A in colon biopsies of patients with ulcerative colitis. Gastroenterology. 2016;150:477–87.

Probiotics, Prebiotics, and Antibiotics in IBD

46

Paolo Gionchetti, Carlo Calabrese, Andrea Calafiore, and Fernando Rizzello

Introduction

The rationale for using probiotics, prebiotics, and antibiotics in IBD is based on convincing evidence that implicates intestinal bacteria in the pathogenesis of the disease. The distal ileum and the colon are the areas with the highest bacterial concentrations and represent the sites of inflammation in IBD. Similarly, pouchitis, the nonspecific inflammation of the ileal reservoir after ileo-anal anastomosis, appears to be associated with bacterial overgrowth and dysbiosis. Enteric bacteria and their products have been found within the inflamed mucosa of patients with Crohn's disease (CD) [1]. The composition of the enteric flora is altered in patients with IBD. Increased numbers of aggressive bacteria, such as Bacteroides, adherent/invasive Escherichia coli, and enterococci, and decreased numbers of protective lactobacilli and bifidobacteria have been observed [2]. Manichanh et al. reported a restriction of biodiversity in the fecal microbiota of CD patients [3]. The phylum Firmicutes and particularly the species *F. prausnitzii* are underrepresented in active CD and UC compared with healthy subjects [4], and reduction of *F. prausnitzii* is associated with higher risk of postoperative recurrence of ileal CD [5]. There is evidence of a loss of immunological tolerance to commensal bacteria in patients with IBD [6]. Patients with CD consistently respond to diversion of fecal stream, with immediate recurrence of inflammation after restoration of intestinal continuity or infusion of luminal content into the bypassed ileum [7, 8]. Furthermore, pouchitis does not occur prior to closure of the ileostomy [9].

P. Gionchetti, M.D. (✉) • C. Calabrese • A. Calafiore • F. Rizzello
Department of Medical and Surgical Sciences (DIMEC), University of Bologna, Policlinico S. Orsola, Via Massarenti 9, 40138 Bologna, Italy
e-mail: paolo.gionchetti@unibo.it

The most compelling evidence that intestinal bacteria play a role in IBD is derived from animal models. Despite great diversity in genetic defects and immunopathology, a consistent feature of many transgenic and knockout mutant murine models of colitis is that the presence of normal enteric flora is required for full expression of inflammation [10].

All of these observations suggest that IBD may be prevented or treated by the manipulation of intestinal microflora, and increasing evidence supports a therapeutic role for probiotics, prebiotics, and antibiotics in IBD [11].

Probiotics

The potential benefit of probiotics in health maintenance and disease prevention has long been acknowledged. At the turn of the last century, the Russian Nobel Prize winner Elie Metchnikoff suggested that high concentrations of lactobacilli in the intestinal flora were important for health and longevity in humans [12]. Probiotics are defined as "living organisms, which upon ingestion in certain numbers, exert health benefits beyond inherent basic nutrition" [13].

The bacteria most commonly associated with probiotic activity are lactobacilli, bifidobacteria, and streptococci, but other, nonpathogenic bacteria (e.g., some strains of *E. coli*) and nonbacterial organisms (e.g., the yeast *Saccharomyces boulardii*) have been used (Table 46.1). It is believed that in order to be clinically useful for probiotics it is important to be: resistant to acid and bile, metabolically active within the luminal flora, where they should survive but not persist in the long term, antagonistic against pathogenic bacteria, safe for human use, and viable following manufacturing processes [14].

Several mechanisms have been proposed to account for the action of probiotics (Table 46.2). These may include modulation of microbiota, enhancement of barrier function,

D.C. Baumgart (ed.), *Crohn's Disease and Ulcerative Colitis*, DOI 10.1007/978-3-319-33703-6_46

Table 46.1 Organisms associated with probiotic activity

Bacteria • Lactobacilli • Bifidobacteria • Streptococci • Enterococci • Nonpathogenic *Escherichia coli*
Nonbacterial organisms • The yeast *Saccharomyces boulardii*

Table 46.2 Mechanisms of action of probiotics

Action	Mechanism
Inhibit pathogenic enteric bacteria	• Decrease luminal pH • Secrete bacteriocidal proteins • Colonization resistance • Block epithelial binding
Improve epithelial and mucosal barrier function	• Produce short-chain fatty acids • Enhance mucus production • Increase barrier integrity
Alter immunoregulation	• Increase IL-10 and TGF-β and decrease TNF-α • Increase immunoglobulin A production

IL-10 interleukin-10, *TGF-β* transforming growth factor-β, *TNF* tumor necrosis factor-α

and immunomodulation through direct effects of probiotic bacteria on different immune and epithelial cell types [15].

Studies in Animal Models

Encouraging results have been obtained with probiotic therapy in experimental colitis. Administration of *Lactobacillus reuteri* has been shown to significantly reduce inflammation in acetic acid- and methotrexate-induced colitis in rats [16, 17]. More recently, a mixture of species of lactobacilli was shown to prevent the development of spontaneous colitis in interleukin-10 (IL-10)-deficient mice [18], and continuous feeding with *Lactobacillus plantarum* was shown to attenuate established colitis in the same knockout model [19]. A strain of Lactobacillus, *Lactobacillus salivarius* subsp. salivarius UCC18, has been reported to reduce the rate of progression from inflammation through dysplasia and colon cancer in IL-10-deficient mice [20]. Furthermore, certain strains of Bifidobacterium infantis and L. salivarius have been shown to attenuate inflammation by reducing T helper type 1 cytokine production in the IL-10 knockout model [21]. Shibolet and colleagues demonstrated that VSL#3 (VSL Pharmaceuticals, Inc., Ft. Laudersdale, FL, USA), a cocktail of probiotic bacteria, significantly attenuates inflammation by decreasing myeloperoxidase and nitric oxide synthase activity in iodoacetamide-induced colitis in rats [22]. Using the same probiotic mixture, Madsen and colleagues reported a significant improvement in inflammation, a reduction in mucosal levels of proinflammatory cytokines, and normalization of colonic barrier integrity in IL-10 knockout mice [23]. More recently Pagnini et al. have shown that VSL#3 was able to promote gut health through stimulation of the innate immune system in a model of chronic CD-like ileitis [24].

Ulcerative Colitis

Tables 46.3 and 46.4 summarize results of clinical trials carried-out with probiotics in UC. Three double-blind, controlled trials have evaluated the efficacy of the probiotic preparation Escherichia coli Nissle 1917 (ECN) in the prevention of relapses of ulcerative colitis (UC). In the first study 120 patients with UC were treated for 12 weeks with either 5×10^{10} colony forming units (cfu) of ECN or 1.5 g/day mesalazine. After 12 weeks 16 % of the patients in ECN group and 11.3 % in the mesalazine group relapsed. The statistical power of this study was low and duration of treatment too short, and therefore the equivalence was not demonstrated [25]. In the second study 116 patients were treated with ECN or mesalazine at lower dose (1.2 g/day) for 1 year. Surprisingly high relapse rate occurred in both the ECN and mesalazine group (67 % versus 73 %) [26]. In the third study 327 patients were treated with either ECN or mesalazine (1.5 g/day) for 1 year. The relapse rate was respectively of 36 % and 34 % in the probiotic group and mesalazine, showing equivalence of the two treatments in an appropriate way [27].

More recently the same preparation has been used as enemas in patients with mild to moderate distal UC in a double-blind study. Ninety patients were randomly assigned to receive 40, 20, or 10 ml containing ECN or placebo for 8 weeks. In the PP analysis ECN rectal application was significantly superior to placebo and well tolerated, in contrast to ITT analysis [28].

In another small randomized controlled trial, Ishikawa et al. evaluated the efficacy of a Bifidobacterium fermented milk as a dietary adjunct in maintaining remission of UC. Twenty-one patients were included in the study; in the group treated with Bifidobacterium fermented milk 3 of (27 %) patients had a relapse of UC compared with 10 of 11 (90 %) of patients in the control group [29]. Similarly, in a 4-week, open-label study, 25 patients with mild to moderate clinical flare-up were treated with the yeast *S. boulardii* at the dose of 250 mg three times/day for 4 weeks; 17 patients (68 %) attained clinical remission [30].

Table 46.3 Probiotics in UC: induction of remission

Study	*N*	Duration	Probiotic	Control	Remission Probiotic/Cont	*P*
Rembacken 1999	116	4 months	Prednisone/ Gentamicin + *E. coli* Nissle	Prednisone/ Gentamicin + 5ASA	68 %; 75 %	Equal to 5ASA? Pred effect
Guslandi 2003	25	1 month	*S. boulardii*	Open label	68 %	
Bibiloni 2005	34	6 week	VSL#3	Open label	63 %	
Sood 2009	147	12 week	VSL#3	Placebo	32.5 %; 10 %	<0.001
Tursi 2010	144	8 week	VSL#3	Placebo	Improvement in UCDAI 60.5 %,	<0.017
Miele 2009	29	1 month	VSL#3	Placebo	92 % 36.4 %	<0.001
Huynh et al. 2009	13	8 week	VSL#3	Open label	56 %	

Table 46.4 Probiotics in UC: maintenance of remission

Study	*N*	Duration	Probiotic	Control	Remission Probiotic; Cont	*P*
Rembacken 1999	116	12 months	*E. coli* Nissle	5ASA	26 %; 25 %	Relapse rates near placebo
Kruis 1997	120	3 months	*E. coli* Nissle	5ASA	84 %; 89 %	Equivalence to 5ASA
Kruis 2004	327	12 months	*E. coli* Nissle	5ASA	64 %; 66 %	Equivalence to 5ASA
Venturi 1999	20	12 months	VSL#3	Open label	75 %	
Ishikawa 2003	21	12 months	Bifidobacterium fermented milk	Placebo	73 %; 10 %	0.018
Miele 2009 Pediatric patients	29	12 months	VSL#3	Mesalamine	79.6 %;26.7 %	0.014

Also VSL#3 has been investigated in the treatment of UC. This product contains cells of four strains of lactobacilli (*L. casei*, *L. plantarum*, *L. acidophilus*, *L. delbrueckii* subsp. bulgaricus), three strains of bifidobacteria (*B. longum*, *B. breve*, *B. infantis*), and one strain of *Streptococcus salivarius* subsp. thermophilus. Each packet of VSL#3 contains 450 billion viable lyophilized bacteria. A pilot study was performed using VSL#3 as a maintenance treatment in UC patients in remission who were either allergic or intolerant to sulfasalazine and mesalazine. Patients ($n=20$) received, 1.8×10^{12} CFU VSL#3 for 12 months and were assessed clinically and endoscopically at baseline, at 6 and 12 months, or if relapse occurred.

Fecal concentrations of lactobacilli, bifidobacteria, and *S. thermophilus* were significantly increased by VSL#3. In total, 15 of the 20 patients (75 %) remained in remission during the study [31]. In an open-label study, high-dose VSL#3 (3.6×10^{12} CFU) induced remission, after 6 weeks, in 63 % of patients with active mild-to-moderate disease, who failed to respond to mesalazine or corticosteroids, and was associated with a positive response in a further 23 % [32]. In a multicenter, double-blind, placebo-controlled trial 147 patients with mild to moderate UC were randomized to receive either 3.6×10^{12} CFU VSL#3 or placebo for 12 weeks. At 6 weeks the rate of patients with >50 % reduction in UCDAI (primary end-point) were respectively 32.5 and 10 % for VSL#3 and placebo ($p=0.001$). At 12 weeks the rate of remission was 42.9 % for VSL#3 and 15.7 % for placebo ($p<0.001$). The VSL# group had significantly greater decreases in UCDAI scores and individual symptoms at weeks 6 and 12 weeks compared with placebo group [33].

More recently, in a multicenter, double-blind, randomized, placebo-controlled study, a total of 144 patients with relapsing UC, while on treatment with salicylates or immunosuppressants, were treated with either VSL#3 (71 patients) at the dose of 3.6×10^{12} CFU/day or placebo (73 patients) for 8 weeks. The decrease of UC activity index (UCDAI) scores of 50 % or more and improvement in rectal bleeding were significantly higher in the VSL#3 treated group, while endoscopic improvement and remission rate did not reach statistical significance. Only few patients reported mild side-effects with placebo and VSL#3 [34].

In two small recent studies, VSL#3 has been reported to achieve remission/response in children with mild to moderate UC. In the first double-blind, placebo-controlled study, 29 patients with newly diagnosed UC were randomized to receive either VSL#3 (weight-based dose, range 0.45×10^{12} CFU -1.8×10^{12} CFU) or placebo both in induction and maintenance of remission in adjunct to standard therapy. Remission was achieved in 13 (92.8 %) treated with VSL#3 and in 4 (36.4 %) treated with placebo ($p<0.001$). VSL#3 was also significantly superior in maintenance of remission [35]. In the second, open-label trial, 18 patients with mild to moderate active UC were treated with VSL#3 in two divided doses (the dose was based on the age of children) for 8 weeks; 10 (56 %) children achieved remission after 8 weeks, and post-VSL#3 treatment demonstrated a bacterial taxonomy change in rectal biopsy. VSL#3 was well tolerated [36].

Pouchitis

Proctocolectomy with ileal pouch-anal anastomosis (IPAA) is the procedure of choice for most patients with ulcerative colitis (UC) requiring colectomy Pouchitis is a nonspecific inflammation of the ileal reservoir and the most common complication of IPAA in patients with UC [37]. Its frequency is related to the duration of follow up, occurring in up to 50 % of patients 10 years after IPAA in large series from major referral centers [38–44]. It is most frequently seen within the first year after ileostomy closure.

Symptoms related to pouchitis include increased stool frequency and liquidity, abdominal cramping, urgency, tenesmus and pelvic discomfort [45]. Rectal bleeding, fever, or extraintestinal manifestations may occur. Fecal incontinence may occur in the absence of pouchitis after IPAA, but is more common in patients with pouchitis. Symptoms of pouch dysfunction in patients with IPAA may be caused by conditions other than pouchitis, including Crohn's disease of the pouch, cuffitis, and an irritable pouch. This is why the diagnosis depends on endoscopic and histological findings in conjunction with symptoms.

On the basis of symptoms and endoscopy, pouchitis can be divided into remission (normal pouch frequency) or active pouchitis (increased frequency with endoscopic appearances and histology consistent with pouchitis) [46, 47]. Active pouchitis may then be divided into acute or chronic, depending on the symptom duration. The threshold for chronicity is a symptom duration of >4 weeks. Up to 10 % of patients develop chronic pouchitis requiring long-term treatment, and a small subgroup has pouchitis refractory to medical treatment [5]. The Pouchitis Disease Activity Index (PDAI) has been developed to standardize diagnostic criteria and assess the severity of pouchitis [48]. The PDAI is a composite score that evaluates symptoms, endoscopy and histology. Each component of the score has a maximum of 6 points. Patients with a total PDAI score ≥7 are classified as having pouchitis although a patient should exhibit both clinical symptoms and endoscopic or histological evidence of pouchitis.

Pouchitis recurs in more than 50 % patients; patients with recurrent pouchitis can broadly be grouped into three categories: infrequent episodes (<1/year), a relapsing course (1–3 episodes/year) or a continuous course. Pouchitis may further be termed treatment responsive or refractory, based on response to antibiotic monotherapy [37, 45].

In the majority of cases the etiology and pathogenesis of pouchitis remains unclear, and patients are labelled as having idiopathic pouchitis. Risk factors, genetic associations, and serological markers of pouchitis suggest that a close interaction between the host immune response and the pouch microbiota plays a relevant role in the etiology of this idiopathic inflammatory condition [49]. Although we do not know the cause of pouchitis, we do believe that the intestinal microbial community plays an important role in maintaining pouch health or driving pouch inflammation [50]. In support of this assumption, it is observed that pouchitis only occurs after restoration of the fecal stream through the pouch [51, 52]. In addition a dysbiosis in pouchitis has been documented [53], and several genes associated with the innate immune response and microbial sensing and recognition have been associated with an increased risk for pouchitis including the NOD2/CARD15 gene [54, 55], Il-1 receptor antagonist gene [56], and Toll-like receptor genes [57].

Table 46.5 summarizes the results of trials carried-out with probiotics in pouchitis. A double-blind study to compare the efficacy of VSL#3 with placebo in the maintenance treatment of chronic pouchitis was carried-out. Patients ($n=40$) who were in clinical and endoscopic remission after 1 month of combined antibiotic treatment (2 g/day of rifaximin plus 1 g/day of ciprofloxacin) were randomized to receive either VSL#3 (1.8×10^{12} CFU) or placebo for 9 months. Patients were assessed clinically every month, and assessed endoscopically and histologically at entry and every 2 months thereafter. Stool culture was performed before and after antibiotic treatment, and monthly during maintenance treatment. Relapse was defined as an increase of at least 2 points in the clinical section of the Pouchitis Disease Activity Index (PDAI) and was confirmed endoscopically and histologically. All 20 patients treated with placebo relapsed during the follow-up period. In contrast, 17 of the 20 (85 %) patients treated with VSL#3 were still in remission after 9 months. Interestingly, all these 17 patients relapsed within 4 months of suspension of the active treatment. Fecal concentrations of lactobacilli, bifidobacteria, and *S. thermophilus* were significantly increased within 1 month of treatment initiation and remained stable throughout the study only in the group treated with VSL#3 [58]. A subsequent double-blind, placebo-controlled study on the effectiveness of VSL#3 (at a daily dose of 1.8×10^{12} CFU) in the maintenance of antibiotic-induced remission in patients with refractory or recurrent pouchitis reported similar results [59]. After 1 year of

Table 46.5 Probiotics in pouchitis

Study	*N*	Duration	Probiotic	Control	Remission Probiotic; Cont	*P*
Gionchetti 2002 [Maintenance: antibiotic–remission]	40	9 months	VSL#3	Placebo	85 %; 0 %	<0.001
Mimura 2004 [Maintenance: antibiotic–remission]	36	12 months	VSL#3	Placebo	85 %; 6 %	<0.001
Gionchetti 2003 [Prevention of onset]	40	12 months	VSL#3	Placebo	90 %; 60 %	<0.05
Shen 2005 [Maintenance antibiotic-dependent]	31	8 months	VSL#3	Open label	19.4 %	ns
Kuisma 2003 [Acute pouchitis]	20	3 months	*Lactobacillus GG*	Placebo	0 %; 0 %	ns
Gionchetti 2007 [Acute pouchitis]	29	4 weeks	VSL#3	Open label	69 %	P<0.01

treatment, 85 % of those in the VSL#3 group were in remission versus only 6 % of those in the placebo group. As regards the mechanism of action of VSL#3 in these patients, continuous administration of VSL#3 decreases matrix metalloproteinase activity, significantly increases tissue levels of IL-10, and significantly decreases tissue levels of the proinflammatory cytokines IL-1, tumor necrosis factor-α, and interferon γ [60].

In contrast, however, a more recent 8-month open-label clinical study reported that less than 20 % of patients treated with were able to maintain remission in clinical practice [61].

The reason for the difference in these results is not clear but differences in the design and protocol of the two studies may have contributed. Particularly, studies by Gionchetti and colleagues and Mimura and colleagues excluded patients who did not achieve complete or near-complete endoscopic remission whereas Shen et al. did not repeat the pouchoscopy after clinical remission. It is known that some patients do not achieve endoscopic remission despite clinical remission following antibiotic treatment, and it is possible that this subset of patients have a more difficult to treat disease which may not respond to probiotics. Gionchetti's and Mimura's groups used a combination of ciprofloxacin and rifaximin or metronidazole for 4 weeks whereas Shen and colleagues used a 2-week course of ciprofloxacin only to induce remission. It is possible that probiotic therapy is more effective following a combination of two different antibiotic agents for a prolonged period. Gionchetti and colleagues' and Mimura and colleagues' studies recruited patients with refractory pouchitis, defined as three or more episodes of pouchitis per year, whereas Shen and colleagues only recruited patients with chronic antibiotic-dependent pouchitis, defined as four or more episodes of pouchitis per year. Therefore, many of the patients included in the studies of Gionchetti's and Mimura's groups had less-aggressive disease in which maintenance of remission may have been easier to achieve. Finally patients had to purchase VSL#3 which was obtained from the company's website; VSL#3 is not covered by insurance and therefore patient's adherence to therapy was a problem; moreover, because VSL#3 was self-administered by patients, medicine counts and prescription records were impossible. Further, fecal bacteriology, as in the previous study, was not done and this further raises the issue of adherence to therapy.

In a 3-month double-blind, placebo-controlled trial *Lactobacillus rhamnosus* strain GG (two gelatin capsules/day of 0.5–1 × 10^{10} CFU/capsule) in patients with a previous history of pouchitis showed that this probiotic was not effective in preventing relapses [62].

Recently, probiotic treatment with Ecologic 825 was able to restore mucosal barrier during maintenance therapy after clinical remission was achieved with combined antibiotic treatment [63].

The efficacy of VSL#3 in the prevention of pouchitis onset was evaluated in a double-blind, placebo-controlled trial [64]. Within 1 week after ileostomy closure, 40 patients were randomized to receive either VSL#3 (0.9 × 10^{12} CFU) or placebo for 12 months. Patients were assessed clinically, endoscopically, and histologically at 1, 3, 6, 9, and 12 months according to PDAI score. During the first year after ileostomy closure, patients treated with VSL#3 had a significantly lower incidence of acute pouchitis compared with those treated with placebo (10 % vs. 40 %; $p<0.05$). Moreover, IBD questionnaire score was significantly improved only in the group treated with VSL#3 and among those who did not develop pouchitis, the median stool frequency was significantly lower in the VSL#3 group. More recently, an open-label study evaluated the efficacy of high-dose of VSL#3

(3.6×10^{12} CFU/day) in the treatment of mild pouchitis, defined as a score between 7 and 12 in the PDAI. Sixteen of 29 patients (69 %) were in remission after 4 weeks [65].

The treatment and prevention of pouchitis has been systematically reviewed in 2010 by a Cochrane analysis [66] In the Cochrane systematic review VSL#3 was more effective than placebo in maintaining remission of chronic pouchitis in patients who achieved remission with antibiotics and VSL#3 was more effective than placebo for the prevention of pouchitis . European Crohn's Colitis (ECCO) guidelines state that VSL#3 is effective in maintaining antibiotic-induced remission and in preventing pouchitis onset [67].

Crohn's Disease

Tables 46.6 and 46.7 summarize the results of clinical trials carried-out in CD. In a small pilot study, E. coli Nissle 1917 was compared with placebo in the maintenance of steroid-induced remission of colonic CD [68]. Twelve patients were treated with *E. coli* Nissle 1917 and 11 were treated with placebo. At the end of the 12-week treatment period, relapse rates were 33 % in the *E. coli* group and 63 % in the placebo group; unfortunately, due the very small number of patients treated, this difference did not reach statistical significance. In a small, comparative, 6-month, open-label study, 32 patients with CD in clinical remission were randomized to receive either combination therapy with the yeast *S. boulardii* (1 g/day) plus mesalamine (2 g/day) or mesalamine (3 g/day). Relapse rates were 37.5 % and 6.25 % respectively in the mesalamine monotherapy group and in the combination group [69]. In a 1-year, double-blind, placebo-controlled trial, Lactobacillus. GG was not effective in the prevention of postoperative recurrence [70]. Similarly in a double-blind trial Lactobacillus GG was shown not be superior than placebo in prolonging remission in children with CD when given as an adjunct to standard therapy [71].

Two randomized double-blind, placebo-controlled study showed *Lactobacillus johnsonii* LA1 (4×10^9 cfu/day) was not superior to placebo to prevent endoscopic recurrence of CD [72, 73].

More recently, in a randomized, placebo-controlled trial, the effects of *Saccharomyces boulardii* in patients with CD who underwent remission after therapy with steroids or salicylates were evaluated. Patients were assigned to placebo or *Saccharomyces boulardii* (1 g/day) for 52 weeks. Relapse rate was not significantly different between the two groups (53.2 % in placebo vs 47.5 % in *Saccharomyces boulardii*), as was the time to relapse [74].

We performed a single-blind study to compare a sequential antibiotic–probiotic treatment with mesalazine in the prevention of postoperative recurrence of CD. Within 1 week after curative surgery, 40 patients were randomized to receive either high-dose rifaximin (a nonabsorbable wide-spectrum antibiotic) for 3 months followed by VSL#3 (1.8×10^{12} CFU/

Table 46.6 Probiotics in CD: maintenance of remission

Study	*N*	Duration	Probiotic	Control	Remission Probiotic; Cont	*P*
Malchow 1997	28	12 months	*E. coli* Nissle 1917	Placebo	70 %; 30 %	ns
Guslandi 2000	32	6 months	*S. boulardii*	5ASA	62.5 %;93.75 %	0.04
Bousvaros 2005	75	24 months	*L. rhamnosus* GG + standard therapy	Placebo + standard therapy	71 %; 83 %	ns
Willert 2010	38	12 months	VSL#3+ standard therapy	Placebo + standard therapy	43 %; 11 %	ns

Table 46.7 Probiotics in CD: prevention of postoperative recurrence

Study	*N*	Duration	Probiotic	Control	Remission Probiotic; Cont	*P*
Campieri 2000	40	12 months	Rifaximin × 3 months followed by VSL#3	5ASA	Endoscopic 80 %; 60 %	Benefit probiotic
Prantera 2002	45	12 months	*L. rhamnosus* GG	Placebo	Clinical 83 %; 89 % Endoscopic 40 %; 65 %	ns
Marteau 2006	98	6 months	*L. johnsonii* LA1	Placebo	Endoscopic 51 %; 36 %	ns
Van Gossum 2006	70	3 months	*L. johnsonii* LA1	Placebo	Endoscopic 21 %; 15 %	ns
Fedorak 2015	119	90 days	VSL#3	Placebo	Endoscopic 10 %; 26.7 %	ns

day) for 9 months, or mesalazine (4 g/day) for 12 months. Patients were assessed clinically and endoscopically at 3 and 12 months. Compared with placebo, the combined antibiotic–probiotic treatment was associated with a significantly lower incidence of severe endoscopic recurrence, both at 3 months (10 % vs. 40 %; $p<0.01$) and 12 months (20 % vs. 40 %; $p<0.01$) [75].

More recently, VSL#3 at the dose of 1.8×10^{12} CFU/day, was shown not to be superior than placebo in maintaining remission in colonic CD, in a 12-month, randomized, double-blind trial [76].

Finally, the ability of VSL#3 to prevent CD recurrence after surgery, was tested in a multicenter, randomized, double-blind, placebo-controlled trial [77].

Patients were randomized, within 30 days after resection, to receive one sachet of VSL#3 (900 billion viable bacteria) ($n=59$) or placebo ($N=60$). Ileocolonoscopy was performed after 90 and 365 days; patients with either no or mild recurrence at day 90 received VSL#3 until day 365. There were no statistical differences in endoscopic recurrence at day 90. Patients receiving VSL#3 ha significantly reduced mucosal inflammatory cytokines levels compared with placebo. This together with the lower rate of recurrence among patients who received early VSL#3 (for all 365 days) suggest a possible beneficial effect of this probiotic for prevention of postoperative CD.

Prebiotics

Prebiotics are dietary substances, usually nondigestible carbohydrates, which beneficially affect the host by selectively stimulating the growth and activity of protective commensal enteric bacteria (Table 46.3) [78]. Fructo-oligosaccharides (FOS), inulin, bran, psyllium, and germinated barley foodstuff (GBF) stimulate the growth of bifidobacteria and lactobacilli, which in turn antagonize pathogenic bacteria by decreasing the luminal pH, inducing colonization resistance, and inhibiting epithelial adhesion and translocation. In addition, these substances increase bacterial fermentation, which produces SCFAs (especially butyrate) that improve epithelial barrier function [79]. These findings suggest that prebiotics are functionally equivalent to probiotic bacteria.

Studies in Animal Models

A variety of different prebiotic preparations have been tested in animal models of colitis. Lactulose has been shown to attenuate inflammation and to stimulate the growth of lactobacilli in IL-10 knockout mice [18], while administration of inulin and GBF has been shown to inhibit dextran sodium sulfate (DSS)-induced colitis in rats by increasing the luminal concentration of SCFAs, lactobacilli, and bifidobacteria [80, 81]. Experiments on FOS have produced conflicting results. Cherbut et al. reported that FOS attenuates the trinitrobenzene sulfonic acid-induced colitis in rats [82], while Moreau et al. reported no benefit of FOS in the DSS rat model of colitis [83]. Furthermore, a combination of inulin and FOS significantly decreased inflammation in HLA-B27 transgenic rats [84]. Taken together, these findings suggest that combination therapy with different prebiotics may be more effective than monotherapy, due to the fact that each agent has specific biological properties.

Human IBD Studies

A few small, controlled studies have investigated the use of prebiotics in UC, whereas there have been no studies on prebiotics in CD or pouchitis. In a small group of UC patients in remission, psyllium (also known as ispaghula or *Plantago ovata*) was shown to be superior to placebo in decreasing symptom severity, and produced a significant increase in the fecal concentration of bifidobacteria [85]. In an open-label, randomized trial, *Plantago ovata* seeds, which have previously been shown to stimulate the production of SCFAs, were tested as a maintenance treatment in UC patients in remission [86]. In this 12-month study, 105 patients were randomized to receive either *Plantago ovata* seeds alone (10 g twice daily), mesalamine alone (500 mg three times daily), or a combination of *Plantago ovata* seeds plus mesalamine at the same doses administered for monotherapy. Rates of remission were similar for the three groups, and a significant increase in the fecal concentration of butyrate was observed after *Plantago ovata* seed administration.

GBF is comprised of the glutamine- and hemicellulose-rich extracts of spent beer-brewing constituents. Use of this probiotic in patients with mild-to-moderate UC has been investigated in a small pilot study and a placebo-controlled trial [87, 88]. At a dose of 25–30 mg/day, GBF decreased clinical and endoscopic activity in these patients and significantly increased fecal concentrations of bifidobacteria. Similar results were reported by a 24-week, open-label trial [89].

Lindsay et al. [90] performed a small, open-label study in 10 patients with active ileo-colonic CD using a combination of 15 g/day of oligofructose and inulin (ratio 70:30 %). They found a significant reduction in disease activity, concomitant with a significant increase in mucosal bifidobacteria. Interestingly prebiotic treatment increased colonic dendritic cells expressing IL-10, Toll-like receptor (TLR)-2 and TLR-4, indicating that these prebiotics affected the innate mucosal immune response. In a small placebo-controlled study oligofructose-enriched inulin was administered as adjunctive treatment to mesalazine 3 g/day for 2 weeks in mild to moderate, active UC. This study showed a significant reduction of the fecal calprotectin in prebiotic treated patients compared to placebo [91].

Antibiotics

Animal Models

In several rodent models the use of broad-spectrum antibiotics can both prevent onset and treat experimental colitis, whereas metronidazole and ciprofloxacin can only prevent experimental colitis but not reverse established disease [92–96]. Broad-spectrum antibiotics are effective in almost all models of acute and chronic colitis [96–99], and, however, have only a transient efficacy in HLA-B27 transgenic rats [100]. Interestingly ciprofloxacin and metronidazole had selective efficacy in different colonic region in IL-10 knockout mice, suggesting that different bacteria cause inflammation indifferent colonic segments [98]. These studies suggest that most clinical forms of IBD may respond if a proper combination of broad-spectrum antibiotics is used.

Ulcerative Colitis

Only few trials of antibacterial agents have been carried out in ulcerative colitis (UC) and results are controversial. Most clinicians have used antibiotics as adjuvant therapy in severe UC. Dickinson et al. have carried out a double-blind controlled trial on the use of oral vancomycin as adjuvant therapy in acute exacerbations of idiopathic colitis. No significant difference was found between the two treatment groups with only a trend towards a reduction in the need for surgery in patients treated with vancomycin [101].

Intravenous metronidazole, used as adjunctive treatment to corticosteroids, was similarly effective than placebo to induce remission in patients with severe UC [102].

In a double blind, placebo controlled trial in patients with acute relapse of UC, 84 patients were randomized to receive corticosteroids plus oral tobramycin or placebo. After 1 week of treatment, 74 % of patient in the tobramycin treatment group vs. 43 % in the placebo group ($p<0.003$) achieved a complete symptomatic remission [103]. Subsequently the combination of tobramycin and metronidazole did not show any beneficial effect when associated to a standard steroid treatment in severely acute UC [104]. Ciprofloxacin has been tested in a randomized, placebo controlled study; 70 patients with mild to moderate active UC were randomized to receive ciprofloxacin 250 mg b.i.d. or placebo for 14 days. At the end of the study, 70.5 % of patients in the ciprofloxacin group vs 72 % in the placebo group achieved remission [105]. Similarly a short course of intravenous ciprofloxacin was not effective as adjunctive treatment to corticosteroids in severe UC in a prospective, randomized, double-blind, placebo-controlled trial [106]. Nevertheless, in a more recent randomized, placebo controlled trial, ciprofloxacin was administered for 6 months to patients with active UC poorly responding to conventional therapy with steroids and mesalamine. At the end of the study, the treatment-failure rate was 21 % in the ciprofloxacin-treated group and 44 % in the placebo group ($p<0.002$). This difference was detected using clinical criteria; while endoscopic and histological findings showed differences only at 3 months but not at 6 months [107].

The nonabsorbable, broad-spectrum antibiotic, rifaximin was tested in a small controlled study to evaluate its efficacy and systemic absorption in patients with moderate to severe active UC refractory to steroid treatment. Twenty-eight patients were randomized to receive rifaximin 400 mg b.i.d. or placebo for 10 days as an adjunct to standard steroid treatment. Although there was no significant difference in clinical efficacy between the two treatments, only rifaximin determined a significant improvement of stool frequency, rectal bleeding, and sigmoidoscopic score [108].

In a more recent systematic review of randomized controlled trials, In active UC, there were nine RCTs with 662 patients and there was a statistically significant benefit for antibiotics inducing remission. However, there was moderate heterogeneity and antibiotics used were all different single or combination drugs [109].

Crohn's Disease

There are several studies looking at the use of antibiotics as primary therapy for luminal CD. Unfortunately, the majority of these are observational, uncontrolled studies or lack sufficient power to truly detect important differences. Metronidazole has been the mostly investigated agent. In 1978, Blichfeldt et al. in a placebo-controlled, double-blind, crossover trial did not found difference between metronidazole and placebo-treated patients, but a positive trend in favor of metronidazole was observed when only the colon was involved [110]. In the National Cooperative Swedish study, metronidazole was compared to sulfasalazine as primary treatment for Crohn's disease; no significant difference was found between the two group, but, interestingly, in the cross-over section of the study, metronidazole was effective in patients not responders to sulfasalazine [111]. Metronidazole was used as single therapy or associated to cotrimoxazole and compared to cotrimoxazole alone and placebo in patients with a symptomatic relapse of Crohn's Disease. At the end of the 4 weeks of treatment there was no difference in response among the three groups [112]. In a Canadian randomized, placebo-controlled trial, Sutherland et al. have shown that treatment with metronidazole for 16 weeks significantly decreased the Crohn's Disease Activity Index (CDAI), but no difference was found in the rates of remission compared with placebo; benefit was dose-dependent with 20 mg/kg having a greater benefit than 10 mg/kg [113]. As in the case of the Swedish study, in the Canadian study metronidazole was effective for colonic and ileocolonic Crohn's disease but not for ileitis. Metronidazole has important side effects that include nausea, anorexia, dysgeusia, dyspepsia, and peripheral neuropathy that limit its use in approximately 20 % of patients. An antibiotic association was used in an Italian randomized controlled study in which metronidazole 250 mg four times daily plus ciprofloxacin 500 mg twice daily were compared to a standard steroid treatment for 12 weeks. No differences were reported in the rates of remission between treatments (46 % with ciprofloxacin plus metronidazole vs 63 % with methylprednisolone) suggesting that this antibiotic association could be an alternative to steroid treatment in acute phases of Crohn's disease [114]. Combination of metronidazole and ciprofloxacin was associated with budesonide 9 mg/day in active Crohn's disease; no difference was registered compared to placebo, but surprisingly the overall response in the two groups was lower than the previous studies on budesonide. Also in this study antibiotic treatment was more effective when the colon was involved than for isolated small bowel disease [115].

Ciprofloxacin 1 g/daily was compared to mesalamine 4 g/daily in a controlled study in mild-to-moderate active CD. After 6 weeks an equivalence in efficacy was registered (remission observed in 56 % and 55 % of patients respectively with ciprofloxacin and mesalamine), offering an alternative treatment in active CD [116]. In a small study ciprofloxacin was shown to be effective in association to standard treatment in patients with resistant disease [117]. Other antibiotics have been tested. Shafran et al. carried out an open-label study on the efficacy and safety of rifaximin 600 mg/day for 16 weeks in the treatment of mild-to-moderate active CD. At the end of the study, 59 % of patients were in remission (CDAI < 150) with a significant reduction of the mean CDAI score compared to baseline ($p<0.0001$) [118]. In an open-label trial, Leiper et al. reported an impressive positive response (64 % patients improved or were in remission after 4 weeks) of clarithromycin in a group of 25 patients with active Crohn's disease, many of whom were unresponsive to other treatments [119]. As stated by European Crohn's Colitis Organization (ECCO), at present, antibiotics are only considered appropriate for septic complications, symptoms attributable to bacterial overgrowth, or perineal disease. Antimycobacterial therapy cannot be recommended on the evidence from controlled trials [120].

Antibiotics have been also tested in prevention of postoperative recurrence. Metronidazole at the dose of 20 mg/kg/day was compared with placebo in double-blind, controlled trial by Rutgeerts et al. [121]. Sixty patients were randomized to receive metronidazole or placebo for 12 weeks. At the end of the treatment, endoscopic relapse was evaluated by Rutgeerts score. Metronidazole significantly decreased the incidence of severe endoscopic relapse (grade 3 or 4) in the neoterminal ileum 6 months after surgery and the clinical recurrence rates at 1 year, with a trend towards a protective effect after 3 years. More recently, the similar antibiotic ornidazole, used continuously for 1 year was significantly more effective than placebo in the prevention of severe endoscopic recurrence in the neoterminal ileum both at 3 and 12 months [122].

Imidazole antibiotics, as suggested by the ECCO Consensus on CD management, may be a therapeutic option after ileocolic resection but are poorly tolerated [120].

Campieri et al. performed a randomized trial to evaluate the efficacy in the prevention of postoperative recurrence of rifaximin 1.8 g daily for 3 months followed by a probiotic preparation (VSL#3) 6 g daily for 9 months versus mesalamine 4 g daily for 12 months in 40 patients after curative resection for CD. After 3 months of treatment, rifaximin determined a significant lower incidence of severe endoscopic recurrence compared to mesalamine [2/20 (10 %) versus 8/20 (40 %)]. This difference was maintained since the end of the study using probiotics [4/20 (20 %) versus 8/20 (40 %)] [75].

A lot of studies have tried to evaluate the efficacy of antimycobacterial drugs in patients with CD, pursuing the possibility that a strain of Mycobacterium might be an etiological agent in CD. Borgaonkar et al. [123] evaluated all randomized controlled trials in which antimycobacterial therapy was compared with placebo, suggesting the efficacy of antimycobacterial therapy only as a maintenance treatment in patients who obtained remission after a combined treatment with corticosteroids and antimycobacterial agents. However, the investigator emphasized the high incidence of side effects, and that, because of the small number of studies included in the meta-analysis, the data were not conclusive and should be taken with caution.

The same antibiotics used to treat luminal Crohn's disease have been reported to be beneficial in the treatment of perianal Crohn's disease, but no controlled trial have been performed [124]. Metronidazole 20 mg/kg has shown rates of fistulae closure from 62 % to 83 % [125, 126]. The combination of metronidazole and ciprofloxacin determined an improvement in 64 % of patients and fistulae closure in 21 % [127]. Unfortunately fistulae tend to recur in most patients after stopping treatment. Although the results of these uncontrolled studies are not conclusive, metronidazole, ciprofloxacin, or their combination are used by most clinicians as first-line treatment in patients with perianal disease, in combination with surgical drainage of abscesses.

A systematic review of randomized controlled trials (RCTs) evaluating antibiotics in IBD was carried-out. Studies with any antibiotics alone or in combination using predefined definitions of remission and relapse were included. For active CD, there was a statistically significant effect of antibiotics being superior to placebo. In perianal CD there were three trials using either ciprofloxacin or metronidazole and there was a statistically significant effect in reducing fistula drainage. For quiescent CD, there were 3 RCTs with different antibiotics combinations (all including antimycobacterials) vs. placebo. There was a statistically significant effect in favor of antibiotics vs. placebo. There was moderate heterogeneity between results and a diverse number of antibiotics were tested either alone or in combination and therefore the data are difficult to interpret [109].

We, more recently, performed a multicenter, randomized, double-blind trial of the efficacy and safety of 400, 800, and 1200 mg rifaximin—Extended Ileal Release (EIR), given twice daily to 402 patients with moderately active CD for 12 weeks, compared with placebo [128].

At the end of the 12-week treatment period, 62 % of patients who received the 800-mg dosage of rifaximin-EIR (61 of 98) were in remission, compared with 43 % of patients who received placebo (*P*_0.005).

Pouchitis

Treatment of pouchitis is largely empirical and only small placebo-controlled trials have been conducted. The awareness of the crucial importance that fecal stasis and the bacterial overgrowth may represent in the pathogenesis of acute pouchitis has led the clinicians to treat patients with antibiotics, which have become the mainstay of treatment, in absence of controlled trials. Table 46.8 summarizes results of trials carried-out with antibiotics in pouchitis. Usually metronidazole and ciprofloxacin are the most common initial approaches, often resulting in a rapid response [129].

However, randomized trials of both metronidazole and ciprofloxacin are small. A double-blind, randomized, placebo-controlled, crossover trial was carried out by Madden et al. to assess the efficacy of 400 mg three times a day of metronidazole per os in 13 patients (11 completed both arms of the study) with chronic, unremitting pouchitis. Patients were treated for 2 weeks, and metronidazole was significantly more effective than placebo in reducing the stool frequency (73 % vs. 9 %), even without improvement of endoscopic appearance and histologic grade of activity. Some patients (55 %) experienced side effects of metronidazole including nausea, vomiting, abdominal discomfort, headache, skin rash, and metallic taste [130].

Metronidazole and ciprofloxacin have been compared in another small randomized trial [131]. Seven patients received ciprofloxacin 1 g/day and nine patients metronidazole 20 mg/kg/day for a period of 2 weeks. Ciprofloxacin lowered the PDAI score from 10.1 ± 2.3 to 3.3 ± 1.7 ($p=0.0001$), whereas metronidazole reduced the PDAI score from 9.7 ± 2.3 to 5.8 ± 1.7 ($p=0.0002$). There was a significantly greater benefit with ciprofloxacin compared to metronidazole in terms of the total PDAI ($p=0.002$), symptom score ($p=0.03$) and endoscopic score ($p=0.03$), as well as fewer adverse events (33 % of metronidazole-treated patients reported side-effects, but none on ciprofloxacin).

The treatment and prevention of pouchitis has been systematically reviewed in 2010 by a Cochrane analysis [66]. For the treatment of acute pouchitis (four RCTS, five agents) ciprofloxacin was more effective at inducing remission than metronidazole.

Patients with chronic, refractory pouchitis do not respond to conventional therapy and often have ongoing symptoms; this is a common cause of pouch failure. Combined antibiotic therapy may be effective [45]. Sixteen consecutive

Table 46.8 Antibiotics in pouchitis

Study	*N*	Duration	Antibiotic	Control	Results Antibiotic; Control
Madden 1994 [acute pouchitis]	11	1 week	Metronidazole	Placebo	79 %; 9 % (reduction of stool frequency)
Gionchetti 1999 [chronic pouchitis]	18	2 weeks	Rifaximin + ciprofloxacin	Open label	88.8 % improvement or remission (total PDAI significant reduction)
Shen 2001 [acute pouchitis]	16	2 weeks	Ciprofloxacin vs metronidazole	Double-blind	Significant reduction in total PDAI in both groups
Mimura 2002 [chronic pouchitis]	44	4 weeks	Ciprofloxacin + metronidazole	Open label	82 % in complete remission (total PDAI significant reduction)
Abdelrazeq 2005 [chronic pouchitis]	8	2 weeks	Rifaximin + ciprofloxacin	Open label	Seven of eight patients in complete remission (total PDAI significant reduction)
Shen 2007 [chronic pouchitis]	16	4 weeks	Tinidazole + ciprofloxacin	Open label	87.5 % in complete remission (total PDAI significant reduction)

PDAI Pouchitis Disease Activity Index

patients with chronic, refractory pouchitis (disease >4 weeks and failure to respond to >4 weeks of single-antibiotic therapy) were treated with ciprofloxacin 1 g/day and tinidazole 15 mg/kg/day for 4 weeks [132]. A historic cohort of ten consecutive patients with chronic refractory pouchitis treated with high dose oral and topical mesalazine daily was used as a comparator. These treatment-refractory patients had a significant reduction in the total PDAI score and a significant improvement in quality-of-life score ($p<0.002$) when taking ciprofloxacin and tinidazole, compared to baseline. The rate of clinical remission in the antibiotic group was 87.5 % and for the mesalazine group was 50 %. In another study, 18 patients refractory to metronidazole, ciprofloxacin or amoxicillin/clavulanic acid for 4 weeks were treated orally with rifaximin 2 g/day (a nonabsorbable, broad-spectrum antibiotic) and ciprofloxacin 1 g/day for 15 days. Improvement was defined as a decrease of at least 3 points in the PDAI and remission as a PDAI score of 0. Sixteen out of 18 patients (88.8 %) either improved ($n=10$) or went into remission ($n=6$) [133]. Median PDAI scores before and after therapy were 11 (range 9–17) and 4 (range 0–16), respectively ($p<0.002$). A British group observed similar benefit in just 8 patients with chronic active refractory pouchitis using the same combination of antibiotics, for the same period, and the same definition of improvement and remission. Seven of the eight patients either went into remission ($n=5$) or improved ($n=2$). The median (range) PDAI scores before and after therapy were 12 (9–18) and 0 (0–15), respectively, ($p=0.018$). All patients were compliant and no side effects were reported [134]. In another combination study, 44 patients with refractory pouchitis received metronidazole 800 mg–1 g/day and ciprofloxacin 1 g/day for 28 days [135]. Remission was defined as a combination of a PDAI clinical score of ≤2, endoscopic score of ≤1 and total score of ≤4. Forty four patients entered the trial and completed treatment. Thirty-six (82 %) went into remission. The median Pouchitis Disease Activity Index scores before and after therapy were 12 (range, 8–17) and 3 (range, 1–10), respectively ($p<0.0001$). The median Inflammatory Bowel Disease Questionnaire score also significantly improved from 96.5 (range, 74–183) to 175 (range, 76–215) with this therapy ($p<0.0001$). The eight patients (five male, three female) who did not go into remission were significantly older (median 47.5 vs. 35 years; $p<0.007$), had a longer history of pouchitis (95.5 vs. 26 months; $p<0.0008$), and tended to have a higher Pouchitis Disease Activity Index score before treatment (median 14.5 vs. 12; $p<0.13$) than those who went into remission.

Conclusions

Many clinical and experimental observations indicate that the intestinal microflora are involved in the pathogenesis of IBD.

Probiotics may provide a simple and attractive way of preventing or treating IBD, and patients find the probiotic concept appealing because it is safe, nontoxic, and natural. VSL#3, a highly concentrated cocktail of probiotics has been shown to be effective in the prevention of pouchitis onset and relapses. Results on the use of this probiotic in UC are promising, both in terms of the prevention of relapses and the treatment of mild-to-moderate attacks. Results with probiotics in CD are poor and there is the need of well-performed studies.

It is important to select a well-characterized probiotic preparation, in view of the fact that the viability and survival of bacteria in many of the currently available preparations are unproven. It should be noted that the beneficial effect of one probiotic preparation does not imply efficacy of other preparations containing different bacterial strains, because each individual probiotic strain has unique biological properties.

Prebiotics are an exciting potential treatment for IBD patients. They offer a safe and cost-effective approach and may be considered for long-term treatment. However, experimental evidence supporting the use of these nutraceuticals is still limited. We need to improve our knowledge on the composition of enteric flora or "the neglected organ" and on the intestinal physiology and its relationship with the luminal ecosystem.

The use of antibiotics in UC is not supported by the available studies, although large studies with broad-spectrum agents are required. Antibiotics have an essential role in treating the septic complications of Crohn's disease, including intrabdominal and perianal abscesses and perianal fistulae.

There is evidence that ciprofloxacin, metronidazole, or their combination are effective in Crohn's colitis and ileocolitis, but not in isolated ileal disease; however, use of antibiotics as primary therapy in Crohn's disease is poorly documented, and large, controlled trials are needed for defining the optimal antibiotic regimens.

The use of antibiotics in pouchitis is largely justified although proper controlled trials have not been conducted.

References

1. Guarner F, Casellas F, Borruel N, Antolín M, Videla S, Vilaseca J, et al. Role of microecology in chronic inflammatory bowel diseases. Eur J Clin Nutr. 2002;56:S34–8.
2. Neut C, Bulois P, Desreumaux P, Membré JM, Lederman E, Gambiez L, et al. Changes in the bacterial flora of the neoterminal ileum after ileocolonic resection for Crohn's disease. Am J Gastroenterol. 2002;97:939–46.
3. Manichanh C, Rigottier-Gois L, Bonnaud E, Gloux K, Pelletier E, Frangeul L, et al. Reduced diversity of faecal microbiota in Crohn's disease revealed by a metagenomic approach. Gut. 2006;55:205–11.
4. Sokol H, Seksik P, Furet JP, Firmesse O, Nion-Larmurier I, Beaugerie L, et al. Low counts of fecalibacterium pausnitzii in colitis microbiota. Inflamm Bowel Dis. 2009;15:1183–9.

5. Sokol H, Pigneur B, Watterlot L, Lakhdari O, Bermúdez-Humarán LG, Gratadoux JJ, et al. Fecalibacterium prausnitzii is an anti-inflammatory commensal bacterium identified by gut microbiota analysis of Crohn' disease patients. Proc Natl Acad Sci U S A. 2008;105:16731–6.
6. Duchmann R, Kaiser I, Hermann E, Mayet W, Ewe K, Meyer zum Büschenfelde KH. Tolerance exist towards resident intestinal flora but is broken in active inflammatory bowel disease (IBD). Clin Exp Immunol. 1995;102:445–7.
7. Janowitz HD, Croen EC, Sachar DB. The role of the faecal stream in Crohn's disease: an historical and analytic perspective. Inflamm Bowel Dis. 1998;4:29–39.
8. D'Haens GR, Geboes K, Peeters M, Baert F, Penninckx F, Rutgeerts P. Early lesions of recurrent Crohn's disease caused by infusion of intestinal contents in excluded ileum. Gastroenterology. 1998;114:771–4.
9. Abdelrazeq AS, Kadiyil N, Botterill ID, Lund JN, Reynolds JR, Holdsworth PJ, et al. Predictors for acute and chronic pouchitis following restorative proctocolectomy for ulcerative colitis. Colorectal Dis. 2007;10:805–13.
10. Sartor RB. Insights into the pathogenesis of inflammatory bowel disease provided by new rodent models of spontaneous colitis. Inflamm Bowel Dis. 1995;1:64–75.
11. Campieri M, Gionchetti P. Probiotics in inflammatory bowel disease: new insight to pathogenesis or a possible therapeutic alternative? Gastroenterology. 1999;116:1246–9.
12. Metchnikoff E. The prolongation of life: optimistic studies. London: William Heinemann; 1907. p. 161–83.
13. Schaafsma G. State of the art concerning probiotic strains in milk products. IDF Nutr Newsl. 1996;5:23–4.
14. Lee YK, Salminen S. The coming age of probiotics. Trends Food Sci Technol. 1995;6:241–5.
15. Ng SC, Hart AL, Kamm MA, Stagg AJ, Knight SC. Mechanism of action of probiotics: recent advances. Inflamm Bowel Dis. 2009;15:300–10.
16. Fabia R, Ar'rajab A, Johansson M-L, Willén R, Andersson R, Molin G, et al. The effect of exogenous administration of Lactobacillus reuteri R2LC and oat fiber on acetic acid-induced colitis in the rat. Scand J Gastroenterol. 1993;28:155–62.
17. Mao Y, Nobaek S, Kasravi B, Adawi D, Stenram U, Molin G, et al. The effects of Lactobacillus strains and oat fibre on methotrexate-induced enterocolitis in rats. Gastroenterology. 1996;111:334–44.
18. Madsen KL, Tavernini MM, Doyle JSG, Tavernini MM, Fedorak RN. Lactobacillus sp. prevents development of enterocolitis in interleukin-10 gene-deficient mice. Gastroenterology. 1999;116:1107–14.
19. Schultz M, Veltkamp C, Dieleman LA, Grenther WB, Wyrick PB, Tonkonogy SL, et al. Lactobacillus plantarum 299 V in the treatment and prevention of spontaneous colitis in interleukin-10 deficient mice. Inflamm Bowel Dis. 2002;8:71–80.
20. O'Mahony L, Feeney M, O'Halloran S, Murphy L, Kiely B, Fitzgibbon J, et al. Probiotic impact on microbial flora, inflammation and tumour development in IL-10 knockout mice. Aliment Pharmacol Ther. 2001;15:1219–25.
21. McCarthy J, O'Mahony L, O'Callaghan L, Murphy L, Kiely B, Fitzgibbon J, et al. Double-blind, placebo-controlled trial of two probiotic strains in interleukin 10 knockout mice and mechanistic link with cytokine balance. Gut. 2003;52:975–80.
22. Shibolet O, Karmeli F, Eliakim R, Swennen E, Brigidi P, Gionchetti P, et al. Variable response to probiotics in two models of experimental colitis in rats. Inflamm Bowel Dis. 2002;8:399–408.
23. Madsen K, Cornish A, Soper P, McKaigney C, Jijon H, Yachimec C, et al. Probiotic bacteria enhance murine and human intestinal epithelial barrier function. Gastroenterology. 2001;121:580–91.
24. Pagnini C, Saeed R, Bamias G, Arseneau KO, Pizarro TT, Cominelli F. Probiotics promotes gut health through stimulation of epithelial innate immunity. Proc Natl Acad Sci U S A. 2010;107:454–9.
25. Kruis W, Schuts E, Fric P, Fixa B, Judmaier G, Stolte M. Double-blind comparison of an oral Escherichia coli preparation and mesalazine in maintaining remission of ulcerative colitis. Aliment Pharmacol Ther. 1997;11:853–8.
26. Rembacken BJ, Snelling AM, Hawkey P, Chalmers DM, Axon AT. Non pathogenic Escherichia coli vs mesalazine for the treatment of ulcerative colitis: a randomized trial. Lancet. 1999;354:635–9.
27. Kruis W, Fric P, Pokrotnieks J, Lukás M, Fixa B, Kascák M, et al. Maintaining remission of ulcerative colitis with Escherichia Coli Nissle 1917 is as effective as with standard mesalazine. Gut. 2004;53:1617–23.
28. Matthes H, Krummenerl T, Giensch M, Wolff C, Schulze J. Clinical trial: probiotic treatment of acute distal ulcerative colitis with rectally administered Escherichia coli Nissle 1917 (EcN). BMC Complement Altern Med. 2010;10:13–20.
29. Ishikawa H, Akedo I, Umesaki Y, Tanaka R, Imaoka A, Otani T. Randomized, controlled trial of the effect of bifidobacteria-fermented milk on ulcerative colitis. J Am Coll Nutr. 2003;22:56–63.
30. Guslandi M, Giollo P, Testoni PA. A pilot trial of Saccharomyces boulardii in ulcerative colitis. Eur J Gastroenterol Hepatol. 2003;15:697–8.
31. Venturi A, Gionchetti P, Rizzello F, Johansson R, Zucconi E, Brigidi P, et al. Impact on the faecal flora composition of a new probiotic preparation. Preliminary data on maintenance treatment of patients with ulcerative colitis (UC) intolerant or allergic to 5-aminosalicylic acid (5 ASA). Aliment Pharmacol Ther. 1999;13:1103–8.
32. Bibiloni R, Fedorak RN, Tannock GW, Madsen KL, Gionchetti P, Campieri M, et al. VSL#3 probiotic mixture induces remission in patients with active ulcerative colitis. Am J Gastroenterol. 2005;100:1539–46.
33. Sood A, Midha V, Makharia GK, Ahuja V, Singal D, Goswami P, et al. The probiotic preparation, VSL#3 induces remission in patients with mild-to-moderately active ulcerative colitis. Clin Gastroenterol Hepatol. 2009;7:1202–9.
34. Tursi A, Brandimarte G, Papa A, Giglio A, Elisei W, Giorgetti GM, et al. Treatment of relapsing mild-to-moderate ulcerative colitis with the probiotic VSL#3 as adjunctive to a standard pharmaceutical treatment: a double-blind, randomized, placebo-controlled study. Am J Gastroenterol. 2010;105(10):2218–27. doi:10.1038/ajg.2010.218. Epub 2010 Jun 1.
35. Miele E, Pascarella F, Riannetti E, Quaglietta L, Baldassano RN, Staiano A. Effect of a probiotic preparation (VSL#3) on induction and maintenance of remission in children with ulcerative colitis. Am J Gastroenterol. 2009;104:437–43.
36. Huynh HQ, de Bruin J, Guan L, Diaz H, Li M, Girgis S, et al. Probiotic preparation VSL#3 induces remission in children with mild to moderate acute ulcerative colitis: a pilot study. Inflamm Bowel Dis. 2009;15:760–8.
37. Pardi DS, D'Haens G, Shen B, Campbell S, Gionchetti P. Clinical guidelines for the management of pouchitis. Inflamm Bowel Dis. 2009;15:1424–31.
38. Fazio VW, Ziv Y, Church JM, Oakley JR, Lavery IC, Milsom JW, et al. Ileal pouch-anal anastomoses complications and function in 1005 patients. Ann Surg. 1995;222:120–7.
39. Sandborn WJ. Pouchitis following ileal pouch-anal anastomosis: definition, pathogenesis, and treatment. Gastroenterology. 1994;107:1856–60.
40. Hurst RD, Molinari M, Chung TP, Rubin M, Michelassi F. Prospective study of the incidence, timing and treatment of

pouchitis in 104 consecutive patients after restorative proctocolectomy. Arch Surg. 1996;131:497–500. discussion 501–2.

41. Meagher AP, Farouk R, Dozois RR, Kelly KA, Pemberton JH. J ileal pouch-anal anastomosis for chronic ulcerative colitis: complications and long-term outcome in 1310 patients. Br J Surg. 1998;85:800–3.
42. Penna C, Dozois R, Tremaine W, Sandborn W, LaRusso N, Schleck C, et al. Pouchitis after ileal pouch-anal anastomosis for ulcerative colitis occurs with increased frequency in patients with associated primary sclerosing cholangitis. Gut. 1996;38:234–9.
43. Simchuk EJ, Thirlby RC. Risk factors and true incidence of pouchitis in patients after ileal pouch-anal anastomoses. World J Surg. 2000;24:851–6.
44. Stahlberg D, Gullberg K, Liljeqvist L, Hellers G, Lofberg R. Pouchitis following pelvic pouch operation for ulcerative colitis. Incidence, cumulative risk, and risk factors. Dis Colon Rectum. 1996;39:1012–8.
45. Shen B. Pouchitis: what every gastroenterologist needs to know. Clin Gastroenterol Hepatol. 2013;11:1538–49.
46. Shen B, Achkar JP, Lashner BA, Ormsby AH, Remzi FH, Bevins CL, et al. Endoscopic and histologic evaluation together with symptom assessment are required to diagnose pouchitis. Gastroenterology. 2001;121:261–7.
47. Pardi DS, Shen B. Endoscopy in the management of patients after ileal pouch surgery for ulcerative colitis. Endoscopy. 2008;40:529–33.
48. Sandborn WJ, Tremaine WJ, Batts KP, Pemberton JH, Phillips SF. Pouchitis after ileal pouch-anal anastomosis: a pouchitis disease activity index. Mayo Clin Proc. 1994;69:409–15.
49. Landy J, Al-Hassi HO, McLaughlin SD, Knight SC, Ciclitira PJ, Nicholls RJ, et al. Etiology of pouchitis. Inflamm Bowel Dis. 2012;18:1146–55.
50. Batista D, Raffals L. Role of intestinal bacteria in the pathogenesis of pouchitis. Inflamm Bowel Dis. 2014;20:1481–6.
51. Nicholls RJ, Belliveau P, Neill M, Wilks M, Tabaqchali S. Restorative proctocolectomy withileal reservoir: a pathophysiological assessment. Gut. 1981;22:462–8.
52. Santavirta J, Mattila J, Kokki M, Matikainen M. Mucosal morphology and fecal bacteriology after ileoanal anastomosis. Int J Colorectal Dis. 1991;6:38.
53. Ruseler-van-Embden JGH, Schouten WR, van Lieshout LMC. Pouchitis: result of microbial imbalance? Gut. 1994;35:658–64.
54. Meier CB, Hegazi RA, Aisenberg J, Legnani PE, Nilubol N, Cobrin GM, et al. Innate immune receptor genetic polymorphisms in pouchitis: is CARD15 a susceptibility factor? Inflamm Bowel Dis. 2005;11:965–71.
55. Tyler AD, Milgrom R, Stempak JM, Xu W, Brumell JH, Muise AM, et al. The NOD2insC polymorphismis associated with worse outcome following ileal pouch-anal anastomosisfor ulcerative colitis. Gut. 2013;62:1433–9.
56. Carter MJ, Di Giovine FS, Cox A, Goodfellow P, Jones S, Shorthouse AJ, et al. The interleukin 1 receptor antagonist gene allele 2 as a predictor of pouchitis following colectomyand IPAA in ulcerative colitis. Gastroenterology. 2001;121:805–11.
57. Lammers KM, Ouburg S, Morre SA, Crusius JB, Gionchett P, Rizzello F, et al. Combined carriership of TLR9-1237C and CD14-260T alleles enhances the risk of developing chronic relapsing pouchitis. World J Gastroenterol. 2005;11:7323–9.
58. Gionchetti P, Rizzello F, Venturi A, Brigidi P, Matteuzzi D, Bazzocchi G, et al. Oral bacteriotherapy as maintenance treatment in patients with chronic pouchitis: a double-blind, placebo-controlled trial. Gastroenterology. 2000;119:305–9.
59. Mimura T, Rizzello F, Helwig U, Poggioli G, Schreiber S, Talbot IC, et al. Once daily high dose probiotic therapy for maintaining remission in recurrent or refractory pouchitis. Gut. 2004;53: 108–14.
60. Ulisse S, Gionchetti P, D'Alò S, Russo FP, Pesce I, Ricci G, et al. Expression of cytokines, inducible nitric oxide synthase, and matrix metalloproteinases in pouchitis: effects of probiotic treatment. Gastroenterology. 2001;96:2691–9.
61. Shen B, Brzezinski A, Fazio VW, Remzi FH, Achkar JP, Bennett AE, et al. Maintenance therapy with a probiotic in antibiotic-dependent pouchitis: experience in clinical practice. Aliment Pharmacol Ther. 2005;22:721–8.
62. Kuisma J, Mentula S, Kahri A, Kahri A, Saxelin M, Farkkila M. Effect of Lactobacillus rhamnosus GG on ileal pouch inflammation and microbial flora. Aliment Pharmacol Ther. 2003;17: 509–15.
63. Persborn M, Gerritsen J, Wallon C, Carlsson A, Akkermans LM, Söderholm JD. The effects of probiotics on barrier function and mucosal pouch microbiota during maintenance treatment for severe pouchitis in patients with ulcerative colitis. Aliment Pharmacol Ther. 2013;38:772–83.
64. Gionchetti P, Rizzello F, Helwig U, Venturi A, Lammers KM, Brigidi P, et al. Prophylaxis of pouchitis onset with probiotic therapy: a double-blind, placebo-controlled trial. Gastroenterology. 2003;124(5):1202–9.
65. Gionchetti P, Rizzello F, Morselli C, Poggioli G, Tambasco R, Calabrese C, et al. High-dose probiotics for the treatment of active pouchitis. Dis Colon Rectum. 2007;50:2075–82.
66. Holubar SD, Cima RR, Sandborn WJ, Pardi DS. Treatment and prevention of pouchitis after ileal-pouch anal anastomosis for ulcerative colitis. Cochrane Database Syst Rev. 2010;6:CD001176.
67. Biancone L, Michetti P, Travis S, Escher JC, Moser G, Forbes A, et al. European evidence-based Consensus in the management of ulcerative colitis: special situations. JCC. 2008;2:63–92.
68. Malchow HA. Crohn's disease and Escherichia coli. A new approach in therapy to maintain remission of colonic Crohn's disease? J Clin Gastroenterol. 1997;25:653–8.
69. Guslandi M, Mezzi G, Sorghi M, Testoni PA. Saccharomyces boulardii in maintenance treatment of Crohn's disease. Dig Dis Sci. 2000;45:1462–4.
70. Prantera C, Scribano ML, Falasco G, Andreoli A, Luzi C. Ineffectiveness of probiotics in preventing recurrence after curative resection for Crohn's disease: a randomized controlled trial with Lactobacillus GG. Gut. 2002;51:405–9.
71. Bousvaros A, Guandalini S, Baldassano RN, Botelho C, Evans J, Ferry GD, et al. A randomized, double-blind trial of Lactobacillus GG versus placebo in addition to standard maintenance therapy for children with Crohn's disease. Inflamm Bowel Dis. 2005;11:833–9.
72. Marteau P, Lemann M, Seksik P, Laharie D, Colombel JF, Bouhnik Y, et al. Ineffectiveness of Lactobacillus johnsonii LA1 for prophylaxis of post-operative recurrence in Crohn's disease: a randomized, double-blind, placebo-controlled GETAID trial. Gut. 2006;55:842–7.
73. Van Gossum A, Dewit O, Louis E, de Hertogh G, Baert F, Fontaine F, et al. Multicenter, randomized-controlled clinical trial (Lactobacillus Johnsonii LA1) on early endoscopic recurrence of Crohn's disease after ileo-caecal resection. Inflamm Bowel Dis. 2007;13:135–42.
74. Bourreille A, Cadiot G, Le Dreau G, Laharie D, Beaugerie L, Dupas JL, et al. *Saccharomyces boulardii d*oes not prevent relapse of Crohn's disease. Clin Gastroenterol Hepatol. 2013;11:982–7.
75. Campieri M, Rizzello F, Venturi A, Poggioli G, Ugolini F. Combination of antibiotic and probiotic treatment is efficacious in prophylaxis of post-operative recurrence of Crohn's disease: a randomized controlled study VS mesalamine. Gastroenterology. 2000;118:A781.
76. Willert RP, Peddi KK, Ombiga J, Bampton PA, Lawrance IC. Randomised, double-blinded, placebo-controlled study of VSL#3 versus placebo in the maintenance of remission in Crohn's disease. Gastroenterology. 2010;138 Suppl 1:T1235.

77. Fedorak RN, Feagan BG, Hotte N, Leddin D, Dieleman LA, Petrunia DM, et al. The probiotic VSL#3 has anti-inflammatory effects and could reduce endoscopic recurrence after surgery for Crohn's Disease. Clin Gastroenterol Hepatol. 2015;13: 928–35.
78. Gibson GR, Roberfroid MB. Dietary modulation of the human colonic microbiota: introducing the concept of prebiotics. J Nutr. 1995;125:1401–12.
79. Jacobasch G, Schmiedl D, Kruschewski M, Schmehl K. Dietary resistant starch and chronic inflammatory bowel diseases. Int J Colorectal Dis. 1999;14:201–11.
80. Videla S, Vilaseca J, Antolin M, García-Lafuente A, Guarner F, Crespo E, et al. Dietary inulin improves distal colitis induced by dextran sodium sulphate in the rat. Am J Gastroenterol. 2001;96:1486–93.
81. Araki Y, Andoh A, Koyama S, Fujiyama Y, Kanauchi O, Bamba T. Effects of germinated barley foodstuff on microflora and short chain fatty acid production in dextran sulfate sodium-induced colitis in rats. Biosci Biotechnol Biochem. 2000;64:1794–800.
82. Cherbut C, Michel C, Lecannu G. The prebiotic characteristics of fructo-oligasaccharides are necessary for necessary for reduction of TNBS-induced colitis in rats. J Nutr. 2003;90:75–85.
83. Moreau NM, Martin LI, Toquet CS, Laboisse CL, Nguyen PG, Siliart BS, et al. Restoration of the integrity of rat caeco-colonic mucosa by resistant starch, but not by fructo-oligosaccharides, in dextran sulfate sodium-induced experimental colitis. Br J Nutr. 2003;90:75–85.
84. Hoentjen F, Welling GW, Harmsen HJ, Zhang X, Snart J, Tannock GW, et al. Reduction of colitis by prebiotics in HLA-B27 transgenic rats is associated with microflora changes and immunomodulation. Inflamm Bowel Dis. 2005;11(11):977–85.
85. Hallert C, Kaldma M, Petersson BG. Ispaghula husk may relieve gastrointestinal symptoms in ulcerative colitis in remission. Scand J Gastroenterol. 1991;26:747–50.
86. Fernandez-Banares F, Hinojosa J, Sanchez-Lombrana JL, Navarro E, Martínez-Salmerón JF, García-Pugés A, et al. Randomized clinical trial of Plantago ovata seeds (dietary fiber) as compared with mesalamine in maintaining remission in ulcerative colitis. Am J Gastroenterol. 1999;94:427–33.
87. Mitsuyama K, Toyonaga A, Sata M. Intestinal microflora as a therapeutic target in inflammatory bowel disease. J Gastroenterol. 2002;37 Suppl 14:73–7.
88. Kanauchi O, Mitsuyama K, Homma T, Hibi T, Naganuma M, Homma T, et al. Treatment of ulcerative colitis by feeding with germinated barley foodstuff: first report of a multicenter open control trial. J Gastroenterol. 2002;37:67–72.
89. Kanauchi O, Mitsuyama K, Homma T, Takahama K, Fujiyama Y, Andoh A, et al. Treatment of ulcerative colitis patients by long-term administration of germinated barley foodstuff: multicenter open trial. Int J Mol Med. 2003;12:701–4.
90. Lindsay JO, Whelan K, Stagg AJ, Gobin P, Al-Hassi HO, Rayment N, et al. Clinical, microbiological, and immunological effects of fructo-oligosaccharide in patients with Crohn's disease. Gut. 2006;55:348–55.
91. Casellas F, Borruel N, Torrejon A, Varela E, Antolin M, Guarner F, et al. Oral oligofructose—enriched inulin supplementation in acute ulcerative colitis is well tolerated and associated with lowered fecal calprotectin. Aliment Pharmacol Ther. 2007;25: 1061–7.
92. Rath HC, Schultz M, Freitag R, Dieleman LA, Li F, Linde HJ, et al. Different subsets of enteric bacteria induce and perpetuate experimental colitis in rats and mice. Infect Immun. 2001;69: 2277–85.
93. Madsen KL, Doyle JS, Tavernini MM, Jewell LD, Rennie RP, Fedorak RN. Antibiotic therapy attenuates colitis in interleukin 10 gene-deficient mice. Gastroenterology. 2000;118:1094–105.
94. Hoentjen F, Harmsen HJ, Braat H, Torrice CD, Mann BA, Sartor RB, et al. Antibiotics with a selective aerobic or anaerobic spectrum have different therapeutic activities in various regions of the colon in interleukin-10 gene deficient mice. Gut. 2003;52: 1721–7.
95. Fiorucci S, Distrutti E, Mencarelli A, Barbanti M, Palazzini E, Morelli A. Inhibition of intestinal bacterial translocation with rifaximin modulates lamina propria monocytic cells reactivity and protects against inflammation in a rodent model of colitis. Digestion. 2002;66:246–56.
96. Bamias G, Marini M, Moskaluk CA, Odashima M, Ross WG, Rivera-Nieves J, et al. Down-regulation of intestinal lymphocyte activation and Th1 cytokine production by antibiotic therapy in a murine model of Crohn's disease. J Immunol. 2002;169:5308–14.
97. Yamada T, Deitch E, Specian RD, Perry MA, Sartor RB, Grisham MB. Mechanisms of acute and chronic intestinal inflammation induced by indomethacin. Inflammation. 1993;17:641–62.
98. Onderdonk AB, Hermos JA, Dzink JL, Bartlett JG. Protective effect of metronidazole in experimental ulcerative colitis. Gastroenterology. 1978;74:521–6.
99. Videla S, Villaseca J, Guarner F, Salas A, Treserra F, Crespo E, et al. Role of intestinal microflora in chronic inflammation and ulceration of the rat colon. Gut. 1994;35:1090–7.
100. Dieleman LA, Goerres M, Arends A, Sprengers D, Torrice C, Hoentjen J, et al. Lactobacillus GG prevents recurrence of colitis in HLA-B27 transgenic rats after antibiotic treatment. Gut. 2003;52:370–6.
101. Dickinson RJ, O'Connor HJ, Pinder I, Hamilton I, Johnston D, Axon AT. Double-blind controlled trial of oral vancomycin as adjunctive treatment in acute exacerbations of idiopathic colitis. Gut. 1985;26:1380–4.
102. Chapman RW, Selby WS, Jewell DP. Controlled trial of intravenous metronidazole as adjunct to corticosteroids in severe ulcerative colitis. Gut. 1986;27:1210–2.
103. Burke DA, Axon ATR, Clayden SA, Dixon MF, Johnston D, Lacey RW. The efficacy of tobramycin in the treatment of ulcerative colitis. Aliment Pharmacol Ther. 1990;4:123–9.
104. Mantzaris GJ, Hatzis A, Kontogiannis P, Triadaphyllou G. Intravenous tobramycin and metronidazole as an adjunct to corticosteroids in acute, severe ulcerative colitis. Am J Gastroenterol. 1994;89:43–6.
105. Mantzaris GJ, Archavlis E, Christoforidis P, Kourtessas D, Amberiadis P, Florakis N, et al. A prospective randomized controlled trial of oral ciprofloxacin in acute ulcerative colitis. Am J Gastroenterol. 1997;92:454–6.
106. Mantzaris GJ, Petraki K, Archavlis E, Amberiadis P, Kourtessas D, Christoforidis P, et al. A prospective randomized controlled trial of intravenous ciprofloxacin as an adjunct to corticosteroids in acute, severe ulcerative colitis. Scand J Gastroenterol. 2001;36:971–4.
107. Turunen UM, Farkkila MA, Hakala K, Seppala K, Sivonen A, Ogren M, et al. Long-term treatment of ulcerative colitis with ciprofloxacin: a prospective, double-blind, placebo-controlled study. Gastroenterology. 1998;115:1072–8.
108. Gionchetti P, Rizzello F, Ferrieri A, Venturi A, Brignola C, Ferretti M, et al. Rifaximin in patients with moderate or severe ulcerative colitis refractory to steroid-treatment: a double-blind, placebo-controlled trial. Dig Dis Sci. 1999;44:1220–1.
109. Khan KJ, Ullman TA, Ford AC, Abreu MT, Abadir A, Marshall JK, et al. Antibiotic therapy in inflammatory bowel disease: a systematic review and meta-analysis. Am J Gastroenterol. 2011;106(4):661–73.
110. Blichfeldt P, Blomhoff JP, Myhre E, Gjone E. Metronidazole in Crohn's disease. A double-blind cross-over clinical trial. Scand J Gastroenterol. 1978;13:123–7.

111. Ursing B, Alm T, Barany F, Bergelin I, Ganrot-Norlin K, Hoevels J, et al. A comparative study of metronidazole and sulfasalazine for active Crohn's disease: the cooperative Crohn's disease study in Sweden: II. Results. Gastroenterology. 1982;83:550–62.
112. Ambrose NS, Allan RN, Keighley MR, Burdon DW, Youngs D, Lennard-Jones JE. Antibiotic therapy for treatment in relapse of intestinal Crohn's disease. A prospective randomized study. Dis Colon Rectum. 1985;28:81–5.
113. Sutherland LR, Singleton J, Sessions J, Hanauer S, Krawitt E, Rankin G, et al. Double blind, placebo controlled trial of metronidazole in Crohn's disease. Gut. 1991;32:1071–5.
114. Prantera C, Zannoni F, Scribano ML, Berto E, Andreoli A, Kohn A, et al. An antibiotic regimen for the treatment of active Crohn's disease: a randomized controlled clinical trial of metronidazole plus ciprofloxacin. Am J Gastroenterol. 1996;91:328–32.
115. Steinhart AH, Feagan BG, Wong CJ, Vandervoort M, Mikolainins S, Croitoru K, et al. Combined budesonide and antibiotic therapy for active Crohn's disease: a randomized controlled trial. Gastroenterology. 2002;123:33–40.
116. Colombel JF, Lemann M, Cassagnou M, Bouhnik Y, Duclols B, Dupas JL, et al. A controlled trial comparing ciprofloxacin with mesalazine for the treatment of active Crohn's disease. Am J Gastroenterol. 1999;94:674–8.
117. Arnold GL, Beaves MR, Prydun VO, Mook WJ. Preliminary study of ciprofloxacin in active Crohn's disease. Inflamm Bowel Dis. 2002;8:10–5.
118. Shafran I, Dondelinger PJ, Johnson LK, Murdock HR. Efficacy and tolerability of rifaximin, a nonabsorbed, gut-selective, oral antibiotic in the treatment of active Crohn's disease: results of an open-label study. Am J Gastroenterol. 2003;98:S250.
119. Leiper K, Morris AI, Rhodes JM. Open label trial of oral clarithromycin in active Crohn's disease. Aliment Pharmacol Ther. 2000;14:801–6.
120. Dignass A, Van Assche G, Lindsay JO, Lémann M, Söderholm J, Colombel JF, et al. The second European evidence-based consensus on the diagnosis and management of Crohn's disease: current management. J Crohns Colitis. 2010;4:28–62.
121. Rutgeerts P, Hiele M, Geboes K, Peeters M, Penninckx F, Aerts R, et al. Controlled trial of metronidazole treatment for prevention of Crohn's recurrence after ileal resection. Gastroenterology. 1995;108:1617–21.
122. Rutgeerts P, Van Assche G, D'Haens G, Baert F, Norman M, Aerden I, et al. Ornidazol for prophilaxis of postoperative Crohn's disease: final results of a double-blind placebo controlled trial. Gastroenterology. 2002;122:A80.
123. Borgaonkar MR, MacIntosh DG, Fardy JM. A meta-analysis of antimycobacterial therapy for Crohn's disease. Am J Gastroenterol. 2000;95:725–9.
124. Schwartz DA, Pemberton JH, Sandborn WJ. Diagnosis and treatment of perianal fistulas in Crohn's disease. Ann Intern Med. 2001;135:906–18.
125. Bernstein LH, Frank MS, Brandt LJ, Boley SJ. Healing of perianal Crohn's disease with metronidazole. Gastroenterology. 1980;79:357–65.
126. Brandt LJ, Bernstein LH, Boley SJ. Metronidazole therapy for perianal Crohn's disease: a follow-up study. Gastroenterology. 1982;83:383–7.
127. Solomon MR, McLeod R. Combination ciprofloxacina and metronidazole in severe perianal Crohn's disease. Can J Gastroenterol. 1993;7:571–3.
128. Prantera C, Lochs H, Grimaldi M, Danese S, Scribano ML, Gionchetti P, et al. Rifaximin-extended intestinal release induces remission in patients with moderately active Crohn's disease. Gastroenterology. 2012;142:473–81.
129. Sandborn WJ, McLeod R, Jewell DP. Medical therapy for induction and maintenance of remission in pouchitis. A systematic review. Inflamm Bowel Dis. 1999;5:33–9.
130. Madden M, McIntyre A, Nicholls RJ. Double- blind cross-over trial of metronidazole versus placebo in chronic unremitting pouchitis. Dig Dis Sci. 1994;39:1193–6.
131. Shen B, Achkar JP, Lashner BA, Ormsby AH, Remzi FH, Brzenzinski A, et al. A randomized clinical trial of ciprofloxacin and metronidazole to treat acute pouchitis. Inflamm Bowel Dis. 2001;7:301–5.
132. Shen B, Fazio VW, Remzi FH, Bennett AE, Lopez R, Brzezinski A, et al. Combined ciprofloxacin and tinidazole therapy in the treatment of chronic refractory pouchitis. Dis Colon Rectum. 2007;50:498–508.
133. Gionchetti P, Rizzello F, Venturi A, Ugolini F, Rossi M, Brigidi P, et al. Antibiotic combination therapy in patients with chronic, treatment-resistant pouchitis. Aliment Pharmacol Ther. 1999;13:713–8.
134. Abdelrazeq AS, Kelly SM, Lund JN, Leveson SH. Rifaximin-ciprofloxacin combination therapy is effective in chronic active refractory pouchitis. Colorectal Dis. 2005;7:182–6.
135. Mimura T, Rizzello F, Helwig U, Poggioli G, Schreiber S, Talbot IC, et al. Four week open-label trial of metronidazole and ciprofloxacin for the treatment of recurrent or refractory pouchitis. Aliment Pharmacol Ther. 2002;16:909–17.

47 Biosimilars in the Treatment of Inflammatory Bowel Disease

Vivian W. Huang and Richard N. Fedorak

Introduction

Inflammatory bowel disease (IBD) constitutes chronic diseases that often require therapy with biologic agents, such as the anti-tumor-necrosis-factor-α antibodies (e.g., infliximab, adalimumab, golimumab), that target specific inflammatory and immune pathways. Initial clinical trials showed these biologic agents to be effective in inducing and maintaining remission for patients with both Crohn's disease (CD) and ulcerative colitis (UC) [1–9]. As the original patents expire, pharmaceutical companies have developed biologic copies that have a similar biologic activity, physicochemical characteristics, efficacy, and safety as the "original" (also termed "innovator" or "reference") biologic agent of interest. These copies are known as "similar biotherapeutic products" by the World Health Organization (WHO) [10], "biosimilars" by the European Medicinal Agency (EMA) [11], "follow-on biologics" by the Federal Drug Agency (FDA) [12], and "subsequent entry biologics (SEB)" by Health Canada [13]. To date biosimilars have been used in the treatment of hematologic, rheumatologic, and dermatologic diseases and includes biosimilars of human growth hormone, granulocyte colony-stimulating factor, erythropoietin. The concept of biosimilar therapy is new for IBD, and focuses on biosimilar monoclonal antibodies for IBD.

What Is a Biosimilar?

Biosimilars are biologic agents developed to have similar biological properties in terms of safety and efficacy as a reference biologic product (often called the "originator" or "innovator" biologic) [10–14]. Biologics such as monoclonal antibodies are structurally complex, may have several functional domains, and may have different pharmacokinetic and pharmacodynamics profiles, and different clinical efficacies in different patient populations. Biologics are large molecules that are produced in complex living systems, and thus any change to cells, processes, equipment, or facilities, can result in changes to the final product. Even innovator biologics are subject to "drift," and over time the final biologic may be different than the innovator biologic [14]. Therefore, biosimilars are distinct from generic compounds for small-molecule chemical drugs.

Development of Biosimilars

The development of a novel biologic starts with preclinical studies on drug development including in vitro studies for analytical characterization; structural and functional assays; mechanistic studies; in vivo animal studies on pharmacokinetic and pharmacodynamics properties; in vivo animal studies on safety and immunogenicity [15]. However, in order for a novel biologic to be approved for clinical use, it must go through significant clinical testing for pharmacokinetics, clinical efficacy, and clinical safety [15]. On the other hand, the development of a biosimilar requires extensive preclinical studies to establish the similarity between the biosimilar and the original biologic, and may not require intensive clinical assessment depending on the clinical indication and the governing bodies [15, 16]. This difference in approach (Table 47.1) has opened up many questions regarding the interchangeability of biosimilars with their reference drug.

Clinical Extrapolation of Biosimilars

Clinical extrapolation of data refers to using available data generated by clinical studies investigating the therapeutic use of one drug for one clinical indication to support the

V.W. Huang, M.Sc., M.D., F.R.C.P.C.
R.N. Fedorak, M.D., F.R.C.P.C., F.R.S.C. (✉)
Department of Medicine, Zeidler Ledcor Centre, University of Alberta, 8540—112 Street, Edmonton, AB T6G 2X8, Canada
e-mail: rfedorak@ualberta.ca

D.C. Baumgart (ed.), *Crohn's Disease and Ulcerative Colitis*, DOI 10.1007/978-3-319-33703-6_47

Table 47.1 Comparison in development of innovator biologics and biosimilars

Phase	Subjects	Development stage	Innovator biologics	Biosimilar
Preclinical	In vitro	Research and development	++	++
		Biochemical structure	+	+++
		Biophysical characteristics	+	+++
		In vitro function assays	++	+++
	In vivo animal	Pharmacokinetic and pharmacodynamic studies (in vivo animal studies)	++	+++
		Toxicology studies (in vivo animal studies)	++	+++
		Immunogenicity	++	++
Clinical	Humans	Pharmacokinetic and pharmacodynamic studies	++	+
		Safety and toxicology studies	+++	+
		Clinical trials	+++	+
		Immunogenicity	+	+

References: [14–18]

therapeutic use of that drug for another clinical indication [17]. This may be appropriate in certain cases where the mechanism of action and target of the biosimilar and the original biologic are the same [17]. However, in the case of more complex biologics or in indications where the pharmacokinetics, pharmacodynamics, efficacy, and immunogenicity may differ from the first indication, further studies may be required. Both the EMA [11] and FDA [12, 19, 20] require comparative clinical trials for pharmacokinetics and efficacy. The appropriateness of clinical extrapolation of biosimilars of innovator biologics used to treat inflammatory disorders such as rheumatoid arthritis and inflammatory bowel disease is still uncertain.

Case: Biosimilar Infliximab, CT-P13 (Remsima; Inflectra)

CT-P13 was the first biosimilar infliximab developed, and is a mouse/human cell hybrid similar to the innovator infliximab) [21]. CT-P13 was initially approved by the EMA in 2013 for therapeutic indications including rheumatoid arthritis, ankylosing spondylitis, Crohn's disease, ulcerative colitis, psoriatic arthritis, and psoriasis [21]. In vitro studies showed that CT-P13 and innovator infliximab have very similar binding affinities for TNF-α (soluble and transmembrane) and Fcγ receptors [22]. Pharmacokinetic and toxicity analyses in animal models showed similar pharmacokinetics and no concerns of toxicity with repeated dosing [23].

Two pivotal clinical studies for CT-P13 include PLANETRA (Program evaluating the autoimmune disease investigational drug cT-p13 in rheumatoid arthritis patients) and PLANETAS (Program evaluating the autoimmune disease investigational drug cT-p13 in ankylosing spondylitis patients) [24, 25]. PLANETRA was designed to compare the efficacy and safety of CT-P13 and innovator infliximab in active rheumatoid arthritis patients with inadequate response to methotrexate treatment [24]. In this phase 3, randomized, double blind parallel-group study, patients with active rheumatoid arthritis despite methotrexate were randomized to 3 mg/kg CT-P13 ($n=302$) or innovator infliximab ($n=304$) with methotrexate and folic acid. CT-P13 demonstrated equivalent efficacy to innovator infliximab at week 30, with primary endpoint of ACR20 (American College of Rheumatology 20 %) response being reached in 60.9 % CT-P13 and 58.6 % innovator infliximab (95 % CI—6 % to 10 %). Pharmacokinetic and pharmacodynamics endpoints were similar for each treatment group. Immunogenicity was similar with 25.4 % and 48.4 % of CT-P13, and 25.8 % and 48.2 % of innovator infliximab treated patients having detectable antibodies to infliximab at weeks 14 and 30, respectively. Similar proportions of patients in each group developed adverse events during treatment (60.1 % CT-P13 and 60.8 % innovator infliximab patients).

PLANETAS was designed to demonstrate pharmacokinetic equivalence and efficacy and safety of CT-P13 compared to innovator infliximab in active ankylosing spondylitis patients [25]. In this phase 1 randomized, double blind, parallel-group study, 250 ankylosing spondylitis patients were randomized to receive 5 mg/kg of CT-P13 ($n=125$) or innovator infliximab ($n=125$). The primary endpoints of area under the concentration-time curve at steady state, and observed maximum steady state serum concentration between weeks 22 and 30, were equivalent. CT-P13 and innovator infliximab had similar efficacy with ASAS20 response achieved in 62.6 % and 70.5 % of CT-P13 and 64.8 % and 72.4 % of innovator infliximab-treated patients at weeks 14 and 30, respectively. Immunogenicity was similar with 9.1 % and 27.4 % of CT-P13, and 11.0 % and 22.5 % of innovator infliximab patients having detectable antibodies to innovator infliximab at weeks 14 and 30, respectively. Similar proportions of patients in each group developed adverse events during treatment (64.8 % CT-P13 and 63.9 % innovator infliximab patients).

In two recent systematic review and meta-analysis reports, biosimilar infliximab was found to have similar clinical efficacy and safety compared with other biologic agents (abatacept, adalimumab, certolizumab pegol, etanercept, golimumab, infliximab, rituximab, and tocilizumab) used to treat rheumatoid arthritis [26] and ankylosing spondylitis [27]. Although these studies would suggest that the use of CT-P13 can be extrapolated to IBD, several points of consideration should be taken. First, the dose of infliximab used for treatment of IBD is higher than for other inflammatory conditions; the PLANETRAS and PLANETRA studies also used different doses for the different rheumatologic conditions [24, 25]. Second, the mechanism of action of an anti-TNF monoclonal antibody in the treatment of IBD is different than in the treatment of rheumatologic conditions. In IBD, antibody-dependent cell-mediated cytotoxicity (ADCC), which requires binding of the antigen through the Fab region and binding to Fcγ receptors on effector cells through the Fc region, is thought to play an important role [28–30]. In contrast, in conditions such as rheumatoid arthritis, it is thought that infliximab's main role is through binding and neutralization of TNFα [28–30]. Third, disease-specific patient populations may exhibit differences in immunogenicity, as it has been shown that patients with ankylosing spondylitis and rheumatoid arthritis show lower incidence of developing antidrug antibodies to infliximab than IBD patients [28–30].

In an attempt to directly compare biosimilar infliximab with innovator infliximab, a phase 3 double-blind comparative effectiveness clinical trial comparing biosimilar infliximab to innovator infliximab in patients with active rheumatoid arthritis, 189 patients with active rheumatoid arthritis on stable doses of oral methotrexate 10–20 mg/w were randomized 2:1 to receive either biosimilar infliximab or innovator infliximab 3 mg/kg IV induction, and then at week 22, responders to biosimilar infliximab were continued on treatment while responders to innovator infliximab were switched to biosimilar infliximab in an open label phase through week 46 [31]. Although still in abstract presentation, the investigators reported that responses after induction, and in the open label phase were similar in both treatment groups.

With respect to biosimilars for the treatment of IBD, Kang et al. [32] report a retrospective case series of eight CD and nine UC patients who were administrated CT-P13 from November 2012 to October 2013. There were three CD and five UC patients who received CT-P13 induction therapy, and at 8 weeks, two CD and all five UC patients achieved clinical response and remission. The CD patient who did not respond to CT-P13 had previously lost response to adalimumab. In a multicenter retrospective study, Jung et al. [33] reported on 59 CD and 51 UC anti-TNF naïve patients who received CT-P13 followed up to 52 weeks. CD patients achieved a 90.6 % (29/32) clinical response rate and 84.4 % (27/32) clinical remission rate at week 8; and 87.5 % (7/8) and 75.0 % (6/8) at week 54, respectively. UC patients achieved slightly lower rates of clinical response 81.0 % (34/42) and clinical remission 38.1 % (16/42) at week 8; and 100 % (12/12) and 50.0 % (6/12) at week 54, respectively. In a prospective case series of 16 CD and 15 UC patients who completed induction therapy with CT-P13, Farkas et al. reported that clinical response and remission was achieved in six (37.5 %) and eight (50 %) of CD patients, and in three (20 %) and ten (66.7 %) of UC patients at week 8; they reported mucosal healing in 11 patients [34]. A prospective, multicenter observational cohort study investigating the safety and efficacy of CT-P13 for the induction and maintenance of remission in CD ($n=126$) and UC ($n=84$) reported a significant decrease in CDAI and in pMAYO score at 2 and 6 weeks of treatment, with numeric decrease in mean CRP level in both CD and UC patients during induction therapy [35]. In a prospective observational single centre study in Norway, 46 CD and 32 UC patients who received induction otherapy with CT-P13 were followed. At week 14, 79% (34/43) of CD patients and 56% (18/32) of UC patients acheived clinical remission with significant reductions in CRP and calprotectin at week 14 [36]. In contrast, in a descriptive study, Murphy et al. compared 14 patients who started CT-P13 to 22 patients who started innovator infliximab and examined rates of surgery, readmission, steroid use, disease activity, and CRP trends [37]. The investigators reported that 29 % of CT-P13 group required surgery vs. 0 % of innovator infliximab group ($p=0.02$); 80 % of CT-P13 group required hospital readmission vs 5 % of innovator infliximab group ($p=0.00004$); 60 % of CT-P13 group required steroid escalation vs 8 % of innovator infliximab group ($p=0.0007$); and 93 % of CT-P13 group had increase in CRP while 100 % of innovator infliximab group had decrease in CRP ($p<0.001$). These conflicting preliminary studies suggest that while CT-P13 has clinical efficacy and safety in induction and maintenance therapy for CD and UC further studies are required to fully clarify the efficacy of the biosimilar in IBD.

Interchangeability of Biosimilar and Innovator Biologics?

Since biosimilars are developed to have similar pharmacokinetics, pharmacodynamics, and efficacy as the innovator drug, they should ideally be interchangeable. Interchangeability is defined as substitution of the biosimilar for the innovator biologic, or vice versa, in clinical practice [18, 38]. Few studies report on the interchangeability between CT-P13 and innovator infliximab. In the rheumatoid arthritis randomized clinical trial open label phase, at week 22, responders to biosimilar infliximab were continued on treatment while responders to innovator infliximab were switched to biosimilar infliximab; Kay et al. reported that rheumatoid arthritis treatment response rates and adverse event rates were similar in both treatment groups [31].

In the IBD series reported by Kang et al. there were five CD and four UC patients who were in maintenance therapy with innovator infliximab and interchanged with CT-P13; one UC discontinued CT-P13 due to arthralgia; one patient lost response [32]. In the retrospective study reported by Jung et al., 25 of 27 (92.6 %) CD patients who had switched from innovator infliximab to CT-P13 (for financial reasons) had similar efficacy although two discontinued CT-P13 due to lack of efficacy [33]. One patient subsequently switched to adalimumab with good response. The other switched back to innovator infliximab, but required high dose steroid and double dose innovator infliximab to achieve complete remission. Of nine UC patients who had switched from innovator infliximab to CT-P13, 6 (66.7 %) maintained similar efficacy compared with innovator infliximab; one discontinued CT-P13 due to lack of efficacy and was switched to adalimumab, and one discontinued CT-P13 due to adverse event. Jarzebicka et al. reported data on 32 pediatric CD patients and 7 paediatric UC patients who were switched from innovator infliximab to CT-P13 [39]. Mean PCDAI dropped to 6.6 (5; 0–30) at the last innovator infliximab infusion, and remained at 5.6 (3.8; 0–30) at the second CT-P13 infusion. Mean PUCAI dropped to 5 (0–9 months) and remained at 11 (0, 0–40) after the second CT-P13 infusion. At the end of the follow up period, 20/32 of the CD patients (63%) remained on maintenance remission therapy, but 5/20 required shorter intervals of infusions. The remaining 12 patients stopped treatment (2 lost therapeutic response, 1 had allergic reaction, 1 developed dermatitis and switched to adaliumab, 5 finished therapy due to finances). Only 4/7 (57%) of the UC patients continued biosimilar at follow up. Of the 3/7 who stopped treatment, 1 had allergic reaction, 1 developed varicella zoster infection, 1 required shorten interval and was switched to adalimumab after loss of response. These case series suggest that CT-P13 may potentially be interchangeable with innovator infliximab without loss of clinical efficacy or increase in adverse events. Currently, Norway is conducting a NOR-SWITCH study to investigate, in an adequately powered clinical trial, the efficacy and safety of switching from innovator infliximab to biosimilar infliximab in patients with rheumatoid arthritis, spondyloarthritis, psoriatic arthritis, CD, UC, and chronic plaque psoriasis [40].

Interchangeability: Is Immunogenicity a Concern?

Regarding interchangeability, there is a concern for immunogenicity and cross-immunogenicity since these are biologic proteins. In the rheumatoid arthritis randomized clinical trial, Kay et al. measured antibody responses to infliximab using sensitive ELISA, and reported that by week 58, similar proportions of patients in each treatment group had developed antidrug antibodies (53.5 % of biosimilar infliximab, and 56.5 % of innovator infliximab group) [31]. Specific to IBD patients, Ben-Horin et al. tested the sera of patients with IBD with or without measurable anti-Remicade antibodies to infliximab for cross-reactivity to two batches of CT-P13 [41]. The sera from all 69 patients who were positive for anti-Remicade® antibodies to infliximab were cross-reactive with CT-P13. Anti-Remicade® antibodies to infliximab neutralized the TNF-α binding capacity of both Remicade® and CT-P13. Findings from these studies emphasize the need for awareness of the potential for generation of antidrug antibodies and cross-reactivity through interchanging biosimilar and original biologic agents.

Why Bother with Biosimilars?

Innovator biologics have been efficacious, but costly, for the management of IBD. Biosimilars were developed with the intent to be less costly. In a budget impact analysis of CT-P13 for the treatment of rheumatoid arthritis in six Central and Eastern European countries, Brodsky et al. compared a reference scenario using no biosimilar with scenario 1 where interchanging biosimilar infliximab and innovator infliximab was not allowed, and scenario 2 where interchanging biosimilar and innovator infliximab was allowed [42]. They reported that over a 3 year time period, scenario 1 and scenario 2 resulted in net savings of euro 15.3M and euro 20.8M, respectively, compared to not using a biosimilar. A similar budget impact analyses of biosimilar infliximab (Remsima(R)) for the treatment of autoimmune diseases (rheumatoid arthritis, ankylosing spondylitis, Crohn's diseas, ulcerative colitis, psoriasis, and psoriatic arthritis) in five European Countries, showed similar drug cost-related savings, reporting a cumulative cost savings of €25.79 million (10% discount) to €77.37 milliion (30% discount) [43]. An important concept to note is that the economics of biosimilars will differ according to the country of interest, and the particular pharmaceutical and health care systems of interest [44]. Currently, there are no IBD specific economic analyses of biosimilar versus innovator biologics.

Current Guidelines and Recommendations

As biosimilars are widely used in many chronic diseases, several international governing bodies have developed guidelines for development of these agents and clinical use. As shown in Table 47.2, governing bodies' requirements for approval of the biosimilar agent and extrapolation to different clinical indications differ depending on the biologic, the clinical indication, and the governing agency [10–13]. Independent of government bodies, clinical practicing gastroenterologists across the world are hesitant to adopt clinical extrapolation and interchangeability of biosimilars to the

Table 47.2 International regulatory authorities definitions and requirements for approval of biosimilar biologics

Governing body	Name of biosimilar	Definition	Requirement for approval/licensing
World Health Organization (WHO) [10]	Similar bio-therapeutic products	A biotherapeutic product that is similar in terms of quality, safety and efficacy to an already licensed reference biotherapeutic product	– Demonstration of structural sameness and bioequivalence of the generic medicine to the reference product – Comparative quality, nonclinical and clinical studies demonstrating similarity to the reference product
European Medicinal Agency (EMA) [11]	Biosimilars	A biological medicine that is similar to another biologic medicine that has already been authorized for use	– Similar to the reference medicine – Does not have any meaningful differences from the reference medicine in terms of quality, safety, or efficacy
Federal Drug Agency (FDA) [12]	Follow-on biologics or Biosimilar	A biologic product that is approved based on a showing that it is highly similar to an FDA-approved biologic product, known as a reference product, and has no clinically meaningful differences in terms of safety and effectiveness from the reference product	– Analytical studies that demonstrate similarity to the reference product – Animal studies (including toxicity assessment) – Clinical study or studies (including assessment of immunogenicity and pharmacokinetics or pharmacodynamics) that demonstrate safety, purity, and potency in one or more appropriate conditions of use for which the reference product is licensed and intended to be used and for which licensure is sought for the biologic product
Health Canada [13]	Subsequent Entry Biologics	A biologic drug that enters the market subsequent to a version previously authorized in Canada, and with demonstrated similarity to a reference biologic drug	– Suitable reference biologic drug exists that was originally authorized for sale based on a complete data package and has significant safety and efficacy data accumulated – SEB can be well characterized by modern analytical methods – SEB can be judged similar to reference biologic drug using predetermined criteria

management of IBD based on rheumatological trials and case series of IBD [45].

A summary of international gastroenterology IBD professional societies clinical practice guidelines and statements is outlined in Table 47.3 [46–51]. The CAG (2013) position statement on biosimilars is that the subsequent entry biologic should be regarded as stand-alone products, and not interchanged with innovator biologics [48]. The ECCO (2013) position statement on biosimilars suggests that more rigorous testing in patients with IBD, with comparison to the appropriate innovator product, is required [50]. The Italian Group for the Study of IBD (IG-IBD) recommends that the biosimilar's efficacy and safety for IBD be obtained prior to marketing [49]. The international guidelines recommend caution with substitution of biosimilars with innovator biologics, and support the need for further clinical trials investigating the efficacy and safety of biosimilars for the management of IBD [46–51].

Conclusion

Inflammatory bowel disease is challenging to treat, and although effective for induction and maintenance of remission, the currently used biologic medications are expensive to the health care system and payer. With the development of biosimilar products that are proposed to have similar efficacy and side effect profile, but at lower costs to the system, health care authorities will pursue these alternatives. Clinicians, therefore, need to be fully aware of the issues relating to extrapolation and interchangeability of innovator and biosimilar products. Until there is complete clarity on the role of biosimilars in the treatment of patients with IBD medical practitioners will need to be vigilant relative to efficacy, loss of response, and adverse events. Finally, the long-term cost-effectiveness of biosimilars in the management of IBD remains to be determined.

Table 47.3 International gastroenterology and IBD professional societies clinical practice guidelines and statements

Clinical practice group	Name of biosimilar	Summary of clinically relevant statements/ recommendations (for full list of statements/ recommendations, please refer to referenced articles)
Brazilian Federation of Gastroenterology and Brazilian Study Group on Inflammatory Bowel Disease [46]	Biosimilar	(1) "Specialists-12 do not allow automatic substitution because it takes place without medical consent"
		(2) "Scientifically grounded proof that a given biosimilar drug is safe and effective against the disease that is the target of extrapolation"
		(3) "The pharmacovigilance of biosimilar products should be mandatorily as rigorous as the pharmacovigilance of innovator biologic products"
British Society of Gastroenterology [47]	Biosimilar	(1) "For patients already on therapy, avoidance of switching from parent drug to biosimilar, or vice versa, at least until we have safety data"
		(2) "Discussion with patients about the choice of anti-TNF"
Canadian Association of Gastroenterology (CAG) [48]	Subsequent entry biologics (SEBs)	(1) "SEBs represent a potentially effective and cost saving option for the management of IBD that may serve to enhance access to biologic therapy"
		(2) "SEBs should be regarded as stand-alone products, and should be supported by well-designed nonclinical and clinical studies in a population relevant to Canadian patients"
		(3) "SEBs cannot be regarded as interchangeable with the RBD"
		(4) "Prescriptions for RBDs should not be automatically substituted for less expensive SEBs by dispensing pharmacies"
		(5) "SEBs should be supported by long-term pharmacovigilance data in a fashion similar to RBDs"
		(6) "Companies bringing SEBs to the Canadian market should be committed to improving patient care by acquiring new scientific data beyond that which is required as a minimum to satisfy regulatory authorities and their commercial imperatives"
European Crohn's Colitis Organization (ECCO) [45]	Biosimilar	(1) "Specific evidence obtained in patients with IBD should be required to establish efficacy and safety for this specific indication, because experience with currently licensed biological medicines has already shown that clinical efficacy in IBD cannot be predicted by effectiveness in other indications, such as rheumatoid arthritis"
		(2) "Clinical trials should be of large enough size to detect common adverse events and powered to show equivalence with a reference biological agent, or conventional superiority"
		(3) "Post-marketing collection of data in both children and adults is necessary to confirm safety by recording less common but important potential adverse effects, as well as identifying any increase in frequency of predictable adverse events contingent on wider access to treatment"
		(4) "Names of biosimilars need clearly to differ from their reference biological medicine in order to facilitate the collection of data on safety and efficacy, which would be impossible if confusion between names will occur"
		(5) "Any decision to substitute a product should only be made with the prescribing health care provider's specific approval and patient's knowledge"

(continued)

Table 47.3 (continued)

Clinical practice group	Name of biosimilar	Summary of clinically relevant statements/ recommendations (for full list of statements/ recommendations, please refer to referenced articles)
Italian Group for the Study of IBD (IG-IBD) [49]	Biosimilar	(1) "Two biosimilars that target the same molecule can be considered equivalent in terms of efficacy and safety only when such equivalence has been demonstrated in preclinical and clinical trials"
		(2) "Adequately powered post marketing clinical trials should be conducted to show/confirm the clinical equivalence of the two agents and to identify similarities and potential differences in their adverse event profiles"
		(3) "A biosimilar agent with proven efficacy and safety for one indication is not necessarily effective and safe for other indications"
		(4) "When the reference drug is used to treat IBD, evidence of the biosimilars efficacy and safety *in this specific setting* be obtained prior to marketing"
		(5) "Due consideration should be given to the markedly heterogeneous clinical presentation and course of these diseases (IBD) and to the current absence of specific, clear-cut biomarkers that can be used to predict IBD patients' responsiveness to these agents and to monitor their short-term efficacy"
		(6) "The regulatory rules and economic assumptions used for generic chemical medicines cannot be applied to biosimilars"
		(7) "An IBD patient being effectively controlled with an original biopharmaceutical should not be switched to a drug claimed to be that drug's biosimilar until preliminary data supporting such changes have been reported"
		(8) "IG-IBD favors the use of biosimilar agents, provided that they meet appropriate quality standards, and that their safety and efficacy has been specifically verified in IBD patients"
		(9) "For biosimilars approved for the use in IBD, post marketing data specifically related to the biosimilar drug (as opposed to its reference product) must be acquired to: (a) detect less common but potentially harmful adverse effects, particularly those associated with long-term use; (b) monitor the actually frequency of expected adverse events"
Spanish Society of Gastroenterology y	Biosimilar	(1) "In order to obtain a given indication a biosimilar should be tested in a clinical trial specifically designed to that end"
		(2) "Substituting a biosimilar for the original drug cannot be an accepted practice"
		(3) "The appropriate use of biosimilar drugs requires interaction by physicians, pharmacists, and regulatory agencies with the aim of favoring the right to health of patients by offering quality, effective, and safe products"

References

1. Hanauer SB, Feagan BG, Lichtenstein GR, Mayer LF, Schreiber S, Colombel JF, et al. Maintenance infliximab for Crohn's disease: the ACCENT I randomized trial. Lancet. 2002;359(9317):1541–9.
2. Sands BE, Anderson FH, Bernstein CN, Chey WY, Feagan BG, Fedorak RN, et al. Infliximab maintenance therapy for fistulising Crohn's disease. N Engl J Med. 2004;350(9):876–85.
3. Rutgeerts P, Sandborn WJ, Feagan BG, Reinisch W, Olson A, Johanns J, et al. Infliximab for induction and maintenance therapy for ulcerative colitis. N Engl J Med. 2005;353(23):2462–76.
4. Hanauer SB, Sandborn WJ, Rutgeerts P, Fedorak RN, Lukas M, MacIntosh D, et al. Human anti-tumor necrosis factor monoclonal antibody (adalimumab) in Crohn's disease: the CLASSIC-I trial. Gastroenterology. 2006;130(2):323–33.
5. Colombel JF, Sandborn WJ, Rutgeerts P, Enns R, Hanauer SB, Pannaccionne R, et al. Adalimumab for maintenance of clinical response and remission in patients with Crohn's disease: the CHARM trial. Gastroenterology. 2007;132(1):52–65.
6. Reinisch W, Sandborn WH, Hommes DW, D'Haens G, Hanauer S, Schreiber S, et al. Adalimumab for induction of clinical remission in moderately to severely active ulcerative colitis: results of a randomized controlled trial. Gut. 2011;60(6):780–7.
7. Sandborn WJ, van Assche G, Reinisch W, Colombel JF, D'Haens G, Wolf DC, et al. Adalimumab induces and maintains clinical remission in patients with moderate-to-severe ulcerative colitis. Gastroenterology. 2012;142:257–265.e13.
8. Sandborn WJ, Feagan BG, Marano C, Zhang H, Strauss R, Johanns J, et al. Subcutaneous golimumab induces clinical response and remission in patients with moderate-to-severe ulcerative colitis. Gastroenterology. 2014;146(1):85–95.
9. Sandborn WJ, Feagan BG, Marano C, Shang H, Strauss R, Johanns J, et al. Subcutaneous golimumab maintains clinical response in patients with moderate-to-severe ulcerative colitis. Gastroenterology. 2014;146(1):96–109.
10. World Health Organization (WHO). Guidelines on evaluation of similar biotherapeutic products (SBPs). Available from: http://www.who.int/biologicals/publications/trs/areas/biological_therapeutics/TRS_977_Annex_2.pdf?ua=1. Cited 26 June 2015.
11. European Medicines Agency (EMA). Guideline on similar biologic medicinal products. Available from: http://www.ema.europa.eu/docs/en_GB/document_library/Scientific_guideline/2014/10/WC500176768.pdf. Cited 26 June 2015.
12. Epstein MS, Ehrenpreis ED, Kulkarni PM. FDA-Related Matters Committee of the American College of Gastroenterology. Biosimilars: the need, the challenge, the future: the FDA perspective. Am J Gastroenterol. 2014;109(12):1856–9.
13. Health Canada. Guidance for Sponsors: Information and Submission Requirements for Subsequent Entry Biologics (SEBs). Available from: http://www.hc-sc.gc.ca/dhp-mps/alt_formats/pdf/brgtherap/applic-demande/guides/seb-pbu/seb-pbu-2010-eng.pdf. Cited 26 June 2015.
14. Ramanan S, Grampp G. Drift, evolution, and divergence in biologics and biosimilars manufacturing. BioDrugs. 2014;28(4):363–72.
15. Bui LA, Hurst S, Finch GL, Ingram B, Jacobs IA, Kirchhoff CF, et al. Key considerations in the preclinical development of biosimilars. Drug Discov Today. 2015;20 Suppl 1:3–15.
16. Van Aerts L, de Smet K, Reichmann G, van der Lann JW, Schneider CK. Biosimilars entering the clinic without animal studies. A paradigm shift in the European Union. MAbs. 2014;6(5):1155–62.
17. Weise M, Kurki P, Wolff-Holz E, Bielsky MC, Schneider CK. Biosimilars: the science of extrapolation. Blood. 2014;124(22):3191–6.
18. McCamish M, Pakulski J, Sattler C, Woolett G. Toward interchangeable biologics. Clin Pharmacol Ther. 2015;97(3):215–7.
19. Federal Drug Agency (FDA). Quality considerations in demonstrating biosimilarity of a therapeutic protein product to a reference product: guidance for industry. Available from: http://www.fda.gov/downloads/Drugs/GuidanceComplianceRegulatoryInformatin/Guidances/UCM291134.pdf. Cited 26 June 2015.
20. Federal Drug Agency (FDA). Scientific considerations in demonstrating biosimilarity to a reference product. Available from: http://www.fda.gov/downloads/Drugs/GuidanceComplianceRegulatoryInformation/Guidances/UCM291128.pdf. Cited 26 June 2015.
21. McKeage K. A review of CT-P13: an infliximab biosimilar. BioDrugs. 2014;28:313–21.
22. Jung SK, Lee KH, Jeon JW, Lee JW, Kwon BO, Kim YJ, et al. Physicochemical characterization of Remsima®. MAbs. 2014;6(5):1163–77.
23. European Medicines Agency (EMA). Committee for Medicinal Products for Human Use (CHMP). Assessment report: Remsima (infliximab); 2013. http://www.ema.europa.eu/docs/en_GB/document_library/EPAR_-_Public_assessment_report/human/002576/WC500151486.pdf. Cited 18 July 2015.
24. Yoo DH, Hrycaj P, Miranda P, Ramiterre E, Piotrowski M, Shevchuk S, et al. A randomized, double-blind, parallel-group study to demonstrate equivalence in efficacy and safety of CT-P13 compared with innovator infliximab when coadministered with methotrexate in patients with active rheumatoid arthritis: the PLANETRA study. Ann Rheum Dis. 2013;72:1613–20.
25. Park W, Hrycaj P, Jeka S, Kovalenko V, Lysenko G, Miranda P, et al. A randomized, double-blind, multicenter, parallel-group, prospective study comparing the pharmacokinetics, safety, and efficacy of CT-P13 and innovator infliximab in patients with ankylosing spondylitis: the PLANETAS study. Ann Rheum Dis. 2013;72:1605–12. doi:10.1136/annrheumdis-2012-203091.
26. Baji P, Pentek M, Czirjak L, Szekanecz Z, Nagy G, Gulacsi L, et al. Efficacy and safety of infliximab-biosimilar compared to other biological drugs in rheumatoid arthritis: a mixed treatment comparison. Eu J Heatlh Econ. 2014;15 Suppl 1:S53–64.
27. Baji P, Pentek M, Szanto S, Geher P, Gulacsi L, Balogh O, et al. Comparative efficacy and safety of biosimilar infliximab and other biological treatments in ankylosing spondylitis: a systematic literature review and meta-analysis. Eur J Health Econ. 2014;15 Suppl 1:S45–52.
28. Feagan BG, Choquette D, Ghosh S, Gladman DD, Ho V, Meibohm B, et al. Review: the challenge of indication extrapolation for infliximab biosimilars. Biologicals. 2014;42:177–83.
29. Hlavaty T, Letkovsky J. Biosimilars in the therapy of inflammatory bowel diseases. Eur J Gastroenterol Hepatol. 2014;26:581–7.
30. Feldman SR. Inflammatory diseases: integrating biosimilars into clinical practice. Semin Arhtritis Rheum. 2015;44:S16–21.
31. Kay J, Wyand M, Chandrashekara S, Olakkengil DJ, Bhojani K, Bhatia G, et al. BOW015, a biosimilar infliximab, in patients with active rheumatoid arthritis on stable methotrexate disease: 54-week results of a randomized, double-blind, active comparator study. In: Bucala RJ, editor. 2014 ACR/ARHP Annual Meeting, Boston, MA. Arthritis Rheumatol. 2014;66(S10):S1–1402.
32. Kang T, Moon H, Lee S, Lim YJ, Kang HW. Clinical experience of the use of CT-P13, a biosimilar to infliximab in patients with inflammatory bowel disease: a case series. Dig Dis Sci. 2015;60(4):951–6.
33. Jung YS, Park DI, Kim YH, Lee JH, Seo PJ, Cheon JH, et al. Efficacy and safety of CT-P13, a biosimilar of infliximab, in patients with inflammatory bowel disease: a retrospective multicenter study. J Gastroenterol Hepatol. 2015;30(12):1705–12.
34. Farkas K, Rutka M, Balint A, Nagy F, Bor R, Milassin A, et al. Efficacy of the new infliximab biosimilar CT-P13 induction therapy in Crohn's disease and ulcerative colitis—experiences from a single center. Expert Opin Biol Ther. 2015;2:1–6.
35. Gecse KB, Lovasz BD, Farkas K, Banai J, Bene L, Gasztonyi B, et al. Efficacy and Safety of the Biosimilar Infliximab CT-P13 Treatment

in Inflammatory Bowel Diseases: A Prospective, Multicentre, Nationwide Cohort. J Crohns Colitis 2016;10(2):133–140.
36. Jahnsen J, Detlie TE, Vatn S, and Ricanek P. Biosimilar infliximab (CT-P13) in the treatment of inflammatory bowel disease: A Norwegian observational study. Expert Rev Gastroenterol Hepatol 2015;9(S1):S45–S52.
37. Murphy C, Sugrue K, Mohamad G, McCarthy J, Buckley M. P505: biosimilar but not the same. In: Egan LJ, editor. 10th congress of ECCO, February 18–21, 2015, Barcelona, Spain. J Crohns Colitis. 2015;9 Suppl 1:S331.
38. Fiorino G, Danese S. The biosimilar road in inflammatory bowel disease: the right way? Best Pract Res Clin Gastroenterol. 2014;28:465–71.
39. Sieczkowksa J, Jarzebicka D, Banaszkiewicz A, Plocek A, Gawronska A, Toporowska-Kowalska E, et al. Switching Between Infliximab Originator and Biosimilar in Paediatric Patients with Inflammatory Bowel Disease. Preliminary Observations. J Crohns Colitis 2016;10(2):127–32.
40. A randomized, double-blind, parallel-group study to evaluate the safety and efficacy of switching from innovator infliximab to biosimilar infliximab compared with continued treatment with innovator infliximab in patients with rheumatoid arthritis, spondyloarthritis, psoriatic arthritis, ulcerative colitis, Crohn's disease and chronic plaque psoriasis—The NOR-SWITCH Study. Available from: https://clinicaltrials.gov/ct2/show/NCT02148640. Cited 26 June 2015.
41. Ben-Horin S, Yavzori M, Benhar I, Fudim E, Picard O, Ungar B, et al. Cross-immunogenicity: antibodies to infliximab in Remicade-treated patients with IBD similarly recognise the biosimilar Remsima. Gut 2015;0:1-7. doi:10.1136gutjnl-2015-309290 (online first).
42. Brodszky V, Baji P, Balogh O, Pentek M. Budget impact analysis of biosimilar infliximab (CT-P13) for the treatment of rheumatoid arthritis in six Central and Easter European countries. Eur J Health Econ. 2014;15 Suppl 1:S65–71.
43. Jha A, Upton A, Dunlop WC, Akehurst R. The Budget Impact of BIosimlar Infliximab (Remsima(R) for the Treatment of Autoimmune Diseases in Five European Countries. Adv Ther 2015;32(8):742–56.
44. Blackstone EA, Fuhr JP. The economics of biosimilars. Am Health Drug Benefits. 2013;6(8):469–78.
45. Baji P, Gulacsi L, Lovascz BD, Golovics PA, Brodsky V, Pentek M, et al. Treatment preferences of originator versus biosimilar drugs in Crohn's disease; discrete choice experiment among gastroenterologists. Scan J Gastroenterol. 2015;10:1–6.
46. Azevedo V, Meirelles E, Kochen J, Mederios A Miszputen S, Teixeira F, et al. Recommendations on the use of biosimilars by the Brazilian Society of Rheumatology, Brazilian Society of Dermatology, Brazilian Federation of Gastroenterology and Brazilian Study Group on Inflammatory Bowel Disease – Focus on clinical evaluation of monoclonal antibodies and fusion proteins used in the treatment of autoimmune diseases. Autoimmun Rev. 2015 May 1. pii: S1568-9972(15)00106-8. doi:10.1016/j.autrev.2015.04.014. [Epub ahead of print].
47. British Society of Gastroenterology. IBD Section Statement on Biosimilar Drugs. Available from: http://www.bsg.org.uk/clinical-guidance/ibd/ibd-section-statement-on-biosimilar-drugs.html. Cited 26 June 2015.
48. Devlin SM, Bressler B, Bernstein CN, Fedorak RN, Bitton A, Singh H, et al. Review: overview of subsequent entry biologics for the management of inflammatory bowel disease and Canadian Association of Gastroenterology position statement on subsequent entry biologics. Can J Gastroenterol. 2013;27(10):567–71.
49. Annese V, Vecchi M. On behalf of the Italian Group for the Study of IBD (IG-IBD). Use of biosimilars in inflammatory bowel disease: Statements of the Italian Group for Inflammatory Bowel Disease. Dig Liver Dis. 2014;46:963–8.
50. Danese S, Gomollon F. ECCO position statement: the use of biosimilar medicines in the treatment of inflammatory bowel disease (IBD). J Crohns Colitis. 2013;87:586–9.
51. Arguelles-Arias F, Barreiro-de-Acosta M, Carballo F, Hinojosa J, Tejerina T. Joint position statement by "Sociedad Espanola de Patologia Digestiva" (Spanish Society of Gastroenterology) and "Sociedad Espanola de Farmacologia" (Spanish Society of Pharmacology) on biosimilar therapy for inflammatory bowel disease. Rev Esp Enferm Dig (Madrid). 2013;105(1):37–43.

Step-Up vs. Top-Down Approach in Crohn's Disease

48

Christine Y. Yu and Daniel W. Hommes

Introduction

Therapy for patients suffering from Crohn's disease (CD) has evolved considerably over the last several years. Through better understanding of the evolution of CD, a robust set of tools for diagnosis, and new insights and data to suggest a more personalized treatment plan based on severity of disease, clinicians are better able to target specific treatment goals. Until the 1990s, treatment was focused on acute flares and symptom control. Current therapeutic aims include: (1) achievement and maintenance of clinical remission, (2) minimization of toxicities and complications, (3) improvement in quality of life, (4) diminution of surgeries and hospitalizations [1–6], and more recently (5) attainment of mucosal healing [6–11].

Traditionally, therapy for all patients with CD revolved around a "step up" approach. Medication regimens with lower risks of toxicity were used early with subsequent therapies added for lack of response. This means that 5-aminosalicylic acids (5-ASA) and corticosteroids were attempted, and once unsuccessful, immunosuppressants and anti-tumor necrosis factor (anti-TNF) agents were introduced in a step-wise fashion. However, each agent has its downfall from poor efficacy with 5-ASA compounds [2] to poor long-term efficacy and side effects with steroids [12–14] and even slow onset of action with thiopurines [15–17]. Overall, despite this eclectic armamentarium, none of these agents have proven to change the natural course of the disease [18–20].

Indirect and direct evidence exists to support early aggressive therapy [21, 22] in which biologics are initiated immediately after diagnosis as first-line therapy for a select patient population. This chapter focuses on the evidence behind early aggressive therapy in selected patients, the "Window of Opportunity" present during the first years after initial diagnosis, safety measures and monitoring that should be taken to prevent (serious) adverse effects, cost-effectiveness of top-down therapy and finally, possible de-escalation therapy once deep remission is achieved.

Top-Down Therapy: Presenting the Data

The association between anti-TNF use and higher rates of mucosal healing indirectly suggest the benefits of early aggressive therapy. As seen in the EXTEND trial, a randomized, double-blind, placebo-controlled trial, 135 adults with moderate to severe ileocolonic CD were randomized to adalimumab or placebo as maintenance after initial induction therapy. At week 52, rates of mucosal healing were 24 % in the adalimumab group as compared to 0 % in the placebo group ($P<.001$) [23]. Higher rates of mucosal healing with early anti-TNF therapy has been supported by a number of other trials [5, 24, 25].

Additionally, shorter durations of disease from time of initial diagnosis to initiation of anti-TNF agents have demonstrated increased efficacy and improved treatment outcomes in patients with moderate to severe CD. Subanalyses of the CHARM (Crohn's trial of the fully Human antibody Adalimumab for Remission Maintenance; maintenance therapy with ADA) trial showed higher clinical remission rates with adalimumab at 52 weeks among patients with shorter disease duration. Patients with disease duration of <2 years had remission rates of 43 % whereas those with disease duration of ≥5 years, remission rates were 28 % ($P<0.001$) [26]. Similarly, in PRECiSE 2 (Pegylated antibody fRagment Evaluation in Crohn's disease Safety and Efficacy; maintenance therapy with certolizumab) subanalysis, response and remission rates with certolizumab pegol at week 26 (CDAI ≤ 150) for patients with disease duration of <1 year were 89 % and 68 %, respectively. In comparison, for those

C.Y. Yu, MD
GI fellow, University of California, Los Angeles, USA

D.W. Hommes, MD, PhD (✉)
Division of Medicine and Gastroenterology, Department of Medicine, Ronald Reagan UCLA Medical Center, 100 UCLA Medical Plaza, Suite 345, Los Angeles, CA 90095, USA
e-mail: DHommes@mednet.ucla.edu

D.C. Baumgart (ed.), *Crohn's Disease and Ulcerative Colitis*, DOI 10.1007/978-3-319-33703-6_48

with disease duration of >5 years, response and remission rates were 57 % and 44 %, respectively [27]. These data suggest a window of opportunity in which early aggressive therapy may have the most impact.

One of the earliest studies to pose a paradigm shift from traditional to early aggressive therapy was a prospective placebo-controlled multicenter trial by Markowitz et al. in which pediatric patients with moderate to severe CD received either combination 6-mercaptopurine (6-MP) and prednisone or prednisone alone. There was a significantly shorter duration of use and lower cumulative dose of steroids in the 6-MP group. Only 9 % of the 6-MP group relapsed compared with 47 % of the placebo group [28]. While, currently early aggressive therapy is now considered primarily with biologic agents, Markowitz and colleagues were amongst the first to demonstrate a more aggressive approach as part of the initial treatment regimen.

Two randomized controlled trials directly examine the relationship between early aggressive and traditional treatment methodologies. The "Step-Up vs. Top-down" study demonstrated improved clinical outcomes. The "top-down" arm received combination anti-TNF and thiopurine induction therapy. If disease flared, they were given additional doses of infliximab and steroids. In comparison, the "step-up" group started with intravenous steroids followed by azathioprine and infliximab if necessary. While improved outcomes at weeks 26 and 52 were seen with the "top-down" group, this early study did not use a regularly scheduled maintenance infliximab as standard of care [10, 22]. In the SONIC trial, Colombel and colleagues studied patients with moderate to severe CD, naïve to immunomodulator or biologic use. Those that were treated with infliximab plus azathioprine or infliximab monotherapy were more likely to achieve steroid-free clinical remission than those treated with azathioprine monotherapy [29].

More recently, an analysis of claims data also found early aggressive therapy to be superior. Patients in the "Early-TNF" group, defined as those that initiated anti-TNF therapy within 30 days of the first prescription for CD, had lower rates of steroid use and CD-related surgeries and more stable dosing of their anti-TNF therapy [30].

Overall, data in the medical literature supports the use of early aggressive therapeutic regimens. Early intensive treatment with combination anti-TNF and thiopurine should be considered in all high-risk patients. More data on newer anti-TNF agents are needed.

Window of Opportunity in CD

CD is a chronic, disabling lifelong condition. Since CD is characterized by progression of inflammatory disease to a more complicated stricturing, penetrating and fibrotic disease, early and late stages of disease should be distinguished [31]. Fibrostenosis and perforation is not associated with early CD; rather patients with recently diagnosed CD tend to

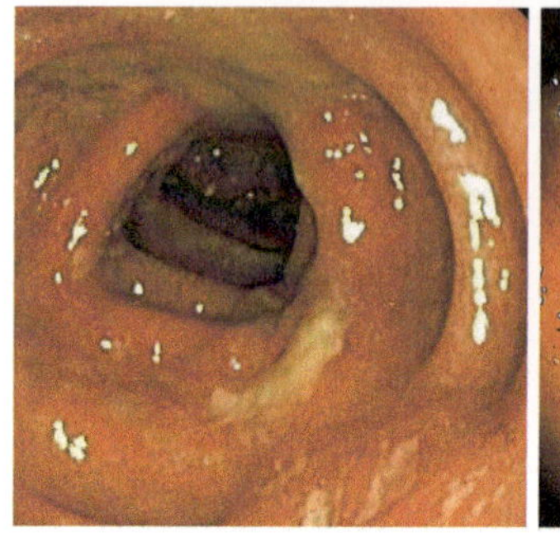

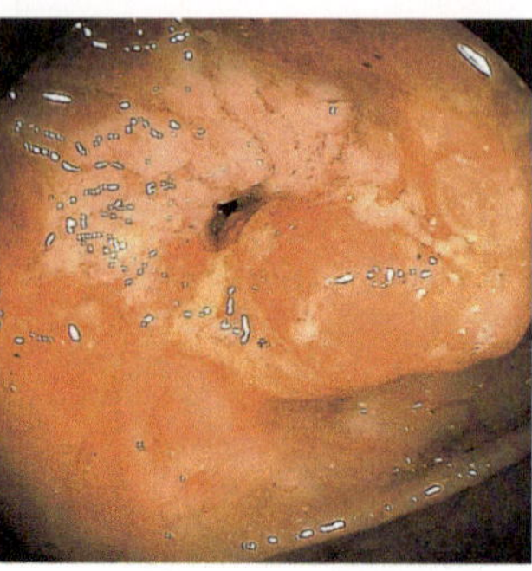

Fig. 48.1 Inflammation (*left panel*) and fibrostenosis (*right panel*)

have purely inflammatory lesions (Fig. 48.1). Repeated episodes of inflammation with subsequent wound healing causing stricture formation, obstruction and eventual penetrating complications are thought to be the cause of intestinal fibrosis. When the disease evolves, the number of complications increases and many patients will develop strictures or fistulae. In this stage, complications caused by tissue remodeling and fibrosis following long-standing disease are irreversible and difficult to treat with the anti-inflammatory agents. Often, surgery cannot be avoided at this stage.

The progression from early to late disease is accompanied by a change in mucosal cytokine profiles. Early CD is characterized by a pronounced Th1 response, whereas in late disease Th2 cytokines are predominating [32]. The concept that mucosal T cell regulation is different in early and late disease, suggests that patients with late disease respond different to therapies.

The progression from early to complicated late disease course has also been reported in rheumatoid arthritis (RA) [33, 34]. In RA patients, therapy is aimed at preventing late disease when complications and bone destruction are irreversible. In this light, intervening in an early stage of the disease has proven to be very effective and superior to treatment in a late disease stage [34–37].

Indeed, superior therapy efficacy is observed in patients with newly diagnosed CD as compared to patients with longer disease durations [29, 38, 39], suggesting that there is a "Window of Opportunity," a particular timeframe in which therapy is most effective (Fig. 48.2). Intervention on early stage disease to prevent progression to a complicated phenotype is essential to the control of symptoms, induction of mucosal healing and induction and maintenance of clinical and endoscopic remission.

Selecting the Right Patient

Top down therapy is particularly important for patients who are likely to develop a complicated, disabling disease course. While varying definitions exist for "complicated" and

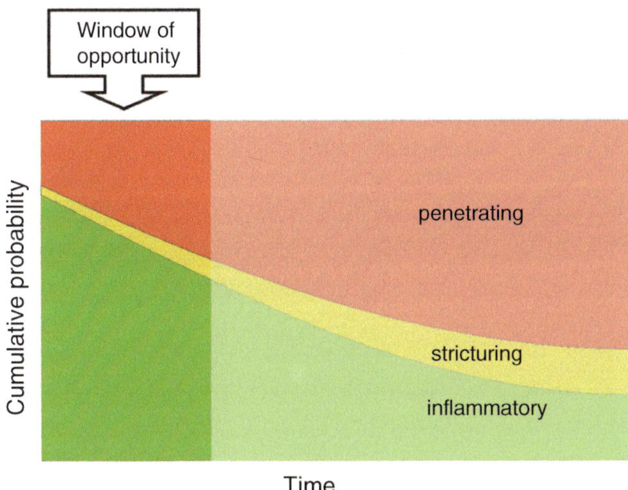

Fig. 48.2 Window of opportunity. Adopted from Cosnes et al. Inflamm Bowel Dis. 2002

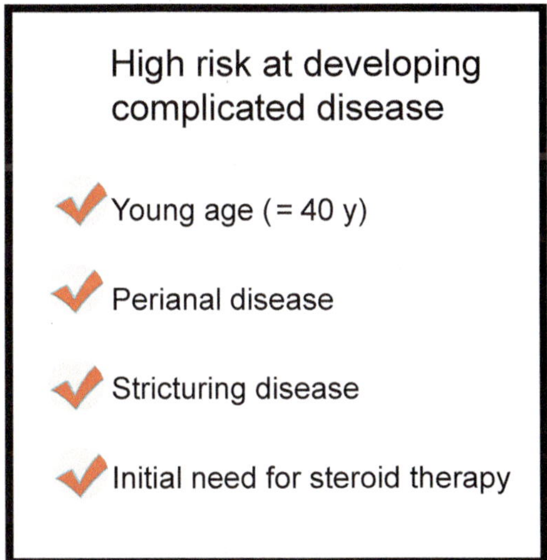

Fig. 48.3 Predictive factors at diagnosis for selection of high-risk patients

"disabling," studies more often use evidence of bowel damage including strictures, fistulas and abscesses, need for hospitalization, immunomodulators, or surgery within the first 5 years of diagnosis [40, 41]. Several studies have identified risk factors that predict progression to disabling disease (Fig. 48.3). Beaugerie and colleagues examined the natural history of over 1100 patients with CD over at least 5 years and identified young age at diagnosis (≤40 years) (OR 2.1), presence of perianal disease at diagnosis (OR 1.6), stricturing disease, and an initial need for corticosteroids (OR 3.1) as predictive factors for progression to disabling disease. When two of these factors were present at diagnosis, 84 % of patients developed disabling disease within 5 years; with three factors, percentage of patients with disabling disease increased to 91 % [40]. Other studies have corroborated perianal disease, stricturing behavior, and need for steroids [41, 42] and have also suggested ileal or ileocolonic location as independent risk factors for surgery ($P<.001$) [31, 42, 43]. Active smoking has been associated with increased risk surgeries and disease complications [44–46].

While predominantly retrospective, data on serologic biomarkers has expanded, particularly regarding biomarkers as potential predictors of CD natural history. Positive anti-Saccharomyces cerevisiae antibody (ASCA) status has been associated with early surgery [47], ileal disease [48], and more severe clinical outcome [49] and might therefore be a useful marker in the selection of patients. Both anti-I2 ($P<0.003$) and anti-outer membrane protein C (anti-OmpC) ($P<0.0006$) were associated with internal penetrating and/or stricturing disease (IP/S) [50]. Additionally, the presence of all four immune responses to ASCA, anti-OmpC, anti-I2, and anti-CBir1 flagellin (anti-CBir1) yielded the highest odds of developing penetrating or stricturing complications and need for intestinal surgery in pediatric patients (OR (95 % CI): 11 (1.5–80.4); $P=0.03$) [50]. In another study, a well-defined correlation was found between triple positive status for ASCA, anti-OmpC as well as anti-I2 and small bowel surgery [51]. Newer markers have been evaluated including antibodies against carbohydrate epitopes [52]. In Reider et al.'s study, positivities for ASCA, anti-mannobioside IgG (AMCA), anti-chitobioside IgG (ACCA), and anti-laminarin IgA (anti-L) were each independently and cumulatively associated with shorter time to disease complications and need for surgery [53].

Data, while lacking, also suggests that genetic predictors exist. Most data have identified mutations to NOD2 locus. The presence of at least 1 NOD2 variant conferred a pooled relative risk for the presence of strictures or fistulas of 1.17 (95 % CI: 1.10–1.24) [54] and was associated with a higher risk of surgery [54–58]. Further studies evaluating the influence of genetics on disease phenotype are needed.

Safety Measures of Early Aggressive Therapy

An important issue related to early intensive treatment is the safety of long-term use of biologics and immunomodulators. Patients are exposed to potentially toxic agents, and therefore appropriate safety measures should be undertaken before immunomodulators and biologics are initiated (Fig. 48.4). Safety measures are aimed at prevention of infections and awareness of several rare complications.

Patients treated with immunomodulators have an increased risk for influenza infections, pneumococcal infections, and Salmonella supp. infections. Therefore, influenza vaccination, pneumococcal vaccination, and appropriate food hygiene (avoiding raw eggs, unpasteurized milk, raw meat) is recommended [59].

Fig. 48.4 Safety measures

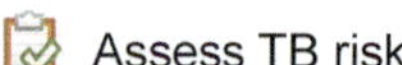

- Assess TB risk
- Vaccination: pneumococcal vaccination, influenza vaccination, Salmonella supsp. prevention (appropriate food hygiene)
- Test for HBV infection
- In case of active infection: treat infection before starting early intervention treatment

Screening for cytomegalovirus (CMV) and herpes simplex virus (HSV) before starting immunomodulator therapy is not recommended. Latent subclinical CMV infection is not a contraindication for starting immunomodulators. However, CMV colitis should be excluded in refractory IBD cases and in case of systemic CMV, immunomodulator therapy should be discontinued. In contrast, given its relationship to lymphoproliferative disease during immunomodulator therapy, Epstein–Barr virus (EBV) screening and antiviral therapy should be considered. In cases of severe EBV infection, immunomodulator therapy should be discontinued. Regular cervical cancer screening and human papilloma virus vaccination are highly recommended for women with IBD, especially if treated with immunomodulators [59].

Also, reactivation of latent hepatitis B (HBV) is considered a serious risk, and therefore all patients with inflammatory bowel disease (IBD) should be tested to exclude HBV. Patients with active chronic HBV infection should be treated according to standard antiviral therapy. Nucleoside/nucleotide analogs are preferred since interferon therapy might exacerbate the colitis. Seronegative patients should receive HBV vaccination. Patients might need a higher dose of immunizing antigen since vaccination efficacy is affected by number of immunomodulators [59].

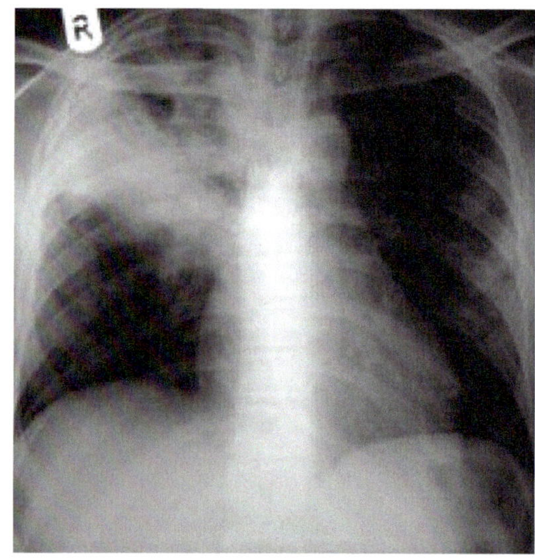

Fig. 48.5 TBC

Anti-TNF use is associated with an approximately 21-fold increased risk of tuberculosis (TB) without appropriate safety measures [60] (Fig. 48.5). TB incidence has decreased with suitable safety measures. Approximately 78% of TB cases present during the first 3 months of treatment and have an atypical presentation, which makes the diagnosis more complicated [61]. For that reason, guidelines advise to assess the risk of TB at the time of diagnosis and before starting treatment with an anti-TNF agent, including patient history, chest X-ray, tuberculin skin test, and interferon-gamma release assays (IGRA). Latent TB may be suspected in case of a positive initial tuberculin skin test and when the patient has recently been exposed to the disease. Physicians should be aware of the possibility of false-negative skin tests, especially when patients are immunocompromised. When the patient is diagnosed with latent TB, treatment with the full therapeutic antituberculous regimen should be initiated and it is advised to delay anti-TNF treatment for at least 3 weeks after initiation of anti-TB regimen. When active TB is diagnosed, anti-TNF treatment is ideally delayed until anti-TB treatment has been completed. However, solid data on the ideal timing during anti-TB treatment are lacking and infectious disease consultation is recommended. When TB is diagnosed during anti-TNF treatment, the anti-TNF agent should be discontinued and TB therapy should be started. Anti-TNF therapy can be resumed if needed after 2 months. All patients should be monitored carefully for signs of cough, fever and weight loss and treating physicians should be aware of uncommon extrapulmonary TB as well as the more common lung disease [59].

After all, when taking appropriate safety measures, anti-TNF and immunomodulator therapy appears to be relatively

Fig. 48.6 Monitoring strategies for patients with early intensive therapy

Assess disease activity and therapy efficacy:
– clinical and serological parameters
– endoscopy

Awareness of side effects:
- fever, malaise, cough → consider and exclude:
- opportunistic infection
- pneumonia
- TB
- fungal infection
- active infection:
- withdraw immunomodulator until resolution of infection
- new presentation of neurological disorders
- exclude PML with MRI and lumbar puncture

safe. Safety data from referral centers and randomized controlled trials do not show an increased risk of malignancies or infections in anti-TNF treated patients. In a large meta-analysis of 21 placebo-controlled trials including 5356 patients, no increased risk of death, serious infection or malignancy compared to controls was reported [62]. In line with this observation, no increased risk was found in infections, mortality or malignancy in 734 anti-TNF treated patients compared to controls, with a median follow-up of 58 months [63]. In addition, no increased risk of malignancy was observed in patients treated with anti-TNF in a large cohort of CD patients [64]. However, long-term safety data are not available yet and therefore awareness of (serious) side effects is warranted.

Monitoring Patients

Monitoring of disease activity is a key component of IBD care. Traditionally, patients are monitored clinically using validated indices including Crohn's Disease Activity Index (CDAI) or the Harvey–Bradshaw Index (HBI). Clinicians are also able to monitor using inflammatory serologic markers such as C-reactive protein, or fecal markers including fecal calprotectin or lactoferrin. Increased levels of calprotectin and lactoferrin have been shown to correlate with the validated Crohn's Disease Endoscopic Index of Severity scores [65, 66], and therefore, these markers might be useful tools to assess disease activity.

Newer evidence in the literature promotes mucosal healing as a method to assess efficacy of ongoing therapy. Mucosal healing predicts long-term outcome and is associated with reduced subsequent disease activity and risk of relapse, increased steroid-free remission rates and less surgery and hospitalization [5–7, 10, 11, 67]. While Bouguen and colleagues noted that fewer than 26 weeks between endoscopic procedures (hazard ratio, 2.35; 95 % confidence interval, 1.15–4.97; $P = .035$) and adjustment to medical therapy when mucosal healing was not observed (hazard ratio, 4.28; 95 % confidence interval, 1.9–11.5; $P = .0003$) are factors associated with mucosal healing [68], further data is needed to determine optimal time intervals between endoscopic assessments for mucosal healing.

To evaluate the risk benefit of early intensive treatment, careful monitoring of potential and sometimes avoidable adverse events is mandatory (Fig. 48.6). Patients on immunosuppressive therapy and with malnutrition are at risk for opportunistic infections [59, 69]. For that reason, patients with fever, cough and systemic illness should be carefully examined and *Mycobacterium tuberculosis* (TB) should be excluded. Patients diagnosed with pneumonia should be treated with an antibiotic covering *S. pneumoniae* [59]. In case of an active infection, it is advised to withdraw immunomodulators until the resolution of infection. Furthermore, about 70 % of the population has latent JC virus, which can cause progressive multifocal leukoencephalopathy upon reactivation. Since reactivation of the JC virus is associated with systemic immunosuppression, treating physicians ought to be aware of this rare situation. PML has been associated with natalizumab with a risk estimate of approximately 1:1000 (0.2–2.8 per thousand) with a mean exposure of 18 months of therapy [70–72]. Patient presenting with new-onset neurological symptoms should receive an MRI scan and lumbar puncture.

Studies show divergent data on the occurrence of malignant lymphoma in IBD patients receiving immunomodulators. Whereas some studies do not show an increased risk, other studies do find a moderately elevated risk, especially in patients on thiopurine therapy [73–77]. Most recently, a meta-analysis by Williams et al. examined 22 randomized controlled trials with over 7000 patients comparing anti-TNF treatment with placebo and found no increased risk of malignancy; however, no trials provided data beyond 1 year of treatment. Hence, long-term risk needs to be further assessed [77]. Nonetheless, the absolute risk appears to be low and should be weighed against the benefits of immunomodulator therapy.

De-escalation Therapy for Deep Remission

Once remission is achieved, it is important to know if, when and how to de-escalate therapy. Although severe adverse events are rare, especially when appropriate safety measures are undertaken and patients are correctly monitored, they can occur and therefore establishing an individualized risk-benefit ratio is encouraged. The disadvantages of discontinuation of therapy should be taken into account, including relapse, possibly lower response to re-induction therapy, infusion reactions and surgery. Particularly important when considering de-escalation is the earlier pattern of the disease and response to therapies. In addition, several factors may predict relapse, including smoking, previous steroid use and elevated fecal calprotectin and CRP.

Anti-TNF and Anti-TNF–Azathioprine Combination Therapy

The proportion of patients with infliximab-induced remission that relapsed after discontinuing infliximab was assessed in a prospective single-center study. In this study, infliximab was stopped in patients who were treated with infliximab for at least 1 year, and who were in steroid-free remission for 6 months. After the median follow up time of 12 months, about 50 % of the patients relapsed and 35 % remained without clinical relapse up to 7 years [78]. Results from an observational study evaluating the long-term effects of infliximab showed maintenance of remission after infliximab discontinuation in 20 % of the patients who experienced a sustained clinical response to infliximab [63].

In a prospective cohort study (STORI) from the GETAID group [67], relapse was assessed in patients on combination infliximab and thiopurine therapy for >1 year and in stable remission for ≥6 months after stopping infliximab therapy. Approximately 44 % of the patients relapsed within 1 year of discontinuation; patients retreated with infliximab after relapse responded well. On multivariable analysis, risk factors for relapse included male sex, the absence of surgical resection, leukocyte counts >6.0 × 10(9)/L, and levels of hemoglobin ≤14.5 g/L, C-reactive protein ≥5.0 mg/L, and fecal calprotectin ≥300 μg/g. Patients with no more than two of these risk had a 15 % risk of relapse within 1 year [67].

In a study investigating the ability to stop immunosuppressives in patients treated with combination therapy, an enduring response was observed after withdrawal of immunosuppressives [79]. Importantly, they reported low infliximab trough levels before immunosuppressive withdrawal as a predictor for surgery. Three risk factors for relapse after azathioprine withdrawal in patients treated with infliximab/azathioprine combination therapy were identified in another study [80]. Infliximab-azathioprine exposure duration of ≤811 days (hazard ratio (HR) = 7.46, $P = 0.01$), C-reactive protein >5 mg/l (HR = 4.79, $P = 0.008$), and platelet count >298 10(9)/l (HR = 4.75, $P = 0.02$) were found to predict infliximab failure, which was defined as disease flare, hypersensitivity reactions leading to infliximab discontinuation or surgery.

Pariente et al. reviewed 11 studies investigating cessation of immunosuppresants (IS) and/or biologics [81]. Patients receiving IS alone had relapse rates at 12 months following immunosuppressant cessation of 20 %. Patients receiving combination therapy with IS and infliximab for at least 6 months had relapse rate following IS cessation of 20 % at 24 months, similar in patients who maintained combination therapy. With anti-TNFs, relapse rates were 40 and 50 % over 1 and 2 years, respectively, after cessation. In summary, decisions on de-escalation of therapy should be made on a case-by-case basis and should be considered in patients with high risk of adverse events and low risk of relapse. Further work in identifying these patients is needed to tailor therapy and to prevent relapse.

Conclusion

Early aggressive therapy in CD is beneficial in selected patients who are likely to develop a severe and disabling disease course. Predictors include young age at diagnosis, the presence of perianal disease, stricturing disease, and the initial need for corticosteroids. This approach appears to be relatively safe, but the risks of opportunistic infections and neoplasm should always be weighed against the benefits of therapy. Patients should be monitored carefully on a regular basis and de-escalation of therapy should be considered for those at high risk of adverse events and those in deep remission. The value of serological, immunologic, and genetic markers in monitoring and predicting disease is currently under investigation, and could be helpful to further optimize therapy.

References

1. Levesque BG, Sandborn WJ, Ruel J, Feagan BG, Sands BE, Colombel JF. Converging goals of treatment of inflammatory bowel disease from clinical trials and practice. Gastroenterology. 2015;148(1):37–51.e1.
2. Lichtenstein GR, Hanauer SB, Sandborn WJ. Management of Crohn's disease in adults. Am J Gastroenterol. 2009;104(2):465–83. quiz 4, 84.
3. Hommes D, Colombel JF, Emery P, Greco M, Sandborn WJ. Changing Crohn's disease management: need for new goals and indices to prevent disability and improve quality of life. J Crohns Colitis. 2012;6 Suppl 2:S224–34.
4. Lichtenstein GR, Yan S, Bala M, Hanauer S. Remission in patients with Crohn's disease is associated with improvement in employment and quality of life and a decrease in hospitalizations and surgeries. Am J Gastroenterol. 2004;99(1):91–6.
5. Rutgeerts P, Diamond RH, Bala M, Olson A, Lichtenstein GR, Bao W, et al. Scheduled maintenance treatment with infliximab is superior to episodic treatment for the healing of mucosal ulceration associated with Crohn's disease. Gastrointest Endosc. 2006;63(3):433–42. quiz 64.
6. Schnitzler F, Fidder H, Ferrante M, Noman M, Arijs I, Van Assche G, et al. Mucosal healing predicts long-term outcome of maintenance therapy with infliximab in Crohn's disease. Inflamm Bowel Dis. 2009;15(9):1295–301.
7. Pineton de Chambrun G, Peyrin-Biroulet L, Lemann M, Colombel JF. Clinical implications of mucosal healing for the management of IBD. Nat Rev Gastroenterol Hepatol. 2010;7(1):15–29.
8. Geboes K, Rutgeerts P, Opdenakker G, Olson A, Patel K, Wagner CL, et al. Endoscopic and histologic evidence of persistent mucosal healing and correlation with clinical improvement following sustained infliximab treatment for Crohn's disease. Curr Med Res Opin. 2005;21(11):1741–54.
9. Sandborn WJ, Hanauer S, Van Assche G, Panes J, Wilson S, Petersson J, et al. Treating beyond symptoms with a view to improving patient outcomes in inflammatory bowel diseases. J Crohns Colitis. 2014;8(9):927–35.
10. Baert F, Moortgat L, Van Assche G, Caenepeel P, Vergauwe P, De Vos M, et al. Mucosal healing predicts sustained clinical remission in patients with early-stage Crohn's disease. Gastroenterology. 2010;138(2):463–8. quiz e10–1.
11. Froslie KF, Jahnsen J, Moum BA, Vatn MH. Mucosal healing in inflammatory bowel disease: results from a Norwegian population-based cohort. Gastroenterology. 2007;133(2):412–22.
12. Steinhart AH, Ewe K, Griffiths AM, Modigliani R, Thomsen OO. Corticosteroids for maintenance of remission in Crohn's disease. Cochrane Database Syst Rev. 2003;(4):Cd000301.
13. Faubion Jr WA, Loftus Jr EV, Harmsen WS, Zinsmeister AR, Sandborn WJ. The natural history of corticosteroid therapy for inflammatory bowel disease: a population-based study. Gastroenterology. 2001;121(2):255–60.
14. Schoon EJ, Bollani S, Mills PR, Israeli E, Felsenberg D, Ljunghall S, et al. Bone mineral density in relation to efficacy and side effects of budesonide and prednisolone in Crohn's disease. Clin Gastroenterol Hepatol. 2005;3(2):113–21.
15. Ardizzone S, Maconi G, Russo A, Imbesi V, Colombo E, Bianchi Porro G. Randomised controlled trial of azathioprine and 5-aminosalicylic acid for treatment of steroid dependent ulcerative colitis. Gut. 2006;55(1):47–53.
16. Candy S, Wright J, Gerber M, Adams G, Gerig M, Goodman R. A controlled double blind study of azathioprine in the management of Crohn's disease. Gut. 1995;37(5):674–8.
17. Holtmann MH, Krummenauer F, Claas C, Kremeyer K, Lorenz D, Rainer O, et al. Long-term effectiveness of azathioprine in IBD beyond 4 years: a European multicenter study in 1176 patients. Dig Dis Sci. 2006;51(9):1516–24.
18. Becker JM. Surgical therapy for ulcerative colitis and Crohn's disease. Gastroenterol Clin North Am. 1999;28(2):371–90. viii–ix.
19. Bouguen G, Peyrin-Biroulet L. Surgery for adult Crohn's disease: what is the actual risk? Gut. 2011;60(9):1178–81.
20. Peyrin-Biroulet L, Harmsen WS, Tremaine WJ, Zinsmeister AR, Sandborn WJ, Loftus Jr EV. Surgery in a population-based cohort of Crohn's disease from Olmsted County, Minnesota (1970–2004). Am J Gastroenterol. 2012;107(11):1693–701.
21. Cosnes J, Nion-Larmurier I, Beaugerie L, Afchain P, Tiret E, Gendre JP. Impact of the increasing use of immunosuppressants in Crohn's disease on the need for intestinal surgery. Gut. 2005; 54(2):237–41.
22. D'Haens G, Baert F, van Assche G, Caenepeel P, Vergauwe P, Tuynman H, et al. Early combined immunosuppression or conventional management in patients with newly diagnosed Crohn's disease: an open randomised trial. Lancet (London, England). 2008;371(9613):660–7.
23. Rutgeerts P, Van Assche G, Sandborn WJ, Wolf DC, Geboes K, Colombel JF, et al. Adalimumab induces and maintains mucosal healing in patients with Crohn's disease: data from the EXTEND trial. Gastroenterology. 2012;142(5):1102–11.e2.
24. Rutgeerts P, Feagan BG, Lichtenstein GR, Mayer LF, Schreiber S, Colombel JF, et al. Comparison of scheduled and episodic treatment strategies of infliximab in Crohn's disease. Gastroenterology. 2004;126(2):402–13.
25. Sandborn WJ. Mucosal healing in inflammatory bowel disease. Rev Gastroenterol Disord. 2008;8(4):271–2.
26. Schreiber S, Reinisch W, Colombel JF, Sandborn WJ, Hommes DW, Robinson AM, et al. Subgroup analysis of the placebo-controlled CHARM trial: increased remission rates through 3 years for adalimumab-treated patients with early Crohn's disease. J Crohns Colitis. 2013;7(3):213–21.
27. Schreiber S, Colombel JF, Bloomfield R, Nikolaus S, Scholmerich J, Panes J, et al. Increased response and remission rates in short-duration Crohn's disease with subcutaneous certolizumab pegol: an analysis of PRECiSE 2 randomized maintenance trial data. Am J Gastroenterol. 2010;105(7):1574–82.
28. Markowitz J, Grancher K, Kohn N, Lesser M, Daum F. A multicenter trial of 6-mercaptopurine and prednisone in children with newly diagnosed Crohn's disease. Gastroenterology. 2000;119(4):895–902.
29. Colombel JF, Sandborn WJ, Reinisch W, Mantzaris GJ, Kornbluth A, Rachmilewitz D, et al. Infliximab, azathioprine, or combination therapy for Crohn's disease. N Engl J Med. 2010;362(15):1383–95.
30. Rubin DT, Uluscu O, Sederman R. Response to biologic therapy in Crohn's disease is improved with early treatment: an analysis of health claims data. Inflamm Bowel Dis. 2012;18(12):2225–31.
31. Cosnes J, Cattan S, Blain A, Beaugerie L, Carbonnel F, Parc R, et al. Long-term evolution of disease behavior of Crohn's disease. Inflamm Bowel Dis. 2002;8(4):244–50.
32. Kugathasan S, Saubermann LJ, Smith L, Kou D, Itoh J, Binion DG, et al. Mucosal T-cell immunoregulation varies in early and late inflammatory bowel disease. Gut. 2007;56(12):1696–705.
33. Quinn MA, Emery P. Window of opportunity in early rheumatoid arthritis: possibility of altering the disease process with early intervention. Clin Exp Rheumatol. 2003;21(5 Suppl 31):S154–7.
34. Roberts LJ, Cleland LG, Thomas R, Proudman SM. Early combination disease modifying antirheumatic drug treatment for rheumatoid arthritis. Med J Aust. 2006;184(3):122–5.
35. Breedveld FC, Emery P, Keystone E, Patel K, Furst DE, Kalden JR, et al. Infliximab in active early rheumatoid arthritis. Ann Rheum Dis. 2004;63(2):149–55.

36. Breedveld FC, Weisman MH, Kavanaugh AF, Cohen SB, Pavelka K, van Vollenhoven R, et al. The PREMIER study: a multicenter, randomized, double-blind clinical trial of combination therapy with adalimumab plus methotrexate versus methotrexate alone or adalimumab alone in patients with early, aggressive rheumatoid arthritis who had not had previous methotrexate treatment. Arthritis Rheum. 2006;54(1):26–37.
37. Durez P, Malghem J, Nzeusseu Toukap A, Depresseux G, Lauwerys BR, Westhovens R, et al. Treatment of early rheumatoid arthritis: a randomized magnetic resonance imaging study comparing the effects of methotrexate alone, methotrexate in combination with infliximab, and methotrexate in combination with intravenous pulse methylprednisolone. Arthritis Rheum. 2007;56(12):3919–27.
38. Kugathasan S, Werlin SL, Martinez A, Rivera MT, Heikenen JB, Binion DG. Prolonged duration of response to infliximab in early but not late pediatric Crohn's disease. Am J Gastroenterol. 2000;95(11):3189–94.
39. Lionetti P, Bronzini F, Salvestrini C, Bascietto C, Canani RB, De Angelis GL, et al. Response to infliximab is related to disease duration in paediatric Crohn's disease. Aliment Pharmacol Ther. 2003;18(4):425–31.
40. Beaugerie L, Seksik P, Nion-Larmurier I, Gendre JP, Cosnes J. Predictors of Crohn's disease. Gastroenterology. 2006;130(3):650–6.
41. Loly C, Belaiche J, Louis E. Predictors of severe Crohn's disease. Scand J Gastroenterol. 2008;43(8):948–54.
42. Thia KT, Sandborn WJ, Harmsen WS, Zinsmeister AR, Loftus Jr EV. Risk factors associated with progression to intestinal complications of Crohn's disease in a population-based cohort. Gastroenterology. 2010;139(4):1147–55.
43. Solberg IC, Vatn MH, Hoie O, Stray N, Sauar J, Jahnsen J, et al. Clinical course in Crohn's disease: results of a Norwegian population-based ten-year follow-up study. Clin Gastroenterol Hepatol. 2007;5(12):1430–8.
44. Cosnes J. Tobacco and IBD: relevance in the understanding of disease mechanisms and clinical practice. Best Pract Res Clin Gastroenterol. 2004;18(3):481–96.
45. Cosnes J. What is the link between the use of tobacco and IBD? Inflamm Bowel Dis. 2008;14 Suppl 2:S14–5.
46. Cosnes J, Beaugerie L, Carbonnel F, Gendre JP. Smoking cessation and the course of Crohn's disease: an intervention study. Gastroenterology. 2001;120(5):1093–9.
47. Forcione DG, Rosen MJ, Kisiel JB, Sands BE. Anti-Saccharomyces cerevisiae antibody (ASCA) positivity is associated with increased risk for early surgery in Crohn's disease. Gut. 2004;53(8):1117–22.
48. Linskens RK, Mallant-Hent RC, Murillo LS, von Blomberg BM, Alizadeh BZ, Pena AS. Genetic and serological markers to identify phenotypic subgroups in a Dutch Crohn' s disease population. Dig Liver Dis. 2004;36(1):29–34.
49. Kim BC, Park S, Han J, Kim JH, Kim TI, Kim WH. Clinical significance of anti-Saccharomyces cerevisiae antibody (ASCA) in Korean patients with Crohn's disease and its relationship to the disease clinical course. Dig Liver Dis. 2007;39(7):610–6.
50. Dubinsky MC, Lin YC, Dutridge D, Picornell Y, Landers CJ, Farrior S, et al. Serum immune responses predict rapid disease progression among children with Crohn's disease: immune responses predict disease progression. Am J Gastroenterol. 2006;101(2):360–7.
51. Mow WS, Vasiliauskas EA, Lin YC, Fleshner PR, Papadakis KA, Taylor KD, et al. Association of antibody responses to microbial antigens and complications of small bowel Crohn's disease. Gastroenterology. 2004;126(2):414–24.
52. Lakatos PL, Papp M, Rieder F. Serologic antiglycan antibodies in inflammatory bowel disease. Am J Gastroenterol. 2011;106(3):406–12.
53. Rieder F, Schleder S, Wolf A, Dirmeier A, Strauch U, Obermeier F, et al. Serum anti-glycan antibodies predict complicated Crohn's disease behavior: a cohort study. Inflamm Bowel Dis. 2010;16(8):1367–75.
54. Adler J, Rangwalla SC, Dwamena BA, Higgins PD. The prognostic power of the NOD2 genotype for complicated Crohn's disease: a meta-analysis. Am J Gastroenterol. 2011;106(4):699–712.
55. Abreu MT, Taylor KD, Lin YC, Hang T, Gaiennie J, Landers CJ, et al. Mutations in NOD2 are associated with fibrostenosing disease in patients with Crohn's disease. Gastroenterology. 2002;123(3):679–88.
56. Kugathasan S, Collins N, Maresso K, Hoffmann RG, Stephens M, Werlin SL, et al. CARD15 gene mutations and risk for early surgery in pediatric-onset Crohn's disease. Clin Gastroenterol Hepatol. 2004;2(11):1003–9.
57. Lichtenstein GR, Targan SR, Dubinsky MC, Rotter JI, Barken DM, Princen F, et al. Combination of genetic and quantitative serological immune markers are associated with complicated Crohn's disease behavior. Inflamm Bowel Dis. 2011;17(12):2488–96.
58. Lacher M, Helmbrecht J, Schroepf S, Koletzko S, Ballauff A, Classen M, et al. NOD2 mutations predict the risk for surgery in pediatric-onset Crohn's disease. J Pediatr Surg. 2010;45(8):1591–7.
59. Rahier JF, Magro F, Abreu C, Armuzzi A, Ben-Horin S, Chowers Y, et al. Second European evidence-based consensus on the prevention, diagnosis and management of opportunistic infections in inflammatory bowel disease. J Crohns Colitis. 2014;8(6):443–68.
60. Carmona L, Gomez-Reino JJ, Rodriguez-Valverde V, Montero D, Pascual-Gomez E, Mola EM, et al. Effectiveness of recommendations to prevent reactivation of latent tuberculosis infection in patients treated with tumor necrosis factor antagonists. Arthritis Rheum. 2005;52(6):1766–72.
61. Gardam MA, Keystone EC, Menzies R, Manners S, Skamene E, Long R, et al. Anti-tumour necrosis factor agents and tuberculosis risk: mechanisms of action and clinical management. Lancet Infect Dis. 2003;3(3):148–55.
62. Lichtenstein GR, Feagan BG, Cohen RD, Salzberg BA, Diamond RH, Chen DM, et al. Serious infections and mortality in association with therapies for Crohn's disease: TREAT registry. Clin Gastroenterol Hepatol. 2006;4(5):621–30.
63. Schnitzler F, Fidder H, Ferrante M, Noman M, Arijs I, Van Assche G, et al. Long-term outcome of treatment with infliximab in 614 patients with Crohn's disease: results from a single-centre cohort. Gut. 2009;58(4):492–500.
64. Biancone L, Orlando A, Kohn A, Colombo E, Sostegni R, Angelucci E, et al. Infliximab and newly diagnosed neoplasia in Crohn's disease: a multicentre matched pair study. Gut. 2006;55(2):228–33.
65. Sipponen T, Karkkainen P, Savilahti E, Kolho KL, Nuutinen H, Turunen U, et al. Correlation of faecal calprotectin and lactoferrin with an endoscopic score for Crohn's disease and histological findings. Aliment Pharmacol Ther. 2008;28(10):1221–9.
66. Sipponen T, Savilahti E, Kolho KL, Nuutinen H, Turunen U, Farkkila M. Crohn's disease activity assessed by fecal calprotectin and lactoferrin: correlation with Crohn's disease activity index and endoscopic findings. Inflamm Bowel Dis. 2008;14(1):40–6.
67. Louis E, Mary JY, Vernier-Massouille G, Grimaud JC, Bouhnik Y, Laharie D, et al. Maintenance of remission among patients with Crohn's disease on antimetabolite therapy after infliximab therapy is stopped. Gastroenterology. 2012;142(1):63–70.e5; quiz e31.
68. Bouguen G, Levesque BG, Pola S, Evans E, Sandborn WJ. Endoscopic assessment and treating to target increase the likelihood of mucosal healing in patients with Crohn's disease. Clin Gastroenterol Hepatol. 2014;12(6):978–85.
69. Toruner M, Loftus Jr EV, Harmsen WS, Zinsmeister AR, Orenstein R, Sandborn WJ, et al. Risk factors for opportunistic infections in

patients with inflammatory bowel disease. Gastroenterology. 2008;134(4):929–36.
70. Bloomgren G, Richman S, Hotermans C, Subramanyam M, Goelz S, Natarajan A, et al. Risk of natalizumab-associated progressive multifocal leukoencephalopathy. N Engl J Med. 2012;366(20): 1870–80.
71. Yousry TA, Major EO, Ryschkewitsch C, Fahle G, Fischer S, Hou J, et al. Evaluation of patients treated with natalizumab for progressive multifocal leukoencephalopathy. N Engl J Med. 2006;354(9): 924–33.
72. Fine AJ, Sorbello A, Kortepeter C, Scarazzini L. Progressive multifocal leukoencephalopathy after natalizumab discontinuation. Ann Neurol. 2014;75(1):108–15.
73. Beaugerie L, Brousse N, Bouvier AM, Colombel JF, Lemann M, Cosnes J, et al. Lymphoproliferative disorders in patients receiving thiopurines for inflammatory bowel disease: a prospective observational cohort study. Lancet (London, England). 2009;374(9701): 1617–25.
74. Farrell RJ, Ang Y, Kileen P, O'Briain DS, Kelleher D, Keeling PW, et al. Increased incidence of non-Hodgkin's lymphoma in inflammatory bowel disease patients on immunosuppressive therapy but overall risk is low. Gut. 2000;47(4):514–9.
75. Kandiel A, Fraser AG, Korelitz BI, Brensinger C, Lewis JD. Increased risk of lymphoma among inflammatory bowel disease patients treated with azathioprine and 6-mercaptopurine. Gut. 2005;54(8):1121–5.
76. Lewis JD, Bilker WB, Brensinger C, Deren JJ, Vaughn DJ, Strom BL. Inflammatory bowel disease is not associated with an increased risk of lymphoma. Gastroenterology. 2001;121(5):1080–7.
77. Williams CJ, Peyrin-Biroulet L, Ford AC. Systematic review with meta-analysis: malignancies with anti-tumour necrosis factor-alpha therapy in inflammatory bowel disease. Aliment Pharmacol Ther. 2014;39(5):447–58.
78. Waugh AW, Garg S, Matic K, Gramlich L, Wong C, Sadowski DC, et al. Maintenance of clinical benefit in Crohn's disease patients after discontinuation of infliximab: long-term follow-up of a single centre cohort. Aliment Pharmacol Ther. 2010;32(9):1129–34.
79. Bossuyt PJJ JM, Ballet V. Discontinuation of immunosuppressives in patients with Crohn's disease treated with scheduled maintenance infliximab: prospective long-term follow-up and influence on infliximab trough levels. Gut. 2010;59(Suppl III):A80.
80. Oussalah A, Chevaux JB, Fay R, Sandborn WJ, Bigard MA, Peyrin-Biroulet L. Predictors of infliximab failure after azathioprine withdrawal in Crohn's disease treated with combination therapy. Am J Gastroenterol. 2010;105(5):1142–9.
81. Pariente B, Laharie D. Review article: why, when and how to de-escalate therapy in inflammatory bowel diseases. Aliment Pharmacol Ther. 2014;40(4):338–53.

Leukocytapheresis Therapy of Inflammatory Bowel Disease

49

Takanori Kanai

Background

Ulcerative colitis (UC) and Crohn's disease (CD) are the two major phenotypes of the idiopathic inflammatory bowel diseases (IBD) of the gut. IBD is characterized by infiltration of a large number of myeloid leukocytes (granulocytes and monocytes) into the intestinal mucosa followed by inflammation, erosions and ulcers. While UC usually is confined to the large intestine (colon and rectum), CD can affect any part of the gut, from the mouth to the perianal region [1–7], and up to 70 % of CD patients may have small intestinal involvement. This difference indicates that the molecular mechanism of immune cell migration to the colon and the small intestine may be different [8]. Both UC and CD run a remitting-relapsing course affected by diverse environmental and genetic predisposing factors [1, 3, 4, 9–13]. IBD is exacerbated and perpetuated by inflammatory cytokines such as tumor necrosis factor (TNF)-α, interleukin (IL)-6, IL-12, interferon (IFN)-γ, and IL-17 [14–20].

Leukocytes have the potential to initiate and exacerbate inflammation by releasing a cascade of proinflammatory cytokines, proteases, and reactive oxygen derivatives, leading to extensive tissue injury [2]. In the face of the evidence for the involvement of various cytokines in the immunopathogenesis of IBD and the fact that infiltrated leukocytes derived from peripheral blood are major sources of these cytokines, the leukocytes appear logical targets in the treatment of IBD. Indeed, histological examination of the mucosal tissue in biopsy specimens from patients with active IBD reveals a spectrum of pathologic manifestations among which presence of an abundance of neutrophils, lymphocytes, and macrophages relates specifically to clinical disease activity and severity of the disease [1–3, 21–23]. Accordingly, several studies have reported that patients with active IBD harbor elevated circulating granulocytes and monocytes [24, 25], which show activation behavior and prolonged survival time [26–33].

Leukocytapheresis is a kind of bloodletting, which dates back to the time of Hippocrates (460–377 BC) in Ancient Greece, from there it reached Europe as a major treatment practice. The perception then was that disease reflected presence of disease-causing substances in the blood and bloodletting was to expel the pathologic agents. Bloodletting was widely practiced for diseases like polycythemia vera, inflammation, fever, hypertension, and other undiagnosed diseases. However, in 1162, the Vatican ruled against bloodletting. In the early 20 century, centrifugation was introduced to separate blood cells from the plasma and exclude the unwanted fraction. Because centrifugation involves removing large volume of blood from the patient, it soon was abandoned in favor of direct hemoperfusion systems. Leukocytapheresis was first introduced to treat patients with chronic myelocytic leukemia [34, 35] and chronic lymphocytic leukemia [36]. In 1975, thoracic duct drainage was associated with clinical improvement in 12 patients with rheumatoid arthritis [37]. In 1979, Tenenbaum and colleagues [38] successfully performed leukocytapheresis for rheumatoid arthritis using an IBM blood cell separator. The logics of leukocytapheresis for autoimmune diseases was based on the suspicion that lymphocytes were producing autoantibody or stimulating antibody production promoting autoimmune disease like rheumatoid arthritis. Recent evidence suggests that the efficacy of the therapy might not simply be attributed to cell removal per se because contact activation of cells with the treatment surface or a change in the proportions of regulatory (suppressor) T cells and pathogenic macrophages might produce immunomodulatory effects. This notion has been further discussed below.

T. Kanai, M.D. (✉)
Division of Gastroenterology and Hepatology, Department of Internal Medicine, Keio University School of Medicine, Tokyo 160-8582, Japan
e-mail: takagast@z2.keio.jp

D.C. Baumgart (ed.), *Crohn's Disease and Ulcerative Colitis*, DOI 10.1007/978-3-319-33703-6_49

Leukocytapheresis for Inflammatory Bowel Disease

The Centrifugation Method

In 1985, Bick et al. [39] reported the first clinical trial of centrifugal leukocytapheresis in IBD for patients with active CD. This uncontrolled trial together with their follow-up studies [40, 41] suggested that leukocytapheresis had efficacy in patients with CD, but their preliminary observations were to be confirmed by subsequent studies in large cohorts of patients. In line with this thinking, in 1994, Lerebours and colleagues [42] assessed the efficacy of centrifugal lymphapheresis to suppress early relapse in patients with CD in clinical remission after steroid treatment for an acute attack. Twenty-eight patients were included in this randomized multicenter prospective study. Before starting steroid tapering, patients were randomly assigned either to lymphapheresis (nine sessions within 4–5 weeks) or to a control group (no lymphapheresis). The primary judgment criterion was the cumulated recurrence rate after steroid discontinuation. All the treated patients (12 of 12) were successfully withdrawn from corticosteroids together with 10 of 15 in the control group. At the end of an 18 months follow-up, the cumulated relapse rate was 83 % in the lymphapheresis group and 62 % in the control group. However, this study [42] is so far the best controlled trial targeting peripheral blood lymphocytes in IBD and showed that lymphapheresis alone is not an effective treatment for patients with CD, it may reactive an otherwise quiescent IBD. The authors' conclusion was "although there was a trend towards a diminished incidence of corticosteroid dependence, centrifugal lymphapheresis did not prevent the occurrence of early relapses".

In 1997, Ayabe et al. [24] reported an open pilot study of centrifugal leukocytapheresis in patients with corticosteroid refractory active UC, with focus on efficacy and safety. Fourteen patients with severe UC were treated by centrifugal leukocytapheresis. Patients received one leukocytapheresis session per week for 3 consecutive weeks. In each session, leukocyte-rich fractions of the buffy coat layer were removed from 2000 to 2400 mL of peripheral blood taken via an antecubital vein. Approximately 180 mL of ACD-A (acid citrate dextrose; 3 % w/v citrate) was used as an anticoagulant. Thirteen patients (92.9 %) achieved clinical remission within 4 weeks after leukocytapheresis and remained in remission for 8 months on average without any additional corticosteroid therapy. Both colonoscopic and histological examinations confirmed the efficacy of the treatment with respect to reduction of severe inflammation in the affected colon. No serious side effect was observed throughout the therapy. Additionally, the expression of L-selectin and VLA4α, which are target molecules on leukocytes for interactions with endothelial cells, was down-modulated. The same group conducted a second pilot study in which 23 patients with severe corticosteroid refractory UC received centrifugal leukocytapheresis [25]. Eighteen of 23 patients (78.3 %) achieved clinical remission. The third study by this group [43] was a multicenter open label trial involving 50 patients with active corticosteroid refractory UC conducted in 14 medical institutions. By using the Haemonectics' Component Collection System (Braintree, MA, USA), leukocytapheresis was done once a week for 5 consecutive weeks, processing 2000–2400 mL of patients' blood per session as in their first study [24]. At the end of the study, stool frequency was decreased to less than 4 times a day in 68.4 % (26 of 38) of patients and C-reactive protein (CRP, an inflammation marker) level was normalized in 56.7 % (17 of 30) of the patients. Similarly, endoscopic remission was achieved in 57.7 % (26 of 45) patients and histological improvement was seen in 54.1 % (20 of 37) of patients tested. Following 5–6 leukocytapheresis sessions, improved disease activity was seen in 74 % (37 of 50) of patients by general assessment criteria, but only 11 patients (22.0 %) achieved clinical remission. It is not clear why this multicenter study revealed lower rate of clinical remission as compared with the earlier two studies.

The Adacolumn Selective Leukocytapheresis System

The Adacolumn (Fig. 49.1a) is an example of a medical device that can selectively remove activated myeloid lineage leukocytes. These include granulocytes, monocytes/macrophages together with significant fraction of platelets. The Adacolumn does not significantly deplete lymphocytes [29, 30, 44, 45]. The leukocytapheresis procedure is simple (Fig. 49.2). Two large cannulas are placed in the antecubital veins of the two arms (or other suitable sites) for direct blood access to the column and blood return to the patient. The blood flows into the column usually at 30 mL/min and returns to the patient from the column outflow. The blood flow can be increased or decreased if necessary. Each session takes on the average 60 min (can be prolonged or decreased if necessary). The column itself (Adacolumn) is filled with specially designed cellulose acetate beads of 2 mm in diameter as leukocytapheresis carriers. Pre and post column blood cell counts have revealed that the carriers adsorb from the blood, which passes through the column about 65 % granulocytes, 55 % of monocytes/macrophages together with a small fraction of lymphocytes [30, 45]. These are the leukocytes that bear the so-called FcγR and complement receptors [44, 45]. These numerical data have been verified by scanning electron microscopy on the beads taken from the column following a leukocytapheresis session (Fig. 49.1). The science and the therapeutic rationale behind the development of the Adacolumn have been broadly presented in two publications [46, 47].

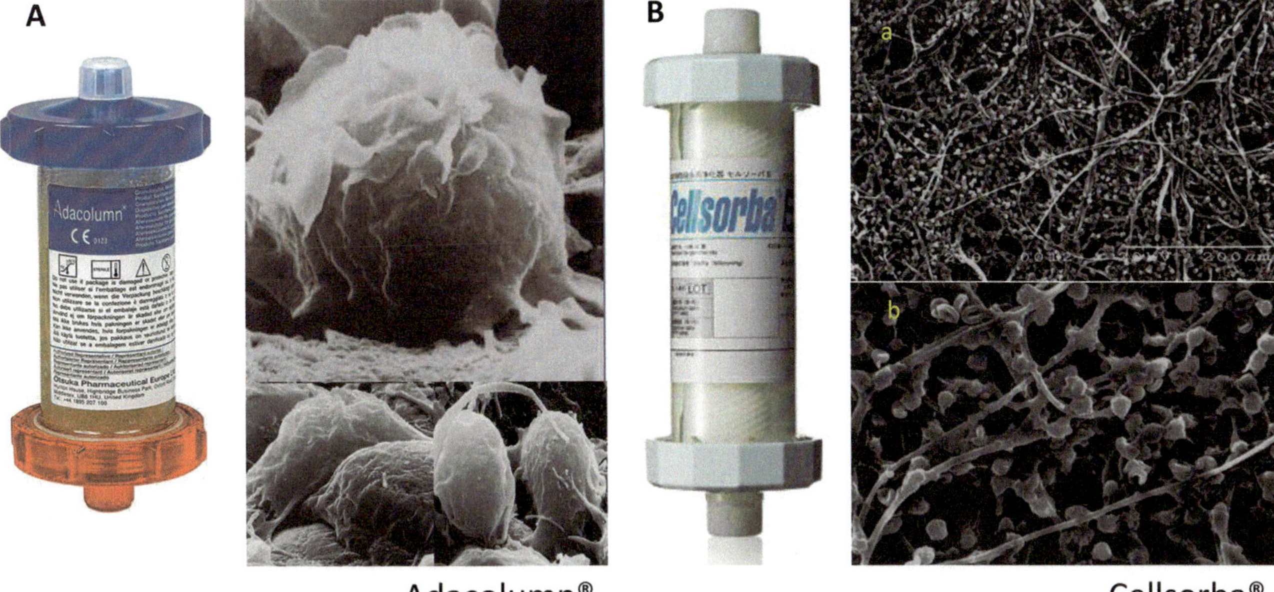

Fig. 49.1 Scanning electron photomicrographs of carriers that have adsorbed leukocytes during leukocytapheresis. (**a**) The Adacolumn is filled with cellulose acetate beads as leukocytapheresis carriers that selectively adsorb granulocytes, monocytes/macrophages, a significant fraction of platelets together with a small number of lymphocytes. These are the leukocytes that bear the FcR and complement receptors. The scanning electron photomicrographs show adsorption of monocytes and granulocytes to a carrier. (**b**) The Cellsorba column is a filter consisting of polyester non-woven fabric that non-selectively removes leukocytes. The scanning photomicrographs show leukocytes trapped in the Cellsorba filter. (**b**) is a higher magnification view of (**a**)

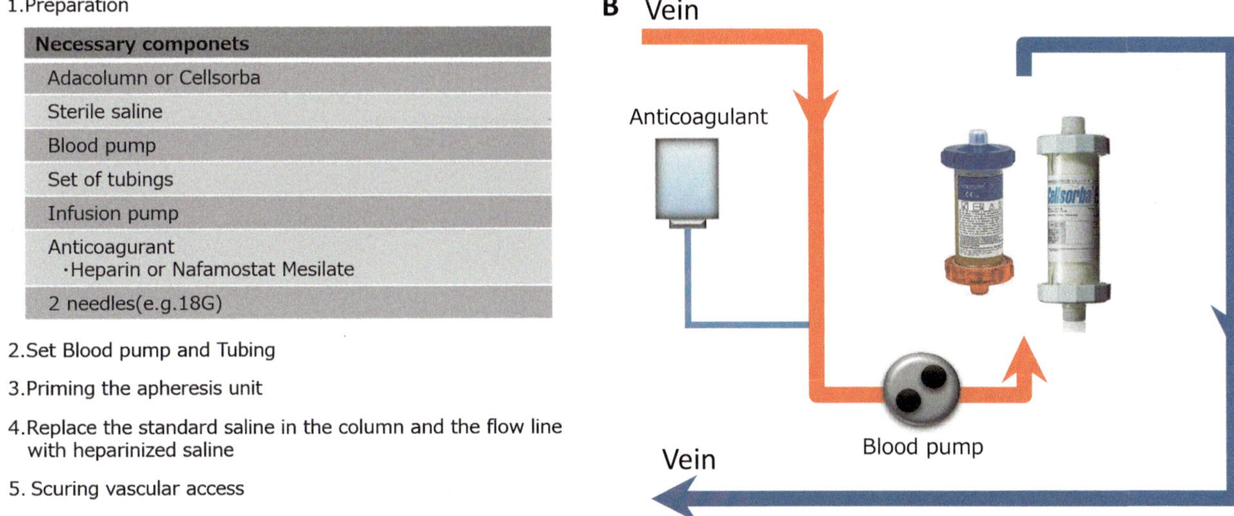

A 1.Preparation
Necessary componets
Adacolumn or Cellsorba
Sterile saline
Blood pump
Set of tubings
Infusion pump
Anticoagurant
·Heparin or Nafamostat Mesilate
2 needles(e.g.18G)
2.Set Blood pump and Tubing
3.Priming the apheresis unit
4.Replace the standard saline in the column and the flow line with heparinized saline
5. Scuring vascular access
6.Run the blood pump
7.Returning residual blood
B Vein
Anticoagulant
Blood pump
Vein

Fig. 49.2 (**a**) The outline of the procedure for leukocytapheresis. (**b**) Extracorporeal blood flow view of the Adacolumn and Cellsorba filter. The direction of blood flow indicated by the *arrows* shows that whereas blood inlet for the Adacolumn is from the lower port, for the Cellsorba is from the upper port

The first clinical trial of Adacolumn in patients with active UC was an open multicenter controlled study conducted at 14 hospitals throughout Japan [48]. Of 105 eligible patients, 53 were in group I for Adacolumn and 52 in group II for conventional drug therapy. According to the study design, in group II, prednisolone (PSL) was increased to 63 ± 13.82 mg/day per patient at week 1 to promote remission compared with 23.5 ± 3.42 mg/day per patient in group I. In both groups, the PSL dose could be reduced if remission or improvement was observed. At week 7 (efficacy assessment time point), the average dose of PSL in group I was 14.2 ± 2.25 mg/day per patient vs 22.9 ± 2.07 mg/day in group II. Overall, 31 of 53 group I patients (58.5 %) responded to Adacolumn leukocytapheresis therapy, 11 achieved remission, 20 had their symptoms improved and 22 did not respond. In group II, 23 of 52 patients (44.2 %) responded to conventional drug therapy, seven had remission, 16 had their symptoms improved and 29 did not respond. Likewise, in group I, a total of eight non serious adverse effects like transient flushing, light headedness in five patients were reported, but no patient discontinued the apheresis treatment due to adverse reactions. In contrast, in group II, 40 adverse events in 24 patients were observed; 21 of 24 patients received medical treatment and three patients discontinued the treatment.

Subsequently, Hanai and colleagues [28, 29] reported treating 41 patients with severe UC by using the Adacolumn to deplete their peripheral blood granulocytes and monocytes/macrophages. No additional drug therapy was initiated while their ongoing medications were tapered as symptoms improved. Pretreatment circulating neutrophil counts were very high, $9.3 \pm 0.5 \times 10^9$/L, about three times the level seen in controls [30] and significant reductions were seen at week 12 of treatment, $4.9 \pm 0.4 \times 10^9$/L. Hemoglobin (Hb) at week 12 relative to baseline had increased by 25 %, which might relate to the cessation of rectal bleeding following remission or improvements of clinical symptoms. Along with a fall in the patients' clinical activity index (CAI), disease activity index (DAI) and peripheral blood neutrophil counts, there was a comparable fall in CRP [29].

In one of the aforementioned studies by Hanai and colleagues [29], a total of 146 patients with active UC were given salicylates as the first-line medication. Ninety-two did not improve and were put on intensive corticosteroid (PSL) therapy. Among these 92 cases, 31 patients did not improve (steroid refractory) and underwent Adacolumn leukocytapheresis therapy. These patients had a CAI of >12, a DAI of >10 and were treated twice weekly for 2–3 consecutive weeks and then at one session per week. At the conclusion of five treatment sessions, 60 % of these steroid refractory patients achieved remission or were significantly improved. At the conclusion of ten treatment sessions, the remission rate was an 80 %. The corticosteroid refractory patients in this study represented a sub-group of patients with severe UC that are at a significant risk of serious complications. Indeed treatment failure after 5–10 days of intensive corticosteroids is often considered to be an indication for colectomy or exposure to CyA [46, 49]. However, only 4 of the 31 (13 %) patients underwent colectomy. At 12 months, 79 % of patients had maintained their remission, which compares with a relapse rate of 60–80 % for CyA [48], but unlike CyA [50] Adacolumn was without major side effects. These initial response rates achieved by Hanai et al. have subsequently been reproduced both in Japan and in Europe [51–55]. In one of these studies, Kanke et al. [51] reported that 90 min per Adacolumn session was significantly better than 60 min per session.

Currently, treatment of ulcerative colitis, Crohn's disease and generalized pustular psoriasis by the Adacolumn are covered by the Japan national health insurance system. Additionally, the Adacolumn is CE-marked for the treatment of ulcerative colitis, Crohn's disease, rheumatoid arthritis, generalized pustular psoriasis, and Behçet's disease in the European Union. In China, the Adacolumn has been approved as medical device by the SFDA of China, and a multicenter clinical study has been undertaken to show efficacy outcomes in active IBD.

Adacolumn Leukocytapheresis as First-Line Medication for Steroid Naïve Patients

In one of the first publications on Adacolumn leukocytapheresis in IBD, Hanai, and colleagues reported treating 41 patients with UC in active stage. Eight of the 41 patients treated by Hanai et al. [29] were steroid naïve at entry. All eight (100 %) went into a clinical remission with the Adacolumn treatment and remained steroid naïve during the treatment and follow-up time. Subsequently, Suzuki et al. [56, 57] reported treating 20 steroid naïve patients with active UC by Adacolumn leukocytapheresis. These patients had moderate to severe UC; mean CAI was 8.8, range 5–17. At entry, all patients were on 5-ASA (1.5–2.25 g/day). Each patient was to receive up to a maximum of ten Adacolumn sessions, at a frequency of two sessions/week. Efficacy was assessed 1 week after the last session. CAI fell to clinical remission levels (CAI < 4) in the majority of patients after six sessions, only two of the 20 patients required all ten sessions. At post treatment, the mean CAI was 3; range 0–12 ($P = 0.0001$) and 17 of 20 patients (85 %) were in clinical remission. There were significant changes in total peripheral white blood cell counts (WBC $\times 10^9$/L), 9.8 ± 1.0 (range 5.9–22.5) vs 7.0 ± 0.6 (range 3.5–15.3) for pre and post treatment, respectively ($P = 0.003$) together with decreases in CRP ($P = 0003$). During the Adacolumn leukocytapheresis therapy, two incidences of transient mild headache were reported. In both cases, the headache receded within 3 h without medication. Further text on this subgroup of UC patients is presented in the subsequent sections of this chapter.

Adacolumn Leukocytapheresis Suppressed Relapse in Asymptomatic Patients

Bjarnason and colleagues in London evaluated the efficacy of Adacolumn leukocytapheresis to suppress relapse in asymptomatic IBD patients at a high risk of experiencing a clinical relapse [58]. This approach reflects a fundamental change in the philosophy of treating IBD. Instead of treating active disease, asymptomatic patients are identified solely on the basis of a very high fecal calprotectin concentration, a neutrophil selective protein that provides quantitative measure of intestinal inflammatory activity [21–23]. The high calprotectin levels (over 250 μg/g) place them in a very high risk group for relapse of their disease [21].

This prospective, randomized controlled study, assigned patients to Adacolumn leukocytapheresis, undergoing 5, once a week leukocytapheresis treatment in an outpatient setting, or to unchanged treatment. Follow-up was monthly for 6 months for clinical relapse. Thirty-one patients who met the inclusion criteria were included from 244 potential subjects who underwent screening. In the Adacolumn group 64 % maintained their remission compared to 24 % in the control group ($P=0.03$). Life table analysis demonstrated the mean survival in the Adacolumn group was 181 days vs 104 days in the control arm ($P=0.01$). It would appear that 5 weekly sessions of Adacolumn in such patients will have a significant effect and potentially avoid the morbidity associated with clinical relapse and subsequent drug therapy.

Adacolumn Leukocytapheresis in the Treatment of Crohn's Disease

The vast majority of studies with the Adacolumn have been in patients with UC. However, there is evidence to suggest that Adacolumn leukocytapheresis is effective in patients with CD as well. The first study in CD was reported by Matsui and colleagues [59]. In that study, seven patients with CD refractory to conventional medication including nutritional therapy, each received five Adacolumn sessions. Five of seven patients achieved remission. It should be relevant to state here that the only two nonresponders in Matsui's study [60] had the CD lesions confined to the small intestine, not a common site to find infiltrated neutrophils. In the follow-up study by Fukuda et al. [61], 21 patients with severe drug and nutritional therapy refractory CD received five Adacolumn sessions each. Efficacy rate was 52.5 % in these severe patients. More recently, Domenech et al. [55] reported treating 12 steroid dependent patients with CD. The remission rate in this study was 70 %, which is higher than in the study reported by Fukuda et al. [61]. Finally, Lofberg and colleagues [62] have reported treating seven patients with CD who were refractory or had relapsed despite medication. Six had received infliximab, but without success. Adacolumn leukocytapheresis was performed at one session per week for 5 weeks. Efficacy was assessed at week 7 and 12 months. The median value of Crohn's disease activity index (CDAI) scores decreased from 290 at week 1 to 184 at week 7 ($P=0.031$). At the 12 months follow-up, CDAI had decreased further to 128.5 ($P=0.0156$).

Immunomodulation Associated with Adacolumn Leukocytapheresis

Although the aim of treatment with the Adacolumn has been to remove excess and activated granulocytes and monocytes from the circulation, it has been difficult to explain why some patients continue to improve long after the treatment is concluded. Also the low relapse rate reported by Hanai et al. [29] cannot be fully explained by our current understanding of neutrophil function per se. Alternative mechanisms of actions have therefore been sought. Adacolumn is filled with cellulose acetate beads to which leukocytes that bear the FcγR and complement receptors adhere [44, 45]. The adsorbed leukocytes release an array of active substances both toxic and nontoxic, but some anti-inflammatory as well. Most of these substances are of short half-life and may not reach the patients' circulation in appreciable amounts. Several investigators have carried out analysis on blood samples taken from the Adacolumn inflow and outflow (blood return line to patients) during leukocytapheresis. Both Hanai et al. [63] and Suzuki et al. [56] found a significant increase in blood levels of soluble TNF-α receptors I and II. Soluble TNF receptors are reported to neutralize TNF without invoking TNF-like actions [64]. Similarly, several studies report a marked decrease in the capacity of peripheral blood leukocytes to release inflammatory cytokines including TNF-α, IL-1β, IL-6, and IL-8 following Adacolumn leukocytapheresis [28, 30, 48, 65]. The procedure appears to produce a similar effect on leukocyte trafficking receptors. Thus the expression of both L selectin [30, 44, 48, 65] and the chemokine receptor, CXCR3 [44] was markedly reduced and was sustained well beyond the last leukocytapheresis session, while the expression of the leukocyte integrin, Mac-1 (CD11b/CD18) was upregulated [30, 45]. These actions should suppress leukocyte extravasation.

Recently, Ishihara et al. [66] reported novel immunomodulatory actions for the Adacolumn by using an experimental model. They established an SCID adoptive transfer model of chronic colitis. Injection of apoptotic cells (ACs) into the model in the presence of B cells led to interesting findings. The ACs-mediated effect was lost in the absence of B cells or presence of regulatory B cells (Breg)-depleted cells. Further, the Adacolumn induced neutrophil apoptosis during passage of blood through the column due to the generation of small amounts of reactive oxygen species (ROS) in the column. Finally, suppression of colitis was seen upon injection of ROS exposed neutrophils into the model. Their results suggested that the Adacolumn not only depletes elevated and activated neutrophils and monocytes (myeloid lineage) from the circulation but also indirectly promotes expansion or activation of Breg, which are involved in maintaining regulatory T cells (Treg) [67]. In clinical settings, the Adacolumn has been associated with expansion of Treg, an increase in interleukin-10 level and a decrease of anti-nuclear antibodies titer [47, 68]. Figure 49.3 summarizes the immunomodulatory actions of the Adacolumn leukocytapheresis.

The Cellsorba Leukocyte Removal System

The Cellsorba leukocyte removal filter column (Fig. 49.1b) is developed by Asahi Kasei Medical in Japan and has been comprehensively described by Sawada et al. [69]. This system is also a direct blood perfusion device (Fig. 49.2). Blood access is from the antecubital vein in one arm and return via

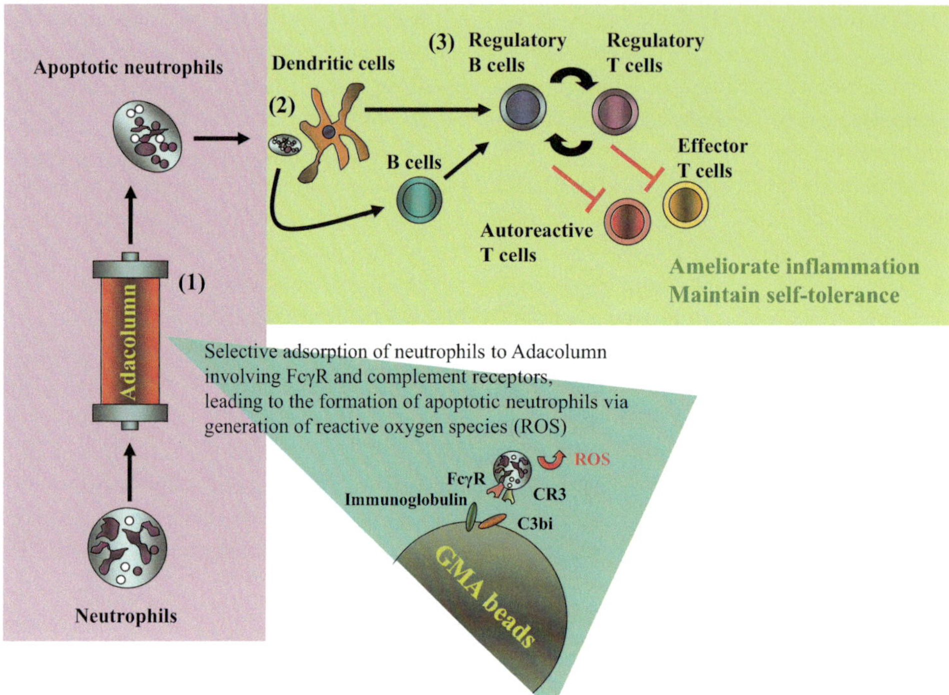

Fig. 49.3 Pathways leading to neutrophil apoptosis and immunoregulation by the Adacolumn. Patients with IBD show inappropriate innate and adaptive immune responses to commensal bacteria due to imbalance of mucosal immune profile. Neutrophil apoptosis is suppressed by elevated levels of endotoxin, and certain inflammatory cytokines as well as by corticosteroids, which are given to most patients with active IBD. (*1*) Selective adsorption of elevated and activated neutrophils to the column carriers (GMA beads) involving FcγR and complement receptors. Ligations of FcγR and complement receptor, leading to the formation of apoptotic neutrophils in the circulation via generation of reactive oxygens. (*2*) Apoptotic neutrophils are taken up by dendritic cells or by direct contact with B cells leading to the generation of regulatory B cells (Breg). (*3*) Breg and regulatory T cells (Treg) are also expanding. Breg and Treg will suppress autoreactive T-cells or effecter T-cells in the intestinal mucosa of IBD patients. *IBD* inflammatory bowel disease, *FcγR* Fc gamma receptor, *CR3* complement receptor 3, *C3bi* inactive C3b component of complement, *ROS* reactive oxygen species

the antecubital vein in the contralateral arm. Alternative access sites may be used if necessary. Cellsorba uses a filter consisting of polyester non-woven fabric that non-selectively removes approximately 13.0×10^9 leukocytes from the circulating blood during one treatment session [70]. The column is capable of removing almost 100 % of neutrophils and monocytes including macrophages and 30–60 % of lymphocytes when measured between the inlet and the outlet of the column [69].

The first major application of Cellsorba for the treatment of UC was undertaken in 1995 by Sawada et al. [71]. Cellsorba leukocytapheresis was administered five times at 1 week intervals for 5 consecutive weeks during intensive therapy and 5 times, at approximately 1 month intervals for 5 months during maintenance therapy to 13 patients with IBD (eight UC and five CD patients). Improved clinical response during the intensive therapy was seen in 11 of 13 patients (84.6 %); 6 of 8 UC patients (75.0 %) and 5 of 5 CD patients (100 %). The remission was maintained in 8 of 13 patients (61.5 %) during the maintenance therapy.

A multicenter trial was carried out in Japan to assess the efficacy and safety of Cellsorba vs corticosteroid therapy in patients with active UC refractory to conventional medication [69]. This was a controlled multicenter study with randomized assignment of 76 patients with UC to two groups. The 39 patients in the Cellsorba group received weekly leukocytapheresis for 5 consecutive weeks as an intensive therapy, which was added to the on-going drug therapy, while steroids were maintained but not increased. Leukocytapheresis was gradually reduced to one session every 4 weeks as maintenance therapy. In the high dose PSL group ($n = 37$), PSL was added or increased to 30–40 mg/day for moderately severe and to 60–80 mg/day for severe patients and was then gradually tapered. The Cellsorba group showed a significantly higher efficacy compared with PSL (74 % vs 38 %; $P = 0.005$) and lower incidence of side effects (24 % vs 68 %; $P < 0.001$).

Further, Sawada and colleagues [72] investigated the efficacy of Cellsorba leukocytapheresis in a multicenter trial using active and sham devices in a double-blind study with focus on assessing the placebo effect of extracorporeal circulation. Twenty-five patients with active UC of severe or moderately severe level were assigned to the active treatment or sham treatment. Six patients who did not meet the inclusion criteria were excluded at screening and 19 (ten in the active group and nine in the sham group) were included. Cellsorba leukocytapheresis was performed once a week for 5 weeks followed by two additional sessions during the following 4 weeks, at 2 weeks intervals. Corticosteroids and other concomitant medications were continued at the same dosage for 4 weeks. CAI showed that the active group achieved a significantly greater improvement (80 %, eight of ten patients) compared with the sham apheresis group (33 %, three of nine patients; $P<0.05$). Although there was a significant advantage in favor of the active treatment, the total number of patients was rather small in this study. Likewise, patients had active UC refractory to conventional drug therapy and most of them were receiving concomitant corticosteroid. A similar study with a large cohort of patients with strict control of their concomitant medications is warranted to verify the results of this study.

Sawada et al. [73] further reported the efficacy and safety of Cellsorba in treating patients with severe or fulminant UC or toxic megacolon. Six patients were included and Cellsorba leukocytapheresis was performed three times per week for 2 weeks, followed by four further sessions in the following 4 weeks. Four of six patients improved and achieved remission, and the remaining two patients had to undergo colectomy while their symptoms had been reduced by Cellsorba. Further larger studies are essential to fully assess the efficacy of Cellsorba in this clinical setting.

In earlier studies, Sawada et al. [74] and Yamaji et al. [75], reported fluctuations in the leukocyte count in the peripheral blood during Cellsorba leukocytapheresis. The count fell to 20–40 % of the baseline level at 20–30 min after the start of each session. Cellsorba itself had a sustained removal performance in excess of 90 % of the baseline value for the circulating blood leukocytes [76]. Therefore, it appears that leukocytes from the marginal pools including the bone marrow, spleen and vessel walls compensate for the lost leukocytes during a session. This finding led to the concept and investigation of Cellsorba as a therapy for UC. It is believed that activated peripheral blood leukocytes serve as "primed reserve cells" which might include leukocytes that originally have been activated in the lymph nodes. During active IBD, this pool provides a sustainable supply of activated leukocytes for infiltration into the colonic mucosa. By depleting this pool, leukocytapheresis can, in effect influence the source of activated leukocytes in the marginal pools as well. Indeed, infiltration of activated leukocytes into the intestinal mucosa has been considered as a major factor in the etiology of IBD [1, 21, 26].

Perhaps a word of caution is warranted in relation to any leukocytapheresis procedure which depletes lymphocytes. Thus, a study by King and colleagues [77] indicates that the state of lymphopenia may promote the development of autoimmunity. Likewise, it is known that human diseases of autoimmune etiology often present with lymphopenia [59]. These findings led us to say that transient lymphopenia during Cellsorba leukocytapheresis potentially may trigger homeostatic T cell expansion-associated autoimmune disease. Accordingly, if a patient with UC develops autoimmune disease following exposure to Cellsorba, the transient lymphopenia can be suspected to have predisposed to the condition. Currently, treatment of ulcerative colitis and rheumatoid arthritis by Cellsorba are covered by the Japan health insurance system. In Europe, Cellsorba has been CE-marked and approved as medical device. In Table 49.1, typical efficacy outcomes for the Adacolumn and the Cellsorba filter column are presented.

Immunomodulation Associated with Cellsorba Leukcocytapheresis

In the first major study by Sawada et al. [71] in patients with IBD, flow cytometry revealed that patients who improved had a higher percentage of HLA-DR$^+$, HLA-DR$^+$CD3$^+$, and HLA-DR$^+$CD8$^+$ cells (pro-inflammatory) at entry. The levels of these cells, CRP and erythrocyte sedimentation rate (ESR) decreased to within the normal range by the end of therapy. In contrast, patients who showed poor response to leukocytapheresis, CRP and ESR did not change. Cellsorba leukocytapheresis also affected the cytokine production [74, 75]. The levels of pro-inflammatory cytokines, TNF-α, IL-1β, IL-2, IL-8, and IFN-α were high in responders at entry and were significantly reduced by leukocytapheresis [85]. These cytokines are mainly secreted by activated peripheral blood leukocytes [86, 87]. Additionally, the level of IL-4, an immunoregulatory cytokine increased after leukocytapheresis [88]. These observations indicate that Cellsorba leukocytapheresis is associated with changes in cytokine profile in the disease state, returning to normality via inhibition of several pro-inflammatory cytokines and by stimulation of an immunoregulatory cytokine.

Andoh et al. [89] evaluated the alterations in circulating T cell subsets after Cellsorba leukocytapheresis therapy in 18 patients with UC. Peripheral blood was obtained within 5 min before and 5 min after leukocytapheresis therapy. The average number of lymphocytes, T and B cells were significantly decreased after Cellsorba ($P<0.01$). The number of CD4$^+$ and CD8$^+$ T cells were also significantly decreased ($P<0.01$), but the CD4$^+$/CD8$^+$ ratio did not change. Also, the number of CD45RO$^+$CD4$^+$ memory T cells significantly decreased. Using intracellular cytokine staining method, they showed that IFN-γ expressing (Th1) cells had significantly decreased after leukocytapheresis while there was no significant change in the number of IL-4-expressing (Th2) cells. The Th1/Th2 ratio was significantly decreased after Cellsorba.

Table 49.1 Typical efficacy outcomes for leukocytapheresis in patients with ulcerative colitis (UC) or with Crohn's disease (CD)

Investigation undertaken	Main findings	Author, Ref.
Prospective study in a mixed population of UC patients	Steroid naive patients remitted after five sessions, severe patients responded to ten sessions	Hanai et al. [29]
Leukocytapheresis vs prednisolone in UC patients	Five sessions had significantly better safety and efficacy than the corticosteroid	Shimoyama et al. [48]
Efficacy of 60 min vs 90 min leukocytapheresis in UC patients	Ten leukocytapheresis sessions at 60 min or at 90 min showed similar clinical efficacy	Kanke et al. [51]
Leukocytapheresis in steroid-refractory or dependent UC patients	Remission rate in patients with severe UC was 20 % vs 70 % in patients with moderate UC	Naganuma et al. [52]
Treatment of active distal UC with leukocytapheresis	In this difficult cohort of 30 cases, 21 patients (70 %) achieved remission	Yamamoto et al. [53]
Leukocytapheresis in 12 steroid-dependent CD patients	Efficacy rate in this small cohort of CD patients was 70 %	Domenech et al. [55]
GMA as a first line treatment in steroid naive UC patients	A remission rate of 85 % was achieved, and 17 patients were spared from drug therapy	Suzuki et al. [56]
The first GMA trial in patients with CD refractory to pharmacologics	Five of seven patients achieved clinical remission, the two nonresponders had small intestinal CD	Matsui et al. [60]
Multicenter, leukocytapheresis in drug refractory CD	CD activity index decreased from 276 to 215 after five sessions ($P=0.0005$)	Fukuda et al. [61]
Looking at mucosal biopsies pre and post GMA in CD and UC patients	Interferon-γ producing leukocytes in the intestinal mucosa were depleted	Muratov et al. [62]
Efficacy of LCAP in UC patients on corticosteroids	This study reported 74 % efficacy for LCAP + concomitant steroid	Sawada et al. [69]
Efficacy of LCAP vs sham apheresis; filter was omitted	The remission rates were 80 % for active therapy and 33 % for sham apheresis	Sawada et al. [72]
LCAP in fulminant UC, toxic megacolon	Four of six patients responded to LCAP after ten sessions	Sawada et al. [73]
The efficacy of GMA in relation to patients' bodyweight	The remission rate for 3 L processed blood per session was better than for 1.8 L/session	Yoshimura et al. [78]
GMA, ten sessions over 10 weeks vs ten sessions over 5 weeks	Intensive GMA produced higher efficacy in a shorter time vs routine, weekly GMA	Sakuraba et al. [79]
Safety and feasibility of daily leukocytapheresis, five sessions in 5 days	Daily leukocytapheresis was safe and well tolerated without any serious adverse event	Yamamoto et al. [80]
Controlled trial in severe UC refractory to available pharmacologics	Efficacy difference between active and sham apheresis did not reach significance level	Sands et al. [81]
Controlled trial in severe CD refractory to available pharmacologics	Efficacy difference between active and sham apheresis did not reach significance level	Sands et al. [82]
Long-term post marketing surveillance on GMA therapy	Efficacy and safety of GMA was reported in a large UC patients population in Japan	Hibi et al. [83]
Long-term post marketing surveillance on LCAP filter column	Efficacy of LCAP was reported in 847 UC patients from Japan	Yokoyama et al. [84]

Leukocytapheresis was done with either Adacolumn (GMA) or with Cellsorba filter (LCAP). Generally, one leukocytapheresis session is 60 min or as indicated

The Science Behind Leukocytapheresis as a Natural Biologic Therapy

IBD may be viewed as the consequence of an exuberant immune profile triggered and maintained by inflammatory cytokines including TNF-α, IL-6, IL-12, IFN-γ, IL-17, and others [19, 20]. This might be a major factor for IBD showing poor response to conventional drug therapy [1, 29, 90, 91]. Indeed, administrations of these agents, often at high doses over long periods of time can produce additional complications [1, 50, 73, 92, 93]. Further, it is true to say that for decades, drug therapy of IBD has been empirical rather than based on sound understanding of the disease mechanisms (poorly understood etiology). The current view is that treatment interventions targeted at inflammatory mediators (like biologicals) should be more effective and produce minimal side effects. Accordingly, the present era of antibody based therapy targeting specific cytokines, chemokines, and adhesion molecules represent some progress, albeit truly effective in a minority of treated patients [91, 94, 95]. Cytokines in particular represent the best validated therapeutic targets and it is logical to view cytokines as major causes of persistent intestinal inflammation. However, major sources of inflammatory cytokines include leukocytes of the myeloid lineage [86, 87], which in IBD are elevated [29, 30] with activation behavior [26], prolonged survival time [33] and are found in vast numbers within the inflamed intestinal mucosa [1, 21]. Granulocyte infiltration into the mucosal tissue indeed can predict relapse of both UC and CD [21, 58]. This indicates that during quiescent IBD, activated leukocytes infiltrate the intestinal mucosa and have a major role in mucosal inflammation, injury and IBD relapse [1, 21, 26, 58]. Indeed, leukocyte activation and prolonged survival is a feature of persistent inflammation and neutrophil mediated mucosal damage has been shown to be associated with the development of IBD [21, 26, 31, 32]. Accordingly, selective depletion of activated peripheral blood leukocytes by centrifugation, the Adacolumn or Cellsorba has been associated with dramatic efficacy and a marked reduction of inflammatory cytokines produced by leukocytes [28, 29, 45, 74, 75].

Naïve T cells preferentially recirculate between blood and secondary lymphoid tissues, entering lymph nodes from the blood by crossing high endothelial venules. After encountering the activated dendritic cells undergoing antigen presentation in the mesenteric lymph nodes, the naïve T cells become activated, proliferate and differentiate into activated effector T cells. These effector T cells then acquire the gut-homing receptors, integrin $\alpha\beta_4\beta_7$. Thus, colitogenic effector T cells, unlike naïve T cells can migrate efficiently to sites of inflammation [96], subsequently entering afferent lymphatic vessels and travel to local lymph nodes [93, 96–99]. In parabiotic mouse models, endogenous memory T cells in most peripheral tissues react in equilibrium with migrating blood-borne donor T cells within a week [100], suggesting that there is rapid recirculation of T cells in peripheral tissues. These recent understandings suggest that selective removal of these colitogenic activated effector T cells by leukocytapheresis should reduce the cellular components of IBD.

Factors believed to contribute to granulocyte activation and its increased survival time in IBD include inflammatory cytokines [101] and paradoxically corticosteroids [85] which are given to most patients with active IBD. Indeed, corticosteroids are known to reactivate quiescent UC and may precipitate the first UC attack [1]. These again in part explain why IBD shows poor response to drug therapy and strengthen our assumption that activated leukocytes are involved in the initiation, exacerbation and perpetuation of IBD. Activated leukocytes and their cytokines together with corticosteroids might constitute a vicious cycle whereby leukocytes produce cytokines which then support the former in addition to promoting inflammation and both are enhanced by corticosteroids. Hence, peripheral blood leukocytes should be the most appropriate target of therapy in IBD. Based on this thinking, leukocytapheresis should be equivalent to removing inflammatory cytokines at the upstream of inflammatory drive.

To continue the above arguments, we could say that the effectiveness of certain cytokine antagonists like infliximab might be viewed as a solid evidence for the involvement of TNF-α (in this case) in the immunopathogenesis of IBD. Hence, given that major sources of TNF-α (and other inflammatory cytokines) include activated leukocytes, depleting these cells from patients' body should represent biologic therapy, a natural medication which is safe and because it removes from the body the effector cells instead of adding, it is not likely to cause refractoriness. Alternatively, leukocytapheresis as an adjunct to conventional medication should spare most patients with active IBD from additional drug therapy and reduce the number of patients who require colectomy.

Effective Dosage of Leukocytapheresis in Patients with IBD

For leukocytapheresis, which is a non-pharmacologic treatment option, dosage would mean the number of sessions, and the processed blood volume per session in one treatment course. The modern day medicine has relied on the outcomes of clinical trials to determine the dosage of drugs with maximum efficacy margin and minimum adverse effect. However, for leukocytapheresis, which is a non-drug treatment strategy, reliance on clinical trials has been less demanding or at least lack of it has not caused serious concern because of its good safety profile. Nonetheless, in clinical settings, physicians need to know the most effective frequency, processed blood volume per session, and the total number of sessions for patients with mild, moderate or severe IBD. The reality is that hitherto, leukocytapheresis therapy has been an empirical practice. Some institutes administer two sessions per week in the first 2–3 weeks and then one session per week up to ten or eleven sessions [45]. Hanai et al. [48] reported that although patients with steroid naïve UC responded well to five GMA sessions, steroid refractory patients with severe UC responded better to ten sessions. In contrast, Suzuki et al. [56] administer two sessions per week and cease when CAI decreases to four or less (clinical remission level); patients who do not improve after several sessions are classified as nonresponders [102]. These treatment regimens are all contrary to the initial clinical trials in which five leukocytapheresis sessions over 5 consecutive weeks were applied [68]. Regarding the duration of one leukocytapheresis session, Kanke et al. [51] found that 90 min was significantly better than the routinely applied 60 min per session. Likewise, Yoshimura, et al. [103] increased the processed blood volume from the conventional 1800 mL per leukocytapheresis session to over 3000 mL per session. In this study, the efficacy rate in the higher processed blood volume group was significantly greater than in the 1800 mL per session group [78]. In a prospective multicenter study, Sakuraba et al. [79] found that intensive leukocytapheresis at two sessions per week induced remission in a shorter time and at a significantly higher rate when compared to weekly leukocytapheresis. The authors assigned 112 patients with moderately active UC to two groups. Group 1 patients received one leukocytapheresis session per week, while group 2 patients received two sessions per week, up to ten sessions in both groups. The remission rate in group 1 was 46.7 %, while in group 2 was 73.1 %. Further, the mean time to remission was 28.1 days, in group 1 and 16.3 days in group 2. In spite of these outcomes, there is evidence to suggest that the efficacy of GMA is time dependent. Recently, Yamamoto, et al. [80] administered one GMA session per day over five consecutive days. There was no safety concern, but the efficacy rate was very much less than in the five leukocytapheresis sessions reported by Shimoyama et al. [48]. Further, as reviewed above, in patients with active IBD, large numbers of myeloid lineage leukocytes are found within the mucosal tissue [104], which may take several weeks to clear in spite of CAI showing clinical remission [105]. Likewise, the immunomodulatory actions of leukocytapheresis are time dependent. In line with this assertion, in rheumatoid arthritis patients, there was a sustained increase in CD4+ T-lymphocytes up to 12 weeks following the last leukocytapheresis session [30]. Similarly, there was a striking down-modulation of the inflammatory chemokine receptor CXCR3 on leukocytes several weeks after the last leukocytapheresis session [45, 67]. Clearly additional studies are warranted for establishing the optimum frequency and duration of leukocytapheresis session.

Predictive Factors of Clinical Response to Leukocytapheresis

Just like knowing the effective dosage of leukocytapheresis is highly desirable in clinical settings, knowing baseline demographic variables, which potentially identify a patient as a responder or otherwise as a nonresponder to leukocytapheresis should help to avoid futile use of medical resources and reduce morbidity time for many patients. As stated above, the best responders to leukocytapheresis are first episode cases [102] followed by steroid naïve patients [29, 56, 57, 106]. Recently, Yokoyama and colleagues looked for predictive factors of clinical response to leukocytapheresis [107, 108]. In their first investigation [109], they reported that patients with a short duration of UC and low cumulative PSL dose in the past respond well to leukocytapheresis. However, the best responders in that study were patients who received leukocytapheresis immediately after a clinical relapse [107]. Additionally, leukocytapheresis was effective in patients with low white blood cell counts at the first treatment session. In their second study [108], Yokoyama and colleagues found a significant fall in myeloid leukocytes and platelets in responders vs nonresponders to leukocytapheresis. Further, baseline CAI was lower in the remission group vs nonremission. After 12 months, 52 of 134 patients had maintained remission. Disease duration was longer in the relapsed group vs maintained remission group [108]. This study also reported that first UC episode, and corticosteroid responder features together with drug naïve patients were significant factors for response to leukocytapheresis, whereas corticosteroid dependent UC was associating with relapse in those who had achieved remission [108]. Patients in who colonoscopy reveals deep ulcers and extensive loss of the mucosal tissue together with those who have a long history of exposure to multiple pharmacologics to which the disease has become refractory may not benefit from leukocytapheresis [81, 82, 104, 106, 110]. However, it is very important and clinically relevant to indicate here that pharmacologics in particular, corticosteroids given to patients when they first develop IBD can lead to a complicated disease course in the long term [1, 80, 111]. Allison et al. [1] comment that corticosteroids may even reactivate an otherwise quiescent IBD (when given as maintenance therapy or for an unrelated condition). Similarly, Yamamoto et al. [112] found that patients who received Adacolumn leukocytapheresis in the early days of their active IBD had a more favorable long term clinical course by avoiding corticosteroids and other pharmacologics at an early stage of IBD. These findings are inconsistent with lack of efficacy outcomes that randomized sham-controlled study reported by Sands et al. in both UC [81] and CD [82] patients. Kruis et al. [113] carried out a post-hoc analysis on randomized sham-controlled study of Adacolumn for active UC [81]. Only 38 % of the patients or 63 of 165 showed microscopic erosion/ulceration at distal sigmoid colon (group P). The remaining 62 % of the patients did not show microscopic erosion/ulceration (group A). Further, group P patients showed significantly higher Mayo endoscopic score together with neutrophil infiltration into the colonic mucosa compared with patients in group A (P=0.0132, P=0.0243 and P<0.0001, respectively). Likewise, group P patients had a significantly (P=0.0275) higher remission rate (11 of 46; 24 %) when treated with Adacolumn than with sham the procedure (0/17; 0 %). They suggested that true disease activity should be specified for further randomized controlled trials. Likewise, a randomized sham-controlled study for CD [114], patients with CDAI score greater than 300 showed higher clinical response rate (35 of 80 patients; 44 %) when treated with the Adacolumn as compared with the sham procedure (13/48; 27 %) [103].

Safety of Leukocytapheresis in Patients with IBD

Safety of leukocytapheresis with the Adacolumn and the Cellsorba filter column has been assessed in two large scale observational reports [83, 84]. In the first of these two reports, Hibi and colleagues [83] compiled all adverse events (AEs) including problems during the Adacolumn procedures (treatment feasibility) on 697 patients who had been treated over several years. The timeline of AEs was from entry, prior to each leukocytapheresis session up to 2 weeks after the last session. AEs were recorded when observed if the patient was under treatment or reported by patients during their visits to the hospital. In case of spontaneously occurring severe AEs, the physician was to be contacted at that time. Physicians were to monitor the patient until the AE resolved or the outcome was known. During a 7-year period, there was no serious AE related to the Adacolumn; all reported events were of mild to moderate severity. Also, there was no report of an event being associated with the product quality. More than half of the reported events were related to the difficulty in performing blood access and adequate flow rate, elevation of system venous pressure, coagulation, blood return problems. The total number of leukocytapheresis sessions in 697 cases were 5287, mean ± SD = 7.6 ± 2.7, range 1–15 sessions. Overall, AEs occurred during 2.3 % of the total 5287 leukocytapheresis sessions. Seven cases were withdrawn due to difficulties of achieving blood access. The causality of other AEs to the device could not be ruled out. However, alanine transaminase (ALT) and aspartate transaminase (AST) elevations were most likely related to the primary disease, while symptoms like headache and light headedness were thought to be associated with extracorporeal circulation. Events were not significantly more frequent in patients who received ≥6 leukocytapheresis sessions compared with patients who received ≤5 sessions. However, female patients and inpatients showed higher events compared with male patients or outpatients ($P<0.05$). Hematology values including leukocyte counts and CRP showed marked deviations from normal ranges at baseline and improved after leukocytapheresis treatment ($P<0.0001$). Further, the rate of AE was not necessarily higher in nonresponders. Overall, the event rate in the 697 was similar to historical observations [48, 51, 52].

In the second report on Cellsorba filter by Yokoyama and colleagues [84], the overall incidence of AEs was 10.3 % (87 of 847 patients), very much higher than 2.3 % reported for the Adacolumn, which included procedure feasibility. The main reported AEs were headache, nausea, and fever. Such AEs are commonly associated with extracorporeal circulation. AEs related to infections were seen only in three patients. Almost all of the adverse events were of mild to moderate severity, and all the patients either recovered from the events or showed significant improvement. Six severe adverse events were reported in five patients. These included deep vein thrombosis, hypotension, anaphylactic shock, and infective endocarditis/candidemia. All the patients recovered from these events after appropriate treatments. Oral corticosteroids were administered to both patients with deep vein thrombosis. For the patient who developed anaphylactic shock, nafamostat mesilate was used as the anticoagulant; after the event, the patient was able to receive leukocytapheresis by changing the anticoagulant to heparin. An episode of candidemia and infective endocarditis was observed in a male patient, who was also treated with sulphasalazine, oral corticosteroids, azathioprine, and CyA; this suggests that the patient was highly immunosuppressed. The patient needed a catheter insertion for vascular access for the leukocytapheresis therapy, which could have also been a cause of infection. Therefore, the infection might not be due to the leukocyte removal. He recovered after removal of the catheter and antifungal therapy.

Conclusion

Patients with active IBD, peripheral leukocytes are elevated with activation behavior, increased survival time and are believed to be major factors in the immunopathogenesis of IBD. Hence, depleting activated leukocytes should be considered as a safe and effective natural biologic therapy, equivalent to reducing inflammatory cytokine release at an upstream point. Published data show leukocytapheresis producing impressive efficacy, strong drug sparing effects with potential to reduce the number of patients with severe disease who must undergo colectomy or be exposed to potent immunosupressors like CyA. Recently, new drugs that similar to the concept of leukocytapheresis are developing to interfere leukocyte trafficking [115–117]. Vedolizumab (Entyvio®) was approved in 2014 by the FDA and EMA for both UC and CD, the therapeutic antibody is blocking the interaction between $\alpha4\beta7$ and anti-mucosal vascular addressin cell adhesion molecule (MAdCAM)-1 [109, 116, 117]. Oral Fingolimod (FTY720) had introduced for to treat patients with multiple sclerosis, which interfere with lymphocytes traffic between lymphoid organs and blood [118, 119]. Also, development of these drugs is ongoing for IBD [116, 120].

Leukocytapheresis is one kind of non-pharmacologic therapeutic method which modulates autologous leukocyte's functions or process these cells during apheresis [65, 66]. There is low possibility in leukocytapheresis to produce serious adverse effects, such as opportunistic infection or allergic reaction, and also to develop loss of response that is a major problem in biologics. Therefore, the method is applicable for maintenance therapy in patients with IBD during pregnancy [114, 121]. However, studies with high levels of evidence to optimize the treatment including duration, interval, and number of session were anticipated.

References

1. Allison MC, Dhillon AP, Lewis WG, Pounder RE, editors. Inflammatory bowel disease. London: Mosby; 1998. p. 9–95.
2. Fiocchi C. Inflammatory bowel disease: etiology and pathogenesis. Gastroenterology. 1998;115:182–205.

3. Podolsky DK. Inflammatory bowel disease. N Engl J Med. 2002;347:417–29.
4. Harris ML, Bayless TM. Dietary antigens as aggravating factors in Crohn's disease. Dig Dis Sci. 1989;34:1613–4.
5. Abraham C, Cho JH. Inflammatory bowel disease. N Engl J Med. 2009;361(21):2066–78.
6. Ordás I, Eckmann L, Talamini M, Baumgart DC, Sandborn WJ. Ulcerative colitis. Lancet. 2012;380(9853):1606–19.
7. Baumgart DC, Sandborn WJ. Crohn's disease. Lancet. 2012; 380(9853):1590–605.
8. Hart AL, Ng SC, Mann E, Al-Hassi HO, Bernardo D, Knight SC. Homing of immune cells: role in homeostasis and intestinal inflammation. Inflamm Bowel Dis. 2010;16(11):1969–77.
9. Khor B, Gardet A, Xavier RJ. Genetics and pathogenesis of inflammatory bowel disease. Nature. 2011;474(7351):307–17.
10. Molodecky NA, Panaccione R, Ghosh S, Barkema HW, Kaplan GG. Alberta Inflammatory Bowel Disease Consortium. Challenges associated with identifying the environmental determinants of the inflammatory bowel diseases. Inflamm Bowel Dis. 2011;17(8): 1792–9.
11. Wlodarska M, Kostic AD, Xavier RJ. An integrative view of microbiome-host interactions in inflammatory bowel diseases. Cell Host Microbe. 2015;17(5):577–91.
12. Dalal SR, Chang EB. The microbial basis of inflammatory bowel diseases. J Clin Invest. 2014;124(10):4190–6.
13. Shanahan F. Crohn's disease. Lancet. 2002;359:62–9.
14. Francescone R, Hou V, Grivennikov SI. Cytokines, IBD, and colitis-associated cancer. Inflamm Bowel Dis. 2015;21(2):409–18.
15. Brenner D, Blaser H, Mak TW. Regulation of tumor necrosis factor signalling: live or let die. Nat Rev Immunol. 2015;15(6):362–74.
16. Hunter CA, Jones SA. IL-6 as a keystone cytokine in health and disease. Nat Immunol. 2015;16(5):448–57.
17. Baumgart DC, Carding SR. Inflammatory bowel disease: cause and immunobiology. Lancet. 2007;369(9573):1627–40.
18. Neurath MF. Cytokines in inflammatory bowel disease. Nat Rev Immunol. 2014;14(5):329–42.
19. Schreaiber S, Nikolaus S, Hampe J, Hämling J, Koop I, Groessner B, et al. Tumour necrosis factor alpha and interleukin 1beta in relapse of Crohn's disease. Lancet. 1999;353:459–61.
20. Papadakis KA, Targan SR. Role of cytokines in the pathogenesis of inflammatory bowel disease. Annu Rev Med. 2000;51:289–98.
21. Tibble JA, Sigthorsson G, Bridger D, Fagerhol MK, Bjarnason I. Surrogate markers of intestinal inflammation are predictive of relapse in patients with inflammatory bowel disease. Gastroenterology. 2000;119:15–22.
22. Limburg P, David M, Ahlquist A, Sandborn WJ. Faecal calprotectin levels predict colorectal inflammation among patients with chronic diarrhoea referred for colonoscopy. Am J Gastroenterol. 2000;95:2831–7.
23. Roseth AG, Schmidt PN, Fagerhol MK. Correlation between fecal excretion of Indium-111-labelled granulocytes and calprotectin, a granulocyte marker. Scand J Gastroenterol. 1999;34:50–4.
24. Ayabe T, Ashida T, Taniguchi M, et al. A pilot study of centrifugal leukocyte apheresis for corticosteroid-resistant active ulcerative colitis. Intern Med. 1997;36:322–6.
25. Ayabe T, Ashida T, Kohgo Y. Centrifugal leukocyte apheresis for ulcerative colitis. Ther Apher. 1998;2:125–8.
26. McCarthy DA, Rampton DS, Liu Y-C. Peripheral blood neutrophils in inflammatory bowel disease: morphological evidence of in vivo activation in active disease. Clin Exp Immunol. 1991;86:489–93.
27. Mahida YR. The key role of macrophages in the immunopathogenesis of inflammatory bowel disease. Inflamm Bowel Dis. 2000;6:21–33.
28. Hanai H, Watanabe F, Saniabadi A, Matsushita I, Takeuchi K, Iida T. Therapeutic efficacy of granulocyte and monocyte adsorption apheresis in severe active ulcerative colitis. Dig Dis Sci. 2002;47: 2349–53.
29. Hanai H, Watanabe F, Takeuchi K, Saniabadi A, Bjarnason I. Leukcocyte adsorptive apheresis for the treatment of active ulcerative colitis: a prospective uncontrolled pilot study. Clin Gastroenterol Hepatol. 2003;1:28–35.
30. Saniabadi AR, Hanai H, Bjarnason I, Lofberg R. Adacolumn, an adsorptive carrier based granulocyte and monocyte apheresis device for the treatment of inflammatory and refractory diseases associated with leukocytes. Ther Apher Dial. 2003;7:48–59.
31. Rugtveit J, Brandtzaeg P, Halstensen TS, Fausa O, Scott H. Increased macrophage subsets in inflammatory bowel disease: apparent recruitment from peripheral blood monocytes. Gut. 1994;35:669–74.
32. Meuret G, Bitzi A, Hammer B. Macrophage turnover in Crohn's disease and ulcerative colitis. Gastroenterology. 1978;74:501–3.
33. Brannigan AE, O'Connell PR, Hurley H. Neutrophil apoptosis is delayed in patients with inflammatory bowel disease. Shock. 2000;13:361–6.
34. Morse EE, Carbone PP, Freireich EJ, Bronson W, Kliman A. Repeated leukapheresis of patients with chronic myelocytic leukemia. Transfusion. 1966;6:175–82.
35. Buckner D, Graw Jr RG, Eisel RJ, Henderson ES, Perry S. Leukapheresis by continuous flow centrifugation CFC; in patients with chronic myelocytic leukemia CML. Blood. 1969;33:353–69.
36. Curtis JE, Hersh EM, Freireich EJ. Leukoapheresis therapy of chronic lymphocytic leukemia. Blood. 1972;39:163–75.
37. Pearson CM, Paulus HE, Machleder HI. The role of the lymphocyte and its products in the propagation of joint disease. Ann N Y Acad Sci. 1975;256:150–68.
38. Tenenbaum J, Urowitz MB, Keystone EC, Dwosh IL, Curtis JE. Leukoapheresis in severe rheumatoid arthritis. Ann Rheum Dis. 1979;38:40–4.
39. Bicks RO, Groshart KW, Chandler RW. The treatment of severe chronically active Crohn's disease by T8 suppressor cell; lymphapheresis. Gastroenterology. 1985;88:1325.
40. Bicks RO, Groshart KW, Chandler RW. The treatment of severe chronically active Crohn's disease by T lymphocyte apheresis. Gastroenterology. 1986;90:A1346.
41. Bicks RO, Groshart KW, Luther RW. Total parenteral nutrition TPN; plus T-lymphocyte apheresis TLA; in the treatment of severe chronic active Crohn's disease. Gastroenterology. 1987;94:A34.
42. Lerebours E, Bussel A, Modigliani R, et al. Treatment of Crohn's disease by lymphocyte apheresis: a randomized controlled trial. Groupe d'Etudes Thérapeutiques des Affections Inflammatoires Digestives. Gastroenterology. 1994;107:357–61.
43. Kohgo Y, Hibi T, Chiba T, Study group for Alternative Therapies in Ulcerastive Colitis Patients. Leukocyte apheresis using a centrifugal cell separator in refractory ulcerative colitis: a multicenter open label trial. Ther Apher. 2002;6:255–60.
44. Hiraishi K, Takeda Y, Saniabadi A, et al. Studies on the mechanisms of leukocyte adhesion to cellulose acetate beads: an in vitro model to assess the efficacy of cellulose acetate carrier-based granulocyte and monocyte adsorptive apheresis. Ther Apher Dial. 2003;7:334–40.
45. Saniabadi AR, Hanai H, Suzuki Y, Bjarnason I, Lofberg R. Adacolumn for selective leukocytapheresis as a non-pharmacological treatment for patients with disorders of the immune system: an adjunct or an alternative to drug therapy? J Clin Apher. 2005;20:171–84.
46. Hyde GM, Thillainayagam AV, Jewell DP. Intravenous cyclosporin as rescue therapy in severe ulcerative colitis: time for a reappraisal? Eur J Gastroenterol Hepatol. 1998;10:411–3.
47. Cuadrado E, Alonso M, De Juan MD, Echaniz P, Arenas JI. Regulatory T cells in patients with inflammatory bowel diseases treated with adacolumn granulocytapheresis. World J Gastroenterol. 2008;14:1521–7.
48. Shimoyama T, Sawada K, Saniabadi A. Safety and efficacy of granulocyte and monocyte apheresis in patients with active ulcerative colitis: a multicenter study. J Clin Apher. 2001;16:1–9.

49. Hanauer SB. Can cyclosporine go it alone in severe ulcerative colitis. Curr Gastroenterol Rep. 2001;3:455–6.
50. Serkova NJ, Christians U, Benet LZ. Biochemical mechanisms of cyclosporine neurotoxicity. Mol Interv. 2004;4:97–107.
51. Kanke K, Nakano M, Hiraishi H, Terano A. Evaluation of granulocyte/monocyte apheresis therapy for active ulcerative colitis. Dig Liver Dis. 2004;36:512–8.
52. Naganuma M, Funakoshi S, Sakuraba A, et al. Granulocytapheresis is useful as an alternative therapy in patients with steroid-refractory or -dependent ulcerative colitis. Inflamm Bowel Dis. 2004;10:251–7.
53. Yamamoto T, Umegae S, Kitagawa T, Yasuda Y, Yamada Y, Takahashi D. Granulocyte and monocyte adsorptive apheresis in the treatment of active distal ulcerative colitis: a prospective, pilot study. Aliment Pharmacol Ther. 2004;20:783–92.
54. Premchand P, Takeuchi K, Bjarnason I. Granulocyte, macrophage, monocyte apheresis for refractory ulcerative proctitis. Eur J Gastroenterol Hepatol. 2004;16:943–5.
55. Domenech E, Hinojosa J, Esteve-Comas M, Gassull A, Spanish Group for the Study of Crohn's Disease and Ulcerative Colitis (GETECCU). Granulocyteaphaeresis in steroid-dependent inflammatory bowel disease: a prospective, open, pilot study. Aliment Pharmacol Ther. 2004;20:1347–52.
56. Suzuki Y, Yoshimura N, Saniabadi AR, Saito Y. Selective neutrophil and monocyte adsorptive apheresis as a first line treatment for steroid naïve patients with active ulcerative colitis: a prospective uncontrolled study. Dig Dis Sci. 2004;49:565–71.
57. Cohen RD. Treating ulcerative colitis without medications—"Look Mom, No Drugs!". Gastroenterology. 2005;128:235–6.
58. Maiden L, Takeuchi K, Bjarnason I, et al. Selective white cell apheresis reduces relapse rates in patients with IBD at significant risk of clinical relapse. Inflamm Bowel Dis. 2008;14:1413–8.
59. Sleasman JW. The association between immunodeficiency and the development of autoimmune disease. Adv Dent Res. 1996;10: 57–61.
60. Matsui T, Nishimura T, Matake H, Ohta T, Sakurai T, Yao T. Granulocytapheresis for Crohn's disease: a report on seven refractory patients. Am J Gastroenterol. 2003;98:511–2.
61. Fukuda Y, Matsui T, Suzuki Y, Kanke K, Hibi T. Adsorptive granulocyte and monocyte apheresis for refractory Crohn's disease: an open multicenter prospective study. J Gastroenterol. 2004;39:1158–64.
62. Muratov V, Lundahl J, Ulfgren AK, et al. Downregulation of interferon-g parallels clinical response to selective leukocyte apheresis in patients with inflammatory bowel disease. A 12-month follow-up study. Int J Colorectal Dis. 2006;21(6):493–504.
63. Hanai H, Watanabe F, Saniabadi A, et al. Correlation of serum soluble TNF-alpha receptors I and II levels with disease activity in patients with ulcerative colitis. Am J Gastroenterol. 2004;99:1532–8.
64. Mohler KM, Torrance DS, Smith GA, Widmer MB. Soluble tumor necrosis factor TNF; receptors are effective therapeutic agents in lethal endotoximia and function simultaneously as both TNF carriers and TNF antagonists. J Immunol. 1993;151:1548–61.
65. Kashiwagi N, Hirata I, Kasukawa R. A role for granulocyte and monocyte apheresis in the treatment of rheumatoid arthritis. Ther Apher. 1998;2:134–41.
66. Ansary MM, Ishihara S, Oka A, Kusunoki R, Oshima N, Yuki T, et al. Apoptotic cells ameliorate chronic intestinal inflammation by enhancing regulatory B-cell function. Inflamm Bowel Dis. 2014;20:2308–20.
67. Flores-Borja F, Bosma A, Ng D, Reddy V, Ehrenstein MR, Isenberg DA, et al. CD19+CD24hiCD38hi B cells maintain regulatory T cells while limiting TH1 and TH17 differentiation. Sci Transl Med. 2013;5:173ra23.
68. Sono K, Yamada A, Yoshimatsu Y, Takada N, Suzuki Y. Factors associated with the loss of response to infliximab in patients with Crohn's disease. Cytokine. 2012;59:410–6.
69. Sawada K, Muto T, Shimoyama T, et al. Multicenter randomized controlled trial for the treatment of ulcerative colitis with a leukocytapheresis colum. Curr Pharm Des. 2003;9:307–21.
70. Shirokaze J. Leukocytapheresis using a leukocyte removal filter. Ther Apher. 2002;6:261–6.
71. Sawada K, Ohnishi K, Fukui S. Leukocytapheresis therapy performed with leukocyte removal filter for inflammatory bowel disease. J Gastroenterol. 1995;30:322–9.
72. Sawada K, Kusugami K, Suzuki Y, et al. Leukocytapheresis in ulcerative colitis: results of a multicenter double-blind prospective case-control study with sham apheresis as placebo treatment. Am J Gastroenterol. 2005;100:1362–9.
73. Sawada K, Egashira A, Ohnishi K, Fukunaga K, Kasuka T, Shimoyama T. Leukocytapheresis LCAP; for management of fulminant ulcerative colitis with toxic megacolon. Dig Dis Sci. 2005;50:767–73.
74. Sawada K, Muto T, Shimoyama T. Leukocytapheresis with leukocyte removal filter as new therapy for ulcerative colitis. Ther Apher. 1997;1:207–11.
75. Yamaji K, Yang K, Tsuda H, Hashimoto H. Fluctuations in the peripheral blood leukocyte and platelet counts in leukocytapheresis in healthy volunteers. Ther Apher. 2002;6:402–12.
76. Shibata H, Kuriyama T, Yamawaki N. Cellsorba. Ther Apher Dial. 2003;7:44–7.
77. King C, Ilic A, Koelsch K, Sarvetnick N. Homeostatic expansion of T cells during immune insufficiency generates autoimmunity. Cell. 2004;117:265–77.
78. Yoshimura N, Tadami T, Kawaguchi T, et al. Processed blood volume impacts clinical efficacy in patients with ulcerative colitis undergoing adsorptive depletion of myeloid lineage leukocytes. J Gastroenterol. 2012;47:49–55.
79. Sakuraba A, Motoya S, Watanabe K, Nishishita M, Kanke K. An open-label prospective randomized multicenter study shows very rapid remission of ulcerative colitis by intensive granulocyte and monocyte adsorptive apheresis as compared with routine weekly treatment. Am J Gastroenterol. 2009;104:2990–5.
80. Yamamoto T, Umegae S, Natsumoto K. Daily granulocyte and monocyte adsorptive apheresis in patients with active ulcerative colitis: a prospective safety and feasibility study. J Gastroenterol. 2011;46:1003–9.
81. Sands BE, Sandborn WJ, Feagan B, Adacolumn Study Group, et al. A randomized, double-blind, sham-controlled study of granulocyte/monocyte apheresis for active ulcerative colitis. Gastroenterology. 2008;135:400–9.
82. Sands BE, Katz S, Wolf DC, et al. A randomized, double-blind, sham-controlled study of granulocyte/monocyte apheresis for moderate to severe Crohn's disease. Gut. 2013;62:1288–94.
83. Hibi T, Sameshima Y, Sekiguchi Y, et al. Treating ulcerative colitis by Adacolumn therapeutic leucocytapheresis: clinical efficacy and safety based on surveillance of 656 patients in 53 centers in Japan. Dig Liver Dis. 2009;41:570–7.
84. Yokoyama Y, Matsuoka K, Kobayashi T, et al. A large-scale, prospective, observational study of leukocytapheresis for ulcerative colitis: treatment outcomes of 847 patients in clinical practice. J Crohns Colitis. 2014;8:981–91.
85. Meagher LC, Cousin JM, Seckl JR, Haslett C. Opposing effects of glucocorticoids on the rate of appoptosis in neutrophilic and eosinophilic granulocytes. J Immunol. 1996;156:4422–8.
86. Cassatella MA. The production of cytokines by polymorphonuclear neutrophils. Immunol Today. 1995;16:21–6.
87. Nikolaus S, Bauditz J, Gionchetti P. Increased secretion of pro-inflammatory cytokines by circulating polymorphonuclear neutrophils and regulation by interleukin-10 during intestinal inflammation. Gut. 1998;42:470–6.
88. Noguchi M, Hiwatashi N, Hayakawa T, Toyota T. Leukocyte removal filter-passed lymphocytes produce large amounts of interleukin-4 in

immunotherapy for inflammatory bowel disease: role of bystander suppression. Ther Apher. 1998;2:109–14.
89. Andoh A, Tsujikawa T, Inatomi O, et al. Leukocytaoheresis therapy modulates circulating T cell subsets in patients with ulcerative colitis. Ther Apher Dial. 2005;9:270–9.
90. Present DH. How to do without steroids in inflammatory bowel disease. Inflamm Bowel Dis. 2000;6:48–57.
91. Hanauer SB. Medical therapy of ulcerative colitis. Gastroenterology. 2004;126:1582–92.
92. Bresnihan B, Cunnane G. Infection complications associated with the use of biologic agents. Rheum Dis Clin North Am. 2003;29: 185–202.
93. Bromley SK, Thomas SY, Luster AD. Chemokine receptor CCR7 guides T cell exit from peripheral tissues and entry into afferent lymphatics. Nat Immunol. 2005;6:895–901.
94. Egan LJ, Sandborn WJ. Advances in the treatment of Crohn's disease. Gastroenterology. 2004;126:1574–81.
95. Shand A, Forbes A. Potential therapeutic role for cytokine or adhesion molecule manipulation in Crohn's disease: in the shadow of infliximab? Int J Colorectal Dis. 2003;18:1–11.
96. Campbell DJ, Debes GF, Johnston B, Wilson E, Butcher EC. Targeting T cell responses by selective chemokine receptor expression. Semin Immunol. 2003;15:277–86.
97. Mackay CR, Marston WL, Dudler L. Naïve and memory T cells show distinct pathways of lymphocyte recirculation. J Exp Med. 1990;171:801–17.
98. Olszewski WL. The lymphatic system in body homeostasis: physiological conditions. Lymphat Res Biol. 2003;1:11–21.
99. Debes GF, Arnold CN, Young AJ, et al. Chemokine receptor CCR7 required for T lymphocyte exit from peripheral tissues. Nat Immunol. 2005;6:889–94.
100. Klonowski KD. Dynamics of blood-borne CD8 memory T cell migration in vivo. Immunity. 2004;20:551–62.
101. Lee A, Whyte M, Haslett C. Inhibition of apoptosis and prolongation of neutrophil functional longevity by inflammatory mediators. J Leukoc Biol. 1993;54:283–8.
102. Suzuki Y, Yoshimura N, Fukuda K, Shirai K, Saito Y, Saniabadi AR. A retrospective search for predictors of clinical response to selective granulocyte and monocyte apheresis in patients with ulcerative colitis. Dig Dis Sci. 2006;51:2031–8.
103. Study for the treatment of Crohn's disease with adacolumn. post-hoc: clinical response in subjects with a CDAI score greater than 300. https://clinicaltrials.gov/ct2/home. Accessed June 2015.
104. Saniabadi AR, Tanaka T, Ohmori T, et al. Treating inflammatory bowel disease by adsorptive leucocytapheresis: a desire to treat without drugs. World J Gastroenterol. 2014;20:9699–715.
105. Hanai H, Takeuchi K, Iida T, et al. Relationship between fecal calprotectin, intestinal inflammation, and peripheral blood neutrophils in patients with active ulcerative colitis. Dig Dis Sci. 2004;49:1438–43.
106. Tanaka T, Okanobu H, Yoshimi S, et al. In patients with ulcerative colitis, adsorptive depletion of granulocytes and monocytes impacts mucosal level of neutrophils and clinically is most effective in steroid naïve patients. Dig Liver Dis. 2008;40:731–6.
107. Yokoyama Y, Kawai M, Fukunaga K, et al. Looking for predictive factors of clinical response to adsorptive granulocyte and monocyte apheresis in patients with ulcerative colitis: markers of response to GMA. BMC Gastroenterol. 2013;13:27.
108. Yokoyama Y, Watanabe K, Ito H, et al. Factors associated with treatment outcome and long-term prognosis of patients with ulcerative colitis undergoing selective depletion of myeloid lineage leukocytes: a prospective multicenter study. Cytotherapy. 2015;17: 680–8.
109. Soler D, Chapman T, Yang LL, Wyant T, Egan R, Fedyk ER. The binding specificity and selective antagonism of vedolizumab, an anti-alpha4beta7 integrin therapeutic antibody in development for inflammatory bowel diseases. J Pharmacol Exp Ther. 2009;330:864–75.
110. Sacco R, Tanaka T, Yamamoto T, Bresci G, Saniabadi AR. Adacolumn leucocytapheresis for ulcerative colitis: clinical and endoscopic features of responders and unresponders. Expert Rev Gastroenterol Hepatol. 2014;27:1–7.
111. Yamamoto T, Umegae S, Matsumoto K. Long-term clinical impact of early introduction of granulocyte and monocyte adsorptive apheresis in new onset, moderately active, extensive ulcerative colitis. J Crohns Colitis. 2012;6:750–5.
112. Evans RC, Clarke L, Heath P, Stephens S, Morris AI, Rhodes JM. Treatment of ulcerative colitis with an engineered human anti-TNF-alpha antibody CDP571. Aliment Pharmacol Ther. 1997;11:1031–5.
113. Kruis W, Nguyen GP, Morgenstern J. Granulocyte/monocyte adsorptive apheresis in moderate to severe ulcerative colitis—effective or not? Digestion. 2015;92:39–44.
114. Takahashi H, Sugawara K, Sugimura M, Iwabuchi M, Mano Y, Ukai K, et al. Flare up of ulcerative colitis during pregnancy treated by adsorptive granulocyte and monocyte apheresis: therapeutic outcomes in three pregnant patients. Arch Gynecol Obstet. 2013;288:341–7.
115. Danese S, Panés J. Development of drugs to target interactions between leukocytes and endothelial cells and treatment algorithms for inflammatory bowel diseases. Gastroenterology. 2014;147(5): 981–9.
116. Bamias G, Clark DJ, Rivera-Nieves J. Leukocyte traffic blockade as a therapeutic strategy in inflammatory bowel disease. Curr Drug Targets. 2013;14:1490–500.
117. Löwenberg M, D'Haens G. Next-generation therapeutics for IBD. Curr Gastroenterol. 2015;17:444.
118. Kappos L, Antel J, Comi G, Montalban X, O'Connor P, Polman CH, et al. Oral fingolimod FTY720 for relapsing multiple sclerosis. N Engl J Med. 2006;14(355):1124–40.
119. Cohen JA, Khatri B, Barkhof F, Comi G, Hartung HP, Montalban X, et al. Long-term up to 4.5 years; treatment with fingolimod in multiple sclerosis: results from the extension of the randomized TRANSFORMS study. J Neurol Neurosurg Psychiatry. 2015 June 25. pii: jnnp-2015-310597.
120. Daniel C, Sartory N, Zahn N, Geisslinger G, Radeke HH, Stein JM. FTY720 ameliorates Th1-mediated colitis in mice by directly affecting the functional activity of CD4+CD25+ regulatory T cells. J Immunol. 2007;178:2458–68.
121. D'Ovidio V, Meo D, Gozer M, Bazuro ME, Vernia P. Ulcerative colitis and granulocyte-monocyte-apheresis: safety and efficacy of maintenance therapy during pregnancy. J Clin Apher. 2015;30(1): 55–7.

Surgical Management of Crohn's Disease and Ulcerative Colitis

50

Robert R. Cima and John H. Pemberton

Introduction

Crohn's disease (CD) and chronic ulcerative colitis (CUC) represent the two ends of the spectrum of inflammatory bowel diseases (IBD). For both diseases, the etiology is unknown [1]. recent research indicates that there are genetic components to both. However, genetics alone does not explain their occurrence. With the growing appreciation of how an individual's microbiome influences both health and disease, the complex interaction between an individual's genotype, diet, and unique gut flora as it relates to the onset and progression of CD and CUC is an area of active research [2]. While both are inflammatory conditions of the intestine, the location, extent, and histologic characteristics of the inflammation define each as distinct disease entities.

There are significant differences in the pattern of intestinal inflammation between CD and CUC that lead to different manifestations of the disease. CD is characterized by transmural inflammation that may occur anywhere along the intestine from mouth to anus. Transmural inflammation leads to a number of complications unique to CD including perforation, abscess, fistula, and stricture. Surgery is not curative in CD, therefore, operations are performed for complications of the disease or to alleviate symptoms. Unlike CD, CUC is an inflammatory disease limited to the mucosa of the colon and rectum. Since the small bowel is not involved by CUC, removal of the colon and rectum cures the intestinal manifestation of the disease. In this chapter, we discuss the indications for and some technical aspects of surgery for CD and CUC.

R.R. Cima, M.D., M.A. (✉) • J.H. Pemberton, M.D.
Division of Colon and Rectal Surgery, Mayo Clinic College of Medicine, 200 First Street SW, Rochester, MN 55905, USA
e-mail: cima.robert@mayo.edu

Surgery for Crohn's Disease

The decision to proceed to elective surgery in a CD patient needs to be a collaborative decision arising from a consensus between the surgeon, the gastroenterologist, and, most importantly, the patient. Prior to elective CD surgery, it is essential that the medical treatment for CD optimized.

Intestinal transmural inflammation results in a number of CD complications that may require surgical intervention. Common indications for operation include: chronic intestinal inflammation, obstruction due to an inflammatory process or chronic stricture formation, perforation, and entero-entero, entero-vesical, entero-vaginal, or entero-cutaneous fistula. Fistulizing CD in the perineum frequently results in anal ulcers, abscesses or complex anal fistulas. The small bowel, particularly the terminal ileum, is most commonly involved with CD. In a large series of patients with CD requiring surgery over an 11-year period, 41 % had disease in the terminal ileum, 16 % had perianal disease, and 16 % colonic disease. Eighteen percent of patients had multiple sites of disease [3, 4]. In these series, the indications for small bowel operation were failure of medical management to control symptoms (50 %), intestinal obstruction (20 %), and fistulous disease (15 %).

Fortunately, CD patients rarely require emergency surgery. This permits the patient to be medically optimized prior to surgery. Optimizing the patient includes ensuring appropriate CD medical therapy, improving the patient's nutritional status and controlling any local sepsis. For patients with intra-abdominal abscesses, radiologic-guided percutaneous drainage should be performed rather than surgical drainage. This is important because it will minimize the inflammation involving non-diseased intestine thus minimizing the amount of bowel that may require resection. Maintaining or improving a CD patient's nutritional status prior to surgery is essential. If the patient cannot be fed via an enteral route, then early institution of parenteral nutrition is appropriate. In preparation for any major CD surgery, it is

D.C. Baumgart (ed.), *Crohn's Disease and Ulcerative Colitis*, DOI 10.1007/978-3-319-33703-6_50

advisable to have the patient marked for a possible stoma by an enterostomal therapist. Since CD patients frequently require subsequent operations for recurrent disease, the scope of surgery should be directed at the specific problem requiring intervention with every attempt made to limit the extent of bowel resection. Extensive or repeated small bowel resections may lead short bowel syndrome and significant nutritional compromise.

Small Bowel Crohn's Disease

As previously mentioned, the small bowel is the most common site of CD activity. Nearly 40 % of patients will have terminal ileum disease [3]. Common symptoms are abdominal discomfort, persistent diarrhea, or obstructive symptoms. Radiographic or endoscopic evaluation often will establish the diagnosis (Fig. 50.1). Fortunately, there are multiple medical therapies for CD. The algorithms used to determine the optimal therapy for an individual patient is beyond the scope of this chapter. However, all CD medical therapies are directed at reducing the local or systemic inflammatory process. The traditional approach to CD therapy was to start with agents directed at reducing local intestinal inflammation to avoid the use of agents with systemic effects, the so called bottom-up approach. Over the last decade there has been a shift in the treatment paradigm of CD favoring an early initiation of biologic agents alone or in combination with immunomodulators [5, 6]. Commonly referred to as a "top down" approach it is hypothesized that early initiation of agents that block mediators of systemic inflammation and promote rapid mucosal healing may alter the natural history of CD. This approach has been shown to significantly increase remission in newly diagnosed CD and reduce the need for hospitalizations and surgery in the short-term (<2 years), as well as be cost-effective in patients with moderate–severe CD [7, 8]. Whether this approach is reasonable in patients with mild disease or truly impacts the long-term course of CD is still debated, but the current approach to moderate–severe disease is early treatment with biologic agents [9].

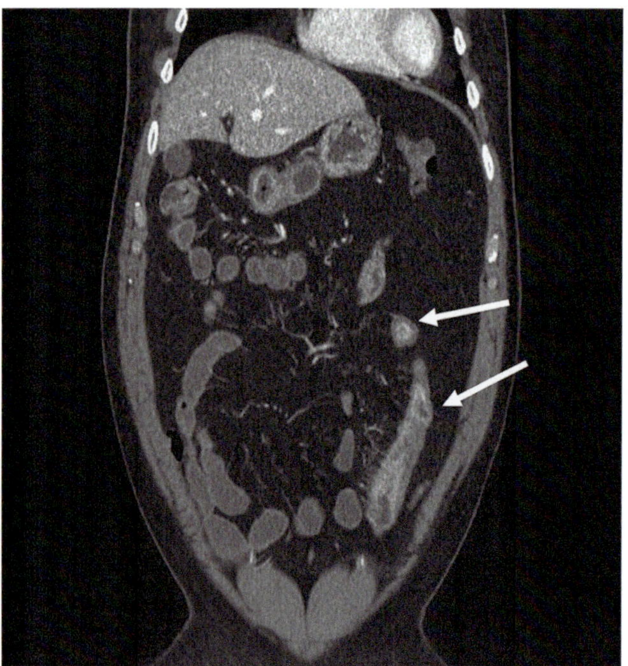

Fig. 50.1 CT image of isolated small bowel Crohn's disease (*arrows*). This image clearly demonstrates the segmental nature CD and the hyper-enhancement of the mesenteric blood vessels and thickened bowel wall characteristic of CD

Surgery for small bowel CD is most commonly performed for medically refractory disease or obstructive symptoms related to terminal ileal disease (Fig. 50.2). The extent of the ileal resection was once a topic of debate. Previously, there was a belief that achieving microscopically negative margins would reduce CD recurrence. However, extended resections lead to excessive loss of small bowel increasing the risk of nutritional compromise in patients that required re-resection. In a prospective randomized, controlled trial, Fazio and colleagues evaluated the extent of resection for focal small bowel CD and found no statistical difference in clinical recurrences between extended and limited resection [10]. Based upon this study and clinical experience the standard is to limit resection of only grossly involved bowel.

Despite medical therapies, recurrence of CD is common after resection. Upwards of 50 % of CD patients who undergo terminal ileal resection will experience endoscopic recurrence of disease in the region of the anastomosis within 1–2 years [11]. However, endoscopic evidence of recurrence does not always translate into recurrent symptoms. McLeod et al. showed that nearly 75 % of patients have endoscopic or

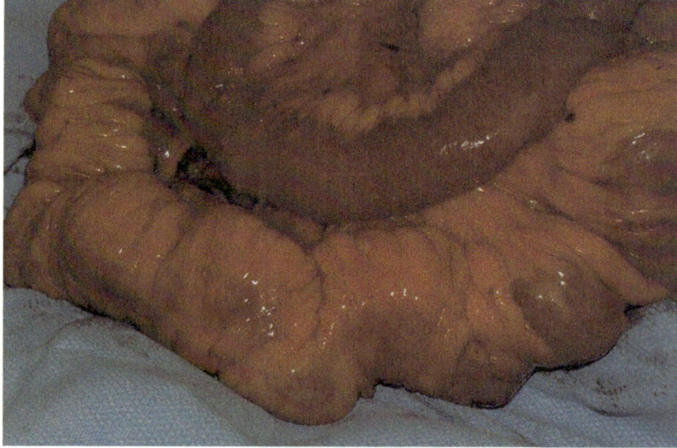

Fig. 50.2 Terminal ileal CD which demonstrates the thickening of the mesentery, creeping fat along the bowel and the increased vascularity of the intestinal serosa which is characteristic of CD

radiologic recurrence by 3 years after surgery but only 40 % had symptoms [12]. With the new "top down" medical treatment strategy the role of medical prophylaxis after CD surgery has also changed towards early initiation or resumption of biologic based therapies to prevent recurrence [13, 14].

Strictureplasty

Another common presentation of small bowel CD is focal stricturing disease which leads to obstructive symptoms. There might be a single area or multiple areas along the length of the small bowel (Fig. 50.3). The strictures are the result of chronic inflammation in which the transmural scarring leads to compromise of the lumen. Previously, areas of multiple strictures were resected or by-passed. Both led to loss of functional bowel length which resulted in nutritional compromise. Furthermore, long segments of by-passed small bowel are associated with bacterial overgrowth and potential increased risk of malignancies in the by-passed segment. The use of strictureplasty in CD was first reported in 1982 [15]. The advantage of this technique is it can be repeated along the length of the bowel without the need for resection. The most commonly used technique is the Heineke–Mikulicz strictureplasty. This technique is useful for strictures up to 4–5 cm in length. The stricture is divided by making a longitudinal enterotomy along the antimesenteric border (Fig. 50.2). The enterotomy is then closed in a transverse fashion which reestablishes and widens the lumen of the bowel. Different types of strictureplasties have been developed for specific situations. For longer strictures (approximately 6–15 cm), the stricture can be folded upon itself and a side to side strictureplasty can be performed. In rare cases, a patient will have a long segment of bowel with multiple strictures or a single long stricture. Traditionally, this situation would have required a resection of the entire involved segment. To address this complex problem, Michellassi developed the long segment side-to-side isoperistaltic strictureplasty [16]. The segment of involved bowel is divided in the middle and then opened along the antimesenteric border. The bowel segments are overlapped in an isoperistaltic fashion and a side-to-side anastomosis is performed.

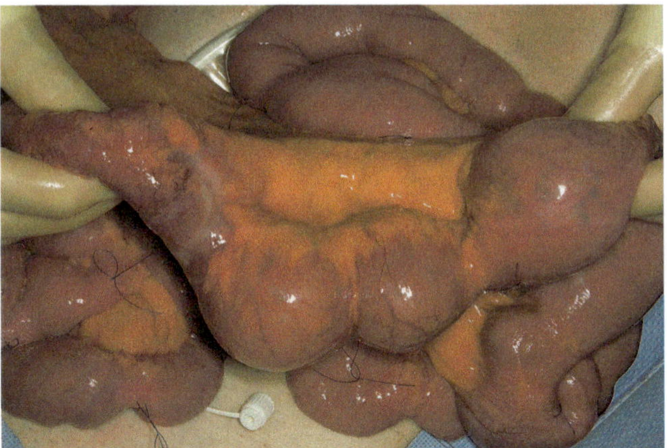

Fig. 50.3 Multiple CD small bowel strictures

Strictureplasty is successful in relieving obstructive symptoms while preserving small bowel length. The Cleveland Clinic reported a large series of 698 strictureplasties performed in 162 patients without any septic complications or deaths [17]. The reoperation rate at 5 years was similar to patients who underwent formal bowel resections. For unclear reasons, in patients requiring reoperation for recurrent strictures, the majority of new strictures occurred at sites remote from the previous strictureplasties [18]. In a recent meta-analysis, strictureplasty is associated with an overall complication rate of 11 % with major complications occurring in 5 % of cases [19]. The median surgical recurrence rate was 24 % after a median follow-up of 46 months.

Treatment of Enteric Fistulas in CD

The transmural inflammation associated with CD results in the fistula formation. Fistulas can occur between different regions of the small and large bowel, adjacent organs, or the abdominal wall. Often, only one side of the fistula is involved with active CD and many entero-enteric fistulas may be asymptomatic. However, if a large segment of bowel is bypassed by the fistula either by connecting to a distal segment of bowel or to the abdominal wall, it may compromise nutrient and fluid absorption to such an extent that surgical division is required.

The initial treatment of a CD enteric fistula is similar to the management of any enteric fistula. Any septic focus needs to be controlled and the anatomy of the fistula delineated. An abdominal CT scan with oral water-soluble contrast is the test of choice because it is both diagnostic and possibly therapeutic. Ideally, any intra-abdominal fluid collection should be drained percutaneously. If the patient has any evidence of systemic infection, broad spectrum antibiotics should be started. Any fluid and electrolyte abnormalities need to be corrected and the patient should be placed on bowel rest. In patients with enterocutaneous fistulas, prompt consultation with a wound or enterostomal therapist is essential in order to avoid skin breakdown and to aid in determining the amount of fistula output with the bowel at rest. Early initiation of intravenous hyper-alimentation is important to prevent further nutritional deterioration. If the patient can be fed orally without significantly increasing the fistula output while maintaining their nutritional state that is preferred to chronic hyper-alimentation. An extended period of intense medical therapy and nutritional support should be attempted prior to surgery. The patient's CD medication management needs to be optimized prior to surgery including the use of biologic therapies. The addition of infliximab to standard medical therapy for enterocutaneous fistulas has resulted in a 68 % closure rate compared to 13 % for placebo [20].

Surgery for CD fistulizing disease requires detailed counseling and operative planning. The patient should be seen and marked by a certified enterostomal therapist for a possible ostomy. At the time of surgery, it is important to distinguish between areas of active CD and "innocent by-stander" bowel. The fistula always originates from the active disease site and extends to non-diseased bowel. The principle in internal fistula surgery is to resect the active disease and repair the non-diseased bowel. If both ends of the fistula are involved with active disease then both segments of bowel are removed. The same strategy is used for fistulas to other organs or the skin. A recent review of the surgical treatment of enterocutaneous fistulas at the Cleveland Clinic reported a 90 day mortality of 3.5 % and a fistula recurrence rate of nearly 21 % over 3 months [21]. However, using the treatment algorithm of controlling sepsis, maximal nutritional and medical therapy and resection of active disease they achieved an 80 % closure rate.

Crohn's Colitis

In some CD patients, the disease is limited to the colon. However, CD is a disease of the entire bowel and patients may present with disease limited to the colon but later develop small bowel disease [22]. The colitis may demonstrate a chronic relapsing course or as a fulminant episode. Indications for surgery in Crohn's colitis include intractable symptoms, fistula formation, stricture formation or severe perianal disease. Fulminant Crohn's colitis may present with massive hemorrhage, free perforation, or systemic toxicity. The surgical management of these patients is similar to patients with fulminant ulcerative colitis. A subtotal colectomy with ileostomy and oversewing of the rectum is the preferred operation. Once the patient's overall medical condition improves and there is no longer evidence of active disease, intestinal continuity can be reestablished by performing an ileorectostomy if the rectum is not involved with Crohn's disease.

In CD patients with segmental involvement of the colon, limited resection is the preferred approach. The Mayo Clinic experience demonstrates that resection of the focal Crohn's colitis leads to 86 % of patients remaining stoma free for more than 10 years [23]. However, nearly 50 % will experience a recurrence in the colon and nearly a third require a second operation for that recurrence. Due to the high recurrence rate, some prefer to offer total proctocolectomy with a permanent end ileostomy as the treatment of choice for segmental Crohn's colitis. Certainly for patients with severe perianal fistulizing CD and segmental colitis a total proctocolectomy and ileostomy should be performed.

Another consideration in Crohn's colitis is the possibility of colon cancer. A meta-analysis by Jess et al. reported nearly a doubling of the standardized incidence ratio for colorectal cancer in Crohn's patients compared to the general public [24]. Any colonic stricture needs to be thoroughly evaluated for a potential malignancy. Furthermore, 10 % of CD patients with a colonic malignancy will have synchronous tumors. In this setting, the preferred operation is a total abdominal colectomy with ileorectostomy.

Perianal Crohn's Disease

Perianal CD is a difficult management problem. Eleven percent of patients will present with perianal disease [22]. There are numerous manifestations of perianal disease including: hypertrophic anal skin tags, ulceration, fissures, anal stenosis, abscesses and fistulas. A patient may have one or multiple manifestations of perianal disease. Common presenting symptoms include severe pain, mucus discharge, bleeding, fecal urgency or incontinence. Surgery for perianal CD is directed at symptom management. Extensive anal operations should be avoided as scarring and recurrent disease may cause irreversible damage to the anal sphincter mechanism resulting in fecal incontinence. Procedures should be limited to controlling local sepsis and preventing recurrent sepsis.

Perianal abscesses need to be drained. Antibiotics alone are not adequate treatment. At the time of abscess drainage if an associated anal fistula is discovered, a loose draining Seton should be placed to provide long-term drainage. If no internal anal opening of a fistula is found, the abscess cavity can be packed as one would a routine perianal abscess. For larger abscess cavities, a mushroom tip rubber catheter can be secured into the cavity to provide long-term drainage.

In patients with complex perianal CD disease, especially fistula disease, imaging is very helpful in guiding management. The combination of endoanal ultrasounds, pelvic MRI and examination under anesthesia will correctly identify 100 % of pathology when at least two of the modalities are used [25]. While surgery is directed at controlling symptoms, newer medical therapies are directed at reducing the initiating inflammatory process and promote fistula healing. All the biologic agents tested to date have excellent efficacy at closing perianal fistulas with success rates between 30 and 100 % either when used alone or combined with surgery [26]. It should be noted that initial surgical control of local sepsis prior to initiation of biologic therapy leads to higher rates of closure. According to the a recent global consensus statement on the treatment of perianal fistulizing CD use of anti-tumor necrosis factor agents as first line therapy is the gold standard of treatment [27]. Once CD medical therapy is optimized and all local sepsis has resolved if there is not spontaneous closure of the fistula an attempt at surgical closure may be attempted.

Complex dissections and flap procedures should be avoided in CD patients with anal fistulas to minimize any unnecessary disruption of the sphincter mechanism. A surgical option for these CD fistulas is to fill the fistula track with a slowly absorbable material. Fibrin glue injected into the tract has been modestly effective in healing perianal fistula tracts [28, 29]. Another option is to place a plug of bioabsorbable material in the tract which permits slow scarring of the tract and eventual closure [30]. Success rates for these procedures are quite variable with most reports closure rates for all patients, not just CD, between 20 and 60 % [31]. The newer ligation of the intersphincteric fistula tract (LIFT) procedure has been shown to have consistently higher fistula closure rates, 70–80 %, in multiple studies of patients with and without CD [32, 33]. An exciting new approach is the use of adipose deprived stem cells as a treatment of Crohn's perianal fistula. After a number of promising small series, recent 2 year follow-up of a phase II trial of 43 patients has demonstrated an 80 % closure rates [34]. Larger trials are now being undertaken to assess this treatment approach.

In patients with extensive medically refractory perianal CD the sphincter mechanism may become impaired leading to fecal incontinence or severe pain such that proctectomy is the only treatment option. Up to 25 % of patients with persistent perianal CD will eventually require proctectomy [35]. Fecal diversion often temporarily improves perianal disease but when reversed, active disease frequently returns. Surgery cannot cure perianal CD. However, conservative surgical management of perianal CD can greatly improve a patient's quality of life.

Despite significant advances in the medical treatment of CD, surgery remains an integral aspect of CD treatment. Although biologic therapies are much more effective at symptom control and reducing the need for hospitalization in CD, population studies have not demonstrated a decrease in the need for surgery [36]. For the foreseeable future, surgery directed at treatment of medically refractory symptoms or complications of CD will continue to be performed ideally by specialist surgeons well versed in the newer aspects of CD care and working in collaboration with the treating gastroenterologist to optimize patient outcomes.

Surgery for Chronic Ulcerative Colitis

Chronic ulcerative colitis (CUC) is a recurring inflammatory condition limited to the colon and rectal mucosa. Since the disease is limited to colon, surgery is curative for the intestinal manifestations of the disease. By definition, the inflammation begins in the rectum and progresses uninterrupted for a variable distance into the colon (Fig. 50.4). The disease course is notable for low level chronic intestinal inflammation with intermittent worsening of the inflammation. These flares of disease activity result in worsening symptoms frequently manifested as by abdominal pain and bloody diarrhea. In a minority of patients, the initial presentation of CUC is a severe acute illness associated with high fever, tachycardia, abdominal pain, distension, and bloody diarrhea. Toxic, or fulminant, colitis is a medical emergency and requires rapid assessment and treatment [37]. Ideally, these patients should be managed by both a gastroenterologist and the surgeon experienced in the care of CUC.

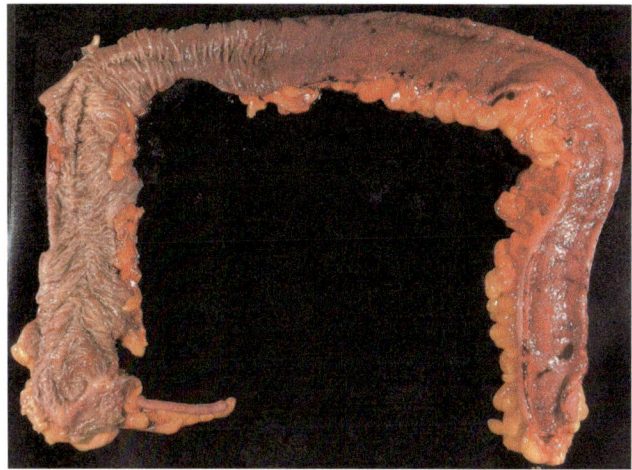

Fig. 50.4 The typical mucosal pattern of CUC which demonstrates contiguous involvement from the low rectum to the transverse colon

Surgery in CUC is divided into two categories, emergent and elective. The operation performed is influenced by the setting in which it is performed. Emergency operations are performed for life threatening complications such as massive hemorrhage or toxic colitis or severe medically refractory disease requiring hospitalization. In this emergency setting, a definitive operation is not recommended. Elective surgery is undertaken to treat intractable symptoms of the disease or for dysplasia or malignancy in the setting of CUC. In appropriate patients a definitive operation can be performed. A definitive operation removes the entire colon and rectum. In many patients, a restorative operation can be performed avoiding the need for a permanent ileostomy.

In appropriately selected patients, the best surgical option is total proctocolectomy with ileal pouch-anal anastomosis (IPAA). IPAA avoids the need for a permanent stoma and maintains the normal route of defecation. This operation is technically demanding and should be performed by surgeons comfortable with the procedure. Long-term follow-up of IPAA patients has demonstrated durable functional results with a high degree of patient satisfaction.

Emergency Surgery for CUC

Emergency surgery is performed in patients with fulminant disease, or toxic megacolon or rarely massive hemorrhage. In the emergency setting, the goal of the operation is to remove the abdominal colon, construct an ileostomy, and leave the rectum undisturbed. Preservation of the rectum maintains the option of a future restorative procedure, such as an ileal pouch anal anastomosis (IPAA). Using this "damage control" approach allows the patient to recover from their acute illness, discontinue any immunosuppressive medication, and improve their nutritional state before a definitive operation is undertaken.

Fulminant colitis is the initial presentation in 10 % of CUC patients [38, 39]. Truelove and Witts defined the clinical syndrome of fulminant colitis [40]. It is characterized by the sudden onset of severe bloody diarrhea (more than ten per day), abdominal pain, dehydration, and anemia. In addition, the patient must have at least two of the following: tachycardia, temperature greater than 38.6 °C, leukocytosis and hypoalbuminemia. These patients are extremely ill and require immediate medical attention. Initial therapy involves aggressive intravenous fluid resuscitation, correction of electrolyte abnormalities and anemia. If the patient has abdominal distension a nasogastric tube should be placed. Stool cultures should be obtained to rule out *C. difficile* or hemorrhagic infectious enteritis. A patient with known CUC may be started on intravenous steroids. In patients without a diagnosis of CUC, an endoscopic evaluation of the colon needs to be performed to help establish the diagnosis. A complete endoscopic evaluation of the colon is not required and may be unsafe in this setting. If the patient is clinically stable, there is no need for antibiotic therapy. However, in the presence of a fever or leukocytosis, broad-spectrum antibiotics should be initiated after cultures are obtained. Close observation for 24–48 h while on maximal medical therapy is crucial. If there is no improvement, or if the patient's condition deteriorates, then surgery is advised. During this observation period, the development of peritonitis or hemodynamic instability requires immediate operation.

Other complications requiring immediate surgical evaluation are toxic megacolon and massive hemorrhage. Toxic megacolon may be seen in the setting of fulminant colitis or in isolation. Transverse colon dilatation greater than 5.5 cm defines the radiographic criteria of toxic megacolon. The entire colon or an isolated segment of the colon (usually transverse) is involved with gaseous distension. Clinically, the patients have significant abdominal distension and pain. They may also have fever and a leukocytosis. These patients are treated in a similar fashion to those with fulminant colitis. Operation is indicated if the patient's clinical or radiographic status worsens, or if there is no improvement after 24–36 h of medical therapy. Profound intestinal hemorrhage is a rare complication of CUC. Aggressive fluid and blood-product resuscitation is required as well as correction of any electrolyte or clotting deficiencies. Ideally, upper intestinal endoscopy needs be performed to rule out a bleeding gastric or duodenal ulcer since these patients are often on steroids at the time of presentation. If the patient remains hemodynamically unstable even after resuscitation, then operation is indicated; medical therapy is too slow to reverse the mucosal inflammation responsible for the bleeding. If the patient responds to resuscitation, then a trial of intravenous steroids may be instituted. Persistent bleeding requiring transfusion after 48–72 h of therapy is an indication for surgery. Perforation outside the setting of toxic megacolon rarely occurs. A patient presenting with a perforation without megacolon should raise concern that the actual diagnosis is Crohn's disease, or that there is another cause for the perforation, such as a gastric or duodenal ulcer. Whatever the cause, there is no role for conservative therapy, and the patient should immediately undergo exploration.

Regardless of the indication for an emergency CUC surgery, the operation of choice is a subtotal colectomy with an end ileostomy. A pelvic dissection is avoided so the planes in the pelvis are not disturbed, making future surgery easier. The rectum should be retained even in patients who are not candidate for a future restorative procedure. Performing the rectal dissection during emergency surgery increases the complexity of the case, lengthens the operation, and increases the risk of bleeding. After the patient recovers and their health status improves the retained rectum can be addressed at a future elective definitive procedure.

Elective Surgery in CUC

The most common indication for elective surgery is intractability, despite medical therapy. Other indications include: colonic dysplasia, a dysplasia associated lesion or mass (DALM), malignancy, or side-effects of the medications. In children, stunting of normal growth is also an indication for surgery. Intractability is a clinical definition. In the chronic disease setting, it refers the inability to discontinue oral steroids completely or the development of severe drug-related side effects.

The presence of colonic dysplasia is an important consideration in CUC patients especially in those with long-standing disease. CUC patients are at high risk of developing colorectal cancer. The cancer risk increases with both duration and extent of the disease. The lifelong risk of colorectal cancer is estimated to be anywhere from 2 % at 20 years after onset of CUC to 43 % at 35 years [41]. The presence of colonic dysplasia on endoscopic biopsies is evidence of epithelial instability. This is considered a premalignant state. Initially reported by Taylor and colleagues and expanded upon recently by Gorfine et al. colon specimens with dysplasia of any grade were 36 times more likely to harbor a cancer [42, 43]. In the Mayo Clinic experience, 18 CUC patients with low-grade dysplasia were observed with serial colonoscopies for a median of 32 months [42]. Nine of the 18 patients developed advanced neoplastic lesions including a cancer. Ullman and colleagues reported a similar high rate of malignancy in the setting of low grade dysplasia without any associated masses [44]. While some recommend increased endoscopic surveillance for low grade dysplasia others consider its presence an indication for surgery. The presence of a polyp not associated with any surrounding dysplasia usually can be managed with endoscopic removal without any increased risk for malignancy [45]. While increased frequency of endoscopic surveillance for low grade dysplasia may be warranted, evidence of recurrent low grade dysplasia or any evidence of moderate or high grade dysplasia is an indication for surgery.

The two primary definitive operations for CUC are total proctocolectomy with end ileostomy (TPC) or total proctocolectomy with ileal-pouch anal anastomosis (IPAA). The TPC can be performed in a single stage with a relatively low morbidity. However, the patient is left with a permanent ileostomy. The IPAA is often a multiple stage procedure and is associated with a higher complication rate. The advantage of IPAA is that it avoids the need for a permanent ileostomy and preserves the normal route of defecation albeit with a higher number of daily bowel movements.

IPAA is the procedure of choice in appropriately selected patients who wish to avoid a permanent ostomy. Due to technical considerations, obese patients and extremely tall patients may not be good IPAA candidates. Our experience is that IPAA needs to be abandoned in less than 4 % of patients intraoperatively due to technical or anatomic problems [46]. Furthermore, advanced age which was once considered a contraindication to IPAA is now considered a relative contra-indication.

Whether IPAA is performed though a traditional open or a minimally invasive approach, the operation involves four steps: (1) removal of the intra-abdominal colon, (2) dissection and removal of the rectum sparing the pelvic nerves and the anal sphincter mechanism, (3) construction of an ileal reservoir, (4) anastomosis of the ileal reservoir to the anal canal. We have previously described our IPAA technique. [47] At our institution, nearly all patients also receive a diverting loop ileostomy at the time of IPAA.

Construction of the ileal pouch requires that the small bowel mesentery be completely mobilized from the retroperitoneum up to the inferior border of the pancreas to ensure there is adequate length mesenteric length to reach the anal canal. To achieve adequate length, it may be necessary to divide either the ileocolic vessel or one of the branches of the superior mesenteric artery. Once the mesentery has been mobilized, the pouch is fashioned. A J-shaped reservoir is constructed from the terminal 30–35 cm of the ileum. The pouch is constructed by folding the terminal ileum into a J-shape. The common wall between the two limbs is divided by repeated firings of a linear cutting stapling device from the apex of the pouch. The pouch is anastomosed to the anal canal by using a circular stapler or alternatively by a hand-sewn pouch to anal canal anastomosis. As mentioned previously, our practice is to construct a proximal diverting loop ileostomy at the time of the pouch operation. However, as will be discussed later, in some select patients omitting the ileostomy can be considered. Eight to twelve weeks after the operation if there is no evidence of a leak from the pouch on a contrast study performed through the anus, the ileostomy is reversed.

While the majority of the literature regarding complications, functional outcomes, and long-term durability of IPAA is based upon IPAAs constructed via an open laparotomy, the last decade has seen a significant transition to IPAA being performed using advanced minimally invasive techniques. In a case matched series reported by Dunker and colleagues, laparoscopic-assisted IPAA as compared to open IPAA resulted in similar functional results and quality of life outcome measurements [48]. Our initial experience at the Mayo Clinic with laparoscopic IPAA was similarly positive [49]. In a report using a large national surgical database, the percentage of minimally invasive IPAA increased from 18.5 % in 2005 to 41.3 % in 2008 and in some individual institution reports as high as 80 % minimally invasive IPAAs [50]. Early reports on minimally invasive IPAA focused on the improved cosmesis, reduced postoperative pain, and decreased length of stay; more recent national studies have also demonstrated significant reductions in major postoperative morbidities [50, 51].

Functional Outcomes

A number of surgeons and institutions have reported their IPAA experience. Across these many studies, the functional results are quite similar [52–54]. The majority of patients report good to excellent function with their IPAA. In the Mayo Clinic IPAA experience, the average number of daytime bowel movements after ileostomy closure was six and one at night. [52] Incontinence was an unusual occurrence during the day with 79 % of patients reporting complete continence, 19 % occasional incontinence and 2 % frequent incontinence episodes. Nocturnal incontinence was more common with 59 % reporting no incontinence episodes and 49 % occasional incontinence episodes. Although long-term follow-up for patients who had minimally invasive IPAA is limited, the 1 and 5 year functional outcomes for 119 patients from the Cleveland Clinic is similar to matched patients who had open IPAA [55].

Thirty years after the introduction of IPAA, the long-term durability of the pouch has been assessed. Hahnloser et al., reported on the functional outcomes of IPAA patients who have had their pouch in place for up to 20 years [56]. Pouch failure is rare even in those who suffer postoperative complications.

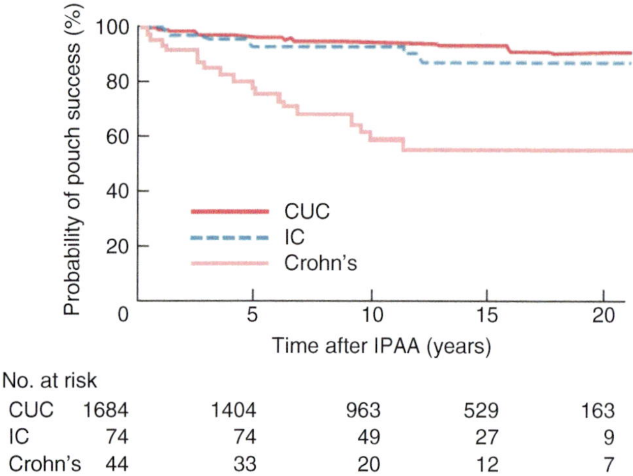

Fig. 50.5 The probability of long-term pouch success over an extended nearly 20 year follow-up period at a single institution, Mayo Clinic, Rochester. (Hahnloser D, et al. Br J Surg 2007;94:333–340)

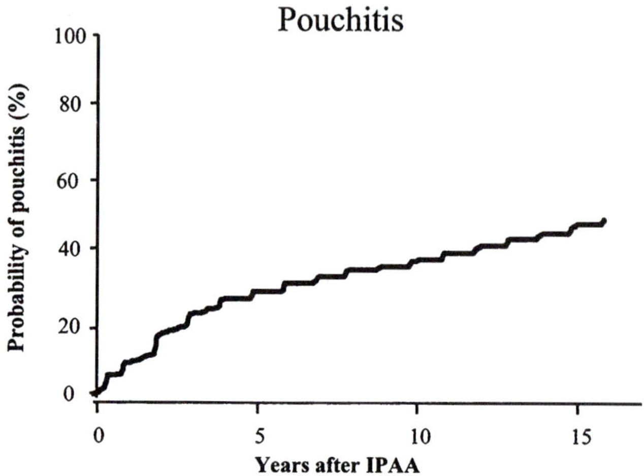

Fig. 50.6 The probability of developing an episode of pouchitis after IPAA for CUC during a 15 year follow-up period as reported from a single center, Mayo Clinic, Rochester, in over 400 patients. (Hahnloser D, et al. Ann Surg. 2004;240:615–21)

The overall pouch success rate is 92 % (Fig. 50.5). Most commonly, permanent diversion or pouch excision were performed for poor pouch function. The strongest association with pouch failure was with postoperative pelvic sepsis. Other reasons for pouch failure were chronic pouchitis and subsequent development of Crohn's disease.

Complications

IPAA is associated with a number of early and late complications. Small bowel obstruction and pelvic abscesses are the most common early complications. Late complications include anastomotic stricture, pouch fistulas, pouchitis, and cuffitis. Delayed presentation (>1 year after reversal of the ileostomy) of a pelvic abscess or fistula raises the concern that the underlying diagnosis is not CUC but rather CD.

Numerous reports of IPAA experience have had similar postoperative complication rates [57–59]. The overall postoperative morbidity rate ranges between 25 % and 30 %. The most worrisome postoperative complication is a pouch leak and associated pelvic sepsis which occurs with a rate between 5–24 %. As discussed later, this rate of pelvis leak does not seem to be influenced by proximal diversion with an ileostomy at the time of pouch construction. Patients with a pelvic phlegmon CT scan respond to broad-spectrum antibiotics. If there is drainable fluid collection, percutaneous CT-guided drainage is the preferred approach. Rarely laparotomy with abdominal washout and drainage is required.

Small bowel obstruction is both a short and long term complication after IPAA. In the Mayo Clinic experience, perioperative small bowel obstruction was 15 % with nearly a quarter requiring operation [60]. The most common site of obstruction was in the pelvis. MacLean reviewed the literature and reported an average incidence of bowel obstruction as 18 % at 1 year, 27 % at 5 years, and 31 % at 10 years [61]. The impact of minimally invasive IPAA on the incidence of bowel obstruction has not been reported. However, in one small series where pelvic adhesions were assessed at the time of ileostomy closure there were significantly reduced [62]. Pouch-anal anastomotic stricture is another common complication after IPAA [60]. There is no correlation between stricture formation and anastomotic technique, hand-sewn versus stapled. Fortunately, these strictures are easily dilated either in the operating room or by the patient using soft dilators.

The most common long-term IPAA complication is pouchitis [63]. The reported incidence of pouchitis is heavily influenced by the diagnostic criteria used. Patients report symptoms similar to colitis including fever, anemia, and diarrhea [64]. An increased number of pouch leakage episodes or fecal incontinence is a common complaint. There are few reliable preoperative or postoperative risk factors that have been associated with development of pouchitis. Fortunately, chronic pouchitis is infrequent and often responds to therapy.

The most common treatment is a 2 week course of oral antibiotics either metronidazole or ciprofloxacin [65]. Patients who suffer frequent recurrent episodes or develop chronic pouchitis may require prolonged antibiotic therapy or even immunomodulator therapy. Rarely, chronic pouchitis requires permanent diversion or pouch excision. In long-term follow-up of IPAA patients, nearly 50 % of patients reported at least one episode at 10 years but it rose to 78 % after 20 years [56] (Fig. 50.6). In this cohort, chronic pouchitis developed in less than 5 % of patients and only 2 % required diversion or pouch removal.

Although the IPAA experience spans three decades, there are a number of technical and outcome issues that continue to be discussed. These include the use of a defunctioning ileostomy, IPAA in older patients, fertility in women after IPAA, and the impact of newer biologic therapies on postoperative IPAA outcomes.

Role of Proximal Diversion

Early in the IPAA experience, the role a proximal ileostomy was to protect the pouch from fecal content while the anastomosis healed. This was deemed to be essential in minimizing the risk of a pelvic leak and sepsis. Over the last decade a number of authors have reported their experience with IPAA without the 'protecting' ileostomy [66–68]. Advocates of this approach believe IPAA can be performed without an increased risk of pelvic sepsis while avoiding the inconvenience of a temporary ileostomy and the need for a second operation. A large single institution report from Sugerman et al., 201 patients underwent a stapled IPAA in which 196 were done without a diverting ileostomy [66]. The majority of these procedures were performed for CUC and nearly all the patients were on steroids at the time of surgery. Anastomotic leaks developed in 12 % of patients with only nine patients requiring operations to construct a proximal ileostomy. In this study, there was no impact on the long-term IPAA function. Others have reported similar outcomes [67]. A small randomized control trial has been performed which found no difference between the standard use of a proximal ileostomy and no ileostomy [68]. Despite some evidence that there is no need for a proximal ileostomy at the time of IPAA, most surgeons prefer constructing one. This is based upon the concern that the severity of complications in patients without ileostomy is greater than those with a proximal ileostomy. This belief is supported by a comparative study between one and two stage IPAA which demonstrated while the complication rates were similar the rate of life-threatening complications were significantly higher in the patients without a proximal ileostomy [69]. Overall, the current evidence suggests that in highly selected patients who have technically uncomplicated procedures performed by experienced IPAA surgeons, a proximal ileostomy may be omitted. However, the surgeon needs to closely monitor the patients for early signs of pelvic sepsis related to a pouch or anastomotic leak.

IPAA and Age

Traditionally, IPAA was offered only to younger CUC patients who required surgery. CUC patients older than 50 who required surgery were not considered candidates for IPAA, because of overconcerns about poor functional outcomes. However, reports from multiple institutions have demonstrated no difference in functional outcomes or quality of life even in their 80s [70]. Overall, the most important consideration is the general health of the patient rather than their chronologic age.

CUC and Fertility

Many CUC patients are diagnosed during their young adulthood years, therefore the impact of both medical and surgical treatment on fertility, especially in women, needs to be considered. Large population based studies conducted in the late 1990s demonstrated that IPAA has a significant negative impact on fertility in young women [71–73]. It is estimated that IPAA reduces a woman's ability to become pregnant by nearly 50 %. Prior to considering the surgery, this issue needs to be thoroughly discussed with the young woman and her family. A detailed analysis of pregnancy rates in Sweden after IPAA revealed a significant reduction in postoperative fertility [71]. Their birth rate was compared to the expected pregnancy and birth rate for age matched Swedish women. There was a no difference in the expected birth rate from the onset of their CUC to the time of surgery. However, after IPAA there was a significant reduction in pregnancy ($P<0.001$). Also, women with IPAA required a much higher rate of in vitro fertilization, 29 % compared to 1 % respectively. In subsequent studies, women who had an ileorectal anastomosis instead of IPAA did not appear to experience a reduction in fertility [74, 75]. While the exact cause of reduced fertility is not known, most assume altered pelvic anatomy and pelvic adhesions play a major role. With the wider adoption of minimally invasive surgery for IPAA, there has been increased interest to determine if that modality influences fertility. In a study performed at the time of diverting ileostomy closure after minimally invasive IPAA, laparoscopic exploration was performed and the presence and density of adhesions in the abdomen, pelvis and adnexa was performed [76]. Using a standardized small bowel and adnexal adhesion scoring system, patients who had a laparoscopic IPAA had significantly fewer adhesions than those that had an open IPAA. Importantly, women had markedly fewer and less dense adnexal adhesions. As an option for young women with CUC who desire to start a family or who are in a stable relationship and might start a family within a few years, total abdominal colectomy and ileostomy is a very reasonable option. This approach removes the majority of the disease, allows medication to be withdrawn and does not disturb the pelvic anatomy. IPAA can be subsequently performed after child-bearing is complete.

After an IPAA, the mode of delivery, either vaginal or cesarean section, should be based upon obstetrical concerns rather than the presence of the pouch [77, 78]. Specific obstetrical issues favoring a cesarean section include: breech position, above gestational age size, prior need for episiotomy, and possible need for an instrument assisted vaginal delivery. However, given the uncertainty of how a labor will progress, many IPAA patients and their obstetricians elect an elective cesarean section to avoid possible injury to the pouch and anal sphincter complex.

Impact of Crohn's Disease after IPAA

CUC and CD likely represent extremes of the inflammatory bowel disease spectrum. However, it may be very difficult to determine prior to performing an IPAA exactly where the patient is on that spectrum. In a review by Shen and colleagues, the reported incidence of CD complications after IPAA performed for CUC is between 3 and 13 % [79]. Early in the IPAA experience, CD development in the pouch was often a devastating complication due to the lack of effective medical treatment options. However, with a better understanding of the disease and biologic based medications pouch retention rate and functional outcomes in these patients is quite reasonable. In a series out of the Cleveland Clinic, nearly 70 % of patients who developed CD after IPAA construction had their pouch in place with excellent functional outcomes at 5 years after diagnosis of CD [80].

Since the limited experience with CD development after IPAA seems to suggest that these patients have very reasonable pouch survivability and functional outcomes, some surgeons offer IPAA to patients with known CD. The ideal candidate would be a patient with a long history of colonic/rectal CD without anal complications or small bowel disease other than limited terminal ileal disease. Regimbeau and colleagues described long-term follow-up in a series of highly select patients with known Crohn's colitis that underwent IPAA in order to avoid a permanent stoma [81]. After a median follow-up of 9 years, 27 % had CD related complications in their pouch. In the 20 patients with greater than 10 years of follow-up, the rate of pouch excision or permanent diversion was 10 %. The functional outcomes were comparable to patients who had IPAA for a diagnosis of IPAA. Other investigators have reported similar outcomes in highly selected CD patients [82]. While the experience with performing IPAA in patients with CD is limited, in highly selected patients at high volume IPAA institutions it could be offered as an alternative to a permanent ostomy with an expectation for a reasonable functional outcome.

The Impact of Biologic Therapies on Surgical Outcomes

In a number of studies, steroid use prior to IPAA and CD has been associated with increased risk of postoperative, particularly infectious, complications [63, 66, 83–85]. With the introduction of anti-TNF and other targeted biologic therapies for inflammatory bowel disease, there has been renewed interest in evaluating the impact of these agents on short-term post-surgical outcomes. The immune system is integral to the initiation and integration of processes that control wound healing. Unlike steroids that impact effector cells' functional capabilities, the biologic agents target messenger or trafficking molecules which prevent propagation and coordination of the immune response. Interference with wound healing, particularly at the intestinal level may manifest as increased intra-abdominal infections from poor or delayed healing of intestinal anastomosis or complete disruptions of anastomoses. The Mayo Clinic was the first to report a possible association between biologic therapy and adverse outcomes in IPAA patients [86]. The outcomes of 47 CUC patients who received preoperative biologic therapy prior to IPAA were compared to 254 who were on therapies other than biologic agents including steroids. The patients who had biologic therapy were statistically more likely to have postoperative infectious complications and pelvic abscesses. Multivariate analysis, including disease severity and steroid use, demonstrated that anti-TNF medication remained independently associated with an increased risk of IPAA-related and infectious complications. A subsequent study from the Cleveland Clinic found a similar association between preoperative biologic therapy and postoperative complications [87]. In some much smaller studies, the association between biologic therapy and postoperative complications in both IPAA and CD patients was not demonstrated [88, 89]. However, in more recent larger and better controlled studies in CD the association of biologic therapy within 2 months of surgery increased intra-abdominal infectious complications was clearly present [90, 91]. The majority of the available literature has come from single institution experiences which always raise some concern for bias. However, numerous recent meta-analyses looking at both CD and CUC surgery have supported the concern that there is a real association between preoperative use of biologic agents and postoperative infectious complications [92–95]. All the studies to date are retrospective making it hard to draw any conclusions regarding the exact role of biologic therapies on postoperative adverse events. Further prospective studies that evaluate the extent and severity of disease, duration of disease activity and medical therapy need to be performed to clarify this important issue. Additionally, as newer agents with different biologic targets start to be used their impact on surgical outcomes should be carefully monitored. Given the uncertainty about the role of biologic therapy and postoperative complications, surgeons should consider the optimal timing of surgery relative to last administration of agents and possibly taking a more conservative surgical approach such as a three stage IPAA.

Conclusion

Successful surgical outcomes for patients with either CD or CUC require a thorough understanding of both the pathophysiology the specific disease-related complications unique to them. Furthermore, close collaboration with a gastroenterologist experienced in caring for inflammatory bowel disease patients will improve the coordination of care for these complex patients. Surgical therapy for Crohn's disease is directed at treating symptoms and complications of the disease as surgical cure is impossible. The nature of CD transmural inflammation leads to a number of complex problems including intra-abdominal abscesses, perforations, fistulas, and strictures. The operative approach to all of these problems is to minimize the resection of non-diseased bowel in order to preserve bowel length and intestinal function. Unlike CD, surgery for CUC cures the patient of the intestinal manifestations of the disease by removing the colon and rectum. During emergent CUC operations, the goal is to remove the abdominal colon leaving the rectum in situ. Leaving the rectum facilitates a future restorative procedure after the patient's health has improved. Ileal-pouch anal anastomosis (IPAA) is a restorative operation that preserves the normal route of defecation, albeit with a different frequency, and avoids a permanent stoma. This is a complex procedure which is associated with a number of short-term and long-term complications which the surgeon needs to be familiar with and capable of addressing. For both CD and CUC, minimally invasive surgery is technically feasible in many circumstances and provides the patients with short-term benefits.

References

1. Schirbel A, Fiocchi C. Inflammatory bowel disease: established and evolving considerations on its etiopathogenesis and therapy. J Dig Dis. 2010;11:266–76.
2. Leone V, Change EB, Devkota S. Diet, microbes, and host genetics: the perfect storm in inflammatory bowel diseases. J Gastroenterol. 2013;48:315–21.
3. Hurst RD, Molinari M, Chung TP, Rubin M, Michelassi F. Prospective study of the features, indications, and surgical treatment in 513 consecutive patients affected by Crohn's disease. Surgery. 1997;122:661–8.
4. Michelassi F, Balestracci T, Chappell R, Block GE. Primary and recurrent Crohn's disease. Experience with 1379 patients. Ann Surg. 1991;214:230–8.
5. Rogler G. Top-down or step-up treatment in Crohn's disease? Dig Dis. 2013;31:83–90.
6. Lin MV, Blonski W, Lichtenstein GR. What is the optimal therapy for Crohn's disease: step-up or top-down? Expert Rev Gastroenterol Hepatol. 2010;4:167–80.
7. Rubin DT, Uluscu O, Sederman R. Response to biologic therapy in Crohn's disease is improved with early treatment: an analysis of health claims data. Inflamm Bowel Dis. 2012;18:2225–31.
8. Marchetti M, Liberato NL, Di Sabatino A, Corazza GR. Cost-effectiveness analysis of top-down versus step-up strategies in patients with newly diagnosed active luminal Crohn's disease. Eur J Health Econ. 2013;14:853–61.
9. Antunes O, Filippi J, Hebuterne X, Peyrin-Biroulet L. Treatment algorithms in Crohn's—up, down, or something else? Best Pract Res Clin Gastroenterol. 2014;28:473–83.
10. Fazio V, Marchetti F, Chruch JM, Goldblum JR. Effect of resection margins on recurrence of Crohn's disease in small bowel: a randomized controlled trial. Ann Surg. 1996;224:563–73.
11. Borely NR, Mortensen NJ, Jewell DP. Preventing postoperative recurrence of Crohn's disease. Br J Surg. 1997;84:1493–502.
12. McLeod RS, Wolff BG, Steinhart AH, Carryer PW, O'Rourke K, Andrews DF, et al. Risk and significance of endoscopic/radiological evidence of recurrent Crohn's disease. Gastroenterology. 1997;113:1823–7.
13. Singh S, Garg SK, Pardi DS, Wang Z, Murad MH, Loftus EV. Comparative efficacy of pharmacologic interventions in preventing relapse of Crohn's disease after surgery: a systematic review and network meta-analysis. Gastroenterology. 2015;148:64–76.
14. De Cruz P, Kamm MA, Hamilton AL, Ritchie KJ, Krejany EO, Gorelik A, et al. Crohn's disease management after intestinal resection: a randomized trial. Lancet. 2015;385:1406–17.
15. Lee EC, Papaionnou N. Minimal surgery for chronic obstruction inpatients with extensive or universal Crohn's disease. Ann R Coll Surg Engl. 1982;64:229–33.
16. Michelassi F. Side-to-side isoperistaltic strictureplasty for multiple Crohn's strictures. Dis Colon Rectum. 1996;39:344–9.
17. Dietz DW, Laureti S, Strong SA, Hull TL, Church J, Remzi FH, et al. Safety and long-term efficacy of strictureplasty in 314 patients with obstructing small bowel Crohn's disease. J Am Coll Surg. 2001;192:330–8.
18. Tichansky D, Cagir B, Yoo E, Marcus SM, Fry RD. Strictureplasty for Crohn's disease: meta-analysis. Dis Colon Rectum. 2000;43:911–9.
19. Wibmer AG, Kroesen AJ, Gröne J, Buhr HJ, Ritz JP. Comparison of strictureplasty and endoscopic balloon dilatation for stricturing Crohn's disease—review of the literature. Int J Colorectal Dis. 2010;25:1149–57.
20. Present DH, Rutgeerts P, Targan S, Hanauer SB, Mayer L, van Hogezand RA, et al. Infliximab for the treatment of fistulas in patients with Crohn's disease. N Engl J Med. 1999;340:1398–405.
21. Lynch AC, Delaney CP, Senagore AJ, Connor JT, Remzi FH, Fazio VW. Clinical outcome and factors predictive of recurrence after enterocutaneous fistula surgery. Ann Surg. 2004;240:825–31.
22. Ramadas AV, Gunesh S, Thomas GA, Williams GT, Hawthorne AB. Natural history of Crohn's disease in a population-based cohort from Cardiff (1986–2003): a study of changes in medical treatment and surgical resection rates. Gut. 2010;59:1200–6.
23. Prabhakar LP, Laramee C, Nelson H, Dozois RR. Avoiding a stoma: role for segmental or abdominal colectomy in Crohn's colitis. Dis Colon Rectum. 1997;40:71–8.
24. Jess T, Gamborg M, Matzen P, Munkholm P, Sorensen TI. Increased risk of intestinal cancer in Crohn's disease: a meta-analysis of population-based cohort studies. Am J Gastroenterol. 2005;100:2724–9.
25. Schwartz DA, Wiersema MJ, Dudiak KM, Fletcher JG, Clain JE, Tremaine WJ, et al. A comparison of endoscopic ultrasound, magnetic resonance imaging, and exam under anesthesia for evaluation of Crohn's perianal fistulas. Gastroenterology. 2001;121:1064–72.
26. Schwartz DA, Ghazi LJ, Regueiro M. Guidelines for medical treatment of Crohn's perianal fistulas: critical evaluation of therapeutic trials. Inflamm Bowel Dis. 2015;21:737–52.
27. Gecse KB, Bemelman W, Kamm MA, Stoker J, Khanna R, Ng SC, et al. World Gastroenterology Organization, International Organisation for Inflammatory Bowel Diseases IOIBD and European Society of Coloproctology and Robarts Clinical Trials: a global

consensus on the classification, diagnosis and multidisciplinary treatment of perianal fistulising Crohn's disease. Gut. 2014;63:1381–92.
28. Grimaud JC, Munoz-Bongrand N, Siproudhis L, Abramowitz L, Sénéjoux A, Vitton V, et al. Fibrin glue is effective healing perianal fistulas in patients with Crohn's disease. Gastroenterology. 2010;138:2275–81.
29. O'Riordan JM, Datta I, Johnston C, Baxter NN. A systematic review of the anal fistula plug for patients with Crohn's and non-Crohn's related fistula-in-ano. Dis Colon Rectum. 2012;55:351–8.
30. O'Connor L, Champagne BJ, Ferguson MA, Orangio GR, Schertzer ME, Armstrong DN. Efficacy of anal fistula plug in closure of Crohn's anorectal fistulas. Dis Colon Rectum. 2006;49:1569–73.
31. Jacob TJ, Perakath B, Keighley MR. Surgical intervention for anorectal fistula. Cochrane Database Syst Rev. 2010;12:CD006319.
32. Hong KD, Kang S, Kalasker S, Wexner SD. Ligation of the intersphincteric fistula tract (LIFT) to treat anal fistula: systematic review and meta-analysis. Tech Coloproctol. 2014;18:685–91.
33. Gingold DS, Murrell ZA, Fleshner PR. A prospective evaluation of the ligation of the intersphincteric tract procedure for complex anal fistula in patients with Crohn's disease. Ann Surg. 2014;260:1057–61.
34. Cho YB, Park KJ, Yoon SN, Song KH, Kim S, Jung SH, et al. Long-term results of adipose-derived stem cell therapy for the treatment of Crohn's fistula. Stem Cell Transl Med. 2015;4:532–7.
35. Figg RE, Church JM. Perineal Crohn's disease: an indicator of poor prognosis and potential proctectomy. Dis Colon Rectum. 2009;52:646–50.
36. Burke JP, Velupillai Y, O'Connell PR, Coffey JC. National trends in intestinal resection for Crohn's disease in the post-biologic era. Int J Colorectal Dis. 2013;28:1401–6.
37. Metcalf AM. Elective and emergent operative management of ulcerative colitis. Surg Clin North Am. 2007;87:633–41.
38. Farmer RG, Easley KA, Rankin GB. Clinical patterns, natural history, and progression of ulcerative colitis. A long-term follow-up of 1116 patients. Dig Dis Sci. 1993;38:1137–46.
39. Cima RR. Timing and indications for colectomy in chronic ulcerative colitis: surgical consideration. Dig Dis. 2010;28:501–7.
40. Truelove SC, Witts LF. Cortisone in ulcerative colitis: final report on a therapeutic trial. Br Med J. 1955;2:1041–8.
41. Kulaylat MN, Dayton MT. Ulcerative colitis and cancer. J Surg Oncol. 2010;101:706–12.
42. Taylor BA, Pemberton JH, Carpenter HA, Levin KE, Schroeder KW, Welling DR, et al. Dysplasia in chronic ulcerative colitis: implications for colonoscopic surveillance. Dis Colon Rectum. 1992;35:950–6.
43. Gorfine SR, Bauer JJ, Harris MT, Kreel I. Dysplasia complicating chronic ulcerative colitis: is immediate colectomy warranted? Dis Colon Rectum. 2000;43:1575–81.
44. Ullman T, Croog V, Harpaz N, Sachar D, Itzkowitz S. Progression of flat low-grade dysplasia to advanced neoplasia in patients with ulcerative colitis. Gastroenterology. 2003;125:1311–9.
45. Odze RD, Farraye FA, Hecht JL, Hornick JL. Long-term follow-up after polypectomy treatment for adenoma-like dysplastic lesions in ulcerative colitis. Clin Gastroenterol Hepatol. 2004;2:534–41.
46. Browning SM, Nivatvongs S. Intraoperative abandonment of ileal pouch to anal anastomosis—the Mayo Clinic experience. J Am Coll Surg. 1998;186:441–5. discussion 445–6.
47. Cima RR, Young-Fadok TM, Pemberton JH. Chapter 27": Procedures for ulcerative colitis. 4. Alimentary tract and abdomen. In: Souba WW, Fink MP, Jurkovich GJ, et al., editors. ACS surgery: principles & practice. New York: WebMD Inc.; 2005. p. 674.
48. Dunker MS, Bemelman WA, Slors JFM, van Duijvendijk P, Gouma DJ. Functional outcome, quality of life, body image, and cosmesis in patients after laparoscopic-assisted and conventional restorative proctocolectomy: a comparative study. Dis Colon Rectum. 2001;44:1800–7.
49. Larson DW, Cima RR, Dozois EJ, Davies M, Piotrowicz K, Barnes SA, et al. Safety, feasibility, and short-term outcomes of laparoscopic ileal-pouch-anal anastomosis: a single institutional case-matched experience. Ann Surg. 2006;243:667–70. discussion 670–2.
50. Causey MW, Stoddard D, Johnson EK, Maykel JA, Martin MJ, Rivadeneira D, et al. Laparoscopy impacts outcomes favorably following colectomy for ulcerative colitis: a critical analysis of the ACS-NSQIP database. Surg Endosc. 2013;27:603–9.
51. Fleming FJ, Francone TD, Kim MJ, Gunzler D, Messing S, Monson JRT. A laparoscopic approach does reduce short-term complications in patients undergoing ileal pouch-anal anastomosis. Dis Colon Rectum. 2011;54:176–82.
52. Meagher AP, Farouk R, Dozois RR, Kelly KA, Pemberton JH. J ileal pouch-anal anastomosis for chronic ulcerative colitis: complications and long-term outcome in 1310 patients. Br J Surg. 1998;85:800–3.
53. Marcello PW, Robert PL, Schoetz Jr DJ, Coller JA, Murray JJ, Veidenheimer MC. Long-term results of ileoanal pouch procedure. Arch Surg. 1993;128:500–3.
54. Romanos J, Samarasekera DN, Stebbing JF, Jewell DP, Kettlewell MG, Mortensen NJ. Outcomes of 200 restorative proctocolectomy operations: the John Radcliffe Hospital experience. Br J Surg. 1997;84:814–8.
55. El-Gazzaz GS, Kiran RP, Remzi FH, Hull TL, Geisler DP. Outcomes for case-matched laparoscopically assisted versus open restorative proctocolectomy. Br J Surg. 2009;96:522–6.
56. Hahnloser D, Pemberton JH, Wolff BG, Larson DR, Crownhart BS, Dozois RR. Results at up to 20 years after ileal pouch-anal anastomosis for chronic ulcerative colitis. Br J Surg. 2007;94:333–40.
57. Bullard KM, Madoff RD, Gemlo BT. Is ileoanal pouch function stable with time? Results of a prospective audit. Dis Colon Rectum. 2002;45:299–304.
58. Fazio VW, Ziv Y, Church JM, Oakley JR, Lavery IC, Milsom JW, et al. Ileal pouch-anal anastomoses complications and function in 1005 patients. Ann Surg. 1995;222:120–7.
59. Fazio VW, O'Riordan MG, Lavery IC, Church JM, Lau P, Strong SA, et al. Long-term functional outcome and quality of life after stapled restorative proctocolectomy. Ann Surg. 1999;230:575–84.
60. Galandiuk S, Scott NA, Dozois RR, Kelly KA, Ilstrup DM, Beart Jr RW, et al. Ileal pouch-anal anastomosis: reoperation for pouch-related complications. Ann Surg. 1990;212:446–52.
61. MacLean AR, Cohen Z, MacRae HM, O'Connor BI, Mukraj D, Kennedy ED, et al. Risk of small bowel obstruction after the ileal pouch-anal anastomosis. Ann Surg. 2002;235:200–6.
62. Indar AA, Efron JE, Young-Fadok TM. Laparoscopic ileal pouch-anal anastomosis reduces abdominal and pelvic adhesions. Surg Endosc. 2009;23:174–7.
63. Ferrante M, Declerck S, De Hertogh G, Van Assche G, Geboes K, Rutgeerts P, et al. Outcome after proctocolectomy with ileal pouch-anal anastomosis for ulcerative colitis. Inflamm Bowel Dis. 2008;14:20–8.
64. Yu ED, Shao Z, Shen B. Pouchitis. World J Gastroenterol. 2007;13:5598–604.
65. Holubar SD, Cima RR, Sandborn WJ, Pardi DS. Treatment and prevention of pouchitis after ileal pouch-anal anastomosis for chronic ulcerative colitis. Cochrane Database Syst Rev. 2010;6:CD001176.
66. Sugarman HJ, Sugerman EL, Meador JG, Newsome Jr HH, Kellum Jr JM, DeMaria EJ. Ileal pouch anal anastomosis without ileal diversion. Ann Surg. 2000;232:530–41.
67. Heuschen UA, Hinz U, Allemeyer EH, Lucas M, Heuschen G, Herfarth C. One- or two-stage procedure for restorative proctocolectomy: rationale for a surgical strategy in ulcerative colitis. Ann Surg. 2002;234:788–94.

68. Grobler SP, Hosie KB, Keighly MRB. Randomized trial of loop ileostomy in restorative proctocolectomy. Br J Surg. 1992;79: 903–6.
69. Williamson MER, Lewis WG, Sagar PM, Holdsworth PJ, Johnston D. One-stage restorative proctocolectomy without temporary ileostomy for ulcerative colitis: a note of caution. Dis Colon Rectum. 1997;40:1019–22.
70. Tan HT, Connolly AB, Morton D, Keighley MR. Results of restorative proctocolectomy in the elderly. Int J Colorectal Dis. 1997;12:319–22.
71. Olsen KØ, Joelsson M, Laurberg S, Järvinen HJ. Fertility after ileal pouch-anal anastomosis in women with ulcerative colitis. Br J Surg. 1999;86:493–5.
72. Lepistö A, Sarna S, Tiitinen A, Järvinen HJ. Female fertility and childbirth after ileal pouch-anal anastomosis for ulcerative colitis. Br J Surg. 2007;94:478–82.
73. Waljee A, Waljee J, Morris AM, Higgins PD. Threefold increased risk of infertility: a meta-analysis of infertility after ileal pouch anal anastomosis in ulcerative colitis. Gut. 2006;55:1575–80.
74. Mortier PE, Gambiez L, Karoui M, Cortot A, Paris JC, Quandalle P, et al. Colectomy with ileorectal anastomosis preserves female fertility in ulcerative colitis. Gastroenterol Clin Biol. 2006;30: 594–7.
75. Olsen KØ, Juul S, Bülow S, Järvinen HJ, Bakka A, Björk J, et al. Female fecundity before and after operation for familial adenomatous polyposis. Br J Surg. 2003;90:227–31.
76. Hull TL, Joyce MR, Geisler DP, Coffey JC. Adhesions after laparoscopic and open ileal pouch-anal anastomosis surgery for ulcerative colitis. Br J Surg. 2012;99:270–5.
77. Scott HJ, McLeod RS, Blair J, O'Connor B, Cohen Z. Ileal pouch-anal anastomosis: pregnancy, delivery and pouch function. Int J Colorectal Dis. 1996;11:84–7.
78. Seligman NS, Sbar W, Berghella V. Pouch function and gastrointestinal complications during pregnancy after ileal pouch-anal anastomosis. J Matern Fetal Neonatal Med. 2011;24: 525–30.
79. Shen B, Patel S, Lian L. Natural history of Crohn's disease in patient who underwent intentional restorative proctocolectomy with ileal pouch-anal anastomosis. Aliment Pharmacol Ther. 2010;31:745–53.
80. Hartley JE, Fazio VW, Remzi FH, Lavery IC, Church JM, Strong SA, et al. Analysis of the outcome of ileal pouch-anal anastomosis in patients with Crohn's disease. Dis Colon Rectum. 2004;47: 1808–15.
81. Regimbeau JM, Panis Y, Pocard M, Bouhnik Y, Lavergne-Stove A, Rufat P, et al. Long-term results of ileal-pouch anal anastomosis of colorectal Crohn's disease. Dis Colon Rectum. 2001;44: 769–76.
82. Le Q, Dubinsky M, McGovern D, Vasiliauskas EA, Ippoliti A, Shih D, et al. Surgical outcomes of ileal pouch-anal anastomosis when used intentionally for well-defined Crohn's disease. Inflamm Bowel Dis. 2013;19:30–6.
83. Yamamoto T, Allan RN, Keighley MR. Risk factors for intra-abdominal sepsis after surgery in Crohn's disease. Dis Colon Rectum. 2000;43:1141–5.
84. Huang W, Tang Y, Nong L, Sun Y. Risk factors for postoperative intra-abdominal septic complications after surgery in Crohn's disease: a meta-analysis of observational studies. J Crohns Colitis. 2015;9:293–301.
85. Farouk R, Pemberton JH, Wolff BG, Dozois RR, Browning S, Larson D. Functional outcomes after ileal pouch-anal anastomosis for chronic ulcerative colitis. Ann Surg. 2000;231:919–26.
86. Selvasekar CR, Cima RR, Larson DW, Dozois EJ, Harrington JR, Harmsen WS, et al. Effect of infliximab on short-term complications in patients undergoing operation for chronic ulcerative colitis. J Am Coll Surg. 2007;204:956–63.
87. Mor IJ, Vogel JD, da Luz Moreira A, Shen B, Hammel J, Remzi FH. Infliximab in ulcerative colitis is associated with an increased risk of postoperative complications after restorative proctocolectomy. Dis Colon Rectum. 2008;51:1202–10.
88. Ferrante M, D'Hoore A, Vermeire S, Declerck S, Norman M, Van Assche G, et al. Corticosteroids but not infliximab increase short-term postoperative infectious complication in patients with ulcerative colitis. Inflamm Bowel Dis. 2009;15:1062–70.
89. Kunitake H, Hodin R, Shellito PC, Sands BE, Korzenik J, Bordeianou L. Perioperative treatment with infliximab in patients with Crohn's disease and ulcerative colitis is not associated with an increased rate of postoperative complications. J Gastrointestinal Surg. 2008;12:1730–7.
90. Myrelid P, Marti-Gallostra MM, Sunde ML, Tholin M, Oresland T, Lovegrove RE, et al. Complications in surgery for Crohn's disease after preoperative antitumour necrosis factor therapy. Br J Surg. 2014;101:539–45.
91. Syed A, Cross RK, Flaser MH. Anti-tumor necrosis factor therapy is associated with infections after abdominal surgery in Crohn's disease patients. Am J Gastroenterol. 2013;108:583–93.
92. Ahmed U, Martin ST, Rao AD, Kiran RP. Impact of preoperative immunosuppressive agents on postoperative outcomes in Crohn's disease. Dis Colon Rectum. 2014;57:663–74.
93. Billious V, ford AC, Tedesco ED, Colombel JF, Roblin X, Peyrin-Biroulet LP. Preoperative use of anti-TNF and postoperative complications in inflammatory bowel diseases: a meta-analysis. J Crohns Colitis. 2013;7:853–67.
94. El-Hussuna A, Krag A, Olaison G, Bendsten F, Gluud LL. The effect of anti-tumor necrosis factor alpha agents on postoperative anastomotic complications in Crohn's disease: a systematic review. Dis Colon Rectum. 2013;56:1423–33.
95. Narula N, Charleton D, Marshall JK. Meta-analysis: peri-operative anti-TNFα treatment and postoperative complications in patients with inflammatory bowel disease. Aliment Pharmacol Ther. 2013;37:1057–64.

Part VI

Extraintestinal Manifestations

Extraintestinal Manifestations: Autoimmune Hepatitis

51

Michael P. Manns and Nora Schweitzer

Definition

The most common liver disease in inflammatory bowel disease (IBD) is primary sclerosing cholangitis (PSC). The main diagnostic tool to confirm PSC is a cholangiography. In case of a normal cholangiography, a small-duct PSC should be considered and can be ruled out by liver biopsy. One important differential diagnosis of liver diseases in IBD is autoimmune hepatitis (AIH) and in some series, 17 % of the AIH-patients had IBD [1].

AIH is a chronic progressive inflammation of the liver of unknown origin. It is characterized by elevated aminotransferases, bilirubin, and γ-globulins, the presence of autoantibodies, and a typical histological picture with interface hepatitis and plasma cell infiltration. Untreated, the prognosis of AIH is poor and studies in the 1970s revealed a 5-year overall survival of 50 %. Notably, these data are limited by the lacking ability to test for HCV at that time. At the time of diagnosis, cirrhosis is present in 30 % of the patients [2]. Albeit pathogenesis is not entirely understood, genetic predisposition, loss of immune tolerance, and environmental factors play important roles in the development of AIH. According to the antibody-pattern, two types of AIH are differentiated. In type1 AIH, antinuclear antibodies (ANA) and smooth muscle antibodies (SMA) are predominant, whereas in type 2 AIH, antibodies to liver/kidney microsome 1 (anti-LKM-1) are characteristic. The latter is mainly seen in children and adolescents. In Norway and Sweden, the point prevalence is 11–17 per 100,000 persons per year and the incidence 1–2 per 100,000 persons per year [3]. Similar data are supposed to be found for the Caucasians in North America.

M.P. Manns, M.D. (✉) • N. Schweitzer, M.D.
Department of Gastroenterology, Hepatology and Endocrinology, Hannover Medical School, Carl-Neuberg-Strasse 1, Hannover 30625, Germany
e-mail: manns.michael@mh-hannover.de

Clinical Presentation

The onset of AIH is usually insidious and up to 34–45 % of patients are asymptomatic. Symptomatic patients often present with nonspecific symptoms as fatigue, jaundice, abdominal pain, weight loss, or arthralgias. In general, the complaints are not specific for AIH and range from asymptomatic individuals to individuals with severe and acute threatening disease with severe liver dysfunction. Other autoimmune disorders, e.g., autoimmune thyroiditis, rheumatoid arthritis, or IBD are common in the medical history of the patient or first-degree family members. AIH can occur at every age and in all ethnical groups. Women are more often affected than men (3.6:1). The main complication of AIH is the progression to liver cirrhosis with severe consequences, e.g., the development of ascites, hepatic encephalopathy, and variceal bleeding. In the case of cirrhosis, patients are at risk for developing hepatocellular carcinoma. Studies in the past revealed that patients with IBD and AIH without signs of cholangitis have a better outcome compared to those with an abnormal cholangiography [1].

Diagnosis

Diagnostic Scores

As there exists no single AIH-specific diagnostic criterion, diagnosis is established by a combination of a typical autoantibody pattern, certain histological findings, and elevated immunoglobulins and aminotransferases. Confirmation of the diagnosis requires the exclusion of other hepatopathies such as viral hepatitis, cholestatic liver diseases or metabolic disorders. In 1993, the International Autoimmune Hepatitis Group (IAIHG) formulated descriptive criteria and a scoring system for diagnosing definite or probable AIH. A review of the scoring system was undertaken in 1999 (Table 51.1) [4, 5]. In clinical practice, the descriptive criteria are sufficient to

D.C. Baumgart (ed.), *Crohn's Disease and Ulcerative Colitis*, DOI 10.1007/978-3-319-33703-6_51

Table 51.1 Revised Original Scoring System of the International Autoimmune Hepatitis Group [4]

Gender	Female	+2	HLA	DR3 or DR4	+1
AP:AST (or ALT) ratio	>3 <1.5	−2 +2	Immune disease	Thyroiditis, colitis, others	+2
γ-Globulin or IgG level above normal	>2.0 1.5–2.0 1.0–1.5 <1.0	+3 +2 +1 0	Other markers	Anti-SLA, actin, LC1, pANCA	+2
ANA, SMA, or anti-LKM1 titers	>1:80 1:80 1:40 <1:40	+3 +2 +1 0	Histological features	Interface hepatitis Plasmacytic Rosettes None of above Biliary changes Other features	+3 +1 +1 −5 −3 −3
AMA	Positive	−4	Treatment response	Complete Relapse	+2 +3
Viral markers	Positive Negative	−3 +3			
Drugs	Yes No	−4 +1	Pretreatment aggregate score: Definite diagnosis >15 Probable diagnosis 10–15		

diagnose AIH in most cases. For more challenging cases, the revised original scoring system, which was originally made for clinical trials, can be applied. This score includes the patient's gender, the ratio between alkaline phosphatase (AP) and AST, the γ-globulin or IgG-level, antibodies, viral markers, drug or alcohol intake, HLA type, other immune diseases, histological features, and the response to treatment. A pretreatment score of 10–15 points or a posttreatment score of 12–17 points are required for the diagnosis "probable AIH," whereas a pretreatment score of 16 or higher and a posttreatment score of more than 17 leads to the diagnosis "definite AIH." The sensitivity of the pretreatment score of 10 points (probable AIH) and pretreatment score of 15 (definite AIH) is 100 % and 95 %, the specificity 73 % and 97 % and the diagnostic accuracy 67 % and 94 %, respectively. In 2006, simplified diagnostic criteria containing only four parameters (autoantibodies, IgG-level, histology, absences of viral hepatitis) were published with 88 % sensitivity and 97 % specificity for probable AIH (≥6 points) and 81 % sensitivity and 99 % specificity for definite AIH (≥7 points) (Table 51.2) [6]. The simplified scoring system showed reliability in worldwide studies, however, prospective studies are lacking [7–10].

Table 51.2 Simplified diagnostic criteria for autoimmune hepatitis, according to Hennes et al., Hepatology (2008) [6][a]

Variable	Cutoff	Points
ANA or SMA	≥1:40	1
ANA or SMA	≥1:80	
or LKM	≥1:40	2[a]
or SLA	Positive	
IgG	>Upper normal limit	1
	>1.10 times upper normal limit	2
Liver histology (evidence of hepatitis is a necessary condition)	Compatible with AIH Typical AIH	1 2
Absence of viral hepatitis	Yes	2
		≥6: probable AIH
		≥7 definite AIH

[a]Addition of points achieved for all autoantibodies (maximum, 2 points)

Biochemical Findings

One characteristic biochemical abnormality of AIH is hypergammaglobulinemia in the absence of cirrhosis with selective elevation of serum IgG. Typically, IgA and IgM remain normal. The elevation of IgG is not only important for diagnosing AIH but also a reliable marker of disease activity. Elevation of liver enzymes shows a hepatitic pattern in most cases. However, aminotransferase activity (ALT, AST) and bilirubinemia may range from just above the upper limit of normal (ULN) to 50-fold ULN, but this level does not correlate to histological inflammatory activity [11]. AP and γ-glutamyl transferase (γGT) usually are only moderately elevated or normal. In patients with liver cirrhosis, thrombopenia, hypalbuminemia, and elevated INR levels may be present.

Autoantibodies

The serological assessment of the diagnosis includes testing ANA, SMA, anti-LKM-1, and anti-liver cytosol type 1-antibodies (anti-LC1). The majority of adult patients show significant titers (>1:40) of ANA, SMA, or both, 3–4 % are positive for anti-LKM1 and up to 20 % present with no antibodies. None of these antibodies is specific for AIH and their presence is not sufficient for affirming the diagnosis nor does their absence preclude AIH. The expression of antibodies can vary during the course of disease, but in contrast to children, the titer level does not correlate to disease activity in adults. In case of seronegativity for ANA, SMA, and anti-LKM-1, testing for atypical perinuclear staining antineutrophil cytoplasmatic antibodies (pANCA) and antibodies to soluble liver antigen (SLA/LP) should be performed. Atypical pANCA were originally considered to be specific for IBD and PSC [12, 13] but are also found in AIH, sometimes as the only positive antibody. Anti-SLA have a limited sensitivity but a high specificity for AIH. Moreover, the presence of anti-SLA is associated with a more severe course of disease and a worse outcome [14, 15]. Serological evaluation should include AMA to preclude PBC. For further investigation of seronegative patients, LKM-2 and -3 antibodies, and LM antibodies (Table 51.3) may be of interest. For a valid diagnosis, the exclusion of other liver diseases is essential. In particular, hereditary disorders as Wilson disease and alpha 1 antitrypsin deficiency, viral hepatitis, steatohepatitis, and drug induced hepatitis should be ruled out. The differentiation between AIH and the autoimmune cholestatic liver diseases PBC or PSC may be difficult, but the effort should be undertaken given the implications for treatment regimen and prognosis.

Histology

A liver biopsy is recommended for establishing the diagnosis and for evaluation of the response to treatment. In patients with coexisting IBD, it is also useful to rule out small duct PSC. Although the histological appearance of AIH is characteristic, there are no pathognomonic features. Typical findings are mononuclear cell infiltrates with infiltration of the limiting plate, also called piece meal necrosis or interface hepatitis, which can progress to lobular hepatitis or central–portal bridging necrosis. Plasma cell infiltrates are regularly seen. Biliary lesions as ductopenia or destructive cholangitis or granulomas are indicative for a different diagnosis. Fibrosis is seen in all but the mildest forms and the degree ranges from mild fibrosis to bridging fibrosis or cirrhosis (Fig.51.1).

Table 51.3 Antibodies in autoimmune hepatitis [43]

Antibody	Target antigen(s)	Liver disease	Value in AIH
ANA*	Multiple targets including: • Chromatin • Ribonucleoproteins • Ribonucleoprotein complexes	AIH PBC PSC Drug-induced: Chronic hepatitis C Chronic hepatitis B Nonalcoholic fatty liver disease	Diagnosis of type 1 AIH
SMA*	Microfilaments (filamentous actin) and intermediate filaments (vimentin, desmin)	Same as ANA	Diagnosis of type 1 AIH
LKM-1*	Cytochrome P450 2D6 (CYP2D6)	Type 2 AIH Chronic hepatitis C	Diagnosis of type 2 AIH
LC-1*	Formiminotransferase cyclodeaminase (FTCD)	Type 2 AIH Chronic hepatitis C	Diagnosis of type 2 AIH Prognostic implications Severe disease
pANCA (atypical)	Nuclear lamina proteins	AIH PSC	Diagnosis of type 1 AIH Reclassification of cryptogenic chronic hepatitis as type 1 AIH
SLA	Soluble liver antigen	AIH Chronic hepatitis C	Diagnosis of AIH Prognostic implications Severe disease Relapse Treatment dependence
LKM3	UDP-glucuronosyl-transferases type 1 (UGT1A)	Chronic hepatitis D Type 2 AIH	Diagnosis of type 2 AIH
ASGPR	Asialoglycoprotein receptor	AIH PBC Drug-induced hepatitis Chronic hepatitis B, C, D	Prognostic implications Severe disease Histological activity Relapse
LKM2	Cytochrome P450 2C9	Ticrynafen-induced hepatitis	None, does not occur after withdrawal of ticrynafen
LM	Cytochrome P450 1A2	Dihydralazine-induced hepatitis APECED hepatitis	Diagnosis of APECED hepatitis

*Antibodies indicating the conventional serological repertoire for the diagnosis of AIH. The other autoantibodes may bese useful in patients who lack the conventional autoantibody markers

AIH autoimmune hepatitis, *ANA* antinuclear antibody, *APECED* autoimmune polyendocrinopathy-candidiasectodermal dystrophy, *ASGPR* antibody to asialoglycoprotein receptor, *LC1* liver cytosol type 1, *LKM* liver kidney/microsome, *LM* liver microsome antibody, *pANCA* perinuclear anti-neutrophil cytoplasmic antibody, *PBC* primary biliary cirrhosis, *PSC* primary sclerosing cholangitis, *SLA* soluble liver antigen, *SMA* smooth muscle antibody, *UGT* uridine diphosphate glucuronosyltransferase

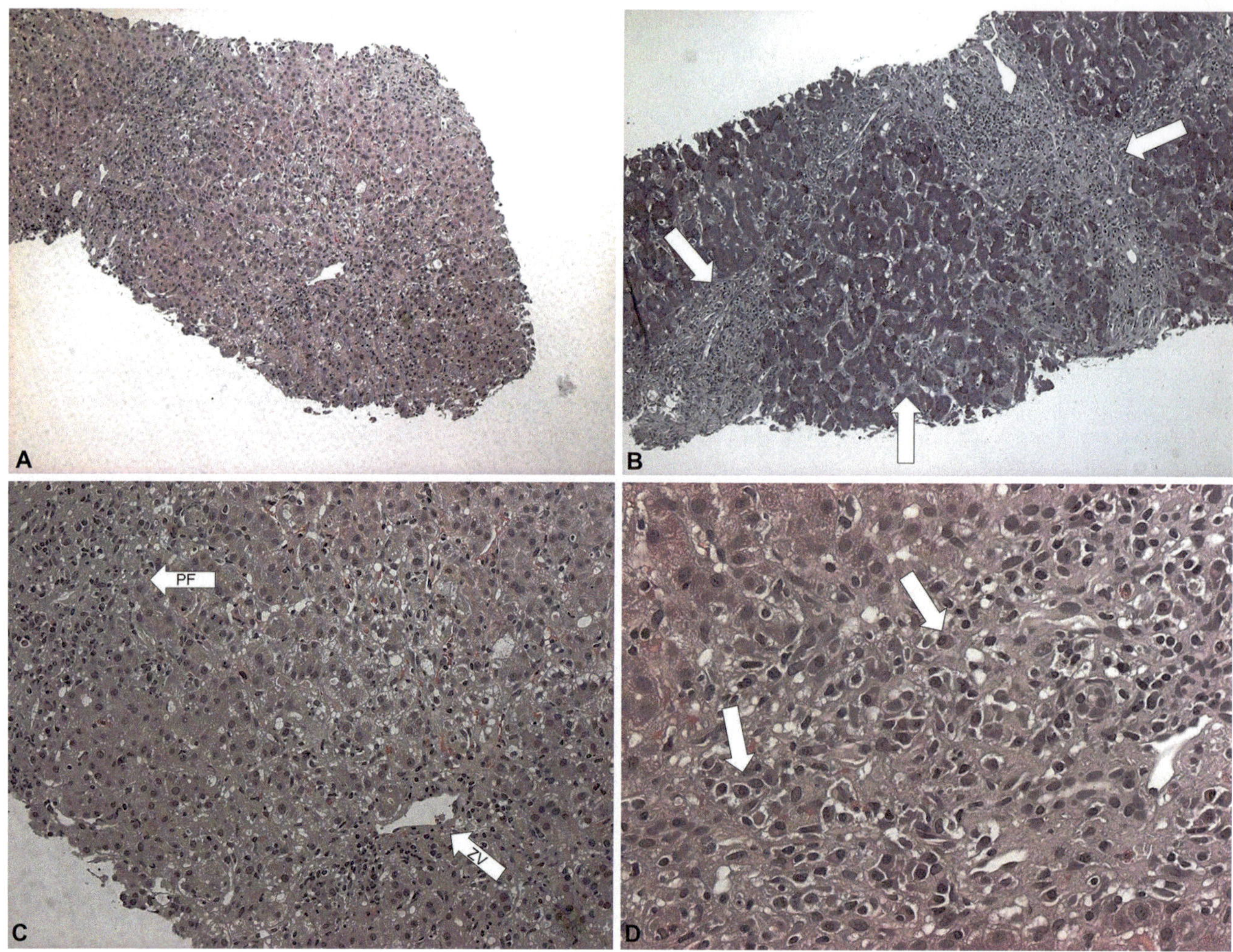

Fig. 51.1 (**a–d**) Histological findings in autoimmune hepatitis A: broadened periportal fields and lobules with lymphocytic infiltration (HE ×100). (**b**) Bridging fibrosis (*arrows*) between remaining parts of lobuli (*lower arrow*) (PAS ×100). (**c**) Lymphoplasmacytic infiltration of periportal field (PF) and lobuli (ZV=central vein) with piecemeal necrosis and single cell necrosis (HE ×200). (**d**) Wide plasmacellular infiltration in a periportal field beside lymphocytes and eosinophilic granulocytes (HE ×400). All figures kindly provided by Prof. H.-P. Kreipe, Medical School Hannover

Diagnostic Difficulties: Overlap Syndrome

Diagnosing AIH is especially delicate in autoantibody-negative patients. If AIH is suspected in an autoantibody-negative patient, a liver biopsy may become of immense importance. Otherwise, the patients are diagnosed and treated late.

Also the setting of autoantibodies or other results matching to more than one autoimmune liver disease may cause confusion. Overlapping features of AIH and PSC or AIH and PBC are not uncommon. Practically, that means for example that a patient with AIH can be AMA-positive, what is highly specific for PBC. Or a patient with AIH presents with an abnormal cholangiography, being indicative for PSC. Some authors also count AMA-negative patients with otherwise typical PBC to AIH-PBC overlap or "autoimmune cholangitis." The overlapping diseases can appear simultaneously or sequentially in one individual patient. However, criteria for diagnosing an overlap are lacking and there are ongoing discussions about the terminology and diagnostic criteria [16]. This is why the estimated prevalence of AIH-PSC overlap ranges from 7.6 % to 53.8 % in different studies [17]. Overlaps of AIH and PBC can be found in 5–10 % of the patients with AIH. In patients with IBD and AIH, an overlap with PSC should always be considered. Particularly children present overlapping signs of AIH and PSC very often (30–50 %) [18]. The AIH-PSC overlap in children is also called "autoimmune sclerosing cholangitis." In clinical practice, patients often require therapy both with anti-inflammatory agents and ursodeoxycholic acid. The prognosis of the AIH-PSC overlap is worse than of AIH alone, mainly because of the risk of developing a malignancy, which is highly elevated in PSC [19]. The outcome of the AIH-PBC overlap is better than in AIH alone [20].

Similar to AIH patients, sera of HCV-infected patients are frequently positive for ANA, SMA, and LKM. LKM-1 antibodies are found in 5–10 % of patients with chronic HCV infection. The clinical relevance of these autoantibodies for HCV patients remains elusive. LKM are regarded as autoimmune phenomena associated with HCV infection, only high titer antibodies are considered to be a sign for a relevant autoimmune reaction. In individual patients, hepatitic flares can occur under interferon based treatment for HCV.

Pathogenesis

Cellular Autoimmunity

The pathogenesis of AIH is not entirely understood. One concept is that in a genetically predisposed individual, environmental factors (e.g., viruses, drugs) can provoke AIH by initiating immune processes. The histological hallmark of AIH is a portal mononuclear cell infiltrate with T and B lymphocytes, macrophages and plasma cells. This massive inflammatory infiltration enables acute and ongoing liver damage. Among the T cells, the majority are CD4 positive. There is evidence for an alteration in T and B cell function in AIH. In particular, the peripheral blood, regulatory T cells (CD4+CD25+ Treg cells) are reduced both in number and function [5, 21] in patients with AIH. In contrast, they accumulate in the liver of untreated adult AIH patients [22, 23]. Under immunosuppression, a loss of intrahepatic Tregs was reported [23]. Tregs are important modulators of CD8+ cells. They control the innate and adaptive immune reaction by inhibition of autoreactive T cells. They go in direct contact with the target cells, reduce interferon production, and increase the secretion of IL-4, IL-10, and TGFß. Studies of Treg function in family members of AIH patients suggest a genetic relation [24].

Autoantigens

Beside self-reactive B and T cells, autoantigens that are presented by MHC class II molecules are required for an autoimmune process in the liver. For a number of autoantibodies found in AIH, the target antigen is known. In AIH type 2, the antigen of anti-LKM-1 antibodies is the enzyme cytochrome P450 2D6 (CYP2D6). Mouse models that express the human antigenic region of CYP2D6 produce antibodies, and develop hepatitis [25]. Anti-LKM-3 antibodies react with UGT [26]. The substrate of anti-SLA is the transfer ribonucleoprotein complex $tRNP^{(Ser)Sec}$, renamed SEPSECS (Sep [O-phosphoserine] tRNA:Sec[selenocysteine] t RNA synthase) [27–29] and anti-LC1 recognizes formiminotransferase cyclodeaminase [30, 31] The target antigen of anti-LM antibodies is CYP1A2 and was first described in patients with a dihydralazine-induced AIH. Furthermore, they are found in patients with APECED (see below). Thus, several specific autoantigens in AIH are known but their role in pathogenesis remains unclear.

Molecular Mimicry

There is growing evidence suggesting that molecular mimicry plays a key role in the generation of liver-specific autoantibodies. Molecular mimicry relies on the similarity of infectious agents with host antigens. Such similarity may lead to an inability of the host immune system to recognize the foreign antigen or it may lead to an autoreactive immune response by cross-reactivity. One well-described example for postinfectious autoimmunity is the acute rheumatic fever, which occurs after contact to antigenic epitopes of streptococcus pyogenes. Sequence homologies between CYP2D6 and HCV, the common viruses herpes simplex virus type 1 (HSV1), cytomegalovirus (CMV), Epstein–Barr virus (EBV), and human adenovirus [32, 33] have been discovered. In mice, AIH can be induced by an infection with an adenovirus carrying human CYP2D6 or FTCD [34]. Also cross-reactivity between HCV, SMA, and ANA were described [35]. According to the "multiple hit-theory," in genetically predisposed patients multiple contacts to viruses might induce a cross-reactive subset of T-cells and permit a loss of immunological self-tolerance.

Genetic Influences

AIH is a complex polygenetic disorder and does not follow a Mendelian pattern. Multiple genetic associations with the major histocompatibility complex (MHC) locus have been described. The MHC region is located on the short arm of chromosome 6 and encodes the human leukocyte antigens (HLA). In Caucasian Europeans and North Americans, HLA DRB1*0301 and DRB1*0401 are associated with a susceptibility to AIH [35, 36]. The significance of this relation lies in the observation that most autoimmune diseases are T cell dependent and that T cell response is MHC restricted [37, 38]. HLA alleles not only cause susceptibility to AIH but also seem to have influence on the course of the disease: patients with DRB1*0301 are younger at diagnosis and have a higher frequency of treatment failure. HLA B8 is associated with a more severe disease and HLA DRB1*0401 develop other autoimmune diseases more often [36, 39]. Beyond that, genes outside the MHC might also contribute to autoimmunity, e.g., the cytotoxic T lymphocyte antigen 4 (CTL4) and a number of SNPs of various genes including cytokines, vitamin D receptor, CD45, and Fas receptor.

One well defined exception is AIH in the setting of the rare autoimmune polyendocrinopathy-candidiasis-ectodermal dystrophy (APECED). APECED is caused by a single-gene mutation on chromosome 21q22.3 which results in a defect autoimmune regulator (AIRE) protein. Patients with this autosomal recessive inherited disease suffer from multiple endocrine organ failure, mucocutaneous candidiasis and ectodermal dystrophy.

Treatment

Treatment Regimens

The outcome of untreated AIH can be fatal. Immunosuppression is the treatment of choice for AIH [40–43]. Treatment goal is the normalization of ALT, AST, and IgG. The complete normalization is a prerequisite for avoiding disease progression. Once remission is achieved, a maintenance therapy for at least 2 years with the lowest possible doses of immunosuppressive agents is the treatment of choice. It is eminently important to diagnose AIH in early stages of the disease to prevent the progression to severe fibrosis or cirrhosis. In fact, cirrhosis at presentation is a predictor for a poor outcome [2]. Around one third of adult patients already present with histological features of cirrhosis at diagnosis [2]. However, consequent treatment can lead to a certain regression of fibrosis [44] and only in a minority, a progress of fibrosis under treatment occurs. Those are mainly patients with treatment failure of corticosteroids.

Two strategies are equally effective in the treatment of AIH:

1. Prednisone alone in a dose of 60 mg per day, or
2. Prednisone in a lower dose (30 mg daily) in combination with azathioprine in a daily dose of 50 mg (or 1–2 mg/kg body weight) [43].

In patients without cirrhosis, in the combined regimen prednisone can be replaced by budesonide, a steroid with a low systemic effect due to a 90 % first pass effect. The starting dose of budesonide is 9 mg/day. In adjunction to azathioprine it was capable to induce complete remission in non-cirrhotic patients while the rate of steroid related side effects was much lower than in the group treated with prednisone and azathioprine [45].

For all three regimens, improvements in biochemical and histological signs of inflammation and an amelioration of symptoms were shown [40–42, 45]. It is evident that immunosuppressive treatment of chronic active hepatitis improves the outcome and the 20-year life expectancy can be enhanced to 80 % [44]. After remission, prednisone can be tapered down to an individual dosage sufficient to maintain remission. It is important not to reduce doses before the goal of treatment is reached. An early titration is associated with a delayed histological improvement and with a prolonged duration of therapy [43]. Until the dose of 20 mg, weekly reduction of 10 mg is adequate, below the dose of 20 mg prednisone, reduction should not exceed 5 mg per week and at a daily dose of 10 mg, 2.5 mg should be reduced weekly until a daily dose of 5 mg. The advantage of the combined therapy regimen is the lower occurrence of steroid related side effects. Therefore, the combination of prednisone/budesonide and azathioprine is the preferred treatment [43]. In Europe, prednisolone is preferred over prednisone. A single therapy with prednisone is appropriate for patients who are at high risk for azathioprine related adverse events. Those are patients with cytopenia, pregnant women or those planning a pregnancy, patients with malignancies and individuals with complete thiopurine methyltransferase deficiency. Furthermore, a sole therapy with prednisone is suggested when a short time of treatment is probable. Patients with increased risk for steroid related side effects should obtain the combined treatment. Those are postmenopausal females, patients with osteoporosis, diabetes or brittle diabetes, obesity or hypertension and last but not least emotional instable individuals.

Independently from the used agent(s), treatment should be continued until remission, treatment failure, incomplete response or drug toxicity [43]. There is no scheduled minimum or maximum duration of immunosuppressive treatment in AIH. It should rather be adapted to the individual course of disease.

Over the last decades it has become evident that an individualized therapy is necessary for optimal treatment.

For example, it is unclear how to manage *asymptomatic patients* best. Asymptomatic patients are most often identified by incidental abnormal liver tests. They tend to be older than symptomatic patients, have a higher frequency of "probable AIH" vs. "definite AIH" but show cirrhosis as often as symptomatic patients. Spontaneous remission is seldom in this group. It is not proven that the outcome of asymptomatic patients ameliorates when treated with corticosteroids and/or azathioprine. For instance, Fedl et al. reported similar prognosis in treated and in untreated asymptomatic patients [2].

Also in *elderlies*, higher stages of fibrosis before treatment than in younger individuals were reported, but this does not result in a higher frequency of definite cirrhosis. Elderly patients have a high percentage of remission [46], but, however, in one study, untreated elder patients had the same prognosis as younger and treated individuals. Thus, it is a matter of debate how to treat elderly patients properly.

Children generally do respond well to treatment but have cirrhosis in almost 50 % at presentation. They need long-term or even lifelong immunosuppressive treatment in most cases and despite that, they require liver transplantation in 15 % before the age of 18 [47].

In patients with end-stage disease without inflammatory activity, meaning *inactive or "burned out" cirrhosis*, a treatment is not indicated and even can be harmful because of higher drug toxicity.

Finally, the clinical picture, treatment response and outcome vary between *ethnic groups*. Black North Americans are younger and present more often with cirrhosis than white North Americans. Also, patients from South America, Africa and Asia have an earlier onset of the disease and are icteric in many cases.

Adjunctive Therapies

In awareness of the patient's individual risk, adjunctive therapies should be applied to reduce treatment-related toxicity. Besides regular weight bearing exercise program, a supplementation of vitamin D and calcium should be standard under therapy with steroids. For individual patients at high risk, the administration of bisphosphonates may be appropriate. In general, people on long-term corticosteroid treatment should be monitored for bone disease [43].

Vaccination against HAV and HBV should be done in every patient with AIH, and if possible, before the initiation of immunosuppression.

Treatment Related Side Effects

During corticosteroid therapy, in up to 80 %, distracting cosmetic changes occur: weight gain, facial rounding, striae distensae, acne, alopecia, and facial hirsutism. More severe adverse effects include opportunistic infections, osteopenia and pathological fractures, brittle diabetes, labile hypertension, and psychosis. 13 % of premature drug withdrawal is attributed to steroid related side effects and nearly half results from intolerable cosmetic changes and obesity [48]. Azathioprine-related toxicity includes nausea and emesis, rash, cholestatic hepatitis, pancreatitis, cytopenia and consecutive opportunistic infections, and malignancies (1.4-fold greater risk than normal) [48, 49]. In total, 10 % of all azathioprine-treated patients suffer from side effects, and in 5 % early adverse events lead to cessation of treatment. In many cases, a reduction of the dose is sufficient to manage the side effects. A rare complication is a diarrheal syndrome with malabsorption and small intestine villus atrophy that improves after discontinuation of azathioprine therapy [50].

At higher risk for adverse events in the treatment of AIH are:

1. *Patients with cirrhosis*. They are more often affected than patients without cirrhosis. Moreover, pretreatment cytopenia due to hepatomegaly is common and thus, patients with cirrhosis are more susceptible for severe cytopenia due to azathioprine.
2. *Pregnant women*. Congenital malformations after treatment with azathioprine have been described in mice but not in humans. The major risk is prematurity and associated with this a higher mortality of the newborn. Fetal loss in women with AIH is higher than in healthy mothers but no greater than in women with other chronic illness. Nevertheless, only anecdotal experience is made with azathioprine during pregnancy, so it is advised to reduce or terminate immunosuppression where possible and to attempt preconception counseling [43].
3. Patients with very low *thiopurine methyltransferase activity* (0.3–0.5 % of the population) have a higher risk for azathioprine related myelosuppression. Patients with a moderate reduction in thiopurine methyltransferase activity commonly tolerate daily doses of 50 mg fairly well and the enzyme activity may increase during treatment [51]. Laboratory testing of the thiopurine methyltransferase activity is only recommended in case of pretreatment cytopenia, new developed cytopenia under treatment or high dose treatment (>150 mg/day) [48].

Treatment Endpoints

Following treatment endpoints are distinguished: remission, treatment failure, incomplete response, drug toxicity.

Remission. The goal of immunosuppressive treatment in AIH is the normalization of liver transaminases, bilirubin and immunoglobulins, as well as the resolution of histological signs of inflammation. The improvement of the objective parameters is accompanied by an amelioration of the symptoms. In adults, a decline in biochemical abnormalities is commonly reached in the first two weeks. Normalization of the named values can be expected in the first 12–24 months. Beyond that period, a complete remission is not likely anymore. Preferably, a discontinuation of treatment should be considered after at least 24 months and at complete remission. 87 % of patients with long-term remission have normal liver tests and immunoglobulins. On the other hand, 60 % relapse despite of resolution of laboratory indices [52]. Indeed, histologically, interface hepatitis is described in more than half of the patients with normal laboratory results. These patients should not terminate treatment because of a high risk for relapse. In general, a liver biopsy is recommended before immunosuppression is stopped.

Treatment failure. A treatment failure is assumed if under an adequate treatment with corticosteroids with or without azathioprine (and under the precondition that the patient is compliant) the symptoms and the laboratory and histological features worsen. Unfortunately, this happens in around 9 % and can be noticed after 3–6 weeks of treatment. In that case, a high dose therapy with prednisone (60 mg) or prednisone (30 mg) in combination with azathioprine 150 mg should be established and maintained for at least 1 month [43]. This strategy results in an improvement of disease activity in 70 % but in a histological remission of only 20 % [53]. Patients with treatment failure must be followed closely to recognize the development of cirrhosis respectively the complications of cirrhosis. Once a patient presents with hepatic encephalopathy, ascites or variceal bleeding, a liver transplantation must be considered.

Incomplete response. Incomplete response means that the patient experiences an improvement but no resolution of the elevated biochemical indices and the histology features under treatment. In these individuals the treatment dose of prednisone may be reduced until the lowest possible level where the aminotransferases remain stable. Azathioprine can also be used to establish stable inflammation parameters.

Drug toxicity. If intolerable adverse effects occur, the treatment must be discontinued or better reduced in dose until side effects diminish or are tolerable.

Relapse. Relapse means a recurrence of inflammatory activity after complete remission and consecutive cessation of treatment. About 80 % of all patients in remission will experience a relapse, so it is a very prevalent event. The management of the relapse should be in first line to reestablish the treatment with prednisone with or without azathioprine. The goal is to gradually reduce and finally to eliminate Prednisone and to increase the dose of azathioprine to 2 mg/kg daily as an indefinite treatment. With this regimen 83 % stay in remission [54].

Salvage Therapies

If treatment failure occurs under high-dose prednisone therapy or 30 mg prednisone in conjunction with 150 mg azathioprine, alternative treatment regimens have to be considered. Most alternative drugs have been used anecdotally, and thus, experience is small. The most promising agent is mycophenolate mofetil [55]. The following agents have also been used for salvage therapy: Cyclosporine, tacrolimus, ursodeoxycholic acid, budesonide, 6-mercaptopurine, methotrexate, and cyclophosphamide. Budesonide and ursodeoxycholic acid were tested in randomized controlled clinic trials and failed as an option for salvage therapy [56, 57] which is no surprise.

Last but not least, liver transplantation is a very effective salvage therapy. Liver transplantation comes into question for patients with (1) acute liver failure, (2) decompensated liver cirrhosis and a MELD-score ≥15, and (3) HCC (within the Milano criteria). The 5-year survival rates after liver transplantation is approximately 78 % [58]. Importantly, a recurrence of AIH in the transplanted organ happens in approximately one-third of the patients [58, 59].

References

1. Perdigoto R, Carpenter HA, Czaja AJ. Frequency and significance of chronic ulcerative colitis in severe corticosteroid-treated autoimmune hepatitis. J Hepatol. 1992;14(2–3):325–31.
2. Feld JJ, Dinh H, Arenovich T, Marcus VA, Wanless IR, Heathcote EJ. Autoimmune hepatitis: effect of symptoms and cirrhosis on natural history and outcome. Hepatology. 2005;42(1):53–62.
3. Boberg KM, Aadland E, Jahnsen J, Raknerud N, Stiris M, Bell H. Incidence and prevalence of primary biliary cirrhosis, primary sclerosing cholangitis, and autoimmune hepatitis in a Norwegian population. Scand J Gastroenterol. 1998;33(1):99–103.
4. Alvarez F, Berg PA, Bianchi FB, Bianchi L, Burroughs AK, Cancado EL, et al. International Autoimmune Hepatitis Group report: review of criteria for diagnosis of autoimmune hepatitis. J Hepatol. 1999;31(5):929–38.
5. Johnson PJ, McFarlane IG. Meeting report: International Autoimmune Hepatitis Group. Hepatology. 1993;18(4):998–1005.
6. Hennes EM, Zeniya M, Czaja AJ, Pares A, Dalekos GN, Krawitt EL, et al. Simplified criteria for the diagnosis of autoimmune hepatitis. Hepatology. 2008;48(1):169–76.
7. Czaja AJ. Performance parameters of the diagnostic scoring systems for autoimmune hepatitis. Hepatology. 2008;48(5):1540–8.
8. Muratori P, Granito A, Pappas G, Muratori L. Validation of simplified diagnostic criteria for autoimmune hepatitis in Italian patients. Hepatology. 2009;49(5):1782–3.
9. Yeoman AD, Westbrook RH, Al Chalabi T, Carey I, Heaton ND, Portmann BC, et al. Diagnostic value and utility of the simplified International Autoimmune Hepatitis Group (IAIHG) criteria in acute and chronic liver disease. Hepatology. 2009;50(2):538–45.
10. Munoz-Espinosa L, Alarcon G, Mercado-Moreira A, Cordero P, Caballero E, Avalos V, et al. Performance of the international classifications criteria for autoimmune hepatitis diagnosis in Mexican patients. Autoimmunity. 2011;44(7):543–8.
11. Vergani D, Longhi MS, Bogdanos DP, Ma Y, Mieli-Vergani G. Autoimmune hepatitis. Semin Immunopathol. 2009;31(3):421–35.
12. Duerr RH, Targan SR, Landers CJ, LaRusso NF, Lindsay KL, Wiesner RH, et al. Neutrophil cytoplasmic antibodies: a link between primary sclerosing cholangitis and ulcerative colitis. Gastroenterology. 1991;100(5 Pt 1):1385–91.
13. Frenzer A, Fierz W, Rundler E, Hammer B, Binek J. Atypical, cytoplasmic and perinuclear anti-neutrophil cytoplasmic antibodies in patients with inflammatory bowel disease. J Gastroenterol Hepatol. 1998;13(9):950–4.
14. Baeres M, Herkel J, Czaja AJ, Wies I, Kanzler S, Cancado EL, et al. Establishment of standardised SLA/LP immunoassays: specificity for autoimmune hepatitis, worldwide occurrence, and clinical characteristics. Gut. 2002;51(2):259–64.
15. Czaja AJ, Shums Z, Norman GL. Nonstandard antibodies as prognostic markers in autoimmune hepatitis. Autoimmunity. 2004;37(3):195–201.
16. Boberg KM, Chapman RW, Hirschfield GM, Lohse AW, Manns MP, Schrumpf E. Overlap syndromes: the International Autoimmune Hepatitis Group (IAIHG) position statement on a controversial issue. J Hepatol. 2011;54(2):374–85.
17. Saich R, Chapman R. Primary sclerosing cholangitis, autoimmune hepatitis and overlap syndromes in inflammatory bowel disease. World J Gastroenterol. 2008;14(3):331–7.
18. Feldstein AE, Perrault J, El Youssif M, Lindor KD, Freese DK, Angulo P. Primary sclerosing cholangitis in children: a long-term follow-up study. Hepatology. 2003;38(1):210–7.
19. Floreani A, Rizzotto ER, Ferrara F, Carderi I, Caroli D, Blasone L, et al. Clinical course and outcome of autoimmune hepatitis/primary sclerosing cholangitis overlap syndrome. Am J Gastroenterol. 2005;100(7):1516–22.

20. Poupon R, Chazouilleres O, Corpechot C, Chretien Y. Development of autoimmune hepatitis in patients with typical primary biliary cirrhosis. Hepatology. 2006;44(1):85–90.
21. Longhi MS, Ma Y, Bogdanos DP, Cheeseman P, Mieli-Vergani G, Vergani D. Impairment of CD4(+)CD25(+) regulatory T-cells in autoimmune liver disease. J Hepatol. 2004;41(1):31–7.
22. Peiseler M, Sebode M, Franke B, Wortmann F, Schwinge D, Quaas A, et al. FOXP3+ regulatory T cells in autoimmune hepatitis are fully functional and not reduced in frequency. J Hepatol. 2012;57(1):125–32.
23. Taubert R, Hardtke-Wolenski M, Noyan F, Wilms A, Baumann AK, Schlue J, et al. Intrahepatic regulatory T cells in autoimmune hepatitis are associated with treatment response and depleted with current therapies. J Hepatol. 2014;61(5):1106–14.
24. Lan RY, Cheng C, Lian ZX, Tsuneyama K, Yang GX, Moritoki Y, et al. Liver-targeted and peripheral blood alterations of regulatory T cells in primary biliary cirrhosis. Hepatology. 2006;43(4):729–37.
25. Holdener M, Hintermann E, Bayer M, Rhode A, Rodrigo E, Hintereder G, et al. Breaking tolerance to the natural human liver autoantigen cytochrome P450 2D6 by virus infection. J Exp Med. 2008;205(6):1409–22.
26. Philipp T, Durazzo M, Trautwein C, Alex B, Straub P, Lamb JG, et al. Recognition of uridine diphosphate glucuronosyl transferases by LKM-3 antibodies in chronic hepatitis D. Lancet. 1994;344(8922):578–81.
27. Costa M, Rodriguez-Sanchez JL, Czaja AJ, Gelpi C. Isolation and characterization of cDNA encoding the antigenic protein of the human tRNP(Ser)Sec complex recognized by autoantibodies from patients withtype-1 autoimmune hepatitis. Clin Exp Immunol. 2000;121(2):364–74.
28. Wies I, Brunner S, Henninger J, Herkel J, Kanzler S, Meyer zum Buschenfelde KH, et al. Identification of target antigen for SLA/LP autoantibodies in autoimmune hepatitis. Lancet. 2000;355(9214):1510–5.
29. Volkmann M, Martin L, Baurle A, Heid H, Strassburg CP, Trautwein C, et al. Soluble liver antigen: isolation of a 35-kd recombinant protein (SLA-p35) specifically recognizing sera from patients with autoimmune hepatitis. Hepatology. 2001;33(3):591–6.
30. Lapierre P, Hajoui O, Homberg JC, Alvarez F. Formiminotransferase cyclodeaminase is an organ-specific autoantigen recognized by sera of patients with autoimmune hepatitis. Gastroenterology. 1999;116(3):643–9.
31. Muratori L, Sztul E, Muratori P, Gao Y, Ripalti A, Ponti C, et al. Distinct epitopes on formiminotransferase cyclodeaminase induce autoimmune liver cytosol antibody type 1. Hepatology. 2001;34(3):494–501.
32. Manns MP, Obermayer-Straub P. Cytochromes P450 and uridine triphosphate-glucuronosyltransferases: model autoantigens to study drug-induced, virus-induced, and autoimmune liver disease. Hepatology. 1997;26(4):1054–66.
33. Wen L, Ma Y, Bogdanos DP, Wong FS, Demaine A, Mieli-Vergani G, et al. Pediatric autoimmune liver diseases: the molecular basis of humoral and cellular immunity. Curr Mol Med. 2001;1(3):379–89.
34. Hardtke-Wolenski M, Fischer K, Noyan F, Schlue J, Falk CS, Stahlhut M, et al. Genetic predisposition and environmental danger signals initiate chronic autoimmune hepatitis driven by CD4+ T cells. Hepatology. 2013;58(2):718–28.
35. Gregorio GV, Choudhuri K, Ma Y, Pensati P, Iorio R, Grant P, et al. Mimicry between the hepatitis C virus polyprotein and antigenic targets of nuclear and smooth muscle antibodies in chronic hepatitis C virus infection. Clin Exp Immunol. 2003;133(3):404–13.
36. Czaja AJ, Strettell MD, Thomson LJ, Santrach PJ, Moore SB, Donaldson PT, et al. Associations between alleles of the major histocompatibility complex and type 1 autoimmune hepatitis. Hepatology. 1997;25(2):317–23.
37. Klein J, Sato A. The HLA system. Second of two parts. N Engl J Med. 2000;343(11):782–6.
38. Klein J, Sato A. The HLA system. First of two parts. N Engl J Med. 2000;343(10):702–9.
39. Czaja AJ, Carpenter HA, Santrach PJ, Moore SB. Significance of HLA DR4 in type 1 autoimmune hepatitis. Gastroenterology. 1993;105(5):1502–7.
40. Cook GC, Mulligan R, Sherlock S. Controlled prospective trial of corticosteroid therapy in active chronic hepatitis. Q J Med. 1971;40(158):159–85.
41. Murray-Lyon IM, Stern RB, Williams R. Controlled trial of prednisone and azathioprine in active chronic hepatitis. Lancet. 1973;1(7806):735–7.
42. Soloway RD, Summerskill WH, Baggenstoss AH, Geall MG, Gitnick GL, Elveback IR, et al. Clinical, biochemical, and histological remission of severe chronic active liver disease: a controlled study of treatments and early prognosis. Gastroenterology. 1972;63(5):820–33.
43. Manns MP, Czaja AJ, Gorham JD, Krawitt EL, Mieli-Vergani G, Vergani D, et al. Diagnosis and management of autoimmune hepatitis. Hepatology. 2010;51(6):2193–213.
44. Czaja AJ, Carpenter HA. Decreased fibrosis during corticosteroid therapy of autoimmune hepatitis. J Hepatol. 2004;40(4):646–52.
45. Manns MP, Woynarowski M, Kreisel W, Lurie Y, Rust C, Zuckerman E, et al. Budesonide induces remission more effectively than prednisone in a controlled trial of patients with autoimmune hepatitis. Gastroenterology. 2010;139(4):1198–206.
46. Czaja AJ, Carpenter HA. Distinctive clinical phenotype and treatment outcome of type 1 autoimmune hepatitis in the elderly. Hepatology. 2006;43(3):532–8.
47. Gregorio GV, Portmann B, Reid F, Donaldson PT, Doherty DG, McCartney M, et al. Autoimmune hepatitis in childhood: a 20-year experience. Hepatology. 1997;25(3):541–7.
48. Czaja AJ. Safety issues in the management of autoimmune hepatitis. Expert Opin Drug Saf. 2008;7(3):319–33.
49. Wang KK, Czaja AJ, Beaver SJ, Go VL. Extrahepatic malignancy following long-term immunosuppressive therapy of severe hepatitis B surface antigen-negative chronic active hepatitis. Hepatology. 1989;10(1):39–43.
50. Ziegler TR, Fernandez-Estivariz C, Gu LH, Fried MW, Leader LM. Severe villus atrophy and chronic malabsorption induced by azathioprine. Gastroenterology. 2003;124(7):1950–7.
51. Czaja AJ, Carpenter HA. Thiopurine methyltransferase deficiency and azathioprine intolerance in autoimmune hepatitis. Dig Dis Sci. 2006;51(5):968–75.
52. Montano-Loza AJ, Carpenter HA, Czaja AJ. Improving the end point of corticosteroid therapy in type 1 autoimmune hepatitis to reduce the frequency of relapse. Am J Gastroenterol. 2007;102(5):1005–12.
53. Montano-Loza AJ, Carpenter HA, Czaja AJ. Features associated with treatment failure in type 1 autoimmune hepatitis and predictive value of the model of end-stage liver disease. Hepatology. 2007;46(4):1138–45.
54. Johnson PJ, McFarlane IG, Williams R. Azathioprine for long-term maintenance of remission in autoimmune hepatitis. N Engl J Med. 1995;333(15):958–63.
55. Richardson PD, James PD, Ryder SD. Mycophenolate mofetil for maintenance of remission in autoimmune hepatitis in patients resistant to or intolerant of azathioprine. J Hepatol. 2000;33(3):371–5.
56. Czaja AJ, Carpenter HA, Lindor KD. Ursodeoxycholic acid as adjunctive therapy for problematic type 1 autoimmune hepatitis: a randomized placebo-controlled treatment trial. Hepatology. 1999;30(6):1381–6.
57. Czaja AJ, Lindor KD. Failure of budesonide in a pilot study of treatment-dependent autoimmune hepatitis. Gastroenterology. 2000;119(5):1312–6.
58. Vogel A, Heinrich E, Bahr MJ, Rifai K, Flemming P, Melter M, et al. Long-term outcome of liver transplantation for autoimmune hepatitis. Clin Transplant. 2004;18(1):62–9.
59. Milkiewicz P, Hubscher SG, Skiba G, Hathaway M, Elias E. Recurrence of autoimmune hepatitis after liver transplantation. Transplantation. 1999;68(2):253–6.

Primary Sclerosing Cholangitis

52

Roger W. Chapman and Kate D. Williamson

Introduction

Primary sclerosing cholangitis (PSC) is a chronic and progressive disease of the biliary tree characterized by concentric, obliterative fibrosis leading to bile duct stricturing and eventually cirrhosis in the majority of cases. The disease course is highly variable between individuals, but most symptomatic patients reach the combined end-point of death or liver transplantation 12–17 years following their diagnosis [1]. Approximately 10–15 % of PSC patients will develop cholangiocarcinoma. Although the underlying etiopathogenesis of PSC is not yet fully elucidated, it is generally accepted to be a condition of immune dysregulation.

Approximately three quarters of the Northern European PSC population have concomitant inflammatory bowel disease (IBD), with the predominant form of IBD being ulcerative colitis (UC). In 1874, only 7 years after PSC was defined, CH Thomas first recognized this association when he described a man who died of a "much enlarged, fatty liver in the presence of ulceration of the colon" [2].

Caring for the PSC patient presents a number of challenges—unfortunately medical therapy remains controversial and the only intervention with proven survival benefit is liver transplantation. Not only is the diagnostic workup and management of PSC complex, but also the treatment of associated conditions such as IBD and cholangiocarcinoma requires expertise that bridges the ever growling divide between hepatology, luminal gastroenterology, and endoscopy.

R.W. Chapman (✉) • K.D. Williamson
Department of Translational Gastroenterology, John Radcliffe, Oxford, UK
e-mail: roger.chapman@ndm.ox.ac.uk

Epidemiology and Clinical Features

Epidemiology

The insidious and slow progression of PSC has made it difficult to obtain accurate data for the true incidence and prevalence of this condition.

A recent study of a population of approximately 1.5 million adults from the Vastra Gotaland region in southern Sweden found a prevalence of 16.2/100,000 and incidence of 1.22/100,000 [3]. This is significantly higher than earlier studies in Northern European descendants that demonstrated the point prevalence and annual incidence of PSC to be approximately 9/100,000 and 0.9–1.3/100,000 years respectively. Similar figures to these lower rates have been demonstrated in a number of population-based studies across Canada, Norway, and Great Britain [4–7]. In the USA, the prevalence has been extrapolated to be 2–7 cases per 100,000 using an assumption that 2.5–7.5 % of the 40–225/100,000 ulcerative colitis patients. This, however, results is an underestimate of the true prevalence, as 20–30 % of patients with PSC have no associated inflammatory bowel disease. Indeed, a study from a population in Olmstead County, MN in the USA estimated a prevalence of 20.9 per 100,000 men and 6.3 per 100,000 women [8].

In addition to the recent Swedish study, data from Spain has also suggested that the incidence of PSC may be increasing [9]. Additionally, a change in disease presentation has been observed over time based on a recent study by Bergquist et al. [10]. This study compared the presentation of patients diagnosed with PSC prior to 1998 ($n = 185$) with those diagnosed after 1998 ($n = 61$). Patients diagnosed after 1998 were significantly older (41 vs. 37 years), had fewer symptoms at presentation (47 % vs. 63 %), and had a lower frequency of concurrent IBD (69 % vs. 82 %). It is likely these apparent historical changes reflect a higher capture of incident and prevalent cases through improved clinician awareness and greater use of diagnostic imaging modalities

D.C. Baumgart (ed.), *Crohn's Disease and Ulcerative Colitis*, DOI 10.1007/978-3-319-33703-6_52

such as MRCP. Higher rates of liver transplantation among prevalent cases (ascertainment bias) may have also contributed to this change.

For as yet unexplained reasons, the reported prevalence of PSC in South East Asia and Southern Europe is 10- to 100-fold less than that of Europe and America [11].

Risk Factors

The median age of onset of PSC is 30–40 years but the disease can present at any age. Interestingly, unlike most immune mediated diseases, two thirds of PSC patients are male. Siblings of PSC patients have a 1.5 % risk of developing PSC and there is a 0.7 % risk in first-degree relatives [12].

Cigarette smoking has long been recognized as a protective factor against the development of ulcerative colitis. Additionally, smoking may also protect against the development of PSC [13–16]. This protective effect is even more marked in patients with primary sclerosing cholangitis than ulcerative colitis and has also been observed in PSC patients who do not have concomitant inflammatory bowel disease. The mechanism by which smoking protects against both disorders is unknown and trials of nicotine therapy have shown no benefit in altering disease progression. Interestingly, a recent study has shown that PSC patients with Crohn's colitis also have a lower prevalence of smoking in contrast to Crohn's colitis patients without PSC, in whom the prevalence of smoking is increased [15, 17].

Etiopathogenesis

In 1991, a PSC review article in GUT hypothesized that PSC is an "Immunologically mediated disease, probably triggered by acquired toxic or infectious agents that may gain access through the colon" [1]. Although current understanding continues to support this, the etiology and pathogenesis of PSC are not yet fully elucidated. Indeed it is likely that a combination of mechanisms result in the development of PSC. Autoimmunity is very likely to play a major role as supported by the strong human specific leukocyte antigen (HLA) haplotype association in PSC, high frequency of other autoimmune diseases such as rheumatoid arthritis, high prevalence of autoantibodies in patient sera, and the link with inflammatory bowel disease [18].

Genetics Factors Predisposing to PSC

The importance of genetic risk in the development of PSC is highlighted by the fact that siblings of PSC patients are 9–39 times more likely to develop PSC than the general population [19]. Additionally, irrespective of whether they develop PSC, siblings have three times the incidence of IBD compared with the general population, suggesting a shared genetic susceptibility for PSC and IBD.

The major histocompatibility complex on the short arm of chromosome 6 encodes the human leukocyte antigen (HLA) molecules. These molecules are highly polymorphic and play a central role in T cell response. As early as 1982 the HLA complex was demonstrated to be a risk locus for PSC [20]. This study demonstrated an association between PSC and HLA-B8 and DR3. HLA-DR2 and DR6 are also associated with PSC whereas HLA DR4 may be protective (Table 52.1). Considering their role in antigen presentation, these HLA associations support the hypothesis that specific (auto-)antigens may be pathogenetically important in PSC.

HLA-B and -C play an additional role as ligands for killer immunoglobulin-like receptors on natural killer cells and some T cell subtypes. More recent data suggests that gene variants may impair these functions and subsequently protect against PSC [22]. This is supported by the fact that these protective variants are less commonly found in Northern European populations where PSC is most prevalent.

Not surprisingly, a recent Genome Wide Association Study (GWAS) of 285 Norwegian PSC patients found strong associations in the HLA complex [23]. There are also other genes outside the HLA region that may play a role in the pathogenesis of PSC. 15 previously established susceptibility loci for UC were evaluated in this GWAS study but only 2 of these (chromosome 3p21, chromosome 2q35) showed any significant association in PSC (Fig. 52.1).

This limited overlap in genetic susceptibility supports data from clinical trials that suggests IBD in association with PSC may represent its own disease phenotype. PSC

Table 52.1 Key HLA haplotypes associated with primary sclerosing cholangitis (PSC) [21]

Haplotype	Significance in PSC
B8-TNF*2-DRB3*0101-DRB1*0301-DQA1*0501-DQB1*0201	Strong association with disease susceptibility
DRB3*0101-DRB1*1301- DQA1*0103-DQB1*0603	Strong association with disease susceptibility
DRB5*0101-DRB1*1501- DQA1*0102-DQB1*0602	Weak association with disease susceptibility
DRB4*0103-DRB1*0401-DQA1*03-DQB1*0302	Strong association with protection against disease
MICA*008	Strong association with disease susceptibility

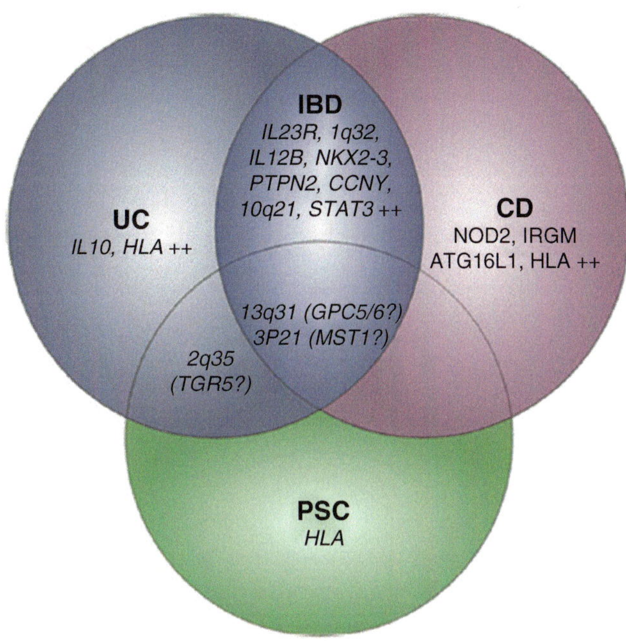

Fig. 52.1 With permission from Karlsen [24]

patients also possess a higher prevalence of the FUT2 gene. FUT2 secretor status and genotype is important in determining the biliary microbial composition ("the biome") in PSC [25].

Autoantibodies

Although autoantigens such as smooth muscle antibodies, antinuclear antibodies, and antineutrophil cytoplasmic antibodies (p-ANCA) are often detected in patient serum, none of these are specific to PSC. The prevalence of p-ANCA approaches 88 % in some studies but it is also found in patients with UC alone (60–87 %), in patients with type I autoimmune hepatitis (50–96 %) and primary biliary cirrhosis (PBC) [18, 26, 27]. Given this lack of specificity it is unlikely pANCA is involved directly in the pathogenesis of PSC and it is not a useful screening test.

Pathogenesis

One hypothesis to explain the association between IBD and liver disease is that PSC is mediated by long-lived memory T cells derived from the inflamed gut that enter the enterohepatic circulation [28]. Aberrant expression of chemokines and adhesion molecules on liver endothelial cells may cause recruitment of these T cells in turn leading to biliary inflammation, fibrosis, and bile duct stricturing.

In support of this, patients with PSC have been demonstrated to aberrantly express adhesion molecules including vascular adhesion protein-1 (VAP-1) and mucosal addressin cell adhesion molecule-1 (MAdCAM1) on biliary epithelium [29]. Additionally, the chemokine CCL25, ordinarily confined to the gut, is upregulated in the liver in PSC, helping recruit CCR9+ T cells. The mechanisms that lead to aberrant expression of adhesion molecules remain unknown but it may be that in genetically susceptible individuals, bacterial antigens, arising from a "leaky gut" from the inflamed colon, act as molecular mimics and cause an immune reaction responsible for initiating PSC. It is possible that specific colonic bacterial species are associated with development of PSC/IBD.

Fickert et al. recently proposed that a process similar to arteriosclerosis may also play a role in the pathogenesis of PSC [30]. Work with multidrug resistance knockout mice (Mdr2–/–) that are unable to produce phospholipids, suggests a subsequent inability to form mixed micelles (bile acids/phospholipids/cholesterol) results in accumulation of hepatotoxic bile acids and cholesterol-supersatured bile. Support for this theory in humans is however lacking. Genetic studies of the human ortholog of Mdr2 (MDR3) have not demonstrated any association between MDR3 genetic variants and susceptibility to PSC.

Clinical Features

The clinical presentation of PSC is variable and typical symptoms are nonspecific including right upper quadrant abdominal pain, fatigue, and pruritus. Up to 55 % of patients are asymptomatic at the time of presentation [7]. It is rare for patients with PSC to present with cholangitis unless they have previously had biliary intervention or have a dominant stricture [31, 32]. Similarly, presentation with jaundice is uncommon and may herald the development of cholangiocarcinoma. Osteopenic bone disease is both a complication of advanced PSC and IBD. Steatorrhea and malabsorption of fat soluble vitamins only occurs after prolonged cholestasis with jaundice.

Few patients present with features of decompensated cirrhosis and portal hypertension such as ascites and variceal hemorrhage. Nevertheless, hepatomegaly and splenomegaly are the most frequent abnormal physical findings at clinical examination at the time of diagnosis in PSC.

Diagnosis of PSC

Laboratory Investigations

Discovery of elevated cholestatic liver biochemistries (alkaline phosphatase and gamma GT) in an asymptomatic IBD patient should always prompt consideration of the diagnosis of PSC. Blood tests typically fluctuate over time and at times may even return completely to normal. Autoantibody tests are of little diagnostic significance. IgM concentrations are increased in about 50 % of patients with advanced PSC.

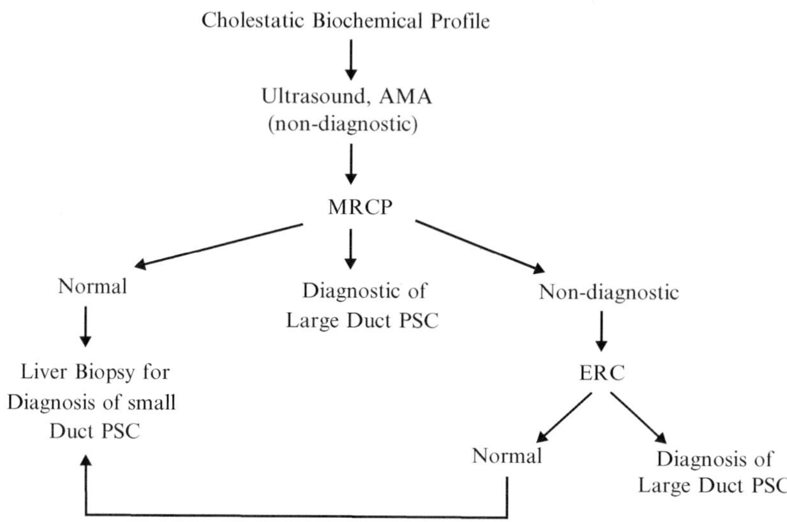

Fig. 52.2 Diagnostic workup for cholestatic liver biochemistry [34]

Serum IgG4 levels should be measured in all patients with suspected PSC. They are elevated in about 9 % of patients and are associated with a worse outcome [33] (see Section Histology).

Radiological Features

The first imaging modality recommended in the workup for a patient with cholestatic LFTS is a transabdominal ultrasound but in the vast majority of PSC patients, this will be nondiagnostic (Fig. 52.2). Usually, a diagnosis of PSC is made when cholangiography (MRCP or endoscopic retrograde pancreatography (ERCP)) demonstrates characteristic bile duct changes of multifocal stricturing and segmental dilatations, causing a "beaded appearance," in the absence of a secondary cause (Fig. 52.3).

Patients with small duct PSC have normal cholangiographic findings—this subgroup, who share similar biochemical and clinical features to large duct PSC, are instead diagnosed when histological changes of PSC are demonstrated on liver biopsy [35] (see Section Laboratory investigations).

Magnetic resonance cholangiopancreatography (MRCP) is now the investigation of choice over endoscopic retrograde cholangiopancreatography (ERCP). MRCP is noninvasive, does not involve radiation, avoids ERCP complications such as pancreatitis and is comparable to ERCP for diagnosis of PSC with good interobserver agreement [36, 37]. ERCP may still have a place in patients where the diagnosis remains uncertain after MRCP and is most useful for imaging subtle abnormalities in the intrahepatic biliary tree. As yet, there is no data on the utility of CT cholangiography for PSC diagnosis.

Histology

When radiological findings support the diagnosis of PSC, histological examination of the liver is not required to confirm this and only exposes patients to unnecessary morbidity.

Histology is diagnostic in only one third of PSC patients, although in another third there may be findings suggestive of biliary disease. The characteristic early biopsy findings of PSC are inflammation with periductal "onion-skin" fibrosis, portal edema, and bile ductular proliferation resulting in expansion of portal tracts (Fig. 52.4). With disease progression, bridging fibrosis eventually leads to cirrhosis. The focal nature of both early and late changes in PSC can make "staging" liver biopsies unreliable [38].

Secondary Sclerosing Cholangitis

When a diagnosis of PSC is suggested by imaging and histology, there are a number of causes of secondary sclerosing cholangitis (SSC) that must be considered (Table 52.2). At times, it can be very difficult to distinguish these from PSC, particularly in PSC patients who have coexisting pathology such as choledocholithiasis. In these patients, the clinical history, presence of IBD, and distribution of cholangiographic abnormalities are most helpful in identifying the predominant disease process [39]. It is particularly important to exclude IgG4-related sclerosing cholangitis.

Special Patient Populations

Small Duct PSC

Small duct PSC is normally diagnosed in the patients with IBD who have cholestatic serum biochemistry with a normal cholangiogram, but it may occur in patients without IBD. It is characterized by histological changes on liver biopsy characteristic of PSC. It occurs in approximately 10 % of the PSC population [40–42]. A recent study from the Calgary health region in Canada has shown an incidence of small duct PSC as 0.15/100,000. In children the incidence rate was 0.23/100,000 compared with 1.11/100,000 in adults [7].

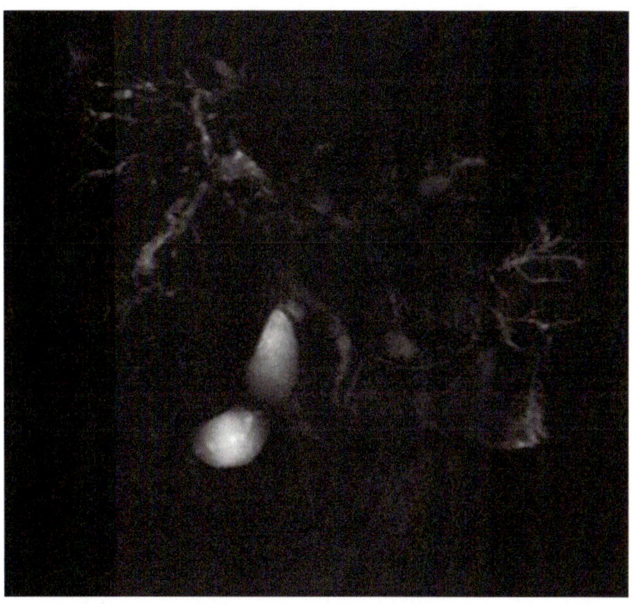

Fig. 52.3 MRCP appearance of PSC

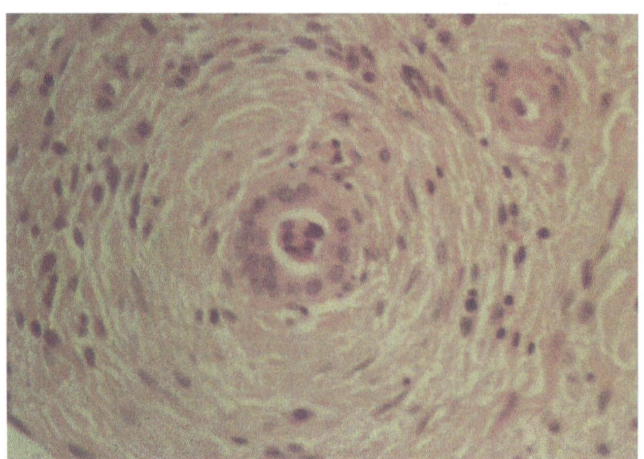

Fig. 52.4 Typical liver histological changes in PSC

Small duct PSC typically runs a milder course than large duct disease with a reduced likelihood of progression to cirrhosis and with a significantly improved survival compared with large duct disease. To date there have been no reports of cholangiocarcinoma in the small duct PSC patient population [43, 44]. Approximately one quarter of small duct PSC patients will subsequently develop large duct disease over a period of 10 years [43–47].

Autoimmune Hepatitis and PSC

Various studies suggest that between 1.4 % and 8 % of PSC patients have coexisting autoimmune liver disease (AIH)—recently defined as PSC-AIH syndrome [48–51]. PSC-AIH is more commonly found in children and young adults and characterized by clinical, biochemical, and histological features of AIH in the presence of cholangiographic findings

Table 52.2 Secondary causes of sclerosing cholangitis

Cholangiocarcinoma
Choledocholithiasis (with sepsis)
Diffuse intrahepatic metastasis
Chemotherapy (e.g., FUDR)
Biliary infections—CMV and immunodeficiency
• Cryptosporidium and immunodeficiency
• Ascariasis
• Ascending cholangitis
Eosinophilic cholangitis
Hepatic inflammatory pseudotumor
Histocytosis X
IgG4-related cholangitis
Ischemic cholangitis
Mast cell cholangiopathy
Portal hypertensive biliopathy
Recurrent pancreatitis
Surgical biliary trauma
AIDS cholangiopathy

identical to PSC [44, 46, 52–55]. PSC-AIH should be considered if the aminotransferase level is elevated more than twice the upper limit of normal and the serum IgG. Rarely, AIH features can develop in patients with established PSC. A liver biopsy should always be performed in these patients to confirm the diagnosis before treating with immunosuppressants. Immunosuppression is only helpful in improving disease progression in this selected group [56–59].

IgG4 Associated Cholangitis

Elevated IgG4 serum levels were first reported more than 10 years ago in patients with autoimmune pancreatitis (AIP) [60]. These patients commonly have associated intra- and extrahepatic biliary stricturing that may mimic PSC. In 2004, a Japanese case series found a subset of PSC patients had a significant infiltrate of IgG4-positive plasma cells isolated to the biliary tree (in the absence of any pancreatic abnormality) [61]. This group is now recognized to represent a distinct clinical entity that, like autoimmune pancreatitis may be responsive to immunosuppression. The term IgG4-related sclerosing cholangitis is used to encompass both this patient group and those patients who have biliary pathology in association with autoimmune pancreatitis [34].

Recent retrospective studies have found elevated serum IgG4 levels in 9–12 % of PSC patients with levels up to twice the upper limit of the normal range [33, 62]. IgG4 positive PSC patients have a reduced incidence of IBD and a more severe disease course when compared with patients who are negative [33].

A recent reevaluation of 98 consecutive liver transplants for patients originally diagnosed with PSC, found that 23 (23 %) of explanted livers stained positive for IgG4. Serum IgG4 levels were elevated in 18 of these patients. Tissue IgG4 positivity was associated with a more aggressive clinical course manifested by shorter time to transplant and a higher likelihood of disease recurrence after liver transplantation [63].

The important clinical implications and potential benefit of immunosuppression in this patient group make it imperative that IgG4 cholangitis is recognized and serum IgG4 levels should be checked in all PSC patients. It is now established that IgG4 disease is a distinct disease entity from PSC patients with and without elevated IgG4 levels [64].

Inflammatory Bowel Disease and PSC

Epidemiology

There is a strong association between IBD and PSC. In patient series from Northern Europe and North America, the prevalence of IBD in people with PSC ranges between 60 and 80 % [65–67]. There are, however, significant geographical variations in the reported prevalence of IBD in PSC with a much weaker association found in certain countries (Table 52.3). This discrepancy may partly be explained because studies reporting a weaker association often only used sigmoidoscopy (and/or no biopsies) subsequently missing a significant proportion of colitis, which may be right sided and microscopic in PSC patients.

IBD in PSC Patients

The predominant form of IBD is ulcerative colitis (UC) with approximately 85 % of IBD/PSC patients affected [67, 74]. IBD can be diagnosed at any time in patients with PSC but most commonly the diagnosis predates PSC by several years [66, 74, 75]. Interestingly, even patients who have received liver transplantation for PSC continue to be at increased risk of developing IBD [76].

All patients with a new diagnosis of PSC should have a full colonoscopy with biopsies, regardless of the presence of gastrointestinal symptoms to evaluate for IBD [34]. Because asymptomatic colitis and rectosigmoid sparing are common

Table 52.3 Prevalence of IBD in PSC patients

Country	Number of pts	IBD (%)	UC	Crohn's
Norway [68]	77	96	74	14
Sweden [65]	305	81	72	
UK [69]	126	73	71	
US [70]	174	71		
Italy [71]	117	54	36	10
Spain [9]	43	46	44	2
India [72]	18	50		
Japan [73]	388	37		

Table 52.4 Clinical characteristics of IBD associated with PSC

Characteristic	UC	UC/PSC
Extend of colitis	54 % (pancolitis)	87 % pancolitis [74]
Rectal sparing	6 %	52 % [74]
Backwash ileitis	7 %	51 % [74]
Pouchitis (following colectomy and ileo-anal pouch formation)	15 %	60 % [78]
Disease course		Typically mild, quiescent [77]
Dysplasia and cancer		RR 4 [79–81] Particularly right sided cancer
Other		Increased risk of peristomal varices in pts undergoing proctocolectomy with ileostomy

features in IBD/PSC, a flexible sigmoidoscopy is insufficient for screening. It is unclear whether interval endoscopies should be performed if a patient remains symptom free following a colonoscopy with normal colonic histology. Some clinicians advocate repeat endoscopy every 5 years.

It is likely that PSC/UC represents a distinct UC genotype and phenotype [74]. The natural history of UC in patients with PSC has a more benign course than in those patients with UC alone despite the fact that the disease usually involves the whole colon [77]. Common features in the PSC/IBD group include: rectal sparing (52 % versus 6 %), backwash ileitis (51 % versus 7 %), and an increased prevalence of pouchitis (following colectomy and ileo-anal pouch formation). The reason for increased rates of pouchitis is unknown (Table 52.4).

Early small, uncontrolled series suggested that PSC/Crohn's typically manifests as extensive colitis and also that isolated small bowel Crohn's is not associated with PSC [67, 82]. A recent case-controlled study specifically examined the course of Crohn's disease in 39 patients with PSC/Crohn's compared with Crohn's patients without PSC. The study confirmed that isolated ileal disease is rare (6 % vs. 31 %). Interestingly, unlike PSC/UC, the two groups followed similar disease courses, as judged by the need for surgical intervention or significant medical therapy (defined as requiring biological therapy with TNFα antagonists or greater than 5 courses of corticosteroids). The PSC/Crohn's patients were more likely to be female than PSC/UC patients (50 % vs. 28 %) and were more likely to have small duct PSC. Interestingly, they were less likely to progress to cancer, liver transplantation and death [17].

PSC in IBD Patients

The true prevalence of PSC within the IBD patient population is unknown because until recently, accurate data have required invasive cholangiography to be carried out on unselected patient groups and PSC patients may have normal liver biochemistry. Work underway using noninvasive MRCP will hopefully provide this data in the near future. Available evidence suggests that approximately 5 % of UC patients have coexisting PSC although this is likely to be an underestimate [83]. This data comes from three major studies (Table 52.5). The largest of these, found that 5 % of a cohort of 1500 UC patients had elevated alkaline phosphatase levels, and in those who subsequently underwent ERCP, 85 % had evidence of PSC [4].

Table 52.5 Prevalence of PSC in patients with UC

Country of origin	Number of pts with UC	Percentage with PSC
Oxford, UK [84]	681	2.9
Oslo, Norway [85]	336	4
Stockholm, Sweden [4]	1500	3.7

The prevalence of PSC in Crohn's disease is significantly less than that of UC, with an estimated percentage of 3–4 % of patients affected [82]. Typically these patients have either ileo-colonic or extensive colonic Crohn's disease.

Both the development of PSC and its outcome are independent of the activity of colitis. It may even occur after proctocolectomy. Interestingly, however, colectomy prior to transplantation for PSC is protective against the development of PSC in the transplanted liver in male patients [86].

PSC and Malignancy

Patients with PSC have a high rate of malignancy and currently more patients die of malignancy than end-stage liver failure (Table 52.6) [87]. The reason for the high rate of malignancy is probably explained by chronic inflammation in the biliary system and the colon, although whether PSC patients have a particular genetic susceptibility to develop cancer is unclear.

Colorectal Cancer

The increased risk of colorectal cancer (CRC) in ulcerative colitis compared with the general population is well estab-

Table 52.6 Standard incidence ration for first cancer after diagnosis of PSC including and excluding first year after diagnosis of PSC [87]

Site of cancer	Observed	Expected	Standard incidence ratio	95 % confidence interval	Excluding
All sites	87	14.3	6.1	(4.9–7.5)	
All sites excluding colorectal and hepatobiliary carcinoma	16	11.8	1.4	(0.8–2.2)	
All gastrointestinal cancers	71	2.5	28.6	(22.4–36.1)	
Esophagus	0	0.1	0.0	(0–30.5)	
Stomach	1	0.4	2.2	(0.1–12.5)	
Small intestine	0	0.1	0.0	(0–50.5)	
Colon–rectum	12	1.2	10.3	(5.3–18.1)	
Hepatobiliary tract	53	0.3	160.6	(120.3–210.1)	
Pancreas	5	0.3	14.3	(4.7–33.4)	
Esophagus	0	0.1	0.0	(0–34.2)	First year
Stomach	1	0.4	2.5	(0.1–14.1)	First year
Small intestine	0	0.1	0.0	(0–56.8)	First year
Colon–rectum	7	1.0	6.8	(2.7–14.0)	First year
Hepatobiliary tract	31	0.3	106.9	(72.6–151.7)	First year
Pancreas	3	0.3	9.7	(2.0–28.4)	First year

lished [79, 88–91]. Based on a meta-analysis of 11 studies, in UC patients with coexisting PSC this risk is elevated five times higher again (OR of 4.79 (95 % CI 3.58–6.41)). This risk increases with time and continues even after liver transplantation [80, 92] (Fig. 52.5).

Although CRC can present at any time in the disease course, the median time from diagnosis of colitis to development of colorectal cancer is 17 years [94]. Interestingly, the majority of these cancers (76 %) are right sided [79]. It has been proposed that this right-sided predominance may result from a carcinogenic effect of increased cecal concentrations of secondary bile acids such as lithocholic acid [88].

Considering the absolute risk for colonic dysplasia or cancer in PSC/UC approaches 31 % after 20 years of colitis [95] it is understandable that guidelines recommend 1–2 year interval colonoscopies with biopsies from the time of diagnosis of PSC/IBD. Patients with Crohn's/PSC are included in this recommendation, although a recent study has shown a low prevalence of dysplasia and cancer in the PSC patients with associated Crohn's colitis compared to PSC/UC [96]. This was not confirmed in a Swedish cohort [97].

Ursodeoxycholic acid (UDCA) treatment in patients with PSC and UC may decrease the risk of colorectal dysplasia and colorectal cancer [98, 99] (see Section Cholangitis).

In patients who develop PSC-associated colorectal malignancy, proctocolectomy with ileo-anal pouch formation is the preferred surgical management as it avoids)the complication of peristomal varices in patients with an ileal stoma.

Cholangiocarcinoma

Cholangiocarcinoma complicates the clinical course of PSC in 10–20 % of patients, with an annual incidence (starting 1 year after diagnosis of PSC) of 0.5–1.5 % [65, 100–103]. Male gender, smoking and a long history of IBD were identified as risk factors for CCA in a case-controlled review of 39 PSC patients presenting with CCA [104].

One third of patients who develop CCA are diagnosed within 1 year of the diagnosis of their PSC. The likely explanation for this is that the development of symptomatic cholangiocarcinoma brings a number of patients with previously unrecognized PSC to medical attention.

The diagnosis of CCA can be challenging in PSC patients and early detection is difficult. Often patients with CCA are asymptomatic and when symptoms develop they are nonspecific, typically indicate metastatic disease and mimic PSC disease progression [105]. Worsening jaundice/bilirubin levels, pruritus, weight loss, and abdominal pain in any PSC patient should always prompt evaluation for CCA. Unfortunately, computed tomography (CT), ultrasonography (US), and MRCP have poor sensitivity for early detection of CCA [106]. Annual MRCP has been advocated as a surveillance method for CCA in patients with large duct PSC, but there is no evidence to support this approach.

Tumor markers play a limited role in the early detection of CCA [34, 103, 107–110]. Using a cut-off level for Carbohydrate Antigen 19-9 (CA19-9) of 130U/ml (normal <55), the sensitivity and specificity is 79 % and 98 %

Fig. 52.5 Risk of colonic neoplasia in PSC [93]

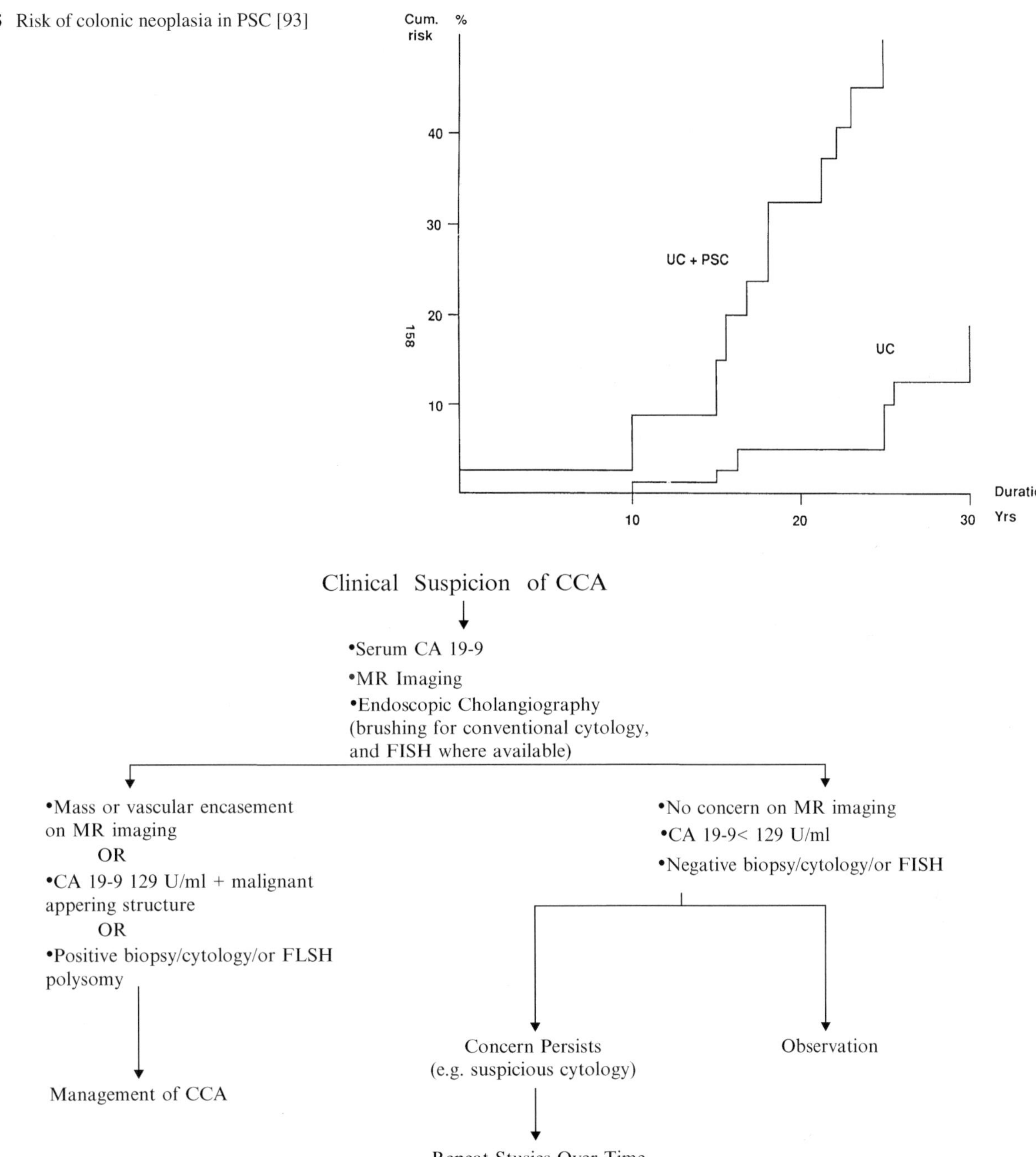

Fig. 52.6 Workup for clinical suspicion of CCA

respectively [108]. CA19-9 can be elevated in benign biliary disease as well as other malignancies including pancreas, colon, stomach, and gynecological cancers. It is important to note that 7 % of the general population (those negative for Lewis antigen) will not produce CA 19-9 regardless of their CCA status. Generally, CA 19-9 has only been useful to identify patients with advanced, unresectable CCA and has no role in cancer surveillance in PSC. Elevated levels of serum trypsinogen-2 were reported to represent an early marker of CCA, but this needs confirmation in a larger study [111].

CCA can develop in any part of the biliary tree. Perihilar CCAs (the so-called Klatskin tumors) are the most common tumor site. These are typically infiltrating, desmoplastic tumors. Mass lesions in the liver make up about 20 % of cancers and distal CBD tumors are uncommon (<10 %) [112].

The discovery of a dominant peripheral stricture on imaging presents a significant diagnostic challenge (Fig. 52.6). The majority of these strictures will be benign. It is uncommon for a coexisting mass to be identified, but if found, this has a virtually 100 % sensitivity and specificity for CCA

[103]. In a recent retrospective study of 89 patients with dominant strictures, MRCP was found to be superior to ERCP for the diagnosis of CCA with a sensitivity, specificity and accuracy of 96 %, 85 %, 81 % compared with 80 %, 75 %, and 78 % respectively [113]. One advantage of ERCP, however, is that it does allow acquisition of cytological specimens using brushings. It is also important to exclude IgG4-related disease in this patient group, as it may mimic PSC and CCA on cholangiography.

Conventional brush cytology specimens obtained through ERCP have poor sensitivity, 18–40 % [103, 110, 114–116]. However, when positive, the specificity approaches 100 %. New diagnostic modalities such as direct image analysis (DIA) and fluorescent in situ hybridization (FISH) have been employed in attempts to increase diagnostic yield on cytological specimens. Early studies indicated a significant improvement in sensitivity [115], but more recently this has been brought into question with the most recent study using FISH polysomy demonstrating a sensitivity of 46 %, only slightly higher than cytology alone [117].

Distinguishing PSC and CCA by direct visualization of the biliary tree with techniques such as endoscopic intraductal US and cholangioscopy is promising. A recent study reported a sensitivity of 92 % and specificity of 93 % for diagnosing malignant strictures compared to 66 % and 51 % respectively using ERCP alone [118]. However, these techniques have not yet been tested in large patient populations. PET is not helpful to distinguish PSC from CCA [119].

Unfortunately, the prognosis for CCA is poor. The median survival is 5–11 months [101, 120, 121]. Most patients are treated palliatively. Even with surgical resection, the 3-year survival is <30 % [122, 123]. The Mayo Clinic in the USA has pioneered the use neoadjuvant chemoradiotherapy, followed by liver transplantation in highly selected patients with nonmetastatic cancers of less than 3 cm in diameter. This approach in this highly selected group, has achieved remarkable 5-year survival rates of up to 82 % [124, 125].

Gallbladder and Pancreatic Cancer

PSC is recognized as a major risk factor for gallbladder carcinoma. In a study examining 286 patients with PSC, 18 (6 %) of patients were found to have gallbladder mass lesions of which 10 were gallbladder cancer [126]. Guidelines recommend annual US surveillance, and that cholecystectomy should be performed for any mass lesion (such as polyps) identified regardless of size.

One study has suggested that the risk of pancreatic carcinomas may also be increased in PSC. This remains to be confirmed [87].

Nonmalignant Complications of PSC and Their Management

Dominant Strictures

Due to an absence of population-based studies, the exact prevalence of dominant strictures is unknown but estimated to occur in approximately 10–58 % of PSC patients during follow-up [71, 127, 128]. The majority of these strictures are benign, but their discovery should always prompt consideration of a CCA (see Section IBD in PSC patients). Dominant strictures are associated with bacterial cholangitis as well as biliary stones.

Patients with symptoms from dominant strictures such as cholangitis, jaundice, pruritus, right upper quadrant pain or worsening biochemical indices are appropriate candidates for therapy. ERCP with sphincterotomy and balloon dilatation (with prophylactic pre-procedural antibiotics) has the best evidence of benefit [129–134]. Stenting should be reserved for strictures that are refractory to repeat dilatation. Large retrospective studies suggest that endoscopic therapy results in clinical improvement and prolonged survival.

Bacterial Cholangitis

It is very unusual for PSC patients to develop cholangitis in the absence of a previous history of instrumentation of the biliary tree or a dominant stricture [135, 136]. The presence of a dominant stricture is thought to predispose to cholangitis through bacterial colonization of stagnant of bile acids.

A recent study demonstrated that 40.5 % of patients with a dominant stricture had bacterial colonization of their biliary tree (In the absence of a stricture, patient bile samples were all sterile) [137]. Most infections are caused by aerobic, enteric organisms such as *E. coli*, Klebsiella, and *E. faecalis* [138]. Unfortunately, short-course antibiotics are poorly effective in eradicating bacteria. However, biliary drainage procedures combined with antibiotics are usually effective. Patients with recurrent bacterial cholangitis may benefit from cyclical prophylactic long-term antibiotics usually quinolones. In patients who fail antibiotic therapy, recurrent cholangitis may be the primary indication for OLTx.

Fatigue and Pruritus

Fatigue is a common problem and has a major impact on the quality of life in PSC patients [138]. It occurs independently of the severity of liver disease. No medical therapy is of proven benefit although the antinarcolepsy agent modenafil has been tried off-label with varying degrees of success.

Pruritus is also common in patients with PSC. 80–90 % of patients will respond to first line therapy with cholestyramine [139].

The antibiotic rifampicin is used as a second line agent for patients who have not responded to cholestyramine. It has shown to be effective treatment for pruritus in cholestatic liver disease [140–142]. The mechanism of action is unknown but it probably induces the hepatic microsomal drug-metabolizing system causing metabolism of endogenous pruritogenic compounds. It may alternatively have a direct antimicrobial effect in the intestinal lumen, causing a change in synthesis of secondary bile acids. It is also a nuclear receptor agonist of PXR.

There is an upregulation of opioid receptors in patients with chronic cholestasis as well as an increased central opioidergic tone and opioid antagonists (nalmefene, naloxone, and naltrexone) have been shown to be effective in pruritus. These drugs can cause a withdrawal-like reaction by preventing binding of endogenous opioids but this complication is transient and settles within the first couple of days [143–145].

A variety of fourth line medications are useful including sertraline. UDCA has not been shown to benefit pruritus. Occasionally, intractable pruritus may be an indication for OLTx [31].

Metabolic Bone Disease

The possibility of Hepatic osteodystrophy should be evaluated in all patients with a new diagnosis of PSC, and every 3–5 years thereafter using bone mineral density scanning [146]. The incidence of osteoporosis is 4–10 % in PSC, with a particularly increased risk in older patients with a long duration of disease, decreased BMI and possibly, worse disease [147, 148]. Calcium and Vitamin D should be prescribed in all PSC patients with osteopenia, and bisphosphonate therapy considered when osteoporosis develops.

Gallstones

PSC patients are predisposed to gallstone disease. In a retrospective review of 286 PSC patients, 25 % of patients had gallstones that were diagnosed at a mean of 5 years following the diagnosis of PSC. Characteristically these stones are small brown bile pigment stones. Ursodeoxycholic acid does not influence the frequency of gallstones [126].

Prognosis and Treatment

Prognosis

The median time to death or liver transplantation in all-comers was thought to be 9.6–18 years [46, 69, 70, 127, 149]. However, a recent study from Holland has shown an increased median survival of 21 years in all-comers whereas the survival was significantly reduced in the transplant centers, due to referral bias [150].

Although the majority of patients who are asymptomatic at the time of diagnosis will eventually develop symptoms, not surprisingly these asymptomatic patients have a better prognosis than the overall PSC population with a survival rate population with a survival rate of 88 % at 5 years and greater than 70 % at 16 years [69, 70]. A study from Germany in 2007 demonstrated that a persistently raised serum bilirubin (>3 months) following initial diagnosis is an independent risk factor correlating with poor outcome and high risk of CCA.

Several prognostic models have been developed to help predict outcomes in advanced PSC. The Mayo score provides the most valid survival information in patients with advanced disease [34]. It uses age, bilirubin, serum AST and Albumin along with a history of variceal bleeding as prognostic parameters to divide patients into low, intermediate and high risk.

The Child–Pugh classification has also been demonstrated to be a satisfactory alternative to disease-specific models in both research studies and clinical decision-making [79].

With the advent of new therapies in development for PSC, the need for accurate surrogate endpoints in place of survival free of liver transplantation or death has become increasingly important. The prognostic models discussed above, using clinical and biochemical data have not proved to be reliable in early stage patients.

There is an increasing evidence base suggesting a valuable role of serum alkaline phosphatase (ALP) as a biomarker in predicting the clinical outcome of PSC [151]. In a recent prospective German study, 215 patients with PSC were followed for over 25 years. Significant reduction of ALP within 6–12 months was shown to be associated with improved median survival free of liver transplantation, compared with no ALP reduction — 15 versus 26 years [152]. Various ALP reductions were evaluated, as previously published, including ALP normalization and ALP reduction to 1.5 times the upper limit of normal (1.5× ULN), with all models proving statistically significant, with the exception of 40 % ALP drop from baseline. This large single center gives further strength to the similar positive findings from PSC cohorts in the UK [153] ($n=139$), Scandinavia [154] ($n=198$), and USA [155] ($n=87$).

With the failure of complicated models to predict the clinical course of PSC, it is perhaps surprising that ALP has emerged as an important prognostic marker in PSC. Interestingly, similar results have been demonstrated in patients with Primary Biliary Cirrhosis treated with Ursodeoxycholic acid.

Other markers of prognosis, including serum biomarkers such as ELF, and newer imaging modalities such as fibroscan, MR Elastography, and multiparametric MR scanning are being evaluated. However, currently ALP appears to be the best surrogate marker to predict the course of PSC [151].

Medical Therapy

Unfortunately, no medical therapy has been proven to improve prognosis in PSC. Advocates of medical therapy appropriately point to a number of reasons why conclusive trial data is lacking; The scarcity of PSC patients, lack of reliable surrogate markers for disease progression, a long time period until primary end-points (such as transplantation/death) and high individual disease variability all make it very difficult to design and carry out trials that are appropriately selective and sufficiently powered to demonstrate a significant benefit.

Ursodeoxycholic acid (UDCA), a naturally occurring bile acid has been extensively studied for the treatment of PSC over the past 20 years. Surprisingly, a trial using high-dose UDCA 28–30 mg/kg day was terminated prematurely because of an increased risk of serious adverse events (death or liver transplantation) compared with placebo [156]. The likely explanation for this unexpected result is that high doses of UDCA result in the conversion of unabsorbed colonic UDCA) into lithocholic acid, a hepatotoxic bile acid. This is supported by data from the original trial that demonstrates markedly elevated serum lithocholic acid levels in the patients treated with high-dose UDCA compared with those who received only placebo [157].

Despite the controversy that stems from the high-dose trial, it remains European practice to prescribe 15–23 mg/kg/day to patients with large duct PSC and coexisting IBD, in keeping with the EASL clinical practice guidelines [34]. This recommendation is made for several reasons:

1. Multiple trials have shown this dose to be safe and effective in improving liver biochemistry [114, 158–160].
2. UDCA has been demonstrated in three clinical studies to reduce rates of colonic dysplasia and colorectal cancer, in patients with coexisting IBD [98, 99, 161].
3. A randomized, double-blind, controlled trial evaluating 219 patients over 5 years found a strong trend towards increased survival using UDCA. (Unfortunately due to few endpoints, this trial was insufficiently powered to reach statistical significance) [160].

Table 52.7 Medical therapies trialed in PSC [32]

No benefit	Possible benefit	Under consideration
Azathioprine	Metronidazole	UDCA
Budesonide	Minocycline	Nor-UDCA
Cladribine	Silymarin	6-EDCA
Colchicine	Tacrolimus	Losartan
Cyclosporine	Vancomycin	Obetocholic acid
Etanercept		Vedolizumab
Infliximab		Simtuzumab
Methotrexate		
Mycophenolate mofetil		
Nicotine		
Penicillamine		
Pentoxifylline		
Pirfenidone		

4. The use of UDCA may reduce the incidence of biliary tract cancers but this needs further study [156, 162].

A number of other medical therapies have been trialed in PSC, none of which have any proven efficacy and these are not recommended in the routine treatment of PSC (Table 52.7). There are a number of novel agents currently being studied in PSC, including bile acids (Nor-Ursodeoxycholic acid); anti-integrins, Vedolizumab, antibiotics, nuclear receptor agonists (obetacholic acid), and antifibrotics. Hopefully one or more of these agents, either alone or in combination will prove to be effective in the future.

In the context of PSC/AIH overlap syndrome, immunosuppressive medications, particularly corticosteroids may have a therapeutic role and a trial of therapy in those circumstances is sometimes indicated [163].

Transplantation

Liver transplantation (LTx) is the only proven lifesaving therapy for end-stage liver disease secondary to PSC. The 5-year survival rate is excellent at approximately 85 % [164–166]. Although in some Scandinavian countries, PSC is the leading indication for liver transplantation, in the USA, it is the fifth leading cause of liver transplantation [167].

Appropriate timing of LTx for PSC is particularly challenging due to the highly variable disease course and unpredictable risk of cholangiocarcinoma. The decision to list a patient for LTx should be made on the basis of clinical signs, biochemical parameters, and cholangiographic findings. There is no justification for performing preemptive LTx to reduce the risk of developing CCA. Traditionally, CCA is regarded as a contraindication to LTx although recent data in highly selected patient groups has been promising (see Section IBD in PSC patients).

The recurrence rate of PSC in a transplanted liver is estimated to be between 20 and 30 % after 5–10 years although it can be very difficult to distinguish recurrent disease from secondary causes of biliary structuring such as peritransplant ductal ischemia [164, 168, 169]. Interestingly the risk of recurrent PSC is reduced in PSC/IBD patients who have had a colectomy prior to or at the time of LTx, compared with those who have not [86, 170]. High-dose post-transplant prednisolone therapy is also associated with an increased risk of recurrent disease.

In IBD/PSC patients, the risk of colorectal dysplasia and cancer persists post-transplantation and ongoing annual colonic surveillance is recommended. Some studies have suggested that this high risk may be increased even further after liver transplantation.

IBD rarely improves post transplantation and up to 30 % of patients will have increased and worsening activity. UC may even develop de novo in patients with PSC after liver transplantation [171, 172].

Conclusion

Over the recent years PSC has been increasingly recognized as an important clinical entity, particularly amongst the IBD population where it is found in up to 10 % of patients. The use of MRCP has simplified the diagnostic process with avoidance of the complications attached to ERCP, without the need for liver biopsy. Indeed, in conjunction with increased clinician awareness, greater application of MRCP has likely led to an increase in the capture of incident and prevalent PSC cases. This may in part explain the changing epidemiology of PSC with an increase in reported prevalence and greater number of PSC patients being asymptomatic at the time of diagnosis.

Patients with PSC/Crohn's appear to have a better prognosis than PSC/UC.

While better insight into the pathogenetic mechanisms underlying the development of PSC has been made, its exact etiology is not yet elucidated and it is likely a number of mechanisms play a role in disease pathogenesis. Genetic studies and evaluation of variations in the constitution of the biome are currently in progress and will hopefully shed further light on this complex process.

No medical treatment has been established to halt the progression of this insidious disease and recent trials on the use of UDCA have raised more questions than they have answered. Trials of new potential therapeutic agents are in progress.

Advances in endoscopic, radiological, and molecular techniques have improved therapeutic options and allowed clinicians to better differentiate benign from malignant biliary disease. Nevertheless, screening for and confirming a suspected diagnosis of cholangiocarcinoma remains one of the significant challenges of managing this complex disease.

References

1. Chapman RW. Aetiology and natural history of primary sclerosing cholangitis: a decade of progress? Gut. 1991;32(12):1433–5.
2. Thomas C. Ulceration of the colon with a much enlarged fatty liver. Trans Pathol Soc Phil. 1873;4:87–8.
3. Lindkvist B et al. Incidence and prevalence of primary sclerosing cholangitis in a defined adult population in Sweden. Hepatology. 2010;52(2):571–7.
4. Olsson R et al. Prevalence of primary sclerosing cholangitis in patients with ulcerative colitis. Gastroenterology. 1991;100(5 Pt 1):1319–23.
5. Boberg KM et al. Incidence and prevalence of primary biliary cirrhosis, primary sclerosing cholangitis, and autoimmune hepatitis in a Norwegian population. Scand J Gastroenterol. 1998;33(1):99–103.
6. Kingham JG, Kochar N, Gravenor MB. Incidence, clinical patterns, and outcomes of primary sclerosing cholangitis in South Wales, United Kingdom. Gastroenterology. 2004;126(7):1929–30.
7. Kaplan GG et al. The burden of large and small duct primary sclerosing cholangitis in adults and children: a population-based analysis. Am J Gastroenterol. 2007;102(5):1042–9.
8. Bambha K et al. Incidence, clinical spectrum, and outcomes of primary sclerosing cholangitis in a United States community. Gastroenterology. 2003;125(5):1364–9.
9. Escorsell A et al. Epidemiology of primary sclerosing cholangitis in Spain. Spanish Association for the Study of the Liver. J Hepatol. 1994;21(5):787–91.
10. Bergquist A, Said K, Broome U. Changes over a 20-year period in the clinical presentation of primary sclerosing cholangitis in Sweden. Scand J Gastroenterol. 2007;42(1):88–93.
11. Ang TL et al. Clinical profile of primary sclerosing cholangitis in Singapore. J Gastroenterol Hepatol. 2002;17(8):908–13.
12. Bergquist A et al. Increased prevalence of primary sclerosing cholangitis among first-degree relatives. J Hepatol. 2005;42(2):252–6.
13. van Erpecum KJ et al. Risk of primary sclerosing cholangitis is associated with nonsmoking behavior. Gastroenterology. 1996;110(5):1503–6.
14. Mitchell SA et al. Cigarette smoking, appendectomy, and tonsillectomy as risk factors for the development of primary sclerosing cholangitis: a case control study. Gut. 2002;51(4):567–73.
15. Loftus Jr EV et al. Primary sclerosing cholangitis is associated with nonsmoking: a case-control study. Gastroenterology. 1996;110(5):1496–502.
16. Eaton J et al. A comprehensive assessment of environmental exposures among 1000 North American patients with primary sclerosing cholangitis, with and without inflammatory bowel disease. Aliment Pharmacol Ther. 2015;41(10):980–90.
17. Halliday JS et al. A unique clinical phenotype of primary sclerosing cholangitis associated with Crohn's disease. J Crohns Colitis. 2012;6(2):174–81.
18. Terjung B, Worman HJ. Anti-neutrophil antibodies in primary sclerosing cholangitis. Best Pract Res Clin Gastroenterol. 2001;15(4):629–42.
19. Bergquist A et al. Increased risk of primary sclerosing cholangitis and ulcerative colitis in first-degree relatives of patients with primary sclerosing cholangitis. Clin Gastroenterol Hepatol. 2008;6(8):939–43.
20. Schrumpf E et al. Sclerosing cholangitis in ulcerative colitis. A follow-up study. Scand J Gastroenterol. 1982;17(1):33–9.
21. Maggs JR, Chapman RW. An update on primary sclerosing cholangitis. Curr Opin Gastroenterol. 2008;24(3):377–83.

22. Hov JR et al. Genetic associations in Italian primary sclerosing cholangitis: heterogeneity across Europe defines a critical role for HLA-C. J Hepatol. 2010;52(5):712–7.
23. Karlsen TH et al. Genome-wide association analysis in primary sclerosing cholangitis. Gastroenterology. 2010;138(3):1102–11.
24. Karlsen TH, Schrumpf E, Boberg KM. Update on primary sclerosing cholangitis. Dig Liver Dis. 2010;42(6):390–400.
25. Folseraas T et al. Extended analysis of a genome-wide association study in primary sclerosing cholangitis detects multiple novel risk loci. J Hepatol. 2012;57(2):366–75.
26. Gow PJ, Fleming KA, Chapman RW. Primary sclerosing cholangitis associated with rheumatoid arthritis and HLA DR4: is the association a marker of patients with progressive liver disease? J Hepatol. 2001;34(4):631–5.
27. Lo SK, Fleming KA, Chapman RW. Prevalence of anti-neutrophil antibody in primary sclerosing cholangitis and ulcerative colitis using an alkaline phosphatase technique. Gut. 1992;33(10):1370–5.
28. Grant AJ et al. Homing of mucosal lymphocytes to the liver in the pathogenesis of hepatic complications of inflammatory bowel disease. Lancet. 2002;359(9301):150–7.
29. Aron JH, Bowlus CL. The immunobiology of primary sclerosing cholangitis. Semin Immunopathol. 2009;31(3):383–97.
30. Fickert P, Moustafa T, Trauner M. Primary sclerosing cholangitis—the arteriosclerosis of the bile duct? Lipids Health Dis. 2007;6:3.
31. Charatcharoenwitthaya P, Lindor KD. Primary sclerosing cholangitis: diagnosis and management. Curr Gastroenterol Rep. 2006;8(1):75–82.
32. Silveira MG, Lindor KD. Clinical features and management of primary sclerosing cholangitis. World J Gastroenterol. 2008;14(21):3338–49.
33. Mendes FD et al. Elevated serum IgG4 concentration in patients with primary sclerosing cholangitis. Am J Gastroenterol. 2006;101(9):2070–5.
34. Chapman R et al. Diagnosis and management of primary sclerosing cholangitis. Hepatology. 2010;51(2):660–78.
35. Bjornsson E et al. The natural history of small-duct primary sclerosing cholangitis. Gastroenterology. 2008;134(4):975–80.
36. Berstad AE et al. Diagnostic accuracy of magnetic resonance and endoscopic retrograde cholangiography in primary sclerosing cholangitis. Clin Gastroenterol Hepatol. 2006;4(4):514–20.
37. Fulcher AS et al. Primary sclerosing cholangitis: evaluation with MR cholangiography—a case-control study. Radiology. 2000;215(1):71–80.
38. Ludwig J. Surgical pathology of the syndrome of primary sclerosing cholangitis. Am J Surg Pathol. 1989;13 Suppl 1:43–9.
39. Abdalian R, Heathcote EJ. Sclerosing cholangitis: a focus on secondary causes. Hepatology. 2006;44(5):1063–74.
40. Bhathal PS, Powell LW. Primary intrahepatic obliterating cholangitis: a possible variant of 'sclerosing cholangitis'. Gut. 1969;10(11):886–93.
41. Ludwig J et al. Morphologic features of chronic hepatitis associated with primary sclerosing cholangitis and chronic ulcerative colitis. Hepatology. 1981;1(6):632–40.
42. Wee A, Ludwig J. Pericholangitis in chronic ulcerative colitis: primary sclerosing cholangitis of the small bile ducts? Ann Intern Med. 1985;102(5):581–7.
43. Angulo P, Maor-Kendler Y, Lindor KD. Small-duct primary sclerosing cholangitis: a long-term follow-up study. Hepatology. 2002;35(6):1494–500.
44. Bjornsson E et al. Patients with small duct primary sclerosing cholangitis have a favourable long term prognosis. Gut. 2002;51(5):731–5.
45. Boberg KM et al. Hepatobiliary disease in ulcerative colitis. An analysis of 18 patients with hepatobiliary lesions classified as small-duct primary sclerosing cholangitis. Scand J Gastroenterol. 1994;29(8):744–52.
46. Broome U et al. Natural history and outcome in 32 Swedish patients with small duct primary sclerosing cholangitis (PSC). J Hepatol. 2002;36(5):586–9.
47. Nikolaidis NL et al. Small-duct primary sclerosing cholangitis. A single-center seven-year experience. Dig Dis Sci. 2005;50(2):324–6.
48. van Buuren HR et al. High prevalence of autoimmune hepatitis among patients with primary sclerosing cholangitis. J Hepatol. 2000;33(4):543–8.
49. Kaya M, Angulo P, Lindor KD. Overlap of autoimmune hepatitis and primary sclerosing cholangitis: an evaluation of a modified scoring system. J Hepatol. 2000;33(4):537–42.
50. Floreani A et al. Clinical course and outcome of autoimmune hepatitis/primary sclerosing cholangitis overlap syndrome. Am J Gastroenterol. 2005;100(7):1516–22.
51. Al-Chalabi T et al. Autoimmune hepatitis overlap syndromes: an evaluation of treatment response, long-term outcome and survival. Aliment Pharmacol Ther. 2008;28(2):209–20.
52. Gohlke F et al. Evidence for an overlap syndrome of autoimmune hepatitis and primary sclerosing cholangitis. J Hepatol. 1996;24(6):699–705.
53. Wilschanski M et al. Primary sclerosing cholangitis in 32 children: clinical, laboratory, and radiographic features, with survival analysis. Hepatology. 1995;22(5):1415–22.
54. Abdalian R et al. Prevalence of sclerosing cholangitis in adults with autoimmune hepatitis: evaluating the role of routine magnetic resonance imaging. Hepatology. 2008;47(3):949–57.
55. Gregorio GV et al. Autoimmune hepatitis/sclerosing cholangitis overlap syndrome in childhood: a 16-year prospective study. Hepatology. 2001;33(3):544–53.
56. Church NI et al. Autoimmune pancreatitis: clinical and radiological features and objective response to steroid therapy in a UK series. Am J Gastroenterol. 2007;102(11):2417–25.
57. Wakabayashi T et al. Duct-narrowing chronic pancreatitis without immunoserologic abnormality: comparison with duct-narrowing chronic pancreatitis with positive serological evidence and its clinical management. Dig Dis Sci. 2005;50(8):1414–21.
58. Hirano K et al. Long-term prognosis of autoimmune pancreatitis with and without corticosteroid treatment. Gut. 2007;56(12): 1719–24.
59. McNair AN et al. Autoimmune hepatitis overlapping with primary sclerosing cholangitis in five cases. Am J Gastroenterol. 1998;93(5):777–84.
60. Yoshida K et al. Chronic pancreatitis caused by an autoimmune abnormality. Proposal of the concept of autoimmune pancreatitis. Dig Dis Sci. 1995;40(7):1561–8.
61. Zen Y et al. IgG4-related sclerosing cholangitis with and without hepatic inflammatory pseudotumor, and sclerosing pancreatitis-associated sclerosing cholangitis: do they belong to a spectrum of sclerosing pancreatitis? Am J Surg Pathol. 2004;28(9):1193–203.
62. Bjornsson E et al. Primary sclerosing cholangitis associated with elevated immunoglobulinG4: clinical characteristics and response to therapy. Am J Ther. 2010;18(3):198–205.
63. Zhang L et al. IgG4+ plasma cell infiltrates in liver explants with primary sclerosing cholangitis. Am J Surg Pathol. 2010;34(1): 88–94.
64. Huggett MT et al. Type 1 autoimmune pancreatitis and IgG4-related sclerosing cholangitis is associated with extrapancreatic organ failure, malignancy, and mortality in a prospective UK cohort. Am J Gastroenterol. 2014;109(10):1675–83.
65. Broome U et al. Natural history and prognostic factors in 305 Swedish patients with primary sclerosing cholangitis. Gut. 1996;38(4):610–5.
66. Chapman RW et al. Primary sclerosing cholangitis: a review of its clinical features, cholangiography, and hepatic histology. Gut. 1980;21(10):870–7.

67. Fausa O, Schrumpf E, Elgjo K. Relationship of inflammatory bowel disease and primary sclerosing cholangitis. Semin Liver Dis. 1991;11(1):31–9.
68. Schrumpf E et al. Risk factors in primary sclerosing cholangitis. J Hepatol. 1994;21(6):1061–6.
69. Farrant JM et al. Natural history and prognostic variables in primary sclerosing cholangitis. Gastroenterology. 1991;100(6):1710–7.
70. Wiesner RH et al. Primary sclerosing cholangitis: natural history, prognostic factors and survival analysis. Hepatology. 1989;10(4):430–6.
71. Okolicsanyi L et al. Primary sclerosing cholangitis: clinical presentation, natural history and prognostic variables: an Italian multicentre study. The Italian PSC Study Group. Eur J Gastroenterol Hepatol. 1996;8(7):685–91.
72. Kochhar R et al. Primary sclerosing cholangitis: an experience from India. J Gastroenterol Hepatol. 1996;11(5):429–33.
73. Takikawa H. Characteristics of primary sclerosing cholangitis in Japan. Hepatol Res. 2007;37 Suppl 3:S470–3.
74. Loftus Jr EV et al. PSC-IBD: a unique form of inflammatory bowel disease associated with primary sclerosing cholangitis. Gut. 2005;54(1):91–6.
75. Aadland E et al. Primary sclerosing cholangitis: a long-term follow-up study. Scand J Gastroenterol. 1987;22(6):655–64.
76. Verdonk RC et al. Inflammatory bowel disease after liver transplantation: risk factors for recurrence and de novo disease. Am J Transplant. 2006;6(6):1422–9.
77. Lundqvist K, Broome U. Differences in colonic disease activity in patients with ulcerative colitis with and without primary sclerosing cholangitis: a case control study. Dis Colon Rectum. 1997;40(4):451–6.
78. Penna C et al. Pouchitis after ileal pouch-anal anastomosis for ulcerative colitis occurs with increased frequency in patients with associated primary sclerosing cholangitis. Gut. 1996;38(2):234–9.
79. Shetty K et al. The risk for cancer or dysplasia in ulcerative colitis patients with primary sclerosing cholangitis. Am J Gastroenterol. 1999;94(6):1643–9.
80. Soetikno RM et al. Increased risk of colorectal neoplasia in patients with primary sclerosing cholangitis and ulcerative colitis: a meta-analysis. Gastrointest Endosc. 2002;56(1):48–54.
81. Marchesa P et al. The risk of cancer and dysplasia among ulcerative colitis patients with primary sclerosing cholangitis. Am J Gastroenterol. 1997;92(8):1285–8.
82. Rasmussen HH et al. Hepatobiliary dysfunction and primary sclerosing cholangitis in patients with Crohn's disease. Scand J Gastroenterol. 1997;32(6):604–10.
83. Saich R, Chapman R. Primary sclerosing cholangitis, autoimmune hepatitis and overlap syndromes in inflammatory bowel disease. World J Gastroenterol. 2008;14(3):331–7.
84. Perrett AD, Higgins G, Johnston HH, Massarella GR, Truelove SC, Wright R. The liver in ulcerative colitis. Q J Med. 1971;40:187–209.
85. Schrumpf E et al. Sclerosing cholangitis in ulcerative colitis. Scand J Gastroenterol. 1980;15(6):689–97.
86. Vera A et al. Risk factors for recurrence of primary sclerosing cholangitis of liver allograft. Lancet. 2002;360(9349):1943–4.
87. Bergquist A et al. Hepatic and extrahepatic malignancies in primary sclerosing cholangitis. J Hepatol. 2002;36(3):321–7.
88. Eaden JA, Mayberry JF. Guidelines for screening and surveillance of asymptomatic colorectal cancer in patients with inflammatory bowel disease. Gut. 2002;51 Suppl 5:V10–2.
89. Bansal P, Sonnenberg A. Risk factors of colorectal cancer in inflammatory bowel disease. Am J Gastroenterol. 1996;91(1):44–8.
90. Brentnall TA et al. Risk and natural history of colonic neoplasia in patients with primary sclerosing cholangitis and ulcerative colitis. Gastroenterology. 1996;110(2):331–8.
91. Kornfeld D, Ekbom A, Ihre T. Is there an excess risk for colorectal cancer in patients with ulcerative colitis and concomitant primary sclerosing cholangitis? A population based study. Gut. 1997;41(4):522–5.
92. Vera A et al. Colorectal cancer in patients with inflammatory bowel disease after liver transplantation for primary sclerosing cholangitis. Transplantation. 2003;75(12):1983–8.
93. Broome U et al. Primary sclerosing cholangitis and ulcerative colitis: evidence for increased neoplastic potential. Hepatology. 1995;22(5):1404–8.
94. Brackmann S et al. Relationship between clinical parameters and the colitis-colorectal cancer interval in a cohort of patients with colorectal cancer in inflammatory bowel disease. Scand J Gastroenterol. 2009;44(1):46–55.
95. Claessen MM et al. High lifetime risk of cancer in primary sclerosing cholangitis. J Hepatol. 2009;50(1):158–64.
96. Braden B et al. Risk for colorectal neoplasia in patients with colonic Crohn's disease and concomitant primary sclerosing cholangitis. Clin Gastroenterol Hepatol. 2012;10(3):303–8.
97. Lindstrom L et al. Increased risk of colorectal cancer and dysplasia in patients with Crohn's colitis and primary sclerosing cholangitis. Dis Colon Rectum. 2011;54(11):1392–7.
98. Pardi DS et al. Ursodeoxycholic acid as a chemopreventive agent in patients with ulcerative colitis and primary sclerosing cholangitis. Gastroenterology. 2003;124(4):889–93.
99. Tung BY et al. Ursodiol use is associated with lower prevalence of colonic neoplasia in patients with ulcerative colitis and primary sclerosing cholangitis. Ann Intern Med. 2001;134(2):89–95.
100. Charatcharoenwitthaya P et al. Impact of inflammatory bowel disease and ursodeoxycholic acid therapy on small-duct primary sclerosing cholangitis. Hepatology. 2008;47(1):133–42.
101. Fevery J et al. Incidence, diagnosis, and therapy of cholangiocarcinoma in patients with primary sclerosing cholangitis. Dig Dis Sci. 2007;52(11):3123–35.
102. Burak K et al. Incidence and risk factors for cholangiocarcinoma in primary sclerosing cholangitis. Am J Gastroenterol. 2004;99(3):523–6.
103. Charatcharoenwitthaya P et al. Utility of serum tumor markers, imaging, and biliary cytology for detecting cholangiocarcinoma in primary sclerosing cholangitis. Hepatology. 2008;48(4):1106–17.
104. Tischendorf JJ et al. Characterization and clinical course of hepatobiliary carcinoma in patients with primary sclerosing cholangitis. Scand J Gastroenterol. 2006;41(10):1227–34.
105. Kaya M et al. Treatment of cholangiocarcinoma complicating primary sclerosing cholangitis: the Mayo Clinic experience. Am J Gastroenterol. 2001;96(4):1164–9.
106. Brandsaeter B et al. Liver transplantation for primary sclerosing cholangitis; predictors and consequences of hepatobiliary malignancy. J Hepatol. 2004;40(5):815–22.
107. Nichols JC et al. Diagnostic role of serum CA 19-9 for cholangiocarcinoma in patients with primary sclerosing cholangitis. Mayo Clin Proc. 1993;68(9):874–9.
108. Levy C et al. The value of serum CA 19-9 in predicting cholangiocarcinomas in patients with primary sclerosing cholangitis. Dig Dis Sci. 2005;50(9):1734–40.
109. Chalasani N et al. Cholangiocarcinoma in patients with primary sclerosing cholangitis: a multicenter case-control study. Hepatology. 2000;31(1):7–11.
110. Siqueira E et al. Detecting cholangiocarcinoma in patients with primary sclerosing cholangitis. Gastrointest Endosc. 2002;56(1):40–7.
111. Lempinen M et al. Enhanced detection of cholangiocarcinoma with serum trypsinogen-2 in patients with severe bile duct strictures. J Hepatol. 2007;47(5):677–83.
112. Blechacz B, Gores GJ. Cholangiocarcinoma: advances in pathogenesis, diagnosis, and treatment. Hepatology. 2008;48(1):308–21.
113. Ashok K. Role of MRCP versus ERCP in bile duct cholangiocarcinoma and benign stricture. Biomed Imaging Interv J. 2007;3:e12–545.

114. Beuers U et al. Ursodeoxycholic acid for treatment of primary sclerosing cholangitis: a placebo-controlled trial. Hepatology. 1992;16(3):707–14.
115. Moreno Luna LE et al. Advanced cytologic techniques for the detection of malignant pancreatobiliary strictures. Gastroenterology. 2006;131(4):1064–72.
116. Boberg KM et al. Diagnostic benefit of biliary brush cytology in cholangiocarcinoma in primary sclerosing cholangitis. J Hepatol. 2006;45(4):568–74.
117. Bangarulingam SY et al. Long-term outcomes of positive fluorescence in situ hybridization tests in primary sclerosing cholangitis. Hepatology. 2010;51(1):174–80.
118. Tischendorf JJ et al. Cholangioscopic characterization of dominant bile duct stenoses in patients with primary sclerosing cholangitis. Endoscopy. 2006;38(7):665–9.
119. El Fouly A, Dechene A, Gerken G. Surveillance and screening of primary sclerosing cholangitis. Dig Dis. 2009;27(4):526–35.
120. Bjornsson E, Angulo P. Cholangiocarcinoma in young individuals with and without primary sclerosing cholangitis. Am J Gastroenterol. 2007;102(8):1677–82.
121. Ahrendt SA et al. Diagnosis and management of cholangiocarcinoma in primary sclerosing cholangitis. J Gastrointest Surg. 1999;3(4):357–67 [discussion 367–8].
122. Rosen CB, Nagorney DM. Cholangiocarcinoma complicating primary sclerosing cholangitis. Semin Liver Dis. 1991;11(1):26–30.
123. Rosen CB et al. Cholangiocarcinoma complicating primary sclerosing cholangitis. Ann Surg. 1991;213(1):21–5.
124. Rosen CB, Heimbach JK, Gores GJ. Surgery for cholangiocarcinoma: the role of liver transplantation. HPB (Oxford). 2008;10(3):186–9.
125. Heimbach JK. Successful liver transplantation for hilar cholangiocarcinoma. Curr Opin Gastroenterol. 2008;24(3):384–8.
126. Said K, Glaumann H, Bergquist A. Gallbladder disease in patients with primary sclerosing cholangitis. J Hepatol. 2008;48(4):598–605.
127. Tischendorf JJ et al. Characterization, outcome, and prognosis in 273 patients with primary sclerosing cholangitis: a single center study. Am J Gastroenterol. 2007;102(1):107–14.
128. Stiehl A et al. Development of dominant bile duct stenoses in patients with primary sclerosing cholangitis treated with ursodeoxycholic acid: outcome after endoscopic treatment. J Hepatol. 2002;36(2):151–6.
129. Kaya M et al. Balloon dilation compared to stenting of dominant strictures in primary sclerosing cholangitis. Am J Gastroenterol. 2001;96(4):1059–66.
130. Ahrendt SA et al. Primary sclerosing cholangitis: resect, dilate, or transplant? Ann Surg. 1998;227(3):412–23.
131. Gaing AA et al. Endoscopic management of primary sclerosing cholangitis: review, and report of an open series. Am J Gastroenterol. 1993;88(12):2000–8.
132. Johnson GK et al. Endoscopic treatment of biliary tract strictures in sclerosing cholangitis: a larger series and recommendations for treatment. Gastrointest Endosc. 1991;37(1):38–43.
133. Baluyut AR et al. Impact of endoscopic therapy on the survival of patients with primary sclerosing cholangitis. Gastrointest Endosc. 2001;53(3):308–12.
134. Gluck M et al. A twenty-year experience with endoscopic therapy for symptomatic primary sclerosing cholangitis. J Clin Gastroenterol. 2008;42(9):1032–9.
135. Bjornsson ES, Kilander AF, Olsson RG. Bile duct bacterial isolates in primary sclerosing cholangitis and certain other forms of cholestasis—a study of bile cultures from ERCP. Hepatogastroenterology. 2000;47(36):1504–8.
136. Boomkens SY et al. The role of Helicobacter spp. in the pathogenesis of primary biliary cirrhosis and primary sclerosing cholangitis. FEMS Immunol Med Microbiol. 2005;44(2):221–5.
137. Pohl J et al. The role of dominant stenoses in bacterial infections of bile ducts in primary sclerosing cholangitis. Eur J Gastroenterol Hepatol. 2006;18(1):69–74.
138. Tabibian N. Rifampin as antipruritic agent in primary sclerosing cholangitis. Am J Gastroenterol. 1989;84(3):340.
139. Polter DE et al. Beneficial effect of cholestyramine in sclerosing cholangitis. Gastroenterology. 1980;79(2):326–33.
140. Ghent CN, Carruthers SG. Treatment of pruritus in primary biliary cirrhosis with rifampin. Results of a double-blind, crossover, randomized trial. Gastroenterology. 1988;94(2):488–93.
141. Bachs L et al. Effects of long-term rifampicin administration in primary biliary cirrhosis. Gastroenterology. 1992;102(6):2077–80.
142. Podesta A et al. Treatment of pruritus of primary biliary cirrhosis with rifampin. Dig Dis Sci. 1991;36(2):216–20.
143. Wolfhagen FH et al. Oral naltrexone treatment for cholestatic pruritus: a double-blind, placebo-controlled study. Gastroenterology. 1997;113(4):1264–9.
144. Mansour-Ghanaei F et al. Effect of oral naltrexone on pruritus in cholestatic patients. World J Gastroenterol. 2006;12(7):1125–8.
145. Bergasa NV et al. Oral nalmefene therapy reduces scratching activity due to the pruritus of cholestasis: a controlled study. J Am Acad Dermatol. 1999;41(3 Pt 1):431–4.
146. Chapman RW. Primary sclerosing cholangitis: what is the role of ursodeoxycholic acid in therapy for PSC? Nat Rev Gastroenterol Hepatol. 2010;7(2):74–5.
147. Angulo P et al. Bone disease in patients with primary sclerosing cholangitis: prevalence, severity and prediction of progression. J Hepatol. 1998;29(5):729–35.
148. Campbell MS et al. Severity of liver disease does not predict osteopenia or low bone mineral density in primary sclerosing cholangitis. Liver Int. 2005;25(2):311–6.
149. Ponsioen CY et al. Natural history of primary sclerosing cholangitis and prognostic value of cholangiography in a Dutch population. Gut. 2002;51(4):562–6.
150. Boonstra K et al. Population-based epidemiology, malignancy risk, and outcome of primary sclerosing cholangitis. Hepatology. 2013;58(6):2045–55.
151. Williamson KD, Chapman RW. Editorial: further evidence for the role of serum alkaline phosphatase as a useful surrogate marker of prognosis in PSC. Aliment Pharmacol Ther. 2015;41(1):149–51.
152. Rupp C et al. Reduction in alkaline phosphatase is associated with longer survival in primary sclerosing cholangitis, independent of dominant stenosis. Aliment Pharmacol Ther. 2014;40(11–12):1292–301.
153. Al Mamari S et al. Improvement of serum alkaline phosphatase to <1.5 upper limit of normal predicts better outcome and reduced risk of cholangiocarcinoma in primary sclerosing cholangitis. J Hepatol. 2013;58(2):329–34.
154. Lindstrom L et al. Association between reduced levels of alkaline phosphatase and survival times of patients with primary sclerosing cholangitis. Clin Gastroenterol Hepatol. 2013;11(7):841–6.
155. Stanich PP et al. Alkaline phosphatase normalization is associated with better prognosis in primary sclerosing cholangitis. Dig Liver Dis. 2011;43(4):309–13.
156. Lindor KD et al. High-dose ursodeoxycholic acid for the treatment of primary sclerosing cholangitis. Hepatology. 2009;50(3):808–14.
157. Sinakos E et al. Bile acid changes after high-dose ursodeoxycholic acid treatment in primary sclerosing cholangitis: relation to disease progression. Hepatology. 2010;52(1):197–203.
158. Mitchell SA et al. A preliminary trial of high-dose ursodeoxycholic acid in primary sclerosing cholangitis. Gastroenterology. 2001;121(4):900–7.
159. Harnois DM et al. High-dose ursodeoxycholic acid as a therapy for patients with primary sclerosing cholangitis. Am J Gastroenterol. 2001;96(5):1558–62.
160. Olsson R et al. High-dose ursodeoxycholic acid in primary sclerosing cholangitis: a 5-year multicenter, randomized, controlled study. Gastroenterology. 2005;129(5):1464–72.
161. Wolf JM, Rybicki LA, Lashner BA. The impact of ursodeoxycholic acid on cancer, dysplasia and mortality in ulcerative colitis patients with primary sclerosing cholangitis. Aliment Pharmacol Ther. 2005;22(9):783–8.

162. Leidenius M et al. Hepatobiliary carcinoma in primary sclerosing cholangitis: a case control study. J Hepatol. 2001;34(6):792–8.
163. Boberg KM, Egeland T, Schrumpf E. Long-term effect of corticosteroid treatment in primary sclerosing cholangitis patients. Scand J Gastroenterol. 2003;38(9):991–5.
164. Graziadei IW et al. Long-term results of patients undergoing liver transplantation for primary sclerosing cholangitis. Hepatology. 1999;30(5):1121–7.
165. Solano E et al. Liver transplantation for primary sclerosing cholangitis. Transplant Proc. 2003;35(7):2431–4.
166. Brandsaeter B et al. Outcome following liver transplantation for primary sclerosing cholangitis in the Nordic countries. Scand J Gastroenterol. 2003;38(11):1176–83.
167. Tischendorf JJ, Geier A, Trautwein C. Current diagnosis and management of primary sclerosing cholangitis. Liver Transpl. 2008;14(6):735–46.
168. Campsen J et al. Clinically recurrent primary sclerosing cholangitis following liver transplantation: a time course. Liver Transpl. 2008;14(2):181–5.
169. Alabraba E et al. A re-evaluation of the risk factors for the recurrence of primary sclerosing cholangitis in liver allografts. Liver Transpl. 2009;15(3):330–40.
170. Cholongitas E et al. Risk factors for recurrence of primary sclerosing cholangitis after liver transplantation. Liver Transpl. 2008;14(2):138–43.
171. MacLean AR et al. Outcome of patients undergoing liver transplantation for primary sclerosing cholangitis. Dis Colon Rectum. 2003;46(8):1124–8.
172. Riley TR et al. A case series of transplant recipients who despite immunosuppression developed inflammatory bowel disease. Am J Gastroenterol. 1997;92(2):279–82.

Autoimmune Pancreatitis and Other Organ Involvement

53

Go Kuwata and Terumi Kamisawa

Abbreviations

AIP	Autoimmune pancreatitis
LPSP	Lymphoplasmacytic sclerosing pancreatitis
IgG4	Immunoglobulin G4
IDCP	Idiopathic duct-centric chronic pancreatitis
GEL	Granulocytic epithelial lesion
ICDC	International consensus diagnostic criteria
CT	Computed tomography
MRI	Magnetic resonance imaging
ERCP	Endoscopic retrograde cholangiopancreatography
MRCP	Magnetic resonance cholangiopancreatography
IgG4-SC	IgG4-related sclerosing cholangitis
PSC	Primary sclerosing cholangitis
IBD	Inflammatory bowel disease
RF	Retroperitoneal fibrosis
IgG4-RF	IgG4-related retroperitoneal fibrosis
ANA	Antinuclear antigen
HPF	High power field
UC	Ulcerative colitis

Introduction

In 1961, Sarles et al. first reported pancreatitis with hypergammaglobulinemia and suggested an autoimmune etiology [1]. In 1995, the term "autoimmune pancreatitis" (AIP) was proposed by Yoshida et al. [2]. Since then, many cases of AIP have been reported in Western countries, as well as in Japan.

The histologic characteristic of almost all AIP cases reported from Japan has been lymphoplasmacytic sclerosing pancreatitis (LPSP). In 2001, Hamano et al. reported that serum immunoglobulin G4 (IgG4) concentrations are specifically elevated in this disease [3]. This type of AIP is frequently associated with various sclerosing extrapancreatic lesions, such as cholangitis, cholecystitis, sialadenitis, dacryoadenitis, and retroperitoneal fibrosis, etc. [4]. These histopathological features of extrapancreatic lesions are similar to the dense infiltration of IgG4-positive plasma cells and lymphocytes and fibrosis detected in the pancreas. Therefore, Kamisawa et al. proposed a clinicopathological entity of "IgG4-related sclerosing diseases" and suggested that AIP represents a pancreatic lesion of this systemic disease [5].

On the other hand, in 2003, Notohara et al. reported that there are two types of histologic groups of AIP. One is LPSP, and the other is idiopathic duct-centric chronic pancreatitis (ICDP) [6]. Zamboni et al. also reported AIP with the histologic finding of a granulocytic epithelial lesion (GEL) [7]. ICDP/GEL is identified on the basis of histological features of neutrophilic infiltration into the epithelium of the pancreatic duct. Case reports of AIP with IDCP/GEL have been mainly from Western countries and are rare from Asia. This type of AIP is sometimes associated with ulcerative colitis or Crohn's disease and shows no relationship to IgG4.

Recently, in 2011, International Consensus Diagnostic Criteria (ICDC) for AIP were proposed [8]. According to these criteria, AIP is classified into two types: type 1 and type 2. The histologic characteristic of type 1 AIP is LPSP, and that of type 2 AIP is IDCP/GEL.

This chapter focuses on the clinicopathological features of each type of AIP and extrapancreatic conditions, especially those involving the alimentary tract.

Type 1 AIP

Clinical Features

A recent nationwide epidemiological survey in Japan reported that the overall prevalence of AIP was estimated as 2.2 cases per 100,000 population [9]. Hart et al. reported the

G. Kuwata, M.D. • T. Kamisawa, M.D., Ph.D. (✉)
Department of Internal Medicine, Tokyo Metropolitan Komagome Hospital, 3-18-22 Honkomagome, Bunkyo-ku, Tokyo 113-8677, Japan
e-mail: kamisawa@cick.jp

D.C. Baumgart (ed.), *Crohn's Disease and Ulcerative Colitis*, DOI 10.1007/978-3-319-33703-6_53

data of 23 institutions from ten different countries; the proportion of type 1 AIP patients was 96 % in Asian countries, 87 % in European countries and 86 % in North American countries [10]. Type 1 AIP occurred predominantly in elderly males. The mean age at diagnosis was 61.6 years, and the proportion of males was 77 %. The major initial symptom was obstructive jaundice induced by associated sclerosing cholangitis.

Serum IgG4 concentrations are elevated frequently in type 1 AIP, although the precise pathogenic role of IgG4 in this disease is unclear. Type 1 AIP represents a systemic disease characterized by extensive IgG4-positive plasma cell and T lymphocyte infiltration of various organs. Clinical manifestations are apparent in organs such as the pancreas, bile duct, gallbladder, salivary glands, and retroperitoneum. Type 1 AIP is not simply a pancreatitis, but rather a pancreatic lesion reflecting an IgG4-related disease. In some cases, only one or two organs are clinically involved, whereas in others, three or four organs are affected.

Diagnosis

Diagnosis of type 1 AIP is definitive in a case with the pancreatic histological features of LPSP. However, since it is difficult to take an adequate specimen from the pancreas, histological confirmation is not usually available. Therefore, the diagnosis requires a combination of other features. According to ICDC (Tables 53.1 and 53.2) [8], type 1 AIP is diagnosed based on the criteria that use a combination of 1 or more cardinal features of AIP as follows:

Imaging of Pancreatic Parenchyma (on Computed Tomography (CT)/Magnetic Resonance Imaging (MRI))

Typical cases show diffuse enlargement, the so-called "sausage-like appearance" (Fig. 53.1). On dynamic CT and MRI, there is delayed enhancement of the enlarged pancreatic parenchyma. It is sometimes associated with a capsule-like low density rim that surrounds the pancreas on CT, which might be induced by inflammatory and fibrous changes involving the peripancreatic adipose tissue that is rather specific to type 1 AIP [11].

Imaging of the Pancreatic Duct (Endoscopic Retrograde Cholangiopancreatography (ERCP) or Magnetic Resonance Cholangiopancreatography (MRCP))

Typical cases shows long segmental (>1/3 length) or multiple strictures of the main pancreatic duct. Cases of type 1 AIP with segmental narrowing of the main pancreatic duct are difficult to differentiate from pancreatic cancer. Derivation of branch ducts from the narrowed portion of the main pancreatic duct and skipped narrowed portions of the main pancreatic duct suggest type 1 AIP rather than pancreatic cancer. Upstream dilatation of the distal pancreatic duct is less in cases of type 1 AIP than of pancreatic cancer [11].

Serology (IgG4 Concentration)

Serological criteria consist of elevated serum IgG4 levels. Although the serum IgG4 level is useful for screening, an elevated serum IgG4 level is neither sufficiently sensitive nor specific. About 20 % of patients with type 1 AIP have normal IgG4 levels at presentation [12]. Some studies have shown that 4–10 % of both healthy and disease controls, including patients with pancreatic cancer, have high serum IgG4 concentrations [12–14].

Other Organ Involvement

Sclerosing Cholangitis

Type 1 AIP is commonly accompanied by sclerosing cholangitis [15]. The histology of IgG4-related sclerosing cholangitis (IgG4-SC) shows obliterative phlebitis and transmural fibrosis with dense infiltration of IgG4-positive plasma cells, which lead to stricture of the bile duct.

IgG4-SC must be differentiated from primary sclerosing cholangitis (PSC). Inflammatory bowel disease (IBD) is frequently seen in PSC patients, whereas it is rare in IgG4-SC. Nakazawa et al. reported that the typical findings of IgG4-SC in ERCP are "segmental stricture," "long stricture with prestenotic dilatation," and "stricture of the lower bile duct," while the typical findings of PSC are "band-like stricture," "beaded appearances," "pruned-tree appearance," and "diverticulum-like appearance" [16]. Whether the limited intrapancreatic bile duct stricture associated with AIP should be regarded as a biliary manifestation of IgG4-related

Table 53.1 Diagnosis of definitive and probable type 1 AIP using ICDC

Diagnosis	Primary basis for diagnosis	Imaging evidence	Collateral evidence
Definitive type 1 AIP	Histology	Typical/indeterminate	Histologically confirmed LPSP (level 1 H)
	Imaging	Typical	Any non-D level 1/level 2
		Indeterminate	Two or more from level 1 (+level 2 D[a])
	Response steroid	Indeterminate	Level 1 S/OOI+Rt or level 1 D+level 2 S/OOI/H+Rt
Probable type 1 AIP		Indeterminate	Level 2 S/OOI/H+Rt

[a]Level 2 D is counted as level 1 in this setting

Table 53.2 Level 1 and level 2 criteria for type 1 AIP

Criterion	Level 1	Level 2
P Parenchymal imaging	Typical: Diffuse enlargement with delayed enhancement (sometimes associate with rim-like enhancement)	Indeterminate (including atypical[b]) Segmental/focal enlargement with delayed enhancement
D Ductal imaging (ERP)	Long (>1/3 length of the main pancreatic duct) or multiple strictures without marked upstream dilatation	Segmental/focal narrowing without marked upstream dilatation (duct size, <5 mm)
S Serology OOI Other organ involvement	IgG4, >2× upper limit of normal value a or b (a). Histology of extrapancreatic organs Any three of the following: (1) Marked lymphoplasmacytic infiltration with fibrosis and without granulocytic infiltration (2) Storiform fibrosis (3) Obliterative phlebitis (4) Abundant (>10 cells/HPF) IgG4-positive cells (b) Typical radiological evidence At least one of the following: (1) Segmental/multiple proximal (hilar/intrahepatic) or proximal and distal bile duct stricture (2) Retroperitoneal fibrosis	IgG4, 1–2× upper limit of normal value a or b (a) Histology of extrapancreatic organs including endoscopic biopsies of bile duct[c] Both of the following: (1) Marked lymphoplasmacytic infiltration without granulocytic infiltration (2) Abundant (>10 cells/HPF) IgG4-positive cells (b) Physical or radiological evidence At least one of the following: (1) Symmetrically enlarged salivary/lachrymal glands (2) Radiological evidence of renal involvement described in association with AIP
H Histology of the pancreas	LPSP (core biopsy/resection) At least three of the following: (1) Periductal lymphoplasmacytic infiltrate without granulocytic infiltration (2) Obliterative phlebitis (3) Storiform fibrosis (4) Abundant (>10 cells/HPF) IgG4-positive cells	LPSP (core biopsy) Any two of the following: (1) Periductal lymphoplasmacytic infiltrate without granulocytic infiltration (2) Obliterative phlebitis (3) Storiform fibrosis (4) Abundant (>10 cells/HPF) IgG4-positive cells
Response to steroid (Rt)[a] Rapid	Diagnostic steroid trial Rapid (≦2 week) radiologically demonstrable resolution or marked improvement in pancreatic/extrapancreatic manifestations	

[a]Diagnostic steroid trial should be conducted carefully by pancreatologists with caveats (see text) only after negative workup for cancer including endoscopic ultrasound-guided fine needle aspiration

[b]Atypical: Some AIP cases may show low-density mass, pancreatic ductal dilatation, or distal atrophy. Such atypical imaging findings in patients with obstructive jaundice and/or pancreatic mass are highly suggestive of pancreatic cancer. Such patients should be managed as pancreatic cancer unless there is strong collateral evidence for AIP, and a thorough workup for cancer is negative (see algorithm)

[c]Endoscopic biopsy of duodenal papilla is a useful adjunctive method because ampulla often is involved pathologically in AIP

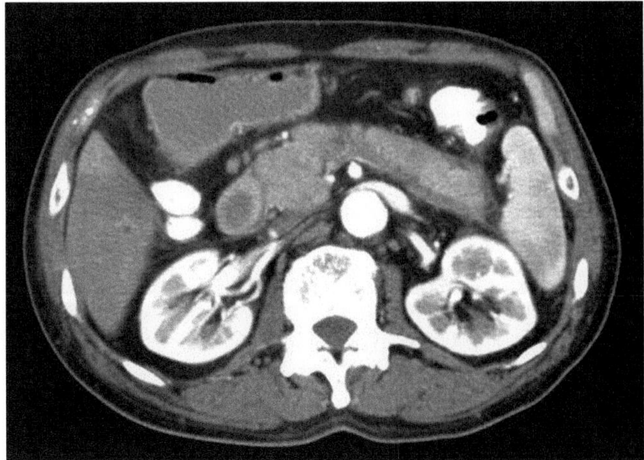

Fig. 53.1 CT imaging of a type 1 AIP case showing diffuse enlargement of pancreatic parenchyma with a capsule-like rim

disease is controversial, because such stenosis can be induced by compression from the swollen pancreas [17].

IgG4-SC must be also differentiated from cholangiocarcinoma. Neither serum IgG4 concentrations nor cholangiographic findings differentiate these disorders clearly [18]. Endoscopic transpapillary biopsy is generally performed. Although cholangiocarcinoma can be excluded by endoscopic biopsy, the superficial nature of samples obtained by this procedure limits their usefulness for diagnosis of IgG4-SC [19].

Cholecystitis can occur with sclerosing cholangitis. Thickening of the gallbladder wall is detected on imaging, but it is asymptomatic in most cases [20].

The major duodenal papilla is frequently swollen in patients with type1 AIP. Endoscopic biopsy from the major papilla is a useful adjunctive method because the papilla is often involved pathologically in AIP [21, 22].

Retroperitoneal Fibrosis

Retroperitoneal fibrosis (RF) is a rare disease characterized by the presence of fibro-inflammatory tissue that develops around the abdominal aorta and iliac arteries. IgG4-related disease is the cause of up to two-thirds of cases of RF [23]. Chiba et al. [24] proposed diagnostic criteria for IgG4-related retroperitoneal fibrosis (IgG4-RF) consisting of three items: typical radiological features, elevation of serum IgG4 levels and the histological finding of an abundant infiltration of IgG4-positive plasma cells at a retroperitoneal mass or extraretroperitoneal sites. In their series of 10 IgG4-RF patients, IgG4-RF showed a predilection for elderly men. Symptoms predominantly related to RF (back pain and edema of the lower extremities) were observed in only two patients, and the remaining patients reported initial symptoms due to associated diseases. Twenty-four other IgG4-related diseases (AIP, sialadenitis, dacryoadenitis, lymphadenopathy, pulmonary pseudotumor, and pituitary pseudotumor) occurred in nine patients. On laboratory examinations, anemia, hypoalbuminemia, increased CRP levels, and antinuclear antigen (ANA) positivity were frequently observed. IgG4-RF responds well to steroids, but malignancies including malignant lymphoma should be ruled out.

Salivary Gland Involvement (Sclerosing Sialadenitis)

Major and minor salivary glands can be affected. This disorder was known for more than a century as Mikulicz's disease, consisting of dacryoadenitis and enlargement of the parotid and submandibular glands, and it is now recognized as an IgG4-related disease [25]. Isolated enlargement of the submandibular glands is common in IgG4-related disease. In contrast, in Sjogren's syndrome, parotid enlargement predominates. Xerostomia commonly accompanies IgG4-related disease, but it is generally less severe than in Sjogren's syndrome, and in contrast to Sjogren's syndrome, it can improve with immunosuppression.

Orbital Involvement (Dacryoadenitis, Orbital Myositis)

The typical presentation of orbital involvement is swelling within the ocular region or frank proptosis, generally caused by lacrimal-gland enlargement (dacryoadenitis) [26, 27]. Proptosis can also result from orbital pseudotumors that do not affect the lacrimal gland, from involvement of extraocular muscles (orbital myositis), and from combinations of these abnormalities.

Tubulointerstitial Nephritis

The most characteristic form of IgG4-related renal involvement is tubulointerstitial nephritis. The histology of this disease is the same as in other organs: lymphoplasmacytic infiltration with IgG4 predominance among plasma cells; storiform fibrosis; and moderate tissue eosinophilia [28].

Many patients with IgG4-related tubulointerstitial nephritis have substantial enlargements of the kidneys and hypodense lesions evident on CT. The clinical presentation can show advanced renal dysfunction and even end-stage renal dysfunction. Substantial proteinuria can develop, but concentrations are generally subnephrotic.

Histopathology of the Pancreas

The histological profile of the pancreas is LPSP, which shows four characteristic features: (1) periductal lymphoplasmacytic infiltrate without granulocytic infiltration; (2) obliterative phlebitis; (3) storiform fibrosis; and (4) abundant (>10 cells/high power field (HPF)) IgG4-positive cells (Fig. 53.2a–c).

Response to Steroid Therapy

Response to steroid therapy is an additional finding that confirms the diagnosis of AIP. Rapid (within 2 weeks) radiologically demonstrable resolution or marked improvement in pancreatic and extrapancreatic manifestations may support the diagnosis. A diagnostic steroid trial should be conducted carefully only after negative workup for cancer [8].

Treatment and Prognosis

Oral steroid therapy is the standard treatment. Indications for steroid therapy in type 1 AIP patients are symptoms such as jaundice and abdominal pain [29]. Before steroid therapy is started, blood glucose levels and jaundice should be controlled. The most commonly used initial dose of prednisolone is 0.6 mg/kg/day, and it is tapered by 5 mg every 1–2 weeks while monitoring the patient's symptoms as well as biochemical, serological, and imaging findings. To prevent relapse, maintenance therapy (5 mg/day) is recommended for 6–12 months [29]. Hart et al. [10] reported that of the 978 subjects with type 1 AIP, 302 (31 %) subjects experienced at least one disease relapse. Most relapses of type 1 AIP occurred in the biliary system or pancreas. Subjects with proximal IgG4-SC showed a relatively high relapse rate (56.1 %) compared with subjects without IgG4-SC (25.7 %). At the time of relapse, readministration or increased doses of steroids are usually effective.

Most AIP patients treated with steroid therapy have good short- and long-term clinical, morphological, and functional outcomes. However, since some patients develop pancreatic stones or malignancy during or after steroid therapy, AIP patients should be rigorously followed up.

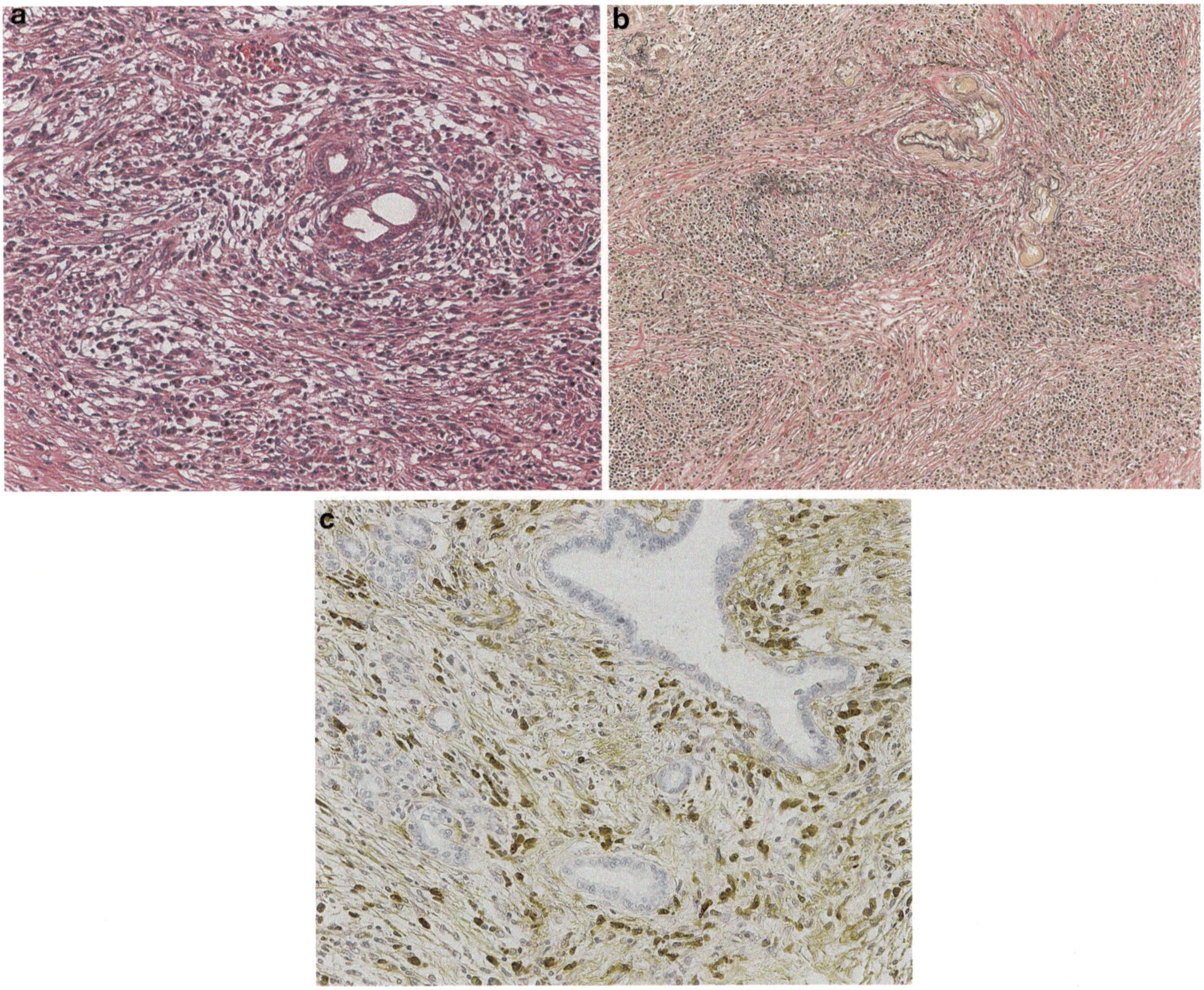

Fig. 53.2 Histopathological findings of the pancreas of a type 1 AIP case. (**a**) Lymphoplasmacytic sclerosing pancreatitis showing abundant infiltration of plasma cells and lymphocytes and storiform fibrosis (H&E stain). (**b**) Obliterative phlebitis (EVG stain). (**c**) Abundant infiltration of IgG4-positive plasma cells (IgG4 immunostaining)

Type 2 AIP

Clinical Features

Type 2 AIP is rare in Asia compared to Europe and North America. Type 2 AIP is seen in younger patients than type 1 AIP, and typical affects males and females equally. Abdominal pain and acute pancreatitis are more frequent in cases of type 2 AIP than of type 1 AIP [10].

Type 2 AIP shows no serological biomarkers, and no extrapancreatic lesions other than ulcerative colitis (UC) or Crohn's disease. Therefore, definitive diagnosis of type 2 AIP requires histological examination of an adequate specimen obtained by core biopsy or resection of the pancreas, which is not frequently available. Type 2 AIP cannot be diagnosed easily, and this may explain the fewer cases of type 2 AIP diagnosed worldwide [30].

Diagnosis

According to ICDC, type 2 AIP is diagnosed based on imaging of the pancreatic parenchyma and pancreatic duct, histology of the pancreas, response to steroid therapy, and coexisting IBD (Tables 53.3 and 53.4) [8].

Criteria of parenchymal imaging are diffuse enlargement with delayed enhancement (Level 1 criterion) and segmental/focal enlargement with delayed enhancement (Level 2).

Histological findings of the pancreas typical for AIP type 2 are (1) GEL with or without granulocytic acinar inflammation, and (2) absent or scant (0–10 cells/HPF) IgG4-positive

Table 53.3 Diagnosis of definitive and probable type 2 AIP using ICDC

Diagnosis	Imaging evidence	Collateral evidence
Definitive type 2 AIP	Typical/indeterminate	Histologically confirmed IDCP (level 1 H) or clinical inflammatory bowel disease + level 2 H + Rt
Probable type 2 AIP	Typical/indeterminate	Level 2 H/clinical inflammatory bowel disease + Rt

Table 53.4 Level 1 and level 2 criteria for type 2 AIP

Criterion	Level 1	Level 2
P Parenchymal imaging	Typical: Diffuse enlargement with delayed enhancement (sometimes associated with rim-like enhancement)	Indeterminate (including atypical[b]): Segmental/focal enlargement with delayed enhancement
D Ductal imaging (ERP)	Long (>1/3 length of the main pancreatic duct) or multiple strictures without marked upstream dilatation	Segmental/focal narrowing without marked upstream dilatation (duct size, <5 mm)
OOI Other organ involvement		Clinically diagnosed inflammatory bowel disease
H Histology of the pancreas (core biopsy/resection)	IDCP: Both of the following: (1) Granulocytic infiltration of duct wall (GEL) with or without granulocytic acinar inflammation (2) Absent or scant (0–10 cells/HPF) IgG4-positive cells	Both of the following: (1) Granulocytic and lymphoplasmacytic acinar infiltrate (2) Absent or scant (0–10 cells/HPF) IgG4-positive cells
Response to steroid (Rt)[a]	Diagnostic steroid trial Rapid (≦2 week) radiologically demonstrable resolution or marked improvement in pancreatic/extrapancreatic manifestations	

[a]Diagnostic steroid trial should be conducted carefully by pancreatologists with caveats only after negative workup for cancer including endoscopic ultrasound-guided fine needle aspiration

[b]Atypical: Some AIP cases may show low-density mass, pancreatic ductal dilatation, or distal atrophy. Such atypical imaging findings in patients with obstructive jaundice and/or pancreatic mass are highly suggestive of pancreatic cancer. Such patients should be managed as pancreatic cancer unless there is strong collateral evidence for AIP, and a thorough workup for cancer is negative

cells (Level 1). Diagnosis of type 2 AIP is definitive in cases with Level 1 or 2 imaging and typical histology of the pancreas. If histology of the pancreas shows only Level 2 criterion, two additional criterions are needed for definitive diagnosis: one is response to steroid therapy and the other is coexisting IBD.

Response to steroid therapy is a finding that confirms the diagnosis of AIP. As in type 1 AIP, a diagnostic steroid trial should be conducted carefully only after a negative workup for cancer. In addition, it does not seem that imaging and response to steroids can distinguish between type 1 and type 2 AIP.

Treatment and Prognosis

Initial reports of type 2 AIP included only patients who had undergone surgical resection. In such patients, no further treatment was required, and no relapse was reported [30]. In the case of type 2 AIP histologically confirmed and medically treated, it appears to either spontaneously resolve or respond promptly to steroid therapy. The initial response rate to steroids was 92.3 % [10]. Common indications for steroid therapy in type 2 AIP patients were symptoms, such as abdominal pain (64 %), and coexisting IBD (48 %). The disease relapse rate in type 2 AIP was only 9 %, and relapses in type 2 AIP were limited to the pancreas [10].

AIP and Inflammatory Bowel Disease

An association between pancreatitis and IBD has been widely accepted, but IBD-associated clinical pancreatitis was found in only 2 % of patients. Recently, increasing evidence has suggested a potential link between AIP and IBD. IBD is frequently associated especially with type 2 AIP. Hart et al. [10] reported that 48 % of type 2 AIP cases have IBD. We had seen a case of probable type 2 AIP coexisting with UC. This case was a 32-year-old male who simultaneously developed both segmental type AIP of the pancreatic body and tail and total colon-type UC (Fig. 53.3a–c). His initial symptoms were upper abdominal pain and bloody diarrhea. AIP occurred as acute pancreatitis with serum amylase elevation (249 IU/L). His serum IgG4 level was within the normal limit (45 mg/dl). Both AIP and UC improved after steroid therapy.

In contrast, only 0.1 % of type 1 AIP cases have IBD. IgG4-positive plasma cell infiltration is sometimes detectable in the colonic mucosa of UC patients [31, 32] (Fig. 53.4), but none of them have storiform fibrosis or obliterative phlebitis. Thus, UC cannot be recognized as a lesion involved in IgG4-related diseases. The IgG4-positive plasma cell count infiltrated in the colonic mucosa of UC patients seems to be related to disease severity [32], but the mechanisms underly-

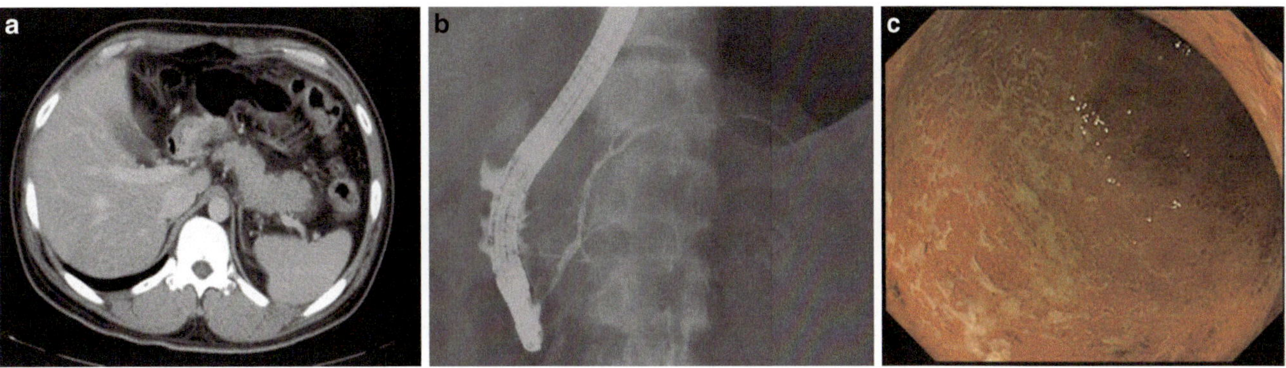

Fig. 53.3 Imaging and endoscopic findings of a type 2 AIP case. (**a**) CT imaging showing enlargement of the pancreatic body and tail. (**b**) ERP showing narrowing of the main pancreatic duct. (**c**) Colonoscopy showing inflamed colonic mucosa suggesting ulcerative colitis

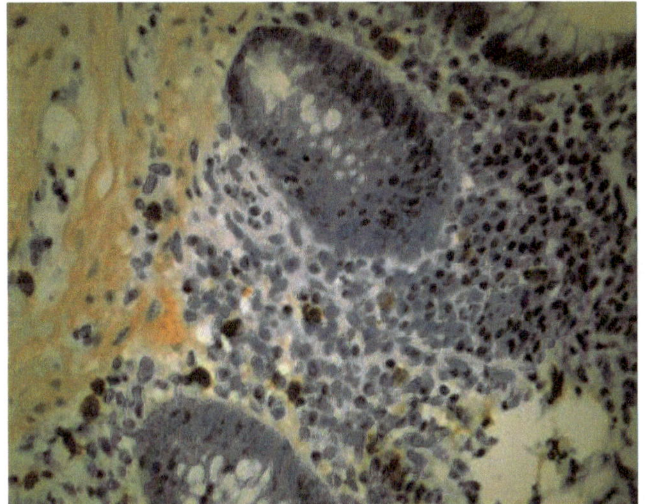

Fig. 53.4 Abundant infiltration of IgG4-positive plasma cells in colonic mucosa of a patient with ulcerative colitis (IgG4-immunostaining)

ing IgG4-positive plasma cell infiltration in the colonic mucosa of UC patients are unknown.

Infiltration of many IgG4-positive plasma cells is detectable in the colonic mucosa of some type 1 AIP patients [33]. However, as neither storiform fibrosis nor obliterative phlebitis was observed in the colonic mucosa, the colonic mucosa cannot be recognized as a colonic lesion involved in IgG4-related diseases. Matsui et al. reported a case of an AIP patient with colonic polyposis containing many IgG4-positive plasma cells that were markedly reduced with steroid therapy [34]. Chetty et al. reported a case of well-circumscribed sclerosing nodular lesions of the cecum and sigmoid colon composed of hyalinized fibrocollagenous tissue with abundant infiltration of IgG4-positive plasma cells [35]. These polypoid or nodular lesions appear to be IgG4-related colonic lesions, but further studies are necessary to confirm this concept.

Summary

AIP is a peculiar form of pancreatitis that should be differentiated from pancreatic cancer. AIP is divided into two subtypes. Type 1 AIP is a pancreatic manifestation of IgG4-related disease and is rarely associated with IBD. Type 2 AIP is not related to IgG4 and is sometimes associated with IBD.

Acknowledgement This chapter was supported by the grant-in-aid for the Refractory Disease from the Ministry of Labor, Health, and Welfare of Japan.

References

1. Sarles H, Sarles JC, Muratore R, Guien C. Chronic inflammatory sclerosis of the pancreas—an autonomous pancreatic disease? Am J Dig Dis. 1961;6:688–98.
2. Yoshida K, Toki F, Takeuchi T, Watanabe S, Shiratori K, Hayashi N. Chronic pancreatitis caused by an autoimmune abnormality. Proposal of the concept of autoimmune pancreatitis. Dig Dis Sci. 1995;40:1561–8.
3. Hamano H, Kawa S, Horiuchi A, Unno H, Furuya N, Akamatsu T, et al. High serum IgG4 concentrations in patients with sclerosing pancreatitis. N Engl J Med. 2001;344:732–8.
4. Kamisawa T, Zen Y, Pillai S, Stone JH. IgG4-related disease. Lancet. 2015;385:1460–71.
5. Kamisawa T, Funata N, Hayashi Y, Eishi Y, Koike M, Tsuruta K, et al. A new clinicopathological entity of IgG4-related autoimmune disease. J Gastroenterol. 2003;38:982–4.
6. Notohara K, Burgart LJ, Yadav D, Chari S, Smyrk TC. Idiopathic chronic pancreatitis with periductal lymphoplasmacytic infiltration: clinicopathologic features of 35 cases. Am J Surg Pathol. 2003;27:1119–27.
7. Zamboni G, Luttges J, Capelli P, Frulloni L, Cavallini G, Pederzoli P, et al. Histopathological features of diagnostic and clinical relevance in autoimmune pancreatitis: a study on 53 resection specimens and 9 biopsy specimens. Virchows Arch. 2004;445:552–63.
8. Shimosegawa T, Chari ST, Frulloni L, Kamisawa T, Kawa S, Mino-Kenudson M, et al. International consensus diagnostic criteria for

autoimmune pancreatitis: guidelines of the International Association of Pancreatology. Pancreas. 2011;40:352–8.
9. Kanno A, Masamune A, Okazaki K, Kamisawa T, Kawa S, Nishimori I, et al. Nationwide epidemiological survey of autoimmune pancreatitis in Japan in 2011. Pancreas. 2015;44:535–9.
10. Hart PA, Kamisawa T, Brugge WR, Chung JB, Culver EL, Czako L, et al. Long-term outcomes of autoimmune pancreatitis: a multicentre, international analysis. Gut. 2013;62:1771–6.
11. Kamisawa T, Imai M, Yui Chen P, Tu Y, Egawa N, Tsuruta K, et al. Strategy for differentiating autoimmune pancreatitis from pancreatic cancer. Pancreas. 2008;37:e62–7.
12. Tabata T, Kamisawa T, Takuma K, Anjiki H, Egawa N, Kurata M, et al. Serum IgG4 concentrations and IgG4-related sclerosing disease. Clin Chim Acta. 2009;408(1–2):25–8.
13. Ghazale A, Chari ST, Smyrk TC, Levy MJ, Topazian MD, Takahashi N, et al. Value of serum IgG4 in the diagnosis of autoimmune pancreatitis and in distinguishing it from pancreatic cancer. Am J Gastroenterol. 2007;102:1646–53.
14. Sadler R, Chapman RW, Simpson D, Soonawalla ZF, Waldegrave EL, Burden JM, et al. The diagnostic significance of serum IgG4 levels in patients with autoimmune pancreatitis: a UK study. Eur J Gastroenterol Hepatol. 2011;23:139–45.
15. Zen Y, Harada K, Sasaki M, Sato Y, Tsuneyama K, Haratake J, et al. IgG4-related sclerosing cholangitis with and without hepatic inflammatory pseudotumor, and sclerosing pancreatitis-associated sclerosing cholangitis: do they belong to a spectrum of sclerosing pancreatitis? Am J Surg Pathol. 2004;28:1193–203.
16. Nakazawa T, Naitoh I, Hayashi K, Miyabe K, Simizu S, Joh T. Diagnosis of IgG4-related sclerosing cholangitis. World J Gastroenterol. 2013;19:7661–70.
17. Hirano K, Tada M, Isayama H, Yamamoto K, Mizuno S, Yagioka H, et al. Endoscopic evaluation of factors contributing to intrapancreatic biliary stricture in autoimmune pancreatitis. Gastrointest Endosc. 2010;71:85–90.
18. Oseini AM, Chaiteerakij R, Shire AM, Ghazale A, Kaiya J, Moser CD, et al. Utility of serum immunoglobulin G4 in distinguishing immunoglobulin G4-associated cholangitis from cholangiocarcinoma. Hepatology. 2011;54:940–8.
19. Nakazawa T, Ando T, Hayashi K, Naitoh I, Ohara H, Joh T. Diagnostic procedures for IgG4-related sclerosing cholangitis. J Hepatobiliary Pancreat Sci. 2011;18:127–36.
20. Kamisawa T, Takuma K, Egawa N, Tsuruta K, Sasaki T. Autoimmune pancreatitis and IgG4-related sclerosing disease. Nat Rev Gastroenterol Hepatol. 2010;7:401–9.
21. Kamisawa T, Tu Y, Nakajima H, Egawa N, Tsuruta K, Okamoto A. Usefulness of biopsying the major duodenal papilla to diagnose autoimmune pancreatitis: a prospective study using IgG4-immunostaining. World J Gastroenterol. 2006;12:2031–3.
22. Chiba K, Kamisawa T, Kuruma S, Iwasaki S, Tabata T, Koizumi S, et al. Major and minor duodenal papillae in autoimmune pancreatitis. Pancreas. 2014;43:1299–302.
23. Zen Y, Onodera M, Inoue D, Kitao A, Matsui O, Nohara T, et al. Retroperitoneal fibrosis: a clinicopathologic study with respect to immunoglobulin G4. Am J Surg Pathol. 2009;33:1833–9.
24. Chiba K, Kamisawa T, Tabata T, Hara S, Kuruma S, Fujiwara T, et al. Clinical features of 10 patients with IgG4-related retroperitoneal fibrosis. Intern Med. 2013;52:1545–51.
25. Geyer JT, Ferry JA, Harris NL, Stone JH, Zukerberg LR, Lauwers GY, et al. Chronic sclerosing sialadenitis (Kuttner tumor) is an IgG4-associated disease. Am J Surg Pathol. 2010;34:202–10.
26. Wallace ZS, Deshpande V, Stone JH. Ophthalmic manifestations of IgG4-related disease: single-center experience and literature review. Semin Arthritis Rheum. 2014;43:806–17.
27. Koizumi S, Kamisawa T, Kuruma S, Tabata T, Iwasaki S, Chiba K, et al. Clinical features of IgG4-related dacryoadenitis. Graefes Arch Clin Exp Ophthalmol. 2014;252:491–7.
28. Saeki T, Nishi S, Imai N, Ito T, Yamazaki H, Kawano M, et al. Clinicopathological characteristics of patients with IgG4-related tubulointerstitial nephritis. Kidney Int. 2010;78:1016–23.
29. Kamisawa T, Okazaki K, Kawa S, Ito T, Inui K, Irie H, et al. Amendment of the Japanese Consensus Guidelines for Autoimmune Pancreatitis, 2013 III. Treatment and prognosis of autoimmune pancreatitis. J Gastroenterol. 2014;49:961–70.
30. Kamisawa T, Chari ST, Lerch MM, Kim MH, Gress TM, Shimosegawa T. Recent advances in autoimmune pancreatitis: type 1 and type 2. Gut. 2013;62:1373–80.
31. Rebours V, Le Baleur Y, Cazals-Hatem D, Stefanescu C, Hentic O, Maire F, et al. Immunoglobulin G4 immunostaining of gastric, duodenal, or colonic biopsies is not helpful for the diagnosis of autoimmune pancreatitis. Clin Gastroenterol Hepatol. 2012;10:91–4.
32. Kuwata G, Kamisawa T, Koizumi K, Tabata T, Hara S, Kuruma S, et al. Ulcerative colitis and immunoglobulin g4. Gut Liver. 2014;8:29–34.
33. Kamisawa T, Egawa N, Nakajima H, Tsuruta K, Okamoto A, Hayashi Y, et al. Gastrointestinal findings in patients with autoimmune pancreatitis. Endoscopy. 2005;37:1127–30.
34. Matsui H, Watanabe T, Ueno K, Ueno S, Tsuji Y, Matsumura K, et al. Colonic polyposis associated with autoimmune pancreatitis. Pancreas. 2009;38:840–2.
35. Chetty R, Serra S, Gauchotte G, Markl B, Agaimy A. Sclerosing nodular lesions of the gastrointestinal tract containing large numbers of IgG4 plasma cells. Pathology. 2011;43:31–5.

Cutaneous and Oral Manifestations of Inflammatory Bowel Disease

54

Caroline P. Allen and Susan M. Burge

Introduction

Cutaneous and oral manifestations occur in 6–30 % of patients with ulcerative colitis and up to 60 % of patients with Crohn disease, but may precede the diagnosis of inflammatory bowel disease (IBD) by several years. The skin or oral mucosa may be affected directly by IBD or indirectly by its treatment, but the prevalence of some inflammatory dermatoses is also increased in IBD (Table 54.1) [1]. Psoriasis is approximately five times more common in patients with Crohn disease and genes in the IL-12/IL-23 pathway have been associated with both diseases [2, 3]. T-helper 17 cells play a key role in the development of psoriasis [4] as well as Crohn disease. The same anti-TNF treatments that have been so successful in severe IBD have revolutionized the treatment of severe psoriasis; however, these have also associated with causing skin conditions, including paradoxically, psoriatic like rashes. Conditions such as aphthous ulcers, erythema nodosum, and some neutrophilic dermatoses (pyoderma gangrenosum, Sweet syndrome, bowel-associated dermatosis–arthritis syndrome) are associated with IBD, but the pathogenesis of the relationship is uncertain. In this chapter we discuss the presentation and management of the more common and important cutaneous and oral problems that may be seen in IBD.

Nutritional Deficiencies

Malnutrition is a well-documented complication of IBD caused by problems such as inadequate diet, malabsorption and chronic inflammation of the gastrointestinal tract with bleeding, diarrhea or bowel fistulae [5]. Patients may be deficient in protein, carbohydrate, vitamins, minerals, and/or essential trace elements, but iron deficiency caused by chronic blood loss is particularly common. Cutaneous features of nutritional deficiency include:

- Itching (iron deficiency may cause itching)
- Pallor (iron deficiency anemia)
- Dryness of the skin with scaling
- Dry hair and brittle nails (fatty acid deficiency)
- Hyperpigmentation (generalized or localized)
- Hair loss (iron deficiency)
- Bruising, petechiae, oral bleeding (vitamin K or vitamin C deficiency)
- Angular stomatitis, cheilitis, glossitis (smooth sore red tongue), mucosal erosions (deficiency of vitamin B complex or folic acid)
- Perifollicular hemorrhage and follicular keratoses on upper arms, back, buttocks and lower extremities containing "corkscrew" coiled hairs (vitamin C deficiency, i.e., scurvy)
- Delayed wound healing
- Follicular hyperkeratosis, mainly affecting the extensor surfaces of extremities (Vitamin A deficiency)

Dry, itchy skin, in the absence of an alternative explanation such as eczema, raises the possibility of nutritional deficiency. Exclude other causes of itch (Table 54.2). Practical steps that may help to relieve itchy dry skin are outlined in Table 54.3.

Zinc Deficiency

Zinc deficiency may be secondary to malabsorption or to parenteral nutrition without zinc [6]. Typical features of deficiency include:

- Scaly erythematous rash resembling psoriasis on hands and feet, but often with the addition of vesicles or pustules
- Pustular paronychia, i.e., pustules and boggy swelling of the nail fold

C.P. Allen, M.A., M.B.B.S., M.R.C.P.
S.M. Burge, B.Sc., D.M., F.R.C.P. (✉)
Department of Dermatology, Oxford University Hospitals NHS Trust, Oxford, UK
e-mail: caroline.allen@gmail.com; sue.burge@ndm.ox.ac.uk

D.C. Baumgart (ed.), *Crohn's Disease and Ulcerative Colitis*, DOI 10.1007/978-3-319-33703-6_54

Table 54.1 Cutaneous manifestations in inflammatory bowel disease

- Nail clubbing and palmar erythema
- Erythema nodosum
- Aphthous ulcers and glossitis
- Thrombophlebitis
- Perianal fissures, fistulae and abscesses—more severe in Crohn disease than ulcerative colitis
- Genital or orofacial Crohn disease
- Peri-stomal dermatitis or folliculitis
- Cutaneous adverse drug reactions
- Manifestations of nutritional deficiency
- Psoriasis (increased prevalence in Crohn disease)
- Neutrophilic dermatoses such as pyoderma gangrenosum, Sweet syndrome, and Bowel-associated dermatosis–arthritis syndrome.
- Vitiligo
- Autoimmune bullous diseases (a rare association): bullous pemphigoid, linear IgA disease, and epidermolysis bullosa acquisita

Table 54.2 Causes of itch

- Primary skin disease, e.g., eczema, psoriasis, urticaria
- Infestation (scabies, fleas, lice)
- Drugs including statins (also cause dryness), ACE inhibitors, opiates, barbiturates, antidepressants
- Systemic disease
  - Iron deficiency
  - Thyroid disease
  - Cholestatic jaundice
  - Chronic renal failure
  - Polycythemia
  - Lymphoma
  - HIV infection

Table 54.3 Management of itchy skin

- Emollients—prescribe 500 g tubs and apply at least twice/day. Creams are preferable for day-time use and greasier oil-based emollients for the evening
- Avoid soap, instead recommend a soap substitute
- Aqueous cream with 1 % menthol may relieve itch if emollients are not effective
- Moderate or potent topical corticosteroid ointments applied once or twice/day may be helpful if skin is inflamed
- Sedating antihistamines may be helpful at night
- Trim nails to reduce damage from scratching

- Periorificial (perioral, periorbital, and perianal) crusted papules and plaques which may be vesicular or pustular
- Photophobia with blepharitis and conjunctivitis
- Slow hair growth or generalized alopecia
- Nail dystrophy with Beau's lines in chronic zinc deficiency
- Delayed healing of wounds
- Secondary bacterial and fungal infections.

Niacin Deficiency

Pellagra caused by niacin deficiency has been reported in Crohn disease. Pellagra is characterized by a symmetrical dermatitis on light-exposed skin (the only sign in one third of patients), diarrhea and dementia. A shiny edematous erythema develops on the exposed skin of nose and cheekbones (malar erythema), anterior neck (Casal necklace), and dorsa of the hands. The rash may blister and the skin becomes scalier with time. Heat, friction or pressure triggers the rash. The acute erythema and superficial scaling fade to leave reddish-brown pigmentation. Typically the lips are dry and cracked, the tongue swollen, and the buccal mucosa dry and smooth.

Cutaneous and Oral Crohn Disease

Definitions

1. Cutaneous Crohn disease: Crohn disease affecting the skin at sites in direct continuity with the gastrointestinal tract, particularly perianal, perineal, vulval, and peristomal sites.
2. Orofacial Crohn disease: Crohn disease affecting the lips and oral mucosa.
3. Metastatic Crohn disease: Crohn disease affecting the skin at sites that are separated from the gastrointestinal tract by normal tissue [7].

Epidemiology and Associations

Cutaneous, orofacial, and metastatic Crohn disease are rare. They usually present after the onset of intestinal Crohn disease, but may precede the onset of intestinal disease by months to years. Mean age at presentation is 34 years and cutaneous disease is more common in woman [7, 8].

Pathogenesis

The pathogenesis of Crohn disease is discussed in the epidemiology and immunobiology chapters of this book.

Clinical Features

The morphology of cutaneous Crohn disease is variable. Patients may have a single lesion or widespread disease, but perianal disease is often an early feature. Signs such as perianal erythema, polypoid tags, moist vegetating plaques, perianal fissures, and sinus tracts occur in around one-third of patients. Aphthous ulcers may involve the anal canal and anal sphincter. Severe disease is associated with abscesses and fistulae that may result in scarring with deformity. Crohn disease may also involve surgical sites including laparotomy scars.

Metastatic Crohn disease affects the genitalia, lower extremities, and flexures. Patients present with dusky erythematous papules, plaques, nodules, or ulcers exuding pus. Genitalia may be erythematous, swollen, and indurated, particularly in children.

Orofacial involvement causes persistent lip or cheek swelling with angular cheilitis, indurated fissuring of the lower lip and gingival erythematous papules. The edematous infiltrated buccal mucosa develops a "cobblestone"—like appearance. Aphthous ulcers are common [7, 8].

Diagnosis and Histopathology

The differential diagnosis in cutaneous or metastatic Crohn disease is broad and includes granulomatous infections (mycobacterial, spirochetal, deep fungal), foreign body reactions and cutaneous sarcoidosis. Genital or inguinal disease may simulate hidradenitis suppurativa (Fig. 54.1), but the grouped open comedones (blackheads) that are a feature of hidradenitis are not present in Crohn disease. Genital swelling may be caused by obstructive lymphedema. Ulcers in Crohn disease may resemble pyoderma gangrenosum.

Orofacial Crohn disease simulates granulomatous cheilitis (orofacial granulomatosis), a poorly understood condition that causes persistent non-tender swelling of the lips. Rarely these patients develop facial nerve palsy and a fissured tongue (Melkersson–Rosenthal syndrome). In some of these patients lip swelling is triggered by an allergic reaction to foods, food additives, or flavorings such as cinnamates, but this is not common.

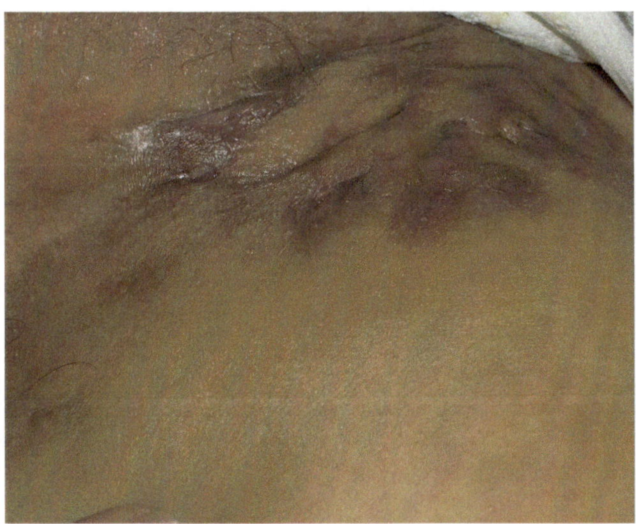

Fig. 54.1 Chronic fistulae, abscesses, and scarring in hidradenitis suppurativa may be difficult to differentiate from cutaneous Crohn disease. Grouped open comedones (*blackheads*) in affected skin suggest hidradenitis and patients with hidradenitis may have a long history of recurrent boils in axillae, breasts, groins, vulva, or perianal skin

Skin biopsy reveals superficial and deep non-caseating granulomas that may be difficult to differentiate from cutaneous sarcoidosis, but the presence of a lymphocyte-rich infiltrate, ulceration and edema favor Crohn disease [7]. Tissue should be cultured to exclude infection.

Chest radiology should be performed to exclude sarcoidosis and patch testing considered in patients with lip swelling.

Treatment

Treatment is difficult and the course tends to be chronic. Medical options include oral metronidazole (250 mg ×3/day), corticosteroids (very potent topical, intralesional or systemic), sulfasalazine, dapsone, azathioprine and TNF-alpha inhibitors (infliximab, adaluminab) [8].

Low dose antibiotics (e.g., penicillin V 250 mg ×2/day for 6 months) may have a role in patients with persistent lip swelling and fissuring to prevent streptococcal infection and lymphatic damage.

Peri-stomal Skin Problems

Skin disorders are reported in >70 % of patients with an abdominal stoma, despite the use of hydrocolloids to secure appliances and protect the skin [9]. Irritant contact dermatitis is common (Fig. 54.2), often with secondary infection, and chronic irritation causes over-granulation or erosions at the mucocutaneous junction. Potent topical corticosteroids settle inflammation, but may impair adhesion of the bag. Betamethasone valerate (0.1 %) aqueous lotion can be applied to the adhesive surface of the stoma

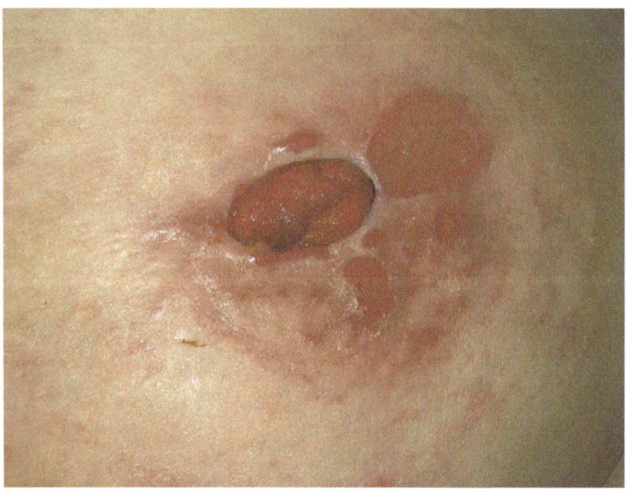

Fig. 54.2 Irritant contact dermatitis is a common problem around stomas

appliance and any alcohol allowed to evaporate before placing the appliance on the skin. Sucralfate powder prevents irritation and may promote healing of erosions [9]. Allergic contact dermatitis is uncommon, but patch testing is sensible to exclude allergy if dermatitis is difficult to control.

Shaving the skin to help the bag to adhere may cause a bacterial folliculitis. Take skin swabs for microbiological culture and treat with antibiotics as well as an antiseptic wash [9].

Peri-stomal psoriasis can usually be controlled with topical corticosteroids. Peri-stomal pyoderma gangrenosum is a rare problem that is discussed below.

Erythema Nodosum

Key Features

- Bilateral tender warm plaques and nodules usually affecting the anterior shins.
- Nodules resolve spontaneously without ulceration or scarring.
- Histopathology reveals a septal panniculitis without vasculitis.
- Associations—numerous underlying conditions
  - Infections particularly streptococcal throat infections and tuberculosis
  - Sarcoidosis
  - Inflammatory bowel disease
  - Pregnancy
  - Drugs including the oral contraceptive pill, bromides and sulfonamides

Definition

Erythema nodosum is a septal panniculitis most commonly affecting the shins.

Epidemiology and Associations

Erythema nodosum is the commonest form of panniculitis. It presents most often in Northern European women. Most cases appear between the second and fourth decades, with a peak incidence between the ages of 20 and 30 years. In the Northern hemisphere the incidence peaks in late winter and early spring suggesting an environmental trigger, perhaps streptococcal infection [10].

Erythema nodosum is common in IBD; studies suggest it is present in up to 15 % of patients with Crohn disease and 10 % of patients with ulcerative colitis. The presence of erythema nodosum may correlate with underlying disease activity. Sarcoidosis is one of the commonest causes in the Western world [11]. Erythema nodosum usually occurs in the acute phase in association with bilateral hilar lymphadenopathy [10]. A strong relationship exists to upper respiratory infections with Group A hemolytic streptococcus—the nodules develop 2–3 weeks after the infection. Tuberculosis (now an uncommon cause in Europe), atypical mycobacterial infections, HIV and hepatitis are among other infectious triggers [11, 12]. Numerous medications have been implicated including the oral contraceptive pill, bromides, sulfonamides, penicillin, granulocyte colony stimulating factor, codeine [11] and BRAF inhibitors [13]. Other associations include celiac disease, rheumatoid arthritis, Behçet's disease and Still's disease. Erythema nodosum has also been reported in association with malignancies, both hematological and solid organ [13].

No underlying cause is found in 40–60 % of patients [11].

Etiology and Pathogenesis

Despite the numerous well-defined provocations, the pathogenesis of erythema nodosum is unclear. The disease may be a hypersensitivity response involving deposition of immune complexes around venues in subcutaneous fat or a type IV delayed hypersensitivity reaction [11].

Clinical Features

Patients develop tender, erythematous, warm nodules, measuring 1–5 cm or more in diameter in a symmetrical distribution on the shins, ankles, and knees (Fig. 54.3). Less frequently, nodules appear on the arms or trunk. Fever, malaise, and headache are common. Some patients complain of abdominal pain, vomiting, or diarrhea.

Nodules do not ulcerate, but fade over 2–6 weeks without loss of fat or scarring, leaving a bruise-like discoloration that resolves more slowly. Resolution is usually more rapid in children.

A chronic migratory variant (subacute nodular migratory panniculitis, erythema nodosum migrans) is much less common; the indurated erythematous plaques are tender and may be asymmetrical.

Diagnosis and Histopathology

Investigations should ensure there is no other underlying cause in patients with IBD. FBC, ESR, urinalysis and chest

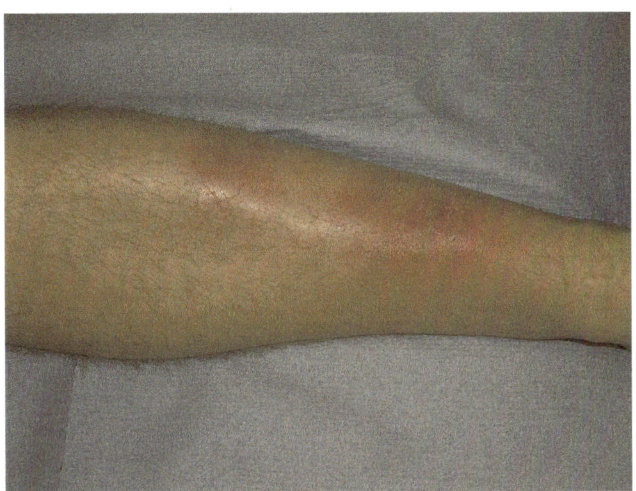

Fig. 54.3 Tender erythematous nodules on the shins in erythema nodosum

radiography should always be performed, but further investigations should be guided by the clinical history and examination. Local prevalence of etiological factors such as bacterial, viral, fungal or protozoal infections should be considered and investigation directed accordingly.

A deep elliptical biopsy including fat is required to demonstrate the typical changes, but is rarely necessary. Histopathology reveals a septal panniculitis, generally with a superficial and deep perivascular lymphocytic infiltrate in the overlying dermis, but no vasculitis [11].

Differential diagnosis includes trauma, cellulitis, insect bites and superficial thrombophlebitis. Nodular vasculitis is another panniculitis, sometimes associated with tuberculosis, that causes symmetrical nodules on the legs; however these nodules tend to be present on the calves rather than the shins and the nodules ulcerate and heal with a depressed scar caused by loss of fat. Histopathology reveals a lobular panniculitis with vasculitis and fat necrosis in contrast to erythema nodosum [12].

Treatment

Most cases resolve spontaneously within 6 weeks. Relapses are more common in patients with idiopathic disease or in those with preceding upper respiratory tract infection than in patients with an underlying problem such as IBD [11].

Pain should be managed with regular non-steroidal anti-inflammatory drugs. Elevation of the legs and support stockings may help to control swelling and speed resolution. Generally oral corticosteroids are not required. Potassium iodide 200–600 mg/day has been recommended in persistent disease, however this is contraindicated in pregnancy, and has been associated with hypothyroidism [11]. Oral tetracylines have been reported to be of benefit in recalcitrant disease [14, 15].

Pyoderma Gangrenosum

Key Features

- Painful ulcer with irregular violaceous undermined border
- Slough or hemorrhagic base
- Purulent discharge
- Rapid enlargement (usually)
- History of minor trauma preceding ulcer
- Sterile pustule preceding ulcer
- Pain out of proportion to the ulcer
- Healing with cribriform scarring
- Responds to systemic corticosteroids

Definition

Pyoderma gangrenosum is an uncommon neutrophilic dermatosis characterized by rapidly enlarging ulcers that are usually extremely painful. The condition was described in 1916 by Broq, and further characterized by Brunstung, Goeckerman, and O'Leary in 1930, who coined the term pyoderma gangrenosum.

Epidemiology and Associations

The annual incidence of pyoderma gangrenosum is estimated at 3–10 patients per million. Pyoderma gangrenosum is most common in middle-aged adults and has an equal sex distribution; however, it has been described in children and in the elderly. Fifty percent of patients with pyoderma gangrenosum have an associated systemic condition and in approximately one-third this is IBD, more often ulcerative colitis than Crohn disease. Other associations include rheumatoid arthritis, seronegative arthritis, and hematological malignancy (particularly myeloid leukemia). Twenty percent of patients have a monoclonal gammopathy of uncertain significance, most commonly an IgA gammopathy [16, 17].

Etiology and Pathogenesis

The etiology and pathogenesis of pyoderma gangrenosum are not well understood, but may be linked to abnormalities in neutrophil function. IgA gammopathies that impair neutrophil function in vitro are associated with pyoderma gangrenosum. Interleukin-8 (IL-8), a leukocyte chemotactant, is overexpressed in pyoderma gangrenosum and ulceration can be induced in xenografts transfected with recombinant human IL-8 [17]. Another clue to the role of neutrophil dysfunction is provided by the dominantly inherited autoinflammatory disorder, PAPA (pyogenic sterile arthritis, pyoderma gangrenosum, and acne). PAPA is caused by mutations in a gene that encodes proline serine threonine phosphatase-interacting protein 1 (PSTPIP-1). PSTPIP-1 co-localizes with pyrin in neutrophils. Normally pyrin downregulates inflammation, but in PAPA, the altered PSTPIP-1 binds more avidly than normal to pyrin, inhibiting its action and leading to activation of IL-1beta and the accumulation of neutrophils [18].

Pathergy (minor trauma triggers ulceration) may play a role in pathogenesis.

Clinical Variants of Pyoderma Gangrenosum

A number of variants have been described—see Table 54.4. The classical and pustular forms of pyoderma gangrenosum are those most often associated with IBD [17].

Classical pyoderma gangrenosum is characterized by a painful ulcer with an irregular, undermined violaceous (bluish-red) border and a necrotic base producing a purulent or hemorrhagic exudate (Fig. 54.4). Patients may have a fever and considerable pain. Typically the ulcers enlarge rapidly. The border may become serpiginous if ulceration extends at different rates in different directions. Healing occurs from the edge resulting in a characteristic pattern of scarring with perforations known as "cribriform" (sieve-like) scarring. Pyoderma gangrenosum triggers neither lymphadenopathy nor lymphangitis, despite the inflammatory appearance. Approximately 20 % of patients demonstrate pathergy (new lesions are initiated by minimal trauma). Pyoderma gangrenosum is most common on the lower limbs, the trunk is affected in 10 % of patients and lesions on the head, groin, genitalia or upper extremities are less common. A sterile neutrophilic infiltrate may be found in other organs, e.g., lungs, heart, liver, spleen, gastrointestinal tract, and lymph nodes.

Table 54.4 Pyoderma gangrenosum: variants

Classical	Painful irregular ulcers with undermined edges. Commonly affects lower limbs. Pathergy seen. Associated with IBD when pyoderma gangrenosum may be peri-stomal
Pustular	Discrete sterile pustules, joint pain, and fever. Associated with IBD. Activity follows activity of IBD
Pyostomatitis vegetans	Mucosal. Associated with ulcerative colitis
Bullous	Painful vesicles and bullae. Associated with hematological malignancy
Superficial granulomatous	Localized, less aggressive. Not usually associated with underlying disease

Rarely pyoderma gangrenosum develops around the stoma of patients with IBD (Fig. 54.5). Peri-stomal pyoderma gangrenosum may present from a few months to many years after the formation of the stoma. Pathergy may play a role in pathogenesis of peri-stomal PG skin may be irritated by leakage of stomal contents or by adhesives used to attach the stoma bag.

A pustular form of pyoderma gangrenosum has been described in association with active IBD. Discrete sterile pustules, 0.5–2 cm in diameter, with a surrounding erythematous halo occur in association with joint pains and fever. Pustules may heal without scarring or progress to the ulcerated lesions of classical pyoderma gangrenosum. The activity of pustular

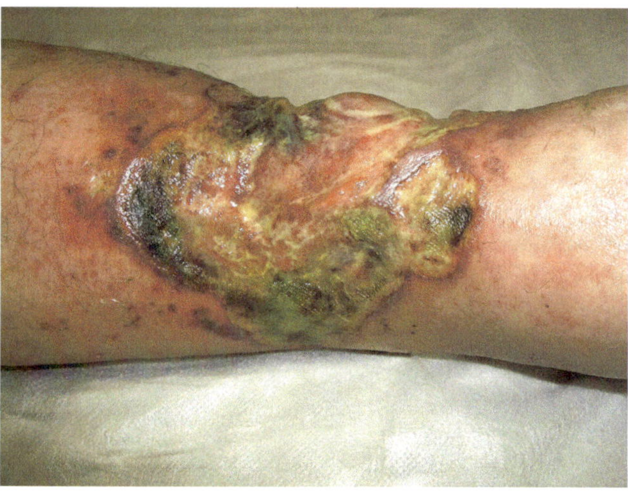

Fig. 54.4 Classical pyoderma gangrenosum. The deep painful ulcer has an irregular, undermined inflammatory border and a necrotic base

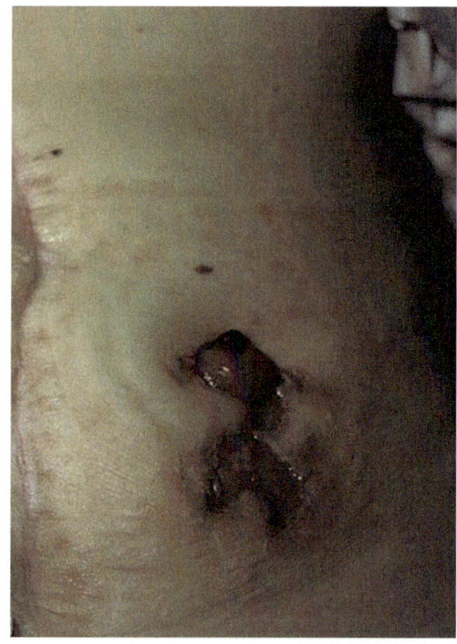

Fig. 54.5 Peri-stomal pyoderma gangrenosum in this patient responded promptly to treatment with a very potent topical corticosteroid

pyoderma gangrenosum tends to follow the activity of the bowel disease and may improve when the underlying disease is treated. Pyostomatitis vegetans may be the mucosal form of pustular pyoderma gangrenosum. This rare condition is associated with ulcerative colitis more often than Crohn disease. Friable grey-yellow pustules may involve oral, vaginal, nasal, and, rarely, periocular mucosa. Ruptured pustules leave vegetating erosions or ulcers. Even extensive oral involvement may be relatively painless [19].

Bullous pyoderma gangrenosum has been recorded in association with hematological malignancy rather than IBD. Painful vesicles and bullae lead to superficial erosions. Sweet syndrome (see below) may have a similar appearance. Superficial granulomatous pyoderma gangrenosum is a localized, less aggressive variant that tends to involve the head and neck. Underlying disease is unusual and some cases may be an atypical form of Wegner's granulomatosis [17, 20].

Differential Diagnosis

Pyoderma gangrenosum may simulate a variety of conditions and the diagnosis can be difficult if the clinical signs are atypical. Nicorandil-induced ulcers simulate pyoderma gangrenosum but infection and malignancy are the most important differentials to exclude—see Table 54.5.

Investigations

- Take a deep cutaneous biopsy from the edge of the ulcer. Tissue should be sent for both histopathological examination and for culture (including atypical mycobacterial and fungal culture). Histopathological findings of follicular or perifollicular inflammation, intradermal abscesses, and/or sterile dermal neutrophilia without vasculitis are supportive of the diagnosis, but are not diagnostic. Clinicopathological correlation is vital.
- Surface swabs are of limited value as bacterial colonization is inevitable, but blood cultures should be performed if systemic infection is suspected.

Table 54.5 Pyoderma gangrenosum: differential diagnosis

Vascular	Venous or arterial insufficiency, occlusive vasculopathy including antiphospholipid antibody syndrome
Infectious	Bacterial including mycobacterial, viral, deep fungal, parasite
Malignancy	Primary cutaneous, lymphoma, metastatic
Medications	Nicorandil, hydroxyurea
Inflammatory	Sweet syndrome, granulomatosis with polyangiitis, panniculitis, autoimmune bullous diseases
Trauma	Bites—insect, spider, snake; dermatitis artefacta

- Blood tests should include FBC, ESR, CRP, protein electrophoresis, and immunoglobulins.

Course and Prognosis

The course of pyoderma gangrenosum is unpredictable; the disease may progress rapidly or be slowly progressive. Lesions may resolve spontaneously and can return for no obvious reason after being quiescent for many years. It was believed that the activity of pyoderma gangrenosum followed that of the underlying bowel disease, but flares of pyoderma gangrenosum have been reported in patients after bowel resection and in patients with inactive ileitis. Severe pyoderma gangrenosum has a mortality of 30 %. Poor prognostic factors include older age at first onset, male sex and bullous disease associated with underlying hematological malignancy [17].

Treatment

Treatment is challenging. Treatment of underlying bowel disease should be optimized, but does not always lead to improvement in pyoderma gangrenosum. It is helpful to monitor the response to treatment objectively by measuring ulcers and by clinical photography [21].

General measures for wound management are important, but surgical debridement may trigger extension of pyoderma gangrenosum and should be avoided. Soaks or wet dressings with 0.01 % potassium permanganate solution may help to reduce bacterial colonization. Moisture retaining wound dressings facilitate wound healing and help with pain control. Alginate dressings absorb exudate and prevent maceration.

Localized pustules, bullae, or small ulcers may be managed with topical treatments such as a very potent topical corticosteroid ointment or 0.1 % tacrolimus ointment. Peri-stomal pyoderma gangrenosum may also respond to a very potent topical corticosteroid or 0.1–0.3 % tacrolimus in carmellose sodium paste [9] take a biopsy if no response after 2 weeks.

Most pyoderma gangrenosum requires systemic treatment. Systemic corticosteroids (prednisolone 0.75–2 mg/kg/day or pulses of intravenous methylprednisolone) or oral cyclosporine (Neoral 4 mg/kg/day in two divided doses) should be started promptly to prevent progression [22]; patient factors should guide the decision as to which to use. Response is usually rapid, but prolonged treatment may be required with combinations of drugs. Other steroid-sparing agents such as methotrexate or dapsone may have a role. Recent data has shown that TNF alpha-blocking agents (infliximab [23] and adalimumab [23]) are very effective for the treatment of PG in patients with underlying IBD. In view of this, anti-TNFs should be considered as first-line treatment [23].

Pain can be severe and require systemic opiates. Pain levels should be documented and can be used as a marker of treatment efficacy. Increasing pain or exudate may indicate secondary bacterial infection.

Sweet Syndrome

Key Features

- Tender erythematous plaques and nodules on the head, neck, and upper extremities
- Fever >38 °C
- Leukocytosis with neutrophilia and raised ESR
- Associations: preceding infection, IBD, malignancy, pregnancy, drugs

Definition

Sweet syndrome is a neutrophilic dermatosis characterized by erythematous papules, nodules, and plaques, fever, and neutrophilia. The syndrome was first described by Robert Sweet in 1964 [24, 25].

Epidemiology and Associations

The disease is more common in women, and classically presents between the ages of 30 and 50 years, with no racial predilection [25].

Sweet syndrome may be precipitated by infection of the upper respiratory tract or gastrointestinal tract. In other cases the syndrome is associated with an underlying systemic disease such as IBD, chronic arthritis, or malignancy, particularly hematological malignancies, e.g., acute myelogenous leukemia and less commonly myeloproliferative disease or myelodysplastic syndromes, lymphoma or paraproteinemias. Solid organ tumors, generally those of the breast, genitourinary system, and gastrointestinal tract, have also been linked to Sweet syndrome. Pregnancy, vaccination, and drugs, including granulocyte colony-stimulating factor (G-CSF), may also trigger the syndrome [24, 25].

Etiology and Pathogenesis

The etiology is unclear. An antigen of infectious or tumor origin may trigger a hypersensitivity reaction. Granulocyte-colony stimulating factor (G-CSF) and interleukin-6 appear to play a role. G-CSF is a known precipitant; tumors that produce G-CSF have been isolated in patients with Sweet syndrome and patients with active Sweet syndrome have been found to have raised levels of serum G-CSF compared to patients in whom the disease was quiescent [25].

Clinical Features

Sweet syndrome is characterized by the abrupt onset of painful erythematous nodules or plaques associated with a high fever (>38 °C). Patients appear unwell and may complain of headache, arthralgia, and myalgia. Other extracutaneous features include iritis, episcleritis and/or conjunctivitis, polyarthritis, and oral mucosal ulcers which mimic aphthae.

The juicy papules and plaques, which present most often on the face and upper trunk, are tender, well-demarcated and edematous (Fig. 54.6). The surface of plaques may appear to be vesicular (pseudo-vesicles), reflecting the intense dermal edema, but it is rare to find discrete vesicles or bullae that can be ruptured. Occasionally plaques become pustular. Like pyoderma gangrenosum, Sweet syndrome demonstrates pathergy i.e., cutaneous lesions may develop at sites of minor trauma such as skin biopsies or venipuncture. Patients may also have pyoderma gangrenosum.

Diagnosis and Histopathology

The diagnosis is suggested by the presence of the typical clinical features, in association with a raised ESR, a raised CRP and a leukocytosis, which is predominantly a neutrophilia. Blood cultures are sterile. See Tables 54.6 and 54.7 for differential diagnoses and investigations.

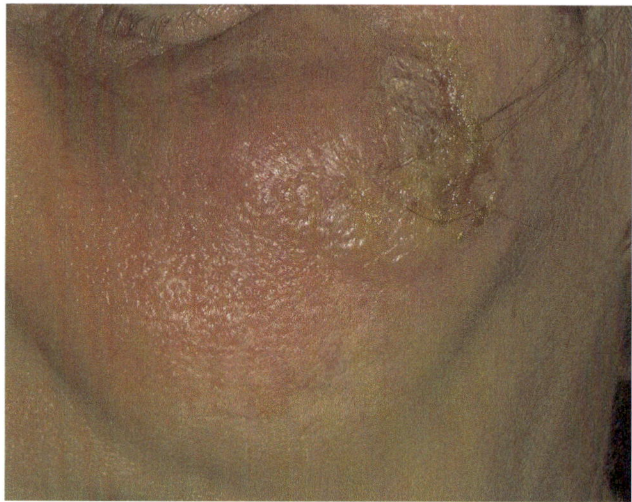

Fig. 54.6 The tender, edematous erythematous plaques of Sweet syndrome are often misdiagnosed as cellulitis

Table 54.6 Sweet syndrome: differential diagnosis

- Infection such as streptococcal cellulitis, bacterial septicemia, herpes simplex infection, deep fungal infection
- Cutaneous vasculitis
- Pustular pyoderma gangrenosum
- Malignancy—primary cutaneous or metastatic
- Urticaria or urticarial vasculitis
- Erythema nodosum
- Insect bites

Table 54.7 Investigations in Sweet syndrome

- FBC and ESR; a neutrophilia and raised ESR are present in Sweet syndrome
- Blood cultures and skin swabs from pustular lesions should be performed to exclude infection
- Take a skin biopsy from a well-developed plaque. Histopathology reveals a dense dermal neutrophilic infiltrate with leukocytoclasis but without vasculitis. Gram stain is negative
- Generally underlying malignancy or inflammatory disease should be excluded, but these are unlikely associations in a patient with IBD

Treatment

Very potent topical corticosteroids (clobetasol propionate 0.05 %) ×2/day may control localized disease. Systemic corticosteroids are the first-line treatment for more widespread disease. A typical regime consists of prednisolone 30 mg/day in conjunction with a very potent topical corticosteroid ×2/day. Recurrences are common. Potassium iodide and colchicine are alternative first-line therapies [26]; second line treatments include indomethacin (indomethacin), clofazimine, cyclosporine (cyclosporine), and dapsone [26].

Bowel-Associated Dermatosis–Arthritis Syndrome

Key Features

- Serum sickness like constitutional signs and symptoms of fever and general malaise.
- Crops of erythematous macules, purpuric papules, and small vesicopustules on upper trunk and extremities.
- Migratory polyarthralgia, non-erosive polyarthritis or tenosynovitis.
- Histopathology reveals a perivascular neutrophilic infiltrate.

Definition

The bowel-associated dermatosis–arthritis syndrome is a neutrophilic dermatosis that is associated with an underlying condition causing an overgrowth of bowel flora. The syndrome comprises cutaneous lesions, non-erosive arthritis, arthralgia, and fever.

Epidemiology and Associations

Early cases were associated with bowel surgery that created a "blind loop", allowing bacterial overgrowth, but subsequently the condition was observed in patients who had not had this type of surgery. Now it is accepted that any condition that predisposes to bowel stasis, including IBD, can precipitate bowel-associated dermatosis–arthritis syndrome [27, 28].

Etiology and Pathogenesis

The overgrowth of bacteria in the bowel with subsequent deposition of immune complexes is thought to trigger disease. *Escherichia coli* and other bacteria are believed to release peptidoglycans that lead to the formation of immune complexes [29].

Clinical Features

Cutaneous lesions generally affect the upper trunk and extremities and consist of crops of erythematous macules, purpuric papules, and crusted vesicopustules. Patients also have a migratory polyarthralgia or a non-erosive polyarthritis in association with fever and malaise.

Diagnosis and Histopathology

Diagnosis is based on the characteristic clinical findings and the history of a predisposing bowel condition. Skin biopsy should be performed to confirm the diagnosis. The histopathological findings resemble Sweet syndrome with dermal edema and a dense neutrophilic infiltrate.

Treatment

The underlying cause should be corrected when possible. Oral antibiotics have been advocated to eradicate bacteria, e.g., oxytetracycline, erythromycin, clindamycin, tetracycline–sulfamethoxazole, or metronidazole. A short course of oral prednisolone may provide symptomatic relief.

Immunobullous Diseases

Definition

The immunobullous diseases are caused by autoantibodies directed against structural proteins in the skin such as keratins, desmosomal proteins, hemidesmosomal proteins, or basement membrane zone proteins. Blisters form because adhesion fails between the keratinocytes (intraepidermal blisters) or within or below the dermo-epidermal junction (subepidermal blisters). Three subepidermal immunobullous diseases have been described in association with IBD: bullous pemphigoid, linear IgA disease (LAD), and epidermolysis bullosa acquisita (EBA).

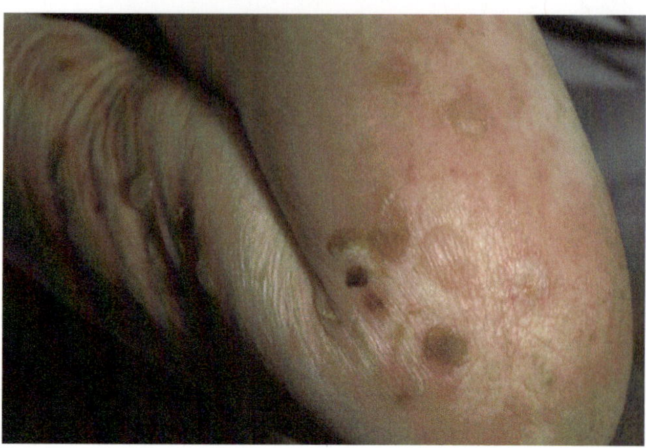

Fig. 54.7 Bullous pemphigoid with urticated papules, tense blisters and crusted erosions on an erythematous background

Etiology and Pathogenesis

The target antigens in bullous pemphigoid, LAD and EBA are in components of the basement membrane zone. In bullous pemphigoid autoantibodies to collagen XVII, a transmembrane component of the hemidesmosomes, appear to initiate disease. The IgA class autoantibodies in LAD are also directed against epitopes in collagen XVII. Type VII collagen, a component of the anchoring fibrils that fasten the lamina densa of the basement membrane to the underlying papillary dermis, is the antigen in EBA [30].

Epidemiology and Associations

Autoimmune blistering diseases are not common and even less common in patients with IBD. Even bullous pemphigoid, the most common immunobullous disease, is rarely reported in IBD. However, the association between IBD and immunobullous diseases appears to be genuine and may reflect a genetically determined susceptibility to develop autoimmune diseases.

Clinical Features

Bullous pemphigoid presents with itchy urticated papules or plaques and tense blisters, 1–3 cm in diameter, on inflamed or normal-appearing skin (Fig. 54.7). Blistering tends to predominate on the lower trunk, flexural surfaces of limbs, axillae and groins. Blisters heal without scarring. Oral blisters are present in about one third of patients.

Blisters in LAD may resemble those in bullous pemphigoid or patients may have small itchy vesicles on extensor surfaces that suggest dermatitis herpetiformis. Patients may have mucosal involvement.

Patients with EBA notice skin fragility or blistering in areas exposed to trauma, e.g., knuckles, elbows, knees, toes. Blisters may be hemorrhagic and underlying skin inflamed or scarred. Patients may develop a nail dystrophy or scarring alopecia. Mucosal lesions are unusual. The signs may suggest porphyria cutanea tarda.

Diagnosis and Histopathology

More common causes of blistering such as infection, acute eczema or a drug eruption should be excluded before considering an autoimmune blistering disease—see Table 54.8.

To confirm the diagnosis of an immunobullous disease, take blood for indirect immunofluorescence microscopy to look for circulating autoantibodies to antigens in the basement membrane zone and biopsy a pre-bullous urticated lesion or a small blister for histology (blisters are subepidermal). Also snap freeze a biopsy from perilesional skin for direct immunofluorescence microscopy to look for deposits of immunoglobulin and complement.

Treatment

The course of these diseases is punctuated by exacerbations and partial remissions. Blistering in bullous pemphigoid is usually controlled by combinations of very potent topical corticosteroids and systemic corticosteroids (30–60 mg/day). Tetracycline (500–2000 mg/day) in combination with nicotinamide (500–2500 mg/day) has been advocated in mild to moderate disease [31]. Systemic corticosteroids,

Table 54.8 Causes of widespread blistering

- Acute eczema
- Cutaneous infections
  - Viral—herpes simplex (may generalize in conditions such as atopic eczema) or varicella-zoster (chickenpox).
  - Bacterial—widespread staphylococcal infection (bullous impetigo)
- Burns
- Staphylococcal scalded skin syndrome caused by a circulating exotoxin produced by Staphylococcus aureus
- Drug reactions
  - Stevens–Johnson syndrome
  - Toxic epidermal necrolysis (TEN)
- Autoimmune blistering diseases
- Cutaneous porphyria
- Epidermolysis bullosa (EB) group of diseases (genetic)

dapsone, intravenous immunoglobulins, plasmapheresis, and rituximab are used with variable success in EBA and LAD. Experimental data suggests that the heat-shock protein-90 (HSP-90) blockers may prove to be a promising alternative for treatment of BP, EBA, and dermatitis herpetiformis [32]; however, clinical data are not yet available.

Cutaneous Adverse Effects of Treatment

Cutaneous adverse drug reactions are common (2–3 % of hospitalized patients), the signs diverse and time courses variable. The predisposition to idiosyncratic drug reactions probably involves both genetic and environmental factors. Reactions may not settle immediately when the drug is withdrawn and some persist for months[1].

Corticosteroids

Cutaneous adverse effects of corticosteroids include cutaneous atrophy, telangiectasia, acne-like pustular rashes and cutaneous infections, both bacterial and candidiasis. Recurrent staphylococcal folliculitis may be a problem in some patients. The nostrils should be swabbed for bacterial culture and nasal carriage of staphylococcus aureus eradicated with mupirocin 2 % ointment. Antiseptic skin cleansers or bath additives containing triclosan may be helpful.

Sulfasalazine

Sulfasalazine is a combination of 5-aminosalicylic acid and sulfapyridine. Photosensitivity may be troublesome, but skin failure caused by reactions such as erythroderma, drug rash with eosinophilia and systemic symptoms (DRESS) or toxic epidermal necrolysis is life-threatening.

Photosensitivity

Patients who are photosensitive develop a scaly erythematous rash on exposed skin. The rash tends to involve the prominences of the forehead, the nose, the cheeks, particularly over the cheekbones, the back of the neck, if not covered by hair, and the upper chest where the shirt sits open. The extensor surfaces of forearms and the backs of the hands may also be affected. Involved skin may pigment. Covered skin is spared. Sparing is usually apparent around the orbit (ask the patient to close his eyes to see the eyelids), on the upper lip, under the nose, below the chin, behind the ears, and under the hair on the forehead or at the back of the neck.

Ideally sulfasalazine should be withdrawn, but it may be possible to reduce the impact of photosensitivity with hats, clothing and regular application of a high-factor sunblock to all exposed skin. A moderate or potent topical corticosteroid ointment will reduce erythema and itch.

Erythroderma

Erythroderma (exfoliative dermatitis) is defined as erythema, with variable amounts of scale, affecting 90 % or more of the body surface. Numerous drugs including sulfasalazine have been reported to cause erythroderma, but erythroderma may also be secondary to primary skin diseases such as eczema or psoriasis and, rarely, to cutaneous T-cell lymphoma.

Most of the skin is itchy, erythematous, and scaly. Sometimes the skin is edematous or blisters and oozes serous fluid. Hair and nails may be lost. Fever, malaise, and lymphadenopathy are common.

Any potentially causative drug should be withdrawn. Patients lose heat and may become hypothermic so temperature should be monitored. The skin barrier is inadequate, increasing the risk of infection as well as loss of fluid and electrolytes. Cardiac failure is another complication, particularly in the elderly. Bland emollients applied 3–4x/day will soothe itchy inflamed skin and soap should be avoided. A sedating antihistamine will reduce irritation. Potent topical corticosteroids or oral corticosteroids are helpful in erythroderma secondary to drugs or eczema.

Stevens–Johnson Syndrome (SJS) and Toxic Epidermal Necrolysis (TEN)

These life-threatening conditions usually develop 2–3 weeks after starting drugs such as sulfonamides, aminopenicillins, antiepileptics, or allopurinol. Vague flu-like symptoms (fever, cough, headache, sore throat, rhinorrhea, and malaise) may precede the onset. Epidermal involvement is more severe and widespread in TEN (>30 % body-surface area) than in SJS (<10 % body surface area).

SJS: Poorly defined, painful erythematous macules evolve rapidly into papules and target lesions, with two or three concentric zones of color change and dark purpuric centers. Large bullae rupture leaving denuded skin. The rash

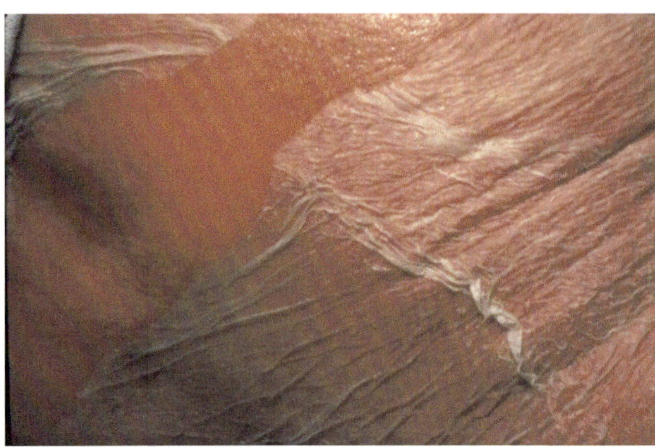

Fig. 54.8 Toxic epidermal necrolysis. Large sheets of necrotic epidermis detach leaving a painful, denuded, oozing dermis

is usually maximal by the fourth day. SJS is characterized by severe mucosal ulceration with involvement of at least two mucosal surfaces (lip, oral cavity, conjunctiva, nasal, urethra, vagina, gastrointestinal tract, respiratory tract). The lips become crusted and hemorrhagic. Painful stomatitis interferes with eating and drinking. Purulent conjunctivitis is associated with photophobia. Late ocular complications include dry eye, scarring, and loss of vision.

TEN: Painful skin or a burning discomfort may herald the onset. The tender dusky erythema progresses to widespread blistering involving <30 % of body-surface area. The thin-walled blisters rupture easily and large sheets of necrotic epidermis detach leaving a painful denuded oozing dermis (Fig. 54.8). Even gentle pressure extends blisters and inadvertent shearing pressure when handling the patient may cause further detachment. Mucosal ulceration may cause dysphagia, photophobia, or painful micturition. Epithelia of trachea, bronchi, and gastrointestinal tract may also be involved. Sequelae include scarring, irregular pigmentation, dry eye, corneal scarring, photophobia, visual impairment, phimosis, and vaginal synechiae.

All systemic drugs started within the preceding 4 weeks should be withdrawn and patients should be admitted to an intensive therapy unit or burn unit for supportive care. IV immunoglobulins, 1 g/kg for 4 days, have been recommended but their role is unproven. Systemic corticosteroids increase the risk of infection and should be avoided [33].

Drug Rash, Eosinophilia, Systemic Symptoms (DRESS)

DRESS (also known as hypersensitivity syndrome) is a life-threatening cutaneous reaction. Typically DRESS presents 2–6 weeks after the drug is started with a morbilliform erythematous rash, facial edema simulating angioedema, lymphadenopathy, a high fever, leukocytosis (often with an eosinophilia), and abnormal liver function tests. Some patients progress to liver failure. Kidneys, lungs, or heart may be affected. Any suspected drugs should be withdrawn. Early treatment with oral prednisolone (0.8–1 mg/kg body weight) or IV methyl prednisolone has been recommended to prevent progression [34].

Tumor Necrosis Factor-Alpha (TNF-α) Antagonists

Although these drugs are used in the treatment of psoriasis, paradoxically TNF-α antagonists induce psoriatic-like rashes in some individuals. Plaque, guttate, and pustular psoriasis have been reported as well as pustular reactions on palms and soles (palmoplantar pustulosis). An alopecia associated with psoriasiform lesions has been described [35]. Other skin problems such as eczema, skin infections, and acneiform rashes have also been observed. Lichen planus, both cutaneous and oral, emerges as a side effect of treatment with TNF-α antagonists [36, 37], and lichen planopilaris has been reported [38]. In one study, 62 % of 50 patients with IBD developed a cutaneous reaction within 12 months of starting adalimumab [39]. In many patients it is possible to continue treatment with the TNF-α antagonist or a substitute from the same class while controlling the skin problem with topical treatments, sometimes in combination with systemic agents, under the guidance of a dermatologist [40].

References

1. Burge S, Wallis D. Oxford handbook of medical dermatology. Oxford: Oxford University Press; 2010.
2. Ferguson LR, Han DY, Fraser AG, Huebner C, Lam WJ, Morgan AR. IL23R and IL12B SNPs and haplotypes strongly associate with Crohn's disease risk in a New Zealand population. Gastroenterol Res Pract. 2010;2010:539461.
3. Einarsdottir E, Koskinen LLE, Dukes E, Kainu K, Suomela S, Lappalainen M, et al. IL23R in the Swedish, Finnish, Hungarian and Italian populations: association with IBD and psoriasis, and linkage to celiac disease. BMC Med Genet. 2009;10:8.
4. Martin DA, Towne JE, Kricorian G, Klekotka P, Gudjonsson JE, Krueger JG, et al. The emerging role of IL-17 in the pathogenesis of psoriasis: preclinical and clinical findings. J Invest Dermatol. 2013;133(1):17–26.
5. Vagianos K, Bector S, McConnell J, Bernstein CN. Nutrition assessment of patients with inflammatory bowel disease. JPEN J Parenter Enteral Nutr. 2007;31(4):311–9.
6. Skrovanek S, DiGuilio K, Bailey R, Huntington W, Urbas R, Mayilvaganan B, et al. Zinc and gastrointestinal disease. World J Gastrointest Pathophysiol. 2014;5(4):496–513.
7. Emanuel PO, Phelps RG. Metastatic Crohn's disease: a histopathologic study of 12 cases. J Cutan Pathol. 2008;35(5):457–61.
8. Lester LU, Rapini RP. Dermatologic manifestations of colonic disorders. Curr Opin Gastroenterol. 2009;25(1):66–73.
9. Lyon CC, Smith AJ, Griffiths CEM, Beck MH. The spectrum of skin disorders in abdominal stoma patients. Br J Dermatol. 2000;143(6):1248–60.

10. Mana J, Marcoval J. Erythema nodosum. Clin Dermatol. 2007; 25(3):288–94.
11. Requena L, Sánchez Yus E. Erythema nodosum. Semin Cutan Med Surg. 2007;26(2):114–25.
12. Gilchrist H, Patterson JW. Erythema nodosum and erythema induratum (nodular vasculitis): diagnosis and management. Dermatol Ther. 2010;23(4):320–7.
13. Mössner R, Zimmer L, Berking C, Hoeller C, Loquai C, Richtig E, et al. Erythema nodosum-like lesions during BRAF inhibitor therapy: report on 16 new cases and review of the literature. J Eur Acad Dermatol Venereol JEADV. 2015;29:1797.
14. Davis MDP. Response of recalcitrant erythema nodosum to tetracyclines. J Am Acad Dermatol. 2011;64(6):1211–2.
15. Rohatgi S, Basavaraj KH, Ashwini PK, Kanthraj GR. Role of tetracycline in recalcitrant erythema nodosum. Indian Dermatol Online J. 2014;5(3):314–5.
16. Hoffman MD. Inflammatory ulcers. Clin Dermatol. 2007;25(1): 131–8.
17. Ruocco E, Sangiuliano S, Gravina A, Miranda A, Nicoletti G. Pyoderma gangrenosum: an updated review. J Eur Acad Dermatol Venereol. 2009;23(9):1008–17.
18. Goldfinger S. The inherited autoinflammatory syndrome: a decade of discovery. Trans Am Clin Climatol Assoc. 2009;120:413–8.
19. Femiano F, Lanza A, Buonaiuto C, Perillo L, Dell'Ermo A, Cirillo N. Pyostomatitis vegetans: a review of the literature. Med Oral Patol Oral Cir Bucal. 2009;14(3):E114–7.
20. Feliciani C, De Simone C, Amerio P. Dermatological signs during inflammatory bowel diseases. Eur Rev Med Pharmacol Sci. 2009;13 Suppl 1:15–21.
21. Miller J, Yentzer BA, Clark A, Jorizzo JL, Feldman SR. Pyoderma gangrenosum: a review and update on new therapies. J Am Acad Dermatol. 2010;62(4):646–54.
22. Ormerod AD, Thomas KS, Craig FE, Mitchell E, Greenlaw N, Norrie J, et al. Comparison of the two most commonly used treatments for pyoderma gangrenosum: results of the STOP GAP randomised controlled trial. BMJ. 2015;350:h2958.
23. Agarwal A, Andrews JM. Systematic review: IBD-associated pyoderma gangrenosum in the biologic era, the response to therapy. Aliment Pharmacol Ther. 2013;38(6):563–72.
24. Wallach D, Vignon-Pennamen M-D. From acute febrile neutrophilic dermatosis to neutrophilic disease: forty years of clinical research. J Am Acad Dermatol. 2006;55(6):1066–71.
25. Cohen PR. Sweet's syndrome—a comprehensive review of an acute febrile neutrophilic dermatosis. Orphanet J Rare Dis. 2007;2:34.
26. Cohen PR. Neutrophilic dermatoses: a review of current treatment options. Am J Clin Dermatol. 2009;10(5):301–12.
27. Jorizzo JL, Apisarnthanarax P, Subrt P, Hebert AA, Henry JC, Raimer SS, et al. Bowel-bypass syndrome without bowel bypass. Bowel-associated dermatosis-arthritis syndrome. Arch Intern Med. 1983;143(3):457–61.
28. Delaney TA, Clay CD, Randell PL. The bowel-associated Dermatosis-Arthritis syndrome. Australas J Dermatol. 1989;30(1): 23–7.
29. Rook A, Burns T. Rook's textbook of dermatology. Chichester, West Sussex/Hoboken, NJ: Wiley-Blackwell; 2010.
30. Fassihi H, Wong T, Wessagowit V, McGrath JA, Mellerio JE. Target proteins in inherited and acquired blistering skin disorders. Clin Exp Dermatol. 2006;31(2):252–9.
31. Venning VA, Taghipour K, Mohd Mustapa MF, Highet AS, Kirtschig G. British Association of Dermatologists' guidelines for the management of bullous pemphigoid 2012. Br J Dermatol. 2012;167(6):1200–14.
32. Tukaj S, Zillikens D, Kasperkiewicz M. Heat shock protein 90: a pathophysiological factor and novel treatment target in autoimmune bullous skin diseases. Exp Dermatol. 2015;24:567.
33. Koh MJ-A, Tay Y-K. An update on Stevens–Johnson syndrome and toxic epidermal necrolysis in children. Curr Opin Pediatr. 2009;21(4):505–10.
34. Walsh SA, Creamer D. Drug reaction with eosinophilia and systemic symptoms (DRESS): a clinical update and review of current thinking. Clin Exp Dermatol. 2011;36(1):6–11.
35. Ribeiro LBP, Rego JCG, Estrada BD, Bastos PR, Piñeiro Maceira JM, Sodré CT. Alopecia secondary to anti-tumor necrosis factor-alpha therapy. An Bras Dermatol. 2015;90(2):232–5.
36. Asarch A, Gottlieb AB, Lee J, Masterpol KS, Scheinman PL, Stadecker MJ, et al. Lichen planus-like eruptions: an emerging side effect of tumor necrosis factor-alpha antagonists. J Am Acad Dermatol. 2009;61(1):104–11.
37. Andrade P, Lopes S, Albuquerque A, Osório F, Pardal J, Macedo G. Oral lichen planus in ibd patients: a paradoxical adverse effect of anti-TNF-α therapy. Dig Dis Sci. 2015;60:2746.
38. Fernández-Torres R, Paradela S, Valbuena L, Fonseca E. Infliximab-induced lichen planopilaris. Ann Pharmacother. 2010;44(9): 1501–3.
39. Baumgart DC, Grittner U, Steingräber A, Azzaro M, Philipp S. Frequency, phenotype, outcome, and therapeutic impact of skin reactions following initiation of adalimumab therapy: experience from a consecutive cohort of inflammatory bowel disease patients. Inflamm Bowel Dis. 2011;17(12):2512–20.
40. Collamer AN, Guerrero KT, Henning JS, Battafarano DF. Psoriatic skin lesions induced by tumor necrosis factor antagonist therapy: a literature review and potential mechanisms of action. Arthritis Care Res. 2008;59(7):996–1001.

Arthritis, Arthropathy, and Osteoporosis in Inflammatory Bowel Disease

55

Alistair Tindell, Hanna Johnsson, and Iain B. McInnes

The most common extraintestinal manifestation in inflammatory bowel disease (IBD) is musculoskeletal disease. Arthritis associated with IBD is distinct from rheumatoid arthritis and is classified with an extended disease group, namely the spondyloarthropathies (SpA). The spondyloarthropathies share common pathophysiology, clinical manifestations, and approaches to investigation and management. Remarkably, they also provide for evolution of the clinical phenotype across tissue compartments, e.g., an IBD dominant presentation may evolve to include significant musculoskeletal or ocular involvement. Such disease developments may impose substantial novel impact on quality of life and require an altered management approach and prioritization. Indeed they may become the dominant clinical issue over time, transiently or in perpetuity. Cross-disciplinary recognition of the propensity for a developing presentation and management of disease evolution is therefore essential. Herein we summarize the key elements of the musculoskeletal elements required for the management of IBD and its wider disease spectrum.

Epidemiology

25–40 % of patients with IBD have extraintestinal manifestations [1], 5–20 % have peripheral arthritis, 1–26 % have spondylitis, and 24 % have asymptomatic sacroilitis found on magnetic resonance imaging (MRI) [1]. Patients recognize this, with arthritis identified by more IBD patients (77 %) as a potential complication of their bowel disease than any other complication—including colon cancer [2]. Peripheral arthritis secondary to IBD occurs equally among the sexes but axial involvement is threefold more common in males [1]. African-Americans are more likely to develop sacroilitis than white Americans [3]. Risk factors for developing an extraintestinal manifestation include the requirement for surgery and the presence of another extraintestinal manifestation in a different system (consistent with the notion of phenotypic and pathophysiologic mobility across tissues). Patients with colonic disease are more likely to develop arthritis, with higher risk in patients with colonic Crohn's disease (CD) than ulcerative colitis (UC) [1]. In CD the risk is also increased by smoking or a young age at diagnosis (<40years) [4]. The arthritis of IBD can be equally, or more, disabling than the underlying bowel disease; or can herald the disease itself—in 10–30 % of patients with IBD-related arthritis, the arthritis presents first [1]. Furthermore, around 60 % of patients with ankylosing spondylitis (AS) have subclinical bowel inflammation [5].

Classification

The conditions collectively referred to as SpA have shared characteristics and can be subdivided dependent on precipitating disease as illustrated in Figs. 55.1 and 55.2.

More recently, it has been considered that the SpA group may instead be different phenotypes of the same disease process and should be subdivided into whether the joints involved are predominantly peripheral or in the axial skeleton. This classification allows for a pragmatic approach to diagnosis and management of the spondyloarthropathies. Furthermore, the previously smaller and less researched groups, such as arthritis associated with IBD (and undifferentiated SpA) can be incorporated into larger studies. At the same time, this collectivization may prevent identification of smaller differences and patient subgroups who may benefit from differing investigation or management. In both classifications there are patients who will not fit into the attempted discrete categorization.

From the Arthritis Research UK Centre of Excellence for Rheumatoid Arthritis Pathogenesis (RACE).

A. Tindell • H. Johnsson • I.B. McInnes (✉)
Institute of Infection, Immunity and Inflammation, College of MVLS, University of Glasgow,
120 University Place, Glasgow G128QQ, UK
e-mail: Iain.McInnes@glasgow.ac.uk

D.C. Baumgart (ed.), *Crohn's Disease and Ulcerative Colitis*, DOI 10.1007/978-3-319-33703-6_55

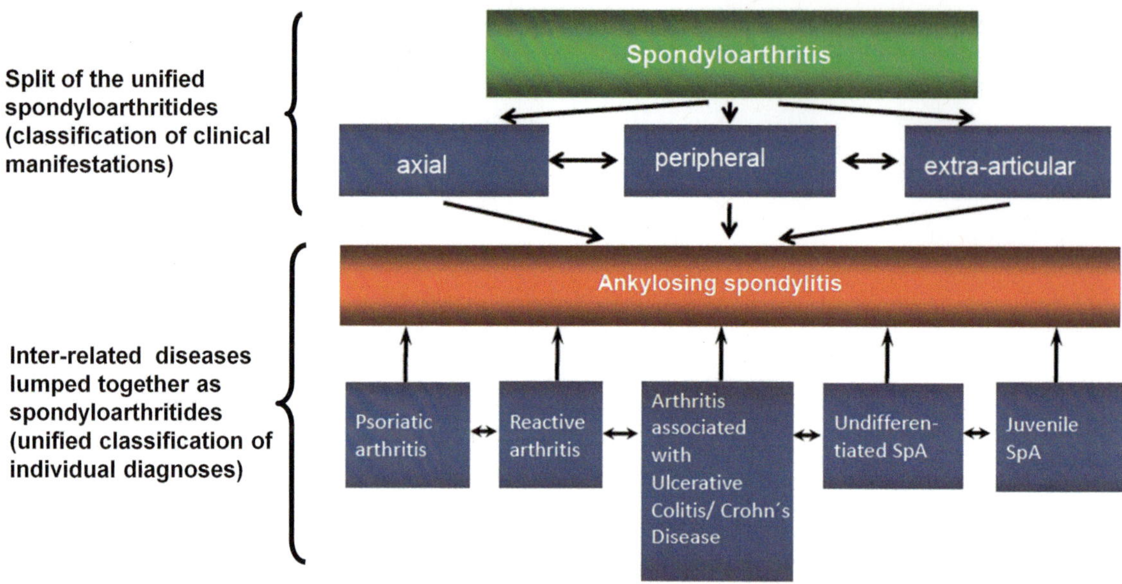

Fig. 55.1 From Zeider H, Amor B. The Assessment in Spondyloarthritis International Society (ASAS) classification criteria for peripheral spondyloarthritis and for spondyloarthritis in general: the spondyloarthritis concept in progress. Ann Rheum Dis. 2011;70:1–3

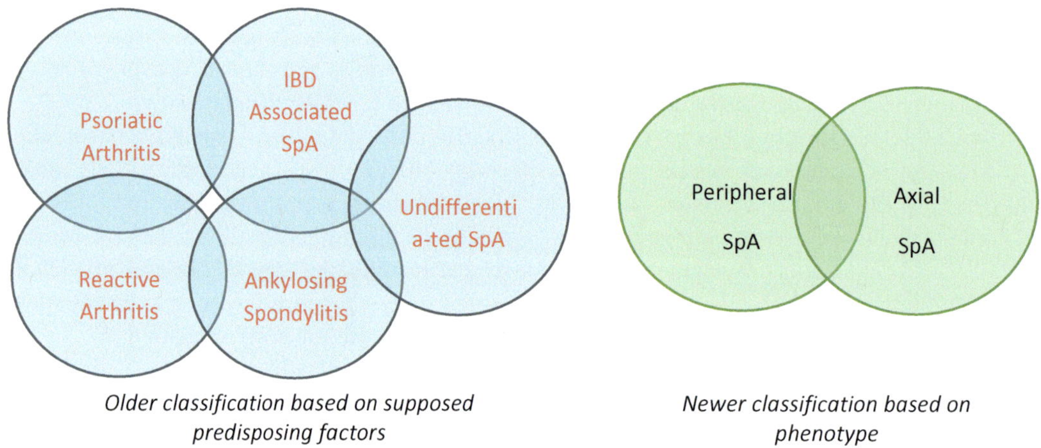

Fig. 55.2 Pragmatic approach to the classification of the spondyloarthropathies. Whichever system is chosen, there are undoubtedly patients who share characteristics with more than one group

Pathogenesis and Pathophysiology

Most of our knowledge of the pathophysiology of IBD related arthritis has been derived from AS and PsA. Roles of genetic and environmental factors have been recognized and an improved understanding of the inflammatory pathways involved has led way to new treatment strategies.

Genetics

Genome-wide association studies (GWAS) have identified genetic factors shared between AS, psoriasis and IBD, as well as disease-specific susceptibility gene loci. The shared genetic factors appear to be predominantly genes with roles in intracellular antigen processing, the type 17 helper T (T_H17) cell pathway and the nuclear factor kappa B pathway. Thus, the immune response is clearly implicated and therefore immune mediated mechanisms in the common features of disease. Of note is that interleukin (IL) 23 receptor variants confer susceptibility to AS, psoriasis, PsA, CD, and UC [6, 7] leading to particular interest in this pathway for therapeutic purposes. The most significant SpA susceptibility gene identified to date is a series of alleles of the human leukocyte antigen (HLA) region of the major histocompatibility complex (MHC). The HLA-B27 allele is present in over 85 % of patients with AS but only 1–5 % of carriers develop the disease [8]. Nearly all patients with IBD who are HLA-B27⁺ develop AS [1] and HLA-B27⁺ individuals are more likely to develop reactive arthritis. The exact mechanism for how HLA-B27 confers a risk is unknown though several mechanisms are proposed. These include some primary pathway whereby antigen presentation is paramount to a class I restricted cell lineage (e.g., CD8 T cells). However, HLA-B27 molecules have the propensity to misfold and as such have been shown to cause endoreticulum stress—this in turn can promote myeloid lineage cytokine production, particularly of IL-23 leading to theoretical amplification of the type 17 immune response that has been associated with disease. Finally it is proposed that HLA-B27 homodimers can form that in turn can activate innate lineage cells via killer receptor recognition. The identification of the endoplasmic reticulum aminopeptidase 1 (ERAP1) gene as a further susceptibility gene for to AS in HLA-B*27⁺ individuals suggest that they work in the same pathway to affect disease susceptibility [8]. ERAP1 trims peptides in the endoplasmic reticulum in preparation for binding to MHC class 1 molecules. This perhaps offers antigen presentation dependent pathways as more likely than misfolding of HLA-B27 as the dominant mechanism. That said none are mutually exclusive and as this is a polygenic disorder there may be several routes to disease susceptibility and progression. Much further work in which GWAS outcomes, detailed clinical phenotyping, and ex vivo immune analyses are combined will assist in resolution of these issues.

Environmental Factors

The most often described example of an environmental factor causing SpA is a bacterial infection preceding reactive arthritis. Although most patients with reactive arthritis have a self-limiting illness, up to 20% develop AS within 10–20 years [9]. However, recently the critical role played by the microbiome in defining risk susceptibility has come to the fore in many autoimmune disorders, with IBD and SpA no exception. Dysbiosis of the intestinal microbiota is a recognized concept in IBD, and has been suggested to play a role in the SpA spectrum as well [9]. Transgenic rats expressing HLA-B27 develop a SpA like illness and colitis and raising the rats in a germ-free environment reduces these phenotypes [9]. In humans, initial studies did not identified any consistent differences between AS and controls [9], but recently a decreased diversity in the gut microbiota with similar microbiota profile to that of IBD, has been identified in PsA [10].

Biomechanical stress is a further factor implicated in the pathogenesis of SpA. Studies have mainly focused on the enthesis, the site of tendon insertion into bones, which are anatomical sites under high biomechanical stress—enthesitis is often one of the first signs of SpA [11, 12]. In animal models, mechanical stress can induce enthesitis with inflammation progressing to adjacent tissues [11]. The same mechanism has not been proposed in human SpA; PsA and PsA nail disease tend to localize to sites of mechanical stress and there are associations between PsA and joint trauma and occupations involving heavy lifting [11].

The IL-23—T_H17 -IL-17 Pathway

The clinical features of SpA are the result of a cascade of proinflammatory adaptive immune cells and the cytokines that they produce. The cascade, as illustrated in Fig. 55.3, is initiated by the interaction of an antigen-presenting cell (APC) with a naive CD4⁺ T cell [13]. The APC is typically a dendritic cell but could comprise a B cell or macrophage. In the presence of

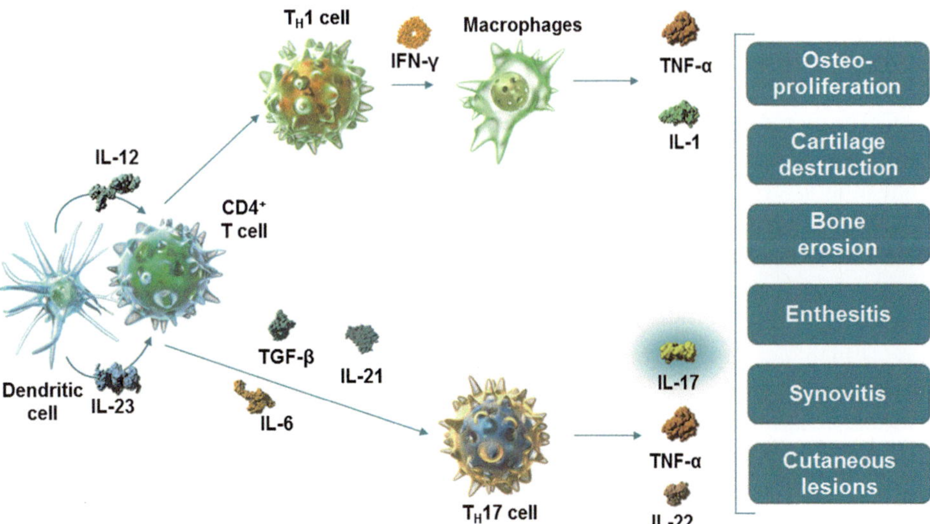

Fig. 55.3 Pro-inflammatory immune cells produce cytokines which can lead to relevant clinical manifestations. Taken from Raychaudhuri SP. Role of IL-17 in psoriasis and psoriatic arthritis. Clin Rev Allergy Immunol. 2013;44(2):183–93

IL-12, naive CD4+ T cells differentiate to T_H1 cells which produce interferon-γ. This can activate macrophages that in turn release additional cytokines, including tumor necrosis factor-α (TNF-α) and IL-1 [13]. If instead IL-6 and TGF-β are expressed, together with IL-1, the antigen-activated precursor T cell develops down the T_H17 pathway by inducing the expression of IL-21 [14]. IL-21 drives the expression of the T_H17-specific transcription factor retinoic acid receptor (RAR)-related orphan receptor (ROR)-γ that in turn induces the expression of the receptor for IL-23, a cytokine that further amplifies T_H17-cell differentiation [14]. T_H17 produce cytokines such as TNF-α, IL-22, and IL-17A and F. The roles of IL-23 and IL-17-secreting T_H17 cells are described below.

IL-23

IL-23 serum levels are elevated in patients with PsA and AS [15]. Dendritic cells and macrophages are the major sources of IL-23, which is produced in response to microbes and also HLA-B*27 receptor misfolding [16, 17]. By inference they likely therefore have a role in the arthropathy of IBD. In experimental mouse models, overexpression of IL-23 activates a group of T_H17 cells, RORγδ$^+$CD3$^+$CD4$^-$CD8$^-$ T cells, in entheseal tissue [16]. These activated T cells can then promote local inflammation and bone remodeling through a variety of effector mediators, including IL-17 and IL-22, which along with TNF-α, contribute to inflammation, osteoproliferation, and bone loss. The result is a SpA like illness in mice with enthesitis, arthritis, psoriasis, and aortic root inflammation [16]. Blocking IL-23 with Ustekinumab (via p40 inhibition) is a licensed treatment for PsA, as described below lending further credence to the role of this pathway in the SpA spectrum.

T_H17 and IL-17

There are several subtypes of IL-17 (IL-17A-F) and they signal through a family of IL-17 receptors (IL-17R). IL-17s are proinflammatory cytokines and IL-17A can act synergistically with TNF-α and IL-1 [1, 18]. In skin psoriasis, the expression of IL-17A, IL-17F, and IL-17C is significantly increased in psoriatic plaques [19] and IL-17RA is expressed on keratinocytes and mediates response to IL-17A and IL-17F. In PsA, high levels of IL-17A may be expressed by T_H17 cells, neutrophils, and synoviocytes [3, 20]. Elevated circulating levels of T_H17 are found in both patients with PsA and AS [15]. There is an increase in IL-17 secreting cells in peripheral blood mononuclear cells and in the facet joints in patients with AS and in synovial fluid of patients with PsA [13, 21–23]. Furthermore, synoviocytes in PsA express high levels of the IL-17A receptor (IL-17RA) [13]. IL-17 signaling promotes attraction of neutrophils, T_H17 cells and dendritic cells, thereby driving a variety of inflammatory cell lineages to amplify the inflammation cascade [24]. Although overexpression of IL-17 alone does not lead to primary pathology [16], blocking IL-17 has proved to be effective in treating SpA models.

New Bone Formation

Ankylosis, new bone formation extending from, and beyond, the normal border of bone [25], is a feature of SpA. This occurs as progenitor cells in the extracellular matrix are committed to developing into osteoblasts and chondrocytes via disruption of bone homeostatic signaling pathways [25]. Two bone protein regulatory families deserve particular attention, namely BMPs and Wnts. These pathways are critical in regulating the extracellular matrix via effects upon cell signaling and transcription promoting chondrogenic differentiation and hypertrophy, and new bone formation via osteoblasts respectively. Critically they appear to operate as a downstream effect of IL-23 [25]. It is not yet understood whether inflammation, and its resolution, results in new bone formation or whether inflammation and bone formation are two separate processes in the same disease [25]. On MRI, sites of ankyloses correlate to previous sites of inflammation, but sites of syndesmophytes do not [25]. TNF-inhibitors appear to have no influence on development of new bone formation; however, it appears NSAIDs do [25]. Control of inflammation does resolve the trabecular bone loss contributing to the osteoporosis seen [25]. In SpA, the contradictory presence of osteoporosis next to new bone formation in ankyloses is seen [25]—trying to understand and target bone metabolism at the molecular biomarker and therapeutic levels is therefore challenging.

Clinical Features

The clinical presentation of SpA can broadly be divided into peripheral or axial disease—certainly this comprises a clinically useful and pragmatic classification. The symptoms can however be overlapping, and enthesitis has been suggested to be the cardinal feature of all forms of SpA [20]. Long-term disability in SpA is caused by pain, fatigue and especially is associated with new bone formation causing disruption of joint function and altered mechanical load leading to chronic pain and functional impairment [25]..

Peripheral SpA

The cardinal features of inflammation with pain, erythema, heat, swelling, and stiffness with subsequent loss of function of peripheral joints are seen in peripheral SpA. Classically, patients describe progressive onset of symptoms with significant morning stiffness in affected joints. Symptoms typically improve with activity. The number and distribution of joints involved can vary. Peripheral SpA associated with IBD can be further divided into types 1 and 2 (see Table 55.1). Dactylitis, inflammation of a digit (which does not obviously localize to an

Table 55.1 Clinical features of spondyloarthropathies in inflammatory bowel disease

Disease	Type 1 peripheral arthritis	Type 2 peripheral arthritis	Axial
Frequency in IBD	5 %	3–4 %	5–12 %
Site	Lower limb	upper limb	Spine
Type	Large Joint	Small Joint, MCPs	Usually sacroiliac
No. of joints	<5 (Oligoarticular)	>5 (Polyarticular)	Also affect costal joints
Duration	<10 weeks, can recur	Months-Years	At least 3 months
Relation to IBD symp	Related	Independent	Independent
Symmetry	Asymmetric	Symmetric	Monolateral
Surgical Cure of IBD	Resolves	Persists	Persists
Erosions	No	Yes	Ankyloses

Table 55.2 Features of inflammatory back pain

• Insidious onset
• Morning stiffness in the spine for more than 30 min
• Improvement of pain and stiffness with exercise and not with rest
• Pain at night, usually in the second half with improvement on getting up
• Alternating buttock pain
The back pain in AS and non-radiographic axial SpA typically starts before 45 years of age and runs a chronic or relapsing course (duration of more than 3 months)

Taken from: Poddubnyy D, Rudwaleit M. Early Spondyloarthritis. Rheumatic Disease Clinics of North America, Vol 38, Iss 2, May 2012, pp. 387–403

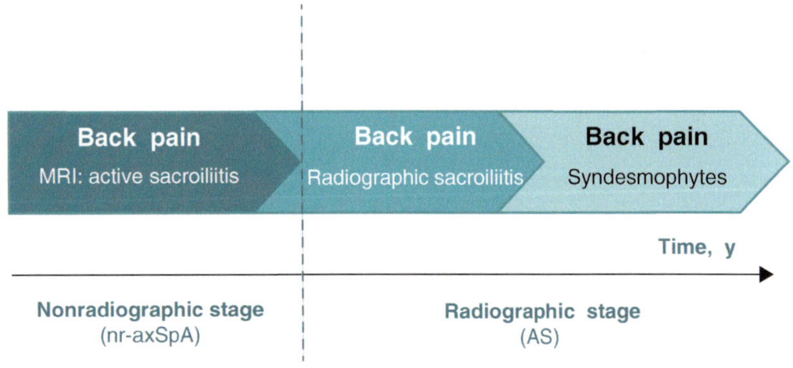

Fig. 55.4 The progression of back pain. Adapted from Rudwaleit M, Sieper J. Referral strategies for early diagnosis of axial spondyloarthritis. Nat Rev Rheumatol. 2012;8(5):262–8

articular structure, but rather to the entire digit), can also be present. Type 1 peripheral arthritis is associated with larger and fewer joints, appears to be related to the course of the inflammatory bowel disease, and causes a self-limiting disease that does not cause erosions [5]. Type 2 peripheral arthritis is a symmetrical polyarticular disease that can last for decades and is associated with destructive (erosive) changes in the joints. It does not appear to be related to the course of the underlying bowel disease [5].

Axial SpA

AS is the model disease of axial SpA. Patients complain of inflammatory back pain (see Table 55.2; Fig. 55.4) with early morning stiffness improving with exercise. Sacroiliitis can cause pain in the buttocks that may radiate to the thighs. Chronicity can result in ankyloses of the spine with irreversibly reduced range of movement. It is now rare however to see the classical deformities of the AS spectrum.

Extra-articular Features and Comorbidities

Extra-articular manifestations of SpA include uveitis and more rarely aortic involvement [4, 26]. Several respiratory, renal, and neurological conditions have been associated with AS. Furthermore, patients with PsA and AS are at increased risk of cardiovascular diseases [27] and good practice is to screen patients with SpA for cardiovascular risk factors [28]. This has been enshrined in the EULAR guidelines for the management of cardiovascular disease in the presence of the common arthropathies. Particular note should be made of the recommendation that the risk for cardiovascular disease be amplified by a factor of 1.5 when applying national risk score attribution for the commencement of statins in vascular protection. It is notable that the association between chronic inflammatory disease and vascular risk is much less secure in the IBD literature and as such the recommendations should be most closely followed in the context of dominant articular or cutaneous disease (psoriasis). Additional comorbidities of note comprise those in the brain (depression, cognitive impairment, anxiety) and in wider metabolic syndrome and development of type II diabetes mellitus (especially in those patients with coincident psoriasis).

Assessment and Diagnosis

There is a broad differential for diagnoses that manifest GI and rheumatic manifestations (see Table 55.3).

There are distinct diagnostic criteria for axial versus peripheral SpA; however, these have primarily been designed for research purposes and neither have the specificity or sensitivity to properly replace diagnosis by an experienced rheumatologist which remains the gold standard. Importantly, in PsA, delayed diagnosis is associated with worse outcomes with development of joint erosion, lower chance of achieving drug-free remission and worse health assessment questionnaire (HAQ) scores [29]. Thus the clinical take home is to refer for assessment any patient with IBD who expresses musculoskeletal features and to expedite those with red flags for inflammation including obvious synovitis, early morning stiffness, and functional decline.

Peripheral SpA

If a patient has only symptoms of peripheral disease, the following criteria are applied.

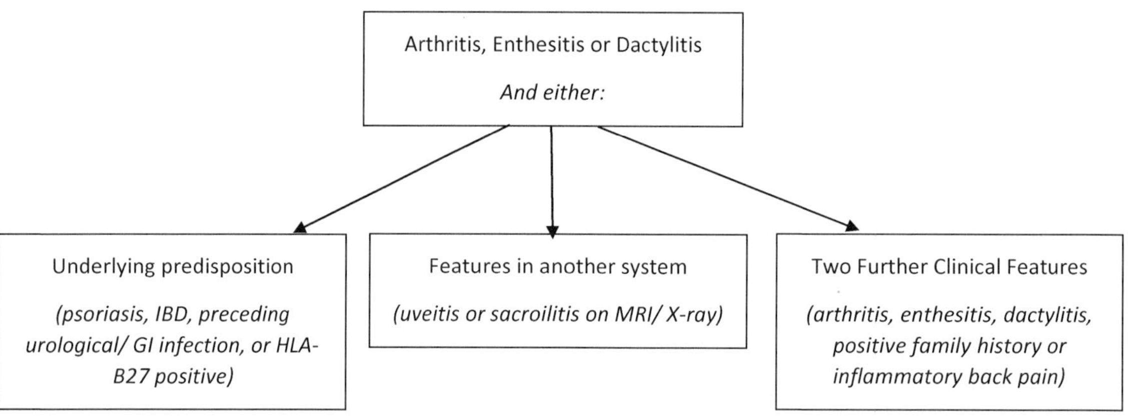

Perhaps given reliance on clinical features, sensitivity is 78% and specificity 82%[25].

Table 55.3 Potential diagnoses that combine GI and rheumatic presentations

IBD related						Non-IBD related			
Disease related			Drug related						
Arthritis	Axial	Enthesitis	Osteoporosis	Septic arthritis	Osteonecrosis	Reactive arthritis	Whipple's disease	Gluten sensitive enteropathy	HIV

Perhaps given reliance on clinical features, sensitivity is 78 % and specificity 82 % [25].

Axial SpA

If a patient has axial disease or peripheral and axial disease the following pathway should be applied [30].

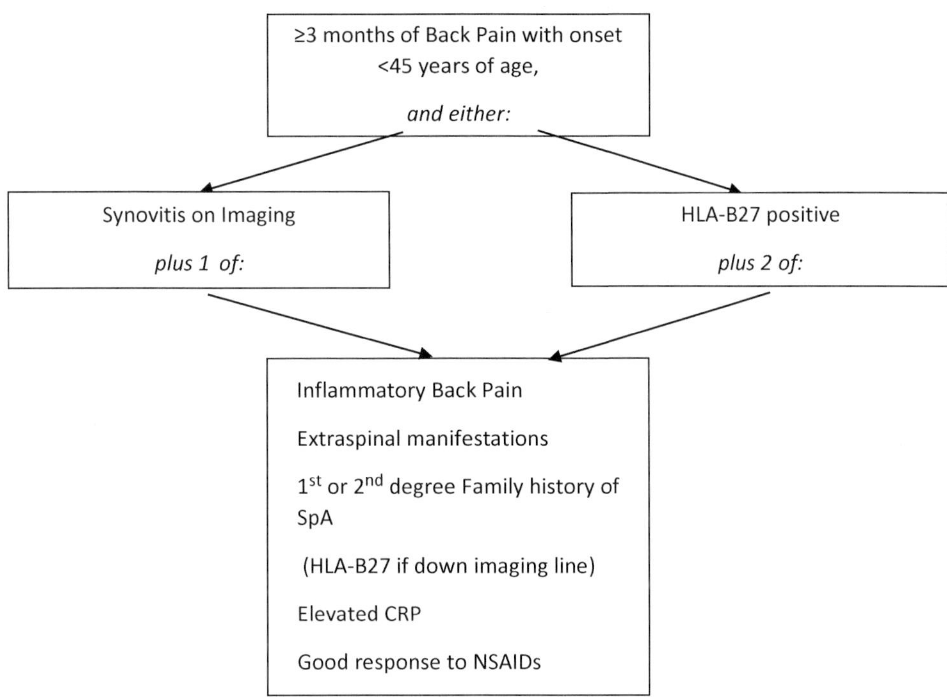

Imaging is an important component of assessment and when positive comprises an important diagnostic clue—with an associated SpA feature it can carry a specificity of 97 %. However, negative imaging does not exclude the diagnosis and in particular may miss early disease—thus the sensitivity of this arm is 66 %, and hence a "clinical arm" has been included which has a lower specificity of 85 % but a higher sensitivity of 83 % [30]. Due to its lower specificity, two rather than one additional features are required. Of note, patients were only used in the criterion if they had had back pain for 3 months and were under 45. It can be expected that, at least, the specificity of the criteria will be reduced when applied in older age groups as other causes of back pain become more prevalent.

Disease scores. There are several scoring systems that can be used to assess disease activity and the functional impact of the disease. They can be used to justify treatment with biologics and serial measurement is a means to formally assess response to treatment. The choice of scoring system depends on the clinical manifestation. In axial SpA, the *Bath Ankylosing Spondylitis Disease Activity Index (BASDAI)* and *Assessment of Spondyloarthritis international Society Health Index (ASAS HI)* are used—the latter is preferred by ASAS (http://www.asas-group.org/clinical-instruments.php?id=01). They are both self-rated scoring systems. For the BASDAI, patients score the severity of their symptoms between 0 and 10. The ASAS HI is a questionnaire of 17 binary responses to statements about ability to perform in everyday situations based on the WHO International Classification of Functioning Disability and Health (ICF) [31]. In peripheral SpA, scoring systems like the Disease Activity Score (DAS) comprising a composite measure of joint examination by a trained assessor, patient assessment of global health and markers of inflammation have been adapted from their use in RA. There are also scoring systems for enthesitis and dactylitis (described in detail by Mease [32, 33]).

Investigations

Blood Tests

C-reactive protein (CRP) and the erythrocyte sedimentation rate have low specificity but can reflect disease activity, and CRP can aid diagnoses. High sensitivity CRP does not provide any further usual information [34]. Other biomarkers are not yet reliable, sensitive, or specific enough to be used out with clinical trials [35]. HLA-B27 should be measured and has an appreciable sensitivity (66–78 %) and specificity (73–94 %) [34]. The acute phase response does not distinguish gut from articular inflammation and cannot replace detailed clinical assessment.

Plain XR

XR can detect destructive changes and bone proliferation [35], both in peripheral and axial SpA. Sacroilitis on XR and with an associated feature carries a specificity of 97 % for AS [30]. Plain anteroposterior X-ray of the pelvis is the recommended view when investigating for axial SpA [34], allowing assessment of both sacroiliac joints and hip joints. XRs are however not sensitive to detect early disease [34] and MRI is then the imaging of choice.

Ultrasound

Imaging by US is useful to assess for inflammation in peripheral joints and enthesis. In PsA, an ultrasound composite score can reliably determine overall disease activity when applied to multiple sites [36]. It can show hypoechoic thickening of the tendon/ligament, erosion, spur formation or fluid collected in adjacent bursa. Power Doppler further increases the sensitivity to inflammation and should constitute part of a routine assessment. US has not been formally tested in the context of IBD—many studies have detected subclinical enthesitis in patients with psoriasis and it is likely that similar analyses of IBD patients will reveal sub clinical enthesial disease. Thus the clinician should have a low index of suspicion and refer to US assessment those patients with clinical features suggestive of enthesitis. This can be very helpful in patients with features also suggestive of fibromyalgia.

MRI

MRI allows direct visualization of inflammation in peripheral and axial joints and entheses [35]. Perientheal osteitis, diffuse bone marrow edema adjacent to enthesial insertion, and soft tissue edema is looked for [20]. However, as the entheses are relatively avascular, fluid may not readily accumulate during inflammation [20]. MRI is of particular importance in axial disease as active sacroiliitis can be detected by MRI but not by XR in the early stages [4, 37]. This is called nonradiographic axial SpA and is defined by the presence of sacroiliac inflammation as detected by MRI or the presence of HLA-B27 in combination with the presence of features typical of SpA [1, 38]. A substantial proportion of patients with nonradiographic axial SpA will develop the radiographic stage of AS over time [37]. The presence of syndesmophytes has the strongest predictive role for further radiographic progression in the spine [37].

To evaluate axial disease, sacroiliac joint MRI with T1 and STIR protocol without gadolinium is the recommended method [34]. There is little value in imaging the rest of the spine; however, this may be useful if other causes of back pain are being investigated [34]. CT is not recommended due to poor sensitivity and significant radiation [34].

Treatment

Collaboration between gastroenterologists and rheumatologists is essential to optimize the treatment of patients with IBD associated arthritis. In our practice we often conduct joint consultations to facilitate combined consistent decision making.

Non-pharmacological

Patient education: Randomized controlled trials in pain and in other medical conditions have consistently shown better outcomes when patients are involved in their management [34]. We highly recommend therefore a shared approach to decision making and follow up. Extend scope practitioners should be engaged in such discussions to consolidate the shared decision approach.

Physiotherapy: Reduces pain and improves function in ankylosing spondylitis [34], as well as preventing deformity and associated respiratory compromise and disability [39]. Extending these findings to all spondyloarthropathies is probably valid.

Pharmacological

NSAIDs are the first line treatment in axial disease and can induce remission [34]. Naproxen appears to have both best efficacy and cardiovascular risk profile [34]. However, NSAIDs can exacerbate bowel inflammation especially in ulcerative colitis; there is no data about COX-2 inhibitors but they could theoretically have the same impact. NSAIDs should thus not be used in active inflammatory bowel disease. They may be used if IBD is in remission but require close monitoring and restriction to minimal effective dose and duration [39]. If there is any indication of bowel disease worsening, they should be discontinued [39].

Glucocorticoids may have a limited role in axial SpA which is refractory to NSAIDs; however, there is a lack of evidence for their use. They provide rapid but short-term relief in symptoms but have multiple medium/ long-term adverse effects including on bone metabolism [34] so should not be used to maintain remission [39].

DMARDs

These are not effective in axial disease [34]. Sulfasalazine can be effective to treat peripheral arthritis and ulcerative colitis but does not affect joint damage progression [39]. It appears to be most effective on peripheral joint symptoms in patients who have active ulcerative colitis [39]. Methotrexate is not routinely used in SpA but may have modest effects on peripheral joint symptoms. It appears to be useful in intestinal symptoms of Crohn's disease (CD) [39]. Azathioprine, leflunomide, and cyclosporine may have some effect in peripheral arthritis but there are few data to support their use [39].

TNF-α Inhibitors

Biologic agents, specifically TNF inhibitors should be initiated when treatment fails (defined in axial disease as ≥2 NSAIDs, and in peripheral disease as DMARDs and steroids) or where there is a poor prognoses (severe disease, high inflammatory markers or bone edema on MRI) [39]. A BASDAI >4 is the basis to start anti-TNF therapy [24]. Distinct health care economies may modify the criteria for the commencement of biologic agents (Table 55.4). TNF inhibitors, including infliximab, etanercept, adalimumab, golimumab, and certolizumab, have shown significant efficacy in the management of axial spondyloarthritis, especially alongside NSAIDs and in early disease [34]. Efficacy appears similar between different anti-TNF agents, and in trials of patients who were otherwise nonresponders to other therapeutic modalities [40]. The INFAST part 1 trial showed that remission rates were significantly higher with infliximab versus naproxen (62 % vs 35 %) in early axial SpA (<3 years) [41]. The INFAST part 2 trial showed if early partial remission was obtained, this was maintained in almost half of patients 6 months after discontinuing the biologic [42]. In established disease, however, almost all those who achieve remission on infliximab relapse within 1 year if treatment is stopped [43]. Given the high response rate to naproxen, and that this response was seen early, a policy of early diagnosis with initial treatment with naproxen, and if no response, then early escalation to anti-TNFs has been suggested [44].

TNF-inhibitors licensed in related conditions are shown below; the first biosimilar has recently been approved for AS and PsA [24]. For the other spondyloarthropathies, recommendations are to an extent extended from these trials, but both the clinical and the immunopathological responses in synovial tissue appear comparable across the different clinical subtypes of peripheral spondyloarthritis [35].

TNF inhibitors however do not appear to affect new bone formation radiologically either axially or peripherally—this is important as bone proliferation and ankylosis leads to long-term, currently irreversible, deformity and loss of function [35, 44, 45]. In addition, in up to 40 % of patients anti-TNF agents are either inefficacious or cause adverse events [35], and efficacy can decrease over time—potentially due to development of antibodies to the drug. Whilst this can be addressed by switching to a different anti-TNF agent, response rate and duration of efficacy appears to decrease with each subsequent agent [35]. Thus novel pathways have more recently been explored and are described below.

Ustekinumab is a human monoclonal antibody that binds to the shared p40 subunit of IL-12 and IL-23, preventing binding to the IL12Rβ1 cell surface receptor. It was initially developed to treat moderate to severe plaque psoriasis. The subsequent PSUMMIT trials showed efficacy in PsA with 20 % or greater improvement in the American College of Rheumatology criteria (ACR20) in up to 50 % of participants [46, 47]. Improvements in dactylitis, enthesitis, and axial symptoms were also observed [46–48], Ustekinumab has effects on reducing radiographic progression [49]. Ustekinumab has also shown efficacy in AS (30 % achieved partial remission and 65 % achieved 40 % reduction [24]); [2] and appears to be effective in intestinal disease in patients with CD, including those who were non-responsive to infliximab [24].

Secukinumab is a human anti-IL-17A monoclonal antibody which has shown efficacy in AS [50] and PsA with ACR20 rates over 50 % [51]. It also reduces dactylitis and enthesitis and inhibits radiographic progression in PsA [51, 52]. Secukinumab was not effective in CD intestinal disease and caused higher adverse events than placebo [24]. Further anti-IL-17 and -23 agents are in different stages of trials and early development [24].

A *phosphodiesterase (PDE4) inhibitor* (apremilast) which acts via inhibition of cAMP intracellular signaling modulates inflammatory mediators and their production, has

Table 55.4 Biologics available for use in each of the spondyloarthopathies

AS and PsA	Psoriasis	IBD	Anterior uveitis
Infliximab, Adalimumab, Certolizumab, Etanercept, Golimumab	Infliximab, Adalimumab, Etanercept Golimumab Certolizumab	Infliximab, Adalimumab (and Golimumab for UC)	Infliximab, Golimumab

shown clinical efficacy in psoriasis and psoriatic arthritis and possibly a trend (not statistically significant) towards efficacy in AS [35, 53, 54]. Further trials are ongoing and discussions are in place to evaluate its place in treatment strategy as it seems to be less effective than TNF inhibitors [24]. *JAK (janus kinase) inhibitors* influence transcription of a variety of effector inflammatory pathways and through this inhibit inflammatory cytokine expression [24]—early studies have shown benefit in psoriasis but no data exists for psoriatic arthritis or any other spondyloarthropathies at present [2].

Tight control: Treating to a defined target has been of fundamental importance in progressing the management of RA. Similar to RA, tight control in PsA produces better outcomes with a treat-to-target approach than with conventional review [55]. Treat-to-target is the policy wherein predefined disease activity levels guide therapeutic changes with patients reviewed 4-weekly and progressed through a protocol of predefined treatment if minimum disease activity is not met [56]. Thus far, no data are available that determine whether such an approach will benefit those with arthropathies associated with IBD—as an interim approach it would be reasonable to measure some element of articular and enthesial disease activity in patients with IBD arthropathy and escalate therapy in the presence of ongoing active disease.

Future questions: The above outlines some of the potential uses of treatment but there remain many unknowns. Questions include [24]:

- What are the effects of treatment on bone development?
- Do subgroups of patients exist to which treatment can be targeted?
- Should another anti-TNF be used if one has already failed or should the patient be switched to a treatment that works via another mode of action?
- What is the optimal order of biologic therapeutics as the new IL-17 and IL-23 inhibitors emerge?
- How safe will IL-17 blockade be in IBD as it becomes established in patients with psoriasis and PsA?
- As in RA, should methotrexate (or should NSAIDs?) be used prior to, or in addition to TNF blockade?
- How should drugs be tailored during remission and will dose reductions and the length of remission be different in different drugs?

Osteoporosis

Epidemiology

The prevalence of osteoporosis is estimated at 14–42 % for patients with IBD, although there are no population based data that has had universal case detection of osteoporosis [57].

Definition

Osteoporosis is defined as a T score ≤2.5 standard deviations below the bone density of an average young healthy adult on DXA scan. The risk of fracture roughly doubles with each standard deviation below the mean [57]. It is asymptomatic, but increases the risk of fractures, which can have significant morbidity and mortality ensuing as a direct result.

Risk Factors

There are multiple compounding factors that may explain the higher prevalence of osteoporosis in IBD patients; however, a Canadian study has shown that after controlling for all other risk factors CD (but not UC) is independently associated with a higher risk of osteoporosis [57]. Low weight, female gender and older age all increase the risk an individual IBD patient may have osteoporosis [57]. Treatments, including azathioprine and anti-TNF agents, have been found to be inconsistently related—this may be because of the confounding factor of high disease activity [57]. Corticosteroid treatment, however, is well known to cause osteoporosis and is commonly used in IBD—50 % of patients have used corticosteroids within 5 years of diagnosis, and 20 % have used at least 3 g of prednisolone in a year [57]. Corticosteroids promote osteoclast survival and osteoblast apoptosis and can cause rapid bone density loss, with effects seen within months of starting corticosteroids. The severity correlates with daily and cumulative doses and duration of therapy [57]. Furthermore, corticosteroids increase the risk of fracture beyond that which can be solely explained by the loss of bone density [57].

Increased systemic inflammation increases bone resorption and decreases new bone formation [57]. TNFα, IL-1 and IL-6 and IFNγ (all of which are increased in IBD) bind receptors on osteoclast progenitors, promoting their maturation and activation, thus increasing bone resorption. This may explain why CD is an independent risk factor for osteoporosis [57]. Low vitamin D is commonly known to cause rickets and osteomalacia, but can also predispose to osteoporosis as it results in a low calcium and subsequent high PTH in response which promotes bone resorption. Up to 65 % of IBD patients have low vitamin D levels [57]. The major source of vitamin D is from exposure to sunlight but dietary intake is also important. It is likely bowel inflammation inhibits absorption. Both calcium and vitamin D are predominantly absorbed in the duodenum and proximal jejunum. In addition, absorption of vitamin D is dependent on dissolution in micelles and the major site of bile acid absorption is the terminal ileum [57]. Thus, patients with UC with terminal ileitis may have impaired vitamin D absorption, but patients with CD can have impaired vitamin D *and* calcium absorption in addition to generalized nutrient deficiencies [57].

Small bowel resection is a risk factor for low vitamin D but osteoporosis does not consistently worsen after surgical resection in CD. This may be because patients who had required surgery had previously high levels of inflammation or were frequently using corticosteroids [57]. There is however an increased prevalence of osteoporosis in patients with UC who have had a total colectomy with an ileo-anal pouch even years after UC has been considered to be cured—perhaps a result of reduced ileal absorption [57].

Screening

This is done with DXA; however, CT can identify osteoporosis if it includes lumbar spine—this may be useful as many IBD patients will undergo scans that will include this area to assess their bowel disease [57]. Systematic population screening for osteoporosis is not recommended in the UK. However, patients taking oral glucocorticoids should be considered for fracture-risk assessment and patients over the age of 50 years with IBD may also be considered for risk assessment, particularly if they have other risk factors [58]. The WHO Fracture Risk Assessment (FRAX) is a freely available online clinical scoring system that utilizes clinical factors to estimate fracture risk without knowledge of BMD and recommends if DXA scanning should be pursued. In addition, once DXA is used, this can be incorporated into the score and a treatment decision advised [58]. The QFracture score is an alternative risk calculator in which the contribution of multiple comorbidities is taken into account.

Therapy

Non-pharmacological

Falls assessment is also a key component of disease management [57]. Exercises such as balance training and strengthening exercises are recommended.

Pharmacological

All patients with IBD should be assessed for low vitamin D and if found, replaced [57].

Bisphosphonates are effective in increasing bone density in IBD patients [57]. The first line treatment in most cases is an oral bisphosphonate, such as weekly Alendronic acid [58]. The second line treatment is with yearly intravenous Zolendronic acid infusions or subcutaneous *denosumab* every 6 months. Zolendronic acid can also be used first line in patients whom the oral route is not an option. Denosumab is a monoclonal antibody against the receptor activator of nuclear factor kappa B ligand and inhibits osteoclastic bone resorption. *Terliparatide* (parathyroid hormone) is recommended in patients with severe osteoporosis and appears to be of particular benefit for vertebral osteoporosis.

Summary

The musculoskeletal manifestations of IBD require a multidisciplinary approach to optimize the assessment and management of patients with this complex combination of chronic inflammatory presentations. Vigilance for phenotypic clinical drift and rapid evaluation of new tissue manifestations of disease should become the norm. Judicious use of imaging combined with clinical communication and assessment will allow early recognition of disease manifestations. It appears that early interventions improve outcomes across the spectrum of inflammatory arthropathies and as such early disease recognition and active intervention seems likely to improve outcomes in the longer term. Similarly the proliferation of pathophysiologic discoveries across the SpA spectrum will facilitate an increasing pipeline of therapeutics with the capacity to alleviate many of the tissue-specific manifestations of the IBD/articular spectrum of disease.

References

1. Levine JS, Burakoff R. Extraintestinal Manifestations of Inflammatory Bowel Disease. Gastroenterol Hepatol (N Y). 2011;7(4):235–41.
2. Huang V, Mishra R, Thanabalan R, Nguyen GC. Patient awareness of extraintestinal manifestations of inflammatory bowel disease. J Crohns Colitis. 2013;7(8):e318–24.
3. Nguyen GC, Torres EA, Regueiro M, et al. Inflammatory bowel disease characteristics among African Americans, Hispanics and non-Hispanic Whites: characterisation of a large North American cohort. Am J Gastroenterol. 2006;101(5):1012–23.
4. Ott C, Takses A, Obermeier F, Schnoy E, Muller M. Smoking increases the risk of extraintestinal manifestations in Crohn's disease. World J Gastroenterol. 2014;20(34):12269–76.
5. Voulgari PV. Rheumatological manifestations in inflammatory bowel disease. Ann Gastroenterol. 2011;24(3):173–80.
6. Reveille JD. Genetics of spondyloarthritis—beyond the MHC. Nat Rev Rheumatol. 2012;8(5):296–304.
7. Bowes J, Budu-Aggrey A, Huffmeier U, Uebe S, Steel K, Hebert HL, et al. Dense genotyping of immune-related susceptibility loci reveals new insights into the genetics of psoriatic arthritis. Nat Commun. 2015;6:6046.
8. Cortes A, Pulit SL, Leo PJ, Pointon JJ, Robinson PC, Weisman MH, et al. Major histocompatibility complex associations of ankylosing spondylitis are complex and involve further epistasis with ERAP1. Nat Commun. 2015;6:7146.
9. Asquith M, Elewaut D, Lin P, Rosenbaum JT, et al. The role of the gut and microbes in the pathogenesis of spondyloarthritis. Best Pract Res Clin Rheumatol. 2014;28(5):687–702.
10. Scher JU, Littman DR, Abramson SB. Microbiome in inflammatory arthritis and human rheumatic diseases. Arthritis Rheumatol. 2015 Sep 2.

11. Jacques P, McGonagle D. The role of mechanical stress in the pathogenesis of spondyloarthritis and how to combat it. Best Pract Res Clin Rheumatol. 2014;28(5):703–10.
12. McGonagle DG, Helliwell P, Veale D. Enthesitis in psoriatic disease. Dermatology. 2012;225(2):100–9.
13. Raychaudhuri SP. Role of IL-17 in psoriasis and psoriatic arthritis. Clin Rev Allergy Immunol. 2013;44(2):183–93.
14. Palmer MT, Weaver CT. Immunology: narcissistic helpers. Nature. 2007;448(7152):416–8.
15. Jandus C, Bioley G, Rivals JP, Dudler J, Speiser D, Romero P. Increased numbers of circulating polyfunctional Th17 memory cells in patients with seronegative spondylarthritides. Arthritis Rheum. 2008;58(8):2307–17.
16. Sherlock JP, Joyce-Shaikh B, Turner SP, et al. IL-23 induces spondyloarthropathy by acting on ROR-γt+CD3+CD4−CD8− entheseal resident T cells. Nat Med. 2012;18(7):1069–76.
17. Smith JA, Colbert RA. The interleukin-23/interleukin-17 axis in spondyloarthritis pathogenesis: Th17 and beyond. Arthritis Rheumatol. 2014;66(2):231–41.
18. Miossec P, Korn T, Kuchroo VK. Interleukin-17 and type 17 helper T cells. N Engl J Med. 2009;361(9):888–98.
19. Johansen C, Usher PA, Kjellerup RB, Lundsgaard D, Iversen L, Kragballe K. Characterization of the interleukin-17 isoforms and receptors in lesional psoriatic skin. Br J Dermatol. 2009;160(2): 319–24.
20. McGonagle D, Benjamin M. Entheses, enthesitis and enthesopathy. Arthritis Research UK Topical Reviews. 2009 Autumn, issue 4, series 6.
21. Shen H, Goodall JC, Hill Gaston JS. Frequency and phenotype of peripheral blood Th17 cells in ankylosing spondylitis and rheumatoid arthritis. Arthritis Rheum. 2009;60(6):1647–56.
22. Menon B, Gullick NJ, Walter GJ, Rajasekhar M, Garrood T, Evans HG, et al. Interleukin-17+CD8+ T cells are enriched in the joints of patients with psoriatic arthritis and correlate with disease activity and joint damage progression. Arthritis Rheumatol. 2014;66(5):1272–81.
23. Appel H, Maier R, Wu P, Scheer R, Hempfing A, Kayser R. Analysis of IL-17(+) cells in facet joints of patients with spondyloarthritis suggests that the innate immune pathway might be of greater relevance than the Th17-mediated adaptive immune response. Arthritis Res Ther. 2011;13(3):R95.
24. Braun J, Klitz U, Heldmann F, Baraliakos X. Emerging drugs for the treatment of axial and peripheral spondyloarthritis. Expert Opin Emerg Drugs. 2015;20(1):1–14.
25. Lories RJ, Schett G. Pathophysiology of new bone formation and ankyloses in spondyloarthritis. Rheum Dis Clin North Am. 2012;38(3):555–67.
26. Moyssakis I, Gialafos E, Vassiliou VA, Boki K, Votteas V, Sfikakis PP, et al. Myocardial performance and aortic elasticity are impaired in patients with ankylosing spondylitis. Scand J Rheumatol. 2009;38(3):216–21.
27. Han C, Robinson Jr DW, Hackett MV, Paramore LC, Fraeman KH, Bala MV. Cardiovascular disease and risk factors in patients with rheumatoid arthritis, psoriatic arthritis, and ankylosing spondylitis. J Rheumatol. 2006;33(11):2167–72.
28. Jamnitski A, Symmons D, Peters MJ, Sattar N, McInnes I, Nurmohamed MT. Cardiovascular comorbidities in patients with psoriatic arthritis: a systemic review. Ann Rheum Dis. 2013;72(2):211–6.
29. Haroon M, Gallagher P, FitzGerald O. Diagnostic delay of more than 6 months contributes to poor radiographic and functional outcome in psoriatic arthritis. Ann Rheum Dis. 2015;74(6):1045–50.
30. Rudwaleit M, van der Heijde D, Landewé R, et al. The development of Assessment of SpondyloArthritis international Society classification criteria for axial spondyloarthritis (part II): validation and final selection. Ann Rheum Dis. 2009;68:777–83.
31. Kiltz U, van der Heijde D, Boonen A, Braun J. The ASAS Health Index (ASAS HI)—a new tool to assess the health status of patients with spondyloarthritis. Clin Exp Rheumatol. 2014;32 Suppl 85:S105–8.
32. Mease PJ, Antoni CE, Gladman DD, Taylor WJ. Psoriatic arthritis assessment tools in clinical trials. Ann Rheum Dis. 2005;64 Suppl 2:ii49–54.
33. Mease P. Psoriatic arthritis and spondyloarthritis assessment and management update. Curr Opin Rheumatol. 2013;25(3):287–96.
34. Robinson PC, Bird P, Lim I, et al. Consensus statement on the investigation and management of non-radiographic axial spondyloarthritis (nr-axSpA). Int J Rheum Dis. 2014;17(5):548–56.
35. Paramrta JE, Baeten D. Spondyloarthritis: from unifying concepts to improved treatment. Rheumatology (Oxford). 2014;53(9): 1547–59.
36. Ficjan A, Husic R, Gretler J, Lackner A, Graninger WB, Gutierrez M, et al. Ultrasound composite scores for the assessment of inflammatory and structural pathologies in Psoriatic Arthritis (PsASon-Score). Arthritis Res Ther. 2014;16(5):476.
37. Rudwaleit M, Sieper J. Referral strategies for early diagnosis of axial spondyloarthritis. Nat Rev Rheumatol. 2012;8(5):262–8.
38. Raychaudhuri SP, Deodhar AJ. The classification and diagnostic criteria of ankylosing spondylitis. J Autoimmun. 2014;48–49:128–33.
39. Peluso R, Manguso F, Vitiello M, Iervolino S, Di Minno MN. Management of arthropathy in inflammatory bowel diseases. Ther Adv Chronic Dis. 2015;6(2):65–77.
40. Zochling J, Braun J. Remission in ankylosing spondylitis. Clin Exp Rheumatol. 2006;24 Suppl 43:S88–92.
41. Sieper J, Lenaerts J, Wollenhaupt J, et al. Efficacy and safety of infliximab plus naproxen versus naproxen alone in patients with early, active spondyloarthritis: results from the double-blind, placebo-controlled INFAST study, Part 1. Ann Rheum Dis. 2014;73(1):101–7.
42. Sieper J, Lenaerts J, Wollenhaupt J, et al. Maintenance of biologic-free remission with naproxen or no treatment in patients with early, active axial spondyloarthritis,: results from a 6-month, randomised, open-label follow-up study, INFAST, Part 2. Ann Rheum Dis. 2014;73(1):108–13.
43. Baraliakos X, Listing J, Brandt J, Rudwaleit M, Sieper J, Braun J. Clinical response to discontinuation of anti-TNF therapy in patients with ankylosing spondylitis after 3 years of continuous treatment with infliximab. Arthritis Res Ther. 2005;7:R439–44.
44. Van der Heijde D, Landewe R, Baraliakos X, et al. Radiographic findings following two years of infliximab therapy in patients with ankylosing spondylitis. Arthritis Rheum. 2008;58(10):3063–70.
45. Van der Heijde D, Landewe R, Einstein S, et al. Radiographic progression of ankylosing spondylitis after up to two years of treatment with etanercept. Arthritis Rheum. 2008;58(5):1324–31.
46. McInnes IB, Kavanaugh A, Gottlieb ABM, et al. Efficacy and safety of ustekinumab in patients with active psoriatic arthritis: 1 year results of the phase 3, multicentre, double-blind, placebo-controlled PSUMMIT 1 trial. Lancet. 2013;382:780–9.
47. Ritchlin C, Rahman P, Kavanaugh A, et al. Efficacy and safety of the anti-IL-12/23 p40 monoclonal antibody, ustekinumab, in patients with active psoriatic arthritis despite conventional non-biological and biological anti-tumour necrosis factor therapy: 6-month and 1-year results of the phase 3, multicentre, double-blind, placebo-controlled, randomised PSUMMIT 2 trial. Ann Rheum Dis. 2014;73:990–9.
48. Kavanaugh A, Puig L, Gottlieb AB, Ritchlin C, You Y, Wang Y, et al. OP0174 efficacy and safety of ustekinumab in psoriatic arthritis patients with spondylitis and peripheral joint involvement: results from a phase 3, multicenter, double-blind, placebo-controlled study. Ann Rheum Dis. 2015;74:136. doi:10.1136/annrheumdis-2015-eular.3096.
49. Kavanaugh A, Ritchlin C, Rahman P, et al. Ustekinumab, an anti-IL-12/23 p40 monoclonal antibody, inhibits radiographic progression in patients with active psoriatic arthritis: results of an integrated

analysis of radiographic data from the phase 3, multicentre, randomised, double-blind, placebo-controlled PSUMMIT-1 and PSUMMIT-2 trials. Ann Rheum Dis. 2014;73:1000–6.

50. Baetan D, Baraliakos X, Braun J, Sieper J, Emery P, van der Heijde D, et al. Anti-interleukin-17A monoclonal antibody secukinumab in treatment of ankylosing spondylitis: a randomised, double-blind, placebo-controlled trial. Lancet. 2013;382(9906):1705–13.
51. McInnes IB, Mease PJ, Kirkham B, et al. Secukinumab, a human anti-interleukin-17A monoclonal antibody, in patients with psoriatic arthritis (FUTURE 2): a randomised, double-blind, placebo-controlled, phase 3 trial. Lancet. 2015; Epub ahead of print. doi: 10.1016/S0140-6736(15)61134-5.
52. van der Heijde D, Landewé R, Mease P, McInnes IB, Conaghan PG, Pricop L, et al. THU0414 secukinumab inhibits radiographic progression in patients with psoriatic arthritis: data from a phase 3 randomized, multicenter, double-blind, placebo-controlled study (Future 1). Ann Rheum Dis. 2015;74:347–8. doi:10.1136/annrheumdis-2015-eular.1806.
53. Edwards C, Blanco F, Crowley J, Hu C, Shah K, Birbara C. THU0416 disease activity and safety during long-term (104-week) treatment with apremilast, an oral phosphodiesterase 4 inhibitor, in patients with psoriatic arthritis: results from a phase III, randomized, controlled trial and open-label extension (Palace 3). Ann Rheum Dis. 2015;74 Suppl 2:348–9. doi:10.1136/annrheumdis-2015-eular.2889.
54. Kavanaugh A, Adebajo A, Gladman D, Gomez-Reino J, Hall S, Lespessailles E, et al. THU0420 long-term (104-week) efficacy and safety profile of apremilast, an oral phosphodiesterase 4 inhibitor, in patients with psoriatic arthritis: results from a phase III, randomised, controlled trial and open-label extension (Palace 1). Ann Rheum Dis. 2015;74 Suppl 2:350–1. doi:10.1136/annrheumdis-2015-eular.2907.
55. Coates L, Moverley A, McParland L, et al. Effect of tight control of inflammation in early psoriatic arthritis (TICOPA): a multicentre, open-label, randomised controlled trial. Lancet. 2014;383:S36.
56. Coates L, Navarro-Coy N, Brown S, et al. The TICOPA protocol (TIghtCOntrol of Psoriatic Arthritis): a randomised controlled trial to compare intensive management versus standard care in early psoriatic arthritis. BMC Musculoskelet Disord. 2013;14:101.
57. Targownik LE, Bernstein CN, Leslie WD. Risk factors and management of osteoporosis in inflammatory bowel disease. Curr Opin Gastroenterol. 2014;30(2):168–74.
58. Scottish Intercollegiate Guidelines Network (SIGN). Management of osteoporosis and the prevention of fragility fractures. Edinburgh: SIGN; 2015. (SIGN publication no. 142). [March 2015]. Available from URL: http://www.sign.ac.uk.

Part VII

Nutrition

Nutrition in Inflammatory Bowel Disease

56

Alan L. Buchman

Malnutrition and Nutrient Deficiencies

It is estimated that as many as 75 % of hospitalized patients with Crohn's disease are malnourished [1]. The prevalence of malnutrition is significant even for patients considered to be in clinical remission. Bin et al. observed decreased handgrip strength of 73 % of subjects who had been in remission at least 3 months [2]. Similar observations were made by Valentini et al. despite the presence of normal body mass index (BMI) and serum albumin concentration [3]. In general, the likelihood of nutritional deficiencies is greater in patients with Crohn's disease than in those with ulcerative colitis. Reduced intake of food because of abdominal cramping, nausea, and nutrient loss in diarrhea are prominent causes of weight loss in patients with IBD. Intestinal malabsorption also contributes to malnutrition in patients with active IBD, primarily those with Crohn's disease involving the small intestine in whom entero-enteric fistulas that bypass large segments of the proximal intestine may also result in substantial nutrient malabsorption. Extensive mucosal disease, bacterial overgrowth proximal to strictures, and surgical resection all contribute to malabsorption and subsequent weight loss. Increased energy expenditure, as seen with fever, abscess or sepsis, or systemic inflammation, can also result in weight loss. Nutrient deficiency can result in altered cellular immunity with increased risk of infection, delayed wound healing, and in children, growth retardation. Therefore, it is important to identify those patients that are at potential risk of malnutrition. Medical and surgical management plans should then include prevention of, and correction of, nutritional deficits.

History and physical examination are probably the best tools currently available to evaluate the gross nutritional status of an individual patient. Those who have lost significant weight (defined as greater than 10 %) and have had reduced oral caloric intake over a 2–24 week period are at risk of both macronutrient and micronutrient deficiencies. The important findings on physical examination besides an accurate weight include loss of subcutaneous fat, muscle wasting, dependent edema, and development of ascites. The subjective global assessment (SGA) is a clinical method for the evaluation of nutritional status, and includes historical, symptomatic, and physical parameters of patients [4]. The findings from a history and physical examination are subjectively weighted to rank patients as well nourished (A), moderately malnourished (B), or severely malnourished (C) (Table 56.1). The SGA provides reproducible results with more than 80 % agreement [4] although undernutrition may still be present despite normal SGA [2, 3].

Vitamin, Mineral, and Trace Metal Deficiencies

Deficiencies of vitamins, minerals, and trace elements may result from either inadequate intake or increased intestinal losses. Deficiencies are more common in Crohn's disease than ulcerative colitis given the majority of micronutrients are absorbed in the small intestine. History and physical examination are useful tools in the diagnosis of specific nutrient deficiencies.

Folic acid and vitamin B-12 are the two most common water-soluble vitamin deficiencies that can occur. Deficiency of other water-soluble vitamins is rare. Folate deficiency may result from intestinal malabsorption when proximal jejunal disease is present, as well as interaction with sulfasalazine which inhibits folate uptake. Approximately 30 % of Crohn's patients may have low serum folate [5]. Replacement can be given with oral folic acid at a dose of 1.0 mg daily. Vitamin B-12 absorption can be impaired if the distal 30–60 cm of the ileum is diseased or resected, which can occur with Crohn's disease [6, 7]. Bacterial overgrowth that occurs proximal to strictures in the small intestine can

A.L. Buchman, M.D., M.S.P.H. (✉)
Department of Surgery, University of Illinois at Chicago, 959 Oak Drive, Glencoe, IL 60022, USA
e-mail: a.buchman@hotmail.com

D.C. Baumgart (ed.), *Crohn's Disease and Ulcerative Colitis*, DOI 10.1007/978-3-319-33703-6_56

Table 56.1 SGA score

A. History

1. Weight change

Overall loss in past 6 months: amount = #_______________kg

Change in past 2 weeks: ___________ increase

___________ no change

___________ decrease

2. Dietary intake change (relative to normal)

________ no change

________ Change: duration = #_____ weeks

type _____ suboptimal solid diet _____ full liquid diet

_____ hypocaloric liquids _____ starvation

3. Gastrointestinal symptoms that persisted > 2 weeks)

____ None ____ Anorexia ____ Nausea ____ Vomiting ____ Diarrhea

4. Functional capacity

__________ No dysfunction (e.g., full capacity)

__________ Dysfunction: duration = # ____________ weeks

____________ working suboptimally

____________ ambulatory

____________ bedridden

5. Disease and its relation to nutritional requirements

Primary diagnosis (specify)

____

Metabolic demand (stress) _____ None _____ Low _____ Moderate _____ High

B. Physical (for each trait specify 0=normal, 1+=mild, 2+=moderate, 3+=severe)

_________ Loss of subcutaneous fat (triceps, chest)

_________ Muscle wasting (quadriceps, deltoids, temporals)

_________ Ankle edema, sacral edema

_________ Ascites

_________ Tongue or skin lesions suggesting nutrient deficiency

C. SGA rating (select one)

______ A = Well nourished (minimal or no restriction of food intake or absorption, minimal change in function, weight stable or increasing)

______ B = Moderately malnourished (food restriction, some function changes, little or no change in body mass)

______ C = Severely malnourished (definitely decreased intake, function, and body mass) also reduce vitamin B-12 absorption. In patients at risk 1000 μg monthly of intramuscular subcutaneous vitamin B-12 should be given. Vitamin B12 can also be absorbed sublingually and intranasally.

Vitamin D is the most common fat-soluble vitamin (vitamins A, D, E, and K) deficiency reported in patients with IBD. Fat-soluble vitamin deficiency results from malabsorption secondary to a reduced bile salt pool resulting from terminal ileal disease or resection. This results in an inability to form sufficient micelles necessary for fat and fat soluble vitamin assimilation. Low serum vitamin D concentration has been associated with more significant Crohn's disease activity and vitamin D concentrations increasing following successful treatment of the Crohn's [8]. A small study of 94 patients suggested that vitamin D supplementation (1200 mg/day) could decrease the likelihood of relapse after 1 year of treatment compared with placebo [9]. Interestingly, only about one third of the patients in each group were vitamin D deficient at study entry. However, it is more likely that active inflammation and more severe disease is the cause of vitamin D malabsorption, accompanied by decreased sun exposure as outdoor activity is often curtailed; absorption and outdoor exposure would increase as disease activity decreases [10]. As an important adjunct to this point, vitamin D concentrations are decreased in the winter time in patients with Crohn's disease who live in temperate areas [9, 11, 12]. Experimental evidence from mice however does suggest artificial colitis induced in vitamin D-deficient animals is more severe [13], and that vitamin D supplementation may decrease severity [14, 15]. Vitamin D-deficient mice were also found to have substantially greater levels of bacteria in colonic tissue, even in the absence of colitis although it should be noted however that vitamin D-deficient mice do not develop colitis spontaneously, suggesting vitamin D does not actually cause colitis, even if it is an environmental contributor to disease activity [15]. Vitamin D deficiency does appear to affect gut barrier function and intestinal permeability is increased [16, 17].

Interestingly, vitamin D deficiency has also been reported in a significant percentage of patients with ulcerative colitis, at least in one study [18], although this may result from the simple fact that individuals who are not feeling well typically do not spend much time outside in the sunlight, which is essential for endogenous vitamin D synthesis.

The combination of vitamin D and calcium malabsorption, as well as corticosteroids (which inhibits calcium absorption) may result in significant metabolic bone disease, including both osteomalacia and osteoporosis. Corticosteroids cause both decreased intestinal absorption and increased urinary excretion of calcium. Patients at risk should receive 1000–1500 mg of elemental calcium daily. Measurement of bone density using dual-energy X-ray absorptiometry (DEXA) should be performed early after the diagnosis of IBD. Supplementation with 1000 IU of daily vitamin D has been reported to prevent bone loss in patients with Crohn's disease [19]. Some patients may require substantially greater doses depending upon their degree of malabsorption and sunlight exposure [11].

Sixteen percent of patients with IBD may also have low serum vitamin A and E concentrations [20]. One study reported a consistent relationship between low vitamin A and E concentrations and disease activity [20]. Deficiencies of these nutrients are uncommon, but have been reported to occur in approximately 16 % and 5 % of patients with Crohn's disease, respectively [21]. On the other hand, deficiency of another fat soluble vitamin, vitamin K, may be very commonly encountered in patients with Crohn's disease [22], although the data is contradictory for ulcerative colitis [6, 22, 23]. Although it is commonly understood that vitamin K if necessary for normal blood clotting via vitamin K-dependent factors, it also has a substantial role in the maintenance of normal bone health [24]. Given that 60 % of the daily vitamin K requirement is synthesized by colonic bacteria, the role of active colonic disease, treatment with antibacterial therapies such as sulfa, and changes in the colonic microbiome in those with colitis, may all be contributing factors although none of these have been specifically investigated to date.

Iron deficiency is common in both active Crohn's disease and ulcerative colitis, and has been reported in 20–40 % of IBD patients; it usually results from gastrointestinal blood loss. Low serum ferritin concentration is the most reliable marker of reduced iron stores, although as an acute phase reactant, serum ferritin may be elevated in the presence of systemic inflammation. Anemia in IBD however is often a result of the chronic disease rather than iron deficiency. Calcium deficiency may develop in part as a result of vitamin D deficiency and deficient calcium absorption, although the diet of many individuals (even those without IBD) may be deficient in calcium to begin with. Magnesium and potassium are electrolytes that may require replaced especially in those patients who have had partial small bowel resections or who have significant diarrhea. Because oral magnesium supplements act as a cathartic, intramuscular or intravenous replacement is often necessary.

Zinc deficiency (40 % of patients with Crohn's disease) may also occur especially in patients with significant diarrhea and small bowel fistula losses [21, 25]. A combination of low serum and urinary zinc concentrations is highly suggestive of zinc deficiency. Zinc deficiency can be corrected with oral zinc sulfate 220 mg twice daily. Selenium deficiency is rare.

Dietary Contributions to the Pathogenesis of IBD

It has been suggested that IBD may at least in part be related to dietary antigens, the interaction of diet with commensal bacteria (which may differ between individuals or between those with and without IBD), or the interaction of diet with genetics—specifically the presence of single of multiple single nucleotide polymorphisms (SNPs), which alone, or in combination, could be a risk factor for the development of IBD in the correct setting with the "wrong" bacteria and/or the "wrong" dietary macronutrient. Further, diet may impact colonization, which itself may be in part dependent upon genetics. Indeed, the role of diet in the development of IBD has never been clarified, and has often been dismissed in recent years. However, diet may indeed play a very important role in the pathogenesis of IBD, albeit indirectly Gene expression against gut flora may be modified based on nutrient-gene interactions [26]. It is also potentially possible the intestinal immune response against gut flora may be regulated in part by diet. The fields of nutrigenomics and nutrigenetics are in their development, but may eventually result in "personalized" diets to prevent or treat IBD. Otherwise, dietary risks for development of IBD are largely based on large epidemiological studies, although the effects of diet within a population may be highly variable [27, 28]. For example, the EPIC study that included 260,686 adults at centers in the UK, Sweden, Denmark, Germany, and Italy, found few specific dietary risk factors for development of ulcerative colitis although a possible association with increased polyunsaturated fat diet intake [29], and more specifically, linoleic fatty acid was found [30].

A link between increasing rates of obesity and IBD has been suggested, although it is not clear whether this observation reflects that fat and adipokines produce inflammatory cytokines [31] and may have a role in the pathogenesis of IBD, or whether the observation of obese patients with Crohn's disease or ulcerative colitis merely represents the increasing rate of obesity in society as a whole [32]. Small studies to date have not shown an increased risk for relapse or disease severity in patients with elevated BMI, although one retrospective study suggested an increased risk of anorectal complications [33]. More recently, new cases of Crohn's disease or ulcerative colitis among obese (BMI ≥ 25) participants in the 300,724 subject European Prospective Investigation into Cancer and Nutrition study were not increased over the incidence among those with lower BMI [34].

Although consumption of a diet with significant intake of refined sugars is not a risk factor for development of IBD [35, 36]. Alun Jones found patients often report similar specific foods that tended to trigger the symptoms of their Crohn's disease [37]. These foods included wheat, dairy products, and some vegetables such as mustard greens and various cruciferous vegetables. In one study, induction of remission was obtained in 20 patients with active Crohn's disease with either TPN or an elemental enteral formula. Subjects were then randomized to receive an unrefined carbohydrate diet or nil per os (npo), with reintroduction of specific foods each day, starting with foods unlikely to induce Crohn's-like symptoms as described by the patients (presumably including diarrhea and abdominal discomfort). The most frequently described food intolerances were wheat, dairy products, and brassicas in descending order of prevalence, all of which contain significant amounts of sulfur. Egg and red meat intolerance was also frequent. During the first month the subjects were also provided with an elemental enteral formula to drink and maintain their nutritional status. 8/10 subjects in the unrefined carbohydrate diet relapsed in the first 2 months (all within the first 6 months), while at 6 months 7/10 subjects in the exclusionary diet group remained in remission [38]. It must be noted however, that these foods may have triggered symptoms that may have been consistent with IBD, but nonetheless, were not manifestations of IBD. For example, lactose intolerance in individuals with lactase deficiency may result in "gas," bloating and diarrhea; wheat bran is an excellent stool bulking agent, and consumption may result in increased fecal excretion. A small study evaluated the continued consumption of an "exclusionary" diet on the maintenance of remission in patients with Crohn's disease [37]. Although median remission time was longer and the likelihood of relapse greater in a group that received corticosteroids, the results were still suboptimal and dropout was significant. Nevertheless, the study suggested a potential role for specific dietary components in either relapse, or the maintenance of remission in Crohn's disease. A more recent, but poorly constructed and uncontrolled, retrospective review of the use of an exclusion diet wherein dairy, gluten, soy, processed/smoked meats, sauces, syrups, and jams, canned products, dried fruits, packaged snacks, soft drinks, fruit juices, alcoholic beverages, coffee, candy, chocolate, cake, cookies, and gum were excluded and a polymeric formula was supplemented in order to achieve up to 50 % of daily energy intake, reported a mean remission rate of approximately 75 % at 6 weeks without the use of medications other than 5-ASA [39]. Although compliance was not reported, this author finds it difficult to imagine the child or young adult in this "study" that would not "cheat" on such a diet. This study is also a good example of the poor study design and lack of scientific rigor that many nutritional studies exhibit—making the results very difficult to interpret. Unfortunately, clinical recommendations are made based on this kind of report, or even less. There have been no elimination diets in ulcerative colitis, although diets high in sulfur have been associated with disease development.

Andresen suggested in 1925 that ulcerative colitis was due to a "food allergy" [40]. He reported in 1942 that cow's milk, wheat, tomatoes, oranges, potatoes, and eggs appeared to be the primary factor in the development of ulcerative colitis in two-thirds of his patients [41]. It is noted that milk, wheat, and eggs all have high sulfur content. Truelove reported the exclusion of milk successfully maintained remission in five subjects, all of whom relapsed within 2 days to 6 weeks following the reintroduction of milk into their diet; lactose intolerance was not investigated [42]. He then prescribed a gluten-free, milk-free diet to 77 subjects and reported a fewer number of relapses (three) in 26 subjects that received that diet and could tolerate it, when compared with those subjects that received no special diet (8 of 24) [43].

Major dietary sources of sulfur and sulfate include cow's milk, cheeses, eggs, red meat (beef, lamb, sausage), pork, salmon, herring, shellfish, cruciferous vegetables, white beans, soy, lentils, corn, white rice, dried fruits and vegetables, tomato juice, tree nuts, sulfited wines, dried fruit, cordial, and San Pellegrino® brand water [44–49]. These were many of the same foods that were associated with symptoms consistent with Crohn's disease in the Alun Jones studies. There is some inconsistency however in the available data concerning sulfate content in food, although commercial breads, dried fruit, and red meat appear consistently to contain significant amounts of sulfate. Sulfate is also produced from methionine transsulfuration to cysteine followed by oxidation of that substrate to pyruvate and inorganic sulfate. Inorganic sulfur (sulfate and sulfite) is then reduced, and sulfur-containing amino acids are fermented by colonic bacteria to sulfide [50], although inorganic sulfur that is oxidized to sulfate is excreted in the urine.

Colono-toxic effects of sulfur have been observed with the development of acute colitis in rodents treated with dextran sodium sulfate [51, 52]. Sulfide compounds appear to be the most toxic to isolated colonocytes [53]. Sulfate-reducing bacteria produce hydrogen sulfide [54], which is an acid at a pH of 6.0, although this in turn is converted to anionic sulfide by colonic bicarbonate [55]. Hydrogen sulfide then impairs colonocyte butyrate utilization [53]. Fecal sulfide concentration increased in normal volunteers after they ate red meat [56]. Some studies have reported increased fecal sulfide concentration in patients with active ulcerative colitis [57], although sulfide concentration is normal in patients whose disease is in remission [56, 57]. In vitro studies of rat and human colonic tissue have shown that perfusion with sulfide leads to apoptosis of epithelial cells, goblet cell depletion, and increased cellular proliferation [50]. Hydrogen sulfide is rapidly absorbed by colonocytes and oxidized to sulfate or methylated by mucosal thiol-S-methyltransferase [58, 59]. This essentially detoxifies the sulfide, although only once it has entered the colonocyte. In addition, 5-ASA drugs inhibit sulfide formation by colonic bacteria [56, 60, 61], and in fact, that may represent one of the mechanisms of action of the 5-aminosalicylate compounds.

There may also be an additional mechanism by which a high sulfur diet promotes endothelial inflammation. A high methionine diet leads to increased plasma homocysteine (1.5 g/day vs. >4.5-6 g/day) [62, 63]. High dietary methionine intake leads to an increase in the serum homocysteine concentration [63], and increased cellular homocysteine has been associated with an increase in vitro in the adhesion of monocytes to endothelial cells [64]. Surface expression of vascular cell adhesion molecule (VCAM-1) is triggered and secretion of monocyte chemo-attractant (MCP-1) is stimulated. Increased plasma homocysteine concentration may also increase monocyte adhesion to endothelial cells,[65] and is associated with increased urinary neopterin, a marker of inflammation [66]. Increased plasma and mucosal (colonic) homocysteine have been observed in patients with IBD [64, 66, 67].

Magee et al. observed that patients with ulcerative colitis who consumed diets that contained "high intakes of sulfite containing foods" were likely to have an increased endoscopic disease severity using a novel food-sigmoidoscopy score [68]. In this study from the UK, bitter and lager beer, red and white wine, burgers and sausage, and soft drinks were the foods most frequently associated with increased endoscopic disease severity, although the investigators did not have data on dried fruit, dehydrated potatoes, and seafood because of the few number of subjects that had consumed these food items. Jowett et al. reported much lower mean daily sulfur and sulfate intakes in patients with ulcerative colitis, but still found those that remained in remission had significantly lower intakes than those that relapsed (396 and 668 mg, respectively versus 350 and 636 mg; $p<0.05$) [44]. In a preliminary study in four subjects with ulcerative colitis in whom medical remission had recently been induced, Roediger found elimination of sulfur-containing foods (eggs, cheese, whole milk, ice cream, mayonnaise, soy milk, mineral water, wine, cordials, nuts, cabbage, broccoli, cauliflower, and brussels sprouts) as well as decreased intake of red-meat lead to prolonged remission (0 relapses over 56 patient months with an expected rate of 22.6% in four subjects) [69].

For most non-hospitalized patients the most important advice is for patients to consume a diet liberal in protein, with sufficient calories to maintain weight, even with the understanding that dietary intake of sulfur may increase. It is important to recognize that the serum albumin concentration will not normalize in the presence of a protein-losing enteropathy and/or a significant acute phase response, during which acute phase proteins are synthesized in the liver at the expense of visceral proteins. Oral intake of 25–35 kcal of ideal body weight per day (40 kcal/kg/day for weight gain) and 1.0–1.5 g per kilogram of protein will meet the requirements of most adults who are normally nourished to begin with. In regard to the specifics of a diet, controlled studies have not shown benefit of low-residue diets except for those patients with intestinal obstruction. There is some, albeit limited data to support the use high soluble fiber diets to maintain remission in patients with ulcerative colitis [70]. Soluble fiber such as pectin is fermented by colonic bacteria to short chain fatty acids, the preferred fuel for the colonocyte.

Lactose intolerance is not commonly associated with IBD unless the individual was lactose intolerant antedating their IBD or they have Crohn's disease that involves the proximal jejunum, where lactase is located. Dietary lactose should therefore only be restricted if patients have symptoms associated with dairy intake and in whom lactose intolerance can be demonstrated by breath hydrogen testing; many patients with symptoms of lactose intolerance are not actually lactose intolerant [71]. Lactose-containing foods are the primary source of dietary calcium. Furthermore, there is no consistent epidemiological data supporting the role of milk as a cause of IBD.

A low oxalate diet may be required in those patients who have had their terminal ileum resected or who have significant fat malabsorption in the presence of residual colon anastomosed in continuity with the small bowel. These patients have a propensity for oxalate kidney stones.

Nutritional Therapy in IBD

Specific Nutritional Supplements

Initial studies with fish oil supplements (n-3 fatty acids) in ulcerative colitis showed decreased disease activity in patients that received these formulas, but larger randomized trials in Crohn's disease have failed to show consistent results [72–74]. Fish oil may have anti-inflammatory activity because n-3 fatty acids are thought to compete in the substrate pool of the lipoxygenase pathway, thus reducing the production of inflammatory leukotrienes [75]. A study by Belluzzi et al. found 2.7 g of n-3 fatty acids administered as an enteric-coated fish oil preparation maintained 59 % of Crohn's patients in remission after 1 year compared to 26 % in the placebo group, $p<0.05$ [72]. Another study by Lorenz-Meyer failed to show a difference in remission rates compared to placebo [73]. In each study large amounts were given which is unpalatable for most people. Feagan et al. reported on the results of two double-blinded, randomized placebo-controlled trials which utilized the same fish oil preparation used in the earlier study of Belluzzi. They found that although fish oil was safe, the rate of relapse at 1 year was virtually identical between the fish oil group and those treated with placebo [74]. It is unclear whether a study of longer duration would have resulted in different results because most studies of maintenance therapy have used the 1 year threshold. It appears the door on fish oils in IBD has been closed.

Studies have not shown any benefit of glutamine supplementation in either patients with Crohn's disease or ulcerative colitis [76–79]. Animal studies have actually suggested glutamine supplementation may worsen IBD [79, 80].

When is Nutritional Support Necessary?

Nutritional support refers to the use of either intravenous/parenteral (PN) or enteral tube feeding and is usually administered to hospitalized patients, although selected patients (usually those with Crohn's disease and short bowel syndrome or patients with short bowel syndrome resulting from mesenteric infarction in the presence of IBD) may require short- or long-term PN at home. Nutritional support of the hospitalized patient should be instituted promptly when it has been determined from daily calorie counts that a patient is not taking sufficient oral intake of food for ≥7 days. After approximately 7–10 days of npo negative nitrogen balance may develop; this increases the risk of infection and interferes with wound healing. Nutritional support may also be considered an adjunctive therapy in malnourished patients in whom sufficient oral intake to promote nutritional repletion is not immediately achievable. For both active Crohn's disease and ulcerative colitis, nutritional therapy therefore has a significant supportive role. The role for nutritional support as *primary therapy* for inflammatory bowel disease is limited as discussed below. The use of preoperative PN has been suggested to improve surgical outcome and limited bowel resection in Crohn's patients undergoing small bowel resections, but not in large bowel resections [81]. The same is not the case in patients with ulcerative colitis [82]. Most of the reports are retrospective and uncontrolled. An analysis of the data shows generally improved indices of nutritional status, but that were not accompanied by reduced postoperative complications. Therefore, routine use of nutritional support in the preoperative patient should be restricted to seriously malnourished patients (SGA "C") who are not candidates for enteral feeding usually because of bowel obstruction. For patients who are significantly nutritionally depleted, longer term nutritional support may be required in order to improve postoperative morbidity. However, surgery should not be delayed in order to administer nutritional support in the majority of patients. Delayed surgery often leads to a further decline in the nutritional reserve of a patient. Nutritional support should be continued, or initiated post operatively if the patient is considered moderately (SGA "B") or severely malnourished (SGA "C") preoperatively.

Indications for parenteral feeding usually include small bowel obstruction, which may develop in Crohn's disease because of adhesions related to prior surgery, severe edema with luminal compromise during an acute flare, or chronic, fibrotic scar tissue; severe diarrhea and malabsorption during active disease; small bowel ileus; gastrointestinal hemorrhage; treatment for entero-cutaneous or entero-enteric fistulae; and as supportive care in patients that are severely malnourished (SGA "C") or who have active disease with compromised absorptive surface. *The cumulative risk of intestinal failure (inability to maintain nutritional autonomy without parenteral fluid and/or nutritional support) was found to be 0.8 % at 5 years, 3.6 % at 10 years, 6.1 % at 15 years, and 8.5 % after 20 years of Crohn's disease among 1703 patients in Japan* [83]. TPN may also be indicated in a patient with ulcerative colitis and toxic mega colon in which enteral nutrition is contraindicated. TPN is not generally indicated in patients that have a nonobstructive gastrointestinal tract or when the duration of nutritional support is expected to be <7 days.

It is dogma that the gut "atrophies," in the absence of enteral nutrition. While this may be the case in animal studies, the data in humans fail to support this concept. It is commonly thought that in the absence of enteral nutrition, bacteria will translocate across the intestinal epithelium, to the mesenteric lymph nodes, and into the systemic circulation, resulting in sepsis and multi organ failure. Although this has been reported in the rat model, it rarely occurs in humans [84]. When bacterial translocation does occur in humans, it is usually in the setting of small bowel obstruction, and unrelated to the route of feeding, and is usually clinically inconsequential [84].

Nutritional Support as Therapy for IBD

Whether the combination of complete bowel rest and total parenteral nutrition (TPN) can be used successfully as *primary therapy* in patients with acute inflammatory bowel disease with or without the addition of other medical therapy including diet is controversial. The consensus of the literature would suggest that patients with Crohn's enteritis can achieve clinical remission with the combination of bowel rest and parenteral nutrition alone [85–90]. The composite results suggest npo and TPN for 3–6 weeks will achieve a clinical response rate of 64 % in patients with acute Crohn's disease [90]. However, in most studies prednisone was administered simultaneously with TPN, which makes it difficult to discern whether the positive effects observed were the result of bowel rest and TPN or the combined effects with prednisone. The consensus of the literature would also suggest that patients with Crohn's colitis and idiopathic ulcerative colitis do not respond any better to TPN and bowel rest (with or without prednisone) than patients treated with prednisone and diet [91–94]. It must also be recognized that 10 % of the patients in these studies developed complications from PN; these included pneumothorax from central catheter placement, catheter sepsis, and various metabolic complications. Therefore, prior to the administration of a therapy with questionable benefit, the potential risk of therapy should be considered. PN is generally reserved for supportive therapy to maintain nutritional reserve rather than as primary treatment.

Intestinal fistula is one circumstance is which npo and bowel rest may serve as primary treatment. A 38 % of fistula closure rate has been reported in Crohn's patients [95]. However, the reported studies lacked a non-TPN control group and there no long-term follow-up was generally reported. Surgery is usually required if fistula closure is not complete after 3 months of nutritional support. For Medicare reimbursement, 3 months or longer of PN is usually required and it must be documented that enteral feeding distal to the fistula is either not possible or would result in significant malabsorption. With newer medications such as infliximab and adalimumab, TPN and bowel rest may serve less of a role in the treatment fistulas. A randomized study comparing TPN with bowel rest to anti-tumor necrosis antibody (TNF) therapy, in addition to an oral diet is needed.

With regard to EN, products may be provided either orally or via a feeding tube, and may have potential benefit as primary treatment in Crohn's patients [96–101]. The composite data suggest that the administration of either an elemental, peptide based or polymeric diet for 3–6 weeks will achieve a remission rate of approximately 68 %, which is similar to the remission rate reported with TPN and bowel rest. There is no advantage of an elemental or semi-elemental formula, which are often more expensive, over a formula that contains intact protein [101]. Remission rates achieved are comparable to that with corticosteroids [101]. The reason patients with active Crohn's disease may respond to polymeric enteral formulas, but not an ad lib regular oral diet is unclear, but may be related to the lipid composition of the enteral formula or the fact the formula diets are all sterile. The mechanism of action for the induction of remission is not clear. All of the formulas however are sterile, as opposed to orally consumed food, which is not. Limited data to date has suggested that fecal bacteria differ by species and levels in patients with Crohn's disease and those without Crohn's disease, although the fecal microbiota appears to be affected only by TPN and not by EN, although in this particular study the population of *Bacteroides fragilis* was decreased [102]. This observation was also made by Gerasimidis et al., who also observed, in a small study, a decrease in the presence of bacteria from the *Prevotella group* [103]. *Formulas* with increased concentrations of long chain triglycerides and polyunsaturated fats may be risk factors for the relapse of Crohn's disease [100, 101], although other data is contradictory [104].

A systematic review of the studies in which EN was used to maintain remission in patients with Crohn's disease is difficult given the limited number (two) of controlled trials, and different study designs [105]. A subsequent systematic review that evaluated one randomized controlled trial, three prospective, non-controlled trials, and six retrospective studies all of which included elemental, semi-elemental, or polymeric formulas for outcomes (EN vs no EN) the clinical remission rate was higher in those patients who received EN in all studies, and remission was also directly related to the amount of formula consumed in the four studies where the quantity of formula consumed was reported [106]. Nevertheless, because of substantial methodological differences between studies, meta-analysis was not possible.

In summary, nutrition plays a prominent role in the treatment of IBD, both directly and indirectly, and may also play an important role in the pathogenesis of IBD.

References

1. Seidman EG. Nutritional management of inflammatory bowel disease. Gastroenterol Clin N Am. 1989;18:129–55.
2. Bin CM, Flores C, Alvares-da-Silva MR, Francesconi CF. Comparison between handgrip strength, subjective global assessment, anthropometry, and biochemical markers in assessing nutritional status of patients with Crohn's disease in clinical remission. Dig Dis Sci. 2010;55:137–44.
3. Valentini L, Schaper L, Buning C, Hengstermann S, Koernicke T, Tillinger W, et al. Malnutrition and impaired muscle strength in patients with Crohn's disease and ulcerative colitis in remission. Nutrition. 2008;24:694–702.
4. Detsky AS, McLaughlin JR, Baker JP, Johnston N, Whittaker S, Mendelson RA, et al. What is subjective global assessment of nutritional status? JPEN J Parenter Enteral Nutr. 1987;11:8–13.
5. Franklin JL, Rosenberg IH. Impaired folic acid absorption in inflammatory bowel disease: effects of salicylazosulfapyridine. Gastroenterology. 1973;64:517–25.
6. Behrend C, Jeppesen PB, Mortensen PB. Vitamin B-12 absorption after ileorectal anastomosis for Crohn's disease: effect of ileal resection and time span after surgery. Eur J Gastroenterol Hepatol. 1995;7:397–400.
7. Battat R, Kopylov U, Szilagyi A, Saxena A, Rosenblatt DS, Warner M, et al. Vitamin B12 deficiency in inflammatory bowel disease: prevalence, risk factors, evaluation, and management. Inflamm Bowel Dis. 2014;20:1120–8.
8. Ham M, Longhi MS, Lahiff C, Cheifetz A, Robson S, Moss AC. Vitamin D levels in adults with Crohn's disease are responsive to activity and treatment. Inflamm Bowel Dis. 2014;20:856–60.
9. Jørgensen SP, Agnholt J, Glerup H, Lyhne S, Villadsen GE, Hvas CL, et al. Clinical trial: vitamin D3 treatment in Crohn's disease - a randomized double-blind placebo-controlled study. Aliment Pharmacol Ther. 2010;32(3):377–83.
10. Kumari M, Khazai NB, Ziegler TR, Nanes MS, Abrams SA, Tangpricha V. Vitamin D-mediated calcium absorption in patients with clinically stable Crohn's disease: a pilot study. Mol Nutr Food Res. 2010;54(8):1085–91.
11. Farraye FA, Nimitphong H, Stucchi A, Dendrinos K, Boulanger AB, Vijjeswarapu A, et al. Use of a novel vitamin D bioavailability test demonstrates that vitamin D absorption is decreased in patients with quiescent Crohn's disease. Inflamm Bowel Dis. 2011;17:2116–21.
12. Bours PH, Wielders JP, Vermeijden JR, van de Wiel A. Seasonal variation of serum 25-hydroxyvitamin D levels in adults patients with inflammatory bowel disease. Osteroporos Int. 2011;22:2857–67.
13. Lagishetty Y, Misharin AV, Liu NQ, et al. Vitamin D deficiency in mice impairs colonic antibacterial activity and predisposes to colitis. Endocrinology. 2010;151:2423–32.
14. Froicu M, Weaver V, Wynn TA, et al. A crucial role for the vitamin D receptor in experimental inflammatory bowel diseases. Mol Endocrinol. 2003;17:2386–92.
15. Cantorna MT, Munsick C, Berniss C, Mahon RD. 1,25-dihydroxycholecalciferol prevents and ameliorates symptoms of experimental murine inflammatory bowel disease. J Nutr. 2000;130:2648–52.
16. Froicu M, Cantorna MT. Vitamin D and vitamin D receptor are critical for control of the innate immune response to colonic injury. BMC Immunol. 2007;8:5.
17. Choi JH, Li Y, Rogers CJ, Cantorna MT. Vitamin D regulates the gut microbiome and protect mice from dextran sodium sulfate-induced colitis. J Nutr. 2013;143:1679–86.
18. Blanck S, Aberra F. Vitamin D deficiency is associated with ulcerative colitis disease activity. Dig Dis Sci. 2013;58:1698–702.
19. Vogelsang H, Ferenci P, Resch H, Kiss A, Gangl A. Prevention of bone mineral loss in patients with Crohn's disease by long term oral vitamin D supplementation. Eur J Gstroenterol Hepatol. 1995;7:609–14.
20. Bousvaros A, Zurakowski D, Duggan C, Law T, Rifai N, Goldberg NE, et al. Vitamins A and E serum levels in children and young adults with inflammatory bowel disease: effect of disease activity. J Pediatr Gastroenterol Nutr. 1998;26:129–34.
21. Alkhouri RH, Hashmi H, Baker RD, et al. Vitamin and mineral status in patients with inflammatory bowel disease. J Pediatr Gastroenterol Nutr. 2013;56:89–92.
22. Nowak JK, Grzybowska-Chlebowczyk U, Landowski P, Szaflarska-Poplawska A, Klincewicz B. Prevalence and correlates of vitamin K deficiency in children with inflammatory bowel disease. Sci Rep. 2014;4:4768.
23. Nakajima S, Iijima H, Egawa S, Shinzaki S, Kondo J, Inoue T, et al. Association of vitamin K deficiency with bone metabolism and clinical disease activity in inflammatory bowel disease. Nutrition. 2011;27:1023–8.
24. Kuwabara A, Tanaka K, Tsugawa N, Nakase H, Tsuji H, Shide K, et al. High prevalence of vitamin K and D deficiency and decreased BMD in inflammatory bowel disease. Osteoporos Int. 2009;20:935–42.
25. Valberg LS, Flanagan PR, Kertesz A, Bondy DC. Zinc absorption in inflammatory bowel disease. Dig Dis Sci. 1986;31:724–31.
26. Lee G, Buchman AL. DNA-driven nutritional therapy of inflammatory bowel disease. Nutrition. 2009;25:885–91.
27. Stover PJ. Influence of human genetic variation on nutritional requirements. Am J Clin Nutr. 2006;83:436S–42.
28. Subbiah MT. Understanding the nutrigenomic definitions and concepts at the food-genome junction. OMICS. 2008;12:229–35.
29. Hart AR, Luben R, Olsen A, Tjonneland A, Linseisen J, Nagel G, et al. Diet in the aetiology of ulcerative colitis: a European prospective cohort study. Digestion. 2008;77:57–64.
30. IBD in EPIC Study Investigators, Tjonneland A, Overvad K, Bergmann MM, Nagel G, Linseisen J, et al. Linoleic acid, a dietary n-6 polyunsaturated fatty acid, and the aetiology of ulcerative colitis: a nested case–control study within a European prospective cohort study. Gut. 2009;58:1606–11.
31. Karmiris K, Koutroubakis IE, Kouroumalis EA. The emerging role of adipocytokines as inflammatory mediators in inflammatory bowel disease. Inflamm Bowel Dis. 2005;11:847–55.
32. Steed H, Walsh S, Reynolds N. A brief report of the epidemiology of obesity in the inflammatory bowel disease population of Tayside, Scotland. Obes Facts. 2009;2:370–2.
33. Blain A, Cattan S, Beaugerie L, et al. Crohn's disease clinical course and severity in obese patients. Clin Nutr. 2002;21:51–7.
34. Chan SS, Luben R, Olsen A, Tjonneland A, Kaaks R, Teucher B, et al. Body mass index and the risk for Crohn's disease and ulcerative colitis: data from a European Prospective Cohort Study (the IBD in EPIC Study). Am J Gastroenterol. 2013;108:575–82.
35. Jarnerot G, Jarnmark I, Nilsson K. Consumption of refined sugar by patients with Crohn's disease, ulcerative colitis, or irritable bowel syndrome. Scand J Gastroenterol. 1983;18:999–1102.

36. Riordan AM, Ruxton CH, Hunter JO. A review of associations between Crohn's disease and consumption of sugars. Eur J Clin Nutr. 1998;52:2229–38.
37. Jones VA, Dickinson RJ, Workman E, Wilson AJ, Freeman AH, Hunter JO. Crohn's disease: maintenance of remission by diet. Lancet. 1985;2:177–81.
38. Riordan AM, Hunter JO, Cowan RE, Crampton JR, Davidson AR, Dickinson RJ, et al. Treatment of active Crohn's disease by exclusion diet. East Angelica multi-centre controlled diet. Lancet. 1993;342:1131–4.
39. Sigall-Boneh R, Pfeffer-Gik T, Segal I, Zangen T, Boaz M, Levine A. Partial enteral nutrition with a Crohn's disease exclusion diet is effective for induction of remission in children and young adults with Crohn's disease. Inflamm Bowel Dis. 2014;20:1353–60.
40. Andresen AFR. Gastrointestinal manifestations of food allergy. Med J Res (Suppl). 1925;122:271–5.
41. Andresen AFR. Ulcerative colitis—an allergic phenomenon. Am J Dig Dis. 1942;9:91–8.
42. Truelove SC. Ulcerative colitis provoked by milk. Br Med J. 1961;1:154–60.
43. Wright R, Truelove SC. A controlled therapeutic trial of various diets in ulcerative colitis. Br Med J. 1965;2:138–41.
44. Jowett SL, Seal CJ, Pearce MS, et al. Influence of dietary factors on the clinical course of ulcerative colitis: a prospective cohort study. Gut. 2004;53:1479–84.
45. Roediger WE, Moore J, Babidge W. Colonic sulfide in pathogenesis and treatment of ulcerative colitis. Dig Dis Sci. 1997;42:1571–9.
46. Florin THJ, Neale G, Gibson GR, et al. Metabolism of dietary sulfate: absorption and excretion in humans. Gut. 1991;32:766–73.
47. Di Buono M, Wykes LJ, Ball RO, Pencharz PB. Total sulfur amino acid requirement in young men as determined by indicator amino acid oxidation with l-[1-13C]phenylalanine. Am J Clin Nutr. 2001;74:756–60.
48. Allen HE, Halley-Henderson MA, Hass CN. Chemical composition of bottled mineral water. Arch Environ Health. 1989;44:102–16.
49. Ingenbleek Y. The nutritional relationship linking sulfur to nitrogen in living organisms. J Nutr. 2006;136:1641S–51.
50. Gibson GR, Cummings JH, MacFarlane GT. Growth and activities sulphate-reducing bacteria in gut contents of healthy subjects and patients with ulcerative colitis. FEMS Microbiol Ecol. 1991;86:103–12.
51. Ohkusa T. Production of experimental ulcerative in hamsters by dextran sulfate sodium and change in intestinal microflora. Jpn J Gastroenterol. 1985;82:1337–47.
52. Ishioka T, Kuwabara N, Oohashi Y, Wakabayashi K. Induction of colorectal tumors in rats by sulfated polysaccharides. CRC Crit Rev Toxicol. 1986;17:215–44.
53. Roediger WE, Duncan A, Kapaniris O, Millard S. Reducing sulfur compounds of the colon impairs colonocyte nutrition: implications for ulcerative colitis. Gastroenterology. 1993;104:802–9.
54. MacFarlane GT, Gibson GR, Cummings JH. Comparison of fermentation reactions in different regions of the human colon. J Appl Bacteriol. 1992;72:57–64.
55. Roediger WE, Lawson MJ, Kwok V, Grant AK, Pannall PR. Colonic bicarbonate output as a test of disease activity in ulcerative colitis. J Clin Pathol. 1984;37:704–7.
56. Magee EA, Richardson CJ, Hughes R, Cummings JH. Contribution of dietary protein to sulfide production in the large intestine: an in vitro and a controlled feeding study in humans. Am J Clin Nutr. 2000;72:1488–94.
57. Pitcher MCL, Beatty ER, Gibson GR, Cummings JH. The contribution of sulphate reducing bacteria and 5-aminosalicylic acid to faecal sulphide in patients with ulcerative colitis. Gut. 2000;46:64–72.
58. Levitt MD, Furne J, Springfield J, Suarez F, DeMaster E. Detoxification of hydrogen sulphide and methanethiol in the cecal mucosa. J Clin Invest. 1999;104:1107–14.
59. Furne J, Springfield J, Koenig T, DeMaster E, Levitt MD. Oxidation of hydrogen sulphide and methanethiol to thiosulfate by rat tissues: a specialized function of the colonic mucosa. Biochem Pharmacol. 2001;62:255–9.
60. Roediger WEW, Duncan A. 5-ASA decreases colonic sulphide formation: implications for ulcerative colitis. Med Sci Res. 1996;24:27–9.
61. Edmond LM, Hopkins MJ, Magee EA, Cummings JH. The effect of 5-aminosalicylic acid-containing drugs on sulfide production by sulfate-reducing and amino acid-fermenting bacteria. Inflamm Bowel Dis. 2003;9:10–7.
62. Ditscheid B, Fünfstück R, Busch M, Schubert R, Gerth J, Jahreis G. Effect of l-methionine supplementation on plasma homocysteine concentrations and other free amino acids: a placebo-controlled, double-blind cross-over study. Eur J Clin Nutr. 2005;59:768–75.
63. Verhoef P, van Vliet T, Olthof MR, Katan MB. A high-protein diet increases postprandial but not fasting total homocysteine concentrations: a dietary controlled crossover trial in healthy volunteers. Am J Clin Nutr. 2005;82:553–8.
64. Danese S, Sgambato A, Papa A, Scaldaferri F, Pola R, Sans M, et al. Homocysteine triggers mucosal microvascular activation in inflammatory bowel disease. Am J Gastroenterol. 2005;100:886–95.
65. Morgenstern I, Raijmakers MT, Peters WH, Hoensch H, Kirch W. Homocysteine, cysteine, and glutathione in human colonic mucosa: elevated levels of homocysteine in patients with inflammatory bowel disease. Dig Dis Sci. 2003;48:2083–90.
66. Koga T, Claycombe K, Meydani M. Homocysteine increases monocyte and T-cell adhesion to human aortic endothelial cells. Athersclerosis. 2002;161:365–74.
67. Romagnuolo J, Fedorak RN, Dias VC, Bamforth F, Teltscher M. Hyperhomocysteinemia and inflammatory bowel disease: prevalence and predictors in a cross-sectional study. Am J Gastroenterol. 2001;96:2143–9.
68. Magee EA, Edmond LM, Tasker SM, Kong SC, Curno R, Cummings JH. Associations between diet and disease activity in ulcerative colitis patients using a novel method of data analysis. Nutr J. 2005;4:7.
69. Roediger WEW. Decreased sulphur amino acid intake in ulcerative colitis (letter). Lancet. 1998;351:1555.
70. Fernández-Bañares F, Hinojosa J, Sánchez-Lombraña JL, Navarro E, Martínez-Salmerón JF, García-Pugés A, et al. Randomized clinical trial of Plantago ovata seeds (dietary fiber) as compared with mesalamine in maintaining remission in ulcerative colitis. Am J Gastroenterol. 1999;94:427–33.
71. Suarez FL, Savaiano DA, Levitt MD. A comparison of symptoms after the consumption of milk or lactose-hydrolyzed milk by people with self-reported severe lactose intolerance. N Engl J Med. 1995;333:1–4.
72. Belluzzi A, Brignola C, Campieri M, Pera A, Boschi S, Miglioli M. Effect of enteric coated fish oil preparations on relapses in Crohn's disease. N Engl J Med. 1996;334:1557–60.
73. Lorenz-Meyer H, Bauer P, Nicolay C, Schulz B, Purrmann J, Fleig WE, et al. Omega 3 fatty acids and low carbohydrate diet for maintenance of remission in Crohn's disease: a randomized controlled multicenter trial. Scand J Gastroenterol. 1996;31:778–85.
74. Feagan BG, Sandborn WJ, Mittmann U, Bar-Meir S, D'Haens G, Bradette M, et al. Omega-3 free fatty acids for the maintenance of remission in Crohn's disease: the EPIC randomized controlled trials. JAMA. 2008;299:1690–7.
75. Caughey GE, Mantzioris E, Gibson RA, Cleland LG, James MJ. The effect on human tumor necrosis factor alpha and interleukin

1B production of diets enriched in n-3 fatty acids from vegetable oil or fish. Am J Clin Nutr. 1996;63:116–22.
76. Akobeng AK, Miller V, Stanton J, Elbadri AM, Thomas AG. Double-blind randomized controlled trial of glutamine-enriched polymeric diet in the treatment of active Crohn's disease. J Pediatr Gastroentrol Nutr. 2000;30:78–84.
77. Cordum NR, Schloerb P, Sutton D, et al. Oral glutamine supplementation in patients with Crohn's disease with or without glucocorticoid treatment. Gastroenterology. 1996;10:A888.
78. Zoli G, Care M, Flaco F, et al. Effect of oral glutamine on intestinal permeability and nutritional status in Crohn's disease. Gut. 1995;37:A13.
79. Den Hond E, Hiele M, Peeters M, Ghoos Y, Rutgeerts P. Effect of long-term oral glutamine supplements on small intestinal permeability in patients with Crohn's disease. JPEN J Parenter Enteral Nutr. 1999;23:7–11.
80. Shinozaki M, Saito H, Muto T. Excess glutamine exacerbates trinitrobenzenesulfonic acid-induced colitis in rats. Dis Colon Rectum. 1997;40:S59–63.
81. Lashner BA, Evans AA, Hanauer SB. Preoperative total parenteral nutrition for bowel resection in Crohn's disease. Dig Dis Sci. 1989;34:741–6.
82. Salinas H, Dursun A, Konstantinidis I, Nguyen D, Shellito P, Hodin R, et al. Does preoperative total parenteral nutrition in patients with ulcerative colitis produce better outcomes? Int J Colorectal Dis. 2012;27:1479–83.
83. Watanabe K, Sasaki I, Fukushima K, Futami K, Ikeuchi H, Sugita A, et al. Long-term incidence and characteristics of intestinal failure in Crohn's disease: a multicenter study. J Gastroenterol. 2014;49:231–8.
84. Sedman PC, MacFie J, Palmer MD, Mitchell CJ, Sagar PM. Preoperative total parenteral nutrition is not associated with mucosal atrophy or bacterial translocation in humans. Br J Surg. 1995;82:1663–7.
85. Ostro MJ, Greenberg GR, Jeejeebhoy KN. Total parenteral nutrition and complete bowel rest in the management of Crohn's disease. JPEN J Parenter Enteral Nutr. 1985;9:280–7.
86. Reilly J, Ryan JA, Strole W, Fischer JE. Hyperalimentation in inflammatory bowel disease. Am J Surg. 1976;131:192–200.
87. Mullen JL, Hargrove WC, Dudrick SJ, Fitts Jr WT, Rosato EF. Ten years experience with intravenous hyperalimentation and inflammatory bowel disease. Ann Surg. 1978;187:523–9.
88. Greenberg GR, Fleming CR, Jeejeebhoy KN. Controlled trial of bowel rest and nutritional support in the management of Crohn's disease. Gut. 1988;29:1309–15.
89. Lochs H, Meryn S, Marosi L, Ferenci P, Hörtnagl H. Has total bowel rest have a beneficial effect in the treatment of Crohn's disease. Clin Nutr. 1983;2:61–4.
90. Greenberg GR. Nutritional management of inflammatory bowel disease. Semin Gastrointest Dis. 1993;4:69–86.
91. Dickinson RJ, Ashton MG, Axon AT, Smith RC, Yeung CK, Hill GL. Controlled trial of intravenous hyperalimentation and bowel rest as an adjunct to routine therapy of acute colitis. Gastroenterology. 1980;79:1199–204.
92. McIntyre PB, Powell-Tuck J, Wood SR. Controlled trial of bowel rest in the treatment of severe acute colitis. Gut. 1986;27:481–5.
93. Sitzmann JV, Converse RL, Bayless TM. Favorable response to parenteral nutrition and medical therapy in Crohn's colitis. Gastroenterology. 1990;99:1647–52.
94. Afzal NA, Davies S, Paintin M, Arnaud-Battandier F, Walker-Smith JA, Murch S, et al. Colonic Crohn's disease in children does not respond well to treatment with enteral nutrition if the ileum is not involved. Dig Dis Sci. 2005;50:1471–5.
95. Afonso JJ, Rombeau JL. Nutritional care for patients with Crohn's disease. Hepatogastroenterology. 1990;37:32–41.
96. O'Morain C, Segal AW, Levi AJ. Elemental diet as primary treatment of acute Crohn's disease: a controlled trial. Br Med J (Clin Res Ed). 1984;288:1859–62.
97. Jones VA. Comparison of total parenteral nutrition and elemental diet in induction of remission of Crohn's disease. Dig Dis Sci. 1987;32:100–7.
98. González-Huix F, de León R, Fernández-Bañares F, Esteve M, Cabré E, Acero D, et al. Polymeric enteral diets as primary treatment of active Crohn's disease: a prospective steroid controlled trial. Gut. 1993;34:778–82.
99. Rigaud D, Cosnes J, Le Quintrec Y, René E, Gendre JP, Mignon M. Controlled trial comparing two types of enteral nutrition in treatment of active Crohn's disease: elemental vs polymeric diet. Gut. 1991;32:1492–7.
100. Miura S, Tsuzuki Y, Hokari R, Ishii H. Modulation of intestinal immune system by dietary fat intake: relevance to Crohn's disease. J Gastroenterol Hepatol. 1998;13:1183–90.
101. Zachos M, Tondeur M, Griffiths AM. Enteral nutritional therapy for the induction of remission in Crohn's disease. Cochrane Database Syst Rev. 2007: CD000542.
102. Shiga H, Kajiura T, Shinozaki J, Takagi S, Kinouchi Y, Takahashi S, et al. Changes of faecal microbiota in patients with Crohn's disease treated with an elemental diet and total parenteral nutrition. Dig Liver Dis. 2012;44:736–42.
103. Gerasimidis K, Bertz M, Hanske L, Junick J, Biskou O, Aguilera M, et al. Decline in presumptively protective gut bacterial species and metabolites are paradoxically associated with disease improvement in pediatric Crohn's disease during enteral nutrition. Inflamm Bowel Dis. 2014;20:861–71.
104. Leiper K, Woolner J, Mullan MM, Parker T, van der Vliet M, Fear S, et al. A randomized controlled trial of high versus low long chain triglyceride whole protein feed in active Crohn's disease. Gut. 2001;49:790–4.
105. Akobeng AK, Thomas AG. Enteral nutrition for maintenance of remission in Crohn's disease. Cochrane Database Syst Rev. 2007: CD005984.
106. Yamamoto T, Nakahigashi M, Umegae S, Matsumoto K. Enteral nutrition for the maintenance of remission in Crohn's disease: a systematic review. Eur J Gastroenterol Hepatol. 2010;22:1–8.

Part VIII

Pregnancy, Family Planning and Pediatric Aspects

Pregnancy and Fertility in Inflammatory Bowel Disease

57

Rebecca Matro and Uma Mahadevan

Abbreviations

IBD	Inflammatory bowel disease
UC	Ulcerative colitis
IPAA	Ileal pouch anal anastomosis
IRA	Ileo-rectal anastomosis
aOR	Adjusted odds ratio
CI	Confidence interval
SGA	Small for gestational age
PIANO	Pregnancy in Inflammatory Bowel Disease and Neonatal Outcomes
ECCO	European Crohn-Colitis Organization
FDA	Federal Drug Administration
MTX	Methotrexate
5-ASAs	Aminosalicylates
AZA	Azathioprine
6-MP	6-Mercaptopurine
TNF	Tumor necrosis factor
IFX	Infliximab
ADA	Adalimumab
CZP	Certolizomab pegol
GOL	Golimumab
Ig	Immunoglobulin
RR	Relative risk
BCG	Bacilli Calmette-Guérin

R. Matro, M.D.
Oregon Health and Sciences University, 3181 SW Sam Jackson Park Rd., L461, Portland, OR 97239, USA
e-mail: matro@ohsu.edu

U. Mahadevan, M.D. (✉)
UCSF Center for Colitis and Crohn's Disease, 1701 Divisadero Street #120, San Francisco, CA 94115, USA
e-mail: uma.mahadevan@ucsf.edu

Inflammatory bowel disease affects men and women in their prime reproductive years, with a peak incidence between 20 and 35 years of age [1]. According to Olmstead County data, the median age of diagnosis for Crohn's disease was 29.5 years and for ulcerative colitis (UC) was 34.9 years. A diagnosis of IBD impacts how women approach fertility and pregnancy. Gastroenterologists and other physicians, such as obstetrician-gynecologists, and primary care providers must take into account special considerations when treating women with IBD during the reproductive years. This chapter will discuss these important considerations for medical specialists who care for women with IBD during the preconception period, pregnancy, and lactation (Table 57.1).

Preconception Care and Fertility

Proper care should begin well before pregnancy with preconception counseling and stabilization of disease. Preconception counseling allows clinicians to address specific patient concerns, optimize control of disease activity and minimize chance of relapse during pregnancy, avoid inappropriate medication cessation, and discontinue medications that may adversely affect pregnancy [2]. Women with IBD have a higher rate of voluntary childlessness, possibly due to misinformation regarding fertility, medications, and their effects on the fetus, and concerns regarding passing the disease on to their children [3].

Women with IBD have the same rate of fertility as age-matched controls [4]. However, women with active disease or with prior surgery in the pelvis have impaired fertility. Infertility is increased with active disease due to inflammation involving the fallopian tubes or ovaries, dyspareunia related to perianal disease, decreased libido, and depression [5–7]. Women with Crohn's disease may also have decreased ovarian reserve [8]. Among women with inactive disease, surgery in the pelvis, particularly an ileal pouch anal anastomosis (IPAA), increases infertility threefold [9]. Pelvic scarring and surgical adhesions may lead to tubal infertility [10].

D.C. Baumgart (ed.), *Crohn's Disease and Ulcerative Colitis*, DOI 10.1007/978-3-319-33703-6_57

Table 57.1 Key points in the management of IBD in pregnant patients

Time period	Important points
Preconception	– Establish care with multidisciplinary team: primary care physician, obstetrician, maternal–fetal specialist, gastroenterologist – Discontinue medications that may be harmful to fetus (i.e. methotrexate) – Update health care maintenance and vaccinations – Check baseline laboratories including blood count, B12, folate, iron, and vitamin D and correct if abnormal – Achieve and confirm remission before attempting pregnancy – Establish medication plan for pregnancy and postpartum period
Conception	– Fertility rates are similar among women with inactive IBD who have not had surgery in the pelvis and women without IBD – Disease activity can adversely affect fertility and miscarriage rates
Pregnancy	– Maintain stable disease—increased disease activity may affect pregnancy outcomes – Continue appropriate maintenance medications through pregnancy – Consider adjusting timing of biologic medication to minimize third trimester placental transfer to fetus but not necessary – Monitoring by a high-risk obstetrician in addition to regular obstetrician given increased rates of pregnancy complications
Delivery	– Mode of delivery should be at the discretion of the team and decision should be made on individual basis after discussion with patient – Women with active perineal disease should have a cesarean delivery – Ileostomy should not be over sewn during cesarean delivery
Postpartum	– Most medications can be safely continued during lactation – Infants exposed to biologic agents should not be given any live vaccines in the first 6 months of life (except with certolizumab) – All other vaccines should be given on schedule

This reduction in fertility is also seen in patients who undergo IPAA for familial adenomatous polyposis syndrome, a non-inflammatory condition. Procedures that do not invade the pelvis and result in fewer abdominal and pelvic adhesions, such as ileo-rectal anastomosis (IRA) and laparoscopic surgery, do not appear to impair fertility [11]. These less invasive procedures may be preferable in female children, adolescents, and women who require surgery but wish to preserve fertility.

Before attempting conception, women should be up to date on health care maintenance, vaccinations (hepatitis A and B, pneumococcal, influenza, tetanus/diphtheria/pertussis, and Human Papilloma Virus), and age-appropriate cancer screening [12]. Routine laboratory testing including complete blood count, vitamin B12, folic acid, and iron levels, should be performed. Patients who are having difficulty conceiving or have had previous miscarriages should be screened for vitamin D deficiency and celiac disease, which have been associated with infertility [13, 14].

IBD should be well controlled at the time of conception, and women should be in a durable remission for at least 6 months before attempting conception. The presence of disease activity is associated with reduced ability to conceive, greater chance of disease activity during pregnancy, and increased risk of adverse pregnancy outcomes, including spontaneous abortion, preterm birth, and low birth weight. A large Swedish cohort study of births among 2500 women with IBD reported an increased risk of preterm birth for both UC (aOR 1.78; 95 % CI 1.49–2.13) and Crohn's disease (aOR 1.65; 95 % CI 1.3–2.06), and the risk was greater with increasing disease activity [15]. The risk of low birth weight was also increased in both UC and Crohn's disease. For women with disease flare, the risk of low birth weight was doubled in UC and tripled in Crohn's disease. Small for gestational age (SGA) infants, low Apgar score, and stillbirth were also more common in women with IBD, and risk was greater with increased disease activity.

Given this data, women and their physicians should have a treatment plan in place before, during, and after pregnancy in order to improve compliance and outcomes [2]. The greatest risk of flare occurs when women discontinue medications [16]. Preconception counseling and education regarding the low risk of most medications used to treat IBD and the high risk of significant flare during pregnancy is important in improving compliance and relieving anxiety during pregnancy. Preconception counseling should also include a discussion of appropriate and effective contraceptive use. Women with IBD use contraception at a lower rate than the general population, and a quarter of women with IBD at risk for unintended pregnancy do not use contraception [17].

Pregnancy

Pregnant women with IBD have the same risk of flare as non-pregnant IBD patients, but disease activity at time of conception affects the risk of flare during pregnancy [18]. Among women with active UC at the time of conception, 45 % will have worsening flare during pregnancy, 24 % will have stable active disease, and 25 % will improve [19]. Among women with active Crohn's disease at the time of conception, one third will have worsening flare, one third will have stable active disease, and one third will achieve remission. Risk of flare is not increased in the postpartum period, except if medication is discontinued [16]. The Pregnancy in Inflammatory Bowel Disease and Neonatal Outcomes (PIANO) registry is an ongoing multicenter national prospective study of pregnancy and neonatal outcomes in women with IBD and their offspring in the United States. The registry records mother's medication exposure, IBD history and disease activity, and pregnancy and postpartum complications. The PIANO registry and the European Crohn-Colitis Organization (ECCO) Study Group of Epidemiology Committee (EpiCom) study found a significantly higher rate of disease activity among women with UC compared with Crohn's disease [20, 21]. This difference may be related to secretion by the placenta of pro-inflammatory cytokines associated with UC or under treatment of UC patients during pregnancy [22].

Pregnant women with IBD are at increased risk of complications, including miscarriage, preterm birth, SGA infants, and complications of labor and delivery compared to age match controls [23]. A 2007 cohort study in Northern California found increased rates of spontaneous abortion and pregnancy complications, including eclampsia/preeclampsia, placental abruption, fetal distress, placenta previa, and prolonged/premature rupture of membranes compared to healthy age-matched controls regardless of disease activity, though the majority of patients had mild to inactive disease [24]. In contrast, a prospective study by ECCO found no significant difference in frequency of preterm birth, cesarean section, birth weight, or abortions among women with IBD compared to age-matched controls [25]. However, 87 % of IBD patients in this study were in remission at conception and 86 % maintained quiescent disease throughout pregnancy. Additionally, inadequate weight gain during pregnancy is associated with adverse pregnancy outcomes including preterm birth, SGA infants and fetal growth restriction, and disease activity correlates with reduced weight gain [26]. Therefore, pregnant women with IBD should be followed by maternal fetal medicine specialists or obstetricians experienced with complicated pregnancies.

If a woman develops a disease flare during pregnancy, the evaluation and management are similar to nonpregnant patients except for a few important considerations unique to pregnancy. Laboratory testing may be difficult to interpret, as low albumin and hemoglobin, and elevated erythrocyte sedimentation rate and alkaline phosphatase are common in pregnancy. Women with IBD in the peripartum period are at increased risk of clostridium difficile infection, and stool studies should be obtained to rule out infection in patients with diarrhea [27]. If imaging is required, magnetic resonance imaging is preferable to computerized tomography scan to avoid radiation exposure to the fetus. Gadolinium should be avoided in the first trimester due to potential teratogenicity [28]. Endoscopic evaluation can be performed safely with an unsedated flexible sigmoidoscopy. If a full colonoscopy is required, it should be performed with anesthesia and fetal monitoring when appropriate. The indications for surgery in a pregnant patient are the same as in the nonpregnant patient and include severe bleeding, medically refractory disease, perforation, or obstruction. Non-emergent but necessary operations should ideally be performed during the second trimester [29].

Delivery

Large population-based studies have shown that women with IBD have a 1.5–2 times the rate of cesarean delivery. In the PIANO registry, 44 % of women had a cesarean section, mainly for elective reasons [30]. The greater frequency of cesarean delivery is likely due to the concern of patients and providers for complications such as anal sphincter damage, worsening perianal disease, or pouch dysfunction in patients with IPAA [31, 32]. However, large studies have shown that vaginal delivery with inactive perianal disease does not lead to worsening disease [33]. Two recent studies found no increased risk in symptomatic perianal flares in women with perianal Crohn's disease who delivered vaginally or by cesarean section [34, 35]. Mode of delivery also did not influence the natural history of IBD. However, patients with *active* perianal disease at the time of delivery should have a cesarean section to avoid trauma that may exacerbate the disease. Some surgeons recommend cesarean section for women with an IPAA in order to avoid anal sphincter damage and preserve continence. However, vaginal delivery does not appear to significantly alter pouch function [36]. An ileostomy should not be oversewn during a cesarean section. Most women can be safely considered for a vaginal delivery. However, cesarean section should not be unnecessarily delayed if labor is prolonged, as uncontrolled tears and forceps delivery can affect pelvic floor function and substantially impact future bowel habits [37]. In general, decision regarding mode of delivery should be based on obstetric indications, and made on an individual basis with discussion of the risks and benefits.

Medication Use in Pregnancy and Lactation

Women who have a medication plan before conception are more likely to adhere to recommended therapies [16]. Discontinuation of medications can lead to active disease flare, which is a greater risk to the pregnancy than any

Table 57.2 Medications for inflammatory bowel disease

Medication	Considerations for pregnancy	Considerations for breastfeeding
Low risk		
Amoxicillin/Clavulanic acid	Low risk	Compatible
Aminosalicylates	Low risk	Compatible
Balsalazide	Low risk	Compatible; enters breast milk
Olsalazine	Low risk	Compatible; enters breast milk
Low risk with special consideration		
Budesonide	Low risk, limited human data	Compatible; enters breast milk
Asacol HD®	DBP coating associated with teratogenicity in animal studies	Probably compatible; enters breast milk
Thiopurines (Azathioprine/6 mercaptopurine)	Low risk; possible increased risk of infant infections as combination therapy	Compatible; wait 4 h after dose if possible
Infliximab	Low risk	Compatible; detected in breast milk
Adalimumab	Low risk	Compatible; detected in breast milk
Certolizumab	Low risk	Compatible; detected in breast milk
Golimumab	Low risk; limited human data	Likely compatible; limited human data
Natalizumab	Low risk; limited human data	Likely compatible; limited human data
Vedolizumab	Likely low risk; limited human data	Likely compatible; no human data
Ustekinumab	Likely low risk; limited human data	Likely compatible; limited human data
Moderate risk		
Ciprofloxacin	Possible musculoskeletal dysfunction; Caution advised	Compatible
Metronidazole	Avoid in first trimester; possible increased risk of cleft lip/palate	Avoid; may cause toxicity; enters breast milk
Prednisone	Possible risk of cleft palate with first trimester exposure; risk of adrenal insufficiency, premature rupture of membranes, gestational diabetes	Compatible; enters breast milk
Contraindicated: High risk		
Methotrexate	Contraindicated; teratogenic	Contraindicated

potential adverse medication effects. In general, most medications used to treat IBD, with the exception of methotrexate, are considered low risk and can be continued during pregnancy and breastfeeding. In 2015, the Federal Drug Administration (FDA) implemented a new rule that removed the previously used pregnancy risk categories A, B, C, D, and X from human prescription drug labeling. New labeling will require a summary of the risks of using a drug during pregnancy and lactation, a discussion of the data supporting that summary, and relevant information to help healthcare providers make prescribing decisions and counsel women about the use of drugs during pregnancy and lactation [38]. Here we will briefly discuss pregnancy specific concerns with common IBD medications (Table 57.2).

Methotrexate

Methotrexate (MTX) is an abortifacient and is contraindicated during conception and pregnancy. When taken during organogenesis, it can cause congenital anomalies [39]. Pregnancy should be avoided if either the woman or her partner is receiving MTX. Because it is a folate antagonist, MTX should always be taken with folic acid supplementation. MTX should be discontinued for a minimum of 3 months for males and for at least 3–6 months for females prior to conception. MTX is excreted in breast milk and can accumulate in neonatal tissue and interfere with cellular metabolism. It is contraindicated in breastfeeding [40].

Antibiotics

Ciprofloxacin and metronidazole are the two antibiotics used most commonly in management of IBD. A prospective study of women exposed to fluoroquinolones during pregnancy showed a low risk of clinically significant major musculoskeletal abnormalities or birth defects [41]. However, it has a high affinity for cartilage and has been associated with arthropathy in animals and human case reports. Ciprofloxacin is excreted in breast milk, but the American Academy of Pediatrics considers it compatible with breastfeeding.

A case–control study of 17,300 women exposed to metronidazole showed that exposure during the first trimester was associated with a small increased incidence of cleft lip and palate [42]. Animal studies have also shown teratogenicity.

Therefore, metronidazole should be avoided in the first trimester. It is excreted in breast milk and is not recommended in breastfeeding due to potential toxicity.

Amoxicillin-clavulanic acid is the preferred antibiotic during pregnancy. A population-based case–control study of exposure to amoxicillin-clavulanic acid during pregnancy did not find an increased risk of congenital malformations, and it is compatible with breastfeeding [43].

Corticosteroids

Prednisone and budesonide may be used in pregnancy when needed to treat disease flares. One study reported a small increased risk of orofacial clefts in infants exposed to corticosteroids in the month before conception and in the first trimester (OR 3.35; 95% CI: 1.97–5.69) [44]. However, this finding has not been replicated in all studies and the overall risk of major malformations is low (OR 1.45; 95% CI: 0.80–2.60). In the PIANO registry, after controlling for disease activity and concurrent immunosuppressive medications, maternal corticosteroid use was associated with a significant increase in low birth weight and gestational diabetes and a nonsignificant increase in preterm birth and infant infections within the first 4 months of life [45]. A small case series showed no increase in rates of adverse pregnancy outcomes or congenital anomalies with budesonide [46]. Thus, steroids should be used minimally in the first trimester and at the lowest effective dose for as short a duration as possible during pregnancy. However, controlling disease activity and treating a flare are essential, and steroids cannot always be avoided. Prednisolone is the metabolite of prednisone and is minimally excreted in breast milk. Both prednisone and budesonide are compatible with breastfeeding [47].

Aminosalicylates

Aminosalicylates (5-ASAs) are commonly used in treatment of IBD and come in multiple formulations. Sulfasalazine, the original formulation that combines sulfapyridine and salicylate, should be given with at least 2 mg of folic acid during pregnancy due to anti-folate effects. Asacol HD® contains dibutylphthalate, a chemical that has been associated with congenital abnormalities in animal studies [48]. These animal studies used doses greater than 190 times what is used in IBD patients and showed skeletal malformations and adverse effects on the male reproductive system. Human studies with Asacol HD® have not demonstrated an increased risk of birth defects. Sulfasalazine and 5-ASAs are compatible with lactation. Two case reports described reversible diarrhea with aminosalicylate use during breastfeeding [49, 50]. While patients should be aware of this rare complication, they may breastfeed unless the infant gets diarrhea.

Thiopurines

Thiopurine immunomodulators, 6-mercaptopurine (6-MP), and the prodrug azathioprine (AZA) show evidence of teratogenicity in animal studies. However, no replicable pattern of birth defects has been seen in humans. In vivo studies have shown that 6-MP does not cross the placenta, but one of its metabolites, 6-thioguanine, has been detected in the blood of infants born to mothers on AZA or 6-MP [51]. Studies of pregnancy outcomes among women exposed to 6-MP or AZA have had inconsistent results. One study of women exposed to AZA early in pregnancy showed a trend toward increased congenital anomalies (OR 1.41; 95% CI: 0.98–2.04) and an increased risk of ventricular and atrial septal defects (OR 3.18; 95% CI: 1.45–6.04) [52]. The exposed women also had increased rates of preterm delivery, low birth weight, and SGA infants; however, these findings are likely due to greater disease severity in the women on AZA. On the other hand, several more recent studies have shown no increased risk of birth defects among infants born to women on 6-MP/AZA. In the PIANO registry, nearly 300 infants born to mothers on AZA have not had an increased rate of congenital malformations [20]. A retrospective multicenter study also did not show an association between thiopurine exposure and perinatal complications [53]. A meta-analysis suggested a relationship between thiopurine exposure and preterm birth, but increased congenital anomalies were not seen [54]. Finally, another small study showed that children of mothers on AZA/6MP had no differences in health status or rates of infections compared to age-matched controls [55]. AZA/6-MP should not be started for the first time during pregnancy because of the time required for response and the small risks of pancreatitis or bone marrow suppression. Finally, AZA/6-MP are excreted at low levels in breast milk, and the greatest levels are seen within four hours of drug ingestion [56]. Both are considered compatible with breastfeeding, but mothers may be advised to wait 4 h after taking the medication before breastfeeding. If this is not possible with a newborn infant, mothers may still breastfeed, as breast milk transfer is very low.

Anti–Tumor Necrosis Factor (TNF) Alpha Agents

Infliximab (IFX), adalimumab (ADA), certolizumab pegol (CZP), and golimumab (GOL) are anti–tumor necrosis factor alpha antagonists used for treatment of IBD. IFX and ADA are immune globulin (Ig) G1 antibodies that are actively transported across the placenta by the FcRn receptor on the placenta. The majority of transfer occurs in the third trimester, but it may begin as early as the beginning of the second trimester [57]. IFX and ADA are detected in infant serum for up to 6 months from birth [58]. Mean infant and cord blood levels at birth are more than 160 % of the mother's serum level at that time. CZP is a pegylated Fab' fragment that is not actively transported across the placenta and is detected in minimal concentrations in infant serum or cord blood. GOL concentrations in infants and mothers at birth have not been reported, but are expected to be similar to IFX and ADA, as it is also an IgG1 antibody.

Numerous case reports, case series, and meta-analyses of pregnancy outcomes with use of anti-TNF agents have been published to date and have not demonstrated an increased incidence of birth defects or adverse pregnancy outcomes. The PIANO registry has reported on 392 women on a biological agent during pregnancy, and 107 women on combination therapy through 2013 [59]. There has been no increase in rates of birth defects, infant growth and development, or achievement of developmental milestones. However, infants born to women on combination therapy did have an increased risk of infection at 12 months of age (RR 1.50 (1.08–2.09)). Since levels of anti-TNF agents are undetectable at that age, concerns remain regarding effects on infant immune development with early exposure. In addition, women with UC on combination therapy had higher rates of preterm birth, low birth weight infant, neonatal intensive care unit stay, and any complication compared to women who were not taking either a biologic agent or an immunomodulator. Based on these data, AZA/6-MP can be continued during pregnancy. However, for a patient with stable disease on combination therapy, a gastroenterologist may carefully consider stopping AZA/6-MP when the immunomodulator is being used purely for purposes of immunogenicity.

Because of infant drug exposure and concern for immune development and infectious risks, the optimal timing of anti-TNF dosing during pregnancy, and if and when to stop it in order to minimize infant exposure have been debated. The potential risks of drug transfer and infant exposure must be weighed against the risk to the mother of stopping the medication, including severe disease flare that may lead to preterm birth and immunization of the mother to the drug so that she cannot use it effectively after delivery.

CZP has minimal placental transfer and can be continued through pregnancy with no adjustment in dose or timing. For patients in remission on IFX, ADA, or GOL, because of the high rate of placental transfer in the third trimester, we may adjust the timing of doses to allow the maximum amount of time between drug dosing and delivery. For IFX, we give the last dose at week 30–32 of gestation. For ADA, we give the last injection at week 36–38; and for GOL, we give the last injection at week 34–36 of gestation. The next infusion or injection is given right after delivery, and can be given 24 h after a vaginal delivery and 48 h after a cesarean delivery, assuming there is no infection or complication.

In utero anti-TNF drug exposure late in pregnancy has raised concerns regarding development of the infant immune system and immunosuppression, and rare cases have been reported of serious infections in infants after birth [60]. One case reported the death of an infant exposed to IFX who developed disseminated bacille Calmette-Guérin (BCG) after administration of the live BCG vaccine [61]. However, Bortlik et al reported 15 children exposed to anti-TNF in utero who had no serious complications after BCG vaccination within 1 week of birth [62]. Immunological development was also evaluated, and 17 children tested had normal cellular immunity. All children had detectable serologic response to vaccinations. This limited data suggests the relative safety of vaccinations in infants exposed to biologics. However, it is still recommended that infants exposed to anti-TNF agents (except CZP) not receive any live vaccinations in the first 6 months of life unless biologic levels are undetectable. All other vaccinations should be given on schedule. This discussion should be part of pre-conception counseling and the information communicated to the pediatrician.

Anti-TNF agents have been detected in breast milk in minute amounts and at significantly lower concentrations than is detected in serum. The PIANO registry reported results of 57 women who submitted breast milk samples at 1, 12, 24, and 48, 72, 96, 120, and 168 h after biologic drug administration (27 infliximab, 15 adalimumab, 10 certolizumab pegol, 1 golimumab) [63]. Maximum IFX concentration (90–591 ng/mL) was detected between 24–48 h after infusion. ADA was detected in 2 of 15 and CZP was detected in 3 of 10 samples. Maximum concentration for both was seen 12–24 h after dosing. GOL was not detected in the one sample reported. In the PIANO registry, rates of growth and milestone achievement and risk of infection were similar in breastfed infants of mothers on biologics compared to breastfed infants of mothers not on biologics. Therefore, these agents are considered compatible with breastfeeding.

Natalizumab, Vedolizumab, Ustekinumab

Natalizumab has been used for many years in the treatment of multiple sclerosis, and most information regarding pregnancy outcomes is derived from those patients. Available data from the Tysabri Pregnancy Exposure Registry of 362 pregnancy outcomes, mostly in women with multiple sclerosis, did not suggest any detrimental effect of natalizumab exposure [64]. A recent prospective controlled observational study of 101 women with multiple sclerosis exposed to natalizumab in the first trimester also did not show an increased risk of adverse pregnancy outcomes [65]. Natalizumab was not detected in breast milk from one woman in the PIANO registry [63].

Since vedolizumab is an IgG1 antibody, the amount of transfer is expected to be similar to other IgG1 monoclonal antibodies with the greatest transfer in the third trimester. Published human safety data during pregnancy is limited.

Women in the vedolizumab clinical development program who became pregnant were discontinued from the study. However, among 24 vedolizumab-treated women, there were 12 live births, five elective terminations, and four spontaneous abortions [66]. Women are currently being enrolled in the PIANO registry and will provide additional long-term safety data of vedolizumab exposure in pregnancy. The half-life of vedolizumab is 25 days, compared to 7 for infliximab. This may have implications for dosing during pregnancy in the future; however, further data are needed.

Finally, little data exists regarding the use of ustekinumab during pregnancy. One case reported an uncomplicated pregnancy and another publication reported spontaneous abortion in two women exposed to ustekinumab [67, 68]. Another report of 26 completed pregnancies showed no increased risk of spontaneous abortion compared to the general population among women exposed to ustekinumab [69]. Three women in the PIANO registry have provided breast milk samples, and UST was detected in one [63].

Conclusion

Women with IBD require a multidisciplinary approach in order to maximize their chances of a successful, healthy pregnancy. Those who have not had pelvic surgery and do not have active disease have similar rates of fertility as women without IBD. However, once pregnant, women with IBD are at increased risk of adverse pregnancy outcomes, even with inactive disease, and should be managed as high-risk obstetric patients. Disease activity and inadequate gestational weight gain are associated with adverse pregnancy outcomes. Thus, women should aim to maintain stable or quiescent disease during pregnancy in order to minimize the risk of miscarriage and preterm birth. Preconception counseling including a discussion of fertility and medication use is essential. Women should have a therapy plan in place prior to conception, and they should be aware of the risks of discontinuing effective medications leading to disease flare. A treatment plan established prior to conception can reduce the chance of discontinuation of effective medications and lead to more successful outcomes. A multidisciplinary team including the obstetrician, maternal–fetal medicine specialist, gastroenterologist, and pediatrician is essential to ensure a healthy pregnancy, healthy mother, and healthy baby with appropriate therapy and precautions during pregnancy and lactation.

References

1. Loftus EV, Shivashankar R, Tremaine WJ, Harmsen WS, Zinsmeiseter AR. Updated incidence and prevalence of Crohn's disease and ulcerative colitis in Olmsted County, Minnesota (1970–2011). Presented at ACG 2014 annual scientific meeting, October 2014.
2. De Lima A, Zelnikova Z, van der Ent C, van der Woude C. Preconception care in IBD women leads to less disease relapses during pregnancy [abstract]. Gastroenterology. 2014;146(Suppl):S-444.
3. Selinger CP, Eaden J, Selby W, Jones DB, Katelaris P, Chapman G, et al. Inflammatory bowel disease and pregnancy: lack of knowledge is associated with negative views. J Crohns Colitis. 2013;7:e206–13.
4. Olsen KO, Juul S, Berndtsson I, Oresland T, Laurberg S. Ulcerative colitis: female fecundity before diagnosis, during disease, and after surgery compared with a population sample. Gastroenterology. 2002;122:15–9.
5. Bajocco PJ, Korelitz BJ. The influence of inflammatory bowel disease and its treatment on pregnancy and fetal outcome. J Clin Gastroenterol. 1984;6:211–6.
6. Fielding JF, Cooke WT. Pregnancy and Crohn's disease. BMJ. 1970;2:76–7.
7. Timmer A, Bauer A, Dignass A, Rogler G. Sexual function in persons with inflammatory bowel disease: a survey with matched controls. Clin Gastroenterol Hepatol. 2007;5:87–94.
8. Şenateş E, Çolak Y, Erdem ED, Yeşil A, Coşkunpınar E, Şahin Ö, et al. Serum anti-Mullerian hormone levels are lower in reproductive age women with Crohn's disease compared to healthy control women. J Crohns Colitis. 2013;7:e29–34.
9. Waljee A, Waljee J, Morris AM, Higgins PDR. Threefold increased risk of infertility: a meta-analysis of infertility after ileal pouch anal anastomosis in ulcerative colitis. Gut. 2006;55:1575–80.
10. Rajaratnam SG, Eglinton TW, Hider P, Fearnhead NS. Impact of ileal pouch-anal anastomosis on female fertility: meta-analysis and systematic review. Int J Colorectal Dis. 2011;26:1365–74.
11. Mortier PE, Gambiez L, Karoui M, Cortot A, Paris JC, Quandalle P, et al. Colectomy with ileorectal anastomosis preserves female fertility in ulcerative colitis. Gastroenterol Clin Biol. 2006;30: 594–7.
12. Moscandrew M, Mahadevan U, Kane S. General health maintenance in IBD. Inflamm Bowel Dis. 2009;15:1399–409.
13. Paffoni A, Ferrari S, Viganò P, Pagliardini L, Papaleo E, Candiani M, et al. Vitamin D deficiency and infertility: insights from in vitro fertilization cycles. J Clin Endocrinol Metab. 2014;99:E2372–6.
14. Choi JM, Lebwohl B, Wang J, Lee SK, Murray JA, Sauer MV, et al. Increased prevalence of celiac disease in patients with unexplained infertility in the United States. J Reprod Med. 2011;56:199–203.
15. Broms G, Granath F, Linder M, Stephansson O, Elmberg M, Kieler H. Birth outcomes in women with inflammatory bowel disease: effects of disease activity and drug exposure. Inflamm Bowel Dis. 2014;20:1091–8.
16. Julsgaard M, Norgaard M, Hvas CL, Grosen A, Hasseriis S, Christensen LA. Self-reported adherence to medical treatment, breast feeding behavior, and disease activity during the postpartum period in women with Crohn's disease. Scand J Gastroenterol. 2014;49:958–66.
17. Gawron LM, Gawron AJ, Kasper A, Hammond C, Keefer L. Contraception method selection by women with inflammatory bowel diseases: a cross-sectional survey. Contraception. 2014;89:419–25.
18. Nielsen OH, Andreasson B, Bondesen S, Jarnum S. Pregnancy in ulcerative colitis. Scand J Gastroenterol. 1983;18:735–42.
19. Miller JP. Inflammatory bowel disease in pregnancy: a review. J R Soc Med. 1986;79:221–5.
20. Mahadevan U, Martin CF, Sandler RS, Kane S, Dubinsky M, Lewis JD, et al. PIANO: A 1000 patient prospective registry of pregnancy outcomes in women with IBD Exposed to immunomodulators and biologic therapy [abstract]. Gastroenterology. 2012;142(Suppl):S-149.
21. Pedersen N, Bortoli A, Duricova D, D'Inca R, Panelli MR, Gisbert JP, et al. The course of inflammatory bowel disease during pregnancy and postpartum: a prospective European ECCO-EpiCom Study of 209 pregnant women. Aliment Pharmacol Ther. 2013;38:501–12.
22. Nasef NA, Ferguson LR. Inflammatory bowel disease and pregnancy: overlapping pathways. Transl Res. 2012;160:65–83.

23. Molnár T, Farkas K, Nagy F, Lakatos PL, Miheller P, Nyari T, et al. Pregnancy outcome in patients with inflammatory bowel disease according to the activity of the disease and the medical treatment: a case–control study. Scand J Gastroenterol. 2010; 45:1302–6.
24. Mahadevan U, Sandborn WJ, Li DK, Hakimian S, Kane S, Corley DA. Pregnancy outcomes in women with inflammatory bowel disease: a large community-based study from Northern California. Gastroenterology. 2007;133:1106–12.
25. Bortoli A, Pedersen N, Duricova D, D'Inca R, Gionchetti P, Panelli MR, et al. Pregnancy outcome in inflammatory bowel disease: prospective European case–control ECCO-EpiCom study, 2003–2006. Aliment Pharmacol Ther. 2011;34:724–34.
26. Oron G, Yogev Y, Shcolnick S, Hod M, Fraser G, Wiznitzer A, et al. Inflammatory bowel disease: risk factors for adverse pregnancy outcome and the impact of maternal weight gain. J Matern Fetal Neonatal Med. 2012;25:2256–60.
27. Unger JA, Whimbey E, Gravett MG, Eschenbach DA. The emergence of Clostridium difficile infection among peripartum women: a case–control study of a C. difficile outbreak on an obstetrical service. Infect Dis Obstet Gynecol. 2011. doi:10.1155/2011/267249.
28. Okuda Y, Sagami F, Tirone P, Morisetti A, Bussi S, Masters RE. Reproductive and developmental toxicity study of gadobenate dimeglumine formulation (E7155) (3): study of embryo-fetal toxicity in rabbits by intravenous administration. J Toxicol Sci. 1999;24(Suppl):79–87.
29. ACOG Committee on Obstetric Practice. ACOG Committee Opinion No. 474: nonobstetric surgery during pregnancy. Obstet Gynecol. 2011;117:420–1.
30. Mahadevan U, Martin C, Dubinsky M, Kane S, Sands B, Sandborn W. Exposure to anti-TNFα therapy in the third trimester of pregnancy is not associated with increased adverse outcomes: results from the PIANO Registry [abstract]. Gastroenterology. 2014;146(Suppl):S-170.
31. Cornish J, Tan E, Teare J, Teoh TG, Rai R, Clark SK, et al. A meta analysis on the influence of inflammatory bowel disease on pregnancy. Gut. 2007;56(6):830–7.
32. Nguyen GC, Boudreau H, Harris ML, Maxwell CV. Outcomes of obstetric hospitalizations among women with inflammatory bowel disease in the United States. Clin Gastroenterol Hepatol. 2009;7: 329–34.
33. Ilnyckyj A, Blanchard JF, Rawsthorne P, Bernstein CN. Perianal Crohn's disease: role of mode of delivery. Am J Gastroenterol. 1999;94:3274–8.
34. Cheng AG, Oxford EC, Sauk J, Nguyen JJ, Yajnik V, Freidman S, et al. Impact of mode of delivery on outcomes in patients with perianal Crohn's disease. Inflamm Bowel Dis. 2014;20:1391–8.
35. Ananthakrishnan A, Cheng A, Cagan A, Cai T, Gainer VS, Shaw SY, et al. Mode of childbirth and long-term outcomes in women with inflammatory bowel disease. Dig Dis Sci. 2015;60:471–7.
36. Ravid A, Richard C, Spencer L, O'Connor BI, Kennedy ED, MacRae HM, et al. Pregnancy, delivery, and pouch function after ileal pouch-anal anastomosis for ulcerative colitis. Dis Colon Rectum. 2002;45:1283–8.
37. Handa VL, Blomquist JL, McDermott KC, Friedman S, Munoz A. Pelvic floor disorders after vaginal birth: effect of episiotomy, perineal laceration, and operative birth. Obstet Gynecol. 2012;119:233–9.
38. Food and Drug Administration. Pregnancy and lactation labeling final rule. http://federalregister.gov/a/2014-28241. Accessed 22 Feb 2015.
39. Food and Drug Administration Access Data. Methotrexate injection, USP. Lake Forest, IL: Hospira Inc. Oct 2011. http://www.accessdata.fda.gov/drugsatfda_docs/label/2011/011719s117lbl.pdf. Accessed 22 Feb 2015.
40. Johns DG, Rutherford LD, Leighton PC, Vogel CL. Secretion of methotrexate into human milk. Am J Obstet Gynecol. 1972;112:978–80.
41. Loebstein R, Addis A, Ho E, Andreou R, Sage S, Donnenfeld AE, et al. Pregnancy outcome following gestational exposure to fluoroquinolones: a multicenter prospective controlled study. Antimicrob Agents Chemother. 1998;42:1336–9.
42. Czeizel AE, Rockenbauer M. A population based case–control teratologic study of oral metronidazole treatment during pregnancy. Br J Obstet Gynaecol. 1998;105:322–7.
43. Czeizel AE, Rockenbauer M, Sorensen HT, Olsen J. Augmentin treatment during pregnancy and the prevalence of congenital abnormalities: a population-based case–control teratologic study. Eur J Obstet Gynecol Reprod Biol. 2001;97:188–92.
44. Park-Wyllie L, Mazzotta P, Pastuszak A, Moretti ME, Beique L, Hunnisett L, et al. Birth defects after maternal exposure to corticosteroids: prospective cohort study and meta-analysis of epidemiological studies. Teratology. 2000;62:385–92.
45. Lin K, Martin C, Dassopoulos T, Esposti SD, Wolf D, Beaulieu D, et al. Pregnancy outcomes amongst mothers with inflammatory bowel disease exposed to systemic corticosteroids: results from the PIANO registry [abstract]. Gastroenterology. 2014;146(Suppl):S-1.
46. Beaulieu DB, Ananthakrishnan AN, Issa M, Rosenbaum L, Skaros S, Newcomer JR, et al. Budesonide induction and maintenance therapy for Crohn's disease during pregnancy. Inflamm Bowel Dis. 2009;15:25–8.
47. Greenberger PA, Odeh YK, Frederiksen MC, Atkinson Jr AJ. Pharmacokinetics of prednisolone transfer to breast milk. Clin Pharmacol Ther. 1993;53:324–8.
48. Gallinger ZR, Nguyen GC. Presence of phthalates in gastrointestinal medications: is there a hidden danger? World J Gastroenterol. 2013;19:7042–7.
49. Branski D, Kerem E, Gross-Kieselstein E, Hurvitz H, Litt R, Abrahamov A. Bloody diarrhea—a possible complication of sulfasalazine transferred through human breast milk. J Pediatr Gastroenterol Nutr. 1986;5:316–7.
50. Nelis GF. Diarrhoea due to 5-aminosalicylic acid in breast milk. Lancet. 1989;1:383.
51. de Boer NK, Jarbandhan SV, de Graaf P, Mulder CJ, van Elburg RM, et al. Azathioprine use during pregnancy: unexpected intrauterine exposure to metabolites. Am J Gastroenterol. 2006;101: 1390–2.
52. Cleary BJ, Källén B. Early pregnancy azathioprine use and pregnancy outcomes. Birth Defects Res A Clin Mol Teratol. 2009;85:647–54.
53. Casanova MJ, Chaparro M, Domenech E, Barreiro-de Acosta M, Bermejo F, Iglesias E, et al. Safety of thiopurines and anti-TNF-alpha drugs during pregnancy in patients with inflammatory bowel disease. Am J Gastroenterol. 2013;108:433–40.
54. Akbari M, Shah S, Velayos FS, Mahadevan U, Cheifetz AS. Systematic review and meta-analysis on the effects of thiopurines on birth outcomes from female and male patients with inflammatory bowel disease. Inflamm Bowel Dis. 2013;19:15–22.
55. de Meij TG, Jharap B, Kneepkens CM, van Bodegraven AA, de Boer NK; Dutch Initiative on Crohn and Colitis. Long-term follow-up of children exposed intrauterine to maternal thiopurine therapy during pregnancy in females with inflammatory bowel disease. Aliment Pharmacol Ther. 2013;38:38–43.
56. Christensen LA, Dahlerup JF, Nielsen MJ, Fallingborg JF, Schmiegelow K. Azathioprine treatment during lactation. Aliment Pharmacol Ther. 2008;28:1209–13.
57. Gisbert JP, Chaparro M. Safety of anti-TNF agents during pregnancy and breastfeeding in women with inflammatory bowel disease. Am J Gastroenterol. 2013;108:1426–38.
58. Mahadevan U, Wolf DC, Dubinsky M, Cortot A, Lee SD, Siegel CA, et al. Placental transfer of anti-tumor necrosis factor agents in

pregnant patients with inflammatory bowel disease. Clin Gastroenterol Hepatol. 2013;11:286–92.

59. Mahadevan U, Martin C, Chambers C, Kane S, Dubinsky M, Sandborn W, et al. Achievement of developmental milestones among offspring of women with inflammatory bowel disease: the PIANO registry [abstract]. Gastroenterology. 2014;146 (Suppl):S-1.
60. Johnsson A, Avlund S, Grosen A, Julsgaard M. Chicken pox infection in a three months old infant exposed in utero to Adalimumab. J Crohns Colitis. 2013;7:e116–7.
61. Cheent K, Nolan J, Shariq S, Kiho L, Pal A, Arnold J. Case report: disseminated BCG infection in an infant born to a mother taking infliximab for Crohn's disease. J Crohns Colitis. 2010;4: 603–5.
62. Bortlik M, Duricova D, Machkova N, Kozeluhova J, Kohout P, Hrdlicka L, et al. Impact of anti-tumor necrosis factor alpha antibodies administered to pregnant women with inflammatory bowel disease on long-term outcome of exposed children. Inflamm Bowel Dis. 2014;20:495–501.
63. Matro R, Martin CF, Wolf D, Samir SA, Mahadevan U. Detection of biologic agents in breast milk and implication for infection, growth and development in infants born to women with inflammatory bowel disease: results from the PIANO Registry [abstract]. Gastroenterology. 2015;148(Suppl):S-141.
64. Cristiano L, Friend S, Bozic C, Bloomren G. Evaluation of pregnancy outcomes from the Tysabri (natalizumab) Pregnancy Exposure Registry [abstract]. Neurology. 2013;80:P02.127.
65. Ebrahimi N, Herbstritt S, Gold R, Amezcua L, Koren G, Hellwigh K. Pregnancy and fetal outcomes following natalziumab exposure in pregnancy: a prospective, controlled observational study. Mult Scler. 2015;21:198–205.
66. Mahadevan U, Dubinsky M, Vermeire S, Abhyandkar B, Lasch K. Vedolizumab exposure in pregnancy: Outcomes from clinical studies in inflammatory bowel disease [abstract]. J Crohns Colitis. 2015;9(Suppl):S-361–2.
67. Andrulonis R, Ferris LK. Treatment of severe psoriasis with ustekinumab during pregnancy. J Drugs Dermatol. 2012;11:1240–1.
68. Fotiadou C, Lazaridou E, Sotiriou E, Ioannides D. Spontaneous abortion during ustekinumab therapy. J Dermatol Case Rep. 2012;6:105–7.
69. Schaufelberg BW, Horn E, Cather JC, Rahawi K. Pregnancy outcomes in women exposed to ustekinumab in the Psoriasis Clinical Development Program [abstract]. J Am Acad Dermatol. 2014;70:AB178.

Pediatric Aspects of Inflammatory Bowel Disease

58

Brendan Boyle and Jeffrey S. Hyams

Introduction

A significant percentage of newly diagnosed individuals with inflammatory bowel disease (IBD) fall within the pediatric age range (≤16 years old). These patients often present a set of issues that differ from adults with IBD and require a good understanding of how the effects of disease and therapy on growth and development must influence care. This chapter will highlight important differences between pediatric and adult IBD. A description of risks and benefits of available therapies will also be reviewed, especially with regard to risks of toxicity with thiopurines as monotherapy or in combination with anti-TNF given the association with lymphoma and HSTCL in younger patients with IBD.

Pediatric Aspects of IBD

Demographics

The Pediatric Inflammatory Bowel Disease Collaborative Research Group Registry, a natural history study started in 2002 enrolled 1928 subjects diagnosed with IBD before their 16th birthday. The age distribution of the cohort at diagnosis was 6 % <5 years, 28 % from 5–9 years, and 66 % from 10–16 years with a slight predominance of males over females (57 % vs. 43 %) [1]. In a population-based state-wide US epidemiologic study, the incidence of IBD in the pediatric population was 7.5 per 100,000 with that of Crohn's disease (4.6 per 100,000) being twice that of ulcerative colitis (2.1 per 100,000). Eighty-nine percent of new cases were nonfamilial [2].

Disease Location

The location or extent of disease differs according to age of disease onset in children newly diagnosed with Crohn's disease. Children under the age of 10 years, and in particular children under the age of 5 years, characteristically present with isolated colitis, whereas ileal disease (with or without accompanying colitis) begins to occur more often in children whose disease is diagnosed after the age of 9–10 years [3, 4]. Upper tract involvement (proximal to the ligament of Treitz) is present most commonly in those children with ileocolonic disease (up to 50–60 %), with esophageal involvement seen in 27 % (macroscopic in 18 %), and gastroduodenal involvement in 56 % (macroscopic 42 %). Isolated UGI involvement is rare [5]. Pediatric onset ulcerative colitis is characterized by extensive colitis or pancolitis in the majority of cases and isolated proctitis is less common than in adult populations [6, 7].

Serology

As in adults antibodies to a variety of microbial antigens have been found in children with Crohn's disease. However, in children there appears to be an age-related expression of these antibodies. In a cohort of 705 children from three prospectively characterized cohorts in North America, the rate of ASCA (both IgG and IgA) positivity was <20 % for children <7years of age compared to 40 % for those 8–15 years of age, likely representing the preponderance of isolated colonic disease in young children. Anti-CBIR1 was detected in 66 % and 54 %, respectively, from the two age groups [8].

B. Boyle, M.D., M.P.H.
Division of Pediatric Gastroenterology, Hepatology, and Nutrition, Nationwide Children's Hospital, The Ohio State University College of Medicine and Public Health, 700 Children's Drive, Columbus, OH 43205, USA
e-mail: brendan.boyle@nationwidechildrens.org

J.S. Hyams, M.D. (✉)
Division of Digestive Diseases, Hepatology, and Nutrition, Connecticut Children's Medical Center, 282 Washington Street, Hartford, CT 06106, USA

University of Connecticut School of Medicine, 282 Washington Street, Hartford, CT 06106, USA
e-mail: jhyams@connecticutchildrens.org

D.C. Baumgart (ed.), *Crohn's Disease and Ulcerative Colitis*, DOI 10.1007/978-3-319-33703-6_58

Clinical Behavior at Diagnosis

In French and North American population-based pediatric studies, disease behavior at diagnosis was inflammatory (B1) in 70–72 % and stricturing (B2) or penetrating (B3) in 22–30 % [9, 10]. A French population-based study of children with ulcerative colitis found 26 % had proctitis, 35 % left-sided disease, and 37 % extensive colitis at diagnosis [7]. This disease distribution is quite different than reported previously from North America where extensive disease at diagnosis has been observed in up to 80 % of children at presentation [2, 11]. More recent studies propose further subdividing children by age of diagnosis, with those diagnosed at age <10 years consider early onset IBD (EOIBD), and those diagnosed age <6 years as very early onset IBD (VEOIBD). Patients in the VEOIBD group are more likely to have monogenic IBD, with increased risk of primary immunodeficiency, autoimmune enteropathy, and primarily colonic disease distribution. These findings are distinct from patients diagnosed after age 7 years that more commonly have conventional, polygenic IBD [12–14]. The discovery of mutations in the genes coding for one of the two IL10 receptors causing loss of function in IL10 signaling has prompted increasing work looking for genetic polymorphisms that produce a severe IBD-like phenotype [15].

Measuring Disease Activity

While measuring the severity of gastrointestinal symptoms and laboratory abnormalities is similar in children and adults, the profound effect of IBD on linear growth is clearly a pediatric-only problem. Growth abnormalities are quite common in pediatric Crohn's disease and may be the major clinical manifestation. Thus, growth data have been incorporated into the most widely used instrument to measure disease activity in children with Crohn's disease, the Pediatric Crohn's Disease Activity Index (PCDAI) [16]. As measuring changes in growth velocity can only be done accurately over periods of 6 months or more, this has led to concerns that the PCDAI might not be sensitive enough to discern changes in clinical activity over the short-term (e.g., 3 months or less); however, this has not been borne out by additional studies [17]. The PCDAI can range in score from 0 to 100 with <10 denoting remission, 10–30 mild disease, and >30 moderate to severe disease. Given the limitations in calculating the complete PCDAI at each visit, more recently the weighted PCDAI (wPCDAI) has also been proposed as a more feasible instrument [18]. Additionally, the short PCDAI, a simplified disease assessment tool excluding need for laboratory and perianal assessment, has been developed and validated against the full and abbreviated PCDAI has been proposed to be utilized in observational and quality improvement research [19].

The Pediatric Ulcerative Colitis Activity Index (PUCAI) has been developed and validated to measure the activity of pediatric ulcerative colitis [20]. It ranges from 0 to 85 points with <10 signifying inactive disease, 10–34 mild disease, 35–64 moderate disease, and 65 or greater severe disease. Debate regarding how to most fully assess clinical remission in IBD exists. Variable definitions of remission in IBD including clinical, serologic, endoscopic, and histologic remission have been proposed and have resulted in the concept of "treat to target", with some centers suggesting histologic remission should be the ultimately therapeutic goal [21].

An expanding body of literature has evaluated the use of biomarkers including fecal calprotectin as an indirect assessment of luminal activity. Recent studies have found that many patients in clinical or even endoscopic remission continue to have histologically active disease. Fecal calprotectin was found to be significantly higher in those with active histologic disease compared to those with histologic healing (median 278 μg/g vs. 68 μg/g ($p=0.002$)), suggesting calprotectin may be a more reliable marker of histologic disease activity [22]. Additional studies have suggested cut off calprotectin values of approximately <200 μg/g correlate well with endoscopic and histologic healing. Use of the calprotectin therefore may reduce the need for repeat endoscopic evaluation [23]. Application of calprotectin as a reliable marker of remission in the pediatric population requires further investigation.

Growth

The effect of disease activity on linear growth is unique to pediatrics. It has been estimated that up to 88 % of children with Crohn's disease have abnormal growth velocity at the time of diagnosis while in pediatric ulcerative colitis this number is <10 % [24]. In our experience the numbers for patients with Crohn's disease are not quite so stark, but certainly still involves well over 30–40 % of newly diagnosed patients. Two excellent review articles on this topic have been published and should be consulted for further detail [25, 26].

Many mechanisms of disturbed growth have been suggested for pediatric IBD. Poor growth appears to relate to a combination of factors including chronic caloric deprivation largely secondary to poor intake [27]. However, the inflammatory process itself leads to the production of cytokines that result in IGF-1 dysregulation by decreasing responsiveness of the growth hormone receptor in the liver to growth hormone diminishing IGF-1 production. Moreover, there is a direct effect of the cytokines on growing bone [28] and decreasing responsiveness to testosterone [29]. Use of corticosteroids even in small daily doses of prednisone (5 mg/m^2) can also impair growth

[30, 31]. The crucial factor in the effect of corticosteroids on growth appears not to be the dose used short-term, but rather whether they are used long-term [32].

Diagnosis of Pediatric IBD

The diagnosis of IBD in children is usually straightforward and the techniques employed are similar to those used in adults including upper and lower endoscopy and small bowel assessment usually performed with radiographic imaging. Ionizing radiation exposure when imaging the small bowel is of special concern given its association with DNA damage. The potential increased likelihood of malignancy following recurrent exposure to ionizing radiation emphasizes the importance of minimizing radiation exposure in the pediatric population [33–35]. Magnetic resonance enterograpy (MRE) is replacing barium imaging and CT scans in many institutions. A 2013 systematic review of 11 studies evaluated the use of MRE to assess the small bowel in a total of 496 pediatric patients with CD. It was concluded that in centers with expertise in MRE, this is the preferred imaging technique over those involving radiation. Rates of detecting small bowel abnormalities were similar while minimizing radiation exposure [36].

Management of Pediatric IBD

There are few controlled trials of medications in the treatment of pediatric IBD; most experience is extrapolated from adult studies though several recent trials have demonstrated the efficacy of biologic therapies with anti-TNF in treating both pediatric CD and UC.

Aminosalicylates

Though data to support the use of aminosalicylates for the treatment of pediatric Crohn's disease or ulcerative colitis are scant, they are commonly used for both. Specific dosing guidelines for children have not been established and therefore in practice there is large variation. The most common dose used is 50 mg/kg/day of mesalamine though anecdotally some clinicians use up to 100 mg/kg/day (maximum 4 g). No pediatric-specific side effects have been identified.

Corticosteroids

Corticosteroids have been the historical mainstay of the treatment of moderate to severe Crohn's disease and ulcerative colitis though no placebo-controlled randomized trials have been published. Nonetheless the ability of corticosteroids to induce remission in most children has been well established [37, 38]. A natural history study of the effect of corticosteroids in pediatric Crohn's disease found that at 1 year, 61 % of patients were corticosteroid responsive, 31 % corticosteroid dependent, and 8 % had gone on to surgery [37]. A similar study published on the use of corticosteroids in newly diagnosed ulcerative colitis disease in children found that by 1 year 45 % of children were corticosteroid dependent and 5 % of the corticosteroid-treated patients had come to colectomy [38]. In both reports the use of immunomodulators (50–75 % of patients) and infliximab (17–25 %) was common in patients with corticosteroid dependence. Two studies have compared budesonide with prednisolone in the treatment of Crohn's disease in children and shown similar efficacy [39, 40], though bias in patient selection (i.e., milder patients) may have influenced the results. Pediatric-specific side effects of corticosteroids are common and effects on growth, bone metabolism, and the cosmetic issues such as Cushingoid appearance and acne are of particular concern.

Immunomodulators

Multiple publications have looked at the use of immunomodulators in the treatment of pediatric Crohn's disease though only one randomized placebo-controlled study has been performed [41]. In this study of 55 newly diagnosed children with moderate to severe CD who all received an initial course of prednisone and then either 6-mercaptopurine or placebo, initial remission rates at 3 months were similar, but by 1 year the 6-mercaptopurine-treated group had received significantly less corticosteroid and had a much lower relapse rate. Largely based on this study, thiopurines became standard of care in the treatment of moderate to severe CD in children and are customarily introduced quite soon after diagnosis. However, several follow-up observational or retrospective studies have found rates of sustained remission to be decreased compared to the original RCT [42–44]. Two recent studies looking at the effect of early introduction of thiopurines in adults with Crohn's disease have shown no beneficial effect [45, 46]. The potential of thiopurines to contribute to lymphoma, skin cancer, as well as hemophagocytic lymphohistiocytosis (HLH) has caused some clinicians to limit their use (see below).

Increased interest has focused on methotrexate as an alternative immunomodulator. Two pediatric studies found that 45–50 % of patients intolerant of thiopurines were in steroid-free remission at 12 months after change from thiopurines to MTX [47, 48]. Furthermore, a recent study evaluating data from a large prospective IBD registry found that the use of MTX as maintenance therapy has been increasing, with 14 %

of patients treated with MTX as first-line immunomodulator therapy in 2002 and expanding to 60 % in 2010 [49]. A 2014 multicenter retrospective cohort study comparing outcomes for patients treated with subcutaneous versus oral MTX found rates of overall steroid free remission to be similar. However, oral MTX use was associated with a longer time to remission, less improvement in linear growth and a trend toward reduced sustained SFR. The authors therefore suggested the subcutaneous route is initially preferred [50]. No head-to-head comparisons of outcomes with thiopurines and methotrexate in pediatric CD have been published.

Biological Therapy

The REACH clinical trial included 112 initial study subjects with moderate/severe disease despite therapy with corticosteroids and immunomodulators who were treated with 5 mg/kg at 0, 2, and 6 weeks. Eighty-eight percent were in response and 59 % in remission at 10 weeks. Patients in response or remission at 10 weeks were then randomized to receive either 5 mg/kg every 8 weeks or every 12 weeks, with an opportunity to step up dose to 10 mg/kg or decrease interval (for those in the 12 week group) in case of loss of response. At week 54, 33 of 52 (64 %) and 29 of 52 (56 %) patients receiving infliximab every 8 weeks did not require dose adjustment and were in clinical response and clinical remission, respectively, compared with 17 of 51 (33 %) and 12 of 51 (24 %) patients receiving treatment every 12 weeks ($p = .002$ and $p < .001$, respectively) [51].

Longer-term follow-up following infliximab therapy in children has also been examined. A multicenter study involving 66 patients in the Netherlands had a mean follow-up of 41 months with 15 % having a prolonged response following episodic therapy, 56 % were infliximab dependent (requiring repeated infusions to maintain efficacy), and 29% lost response [52]. A second multicenter study examined the long-term course of 202 children with follow-up periods ranging up to 3 years. One hundred twenty-eight of the study cohort were treated with maintenance therapy and had follow-up of ≥1 year. The likelihood of continuing infliximab was 93 %, 78 %, and 67 % at 1, 2, and 3 years respectively (Kaplan Meier analysis). A step-up in therapy (either increased dose or decreased interval) was needed in about half the patients. Corticosteroid-free clinical remission for the periods from 0–1, 1–2, and 2–3 years after starting infliximab was 26 %, 44 %, and 33 % [53].

Recent adult studies have identified the relationship between sustained remission and infliximab trough and antibody to infliximab levels (ATI) [54]. Similar associations are found in pediatric IBD. A prospective cohort study of pediatric patients with IBD found that higher infliximab levels and lower CRP at week 14 were associated with week 54 efficacy and rates of remission [55]. A retrospective pediatric study of 134 patients with IBD found similar associations. ATI ≥ 5 was associated with lower infliximab trough levels than those with ATI < 5 ($p < 0.001$). Additionally, ATI ≥ 12 was associated with need for surgical resection compared to those with ATI < 12 ($p = 0.01$) [56].

The use of adalimumab in pediatric Crohn's disease was initially reported in multiple small single center series and one larger retrospective report of 115 patients. Nearly all patients had previously been treated with infliximab. The majority of children received induction dosing of 80 and 40 mg separated by 2 weeks followed by 40 mg every other week . Corticosteroid-free remission was noted in 22 %, 33 %, and 42 % of patients at 3, 6, and 12 months, respectively [57]. More recently, the open-label IMAgINE 1 study evaluated the efficacy of adalimumab with moderate to severe Crohn's disease. Study design evaluated outcomes for groups treated with high- or low-dosage after 26 weeks. In total, adalimumab was found to induce and maintain remission in 33 % of patients at 26 weeks. In patients that were infliximab naïve at the initiation of the trial, clinical remission rates at 26 weeks were significantly increased in the high dose versus low dose groups (57 % vs. 35 % $p = 0.026$) [58].

Outcomes with the use of infliximab in children with ulcerative colitis from a large multicenter pediatric IBD Registry have been reported. Corticosteroid-free inactive disease by physician global assessment was noted in 12/44 at 6 months (27 %), 15/39 at 12 months (38 %), and 6/28 (21 %) at 24 months. Kaplan-Meier analysis showed the likelihood of remaining colectomy-free following infliximab was 75 % at 6 months, 72 % at 12 months, and 61 % at 2 years [59]. In a more recent prospective pediatric UC trial including patients with moderate to severe UC, 73 % of patients responded to infliximab by week 8 after induction dosing of 5 mg/kg at weeks 0, 2, and 6. At week 54, 38 % of responders that continued to receive standard dosing maintenance infliximab therapy remained in remission [60].

The landmark SONIC study included adults with Crohn's disease and demonstrated significantly improved corticosteroid-free remission rates in anti-TNFα naive patients treated with azathioprine plus infliximab versus infliximab alone or azathioprine alone, and therefore use of dual therapy in this population greatly increased [61]. However, there are also convincing data that adult patients who have failed thiopurines and move on to infliximab do not have additional success by maintaining the thiopurine [62]. Moreover, the recently published COMMIT study in adults with Crohn's disease showed no added efficacy when comparing infliximab alone to infliximab plus methotrexate with both groups having clinical remission rates near 70 % at week 50. However, antibodies to infliximab were higher in the monotherapy group compared to combination (20 % vs. 4 % $p = 0.01$) [63].

The impressive remission rates and potential promise of mucosal healing have prompted early consideration for biological therapy in treating IBD. For pediatric patients in particular, establishing corticosteroid-free remission prior to or during the years of rapid linear growth and sexual development is very important. The use of an anti-TNFα agent as primary therapy in the setting of extensive disease, complicated early disease, severe fistula, or disease onset in an adolescent with growth failure already showing signs of puberty in whom the window for growth is short has become increasingly common. Data have also suggested that antibody titers to specific microbial antigens measured at the time of diagnosis may predict the development of complicated disease requiring surgery (obstruction, perforation) and may play a role in helping identify subjects more likely to benefit from biological therapy at the time of diagnosis [64].

The striking impact of early anti-TNF use upon growth in inflammatory CD was recently demonstrated using data from a large observational cohort study, which included patients newly diagnosed with Crohn's disease at age <17. Twelve month outcomes for 3 groups of propensity-matched patients were compared: early infliximab, early immunomodulator therapy (IM), or no IM or infliximab therapy in the first 3 months. Clinical and growth outcomes were both found to be superior in those treated with early infliximab therapy compared to those with early IM or no early IM or infliximab therapy. In patients treated with early infliximab, 85 % were in remission at month 12 compared to 60 % in the early IM and 54 % in the no early IM or infliximab groups ($p=0.0003$). Normalization of C-reactive protein was most frequent in the early infliximab group. Further data are needed to determine which patients should be considered for anti-TNF therapy at the time of diagnosis [65].

Pediatric trials evaluating combination versus monotherapy with anti-TNF have not been performed. However, recently published observational data evaluated durability of infliximab therapy in 502 patients with Crohn's disease. In total, approximately 60 % of patients remained on infliximab 5 years after its initiation. The probability ± standard error that patients remained on infliximab 5 years after initiating treatment was significantly higher for those receiving concomitant therapy for >6 months compared to both anti-TNF monotherapy or those treated with combination therapy for <6 months (0.7 ± 0.04 vs. 0.48 ± 0.08 vs. 0.55 ± 0.06 ($p<0.001$)). Importantly, the durability of infliximab therapy in males treated for >6 months with combination therapy was greater in those treated with infliximab/MTX than those treated with infliximab/thiopurines (0.97 ± 0.03 vs. 0.58 ± 0.08 $p<0.01$) [66].

Clinical experience with anti-integrin therapy including natalizumab and more recently vedolizumab is emerging. There is a single report on the use of natalizumab in adolescents with moderate to severe Crohn's disease. Using an open-label dosing schedule of 3 mg/kg at weeks 0, 4, and 8 weeks in 31 subjects, 55 % had a clinical response and 29 % were in remission at 10 weeks [67]. Natalizumab targets both alpha4beta1 and alpha4beta7 integrin therefore modulating both brain and gut lymphocyte migration. Its use has been associated with progressive multifocal leukoencephalopathy (PML) caused by reactivation of latent JC virus. In contrast to natalizumab, vedolizumab targets only alpha4beta7 integrin and thus acts only upon gut, not brain lymphocytes and should therefore have reduced risk of PML. The adult 2013 RCTs in both CD and UC found vedolizumab to be effective toward inducing remission and has been recently approved for treatment of both UC and CD in adults [68, 69]. Currently, pediatric data with the use of vedolizumab is limited to abstract presentations.

Toxicity and Risk

It is known that both immunomodulators and anti-TNF therapies have potential risks of toxicity and these are of particular concern in pediatric patients. The risks of chronic thiopurine toxicity are being increasingly recognized. Bone marrow suppression, hepatotoxicity, and infectious risks including viral, bacterial, and opportunistic have been previously well described [70]. More recent publications have described the risk of hemophagocytic lymphohistiocytosis (HLH) and EBV associated lymphoproliferative disorders, especially in association with primary EBV infection in patients treated with thiopurines [71, 72]. Lymphoma risk with thiopurines is also greatest in patients <30 years having a standardized incidence ratio of 6.99 (95 % CI 2.99–16.4). The risk in males appears greater than females [73].

Of particular concern in pediatrics, especially in males, is the decision regarding whether combination therapy with anti-TNF and thiopurines is contraindicated. This dilemma stems from the association of hepatosplenic T cell lymphoma (HSTCL) occurring in young patients (primarily males) treated with concomitant therapy [74]. No cases of HSTCL have been noted in adult or pediatric patients treated with infliximab monotherapy, however, in nearly all cases of HSTCL, the unifying drug exposure has been thiopurines.

Given the predilection of this invariably fatal lymphoma for young males, most pediatric gastroenterologists do not use combined anti-TNF/thiopurine therapy in young male patients. If there is a need to use combined therapy, methotrexate has become the immunomodulator of choice in low dosage to decrease anti-infliximab antibody production. No consensus exists as to whether young females can or cannot be treated with combined therapy with thiopurines and anti-TNFα agents as HSTCL has rarely been reported in females as well [74] . The recently described improved durability of infliximab when used in combination with MTX provides a promising alternative to combination therapy with thiopurines or treatment with anti-TNF monotherapy [66].

Enteral Nutritional Support

There is considerable variation in the frequency with which primary enteral nutrition is used as an induction strategy in children newly diagnosed with Crohn's disease. While commonly used in Europe, it is utilized much less frequently in most of North America despite its favorable side effect profile, positive impact upon growth/nutritional deficiencies and lack of toxicity risk. There are several older published trials comparing the relative efficacy of enteral nutrition versus corticosteroids and in whole there is fairly equivalent efficacy [75–77]. A recent prospective study compared 8 week outcomes in three groups of pediatric patients with active disease: anti-TNF therapy, exclusive enteral nutrition (EEN) or partial enteral nutrition (PEN). Improvement in mucosal inflammation was found to be superior for both the EEN and anti-TNF groups compared to PEN, thus adding further support for expanded use of this treatment approach [78].

There are situations in which enteral nutrition should be the initial intervention of choice including patients with primarily small bowel disease and growth failure. In these patients, primary enteral nutritional therapy can both induce remission and also reverse nutritional deficiencies and promote improved linear growth. A challenge unique to treatment with exclusive enteral therapy is to successfully motivate the child and family to maintain treatment by drinking the formula or using a nasogastric tube. In some patients enteral therapy has been used for several months initially to then be followed by scheduled periods of re-administration after allowing a regular diet [79]. For many patients who start primary enteral nutrition therapy, an immunomodulator is concomitantly initiated as the long-term maintenance strategy.

Severe/Fulminant Ulcerative Colitis

The management of fulminant colitis in children presents a particular challenge. Frequently these are children at or shortly following diagnosis when understanding of the disease itself may be limited, and a willingness to proceed to colectomy if necessary has not been established. A prospective study of children with fulminant ulcerative colitis has given additional insight into disease management in this situation. In this study, 126 children hospitalized with severe ulcerative colitis were followed for up to 1 year. Approximately one third failed therapy with intravenous steroids and required rescue with either infliximab, cyclosporine, or colectomy. The most sensitive predictor of the failure of intravenous corticosteroids was a PUCAI score of 45 or higher on day 3 of hospitalization. Overall 9% and 19% of children hospitalized with severe/fulminant colitis required colectomy by initial discharge or 1 year, respectively [80]. More recent studies have focused upon dose optimization with infliximab in treating acute severe UC (ASUC). A recent adult and pediatric review concluded that standard weight-base infliximab dosing may not be equally effective for ASUC. Potential contributors to the need for dose optimization in this population include high TNF burden, highly active reticuloendothelial system, and marked infliximab stool losses related to protein losing enteropathy [81]. Prospective studies will be needed to better understand targeted management with infliximab in pediatric ASUC.

Most pediatric gastroenterologists will use infliximab as their preferred rescue medication for corticosteroid failures, though some still prefer calcineurin inhibitors. Small case series have been published on the use of cyclosporine and tacrolimus for severe colitis in children [82, 83]. Though the results of these studies have suggested a delay in the need for colectomy following calcineurin inhibitor treatment, the overall long-term prognosis for avoiding colectomy is low. Failure of one of these agents should not lead to use of the other because of concerns of increased risk of serious infection. In the authors' view saving a life is more important than saving a colon. Results of colectomy and ileal pouch anal anastomosis (IPAA) in children are similar to those of adults. The issue of possible impaired fecundity later in life for adolescent girls who may be subject to IPAA should be raised before this procedure is done.

Summary

It is crucial that clinicians caring for children and adolescents with IBD be fully informed about the relationship of disease activity and therapy to growth and development, each of which need to be considered when planning various medical and surgical therapies. The balance between risks and benefits of therapies, especially regarding potential toxicities with thiopurine monotherapy and in combination with anti-TNF therapy is increasingly recognized.

References

1. Oliva-Hemker M, Hutfless S, Al Kazzi ES, Lerer T, Mack D, LeLeiko N, et al. Clinical presentation and five-year therapeutic management of very early-onset inflammatory bowel disease in a large north American cohort. J Pediatr. 2015.doi:10.1016/s0022-3476-00429-1.
2. Kugathasan S, Judd RH, Hoffmann RG, Heikenen J, Telega G, Khan F, et al. Epidemiologic and clinical characteristics of children with newly diagnosed inflammatory bowel disease in Wisconsin: a statewide population-based study. J Pediatr. 2003;143:525–31.

3. Heyman MB, Kirschner BS, Gold BD, Ferry G, Baldassano R, Cohen SA, et al. Children with early-onset inflammatory bowel disease (IBD): analysis of a pediatric IBD consortium registry. J Pediatr. 2005;146:35–40.
4. Meinzer U, Ideström M, Alberti C, Peuchmaur M, Belarbi N, Bellaïche M, et al. Ileal involvement is age dependent in pediatric Crohn's disease. Inflamm Bowel Dis. 2005;11:639–44.
5. Mack D, Markowitz J, Lerer T, Griffiths A, Evans J, Otley A, et al. S1189 Upper gastrointestinal involvement in pediatric Crohn's disease: experience of a large multicenter inception cohort. Gastroenterology. 2010;138(5):S-200.
6. Van Limbergen J, Russell RK, Drummond HE, Aldhous MC, Round NK, Nimmo ER, et al. Definition of phenotypic characteristics of childhood-onset inflammatory bowel disease. Gastroenterology. 2008;135:1114–22.
7. Gower-Rousseau C, Dauchet L, Vernier-Massouille G, Tilloy E, Brazier F, Merle V, et al. The natural history of pediatric ulcerative colitis: a population-based cohort study. Am J Gastroenterol. 2009;104:2080–8.
8. Markowitz J, Kugathasan S, Dubinsky M, Mei L, Crandall W, Leleiko N, et al. Age of diagnosis influences serologic responses in children with Crohn's disease: a possible clue to etiology? Inflamm Bowel Dis. 2009;15:714–9.
9. Vernier-Massouille G, Balde M, Salleron J, Turck D, Dupas JL, Mouterde O, et al. Natural history of pediatric Crohn's disease: a population-based cohort study. Gastroenterology. 2008;135:1106–13.
10. Dubinsky MC, Lin YC, Dutridge D, Picornell Y, Landers CJ, Farrior S, et al. Serum immune responses predict rapid disease progression among children with Crohn's disease: immune responses predict disease progression. Am J Gastroenterol. 2006;101:360–7.
11. Hyams JS, Davis P, Grancher K, Lerer T, Justinich CJ, Markowitz J. Clinical outcome of ulcerative colitis in children. J Pediatr. 1996;129:81–8.
12. Ruemmele FM, El Khoury MG, Talbotec C, Maurage C, Mougenot JF, Schmitz J, et al. Characteristics of inflammatory bowel disease with onset during the first year of life. J Pediatr Gastroenterol Nutr. 2006;43:603–9.
13. Benchimol E, Mack DR, Nguyen GC, Snapper SB, Li W, Mojaverian N, et al. Incidence, outcomes, and health services burden of very early onset inflammatory bowel disease. Gastroenterology. 2014;147:803–13.
14. Uhlig HH, Schwerd T, Koletzko S, Shah N, Kammermeier J, Elkadri A, et al. The diagnostic approach to monogenic very early onset inflammatory bowel disease. Gastroenterology. 2014;147:990–1007.
15. Glocker EO, Kotlarz D, Boztug K, Gertz EM, Schaffer AA, Noyan F, et al. Inflammatory bowel disease and mutations affecting the interleukin-10 receptor. N Engl J Med. 2009;361:2033–45.
16. Hyams JS, Ferry GD, Mandel FS, Gryboski JD, Kibort PM, Kirschner BS, et al. Development and validation of a pediatric Crohn's disease activity index. J Pediatr Gastroenterol Nutr. 1991;12:439–47.
17. Hyams J, Markowitz J, Otley A, Rosh J, Mack D, Bousvaros A, et al. Evaluation of the pediatric Crohn disease activity index: a prospective multicenter experience. J Pediatr Gastroenterol Nutr. 2005;41:416–21.
18. Turner D, Griffiths AM, Walters TD, Seah T, Markowitz J, Pfefferkorn M, et al. Mathematical weighting of the pediatric Crohn's disease activity index (PCDAI) and comparison with its other short versions. Inflamm Bowel Dis. 2012;18:55–62.
19. Kappelman MD, Crandall WV, Colletti RB, Goudie A, Leibowitz IH, Duffy L, et al. Short pediatric Crohn's disease activity index for quality improvement and observational research. Inflamm Bowel Dis. 2011;17:112–7.
20. Turner D, Otley AR, Mack D, Hyams J, de Bruijne J, Uusoue K, et al. Development, validation, and evaluation of a pediatric ulcerative colitis activity index: a prospective multicenter study. Gastroenterology. 2007;133:423–32.
21. Bryant RV, Burger DC, Delo J, Walsh AJ, Thomas S, von Herbay A, et al. Beyond endoscopic mucosal healing in UC: histological remission better predicts corticosteroid use and hospitalisation over 6 years of follow-up. Gut. 2015. doi:10.1136/gutjnl-2015-309598.
22. Guardiola J, Lobatón T, Rodríguez-Alonso L, Ruiz-Cerulla A, Arajol C, Loayza C, et al. Fecal level of calprotectin identifies histologic inflammation in patients with ulcerative colitis in clinical and endoscopic remission. Clin Gastroenterol Hepatol. 2014;12:1865–70.
23. Theede K, Holck S, Ibsen P, Ladelund S, Nordgaard-Lassen I, Mertz Nielsen A. Level of fecal calprotectin correlates with endoscopic and histologic inflammation and identifies patients with mucosal healing of ulcerative colitis. Clin Gastroenterol Hepatol. 2015. doi:10.1016/s1542-3565-00773-9.
24. Kanof ME, Lake AM, Bayless TM. Decreased height velocity in children and adolescents before the diagnosis of Crohn's disease. Gastroenterology. 1988;95:1523–7.
25. Walters TD, Griffiths AM. Mechanisms of growth impairment in pediatric Crohn's disease. Nat Rev Gastroenterol Hepatol. 2009;6:513–23.
26. Heuschkel R, Salvestrini C, Beattie RM, Hildebrand H, Walters T, Griffiths A. Guidelines for the management of growth failure in childhood inflammatory bowel disease. Inflamm Bowel Dis. 2008;14:839–49.
27. Motil KJ, Grand RJ. Nutritional management of inflammatory bowel disease. Pediatr Clin North Am. 1985;32:447–69.
28. Varghese S, Wyzga N, Griffiths AM, Sylvester FA. Effects of serum from children with newly diagnosed Crohn disease on primary cultures of rat osteoblasts. J Pediatr Gastroenterol Nutr. 2002;35:641–8.
29. Mauras N. Growth hormone therapy in the glucocorticosteroid-dependent child: metabolic and linear growth effects. Horm Res. 2001;56 Suppl 1:13–8.
30. Hyams JS, Moore RE, Leichtner AM, Carey DE, Goldberg BD. Relationship of type I procollagen to corticosteroid therapy in children with inflammatory bowel disease. J Pediatr. 1988;112:893–8.
31. Allen DB. Influence of inhaled corticosteroids on growth: a pediatric endocrinologist's perspective. Acta Paediatr. 1998;87:123–9.
32. Pfefferkorn M, Burke G, Griffiths A, Markowitz J, Rosh J, Mack D, et al. Growth abnormalities persist in newly diagnosed children with Crohn disease despite current treatment paradigms. J Pediatr Gastroenterol Nutr. 2009;48:168–74.
33. Brody AS, Frush DP, Huda W, Brent RL. Radiation risk to children from computed tomography. Pediatrics. 2007;120:677–82.
34. Brenner DJ, Sachs RK. Estimating radiation-induced cancer risks at very low doses: rationale for using a linear no-threshold approach. Radiat Environ Biophys. 2006;44:253–6.
35. Mazrani W, McHugh K, Marsden PJ. The radiation burden of radiological investigations. Arch Dis Child. 2007;92:1127–31.
36. Giles E, Barclay AR, Wilson DC, Chippington S. Systematic review: MRI enterography for assessment of small bowel involvement in paediatric Crohn's disease. Aliment Pharmacol Ther. 2013;37:1121–31.
37. Markowitz J, Hyams J, Mack D, Leleiko N, Evans J, Kugathasan S, et al. Corticosteroid therapy in the age of infliximab: acute and 1-year outcomes in newly diagnosed children with Crohn's disease. Clin Gastroenterol Hepatol. 2006;4:1124–9.
38. Hyams J, Markowitz J, Lerer T, Griffiths A, Mack D, Bousvaros A, et al. The natural history of corticosteroid therapy for ulcerative colitis in children. Clin Gastroenterol Hepatol. 2006;4:1118–23.
39. Levine A, Weizman Z, Broide E, Shamir R, Shaoul R, Pacht A, et al. A comparison of budesonide and prednisone for the treatment of

active pediatric Crohn disease. J Pediatr Gastroenterol Nutr. 2003;36:248–52.

40. Escher JC. Budesonide versus prednisolone for the treatment of active Crohn's disease in children: a randomized, double-blind, controlled, multicentre trial. Eur J Gastroenterol Hepatol. 2004;16:47–54.
41. Markowitz J, Grancher K, Kohn N, Lesser M, Daum F. A multicenter trial of 6-mercaptopurine and prednisone in children with newly diagnosed Crohn's disease. Gastroenterology. 2000;119:895–902.
42. Boyle BM, Kappelman MD, Colletti RB, Baldassano RN, Milov DE, Crandall WV. Routine use of thiopurines in maintaining remission in pediatric Crohn's disease. World J Gastroenterol. 2014;20:9185–90.
43. Riello L, Talbotec C, Garnier-Lengliné H, Pigneur B, Svahn J, Canioni D, et al. Tolerance and efficacy of azathioprine in pediatric Crohn's disease. Inflamm Bowel Dis. 2011;17:2138–43.
44. Goodhand JR, Tshuma N, Rao A, Kotta S, Wahed M, Croft NM, et al. Do children with IBD really respond better than adults to thiopurines? J Pediatr Gastroenterol Nutr. 2011;52:702–7.
45. Panés J, López-Sanromán A, Bermejo F, García-Sánchez V, Esteve M, Torres Y, et al. Early azathioprine therapy is no more effective than placebo for newly diagnosed Crohn's disease. Gastroenterology. 2013;145:766–74.
46. Cosnes J, Bourrier A, Laharie D, Nahon S, Bouhnik Y, Carbonnel F, et al. Early administration of azathioprine vs conventional management of Crohn's disease: a randomized controlled trial. Gastroenterology. 2013;145:758–65.
47. Turner D, Grossman AB, Rosh J, Kugathasan S, Gilman AR, Baldassano R, et al. Methotrexate following unsuccessful thiopurine therapy in pediatric Crohn's disease. Am J Gastroenterol. 2007;102:2804–12.
48. Uhlen S, Belbouab R, Narebski K, Goulet O, Schmitz J, Cézard JP, et al. Efficacy of methotrexate in pediatric Crohn's disease: a French multicenter study. Inflamm Bowel Dis. 2006;12:1053–7.
49. Sunseri W, Hyams JS, Lerer T, Mack DR, Griffiths AM, Otley AR, et al. Retrospective cohort study of methotrexate use in the treatment of pediatric Crohn's disease. Inflamm Bowel Dis. 2014;20:1341–5.
50. Turner D, Doveh E, Cohen A, Wilson ML, Grossman AB, Rosh JR, et al. Efficacy of oral methotrexate in paediatric Crohn's disease: a multicentre propensity score study. Gut. 2014. doi:10.1136/gutjnl-2014-307964.
51. Hyams J, Crandall W, Kugathasan S, Griffiths A, Olson A, Johanns J, et al. Induction and maintenance infliximab therapy for the treatment of moderate-to-severe Crohn's disease in children. Gastroenterology. 2007;132:863–73.
52. de Ridder L, Rings EH, Damen GM, Kneepkens CM, Schweizer JJ, Kokke FT, et al. Infliximab dependency in pediatric Crohn's disease: long-term follow-up of an unselected cohort. Inflamm Bowel Dis. 2008;14:353–8.
53. Hyams JS, Lerer T, Griffiths A, Pfefferkorn M, Kugathasan S, Evans J, et al. Long-term outcome of maintenance infliximab therapy in children with Crohn's disease. Inflamm Bowel Dis. 2009;15:816–22.
54. Vande Casteele N, Ferrante M, Van Assche G, Ballet V, Compernolle G, Van Steen K, et al. Trough concentrations of infliximab guide dosing for patients with inflammatory bowel disease. Gastroenterology. 2015;148:1320–9.
55. Singh N, Rosenthal CJ, Melmed GY, Mirocha J, Farrior S, Callejas S, et al. Early infliximab trough levels are associated with persistent remission in pediatric patients with inflammatory bowel disease. Inflamm Bowel Dis. 2014;20:1708–13.
56. Zitomersky NL, Atkinson BJ, Fournier K, Mitchell PD, Stern JB, Butler MC, et al. Antibodies to infliximab are associated with lower infliximab levels and increased likelihood of surgery in pediatric IBD. Inflamm Bowel Dis. 2015;21:307–14.
57. Rosh JR, Lerer T, Markowitz J, Goli SR, Mamula P, Noe JD, et al. Retrospective evaluation of the safety and effect of adalimumab therapy (RESEAT) in pediatric Crohn's disease. Am J Gastroenterol. 2009;104:3042–9.
58. Hyams JS, Griffiths A, Markowitz J, Baldassano RN, Faubion Jr WA, Colletti RB, et al. Safety and efficacy of adalimumab for moderate to severe Crohn's disease in children. Gastroenterology. 2012;143:365–74.
59. Hyams JS, Lerer T, Griffiths A, Pfefferkorn M, Stephens M, Evans J, et al. Outcome following infliximab therapy in children with ulcerative colitis. Am J Gastroenterol. 2010;105:1430–6.
60. Hyams J, Damaraju L, Blank M, Johanns J, Guzzo C, Winter HS, et al. Induction and maintenance therapy with infliximab for children with moderate to severe ulcerative colitis. Clin Gastroenterol Hepatol. 2012;10:391–9.
61. Colombel JF, Sandborn WJ, Reinisch W, Mantzaris GJ, Kornbluth A, Rachmilewitz D, et al. Infliximab, azathioprine, or combination therapy for Crohn's disease. N Engl J Med. 2010;362:1383–95.
62. Lichtenstein GR, Diamond RH, Wagner CL, Fasanmade AA, Olson AD, Marano CW, et al. Clinical trial: benefits and risks of immunomodulators and maintenance infliximab for IBD-subgroup analyses across four randomized trials. Aliment Pharmacol Ther. 2009;30:210–26.
63. Feagan BG, McDonald JW, Panaccione R, Enns RA, Bernstein CN, Ponich TP, et al. Methotrexate in combination with infliximab is no more effective than infliximab alone in patients with Crohn's disease. Gastroenterology. 2014;146:681–8.
64. Dubinsky MC, Kugathasan S, Mei L, Picornell Y, Nebel J, Wrobel I, et al. Increased immune reactivity predicts aggressive complicating Crohn's disease in children. Clin Gastroenterol Hepatol. 2008;6:1105–11.
65. Walters TD, Kim MO, Denson LA, Griffiths AM, Dubinsky M, Markowitz J, et al. Increased effectiveness of early therapy with anti-tumor necrosis factor-α vs an immunomodulator in children with Crohn's disease. Gastroenterology. 2014;146:383–91.
66. Grossi V, Lerer T, Griffiths A, LeLeiko N, Cabrera J, Otley A, et al. Concomitant use of immunomodulators affects the durability of infliximab therapy in children with Crohn's disease. Clin Gastroenterol Hepatol. 2015. doi:10.1016/s.1542-3565-00412-7.
67. Hyams JS, Wilson DC, Thomas A, Heuschkel R, Mitton S, Mitchell B, et al. Natalizumab therapy for moderate to severe Crohn disease in adolescents. J Pediatr Gastroenterol Nutr. 2007;44:185–91.
68. Sandborn WJ, Feagan BG, Rutgeerts P, Hanauer S, Colombel JF, Sands BE, et al. Vedolizumab as induction and maintenance therapy for Crohn's disease. N Engl J Med. 2013;369:711–21.
69. Feagan BG, Rutgeerts P, Sands BE, Hanauer S, Colombel JF, Sandborn WJ, et al. Vedolizumab as induction and maintenance therapy for ulcerative colitis. N Engl J Med. 2013;369:699–710.
70. Warman JI, Korelitz BI, Fleisher MR, Janardhanam R. Cumulative experience with short- and long-term toxicity to 6-mercaptopurine in the treatment of Crohn's disease and ulcerative colitis. J Clin Gastroenterol. 2003;37:220–5.
71. James DG, Stone CD, Wang HL, Stenson WF. Reactive hemophagocytic syndrome complicating the treatment of inflammatory bowel disease. Inflamm Bowel Dis. 2006;12:573–80.
72. Beaugerie L, Brousse N, Bouvier AM, Colombel JF, Lémann M, Cosnes J, et al. Lymphoproliferative disorders in patients receiving thiopurines for inflammatory bowel disease: a prospective observational cohort study. Lancet. 2009;374:1617–25.
73. Kotlyar DS, Lewis JD, Beaugerie L, Tierney A, Brensinger CM, Gisbert JP, et al. Risk of lymphoma in patients with inflammatory bowel disease treated with azathioprine and 6-mercaptopurine: a meta-analysis. Clin Gastroenterol Hepatol. 2015;13:847–58.
74. Kotlyar DS, Osterman MT, Diamond RH, Porter D, Blonski WC, Wasik M, et al. A systematic review of factors that contribute to hepatosplenic T-cell lymphoma in patients with inflammatory bowel disease. Clin Gastroenterol Hepatol. 2011;9:36–41.

75. Heuschkel RB, Menache CC, Megerian JT, Baird AE. Enteral nutrition and corticosteroids in the treatment of acute Crohn's disease in children. J Pediatr Gastroenterol Nutr. 2000;31:8–15.
76. Sanderson IR, Udeen S, Davies PS, Savage MO, Walker-Smith JA. Remission induced by an elemental diet in small bowel Crohn's disease. Arch Dis Child. 1987;62:123–7.
77. Ruuska T, Savilahti E, Maki M, Ormala T, Visakorpi JK. Exclusive whole protein enteral diet versus prednisolone in the treatment of acute Crohn's disease in children. J Pediatr Gastroenterol Nutr. 1994;19:175–80.
78. Lee D, Baldassano RN, Otley AR, Albenberg L, Griffiths AM, Compher C, et al. Comparative effectiveness of nutritional and biological therapy in North American children with active Crohn's disease. Inflamm Bowel Dis. 2015;21:1786–93.
79. Belli DC, Seidman E, Bouthillier L, Weber AM, Roy CC, Pletincx M, et al. Chronic intermittent elemental diet improves growth failure in children with Crohn's disease. Gastroenterology. 1988;94:603–10.
80. Turner D, Mack D, Leleiko N, Walters TD, Uusoue K, Leach ST, et al. Severe pediatric ulcerative colitis: a prospective multicenter study of outcomes and predictors of response. Gastroenterology. 2010;138:2282–91.
81. Rosen MJ, Minar P, Vinks AA. Review article: applying pharmacokinetics to optimise dosing of anti-TNF biologics in acute severe ulcerative colitis. Aliment Pharmacol Ther. 2015;41:1094–103.
82. Treem WR, Cohen J, Davis PM, Justinich CJ, Hyams JS. Cyclosporine for the treatment of fulminant ulcerative colitis in children. Immediate response, long-term results, and impact on surgery. Dis Colon Rectum. 1995;38:474–9.
83. Bousvaros A, Kirschner BS, Werlin SL, Parker-Hartigan L, Daum F, Freeman KB, et al. Oral tacrolimus treatment of severe colitis in children. J Pediatr. 2000;137:794–9.

Part IX

Surveillance and Prevention

Management and Prevention of Infectious Diseases in IBD Patients

59

Kristine Macartney and Nigel Crawford

Introduction

One of the most challenging aspects of the care of IBD patients is the management of infectious diseases and their associated morbidity and mortality. Although there are a number of factors that contribute to the prevalence of infectious diseases in IBD patients, it has become clear that those taking multiple immunomodulatory drugs are at greatest risk. There is also increasing evidence of the role of the aberrant mucosal innate and adaptive immune responses to commensal microbiota [1, 2] in the pathogenesis of IBD that is not reviewed in detail in this chapter as it remains unclear to what extent this contributes to the risk of infectious disease overall. However, relapse of IBD can be associated with infection, particularly from enteric pathogens, and treatment of coexistent infection in patients with active IBD can facilitate resolution of an IBD flare. This chapter reviews the increased risk of infection in IBD patients, the most common infections encountered, and the approach to management and prevention, with a particular focus on vaccination of IBD patients.

Risk of Infection in IBD Patients

Mortality and morbidity from infections are overrepresented in those with IBD compared with other patient populations [3–5]. The greatest risk is associated with higher degrees of immunosuppression and disease severity [6, 7]. Patients with IBD are most significantly at increased risk of infection due to treatment with immunomodulatory medications [8]. Other factors also contribute and are described below. It is important to note that there is no clear correlate or measure to determine the extent of immunosuppression in IBD or other immune-mediated inflammatory diseases [9]. Patients with should generally not be considered to have a systemic immune deficit in the absence of immunotherapeutic medications or malnutrition [9].

The Disease Process

Patients with Crohn's disease (CD) have a higher risk of bowel-related infectious diseases due to the transmural and extensive nature of their disease, particularly the formation of fistulae and abscesses, than patients with ulcerative colitis (UC) [6, 10]. Disease severity, including the need for frequent outpatient visits, hospitalization, parenteral nutrition, and surgery, also add to the overall infection risk for IBD patients, including from nosocomial infections [7, 11–13]. Patients can also be at increased infection risk because of chronic conditions related to IBD, including chronic airways disease, nephrolithiasis and primary sclerosing cholangitis [6].

Malnutrition

The presence of malnutrition is a key factor that has been shown to correlate with increased morbidity and mortality in IBD [9]. Malnutrition is common in patients with IBD, especially in active CD in whom 70–80 % of hospitalized and 20–40 % of outpatients have weight loss [14]. Malnutrition is less common in UC patients but can develop rapidly in periods of active disease. Malnutrition appears to impair various components of the immune system and has, in turn, been associated with increased risk of infection, cancer, and suboptimal responses to vaccination [6, 9, 15–17].

K. Macartney, M.D., F.R.A.C.P. (✉)
The Children's Hospital of Westmead, The National Centre for Immunisation Research and Surveillance, P.O. Box 4000, Westmead, NSW 2145, Australia
e-mail: Kristine.macartney@health.nsw.gov.au

N. Crawford, Ph.D., F.R.A.C.P.
Department of General Medicine, Royal Children's Hospital Melbourne, 50 Flemington Road, Parkville, VIC 3052, Australia
e-mail: nigel.crawford@rch.org.au

D.C. Baumgart (ed.), *Crohn's Disease and Ulcerative Colitis*, DOI 10.1007/978-3-319-33703-6_59

Infection and Immunomodulatory Therapy

Drug therapy used for IBD has been identified as one of the most significant factors influencing the risk of developing infection and its severity, whether from a common infectious agent, an opportunistic pathogen, or reactivation of latent infection. The risks for single agent and combination therapy have been more closely studied since the introduction of anti-TNF monoclonal antibodies over a decade ago [6]. However, studies reporting infection rates need to be carefully assessed for inherent biases and limitations, particularly in applying risk estimates to individual settings [18].

Initial results from large multicenter observational cohort registries such as TREAT (a prospective, multicenter, long-term registry of the treatment of Crohn)'s disease) [19] and ENCORE did not suggest that infliximab was an independent cause of increased infection. However, follow-up of 6273 CD patients in the TREAT observational study for a mean duration of 5.2 years did find that treatment with infliximab and prednisone were independently associated with an increased risk of serious infection [7]. In addition, patients treated with prednisone, but not infliximab, had an increased risk of mortality, when compared with "other treatment" only patients [7]. Pooled data from company-sponsored clinical trials found a 36 % risk of infection for infliximab-treated patients, compared with 28 % for non-infliximab treated patients [6, 20–22]. Another meta-analysis of 22 separate randomized controlled trials found an increased risk of opportunistic infection (RR 2.05, 95 % CI 1.10–3.85) in adults with active or quiescent UC or CD who were treated with anti-TNF therapy (compared with placebo) [23]. Data on infection risks in children are more sparse [24]. Where data in IBD patients on the use of these medications has been lacking, studies of their use in patients with other autoimmune diseases, such as rheumatoid arthritis, have been of value [25, 26]. A Cochrane systematic review of the biologic therapies in all diseases (other than HIV) found an overall increased risk of tuberculosis for patients treated with biologics. One particular therapy (certolizumab pegol-interleukin (IL) 1 antagonist) was identified as associated with a higher risk of infections than other biologics [27].

Although certain types of drugs have been associated with different types of infections, strict correlations between a specific agent and pathogen should not be relied upon in clinical practice [9]. The tendency for one drug therapy to predispose to certain infections is related to the drug's mechanism of action [17]. Table 59.1 summarizes data regarding individual therapies. For example, azathioprine and 6-mercaptopurine impact upon T-cell function and are more likely to be associated with viral infections (cytomegalovirus [CMV], varicella-zoster virus [VZV], herpes simplex virus [HSV]), whereas anti-TNF therapy appears to increase the risk for granulomatous infections from mycobacterial or fungal pathogens, such as tuberculosis (TB) or histoplasmosis [7, 10, 17]. Other granulomatous infections have also been reported to occur with anti-TNF therapy [26, 35]. One retrospective review of drug therapy and infection in IBD patients found that corticosteroid use was more commonly associated with fungal infections, especially with *Candida* species [10].

Combinations of immunomodulatory therapy are associated with an increased risk of infection [10]. In a retrospective study of IBD patients from the Mayo Clinic, treatment with a single immunomodulation increased the risk of infection almost threefold (odds ratio [OR] 2.9; 95 % confidence interval [CI] 1.5–7.3). A more substantial increase in the likelihood of infection occurred in patients receiving two or more drugs in combination (OR 14.5; 95 % CI 4.9–43). Cumulative doses of corticosteroids, but not other drugs, were associated with an increased risk of infection.

Other Factors

Increasing age is a risk factor for infection in general, and the age at diagnosis of IBD is a factor related to increased morbidity and mortality in IBD patients [7], even after adjusting for use of immunosuppressive therapy [10, 13, 37]. Longer IBD disease duration has also been identified as a risk factor [7, 38]. Preexisting comorbidities, such as chronic lung disease, have been identified as contributing factors in studies of patients with rheumatologic disease, and, although such conditions have not been widely studied in IBD, they still should be noted. It is important to view the infectious risk of an IBD patient as that related to their lifetime exposures including consideration of infectious agents endemic for their places of residence [17] and exposures due to occupation and lifestyle [17].

Prevention, Diagnosis, and Management

Prevention of infection in IBD patients is best managed through a range of activities, including: (a) thorough clinical and laboratory investigations before starting immunomodulatory therapy, preferably at the time of IBD diagnosis; (b) vaccination and chemoprophylaxis when appropriate; (c) treatment of preexisting viral infections, such as chronic active hepatitis B infection; (d) investigation for concomitant infection during episodes of disease relapse; (e) adjustment of immunotherapy when infection occurs; and (f) patient education. Other factors inherent in the overall good clinical management of IBD patients, such as minimizing risk of malnutrition through institution of nutritional therapies, have also been shown to impact on the prevention of infection.

Table 59.1 Risk of infection for certain immunomodulatory agents used to treat IBD

Drug	Risk of Infection	Comments
Corticosteroids	• Serious infections OR 2.21 (1.46–3.34) from TREAT registry of Crohn's disease patients [7, 19] • Independently associated with serious infections [28] • Infections reported: fungal [10], TB reactivation, post-surgical [29]	• Risk of infection particularly with prolonged high doses, e.g., daily doses >20 mg (or 1–2 mg/kg/day in pediatric patients) for >1–2 weeks
Thiopurines	• Myelosuppression: predictable in thiopurine-S-methyltransferase (TPMT) deficient patients, unpredictable in ~5 % of patients [30] • Infections reported: viral, fungal, bacterial [31]. Precise infection risk unclear. Infections in 7.4 %, serious infection in 1.8 % of 386 patients over 18 years [32] • No increased risk in TREAT registry [19]	• TPMT testing prior to treatment recommended • Routine FBC monitoring recommended
Methotrexate	• Increase in pneumonia in rheumatoid arthritis population (RR: 1.16; 95 % CI: 1.02–1.33) [25]	• Infection risk in IBD patients not well defined
Cyclosporin	• Association with opportunistic infections (*Aspergillus* and *Pneumocystis*) and catheter related sepsis [33]. Infection risk in IBD patients not well studied	• Monitor levels and FBC • Pneumocystis prophylaxis recommended with lymphopenia
Biologics *Anti-TNF monoclonal antibodies* – infliximab – adalimumab – certolozimab pegol *Anti-adhesion molecules* – natalizumab	• Overall twofold increase in risk of infection compared with placebo in adults with UC or CD [23] • Increased risk of infection in TREAT study over 5.2 year follow-up [7] • Increased risk of TB reactivation (OR 4.68, 95 % CI 1.18–18.60; NNTH = 681, 95 % CI 143–14,706) for nine biologics reviewed in Cochrane analysis, compared to control [27] • Risk of serious infections: Certolizumab pegol associated with significantly higher risk compared to control treatment and other biologics (OR 3.51, 95 % CI 1.59–7.79; NNTH = 17, 95 % CI 7–68). Trend toward increased risk of serious infections for all biologics (OR 1.19, 95 % CI 0.94–1.52) [27] • Reactivation of latent hepatitis B infection [34] • Other granulomatous infections [26, 35] • Natalizumab (anti-CD20): risk of JC virus reactivation [36]	• Pretreatment screening for – latent TB – hepatitis B and hepatitis C – other chronic/endemic infections as discussed • Natalizumab: strict restrictions on use

Patient Assessment Prior to Immunomodulatory Therapy

The ideal time to fully evaluate IBD patients for their history and risk of infectious diseases is at diagnosis, prior to commencement of significant immunomodulatory therapy. As described in Table 59.2, a thorough and specific clinical history, physical examination, laboratory tests, and other investigations, where warranted, are indicated [9, 17, 21, 22]. This assessment should be followed by a plan for vaccination (see detailed section below) and treatment, if indicated, for any preexisting infections such as tuberculosis or hepatitis B (also discussed below). Local guidelines for the use of directed antimicrobial therapy should generally be observed, as they take into account drug availability and local antimicrobial resistance patterns. Detailed recommendations for the management of infections in IBD patients have been incorporated in European consensus guidelines [9] and detailed clinical practice reviews and commentaries [17, 22, 24] which are recommended reading for all specialists treating IBD patients. Clinicians managing patients with IBD should consider implementing a systematic approach to support clinician and patient compliance with these guideline recommendations, such as screening and vaccination checklists, which have been shown to improve uptake [39, 40].

Identification and Treatment of Acute Infection

Relapse of IBD is clearly associated with intercurrent infection. A number of studies suggest that infection, most commonly gastrointestinal infection, is present in approximately

Table 59.2 Recommended review of IBD patients prior to initiation of immunomodulatory therapy (see also [9, 17])

Detailed interview
• History of travel and/or living in tropical areas or countries with endemic infections
• History of previous infections
– Bacterial
– VZV infection: age, reactivation to zoster?
– HSV infection: sites, frequency and severity of recurrences
– Fungal infections: oral and vaginal candidiasis, intertrigo, nail infections
• Risk of latent or active tuberculosis
– Country of origin, prolonged stay in countries where TB is endemic, history of contact with TB patients
– Prior BCG vaccination? (date)
– History of latent or active tuberculosis and treatment given
• Immunization status and documentation of vaccination (dates, number of doses, post-vaccination serology—if done)
– Tetanus, diphtheria, poliomyelitis, pneumococcus, meningococcus, BCG
– Rubella, measles, and mumps, hepatitis B[a], HPV
– Others?
• Future plans to travel abroad to endemic areas
Clinical examination
• Identification of systemic and/or local current infections
• Evaluation of dental status (dentist review)
• Gynecological visit and Pap smear (then regularly as per local screening guidelines)
Routine laboratory and other investigations
• Neutrophil count, lymphocyte count and, in the case of lymphopenia, CD4 lymphocyte count
• Urine analysis in patients with a history of urinary tract infection and urinary symptoms
• Serology
– VZV in patients without a clear history of varicella immunization
– HBV[a], HCV, CMV, and HIV serology
• In patients with chronic HCV or HBV infection, alanine aminotransferase (ALT) assay, and assessment of liver disease
• For patients having lived in tropical/endemic areas: *Strongyloides* serology, eosinophil count, and stool examination
• Tuberculin skin test (TST) or Interferon Gamma Release Assay (IGRA)—according to each country's specific guidelines
• Chest X-ray

[a]Patients with a history of hepatitis B vaccination should be tested for the presence of hepatitis B antibodies

10 % of disease relapses [41–43]. With acute presentations, a high index of suspicion is important as the symptoms and signs of typical infection may be attenuated due to the blunted immune response [17]. For example, stool testing for enteric pathogens should be a routine undertaking in patients who present with a relapse of IBD [6, 9]. Treatment of active infection might avoid inappropriate or unnecessary use of steroids or other immunomodulatory therapy [6].

A multidisciplinary approach to management from the patient's gastroenterologist, infectious diseases specialist and organ specific specialist(s) is ideal [17]. Decisions regarding the need for reduction or withdrawal of immunosuppressive therapy will vary, depending on the type of infection and available evidence [9]. While it is optimal to withdraw certain therapies, particularly corticosteroids, in the setting of most types of infections, in certain situations, such as non-serious bacterial infections, a response to appropriate treatment without change in immunomodulatory therapy may occur.

Patient Education

Patient education is essential to minimizing the risk of infectious diseases [9, 17]. Patients should be counseled regarding early recognition of symptoms and presentation for medical care. Advice regarding the avoidance of high-risk foods, such as unpasteurized milk, soft cheeses and cold meats (for *Listeria*), and raw or undercooked poultry/eggs (for *Salmonella*), is also important. As discussed in detail below, the risk of vaccine preventable diseases (VPD) and the benefits of vaccination for both the patient and their family need to be explained. It is very important that IBD patients are provided with travel advice, around both infection risk and specific and appropriate preventative measures for their intended destinations, as well as vaccination (see below).

Specific Infections

Site-Specific Infections

Skin, respiratory tract and urinary tract infections are all more likely in those with IBD. For example, patients with CD appear to be at increased risk of urinary tract infections [12, 44], possibly related to the transmural and fistulating nature of their disease. There is a risk of post-operative infections, such as surgical site infection, pneumonia, or catheter-related infection, which appears particularly high in patients on concurrent and high-dose corticosteroids [11, 13, 45, 46]. Other specific sites for more occult bacterial infections, such as bone/joint and dental sites, need to be considered in ill patients [47].

Viral Infections

Herpes Viruses (Cytomegalovirus, Herpes Simplex Viruses, Varicella-Zoster Virus, and Epstein–Barr Virus)

These human herpes viruses are all unique for their ability to exist in a state of latency in human tissues following primary infection, and the potential to reactivate, with or without disease sequelae. In immunocompromised patients, including those with IBD, severe and disseminated herpes virus infections have been reported. For example, primary infection or reactivation of cytomegalovirus (CMV) can cause disease in almost any organ in immunosuppressed patients. CMV mimicking an acute exacerbation of IBD has been associated with increased morbidity, mortality and surgical intervention [48, 49]. Not all CMV reactivation results in clinical disease and because of the high prevalence of infection, screening for CMV infection prior to introducing immunomodulatory therapy is not recommended [9]. Use of antiviral therapy (such as ganciclovir) is recommended for severe or systemic disease, together with reduction or discontinuation of immunomodulatory therapy [9].

More frequent and severe reactivation of herpes simplex virus (HSV) infection is reported in IBD patients, particularly those on multiple immunosuppressives [9, 10]. Serological screening for past infection is not necessary. However, antiviral treatment of acute disease (using acyclovir, famcyclovir, and valacyclovir) in high-risk patients should occur, and preemptive or prophylactic therapy can also be considered in patients with frequent or severe recurrences [9].

Varicella-zoster virus (VZV) is characterized by its ability to cause more severe primary infection (chickenpox), or to reactivate to cause herpes zoster with greater frequency or morbidity, in immunocompromised hosts [47]. Morbidity and mortality from VZV disease has been reported in IBD patients on immunosuppressive agents, particularly anti-TNF therapy [50–53]. Although antiviral therapy can be helpful in ameliorating disease, prevention via vaccination, ideally prior to immunosuppression, is recommended (see vaccination section below).

Severe clinical Epstein–Barr virus (EBV) infection has been reported in patients with IBD, but EBV is more notably associated with lymphoproliferative disease, particularly primary intestinal lymphoma, due to impaired T-cell immunosurveillance, in immunocompromised patients [54, 55]. Screening prior to initiation of immunomodulatory therapy should be considered, although seroprevalence is high and frequent, usually self-limited or subclinical, reactivation can occur [20].

Viral Hepatitis and Human Immunodeficiency Virus Infection

Two large cohort studies found that most HBV infected patients who had reactivation in the context of IBD therapy were on two or more immunomodulators and/or had detectable HBV-DNA, as well as not receiving antiviral prophylaxis [9, 56, 57]. Screening for preexisting hepatitis B infection is essential in IBD patients; guidelines have been published for the treatment of hepatitis B infection with advice on management of immunosuppressive therapy in IBD patients [9, 22]. Antiviral therapy, regardless of the extent of viremia, is recommended before, during and after immunomodulator treatment, in patients who are hepatitis B surface antigen positive [9, 34].

In patients with preexisting hepatitis C infection, use of immunomodulators including TNF inhibitors appears relatively safe; however, more data are needed [47]. Antiviral therapy for hepatitis C infection may increase toxicity of drugs used for management of IBD, and thus should be used with caution [9]. Similarly, patients with preexisting HIV infection and IBD have not been well studied, and management of HIV should probably be commenced according to usual protocols initially [17]. Most patients, particularly those stabilized on highly active antiretroviral therapy (HAART), can be treated with TNF inhibitors if required [9]. These viruses have not been identified as causing opportunistic infection in IBD patients; however, patients should take every step to prevent their acquisition.

Influenza and Other Viruses (Human Papillomavirus, JC Virus)

There is a lack of specific data on the incidence and severity of influenza in IBD patients. However, immunomodulatory therapy is generally considered to increase the risk of influenza complications, including secondary bacterial infection [9]. IBD patients are therefore recommended to have annual influenza vaccination [20]. In addition, IBD patients should be offered diagnostic testing and early treatment with antiviral agents (oseltamivir or zanamivir) for suspected influenza [20].

There is evidence of a higher incidence of HPV-related cervical dysplasia in female IBD patients, which emphasizes the need for regular cervical screening and vaccination (discussed below) [58, 59]. Reactivation of latent JC virus causing fatal progressive multifocal leukoencephalopathy (PML) has been described in immunosuppressed patients treated with biologics, including the monoclonal antibody against alpha-4 integrin (natalizumab) which has been used to treat refractory Crohn)'s disease. There are no screening tests, treatment or vaccination for this virus, which, although rare, highlights the potentially serious consequences of immunosuppressive therapy.

Bacterial Infections

As discussed earlier, enteric bacterial infections are associated with relapse of IBD, most commonly *Clostridium difficile*, *Campylobacter jejuni*, and *Salmonella* species. *C. difficile* particularly affects those with preexisting extensive colonic involvement, with UC patients infected more commonly than those with CD [6, 60]. Asymptomatic carriage rates in IBD patients appear higher than in the general population [60, 61]. There are high rates of detection at presentation, and recurrence rates ranging from 9 % to 57 % [60]. *C. difficile* infections are recognized to cause increased morbidity and mortality in IBD patients, including a need for surgical treatment; however, more data on risk factors and outcomes, including the association with IBD medications, are needed, particularly since the emergence of the hypervirulent strain B1NNAPI/027 [60, 61].

IBD patients are also considered to be at increased risk of invasive pneumococcal disease, and should be offered vaccination (discussed below). There is evidence for a strong relationship between TNF inhibitors and an increased risk for listeriosis, with age and concomitant use of other immunomodulatory medications playing a role. *Nocardia* species have also caused infections (skin, soft tissue, pulmonary and central nervous system) in patients on immunomodulatory therapy. Severe infection with other bacterial pathogens, such as *Legionella pneumophila* (causing atypical pneumonia or "Legionnaires' disease"), has also been reported in IBD patients on anti-TNF medications [9, 20].

Tuberculosis and Other Mycobacterial Infections

Tuberculosis (TB) affects nearly one-third of the world's population. The lifetime reactivation risk of latent infection (LTBI) is approximately 10%, but is almost certainly higher in immunocompromised persons [47]. Of interest is evidence emerging of the considerable overlap between susceptibility loci for IBD and mycobacterial infection and shared pathways between host responses to mycobacteria and those predisposing to IBD [2]. IBD patients appear to be at increased risk of reactivation of LTBI, on standard immunomodulatory therapy, with risk increased even further on anti-TNF therapy [17]. A Cochrane review of over 200 studies of the use of biologics given for any disease found that, overall, there was an almost fivefold increased risk of TB reactivation compared to controls (OR 4.68, 95% CI 1.18–18.60) [27]. TB reactivation has been seen particularly with infliximab, although other biologics including adalimumab may carry a similar risk [27, 47]. The likelihood of extrapulmonary and disseminated TB appears to be higher in patients on TNF inhibitors [9]. Two studies, in Spain and Japan, have demonstrated that screening for, and treating, LTBI prior to commencement of infliximab decreased the incidence of TB in patients with autoimmune diseases [9, 62, 63]. A thorough clinical history and examination, chest X-ray and screening test for LTBI (either by a tuberculin skin test [TST] or "Mantoux," and/or a blood sample for interferon gamma release assay [IGRA]) are essential prior to starting immunotherapy in IBD patients (see Table 59.2). Both of these methods of screening have limitations, however, and should be interpreted with caution and expert input, particularly in high-risk patients. Guidelines for treatment of LTBI, and of suspected or confirmed TB disease in immunocompromised patients, including those with IBD, have been published, and should be considered in consultation with specialist advice [9].

Parasitic and Fungal Infections

IBD patients also appear to be at increased risk of certain fungal and parasitic infections, although these are relatively rare overall. Histoplasmosis may lead to life-threatening illness in patients undergoing TNF therapy, but has mainly been identified in those who have lived in endemic areas [47]. Coccidioidomycosis also appears to occur more commonly in patients living in endemic areas who are on TNF therapy, but mostly as acute infection rather than reactivation [47]. *Cryptococcus neoformans* is another opportunistic fungal pathogen that can cause serious infections in immunocompromised patients. Infections with *Candida* species were among the most common identified in IBD patients on corticosteroids alone [10]. Invasive aspergillosis, due to this ubiquitous fungus, is predominantly seen in severely immunocompromised hosts. Aspergillosis has been reported in IBD patients using TNF inhibitors, although the exact risk has not been well defined [20].

Pneumocystis carinii (*jiroveci*) can cause severe pneumonia (PCP) in immunocompromised patients, with risk factors including older age, coexisting pulmonary disease and lymphopenia, although the overall incidence is low at 10.6 per 100,000 [64]. In a review of over 5500 patients in Australia and New Zealand, PCP occurred most commonly within the first few months of taking combination therapy [38]. Antibiotic prophylaxis should be strongly considered for patients with lymphopenia, and in those taking TNF inhibitors, high dose corticosteroids or a calcineurin inhibitor [6, 9, 64, 65].

The risks for parasitic infections, such as *Toxoplasma gondii* and *Strongyloides stercoralis*, have not been well quantified, but both these organisms are known to cause severe disease in immunocompromised hosts. Toxoplasmosis most commonly presents as a focal encephalitis, and has been reported in IBD patients on immunomodulatory therapy [20]. Infection with the nematode *Strongyloides stercoralis* is common in developing countries with poor sanitation. Reactivation of infection in immunocompromised hosts can cause disseminated disease, with a high case fatality rate. Screening and preemptive therapy are recommended for those from endemic areas (see Table 59.2).

Vaccine Preventable Diseases and Responses to Immunization

A number of the infections detailed above are vaccine preventable diseases (VPD). The key factors that contribute to increased risk of VPD in IBD patients are described above and are also depicted in Fig. 59.1. This section will review the utility, immunogenicity and safety of vaccines in IBD patients, and present strategies for optimizing immunization in these patients. This includes reviewing and documenting

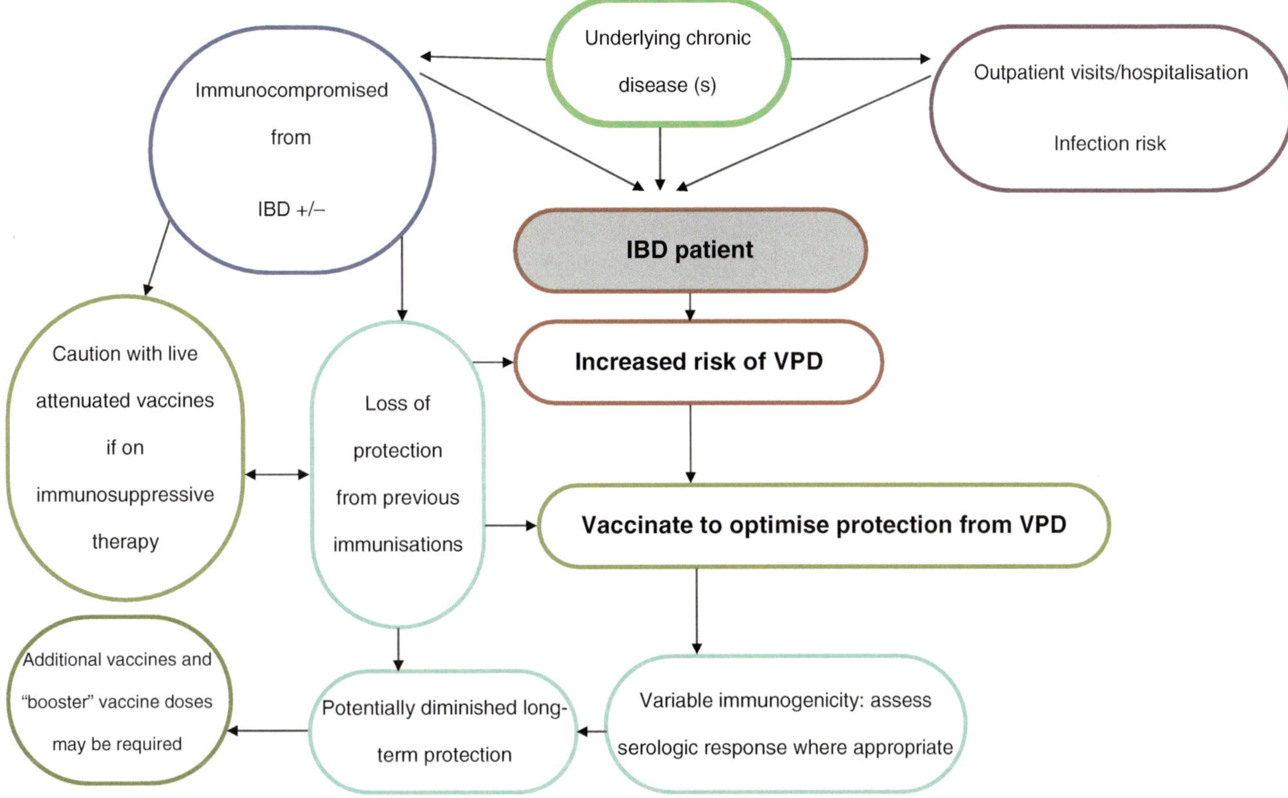

Fig. 59.1 Key factors contributing to increased risk of vaccine preventable diseases (VPD) in IBD patients. Adapted from Crawford et al. Expert Review of Vaccines. 2011;10(2):175–86 (with permission)

vaccines already received, giving "booster" doses of vaccines that may have been previously)administered, and the use of additional vaccines to be considered in IBD patients.

Vaccines are categorized as inactivated (a killed or non-replicating whole or part of the organism or "antigen") or live attenuated (containing a modified or weakened form of the virus or bacteria, which actively replicates in the host to generate an immune response). Inactivated vaccines can be given to patients with IBD, even those on immunosuppressive therapy. Although there are some studies which suggest that the immune response to vaccination may be less optimal in patients with IBD than in healthy individuals, in other studies vaccine responses in IBD patients are not different to healthy controls. Overall, the immune response to vaccination is still very likely to provide significant protection in this vulnerable population.

Live attenuated viral vaccines, are generally considered to be contraindicated in patients on immunosuppressive therapy, although there are some exceptions. For example, measles-mumps-rubella (MMR) vaccine should not be administered to IBD patients on immunosuppressive therapies due to the risk of unchecked vaccine virus replication causing disease [66]. There have been case reports of measles vaccine virus causing severe morbidity and mortality in patients taking immunosuppressive therapy. Other live attenuated vaccines, such as varicella, herpes zoster, and yellow fever vaccines, although generally not recommended, can be considered on a case by case basis, taking account of the specific vaccine and the patient characteristics detailed below. Household contacts of IBD patients should not be administered the live attenuated oral polio vaccine (OPV), but can receive inactivated polio vaccine (IPV). It is also recommended that household contacts are immunized against VPDs such as influenza, pertussis, and varicella to prevent disease transmission to IBD patients [67, 68].

Table 59.3 provides a summary of recommendations from current guidelines and expert reviews for many vaccines in IBD patients.

Vaccine Safety in IBD Patients

Inactivated vaccines in IBD patients are generally considered to have a similar safety profile to that in non-IBD patients [72]. The suggestion of a potential temporal association between vaccines and the onset of autoimmune diseases is long-standing, but the weight of evidence does not support a causative effect [73–75].

Table 59.3 Recommendations for immunization of IBD patients [alphabetical]

Vaccine preventable disease	Vaccine type	Recommendations for use in IBD patients[a] Based on US, European, and Australian guidelines and selected expert reviews [9, 67, 69–71]
Routine		
Diphtheria Tetanus Pertussis	Inactivated (also separate Tetanus, and Diphtheria/Tetanus vaccines)	Recommended in childhood, with boosters in adulthood (frequency depending on local guidelines)
Hepatitis B (also see hepatitis A vaccine below)	Inactivated	Routinely recommended at birth /in childhood in many countries. Check serology, and consider vaccination if non-immune (evidence for fulminant hepatitis B disease in immunosuppressed IBD patients)
Haemophilus influenzae type b (Hib)	Inactivated	Routinely recommended in childhood in some countries. Consider single dose if not given in childhood
Human papillomavirus	Inactivated	Routinely recommended in childhood in some countries. Serology not useful in clinical setting. Consider vaccination if age-eligible and not previously vaccinated
Influenza	Inactivated or Live attenuated intranasal	Recommended annually in IBD patients. Use inactivated vaccine
Measles Mumps Rubella	Live attenuated (also available as single Measles, Rubella and Measles/Rubella vaccines)	Routinely recommended in childhood. Two doses needed for adequate protection. Do not use in significantly immunosuppressed IBD patients
Meningococcal	Inactivated (conjugated, recombinant multicomponent and polysaccharide formulations with different serotypes)	Conjugate vaccines recommended routinely in some countries. Consider use of conjugate vaccine (4-valent) and/or use of recombinant meningococcal B vaccine, depending on local epidemiology and/or travel
Pneumococcal	Inactivated (conjugated and polysaccharide formulations with different serotypes)	Routinely recommended in childhood in some countries. Additional doses and/or primary vaccination recommended in IBD patients. Recommendations for use and number of doses of conjugate (7-valent, 10-valent, or 13-valent) or polysaccharide (23-valent) vary by country
Poliomyelitis	Inactivated trivalent (IPV) or oral live attenuated (OPV)	Routinely recommended in childhood. Serology not required. If booster indicated use IPV. OPV contraindicated in immunosuppressed patients and their household contacts
Rotavirus	Oral live attenuated	Only indicated for infants. Not applicable for IBD patients
Varicella Herpes zoster	Live attenuated Live attenuated (high titer VZV)	Both vaccines contraindicated in immunosuppressed patients. Check serology for previous natural VZV infection. If negative, and not previously immunized, varicella vaccine can be considered if not immunosuppressed (adolescents and adults need 2-dose schedule). Zoster vaccine for use in those aged >50 years
Travel-related and other selected vaccines		
Hepatitis A	Inactivated	Routinely recommended in childhood in some countries. Recommended for travellers to hepatitis A endemic countries. Consider for IBD patients

(continued)

Table 59.3 (continued)

Vaccine preventable disease	Vaccine type	Recommendations for use in IBD patients[a] Based on US, European, and Australian guidelines and selected expert reviews [9, 67, 69–71]
Typhoid fever	Oral live attenuated or inactivated	For travel/residence in endemic areas. Use inactivated (Vi polysaccharide vaccine), not oral live attenuated
Yellow fever	Live attenuated	Contraindicated in immunosuppressed. Waiver for certificate of vaccination for travel is available for medically ineligible persons. Need alternative measures to protect against mosquito bites or consider not travelling to YF endemic areas
Cholera	Inactivated	Rarely indicated. Efficacy modest
Japanese encephalitis	Inactivated	Recommended for travel/prolonged stay in endemic areas
Rabies	Inactivated	Not generally indicated in IBD patients
BCG (Bacillus Calmette-Guérin)	Live attenuated	Contraindicated in immunosuppressed. BCG efficacious for protection against severe TB when given in infancy. Not indicated in IBD patients

[a]Based on selected country-based guidelines and reviews. Country-specific immunization guidelines should also be consulted

In addition, a number of studies have investigated the temporal link between immunization and the onset of autoimmune conditions, such as multiple sclerosis and rheumatoid arthritis, with no link found [76, 77].

Although there have been case reports of flares of disease activity post vaccination, including UC flares post influenza vaccine [78], overwhelmingly the data available from well-designed controlled studies does not support a causal relationship between vaccination and disease flares. Some of this evidence comes from vaccine immunogenicity and safety trials in the IBD population [79–83].

Although no large observational studies in IBD have been performed studies of vaccination and disease relapse in patients with rheumatoid arthritis, systemic lupus erythematosis and multiple sclerosis have not shown any evidence for an association [84, 85]. It is important that exacerbations of chronic diseases are included as conditions of interest for vaccine post-marketing surveillance, using appropriate active surveillance methodologies at a population level [86].

Strategies to Promote Immunization

Although there is increasing awareness among gastroenterologists of the increased risk of VPD [18] low levels of vaccine coverage have been found in outpatient surveys of IBD patients [87]. This emphasizes the important role of gastroenterologists in recommending and, when possible, planning for and delivering vaccines to the IBD population [88]. One survey of adult gastroenterologists found that 39 % (17 out of 44) of respondents did not routinely vaccinate IBD patients [89]. Many respondents only reviewed whether routine childhood vaccinations were up to date, and only 11 % clarified vaccination status prior to TNF inhibitor use. Even if vaccination is a shared care responsibility between the patient's primary care doctor and gastroenterologist, close collaboration and communication between all physicians is essential. The use of electronic reminder systems and "flags" has been identified as one method to clarify the immunization status and make a vaccination plan [18, 89]. Implementation of an IBD patient-specific screening tool based upon established guidelines can also increase the proportion of patients who undergo recommended screening and vaccination [40]. Individual patient vaccination plans should take into account existing guidelines relevant to the patient's location, and also account for any preexisting risk factors [72].

Assessment of Immunization Status in IBD Patients

All immunization guidelines have in common the recommendation that IBD patients should be reviewed at diagnosis to ensure that all routine vaccinations have been received according to their local immunization schedule [72]. Consideration should also be given to additional vaccines, such as pneumococcal, influenza (annual), varicella, and HPV vaccines, and other immunizations depending on the availability and national schedule [67, 69, 72, 90]. The few published studies on compliance with immunization guidelines in IBD patients suggest that vaccine coverage among

IBD patients is low and not well documented [40, 88]. A US survey of 169 adolescents and adults diagnosed with IBD attending an IBD specialty clinic identified that 86 % were on immunosuppressive therapies [88]. On recall of immunization status, only 28 % of patients reported having received influenza vaccine and 9 % pneumococcal vaccine. Serological assessment for hepatitis B virus indicated that only 47 (28 %) had been vaccinated. This study also found most patients (81 %) had a history of varicella (chickenpox) but 31 patients were uncertain and only 12 reported varicella vaccination, leaving 19 (11 %) potentially "at risk" of varicella infection [88]. In these 19 patients, seven had varicella serology performed and 57 % (four out of seven) were confirmed to be seronegative.

One of the difficulties in obtaining a good vaccination history at IBD diagnosis is relying on recall as a measure of vaccination status. In a number of studies self-reporting of vaccination status has been found to be a relatively sensitive tool, but of low specificity. A cross-sectional survey of patients of a US Veteran Affairs Medical Center found self-reported influenza vaccination had a sensitivity of 1.0 and specificity of 0.79. Self-reported pneumococcal vaccination status had a sensitivity of 0.97 and a specificity of 0.53. This may reflect the fact that influenza vaccine is recommended annually and recalled more readily, whereas other vaccines, such as pneumococcal polysaccharide vaccine, may have been administered a number of years previously and forgotten [91]. Similarly, an Australian hospital-based study of nearly 5000 adults aged ≥65 years had high sensitivity (98 %) for self-reported influenza vaccination status but low specificity (56 %) [92]. This highlights that vaccine history needs to be carefully clarified and should be verified whenever possible with the patient's primary care provider. While there are some population-based immunization registers, they exist variably in most regions of the world, and are often for children rather than adults [93].

Role of Serologic Testing

In certain instances, serology can be used to measure the response to vaccination; however, the tests performed are laboratory dependent and may only be suitable for use as a research tool, or for detecting antibody from prior natural infection (not vaccination). Serology can be helpful, such as when there is a clear correlate of protection, such as the presence of hepatitis B surface antibody 6 weeks post hepatitis B vaccination. Other vaccine antibody responses for which routine serology is generally considered reliable as a test of seroconversion (and likely protection) include measles, mumps, and tetanus. However, for most VPD, even the best serologic marker does not provide a strict correlate of protection, and so, if doubt exists as to whether a patient has previously had the recommended number of vaccine doses, revaccination is generally recommended. Individual physicians may consider using serology to guide decision making regarding vaccination of IBD patients for VPD such as varicella [88, 94].

Maternal Vaccination and IBD

Inflammatory bowel disease in pregnancy is increasingly identified as an important area of management [95]. Pregnancy is also a time of increased risk of vaccine preventable diseases such as influenza [96] so optimizing protection via vaccination is important. Other vaccines that can be administered in pregnancy include pertussis, both to protect the mother and the infant [97]. If female IBD patients are on biologics during pregnancy, it is important to avoid live vaccines in infants for the first 6 months, particularly BCG vaccine as there is a risk of infant mortality [9, 98, 99].

Vaccines for IBD Patients

Hepatitis A Vaccine

Hepatitis A is an important vaccine preventable disease, with protection recommended in medical conditions such as IBD [9, 100]. A two-dose schedule at 0 and 6–12 months is recommended and may be administered as a combined hepatitis A–hepatitis B vaccine (see Table 59.3) [101]. The serum immune response to hepatitis A vaccine is adequate in some studies [102] but in others is reduced in patients on two or more immunosuppressive agents (92.6 % [50/54] versus 98.4 % [359/365], $p=0.03$) [103].

Hepatitis B Vaccine

There is a risk of reactivation of hepatitis B infection with the use of immunosuppressive therapies in IBD as detailed above [104–107], so excluding latent infection and ensuring satisfactory response to hepatitis B vaccination in patients with IBD is crucial and should be conducted at diagnosis. Populations vary widely in the seroprevalence of hepatitis B, which is impacted by both disease epidemiology in the country of residence and vaccination policy. In one IBD outpatient serosurvey only 28 % had serological evidence of hepatitis B protection [88]. Similarly, a detailed hepatitis status review of 315 IBD patients (252 Crohn's)disease and 63 ulcerative colitis) who had been vaccinated as part of the routine immunization schedule in France years earlier revealed an adequate post-vaccination anti-Hep B surface antibody (anti-HepBsAb of >10 IU/mL) in 49 % of patients

[105]. In a multivariate analysis, age at diagnosis of >31 years ($p=0.005$) and disease duration of >7 years ($p=0.005$) were associated with a lack of effective vaccination protection [105]. This was similar to a cross-sectional multicenter study in Spain [108]. The response has also been found to be lower in individuals with long-term IBD progression, low serum albumin levels, and corticosteroid therapy [109].

Importantly, a high proportion of IBD patients with protective anti-HepB surface antibody titers can lose them over time, with one study finding 18 % loss of protection per patient year of follow-up and threefold higher in those on anti-TNF therapy [110].

As a non-live vaccine, hepatitis B vaccine can be given to IBD patients irrespective of whether they are receiving immunosuppressive therapy. Vaccination is generally in a three-dose course over a 6-month period [67, 69]. If a previously fully immunized person is shown to be non-immune, an additional "booster" dose should be administered, and confirmation of serological response (>10 mIU/mL) should be undertaken 4–6 weeks after the dose. If the patient continues to show non-response to a booster dose, strategies such as high dose vaccination, repeat boosting and/or intradermal administration can be considered, as these approaches have been successful in other high-risk populations such as hemodialysis patients [111]. A double dose of a combined hepatitis B vaccine is a strategy that has also been shown to improve seroconversion rates, with an OR of 4 (95 % CI 2–8; $p<0.001$) in multivariate analysis, compared with standard dosing [112].

Human Papillomavirus (HPV) Vaccine

Female IBD patients are at increased risk of HPV-related precancerous cervical changes [58, 59]. Approximately 70 % of cervical cancers are associated with HPV serotypes 16 and 18. Two other types, 6 and 11, are the major cause of anogenital warts [113]. There are two inactivated HPV vaccines available; both offer protection against types 16 and 18, with one also containing types 6 and 11. In healthy females both vaccines have been shown to be highly immunogenic and efficacious against cervical carcinoma-in-situ (CIN) ([114, 115], #54). Vaccination is also immunogenic in males and can protect against HPV-related cancers (anogenital and oropharyngeal) in males [116, 117].

The vaccines should ideally be administered before exposure to HPV through sexual contact; most national HPV vaccination programs)administer the vaccines between 9 and 13 years of age [67, 69]. Regular screening for cervical changes is still recommended for all women with IBD who have been vaccinated as vaccination does not protect against all cervical cancer causing strains.

There is currently no serological correlate of protection for HPV vaccines and follow-up has not been long enough to measure the impact on cervical cancer rates. HPV vaccines appear to be more immunogenic than natural infection and high antibody titers have persisted for greater than 6 years of follow-up of original trial patients [115, 118, 119]. In a study of 37 female IBD patients on immunosuppressive therapy, the quadrivalent HPV vaccine was immunogenic, with no serious adverse events reported [120].

The vaccine has also been shown to be immunogenic in females with pediatric rheumatological conditions on biologic therapies [121].

Influenza Vaccine

As the risk of morbidity and mortality from influenza infection is higher in IBD patients [9], it is universally recommended they receive an annual inactivated (non-live) seasonal trivalent influenza vaccine [67, 69]. If the diagnosis of IBD is made in childhood (<9 years of age) and the child has not previously received at least two doses of influenza vaccine (<9 years of age) it is recommended they receive two doses in the first year they receive the vaccine (minimum 1 month apart) and then annual vaccination thereafter [67, 69].

The response to influenza vaccine in patients receiving immunomodulatory therapy appears variable. One study of the trivalent influenza vaccine (TIV) in 146 IBD patients found better immunogenicity against A/H1N1 and A/H3N2 than the B strain ($p<0.02$), independent of immunosuppression status, although anti-TNF therapy diminished the response to one of the three vaccine strains [81]. Anti-TNF therapy was also associated with a reduced response to the pandemic influenza A H1N1/09 vaccine [122].

Other studies have found immunosuppressive treatment impacts on influenza vaccine immunogenicity response in IBD patients [82]. In one study of 80 subjects (29 healthy controls, 50 IBD patients) the 16 patients receiving infliximab and immunomodulatory therapy were less likely to respond to two influenza vaccine antigens (A/New Caledonia/20/99 and B/Hong Kong/330/2001 ($p=0.018$ and $p=0.0002$, respectively). This decreased immunogenicity may potentially be overcome in selected circumstances by administering an additional dose of vaccine, as seen in some special risk group studies of pandemic H1N1 vaccination [123].

Studies to specifically assess efficacy of the trivalent influenza vaccine (TIV) in preventing influenza disease are generally lacking in special risk groups, including patients with IBD [124]. One small randomized trial in HIV ($N=103$) patients found a high efficacy in those receiving TIV [125]. This study, as with many immunogenicity trials in high-risk groups such as IBD patients, was limited by a small sample size and highlights the need for further research including new vaccine delivery methods, such as intradermal vaccination, that could potentially be more immunogenic and hence produce better clinical protection [126, 127]. New vaccine adjuvants may also prove to be more immunogenic in immunocompromised patients such as those with IBD [126, 127].

Measles Vaccine

Protection against measles is variable in IBD patients. One serosurvey found that only 30 % of patients were seropositive [128] and a German study demonstrated that 45 % of IBD patients had not been vaccinated against measles [129].

The ideal time to review protection from measles is at diagnosis and before commencement of any immunosuppressive therapies. A two-dose schedule (minimum 1 month apart) is recommended if not previously vaccinated and can be administered as combined measles–mumps–rubella (MMR) vaccine (see Table 59.3).

It is generally contraindicated to administer primary vaccine doses in immunosuppressed patients, but booster MMR doses have been safely administered in rheumatology patients on biologic therapies [130].

Meningococcal Vaccines

Up to 25 % of IBD patients are diagnosed in adolescence or early adulthood [131] and the incidence in the pediatric population is increasing [132]. The risk of meningococcal disease is highest in this age group and many countries now recommend conjugate meningococcal vaccines, either against meningococcal C vaccine alone or the 4-valent (A, C, W135, Y) vaccine for adolescents [133]. Two vaccines are now also available to protect against meningococcal serogroup B, the most prevalent serogroup in a number of countries, including the UK and Australia [134–136]. Meningococcal B vaccines have been used as an outbreak control measure in US university outbreaks [137], and will be included on the routine immunization schedule for infants in the UK from 2016 onwards. The choice of vaccines against meningococcus should be guided by local disease epidemiology as endemic strains vary by setting [67].

Although there are no studies of the immunogenicity of meningococcal conjugate vaccines in IBD patients, a multicenter cohort study of JIA patients (aged 1–19 years) found the overwhelming majority were able to mount a satisfactory immune response, including patients on high dose immunosuppressive medication [138]. Importantly there was no increase in JIA disease activity or relapse frequency. Meningococcal vaccination, using vaccine(s) relevant for the local epidemiology should therefore be considered as part of standard prototection in both males and females with IBD.

Pertussis Vaccine

Bordetella pertussis (whooping cough) is an important VPD, that requires regular booster doses to ensure ongoing protection. Vaccination is now also recommended in a number of countries during pregnancy to provide protection for both the mother and infant. Pertussis infection in elderly patients with IBD can also cause significant morbidity [139].

A small study in 71 IBD patients, showed that those on immune modulators had an impaired response to pertussis vaccination [140]. Pertussis vaccines are also combined with diphtheria and tetanus, and should be considered in all IBD patients every 10 years.

Pneumococcal Vaccines

Vaccination against pneumococcal disease with conjugate vaccines (containing either 10 or 13 serotypes) is generally recommended for patients with IBD, depending on their age and past history of immunization [141, 142]. There is limited data specifically examining the use of these conjugate pneumococcal vaccines in IBD patients, but a study of juvenile idiopathic arthritis patients on biologic therapies showed excellent immunogenicity [143]. Children receiving anti-TNF inhibitors produced mean antibody titers above the threshold level, but had significantly lower titers against serotypes 4, 14 and 23F ($p<0.05$) than controls [143]. A recent study showed the 13-valent pneumococcal conjugate vaccine provided protection against community acquired pneumococcal pneumonia in older adults in the Netherlands [144].

In adults known to be at high risk of IPD, including IBD patients on immunosuppressive therapies, some guidelines recommend the pneumococcal polysaccharide vaccine (23vPPV) as well [67, 145]. However, the immunogenic response to the 23vPPV in patients on immunosuppressive therapies such as biologic agents is reduced [146]. Variable immunogenicity response to 23vPPV has also been seen in other high (special) risk groups such as patients with rheumatoid arthritis, again particularly those on combination therapies [147]. The 23vPPV vaccine should ideally be administered more than 6–12 months following a pneumococcal conjugate vaccine dose [141].

Varicella Vaccine

Live attenuated vaccines such as varicella must be considered with caution in patients who are immunosuppressed due to risk of unchecked vaccine virus replication and complications [148]. This needs to be balanced with the risk of wild-type varicella infection; in an adult IBD study using a detailed history and serological assessment, approximately 10 % were found to not be protected from varicella [88]. The best approach to preventing varicella in IBD patients is to review the clinical history and immunization status at diagnosis and, if unclear, undertake varicella serology, for evidence of past infection. Varicella vaccination should ideally be given as two doses (minimum 1 month apart), at least 4 weeks before commencing immunosuppressive therapy. This "window of opportunity" is becoming smaller with the earlier use of immunomodulatory therapy in IBD and may not always be possible [148].

A small case series of six children with IBD safely received varicella vaccination while on infliximab therapy [80]. However, larger prospective studies are required before varicella vaccination of persons [149]. Larger studies of live attenuated varicella vaccine have been conducted in other immunocompromised patients, such as children with leukemia on maintenance therapy. However, although the incidence of varicella and later herpes zoster was reduced, vaccine associated rash was common (40 %) and 4 % of patients required antiviral therapy [150]. At follow-up these children were found to have a decreased incidence of herpes zoster ($p<0.05$) [150, 151] but these studies did not lead to routine recommendations of varicella immunization in children on chemotherapy. In summary, the administration of live vaccines needs to be made on a case by case basis with input from gastroenterologists, infectious disease specialists and vaccinologists as required.

Zoster Vaccine

A high titer varicella-zoster virus (VZV) vaccine for the prevention of herpes zoster is now registered in many countries for persons >50 years of age who have previously had varicella infection. This booster dose stimulates cell-mediated immunity to suppress varicella virus reactivation, and hence the development of a "shingles" rash and associated neuralgia. In a single placebo-controlled trial of >38,000 healthy adults aged >60 years followed up with a median of 3.1 years, vaccination reduced the burden of illness due to herpes zoster by 61 % ($p<0.001$) [152]. It also reduced the incidence of post-herpetic neuralgia by 67 % ($p<0.001$) [152]. Ideally, the vaccine should be administered at least 4 weeks before immunosuppressive medication is commenced [153].

An inactivated herpes zoster subunit vaccine has shown high efficacy in a phase 3 clinic trial [154]. In over 15,000 healthy participants aged 50 years or older, overall vaccine efficacy against herpes zoster was 97.2 % (95 % CI 93.7–99.0; $p<0.001$). As an inactivated vaccine, this would not be contraindicated in immunosuppressed IBD patients. Evidence around immunogenicity and efficacy in special risk populations is required, but this vaccine may hold promise for IBD patients.

Future Studies of VPD and Vaccines

There is a requirement to derive more data on the immunogenicity, efficacy, and safety of vaccination in individuals with IBD, particularly those on immunosuppressive therapies. This needs to be collated with other special risk groups on similar therapeutic regimens, such as patients with arthritis on biologic therapies. Immune persistence studies will help determine whether "booster" doses are required in the future. More trials into novel vaccine delivery methods (e.g., intradermal influenza vaccine) [126] and increased valencies of currently available vaccines (e.g., pneumococcal conjugate vaccines) are required to optimize protection in vulnerable IBD patients.

Travel Vaccines

As IBD patients' quality of life improves with advances in disease-modifying therapies and nutritional strategies, more patients will travel. Travel may place IBD patients at risk of infections, including some additional vaccine preventable diseases. Physicians need to explore the destination of travel and provide opportunities for advice at least 4–6 weeks prior to travel (see Table 59.3) [155, 156].

Conclusions

Patients with IBD disease, particularly those on immunosuppressive therapies, are at increased risk of infection, including VPDs. The increased risk of infection in IBD patients impacts on their associated morbidity and mortality. Preventative medicine for IBD patients is crucial to improving quality of life [20]. This should include a comprehensive and ongoing risk assessment for infectious disease risk in all IBD patients that incorporates screening for and treatment of underlying infection(s), patient education, vaccination, chemoprophylaxis, and careful monitoring while on immunosuppressive therapy. Implementation of these preventative strategies will have an appreciable impact on the well-being of all IBD patients.

Acknowledgements A/Professor Kristine Macartney acknowledges Donna Armstrong, Edward Jacyna, and Catherine King for assistance with preparation of this chapter.

Conflict of interest: Murdoch Children's Research Institute research fund has received honoraria for NC sitting on a Wyeth/Pfizer advisory board for pneumococcal vaccines and presentations at conferences and NC investigator-led research project support from CSL for active surveillance of Guillain-Barré syndrome following H1N1 vaccination. KM reports no conflicts of interest

References

1. Baumgart DC, Sandborn WJ. Crohn's disease. Lancet. 2012;380(9853):1590–605. doi:10.1016/s0140-6736(12)60026-9.
2. Jostins L, Ripke S, Weersma RK, Duerr RH, McGovern DP, Hui KY, et al. Host-microbe interactions have shaped the genetic

architecture of inflammatory bowel disease [letter]. Nature. 2012;491(7422):119–24. doi:10.1038/nature11582.

3. Ananthakrishnan AN, McGinley EL. Infection-related hospitalizations are associated with increased mortality in patients with inflammatory bowel diseases. J Crohns Colitis. 2013;7(2):107–12. doi:10.1016/j.crohns.2012.02.015.
4. Jess T, Winther KV, Munkholm P, Langholz E, Binder V. Mortality and causes of death in Crohn's disease: follow-up of a population-based cohort in Copenhagen County, Denmark. Gastroenterology. 2002;122(7):1808–14.
5. Winther KV, Jess T, Langholz E, Munkholm P, Binder V. Survival and cause-specific mortality in ulcerative colitis: follow-up of a population-based cohort in Copenhagen County. Gastroenterology. 2003;125(6):1576–82.
6. Irving PM, Gibson PR. Infections and IBD. Nat Clin Pract Gastroenterol Hepatol. 2008;5(1):18–27.
7. Lichtenstein GR, Feagan BG, Cohen RD, Salzberg BA, Diamond RH, Price S, et al. Serious infection and mortality in patients with Crohn's disease: more than 5 years of follow-up in the TREAT™ registry. Am J Gastroenterol. 2012;107(9):1409–22. doi:10.1038/ajg.2012.218.
8. Aberra FN, Lichtenstein GR. Methods to avoid infections in patients with inflammatory bowel disease. Inflamm Bowel Dis. 2005;11(7):685–95.
9. Rahier JF, Magro F, Abreu C, Armuzzi A, Ben-Horin S, Chowers Y, et al. Second European evidence-based consensus on the prevention, diagnosis and management of opportunistic infections in inflammatory bowel disease. J Crohns Colitis. 2014;8(6):443–68. doi:10.1016/j.crohns.2013.12.013.
10. Toruner M, Loftus Jr EV, Harmsen WS, Zinsmeister AR, Orenstein R, Sandborn WJ, et al. Risk factors for opportunistic infections in patients with inflammatory bowel disease. Gastroenterology. 2008;134(4):929–36.
11. Aberra FN, Lewis JD, Hass D, Rombeau JL, Osborne B, Lichtenstein GR. Corticosteroids and immunomodulators: postoperative infectious complication risk in inflammatory bowel disease patients. Gastroenterology. 2003;125(2):320–7.
12. Karagozian R, Johannes RS, Sun X, Burakoff R. Increased mortality and length of stay among patients with inflammatory bowel disease and hospital-acquired infections. Clin Gastroenterol Hepatol. 2010;8(11):961–5.
13. Serradori T, Germain A, Scherrer ML, Ayav C, Perez M, Romain B, et al. The effect of immune therapy on surgical site infection following Crohn's disease resection. Br JSurg. 2013;100(8):1089–93. doi:10.1002/bjs.9152.
14. Hartman C, Eliakim R, Shamir R. Nutritional status and nutritional therapy in inflammatory bowel diseases. World J Gastroenterol. 2009;15(21):2570–8.
15. Colombel JF, Loftus Jr EV, Tremaine WJ, Egan LJ, Harmsen WS, Schleck CD, et al. The safety profile of infliximab in patients with Crohn's disease: the Mayo clinic experience in 500 patients. Gastroenterology. 2004;126(1):19–31.
16. Gershwin ME, Borchers AT, Keen CL. Phenotypic and functional considerations in the evaluation of immunity in nutritionally compromised hosts. J Infect Dis. 2000;182 Suppl 1:S108–114. doi:10.1086/315905.
17. Viget N, Vernier-Massouille G, Salmon-Ceron D, Yazdanpanah Y, Colombel JF. Opportunistic infections in patients with inflammatory bowel disease: prevention and diagnosis. Gut. 2008;57(4):549–58.
18. de Silva S, Devlin S, Panaccione R. Optimizing the safety of biologic therapy for IBD. Nat Rev Gastroenterol Hepatol. 2010;7(2):93–101.
19. Lichtenstein GR, Feagan BG, Cohen RD, Salzberg BA, Diamond RH, Chen DM, et al. Serious infections and mortality in association with therapies for Crohn's disease: TREAT registry. [Erratum appears in Clin Gastroenterol Hepatol. 2006 Jul;4(7):931]. Clin Gastroenterol Hepatol. 2006;4(5):621–30.
20. Culver EL, Travis SP. How to manage the infectious risk under anti-TNF in inflammatory bowel disease. Curr Drug Targets. 2010;11(2):198–218.
21. Garcia-Vidal C, Rodríguez-Fernández S, Teijón S, Esteve M, Rodríguez-Carballeira M, Lacasa JM, et al. Risk factors for opportunistic infections in infliximab-treated patients: the importance of screening in prevention. Eur J Clin Microbiol Infect Dis. 2009;28(4):331–7.
22. Papa A, Mocci G, Bonizzi M, Felice C, Andrisani G, De Vitis I, et al. Use of infliximab in particular clinical settings: management based on current evidence. Am J Gastroenterol. 2009;104(6):1575–86.
23. Ford AC, Peyrin-Biroulet L. Opportunistic infections with anti-tumor necrosis factor-α therapy in inflammatory bowel disease: meta-analysis of randomized controlled trials. Am J Gastroenterol. 2013;108(8):1268–76. doi:10.1038/ajg.2013.138.
24. Veereman-Wauters G, de Ridder L, Veres G, Kolacek S, Fell J, Malmborg P, et al. Risk of infection and prevention in pediatric patients with IBD: ESPGHAN IBD Porto Group commentary. J Pediatr Gastroenterol Nutr. 2012;54(6):830–7. doi:10.1097/MPG.0b013e31824d1438.
25. Bernatsky S, Hudson M, Suissa S. Anti-rheumatic drug use and risk of serious infections in rheumatoid arthritis. Rheumatology. 2007;46(7):1157–60.
26. Bongartz T, Sutton AJ, Sweeting MJ, Buchan I, Matteson EL, Montori V. Anti-TNF antibody therapy in rheumatoid arthritis and the risk of serious infections and malignancies: systematic review and meta-analysis of rare harmful effects in randomized controlled trials. JAMA. 2006;295(19):2275–85.
27. Singh JA, Wells GA, Christensen R, Tanjong Ghogomu E, Maxwell L, Macdonald JK, et al. Adverse effects of biologics: a network meta-analysis and Cochrane overview. Cochrane Database Syst Rev. 2011;2:CD008794.
28. Afif W, Loftus Jr EV. Safety profile of IBD therapeutics: infectious risks. Gastroenterol Clin North Am. 2009;38(4):691–709.
29. Irving PM, Gearry RB, Sparrow MP, Gibson PR. Review article: appropriate use of corticosteroids in Crohn's disease. Aliment Pharmacol Ther. 2007;26(3):313–29.
30. Connell WR, Kamm MA, Ritchie JK, Lennard-Jones JE. Bone marrow toxicity caused by azathioprine in inflammatory bowel disease: 27 years of experience. Gut. 1993;34(8):1081–5.
31. Lamers CB, Griffioen G, van Hogezand RA, Veenendaal RA. Azathioprine: an update on clinical efficacy and safety in inflammatory bowel disease. Scand J Gastroenterol Suppl. 1999;230:111–5.
32. Present DH, Meltzer SJ, Krumholz MP, Wolke A, Korelitz BI. 6-Mercaptopurine in the management of inflammatory bowel disease: short- and long-term toxicity. Ann Intern Med. 1989;111(8):641–9.
33. Arts J, D'Haens G, Zeegers M, Van Assche G, Hiele M, D'Hoore A, et al. Long-term outcome of treatment with intravenous cyclosporin in patients with severe ulcerative colitis. Inflamm Bowel Dis. 2004;10(2):73–8.
34. Morisco F, Castiglione F, Rispo A, Stroffolini T, Vitale R, Sansone S, et al. Hepatitis B virus infection and immunosuppressive therapy in patients with inflammatory bowel disease. Dig Liver Dis. 2011;43 Suppl 1:S40–48.
35. Wallis RS, Broder MS, Wong JY, Hanson ME, Beenhouwer DO. Granulomatous infectious diseases associated with tumor necrosis factor antagonists. Clin Infect Dis. 2004;38(9):1261–5.
36. Van Assche G, Van Ranst M, Sciot R, Dubois B, Vermeire S, Noman M, et al. Progressive multifocal leukoencephalopathy after natalizumab therapy for Crohn's disease. N Engl J Med. 2005;353(4):362–8.

37. D'Haens GR, Vermeire S, Van Assche G, Noman M, Aerden I, Van Olmen G, et al. Therapy of metronidazole with azathioprine to prevent postoperative recurrence of Crohn's disease: a controlled randomized trial. Gastroenterology. 2008;135(4):1123–9.
38. Lawrance IC, Radford-Smith GL, Bampton PA, Andrews JM, Tan PK, Croft A, et al. Serious infections in patients with inflammatory bowel disease receiving anti-tumor-necrosis-factor-alpha therapy: an Australian and New Zealand experience. J Gastroenterol Hepatol. 2010;25(11):1732–8.
39. Parker S, Chambers White L, Spangler C, Rosenblum J, Sweeney S, Homan E, et al. A quality improvement project significantly increased the vaccination rate for immunosuppressed patients with IBD. Inflamm Bowel Dis. 2013;19(9):1809–14. doi:10.1097/MIB.0b013e31828c8512.
40. Walsh AJ, Weltman M, Burger D, Vivekanandarajah S, Connor S, Howlett M, et al. Implementing guidelines on the prevention of opportunistic infections in inflammatory bowel disease. J Crohns Colitis. 2013;7(10):e449–456. doi:10.1016/j.crohns.2013.02.019.
41. Epple HJ. Therapy- and non-therapy-dependent infectious complications in inflammatory bowel disease. Dig Dis. 2009;27(4):555–9.
42. Mylonaki M, Langmead L, Pantes A, Johnson F, Rampton DS. Enteric infection in relapse of inflammatory bowel disease: importance of microbiological examination of stool. Eur J Gastroenterol Hepatol. 2004;16(8):775–8.
43. Navarro-Llavat M, Domenech E, Bernal I, Sanchez-Delgado J, Manterola JM, Garcia-Planella E, et al. Prospective, observational, cross-sectional study of intestinal infections among acutely active inflammatory bowel disease patients. Digestion. 2009;80(1):25–9.
44. Ben-Ami H, Ginesin Y, Behar DM, Fischer D, Edoute Y, Lavy A. Diagnosis and treatment of urinary tract complications in Crohn's disease: an experience over 15 years. Can J Gastroenterol. 2002;16(4):225–9.
45. Billioud V, Ford AC, Tedesco ED, Colombel JF, Roblin X, Peyrin-Biroulet L. Preoperative use of anti-TNF therapy and postoperative complications in inflammatory bowel diseases: a meta-analysis. J Crohns Colitis. 2013;7(11):853–67. doi:10.1016/j.crohns.2013.01.014.
46. Rosenfeld G, Qian H, Bressler B. The risks of post-operative complications following pre-operative infliximab therapy for Crohn's disease in patients undergoing abdominal surgery: a systematic review and meta-analysis. J Crohns Colitis. 2013;7(11):868–77. doi:10.1016/j.crohns.2013.01.019.
47. Raychaudhuri SP, Nguyen CT, Raychaudhuri SK, Gershwin ME. Incidence and nature of infectious disease in patients treated with anti-TNF agents. Autoimmun Rev. 2009;9(2):67–81.
48. Kishore J, Ghoshal U, Ghoshal UC, Krishnani N, Kumar S, Singh M, et al. Infection with cytomegalovirus in patients with inflammatory bowel disease: prevalence, clinical significance and outcome. J Med Microbiol. 2004;53(Pt 11):1155–60.
49. Papadakis KA, Tung JK, Binder SW, Kam LY, Abreu MT, Targan SR, et al. Outcome of cytomegalovirus infections in patients with inflammatory bowel disease. Am J Gastroenterol. 2001;96(7):2137–42.
50. Gupta G, Lautenbach E, Lewis JD. Incidence and risk factors for herpes zoster among patients with inflammatory bowel disease. Clin Gastroenterol Hepatol. 2006;4(12):1483–90.
51. Korelitz BI, Fuller SR, Warman JI, Goldberg MD. Shingles during the course of treatment with 6-mercaptopurine for inflammatory bowel disease. Am J Gastroenterol. 1999;94(2):424–6.
52. Mouzas IA, Greenstein AJ, Giannadaki E, Balasubramanian S, Manousos ON, Sachar DB. Management of varicella infection during the course of inflammatory bowel disease. Am J Gastroenterol. 1997;92(9):1534–7.
53. Vonkeman H, ten Napel C, Rasker H, van de Laar M. Disseminated primary varicella infection during infliximab treatment. J Rheumatol. 2004;31(12):2517–8.
54. Smith MA, Irving PM, Marinaki AM, Sanderson JD. Review article: malignancy on thiopurine treatment with special reference to inflammatory bowel disease. Aliment Pharmacol Ther. 2010;32(2):119–30. doi:10.1111/j.1365-2036.2010.04330.x.
55. Sokol H, Beaugerie L, Maynadié M, Laharie D, Dupas JL, Flourié B, et al. Excess primary intestinal lymphoproliferative disorders in patients with inflammatory bowel disease. Inflamm Bowel Dis. 2012;18(11):2063–71. doi:10.1002/ibd.22889.
56. Loras C, Gisbert JP, Minguez M, Merino O, Bujanda L, Saro C, et al. Liver dysfunction related to hepatitis B and C in patients with inflammatory bowel disease treated with immunosuppressive therapy. Gut. 2010;59(10):1340–6. doi:10.1136/gut.2010.208413.
57. Park SH, Yang SK, Lim YS, Shim JH, Yang DH, Jung KW, et al. Clinical courses of chronic hepatitis B virus infection and inflammatory bowel disease in patients with both diseases. Inflamm Bowel Dis. 2012;18(11):2004–10. doi:10.1002/ibd.22905.
58. Bhatia J, Bratcher J, Korelitz B, Vakher K, Mannor S, Shevchuk M, et al. Abnormalities of uterine cervix in women with inflammatory bowel disease. World J Gastroenterol. 2006;12(38):6167–71.
59. Kane S, Khatibi B, Reddy D. Higher incidence of abnormal Pap smears in women with inflammatory bowel disease. Am J Gastroenterol. 2008;103(3):631–6.
60. Musa S, Thomson S, Cowan M, Rahman T. *Clostridium difficile* infection and inflammatory bowel disease. Scand J Gastroenterol. 2010;45(3):261–72.
61. Berg AM, Kelly CP, Farraye FA. *Clostridium difficile* infection in the inflammatory bowel disease patient. Inflamm Bowel Dis. 2013;19(1):194–204. doi:10.1002/ibd.22964.
62. Carmona L, Gomez-Reino JJ, Rodriguez-Valverde V, Montero D, Pascual-Gomez E, Mola EM, et al. Effectiveness of recommendations to prevent reactivation of latent tuberculosis infection in patients treated with tumor necrosis factor antagonists. Arthritis Rheum. 2005;52(6):1766–72.
63. Takeuchi T, Tatsuki Y, Nogami Y, Ishiguro N, Tanaka Y, Yamanaka H, et al. Postmarketing surveillance of the safety profile of infliximab in 5000 Japanese patients with rheumatoid arthritis. Ann Rheum Dis. 2008;67(2):189–94.
64. Long MD, Farraye FA, Okafor PN, Martin C, Sandler RS, Kappelman MD. Increased risk of *Pneumocystis jiroveci* pneumonia among patients with inflammatory bowel disease. Inflamm Bowel Dis. 2013;19(5):1018–24. doi:10.1097/MIB.0b013e3182802a9b.
65. Harigai M, Koike R, Miyasaka N. Pneumocystis pneumonia associated with infliximab in Japan [letter]. N Engl J Med. 2007;357(18):1874–6.
66. Monafo WJ, Haslam DB, Roberts RL, Zaki SR, Bellini WJ, Coffin CM. Disseminated measles infection after vaccination in a child with a congenital immunodeficiency. J Pediatr. 1994;124(2):273–6.
67. Australian Technical Advisory Group on Immunisation (ATAGI). The Australian immunisation handbook. 10th ed. Canberra: Australian Government Department of Health and Ageing; 2013.
68. Kappagoda C, Shaw PJ, Burgess MA, Botham SJ, Cramer LD. Varicella vaccine in non-immune household contacts of children with cancer or leukaemia. J Paediatr Child Health. 1999;35(4):341–5.
69. Advisory Committee on Immunization Practices (ACIP). (2011, January). General recommendations on immunization Retrieved March 4, 2011, from http://www.cdc.gov/vaccines/pubs/ACIP-list.htm
70. Rahier JF, Moutschen M, Van Gompel A, Van Ranst M, Louis E, Segaert S, et al. Vaccinations in patients with immune-mediated inflammatory diseases. Rheumatology. 2010;49(10):1815–27.
71. Wasan SK, Baker SE, Skolnik PR, Farraye FA. A practical guide to vaccinating the inflammatory bowel disease patient. Am J Gastroenterol. 2010;105(6):1231–8.
72. Sands BE, Cuffari C, Katz J, Kugathasan S, Onken J, Vitek C, et al. Guidelines for immunizations in patients with inflammatory bowel disease. Inflamm Bowel Dis. 2004;10(5):677–92.

73. Demicheli V, Jefferson T, Rivetti A, Price D. Vaccines for measles, mumps and rubella in children. Cochrane Database Syst Rev. 2005;4, CD004407. doi:10.1002/14651858.CD004407.pub2.
74. Offit PA, Hackett CJ. Addressing parents' concerns: do vaccines cause allergic or autoimmune diseases? Pediatrics. 2003;111(3):653–9. doi:10.1542/peds.111.3.653.
75. Villumsen M, Jess T, Sørup S, Ravn H, Sturegård E, Benn CS, et al. Risk of inflammatory bowel disease following Bacille Calmette-Guérin and smallpox vaccination: a population-based Danish case-cohort study. Inflamm Bowel Dis. 2013;19(8):1717–24. doi:10.1097/MIB.0b013e318281f34e.
76. Bengtsson C, Kapetanovic MC, Källberg H, Sverdrup B, Nordmark B, Klareskog L, et al. Common vaccinations among adults do not increase the risk of developing rheumatoid arthritis: results from the Swedish EIRA study. Ann Rheum Dis. 2010;69(10):1831–3.
77. Scheller NM, Svanström H, Pasternak B, Arnheim-Dahlström L, Sundström K, Fink K, et al. Quadrivalent HPV vaccination and risk of multiple sclerosis and other demyelinating diseases of the central nervous system. JAMA. 2015;313(1):54–61. doi:10.1001/jama.2014.16946.
78. Kwon OS, Park YS, Choi JH, Kim SH, Song MH, Lee HH, et al. A case of ulcerative colitis relapsed by influenza vaccination. Korean J Gastroenterol. 2007;49(5):327–30.
79. Lee CK, Kim HS, Ye BD, Lee KM, Kim YS, Rhee SY, et al. Patients with Crohn's disease on anti-tumor necrosis factor therapy are at significant risk of inadequate response to the 23-valent pneumococcal polysaccharide vaccine. J Crohns Colitis. 2014;8(5):384–91. doi:10.1016/j.crohns.2013.09.022.
80. Lu Y, Bousvaros A. Varicella vaccination in children with inflammatory bowel disease receiving immunosuppressive therapy. J Pediatr Gastroenterol Nutr. 2010;50(5):562–5.
81. Lu Y, Jacobson DL, Ashworth LA, Grand RJ, Meyer AL, McNeal MM, et al. Immune response to influenza vaccine in children with inflammatory bowel disease. Am J Gastroenterol. 2009;104(2):444–53.
82. Mamula P, Markowitz JE, Piccoli DA, Klimov A, Cohen L, Baldassano RN. Immune response to influenza vaccine in pediatric patients with inflammatory bowel disease. Clin Gastroenterol Hepatol. 2007;5(7):851–6.
83. Rahier JF, Papay P, Salleron J, Sebastian S, Marzo M, Peyrin-Biroulet L, et al. H1N1 vaccines in a large observational cohort of patients with inflammatory bowel disease treated with immunomodulators and biological therapy. Gut. 2011;60(4):456–62. doi:10.1136/gut.2010.233981.
84. Confavreux C, Suissa S, Saddier P, Bourdès V, Vukusic S. Vaccinations and the risk of relapse in multiple sclerosis. N Engl J Med. 2001;344(5):319–26.
85. Stojanovich L. Influenza vaccination of patients with systemic lupus erythematosus (SLE) and rheumatoid arthritis (RA). Clin Dev Immunol. 2006;13(2-4):373–5.
86. Crawford NW, Clothier H, Hodgson K, Selvaraj G, Easton ML, Buttery JP. Active surveillance for adverse events following immunization. Expert Rev Vaccines. 2014;13(2):265–76. doi:10.1586/14760584.2014.866895.
87. Crawford N, Catto-Smith A, Oliver M, Cameron D, Buttery J. An Australian audit of vaccination status in children and adolescents with inflammatory bowel disease. BMC Gastroenterol. 2011;11(1):87.
88. Melmed GY, Ippoliti AF, Papadakis KA, Tran TT, Birt JL, Lee SK, et al. Patients with inflammatory bowel disease are at risk for vaccine-preventable illnesses. Am J Gastroenterol. 2006;101(8):1834–40.
89. Gupta A, Macrae FA, Gibson PR. Vaccination and screening for infections in patients with inflammatory bowel disease: a survey of Australian gastroenterologists. Intern Med J 2009. doi:10.1111/j.1445-5994.2009.02114.x [Epub ahead of print].
90. Department of Health United Kingdom. (2006). Immunisation against infectious disease—`The Green Book'. Chapter 7: Immunisation of individuals with underlying medical conditions. Retrieved March 4, 2011, from http://www.dh.gov.uk/en/publichealth/Healthprotection/Immunisation/Greenbook/index.htm
91. Mac Donald R, Baken L, Nelson A, Nichol KL. Validation of self-report of influenza and pneumococcal vaccination status in elderly outpatients. Am J Prev Med. 1999;16(3):173–7.
92. Skull SA, Andrews RM, Byrnes GB, Kelly HA, Nolan TM, Brown GV, et al. Validity of self-reported influenza and pneumococcal vaccination status among a cohort of hospitalized elderly inpatients. Vaccine. 2007;25(25):4775–83.
93. Hull BP, Deeks SL, McIntyre PB. The Australian Childhood Immunisation Register—a model for universal immunisation registers? Vaccine. 2009;27(37):5054–60.
94. Kopylov U, Levin A, Mendelson E, Dovrat S, Book M, Eliakim R, et al. Prior varicella zoster virus exposure in IBD patients treated by anti-TNFs and other immunomodulators: implications for serological testing and vaccination guidelines. Aliment Pharmacol Ther. 2012;36(2):145–50. doi:10.1111/j.1365-2036.2012.05150.x.
95. Beaulieu DB, Kane S. Inflammatory bowel disease in pregnancy. World J Gastroenterol. 2011;17(22):2696–701. doi:10.3748/wjg.v17.i22.2696.
96. Creanga AA, Johnson TF, Graitcer SB, Hartman LK, Al-Samarrai T, Schwarz AG, et al. Severity of 2009 pandemic influenza A (H1N1) virus infection in pregnant women. Obstet Gynecol. 2010;115(4):717–26. doi:10.1097/AOG.0b013e3181d57947.
97. Amirthalingam G, Andrews N, Campbell H, Ribeiro S, Kara E, Donegan K, et al. Effectiveness of maternal pertussis vaccination in England: an observational study. Lancet. 2014;384(9953):1521–8. doi:10.1016/s0140-6736(14)60686-3.
98. Cheent K, Nolan J, Shariq S, Kiho L, Pal A, Arnold J. Case report: Fatal case of disseminated BCG infection in an infant born to a mother taking infliximab for Crohn's disease. J Crohns Colitis. 2010;4(5):603–5. doi:10.1016/j.crohns.2010.05.001.
99. Mahadevan U, Wolf DC, Dubinsky M, Cortot A, Lee SD, Siegel CA, et al. Placental transfer of anti-tumor necrosis factor agents in pregnant patients with inflammatory bowel disease. Clin Gastroenterol Hepatol. 2013;11(3):286–92. doi:10.1016/j.cgh.2012.11.011.
100. Centers for Disease Control and Prevention (CDC). Vaccines that might be indicated for adults based on medical and other indications, United States, 2015. Retrieved July 22, 2015, from http://www.cdc.gov/vaccines/schedules/hcp/imz/adult-conditions.html
101. Urganci N, Kalyoncu D. Immunogenecity of hepatitis A and B vaccination in pediatric patients with inflammatory bowel disease. J Pediatr Gastroenterol Nutr. 2013;56(4):412–5. doi:10.1097/MPG.0b013e31827dd87d.
102. Radzikowski A, Banaszkiewicz A, Lazowska-Przeorek I, Grzybowska-Chlebowczyk U, Woś H, Pytrus T, et al. Immunogenecity of hepatitis A vaccine in pediatric patients with inflammatory bowel disease. Inflamm Bowel Dis. 2011;17(5):1117–24. doi:10.1002/ibd.21465.
103. Park SH, Yang SK, Park SK, Kim JW, Yang DH, Jung KW, et al. Efficacy of hepatitis A vaccination and factors impacting on seroconversion in patients with inflammatory bowel disease. Inflamm Bowel Dis. 2014;20(1):69–74. doi:10.1097/01.MIB.0000437736.91712.a1.
104. Biancone L, Pavia M, Del Vecchio Blanco G, D'Incà R, Castiglione F, De Nigris F. The Italian Group for the Study of the Colon and Rectum Hepatitis B and C virus infection in Crohn's disease. Inflamm Bowel Dis. 2001;7(4):287–94.
105. Chevaux J-B, Nani A, Oussalah A, Venard V, Bensenane M, Belle A, et al. Prevalence of hepatitis B and C and risk factors for nonvaccination in inflammatory bowel disease patients in Northeast France. Inflamm Bowel Dis. 2010;16(6):916–24.

106. Hou JK, Velayos F, Terrault N, Mahadevan U. Viral hepatitis and inflammatory bowel disease. Inflamm Bowel Dis. 2010;16(6):925–32.
107. Shale MJ. The implications of anti-tumour necrosis factor therapy for viral infection in patients with inflammatory bowel disease. Br Med Bull. 2009;92(1):61–77. doi:10.1093/bmb/ldp036.
108. Loras C, Saro C, Gonzalez-Huix F, Minguez M, Merino O, Gisbert JP, et al. Prevalence and factors related to hepatitis B and C in inflammatory bowel disease patients in Spain: a nationwide, multicenter study. [Erratum appears in Am J Gastroenterol 2009 Mar;104(3):801]. Am J Gastroenterol. 2009;104(1):57–63.
109. Sempere L, Almenta I, Barrenengoa J, Gutiérrez A, Villanueva CO, de-Madaria E, et al. Factors predicting response to hepatitis B vaccination in patients with inflammatory bowel disease. Vaccine. 2013;31(30):3065–71. doi:10.1016/j.vaccine.2013.04.059.
110. Gisbert JP, Villagrasa JR, Rodríguez-Nogueiras A, Chaparro M. Kinetics of anti-hepatitis B surface antigen titers after hepatitis B vaccination in patients with inflammatory bowel disease. Inflamm Bowel Dis. 2013;19(3):554–8. doi:10.1097/MIB.0b013e31827febe9.
111. Fabrizi F, Dixit V, Messa P, Martin P. Intradermal vs intramuscular vaccine against hepatitis B infection in dialysis patients: a meta-analysis of randomized trials. J Viral Hepat. 2010. doi:10.1111/j.1365-2893.2010.01354.x [Epub ahead of print].
112. Gisbert JP, Menchén L, García-Sánchez V, Marín I, Villagrasa JR, Chaparro M. Comparison of the effectiveness of two protocols for vaccination (standard and double dosage) against hepatitis B virus in patients with inflammatory bowel disease. Aliment Pharmacol Ther. 2012;35(12):1379–85. doi:10.1111/j.1365-2036.2012.05110.x.
113. Frazer IH, Cox JT, Mayeaux Jr EJ, Franco EL, Moscicki AB, Palefsky JM, et al. Advances in prevention of cervical cancer and other human papillomavirus-related diseases. Pediatr Infect Dis J. 2006;25(2 Suppl):S65–81.
114. Joura EA, Leodolter S, Hernandez-Avila M, Wheeler CM, Perez G, Koutsky LA, et al. Efficacy of a quadrivalent prophylactic human papillomavirus (types 6, 11, 16, and 18) L1 virus-like-particle vaccine against high-grade vulval and vaginal lesions: a combined analysis of three randomised clinical trials. Lancet. 2007;369(9574):1693–702.
115. The GlaxoSmithKline Vaccine HPV-007 Study Group. Sustained efficacy and immunogenicity of the human papillomavirus (HPV)-16/18 AS04-adjuvanted vaccine: analysis of a randomised placebo-controlled trial up to 6·4 years. Lancet. 2009;374(9706):1975–85.
116. Block SL, Nolan T, Sattler C, Barr E, Giacoletti KE, Marchant CD, et al. Comparison of the immunogenicity and reactogenicity of a prophylactic quadrivalent human papillomavirus (types 6, 11, 16, and 18) L1 virus-like particle vaccine in male and female adolescents and young adult women. Pediatrics. 2006;118(5):2135–45.
117. Giuliano AR, Palefsky JM, Goldstone S, Moreira Jr ED, Penny ME, Aranda C, et al. Efficacy of quadrivalent HPV vaccine against HPV Infection and disease in males. N Engl J Med. 2011;364(5):401–11.
118. Baylor NW, Wharton M. Efficacy data and HPV vaccination studies. JAMA. 2009;302(24):2658–9. doi:10.1001/jama.2009.1882.
119. Bonanni P, Boccalini S, Bechini A. Efficacy, duration of immunity and cross protection after HPV vaccination: a review of the evidence. Vaccine. 2009;27 Suppl 1:A46–53. doi:10.1016/j.vaccine.2008.10.085.
120. Jacobson DL, Bousvaros A, Ashworth L, Carey R, Shrier LA, Burchett SK, et al. Immunogenicity and tolerability to human papillomavirus-like particle vaccine in girls and young women with inflammatory bowel disease. Inflamm Bowel Dis. 2013;19(7):1441–9. doi:10.1097/MIB.0b013e318281341b.
121. Akikusa JD, Crawford NW. Vaccination in paediatric rheumatology. Curr Rheumatol Rep. 2014;16(8):432. doi:10.1007/s11926-014-0432-9.
122. Andrisani G, Frasca D, Romero M, Armuzzi A, Felice C, Marzo M, et al. Immune response to influenza A/H1N1 vaccine in inflammatory bowel disease patients treated with anti TNF-α agents: effects of combined therapy with immunosuppressants. J Crohns Colitis. 2013;7(4):301–7. doi:10.1016/j.crohns.2012.05.011.
123. de Lavallade H, Garland P, Sekine T, Hoschler K, Marin D, Stringaris K, et al. Repeated vaccination is required to optimise seroprotection against H1N1 in the immunocompromised host. Haematologica. 2010. doi:10.3324/haematol.2010.032664 [Epub ahead of print].
124. Kunisaki KM, Janoff EN. Influenza in immunosuppressed populations: a review of infection frequency, morbidity, mortality, and vaccine responses. Lancet Infect Dis. 2009;9(8):493–504.
125. Tasker SA, Treanor JJ, Paxton WB, Wallace MR. Efficacy of influenza vaccination in HIV-infected persons. Ann Intern Med. 1999;131(6):430–3.
126. Gelinck LB, van den Bemt BJ, Marijt WA, van der Bijl AE, Visser LG, Cats HA, et al. Intradermal influenza vaccination in immunocompromized patients is immunogenic and feasible. Vaccine. 2009;27(18):2469–74.
127. Morelon E, Noble CP, Daoud S, Cahen R, Goujon-Henry C, Weber F, et al. Immunogenicity and safety of intradermal influenza vaccination in renal transplant patients who were non-responders to conventional influenza vaccination. Vaccine. 2010;28(42):6885–90.
128. Naganuma M, Nagahori M, Fujii T, Morio J, Saito E, Watanabe M. Poor recall of prior exposure to varicella zoster, rubella, measles, or mumps in patients with IBD. Inflamm Bowel Dis. 2013;19(2):418–22. doi:10.1002/ibd.23027.
129. Wilckens V, Kannengiesser K, Hoxhold K, Frenkel C, Kucharzik T, Maaser C. The immunization status of patients with IBD is alarmingly poor before the introduction of specific guidelines. Scand J Gastroenterol. 2011;46(7-8):855–61. doi:10.3109/00365521.2011.574734.
130. Heijstek MW, Pileggi GC, Zonneveld-Huijssoon E, Armbrust W, Hoppenreijs EP, Uiterwaal CS, et al. Safety of measles, mumps and rubella vaccination in juvenile idiopathic arthritis. Ann Rheum Dis. 2007;66(10):1384–7. doi:10.1136/ard.2006.063586.
131. Beattie RM, Croft NM, Fell JM, Afzal NA, Heuschkel RB. Inflammatory bowel disease. Arch Dis Child. 2006;91(5):426–32.
132. Phavichitr N, Cameron DJ, Catto-Smith AG. Increasing incidence of Crohn's disease in Victorian children. J Gastroenterol Hepatol. 2003;18(3):329–32.
133. Centers for Disease Control and Prevention (CDC). Updated recommendations for use of meningococcal conjugate vaccines - Advisory Committee on Immunization Practices (ACIP), 2010. MMWR Morb Mortal Wkly Rep. 2011;60(3):72–6.
134. ClinicalTrials.gov. (2015). A trial to assess the safety, tolerability and immunogenicity of Repevax and rLP2086 vaccine when given together in healthy subjects aged >=11 to <19 years (NCT01323270). Retrieved July 22, 2015, from http://clinicaltrials.gov/ct2/show/NCT01323270?term=B1971010&rank=1
135. Snape MD, Pollard AJ. The beginning of the end for serogroup B meningococcus? Lancet. 2013;381(9869):785–7. doi:10.1016/S0140-6736(12)62194-1.
136. Vesikari T, Esposito S, Prymula R, Ypma E, Kohl I, Toneatto D, et al. Immunogenicity and safety of an investigational multicomponent, recombinant, meningococcal serogroup B vaccine (4CMenB) administered concomitantly with routine infant and child vaccinations: results of two randomised trials. Lancet. 2013;381(9869):825–35. doi:10.1016/S0140-6736(12)61961-8.
137. McNamara LA, Shumate AM, Johnsen P, MacNeil JR, Patel M, Bhavsar T, et al. First use of a serogroup B meningococcal vaccine in the US in response to a university outbreak. Pediatrics. 2015;135(5):798–804. doi:10.1542/peds.2014-4015.
138. Zonneveld-Huijssoon E, Ronaghy A, Van Rossum MAJ, Rijkers GT, Van Der Klis FRM, Sanders EAM, et al. Safety and efficacy

of meningococcal C vaccination in juvenile idiopathic arthritis. Arthritis Rheum. 2007;56(2):639–46.

139. Horton HA, Kim H, Melmed GY. Vaccinations in older adults with gastrointestinal diseases. Clin Geriatr Med. 2014;30(1):17–28. doi:10.1016/j.cger.2013.10.002.

140. Dezfoli S, Horton HA, Berel D, Targan SR, Vasiliauskas EA, Dubinsky M, et al. Immunomodulators, but not anti-TNF monotherapy, impair pertussis and tetanus booster vaccine responses in adults with inflammatory bowel disease (IBD) [abstract; Su2081]. Gastroenterology. 2012;142(5 Suppl 1):S564–565. doi:10.1016/S0016-5085(12)62169-6.

141. Centers for Disease Control and Prevention (CDC). (2014). Pneumococcal ACIP vaccine recommendations. Advisory Committee for Immunization Practices (ACIP). Retrieved July 22, 2015, from http://www.cdc.gov/vaccines/hcp/acip-recs/vacc-specific/pneumo.html

142. Steens A, Vestrheim DF, Aaberge IS, Wiklund BS, Storsaeter J, Riise Bergsaker MA, et al. A review of the evidence to inform pneumococcal vaccine recommendations for risk groups aged 2 years and older. Epidemiol Infect. 2014;142(12):2471–82. doi:10.1017/S0950268814001514.

143. Farmaki E, Kanakoudi-Tsakalidou F, Spoulou V, Trachana M, Pratsidou-Gertsi P, Tritsoni M, et al. The effect of anti-TNF treatment on the immunogenicity and safety of the 7-valent conjugate pneumococcal vaccine in children with juvenile idiopathic arthritis. Vaccine. 2010;28(31):5109–13.

144. Bonten MJM, Huijts SM, Bolkenbaas M, Webber C, Patterson S, Gault S, et al. Polysaccharide conjugate vaccine against pneumococcal pneumonia in adults. N Engl J Med. 2015;372(12):1114–25. doi:10.1056/NEJMoa1408544.

145. Centers for Disease Control and Prevention (CDC). Updated recommendations for prevention of invasive pneumococcal disease among adults using the 23-valent pneumococcal polysaccharide vaccine (PPSV23). JAMA. 2010;304(15):1660–2.

146. Melmed GY, Agarwal N, Frenck RW, Ippoliti AF, Ibanez P, Papadakis KA, et al. Immunosuppression impairs response to pneumococcal polysaccharide vaccination in patients with inflammatory bowel disease. Am J Gastroenterol. 2009;105(1):148–54.

147. Bingham 3rd CO, Looney RJ, Deodhar A, Halsey N, Greenwald M, Codding C, et al. Immunization responses in rheumatoid arthritis patients treated with rituximab: results from a controlled clinical trial. Arthritis Rheum. 2010;62(1):64–74.

148. Levin MJ. Varicella vaccination of immunocompromised children. J Infect Dis. 2008;197 Suppl 2:S200–206.

149. Galea SA, Sweet A, Beninger P, Steinberg SP, Larussa PS, Gershon AA, et al. The safety profile of varicella vaccine: a 10-year review. J Infect Dis. 2008;197 Suppl 2:S165–169.

150. Gershon AA, Steinberg SP. Persistence of immunity to varicella in children with leukemia immunized with live attenuated varicella vaccine. N Engl J Med. 1989;320(14):892–7. doi:10.1056/NEJM198904063201403.

151. Gershon AA, LaRussa P, Steinberg S, Mervish N, Lo SH, Meier P. The protective effect of immunologic boosting against zoster: an analysis in leukemic children who were vaccinated against chickenpox. J Infect Dis. 1996;173(2):450–3.

152. Oxman MN, Levin MJ, Johnson GR, Schmader KE, Straus SE, Gelb LD, et al. A vaccine to prevent herpes zoster and postherpetic neuralgia in older adults. N Engl J Med. 2005;352(22):2271–84. doi:10.1056/NEJMoa051016.

153. Cohen JI. Strategies for herpes zoster vaccination of immunocompromised patients. J Infect Dis. 2008;197 Suppl 2:S237–241. doi:10.1086/522129.

154. Lal H, Cunningham AL, Godeaux O, Chlibek R, Diez-Domingo J, Hwang S-J, et al. Efficacy of an adjuvanted herpes zoster subunit vaccine in older adults. N Engl J Med. 2015;372(22):2087–960. doi:10.1056/NEJMoa1501184.

155. Esteve M, Loras C, García-Planella E. Inflammatory bowel disease in travelers: choosing the right vaccines and check-ups. World J Gastroenterol. 2011;17(22):2708–14. doi:10.3748/wjg.v17.i22.2708.

156. Greveson K, Shepherd T, Mulligan JP, Hamilton M, Woodward S, Norton C. et al. Travel health and pretravel preparation in the patient with inflammatory bowel disease. Frontline Gastroenterol. 2015. doi:10.1136/flgastro-2014-100548 [Epub ahead of print].

Incidence of Cancer and Screening in Inflammatory Bowel Disease

60

Jimmy K. Limdi and Francis A. Farraye

Patients with long-standing ulcerative colitis (UC) or Crohn's colitis are at an increased risk for development of colorectal cancer (CRC). Although several risk factors for the development of CRC have been recognized, colitis-related dysplasia confers the greatest risk and colonoscopic surveillance to detect dysplasia has been advocated by gastrointestinal societies [1–9]. The goal of endoscopic surveillance is to reduce mortality and morbidity of CRC by either detecting and resecting dysplasia or detecting CRC at earlier and potentially curable stages [10]. Although recent literature has been conflicting on whether there have been changes in the risk of CRC in IBD patients, the majority of emerging studies from diverse population-based cohorts suggest that there has been a reduction in the risk of CRC in IBD patients [11–13]. The implementation of surveillance colonoscopy, allowing detection and endoscopic resection of dysplastic lesions before the development of CRC and appropriate timing of colectomy and more effective treatments resulting in mucosal healing may explain this temporal reduction [14].

Surveillance strategies have traditionally relied on examination of the mucosa with targeted biopsies of visible lesions and random biopsy sampling based on the presumption that dysplasia is frequently not associated with visible mucosal abnormalities [15, 16]. Meanwhile, advances in optical technology allowing for greater endoscopic resolution of dysplasia and consensus that most dysplasia in patients with IBD is visible, has led to a paradigm shift in the approach to surveillance and management of dysplasia [17, 18]. This chapter will review the epidemiology and risk factors for CRC in patients with IBD, outline the most recent surveillance guidelines from scientific societies, discuss the management of dysplasia and briefly summarize chemoprevention.

J.K. Limdi, M.B.B.S., F.R.C.P.
Division of Gastroenterology, The Pennine Acute Hospitals NHS Trust, Manchester, UK

Institute of Inflammation and Repair, University of Manchester, Manchester, UK
e-mail: jimmy.limdi@nhs.net

F.A. Farraye, M.D., M.Sc. (✉)
Department of Gastroenterology, Boston Medical Center, Boston University School of Medicine, 85 East Concord Street, Boston, MA, USA
e-mail: francis.farraye@bmc.org

Epidemiology

The association between IBD and CRC has been recognized for nearly 100 years since the first sigmoidoscopic descriptions of polyps in cancer in the setting of colitis in the 1920s [19]. The precise level of risk however remains unknown with controversy surrounding aspects of our current surveillance strategies for patients with IBD. Indeed, the traditional adenoma-carcinoma sequence, which forms the basis of surveillance strategies for sporadic CRC, does not apply to colitis-associated cancers [20, 21]. The pathogenesis of CRC in IBD is less certain and is believed to be a consequence of the cytokine milieu and free radicals associated with inflammation creating or superimposing upon molecular alterations [22]. Some features that distinguish the colitis-related CRC from sporadic CRC include:

1. An increased risk of CRC in patients with chronic colitis compared to the general population.
2. The rate of synchronous tumors in IBD is higher than in sporadic CRC [12 % versus 3–5 %] [23].
3. Absence of a preceding adenomatous lesion.
4. The dysplasia to carcinoma sequence may be accelerated compared to non-colitis patients with estimates running from 2 to 5 years [24]. Genetic alterations are similar to sporadic CRC but seem to occur in a different sequence, with p53 mutated early and APC and GSK3β mutations occurring late and over a shorter time frame [25].
5. Morphological features of CRC in IBD are more varied with serrated or flatter and often multifocal lesions affecting broad segments of mucosa.

The risk of CRC in IBD (and UC in particular) increases with time but risk estimates are difficult to quantify, often

D.C. Baumgart (ed.), *Crohn's Disease and Ulcerative Colitis*, DOI 10.1007/978-3-319-33703-6_60

handicapped by heterogeneity in the retrospective cohorts used in the analysis.

A large meta-analysis by Eaden et al. estimated a cumulative CRC risk of 2 % at 10 years, 8 % at 20 years and 18 % after 30 years of colitis [26]. Herrinton and colleagues in a closed health maintenance organization (HMO] study from Northern California found in excess CRC incidence and mortality in IBD patients similar to a previous population-based study from Olmsted County, Minnesota [13, 14]. It is noteworthy that adoption of surveillance colonoscopy in at-risk IBD patients from the HMO in Northern California was low although to what extent this was driven by patient choice or indeed physician practice is open to speculation [27]. A recent population-based study from Copenhagen County, Denmark, demonstrated a decreasing incidence of CRC in IBD patients over the last few decades [28]. A 40-year colonoscopic surveillance program from St. Mark's Hospital, UK reported a cumulative incidence of developing CRC in IBD patients at 0.1 % in the first decade since UC symptom onset, followed by 2.9 %, 6.7 % and 10 % by the second, third, and fourth decade respectively [29]. Of 1375 UC patients followed for 15,234 patient-years (median 11 years per patient) CRC was detected in 72 patients [28]. There was a significant decrease in the incidence of colectomy for dysplasia and a reduction in the incidence rate (IR) of advanced CRC and interval cancers over 4 decades of surveillance. Although IR for early CRC increased 2.5-fold in the current decade a high 10-year survival (79.6 %) was reported. Furthermore, IR of dysplasia was also noted to be increased, likely attributable to the use of chromoendoscopy which was noted to be twice as effective at dysplasia detection as white light endoscopy ($p<0.001$) [29]. The rate of progression from indefinite and low-grade dysplasia to cancer observed in high-risk cohorts from academic centers appears low even when variables such as primary sclerosing cholangitis and previous advanced dysplasia are factored in [30–33]. Such controversy notwithstanding, recent studies suggest a decrease in the risk of CRC in IBD, a temporal reduction that could be explained by more aggressive control of inflammation through medication, the greater uptake of surveillance colonoscopy allowing detection and resection of dysplastic lesions before the development of CRC and appropriate timing of colectomy [14, 34, 35].

The data is less clear in CD with many earlier studies having failed to adjust for variables such as disease location (colonic or small bowel), history of colonic resection or disease duration. In patients with Crohn's colitis who did not have a colectomy, an increased incidence of CRC has been noted [36–39]. In a large population-based study, Bernstein et al. confirmed an increased incidence of CRC in CD patients equal to the risk for UC patients [40]. A subsequent meta-analysis of 12 studies reported an overall CRC relative risk (RR) in CD patients of 2.5 (95 % CI, 1.3–4.7). The RR increased to 4.5 (95 % CI, 1.3–1.49) in patients with colonic Crohn's disease, but was less for ileal disease (RR 1.1, CI 0.8–1.5) [41]. The risk of developing CRC therefore appears to be equivalent in patients with Crohn's colitis and UC.

Risk Factors for CRC in IBD

Several risk factors are associated with increased risk of development of colorectal neoplasia in patients with IBD. These include young age of disease onset, longer duration of disease, extent of colitis, family history of CRC in a first-degree relative diagnosed before 50 years of age, personal history of primary sclerosing cholangitis (PSC), a personal history of dysplasia, stricturing disease in UC patients, active endoscopic or histological inflammation, inflammatory ("pseudo") polyps and possibly male gender [2–9, 42, 43]. Patients with subtotal colitis or pancolitis have the highest risk of developing CRC and patients with colonic CD disease involving more than a third of the colon are also at increased risk of CRC [36, 44, 45]. The extent of colonic involvement must be based on both endoscopic and histological criteria and on whichever reveals more extensive disease [2, 4, 46–48]. Although patients with proctitis or proctosigmoiditis alone are at no increased risk compared with the general population, many patients with proctitis will develop more proximal disease over the course of their lifetime and a screening colonoscopy is recommended 8 years after the onset of symptoms even in patients with previously isolated proctitis to confirm extent of disease [5, 44, 49, 50]. There is insufficient evidence to support the presence of backwash ileitis as an independent risk factor for developing CRC [2]. Longer duration of disease increases the risk of CRC; specifically the RR rises of 8–10 years of disease which forms the rationale behind the initiation of surveillance colonoscopy [28, 51].

A concurrent diagnosis of PSC is an indisputable risk factor for the development of CRC. A meta-analysis of 11 trials by Soetikno et al. reported a fourfold increased risk of developing colonic neoplasia patients with PSC and UC compared to those with UC alone [52]. In addition, several clinical trials have demonstrated a persistently elevated risk of CRC despite undergoing orthotopic liver transplantation [53–55]. Thus, patients with IBD and PSC should undergo surveillance colonoscopy annually beginning at the time PSC is diagnosed.

A family history of CRC in a first-degree relative under 50 years of age is a high-risk factor developing CRC in IBD patients. A case-control study of 297 patients from the Mayo Clinic found that a family history of CRC was twice as common in patients with UC and CRC compared to those patients with UC alone [56]. In another study by Askling and colleagues, family history of CRC was associated with a greater than twofold increased risk of CRC in patients with IBD [57]. Although disease duration has been proven to increase the risk of developing CRC, studies examining a link between early age of onset of IBD and CRC are conflicting. Thus, according to AGA guidelines, surveillance should be based on duration of illness, not chronological age [2]. A population-based cohort study of 7607 patients diagnosed with IBD assessed the sex-specific incidence of CRC and found that IBD confers a lower risk of CRC to females than to males [58].

The known risk factors for CRC in IBD are almost all nonmodifiable with the possible exception of inflammation [42, 43, 59]. In a case control study of 68 patients, Rutter and colleagues found that the degree of histological inflammation positively correlated with an increased risk of neoplasia [42]. A cohort study of 418 patients with UC found a positive association between degree of microscopic inflammation and advanced neoplasia [43]. Two other studies have similarly noted an increased risk of CRC in individuals with higher rates of endoscopic or histologic inflammation [59, 60]. Colonoscopic features such as strictures are considered a risk factor for CRC in UC but not in CD [60, 61]. A shortened tubular colon and multiple pseudopolyps also increase CRC risk, the latter also significantly limiting the ability to adequately survey the colon [62]. These clinically important associations should be considered when counseling a patient about their risk of developing CRC.

Surveillance

The goal of endoscopic surveillance is to reduce mortality and morbidity of CRC by either detecting and resecting dysplasia or detecting CRC at earlier and potentially curable stage [10]. Although no randomized controlled trials have evaluated the efficacy of surveillance colonoscopy, endoscopic surveillance has been shown to reduce the risk of death from CRC in the IBD population and also to be cost-effective in various case-series, case-control studies, and population-based cohort studies [11, 12, 63–66]. Thus, the invasive nature of colonoscopy and considerable utilization of societal resources notwithstanding, surveillance colonoscopy in IBD patients has been endorsed by multiple societies [2–9]. Most societies agree that all patients with a history of UC (including isolated proctitis) and Crohn's colitis should be offered screening colonoscopy approximately 8–10 years after onset of clinical symptoms to restage disease extent and evaluate features that may confer a higher risk for IBD–CRN. An exception is the NICE guidance, which recommends surveillance in patients with Crohn's colitis involving more than one segment, those with left-sided or more extensive UC but not isolated ulcerative proctitis [7].

Optimal surveillance intervals have not been defined in prospective studies and societies thus differ in their recommendations with surveillance intervals after a screening colonoscopy. All societies agree and recommend that patients with the highest risk of IBD-CRN have annual screening. These include concomitant PSC, extensive colitis with active endoscopic or histological inflammation, a family history of CRC in a first-degree relative under the age of 50, a personal history of dysplasia, and stricturing disease in UC patients [2–9]. Normal appearing mucosa appears to be associated with a lower risk of IBD-CRN [61]. Thus, patients with lower risk are recommended surveillance between 2–5 years. The BSG, ECCO, NICE, and CCA support a risk-stratification approach, increasing surveillance intervals to 5 years in lowest risk patients [6–9]. United States societies have not yet recommended lengthening of surveillance intervals beyond 3 years [2, 4, 5]. Specific recommendations from the 2010 AGA Technical Review on the Diagnosis and Management of Colorectal Neoplasia in IBD are outlined in Table 60.1. Recommendations from the British Society of

Table 60.1 AGA surveillance guidelines for CRC in IBD

- All patients, regardless of extent of disease at initial diagnosis, should undergo a screening colonoscopy a maximum of 8 years after onset of symptoms, with multiple biopsy obtained throughout the entire colon, to assess the microscopic extent if inflammation
- Patients with ulcerative proctitis or ulcerative proctosigmoiditis are not considered at increased risk for IBD-related CRC and thus may be managed on the basis of average risk recommendations
- Patients with extensive left-sided colitis should begin surveillance with 1–2 years after the initial screening endoscopy
- After two negative exams (no dysplasia or cancer), further surveillance exams should be performed every 1–3 years
- Patients with PSC should begin surveillance colonoscopy at the time of PSC diagnosis and then yearly
- Patients with a history of CRC in a first-degree relative, ongoing active endoscopic or histologic inflammation, or anatomic abnormalities (shortened colon, multiple pseudopolyps, or stricture), may from more frequent surveillance colonoscopy
- Representative biopsy specimens from each anatomic section of the colon is recommended. Though no prospective trails have determined the optimal number of biopsies to take, one study has recommended a minimum of 33 biopsy specimens
- Surveillance colonoscopy should ideally be performed when patient is in remission
- These recommendations apply to Crohn's colitis who have disease involving at least one-third of their colon

Table 60.2 Recommendations from the British Society of Gastroenterology

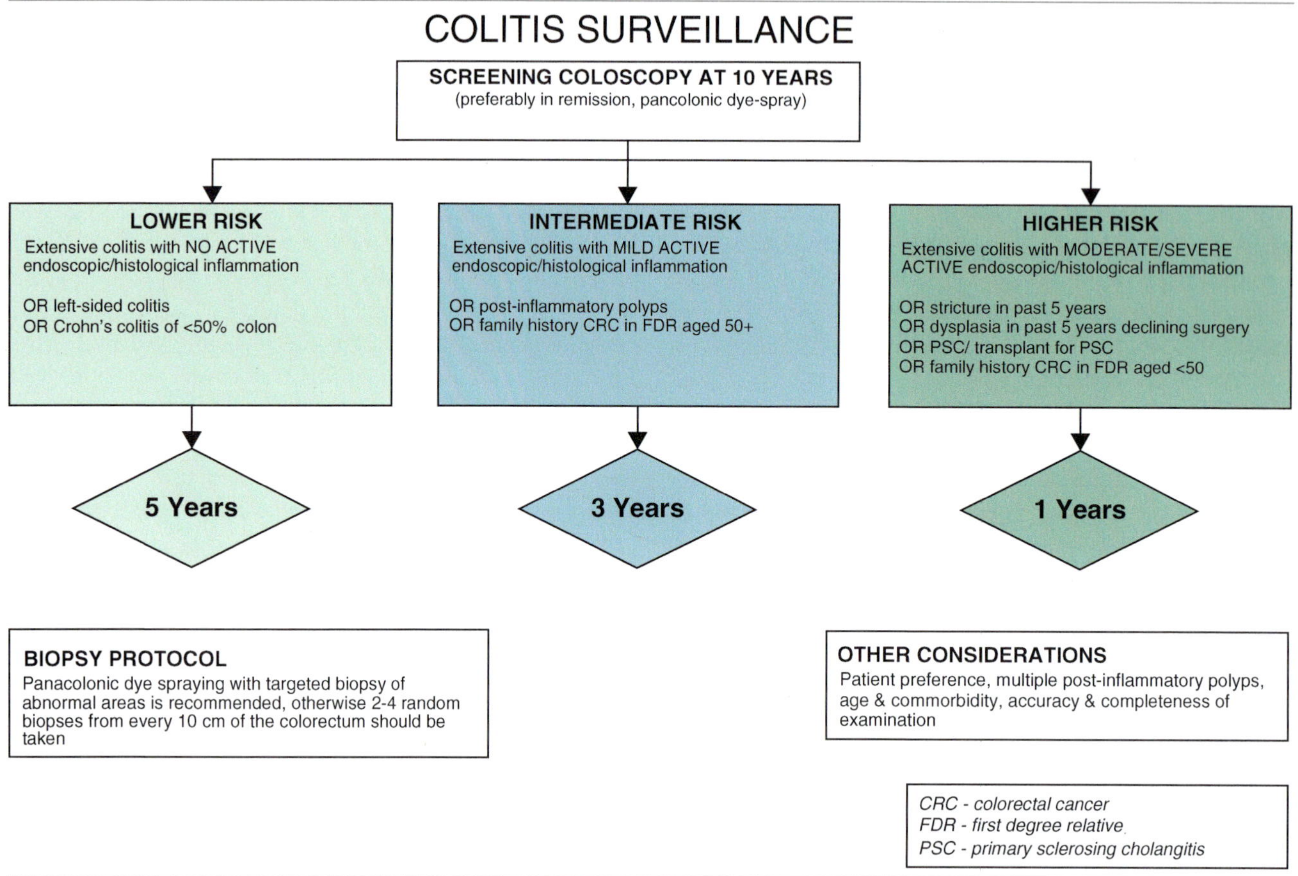
COLITIS SURVEILLANCE
SCREENING COLOSCOPY AT 10 YEARS
(preferably in remission, pancolonic dye-spray)
LOWER RISK
Extensive colitis with NO ACTIVE endoscopic/histological inflammation
OR left-sided colitis
OR Crohn's colitis of <50% colon
INTERMEDIATE RISK
Extensive colitis with MILD ACTIVE endoscopic/histological inflammation
OR post-inflammatory polyps
OR family history CRC in FDR aged 50+
HIGHER RISK
Extensive colitis with MODERATE/SEVERE ACTIVE endoscopic/histological inflammation
OR stricture in past 5 years
OR dysplasia in past 5 years declining surgery
OR PSC/ transplant for PSC
OR family history CRC in FDR aged <50
5 Years
3 Years
1 Years
BIOPSY PROTOCOL
Panacolonic dye spraying with targeted biopsy of abnormal areas is recommended, otherwise 2-4 random biopses from every 10 cm of the colorectum should be taken
OTHER CONSIDERATIONS
Patient preference, multiple post-inflammatory polyps, age & commorbidity, accuracy & completeness of examination
CRC - colorectal cancer
FDR - first degree relative
PSC - primary sclerosing cholangitis

Reproduced from Gut. Cairns SR, Scholefield JH, Steele RJ, et al. 59:666–89. ©2010 with permission from BMJ Publishing from BMJ Publishing Group Ltd

Gastroenterology from 2010 incorporate risk factors and newer imaging techniques and are outlined in Table 60.2.

Several factors influence the success of surveillance. Firstly, the ability to detect dysplasia may be variable. Random biopsy sampling was based on the presumption that dysplasia is frequently not associated with visible mucosal abnormalities. To detect dysplasia with 90 % probability, 33 serial colonic biopsies from four quadrant biopsy specimens need to be obtained every 10 cm from each anatomical segment of the colon [67]. This practice has been endorsed by multiple societies [2–4]. Although possibly true at the inception of surveillance, evolution in endoscopic technology over the years, through standard definition colonoscopy using video chips to high-definition colonoscopy and indeed evidence that most dysplasia is visible at standard white light colonoscopy has challenged this view [17, 68]. Furthermore, random biopsies sample well less than 1 % of total colonic mucosa and one study suggested that up to 1266 random biopsies would be needed to detect one additional episode of dysplasia [69, 70]. In a study in which UC patients underwent colonoscopy every 2 years, interval cancers were observed to develop between 10 and 28 months after dysplasia-free examination [71]. Dysplasia can still be present in a normal appearing colon [17]. Additional aspects such as resectability of dysplasia, anatomical features such as pseudopolyps and a shortened tubular colon may pose difficulties with dysplasia detection. Colonic inflammation can also make pathologic discrimination of dysplasia difficult, thus surveillance should ideally take place when the patient is in clinical remission. All this should be discussed carefully with patients when committing to a surveillance program. Despite this, evidence suggests that patients do not wish to consider colectomy until there is a relatively high certainty of cancer underpinning the importance of careful considerations and meticulous assessment using the best available technology and skill to detect and reset dysplasia to avoid IBD-CRN and colectomy [72].

Meanwhile, new imaging techniques such as chromoendoscopy, narrow band imaging, and confocal endomicroscopy have been developed as an adjunctive technique to detect more subtle mucosal abnormalities. Multiple studies have demonstrated a superior diagnostic yield and therapeutic advantage with chromoendoscopy when compared with standard random biopsy and white light technique for index screening of dysplasia in colitis [73–78]. Meta-analysis of these trials supports the use of chromoendoscopy with targeted biopsies for detecting dysplasia being 8.9 times more likely to detect any dysplasia and 5.2 times more likely to detect non-polypoid dysplasia than white light endoscopy with random biopsy [79, 80]. Such evolution in knowledge has seen cautious translation in societal recommendations over the years. Thus, the ACG 2010 guidelines considered it premature to endorse chromoendoscopy in low-risk patients [4]. The CCFA 2004 and AGA 2010 guidelines, however consider chromoendoscopy with targeted biopsies as a reasonable alternative to white light endoscopy for endoscopists experienced in this technique [2, 3]. All recent European guidelines (ECCO, BSG, NICE) and recent ASGE guidance endorse chromoendoscopy with targeted biopsies as a surveillance protocol of choice [5–8]. The recently published SCENIC international consensus statements recommend chromoendoscopy over standard white light colonoscopy and suggest chromoendoscopy over high-definition colonoscopy for dysplasia surveillance in IBD [68]. Meta-analysis showed a significantly greater proportion of dysplasia detection at chromoendoscopy (RR 1.8, absolute risk increase 6 %) then white light colonoscopy alone [68]. This strategy has also been shown to be cost-effective especially with increasing surveillance interval based on the risk of CRC [81]. Although the SCENIC consensus recommends chromoendoscopy over high-definition white light colonoscopy it was acknowledged that this recommendation is conditional being based on a small observational study [68, 82]. Where chromoendoscopy expertise is not available SCENIC recommends high-definition over standard white light colonoscopy [68]. Chromoendoscopy involves the use of topical contrast agents, either 0.1 % methylene blue or 0.03–0.5 % indigo carmine. Excellent bowel preparation is a prerequisite. Colonic mucosa is segmentally sprayed with contrast agent after cecal intubation and upon withdrawal, using a spray catheter or through the forward water–jet channel using an automated pump [73–75, 80, 81, 83]. Chromoendoscopy enhances mucosal irregularities and helps to delineate the lesion morphology, size, and border to evaluate for endoscopic features of submucosal invasion. Thus, endoscopically resectable lesions may be resected if feasible or tattooed and referred to an endoscopist with expertise in endoscopic mucosal resection or dissection as appropriate. Targeted biopsies should be taken from lesions deemed unresectable endoscopically and lesions of uncertain significance. Furthermore, at least two histological staging biopsies from each colonic segment are recommended to determine histological extent and severity of disease, which in turn affects the risk of dysplasia [5, 6, 8, 9]. Random biopsies however, are not recommended if chromoendoscopy is used for dysplasia surveillance [1, 5, 6, 8, 48]. Successful delivery of dysplasia surveillance using chromoendoscopy hinges on several factors. These include appropriate training (endoscopist and nurses), lesion recognition and its associated learning curve, inter-observer variability amongst pathologists in identifying and grading dysplasia and indeed operational barriers such as availability of dye and equipment, procedural time resulting in some hesitancy amongst gastroenterologists in adopting this modality and in some instances referral to "experts" to provide this [68]. Furthermore, heightened sensitivity of chromoendoscopy in detecting dysplastic foci notwithstanding, the natural history of additional, smaller, flatter lesions identified at chromoendoscopy is poorly understood [84]. The rate of progression from indefinite and low-grade dysplasia to cancer appears to be low some in high-risk cohorts even when variables such as primary sclerosing cholangitis and previous advanced dysplasia are factored in [30–33]. To add to this conundrum, data from the Surveillance, Epidemiology and End results Medicare-linked database of patients over 67 years showed that interval cancers 6–36 months after colonoscopy occurred in much higher proportion of patients with IBD (15.1 % with Crohn's disease and 15.8 % with ulcerative colitis) than patients without IBD (5.8 %) suggesting that clinically relevant areas of neoplasia may be missed with current colonoscopy surveillance [85]. However, the futility of random biopsy has been demonstrated repeatedly in prospective studies. Meanwhile, the evolution in our knowledge of the natural history of dysplasia and the clinical implications of dysplasia found by chromoendoscopy through its wider adoption may close many gaps in our understanding of its true utility. The bulk of evidence favors chromoendoscopy for surveillance and is backed by several scientific societies and international consensus opinion [5, 6, 8, 9, 68]. Several organizations elected not to endorse the SCENIC recommendations feeling that additional studies are needed to confirm that clinical outcomes are improved with chromoendoscopy. A summary of recommendations from the SCENIC consensus for surveillance and management of dysplasia in patients with IBD is outlined in Table 60.3.

Other techniques for image-enhanced endoscopy are under investigation. Narrow-band imaging (NBI), an optical chromoendoscopy technology that uses filters to enhance the contrast of the mucosa and vasculature has not demonstrated an increased yield for dysplasia detection in randomized studies comparing NBI to either standard definition white light endoscopy (WLE) or high definition WLE [86–89]. Studies comparing NBI with chromoendoscopy have reported a numerically higher detection rate with chromoendoscopy but at meta-analysis the difference was not statistically significant. The SCENIC consensus, therefore, does not recommend NBI over dye spray chromoendoscopy [68]. Autofluorescence and confocal laser endomicroscopy are under study but current data do not support their routine use [5, 68].

Table 60.3 Summary of recommendations for surveillance and management of dysplasia in patients with inflammatory bowel disease

	Detection of dysplasia on surveillance colonoscopy
1.	When performing surveillance with white-light colonoscopy, high definition is recommended rather than standard definition (strong recommendation, low-quality evidence)
2.	When performing surveillance with standard-definition colonoscopy, chromoendoscopy is recommended rather than white-light colonoscopy (strong recommendation, moderate-quality evidence)
3.	When performing surveillance with high-definition colonoscopy, chromoendoscopy is suggested rather than white-light colonoscopy (conditional recommendation, low-quality evidence)
4.	When performing surveillance with standard-definition colonoscopy, narrow-band imaging is not suggested is place of white-light colonoscopy (conditional recommendation, low-quality evidence)
5.	When performing surveillance with high-definition colonoscopy, narrow-band imaging is not suggested in place of white-light colonoscopy (conditional recommendation, moderate-quality evidence)
6.	When performing surveillance with image-enhanced high-definition colonoscopy, narrow-band imaging is not suggested in place of chromoendoscopy (conditional recommendation, moderate-quality evidence)
	Management of dysplasis discovered on surveillance colonoscopy
7.	After complete removal of endoscopically resectable polypoid dysplastic lesions, surveillance colonoscopy is recommended rather than colectomy (strong recommendation, very low-quality evidence)
8.	After complete removal of endoscopically resectable nonpolypoid dysplastic lesions, surveillance colonoscopy is suggested rather than colectomy (conditional recommendation, very low-quality evidence)
9.	For patients with endoscopically invisible dysplasis (confirmed by a GI pathologist) referral is suggested to an endoscopist with expertise in IBD surveillance using chromoendoscopy with high-definition colonoscopy (conditional recommendation, very low-quality evidence)

Dysplasia

Detection of dysplasia is the immediate goal of surveillance colonoscopy and in turn the best marker of CRC risk in IBD patients although its detection has not clearly been documented to improve clinical outcomes such as CRC incidence or mortality [68]. Biopsies taken at surveillance colonoscopy must be graded as (1) positive for dysplasia, (2) negative for dysplasia, or (3) indefinite for dysplasia. These are further classified as (1) low-grade dysplasia (LGD), (2) high-grade dysplasia (HGD), or (3) carcinoma [90]. There is considerable inter-observer variability amongst pathologists around interpretation of low-grade dysplasia and "indefinite for dysplasia" categories [91]. Thus, once dysplasia is detected, a second opinion should be obtained from a specialist gastrointestinal pathologist to confirm the diagnosis [91].

Dysplasia is characterized as an endoscopically visible dysplastic lesion detected via targeted biopsies or via resection or indeed endoscopically invisible dysplasia detected by random biopsies [5]. Older guidelines recommended characterizing detected lesions as sporadic adenomas if found outside an area of known colitis or as dysplasia-associated lesion or mass (DALM) if detected within an area of colitis [10]. DALM's were further sub characterized as adenoma like (if raised or had an endoscopic appearance of a sporadic adenoma), or non-adenoma like [2]. Adenoma like DALM's were amenable to endoscopic resection with close follow-up, whereas non-adenoma like DALM's were an indication for surgery, with colectomy being traditionally indicated for high-grade dysplasia detected by random biopsy and multifocal low-grade dysplasia detected at random biopsies [2]. Recent guidelines recommend that the terms DALM, adenoma-like, and non-adenoma like lesion should be abandoned with the addition of terms for ulceration and border of the lesion [48, 68, 80, 92]. Thus, the term endoscopically resectable indicates that (1) distinct margins lesion can be identified, (2) lesion appears completely excised on visual inspection after endoscopic resection, (3) histological assessment of the restricted specimen is consistent with complete removal, and (4) biopsy specimens taken from mucosa immediately adjacent to the resection site are free of dysplasia on histological assessment [68]. Figures 60.1, 60.2, and 60.3 are examples of pseudopolyps, polypoid dysplasia, and non-polypoid dysplasia respectively.

Management of Dysplasia

The ability to accurately identify dysplasia and determine its potential resectability is key to further management [68]. The use of chromoendoscopy and other image enhancing techniques have enhanced dysplasia detection and lesion delineation as described above. Lesion morphology should be described as being polypoid (pedunculated or sessile) or non-polypoid (slightly elevated, flat, or depressed) and lesion borders classified as distinct or indistinct [5, 68, 93]. Any presence of overlying ulceration or features of sub mucosal invasion (such as depression or failure to lift with submucosal injection) may be indicative of underlying malignancy [80].

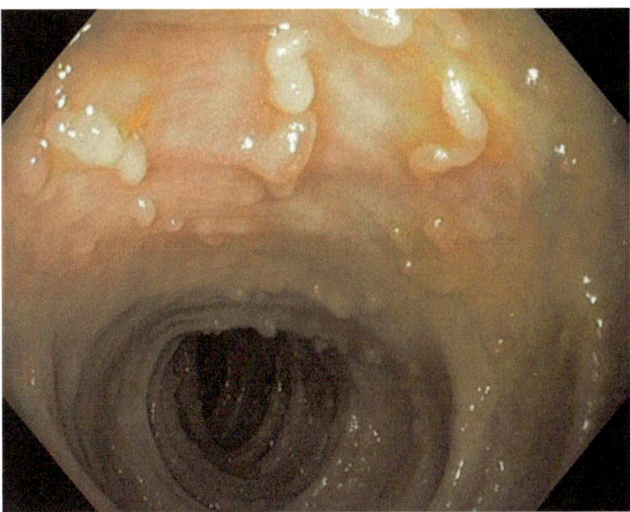

Fig. 60.1 Pseudopolyp

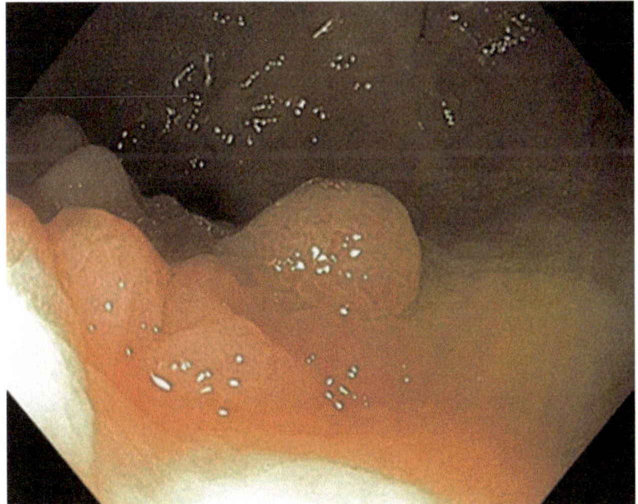

Fig. 60.2 Polypoid dysplasia

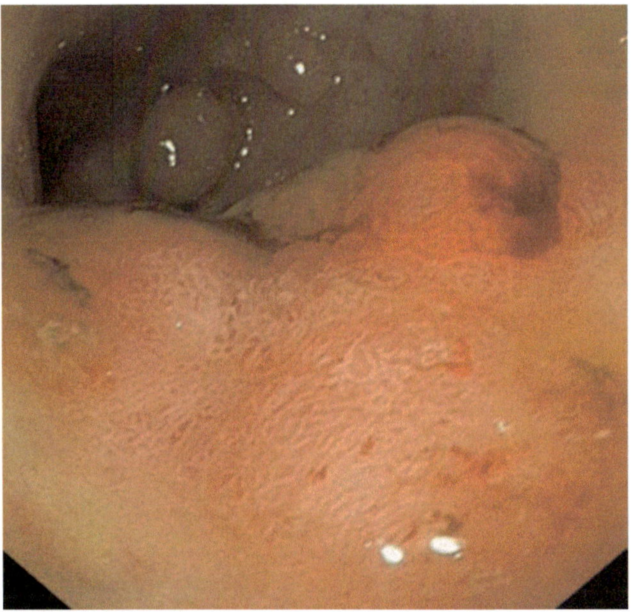

Fig. 60.3 Non-polypoid dysplasia

A lesion detected at endoscopy should be identified as being within or outside an area of known colitis. Lesions in segments outside an area of known colitis should be treated as sporadic adenomas with standard post-polypectomy surveillance recommendations [2, 48, 94, 95]. Lesions in an area of known colitis should be assessed for endoscopic resectability and if possible completely resected by an experienced endoscopist regardless of underlying colitis or grade of dysplasia, acknowledging that inflammation, friability and scarring can make such resection technically more difficult in which case tattooing and photo documentation should be considered to aid subsequent surveillance or resection [5, 48, 68]. Colonic mucosa adjacent to the raised lesion should also be biopsied to evaluate for dysplasia and if complete resection is achieved with dysplasia free margins and no invisible dysplasia elsewhere in the colon, surveillance colonoscopy is recommended rather than colectomy [48, 68]. ECCO recommends surveillance with chromoendoscopy at 3 months and then at least annually whereas US Multi-Society guidelines suggest a 3–6 month check for larger sessile lesions removed in piecemeal fashion or via EMR or ESD with longer surveillance intervals if the initial repeat colonoscopy result is negative [94, 95]. Long-term follow-up studies of endoscopically resectable polypoid lesions are reassuring demonstrating a low risk of developing dysplasia or carcinoma over follow-up [96–100]. A recent meta-analysis also demonstrates a low risk of IBD-CRN following resection of polypoid dysplasia [101]. Indeed patients diagnosed with dysplasia themselves are more likely to refuse or delay colectomy and prefer surveillance colonoscopy [68]. A recent study showed that patients would agree to immediate colectomy only when the risk of synchronous CRC rose to above 73 % [72].

Management of non-polypoid dysplastic lesions is more challenging. Two studies have demonstrated high cure rates after complete resection of circumscribed lateral spreading lesions and lesions with high-grade dysplasia (HGD) [102, 103]. The SCENIC consensus supports surveillance colonoscopy after complete removal of endoscopically resectable non-polypoid dysplastic lesions [68]. This recommendation is conditional recognizing the higher CRC risk and greater endoscopic difficulty with resectability conferred by non-polypoid lesions. Other recent guidelines recommend colectomy for non-polypoid dysplastic lesions because they considered such lesions generally not amenable to endoscopic resection [2, 8, 9].

The management of endoscopically invisible dysplasia detected by random biopsies alone has evolved considerably. Invisible dysplasia was defined in the SCENIC paper as dysplasia identified on random (nontargeted) biopsies of colon mucosa without a visible lesion. Data from St Mark's Hospital indicates that 20 % of patients with flat LGD detected by random biopsies had CRC at the time of immediate colectomy [28]. Ullman et al. found synchronous advanced lesions including flat HGD or CRC in 23 % of patients undergoing colectomy for flat LGD detected on random biopsies [24]. A systematic review of 20 studies and 477 patients with invisible low-grade dysplasia found that 22 % of patients with invisible low-grade dysplasia who had colectomy had CRC [104]. Other studies however have challenged this rate of progression [105–107]. One study showed a 3 % initial and 10 % subsequent rate of progression from LGD to CRC in a 10-year period. Recognition that most dysplasia is visible and evolution in endoscopic technology suggest that random biopsies showing invisible dysplasia in previous studies may have been taken from previously unrecognizable lesions that can now be visualized with modern endoscopic techniques [68]. More recent studies of chromoendoscopy or high-definition white light colonoscopy have reported a 10 % incidence of invisible dysplasia [68]. The AGA recommends colectomy for multifocal flat LGD [2]. The BSG also considers colectomy the best option for LGD but suggests chromoendoscopy if there is uncertainty with the diagnosis and regular surveillance for patients who decline colectomy [6]. The SCENIC consensus supports confirmation of dysplasia by a second GI pathologist and referral to an endoscopist with expertise in IBD surveillance and chromoendoscopy and with high-definition to better inform subsequent decisions regarding surveillance versus colectomy [68]. If a visible dysplastic lesion is identified in the same region of the colon as the invisible dysplasia and the lesion can be resected endoscopically, such patients may remain in a surveillance program. If dysplasia is not found, individualized discussions involving the risks and benefits of surveillance versus colectomy are suggested [68].

Colectomy is the treatment of choice when flat HGD is confirmed by a second GI pathologist or incompletely resected raised dysplasia is discovered. In a review from 1992 of ten prospective surveillance trials including 1225 patients, the prevalence of synchronous CRC in patients with flat HGD was 42 % [15]. In the St Mark's study of 600 patients in a surveillance program over 30 years, 45.5 % of patients with flat HGD detected on random biopsies who underwent immediate colectomy had evidence of CRC in the colectomy specimen. Of those who deferred colectomy and continued surveillance, 25 % later developed CRC [28]. Given the high rate of synchronous carcinomas, colectomy is indicated when flat HGD is found [2]. An endoscopically unresectable lesion or a lesion with dysplasia in the adjacent mucosa is an indication for colectomy [5, 48, 68, 80].

In the presence of chronic active inflammation it is difficult to distinguish regeneration and repair from dysplasia frequently resulting in a pathological finding that is indefinite for dysplasia. Less is known about its significance in assessing CRC risk. In a study of 56 patients with biopsies indefinite for dysplasia, a 9 % 5-year progression rate to HGD or CRC was observed [24]. Aggressive treatment of the underlying inflammation followed by endoscopic reevaluation preferably with chromoendoscopy is recommended [5, 33]. Since the risk of progression to CRC is higher compared to no dysplasia, a follow-up surveillance examination should take place within 3–6 months [2]. See Table 60.4 for a summary of societal guidelines for the management of dysplasia detected at endoscopic surveillance. The updated 2015 algorithm suggested by the American Society for Gastrointestinal Endoscopy for endoscopically visible lesions is shown in Table 60.5.

Chemoprevention

Several chemopreventive agents have been studied for their potential role in the primary prevention of CRC in IBD but none provide resounding proof of a significant effect. These include mesalamine-based agents (5-ASA's), corticosteroids, thiopurine analogues, folic acid, and ursodeoxycholic acid (UDCA). Several lines of evidence including a systematic review suggest a protective effect from 5-ASA's but the results are limited by marked heterogeneity in the studies [108]. Although a chemoprotective effect independent of histological inflammation has not been shown, their utility in maintaining remission warrants continued use [42, 59]. Thiopurine analogues exert chemopreventive activity by reducing inflammation and will often be indicated for disease control [109]. Its use was recently shown to be associated with a 3.5-fold reduction of advanced neoplasia (CRC or high-grade dysplasia) in a cohort of 2841 patients with long-standing extensive UC [110]. Folic acid supplementation has shown a trend towards protection against CRC [111, 112]. The adjusted RR of neoplasia for patients taking folate was 0.72 (95 % CI 0.28–1.83). The risk of neoplasia varied with folate dose (RR, 0.54 for 1.0 mg folate; RR, 0.76 for 0.4 mg folate in a multivitamin, compared with no folate). The degree of dysplasia also varied with folate use (RR for cancer, 0.45; RR for high-grade dysplasia, 0.52; RR for

Table 60.4 Society guidelines for detected dysplasia

	Visible dysplastic lesion, endoscopically resectable with negative biopsies from adjacent mucosa	Visible dysplastic lesion, endoscopically unresectable, or biopsies from adjacent mucosa with dysplasia	Invisible high-grade dypslasia detected by random biopsies	Invisible low-grade dysplasia detected by random biopsies
ECCO,[8] 2013	Surveillance at 3 months and then yearly, regardless of degree of dysplasia	Colectomy	Confirm by expert GI pathologist Rule out visible lesion with repeat chromoendoscopy surveillance Colectomy if confirmed	Confirm by expert GI pathologist Rule out visible lesion with chromoendoscopy surveillance Consider colectomy vs. intensified surveillance with random biopsies
CCA,[9] 2011	Surveillance	Colectomy	Confirm by expert GI pathologist Colectomy	Confirm by expect GI pathologist Multifocal: colectomy vs. intensified surveillance at 3–6 months with chromoendoscopy, then annually Unifocal: consider surgery vs. surveillance at 6 months then annually
BSG,[1] 2010	Surveillance	Colectomy	Not specifically mentioned	Confirm by expect GI pathologist Consider colectomy vs. intensified surveillance
ACG,[4] 2010	Surveillance	Colectomy	Confirm by expert GI pathologist Colectomy	Confirm by expert GI pathologist Colectomy vs. intensified surveillance
AGA,[2] 2010	Adenoma-like DALM: surveillance (6 months)	Non-adenoma-like DALM: colectomy	Confirm by expert GI pathologist Colectomy	Confirm by expert GI pathologist Colectomy vs. intensified surveillance
ASGE,[5] 2006	Surveillance	DALM: colectomy	Confirm by expert GI pathologist Colectomy	Confirm by expert GI pathologist Mutlifocal: colectomy Unifocal: consider colectomy vs. surveillance at 6 months then annually
CCFA,[3] 2005				Confirm by expert GI pathologist Multifocal or repetitive: colectomy Unifocal: colectomy: if patient opts for surveillance, then <6-month intervals recommended

Abbreviations: *ACG* American College of Gastroenterology, *AGA* American Gastroenterological Society, *ASGE* American Society for Gastrointestinal for Gastrointestinal Endoscopy, *BSG* British Society for Gastroenterology, *CCA* Cancer Council of Australia, *CCFA* Crohn's and Colitis Foundation of America, *DALM* dysplasis-associated lesion or mass, *ECCO* European Crohn's and Colitis Organization, *GI* gastrointestinal

low-grade dysplasia, 0.75, compared with patients without dysplasia) ($p = 0.08$). The role of folic acid has not yet been tested in large randomized controlled trials.

Overall, while there is no clear data to support routine the use of folic acid, there appears to be a trend towards benefit and it may be considered in selected patients at the clinician's discretion [113].

The use of UDCA in UC patients with PSC was associated with a decreased risk of colonic dysplasia (odds ratio of 0.18, 95 % CI 0.05–0.61) [114]. The effect of UDCA was noted after controlling for sex, age at onset of UC, duration of UC, duration of PSC, Child-Pugh class, and use of other medications. Another randomized clinical trial of high-dose UDCA demonstrated a 74 % reduction in dysplasia or CRC [115]. In a recent nested cohort study using data from a double-blind, placebo-controlled trial of high-dose UDCA (28–30 mg/kg/day), patients who received high doses of UDCA had a significantly increased risk of developing colorectal neoplasia (dysplasia or cancer) compared to placebo (hazard ratio 4.4, 95 % CI 1.3–20.1) [116].

The American Association for the Study of Liver diseases guideline recommends against use of UDCA for chemoprevention in patients with primary sclerosing cholangitis [117].

Conclusion

Colorectal cancer remains a dreaded complication of long-standing and extensive UC and colonic Crohn's disease. All patients with IBD should undergo an initial surveillance

Table 60.5 ASGE algorithm

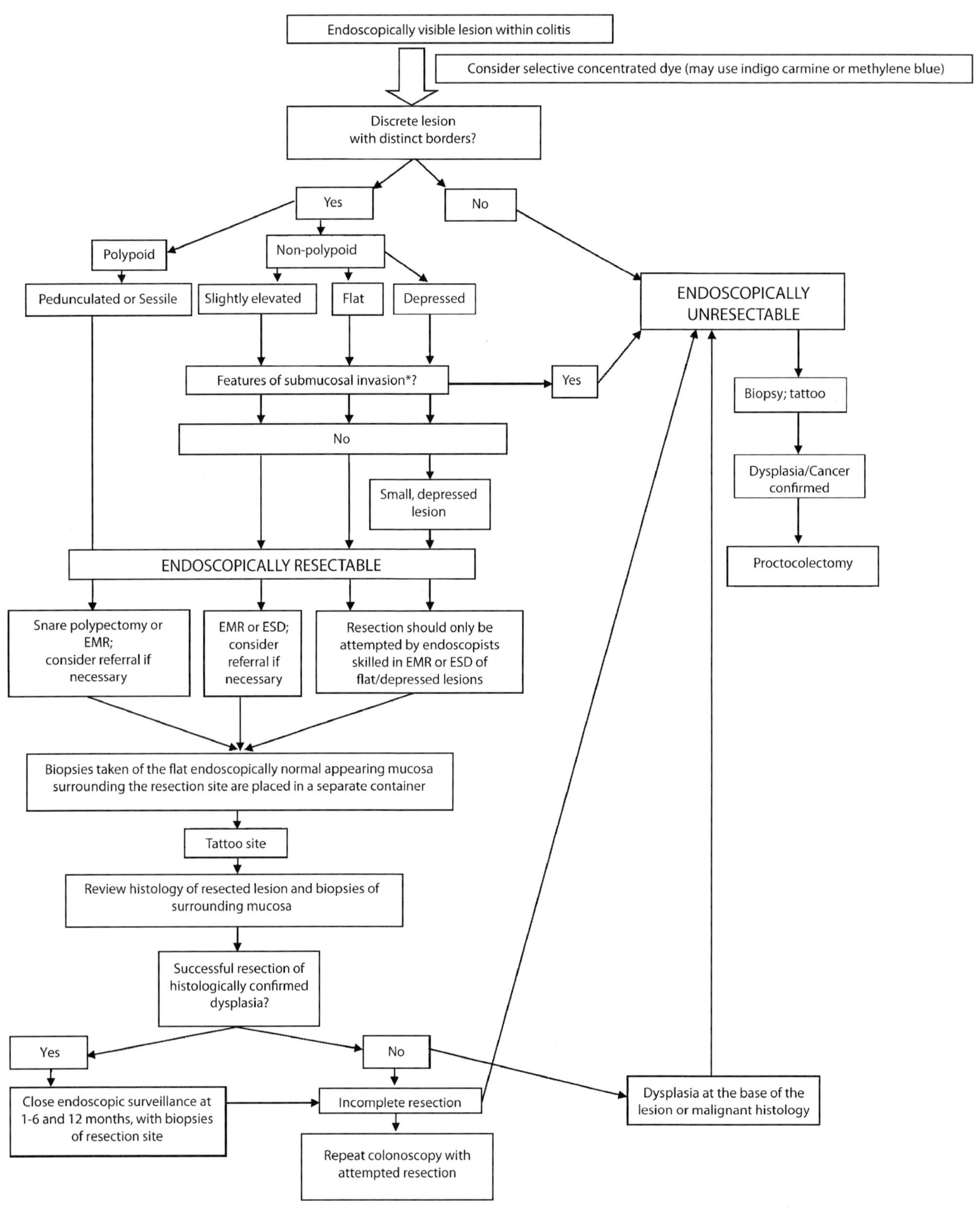

colonoscopy 8–10 years after disease onset to assess the extent of colonic involvement. Most dysplasia is visible at colonoscopy and although random pan colonic biopsies are still recommended by some, newer guidelines endorse high-definition white light colonoscopy and chromoendoscopy as preferred techniques for dysplasia surveillance where appropriate expertise exists. The finding of dysplasia at surveillance warrants an opinion from a second GI pathologist for confirmation. Flat high-grade dysplasia and multifocal flat low-grade dysplasia require evaluation by chromoendoscopy and if no lesion is identified remain indications for colectomy. After complete excision of resectable polypoid or non-polypoid dysplastic lesions surveillance colonoscopy preferably with chromoendoscopy is suggested rather than colectomy. Endoscopically invisible low-grade dysplasia should be confirmed by an endoscopist with expertise in chromoendoscopy and if confirmed options include colectomy or in some instances close surveillance after carefully discussing options with patients. Not all dysplasia progresses to CRC and the clinical implications of dysplasia detected at chromoendoscopy will be unraveled through further prospective and well-designed studies. Meanwhile, evolving definitions of disease control treating to target aiming to achieve mucosal and even histological healing may reduce the risk of dysplasia in IBD through reduction in inflammation, a known risk factor for dysplasia. There is some evidence that mesalazine and thiopurine may reduce the incidence of CRC. Recent evidence suggests that UDCA in higher doses may increase risk and is no longer recommended. Future strategies involving manipulation of the microbiome through probiotics, and antibiotics and other anti-inflammatory agents may alter inflammatory processes and avoid the barrier dysfunction, which promotes dysbiosis and carcinogenesis.

References

1. Mowat C, Cole A, Windsor A, Ahmad T, Arnott I, Driscoll R, et al. Guidelines for the management of inflammatory bowel disease in adults. Gut. 2011;60(5):571–607.
2. Farraye FA, Odze RD, Eaden J, Itzkowitz SH. AGA technical review on the diagnosis and management of colorectal neoplasia in inflammatory bowel disease. Gastroenterology. 2010;138(2): 746–74.
3. Itzkowitz SH, Present DH. Consensus conference: colorectal cancer screening and surveillance in inflammatory bowel disease. Inflamm Bowel Dis. 2005;11:314–21.
4. Kornbluth A, Sachar DB. Ulcerative colitis practice guidelines in adults: American College of Gastroenterology, Practice Parameters Committee. Am J Gastroenterol. 2010;105:501–23 [quiz: 24].
5. ASGE Standards of Practice Committee, Shergill AK, Lightdale JR, Bruining DH, Acosta RD, Chandrasekhara V, Chathadi KV, et al. The role of endoscopy in inflammatory bowel disease. Gastrointest Endosc. 2015;81(5):1101–21.e13.
6. Cairns SR, Scholefield JH, Steele RJ, Dunlop MG, Thomas HJ, Evans GD, et al. British Society of Gastroenterology; Association of Coloproctology for Great Britain and Ireland. Guidelines for colorectal cancer screening and surveillance in moderate and high risk groups (update from 2002). Gut. 2010;59(5):666–89.
7. National Institute for Health and Clinical Excellence. Colonoscopic surveillance for prevention of colorectal cancer in people with ulcerative colitis, Crohn's disease or adenomas. Clinical Guidelines, No. 118. London 2011.
8. Van Assche G, Dignass A, Bokemeyer B, Danese S, Gionchetti P, Moser G, et al. Second European evidence-based consensus on the diagnosis and management of ulcerative colitis part 3: special situations. J Crohns Colitis. 2013;7(1):1–33.
9. Cancer Council Australia Colonoscopy Surveillance Working Party. Clinical Practice Guidelines for Surveillance Colonoscopy—in adenoma follow-up; following curative resection of colorectal cancer; and for cancer surveillance in inflammatory bowel disease. Sydney, Australia: Cancer Council Australia; December, 2011. p. 48–62.
10. Rutter MD, Riddell RH. Colorectal dysplasia in inflammatory bowel disease: a clinicopathologic perspective. Clin Gastroenterol Hepatol. 2013;12:359–67.
11. Karlén P, Kornfeld D, Broström O, Löfberg R, Persson PG, Ekbom A. Is colonoscopic surveillance reducing colorectal cancer mortality in ulcerative colitis? A population based case control study. Gut. 1998;42(5):711–4.
12. Lutgens MW, Oldenburg B, Siersema PD, van Bodegraven AA, Dijkstra G, Hommes DW, et al. Colonoscopic surveillance improves survival after colorectal cancer diagnosis in inflammatory bowel disease. Br J Cancer. 2009;101(10):1671–5.
13. Herrinton LJ, Liu L, Levin TR, Allison JE, Lewis JD, Velayos F. Incidence and mortality of colorectal adenocarcinoma in persons with inflammatory bowel disease from 1998 to 2010. Gastroenterology. 2012;143(2):382–9.
14. Jess T, Loftus Jr EV, Velayos FS, Harmsen WS, Zinsmeister AR, Smyrk TC, et al. Incidence and prognosis of colorectal dysplasia in inflammatory bowel disease: a population-based study from Olmsted County. Minnesota Inflamm Bowel Dis. 2006;12(8): 669–76.
15. Bernstein CN, Shanahan F, Weinstein WM. Are we telling patients the truth about surveillance colonoscopy in ulcerative colitis? Lancet. 1994;343:71–4.
16. Dyson JK, Rutter MD. Colorectal cancer in inflammatory bowel disease: what is the real magnitude of the risk? World J Gastroenterol. 2012;18:3839–48.
17. Rutter MD, Saunders BP, Wilkinson KH, Kamm MA, Williams CB, Forbes A. Most dysplasia in ulcerative colitis is visible at colonoscopy. Gastrointest Endosc. 2004;60(3):334–9.
18. Rubin DT, Rothe JA, Hetzel JT, Cohen RD, Hanauer SB. Are dysplasia and colorectal cancer endoscopically visible in patients with ulcerative colitis? Gastrointest Endosc. 2007;65(7): 998–1004.
19. Crohn BB, Rosenberg H. The sigmoidoscopic picture of chronic ulcerative colitis (non-specific). Am J Med Sci. 1925; 170:220–7.
20. Burstein E, Fearon ER. Colitis and cancer: a tale of inflammatory cells and their cytokines. J Clin Invest. 2008;118:464–7.
21. Grivennikov SI. Inflammation and colorectal cancer: colitis-associated neoplasia. Semin Immunopathol. 2013;35:229–44.
22. Cooks T, Pateras IS, Tarcic O, Solomon H, Schetter AJ, Wilder S, et al. Mutant p53 prolongs NF-κB activation and promotes chronic inflammation and inflammation-associated colorectal cancer. Cancer Cell. 2013;23(5):634–46.
23. Itzkowitz SH. Inflammatory bowel disease and cancer. Gastroenterol Clin North Am. 1997;26:129–39.
24. Ullman T, Croog V, Harpaz N, Sachar D, Itzkowitz S. Progression of flat low-grade dysplasia to advanced neoplasia in patients with ulcerative colitis. Gastroenterology. 2003;125(5):1311–9.

25. Foersch S, Neurath MF. Colitis-associated neoplasia: molecular basis and clinical translation. Cell Mol Life Sci. 2014;71: 3523–35.
26. Eaden JA, Abrams KR, Mayberry JF. The risk of colorectal cancer in ulcerative colitis: a meta-analysis. Gut. 2001;48(4):526–35.
27. Velayos FS, Liu L, Lewis JD, Allison JE, Flowers N, Hutfless S, et al. Prevalence of colorectal cancer surveillance for ulcerative colitis in an integrated health care delivery system. Gastroenterology. 2010;139(5):1511–8.
28. Jess T, Simonsen J, Jørgensen KT, Pedersen BV, Nielsen NM, Frisch M. Decreasing risk of colorectal cancer in patients with inflammatory bowel disease over 30 years. Gastroenterology. 2012;143(2):375–81.
29. Choi CH, Rutter MD, Askari A, Lee GH, Warusavitarne J, Moorghen M, et al. Forty-year analysis of colonoscopic surveillance program for neoplasia in ulcerative colitis: an updated overview. Am J Gastroenterol. 2015;31.
30. Goldstone R, Itzkowitz S, Harpaz N, Ullman T. Progression of low-grade dysplasia in ulcerative colitis: effect of colonic location. Gastrointest Endosc. 2011;74(5):1087–93.
31. Navaneethan U, Jegadeesan R, Gutierrez NG, Venkatesh PG, Hammel JP, Shen B, et al. Progression of low-grade dysplasia to advanced neoplasia based on the location and morphology of dysplasia in ulcerative colitis patients with extensive colitis under colonoscopic surveillance. J Crohns Colitis. 2013;7(12):e684–91.
32. Venkatesh PG, Jegadeesan R, Gutierrez NG, Sanaka MR, Navaneethan U. Natural history of low grade dysplasia in patients with primary sclerosing cholangitis and ulcerative colitis. J Crohns Colitis. 2013;7(12):968–73.
33. Pekow JR, Hetzel JT, Rothe JA, Hanauer SB, Turner JR, Hart J, et al. Outcome after surveillance of low-grade and indefinite dysplasia in patients with ulcerative colitis. Inflamm Bowel Dis. 2010;16(8):1352–6.
34. Jess T, Lopez A, Andersson M, Beaugerie L, Peyrin-Biroulet L. Thiopurines and risk of colorectal neoplasia in patients with inflammatory bowel disease: a meta-analysis. Clin Gastroenterol Hepatol. 2014;12(11):1793–800.
35. Jess T, Riis L, Vind I, Winther KV, Borg S, Binder V, et al. Changes in clinical characteristics, course, and prognosis of inflammatory bowel disease during the last 5 decades: a population-based study from Copenhagen. Denmark Inflamm Bowel Dis. 2007;13(4):481–9.
36. Ekbom A, Helmick C, Zack M, Adami HO. Increased risk of large-bowel cancer in Crohn's disease with colonic involvement. Lancet. 1990;336(8711):357–9.
37. Munkholm P, Langholz E, Davidsen M, Binder V. Intestinal cancer risk and mortality in patients with Crohn's disease. Gastroenterology. 1993;105(6):1716–23.
38. Gillen CD, Walmsley RS, Prior P, Andrews HA, Allan RN. Ulcerative colitis and Crohn's disease: a comparison of the colorectal cancer risk in extensive colitis. Gut. 1994;35(11): 1590–2.
39. Sachar DB. Cancer in Crohn's disease: dispelling the myths. Gut. 1994;35(11):1507–8.
40. Bernstein CN, Blanchard JF, Kliewer E, Wajda A. Cancer risk in patients with inflammatory bowel disease: a population-based study. Cancer. 2001;91(4):854–62.
41. Canavan C, Abrams KR, Mayberry J. Meta-analysis: colorectal and small bowel cancer risk in patients with Crohn's disease. Aliment Pharmacol Ther. 2006;23(8):1097–104.
42. Rutter M, Saunders B, Wilkinson K, Rumbles S, Schofield G, Kamm M, et al. Severity of inflammation is a risk factor for colorectal neoplasia in ulcerative colitis. Gastroenterology. 2004;126(2):451–9.
43. Velayos FS, Loftus Jr EV, Jess T, Harmsen WS, Bida J, Zinsmeister AR, et al. Predictive and protective factors associated with colorectal cancer in ulcerative colitis: a case–control study. Gastroenterology. 2006;130(7):1941–9.
44. Ekbom A, Helmick C, Zack M, et al. Ulcerative colitis and colorectal cancer. A population-based study. N Engl J Med. 1990;323:1228–33.
45. Friedman S, Rubin PH, Bodian C, Harpaz N, Present DH. Screening and surveillance colonoscopy in chronic Crohn's colitis: results of a surveillance program spanning 25 years. Clin Gastroenterol Hepatol. 2008;6(9):993–8.
46. Florén CH, Benoni C, Willén R. Histologic and colonoscopic assessment of disease extension in ulcerative colitis. Scand J Gastroenterol. 1987;22(4):459–62.
47. Sugita A, Sachar DB, Bodian C, Ribeiro MB, Aufses Jr AH, Greenstein AJ. Colorectal cancer in ulcerative colitis. Influence of anatomical extent and age at onset on colitis-cancer interval. Gut. 1991;32(2):167–9.
48. Annese V, Daperno M, Rutter MD, Amiot A, Bossuyt P, East J, et al. European evidence based consensus for endoscopy in inflammatory bowel disease. J Crohns Colitis. 2013;7(12):982–1018.
49. Langholz E, Munkholm P, Davidsen M, Nielsen OH, Binder V. Changes in extent of ulcerative colitis: a study on the course and prognostic factors. Scand J Gastroenterol. 1996;31(3):260–6.
50. Meucci G, Vecchi M, Astegiano M, Beretta L, Cesari P, Dizioli P, et al. The natural history of ulcerative proctitis: a multicenter, retrospective study. Gruppo di Studio per le Malattie Infiammatorie Intestinali (GSMII). Am J Gastroenterol. 2000;95(2):469–73.
51. Jess T, Loftus Jr EV, Velayos FS, Harmsen WS, Zinsmeister AR, Smyrk TC, et al. Risk of intestinal cancer in inflammatory bowel disease: a population-based study from olmsted county, Minnesota. Gastroenterology. 2006;130(4):1039–46.
52. Soetikno RM, Lin OS, Heidenreich PA, Young HS, Blackstone MO. Increased risk of colorectal neoplasia in patients with primary sclerosing cholangitis and ulcerative colitis: a meta-analysis. Gastrointest Endosc. 2002;56(1):48–54.
53. Bleday R, Lee E, Jessurun J, Heine J, Wong WD. Increased risk of early colorectal neoplasms after hepatic transplant in patients with inflammatory bowel disease. Dis Colon Rectum. 1993;36(10): 908–12.
54. Higashi H, Yanaga K, Marsh JW, Tzakis A, Kakizoe S, Starzl TE. Development of colon cancer after liver transplantation for primary sclerosing cholangitis associated with ulcerative colitis. Hepatology. 1990;11(3):477–80.
55. Loftus Jr EV, Aguilar HI, Sandborn WJ, Tremaine WJ, Krom RA, Zinsmeister AR, et al. Risk of colorectal neoplasia in patients with primary sclerosing cholangitis and ulcerative colitis following orthotopic liver transplantation. Hepatology. 1998;27(3):685–90.
56. Nuako KW, Ahlquist DA, Mahoney DW, Schaid DJ, Siems DM, Lindor NM. Familial predisposition for colorectal cancer in chronic ulcerative colitis: a case-control study. Gastroenterology. 1998;115(5):1079–83.
57. Askling J, Dickman PW, Karlén P, Broström O, Lapidus A, Löfberg R, et al. Family history as a risk factor for colorectal cancer in inflammatory bowel disease. Gastroenterology. 2001;120(6):1356–62.
58. Söderlund S, Granath F, Broström O, Karlén P, Löfberg R, Ekbom A, et al. Inflammatory bowel disease confers a lower risk of colorectal cancer to females than to males. Gastroenterology. 2010;138(5):1697–703.
59. Gupta RB, Harpaz N, Itzkowitz S, Hossain S, Matula S, Kornbluth A, et al. Histologic inflammation is a risk factor for progression to colorectal neoplasia in ulcerative colitis: a cohort study. Gastroenterology. 2007;133(4):1099–105.
60. Rubin DT, Huo D, Kinnucan JA, Sedrak MS, McCullom NE, Bunnag AP, et al. Inflammation is an independent risk factor for colonic neoplasia in patients with ulcerative colitis: a case-control study. Clin Gastroenterol Hepatol. 2013;11(12):1601–8.

61. Reiser JR, Waye JD, Janowitz HD, Harpaz N. Adenocarcinoma in strictures of ulcerative colitis without antecedent dysplasia by colonoscopy. Am J Gastroenterol. 1994;89(1):119–22.
62. Rutter MD, Saunders BP, Wilkinson KH, Rumbles S, Schofield G, Kamm MA, et al. Cancer surveillance in longstanding ulcerative colitis: endoscopic appearances help predict cancer risk. Gut. 2004;53(12):1813–6.
63. Choi PM, Nugent FW, Schoetz Jr DJ, Silverman ML, Haggitt RC. Colonoscopic surveillance reduces mortality from colorectal cancer in ulcerative colitis. Gastroenterology. 1993;105(2):418–24.
64. Eaden J, Abrams K, Ekbom A, Jackson E, Mayberry J. Colorectal cancer prevention in ulcerative colitis: a case–control study. Aliment Pharmacol Ther. 2000;14(2):145–53.
65. Lashner BA, Kane SV, Hanauer SB. Colon cancer surveillance in chronic ulcerative colitis: historical cohort study. Am J Gastroenterol. 1990;85:1083–7.
66. Howdle P, Atkin W, Rutter M. Colonoscopic surveillance for prevention of colorectal cancer in people with ulcerative colitis, Crohn's disease or adenomas. National Institute for Health and Clinical Excellence (NICE) Clinical guideline 118. London, UK: National Institute for Health and Clinical Excellence; 2011.
67. Rubin CE, Haggitt RC, Burmer GC, Brentnall TA, Stevens AC, Levine DS, et al. DNA aneuploidy in colonic biopsies predicts future development of dysplasia in ulcerative colitis. Gastroenterology. 1992;103(5):1611–20.
68. Laine L, Kaltenbach T, Barkun A, McQuaid KR, Subramanian V, Soetikno R; SCENIC Guideline Development Panel. SCENIC international consensus statement on surveillance and management of dysplasia in inflammatory bowel disease. Gastroenterology. 2015;148(3):639–51.e28.
69. East JE. Colonoscopic cancer surveillance in inflammatory bowel disease: what's new beyond random biopsy? Clin Endosc. 2012;45:274–7.
70. Rutter MD. Surveillance programmes for neoplasia in colitis. J Gastroenterol. 2011;46 Suppl 1:1–5.
71. Connell WR, Lennard-Jones JE, Williams CB, Talbot IC, Price AB, Wilkinson KH. Factors affecting the outcome of endoscopic surveillance for cancer in ulcerative colitis. Gastroenterology. 1994;107(4):934–44.
72. Siegel CA, Schwartz LM, Woloshin S, Cole EB, Rubin DT, Vay T, et al. When should ulcerative colitis patients undergo colectomy for dysplasia? Mismatch between patient preferences and physician recommendations. Inflamm Bowel Dis. 2010;16(10):1658–62.
73. Kiesslich R, Fritsch J, Holtmann M, Koehler HH, Stolte M, Kanzler S, et al. Methylene blue-aided chromoendoscopy for the detection of intraepithelial neoplasia and colon cancer in ulcerative colitis. Gastroenterology. 2003;124(4):880–8.
74. Rutter MD, Saunders BP, Schofield G, Forbes A, Price AB, Talbot IC. Pancolonic indigo carmine dye spraying for the detection of dysplasia in ulcerative colitis. Gut. 2004;53(2):256–60.
75. Matsumoto T, Nakamura S, Jo Y, Yao T, Iida M. Chromoscopy might improve diagnostic accuracy in cancer surveillance for ulcerative colitis. Am J Gastroenterol. 2003;98(8):1827–33.
76. Hurlstone DP, McAlindon ME, Sanders DS, Koegh R, Lobo AJ, Cross SS. Further validation of high-magnification chromoscopic colonoscopy for the detection of intra- epithelial neoplasia and colon cancer in ulcerative colitis. Gastroenterology. 2004;126:376–8.
77. Hurlstone DP, Sanders DS, Atkinson R, Hunter MD, McAlindon ME, Lobo AJ, et al. Endoscopic mucosal resection for flat neoplasia in chronic ulcerative colitis: can we change the endoscopic management paradigm? Gut. 2007;56(6):838–46.
78. Marion JF, Waye JD, Present DH, Israel Y, Bodian C, Harpaz N, et al. Chromoendoscopy-targeted biopsies are superior to standard colonoscopic surveillance for detecting dysplasia in inflammatory bowel disease patients: a prospective endoscopic trial. Am J Gastroenterol. 2008;103(9):2342–9.
79. Subramanian V, Mannath J, Ragunath K, Hawkey CJ. Meta-analysis: the diagnostic yield of chromoendoscopy for detecting dysplasia in patients with colonic inflammatory bowel disease. Aliment Pharmacol Ther. 2011;33(3):304–12.
80. Soetikno R, Subramanian V, Kaltenbach T, Rouse RV, Sanduleanu S, Suzuki N, et al. The detection of nonpolypoid (flat and depressed) colorectal neoplasms in patients with inflammatory bowel disease. Gastroenterology. 2013;144(7):1349–52.
81. Konijeti GG, Shrime MG, Ananthakrishnan AN, Chan AT. Cost-effectiveness analysis of chromoendoscopy for colorectal cancer surveillance in patients with ulcerative colitis. Gastrointest Endosc. 2014;79(3):455–65.
82. Picco MF, Pasha S, Leighton JA, Bruining D, Loftus Jr EV, Thomas CS, et al. Procedure time and the determination of polypoid abnormalities with experience: implementation of a chromoendoscopy program for surveillance colonoscopy for ulcerative colitis. Inflamm Bowel Dis. 2013;19(9):1913–20.
83. Tsiamoulos ZP, Saunders BP. Easy dye application at surveillance colonoscopy: modified use of a washing pump. Gut. 2011;60:740.
84. Marion JF, Sands BE. The SCENIC consensus statement on surveillance and management of dysplasia in inflammatory bowel disease: praise and words of caution. Gastroenterology. 2015;148(3):462–7.
85. Wang YR, Cangemi JR, Loftus Jr EV, Picco MF. Rate of early/missed colorectal cancers after colonoscopy in older patients with or without inflammatory bowel disease in the United States. Am J Gastroenterol. 2013;108(3):444–9.
86. Dekker E, van den Broek FJ, Reitsma JB, Hardwick JC, Offerhaus GJ, van Deventer SJ, et al. Narrow-band imaging compared with conventional colonoscopy for the detection of dysplasia in patients with longstanding ulcerative colitis. Endoscopy. 2007;39(3):216–21.
87. Ignjatovic A, East JE, Subramanian V, Suzuki N, Guenther T, Palmer N, et al. Narrow band imaging for detection of dysplasia in colitis: a randomized controlled trial. Am J Gastroenterol. 2012;107(6):885–90.
88. van den Broek FJ, Fockens P, van Eeden S, Stokkers PC, Ponsioen CY, Reitsma JB, et al. Narrow-band imaging versus high-definition endoscopy for the diagnosis of neoplasia in ulcerative colitis. Endoscopy. 2011;43(2):108–15.
89. Pellisé M, López-Cerón M, de Rodríguez Miguel C, Jimeno M, Zabalza M, Ricart E, et al. Narrow-band imaging as an alternative to chromoendoscopy for the detection of dysplasia in long-standing inflammatory bowel disease: a prospective, randomized, crossover study. Gastrointest Endosc. 2011;74(4):840–8.
90. Riddell RH, Goldman H, Ransohoff DF, Appelman HD, Fenoglio CM, Haggitt RC, et al. Dysplasia in inflammatory bowel disease: standardized classification with provisional clinical applications. Hum Pathol. 1983;14(11):931–68.
91. Eaden J, Abrams K, McKay H, Denley H, Mayberry J. Inter-observer variation between general and specialist gastrointestinal pathologists when grading dysplasia in ulcerative colitis. J Pathol. 2001;194(2):152–7.
92. The Paris endoscopic classification of superficial neoplastic lesions: esophagus, stomach, and colon: November 30 to December 1, 2002. Gastrointest Endosc. 2003;58(Suppl 6):S3–43.
93. Kamiński MF, Hassan C, Bisschops R, Pohl J, Pellisé M, Dekker E, et al. Advanced imaging for detection and differentiation of colorectal neoplasia: European Society of Gastrointestinal Endoscopy (ESGE) Guideline. Endoscopy. 2014;46(5):435–49.
94. Lieberman DA, Rex DK, Winawer SJ, Giardiello FM, Johnson DA, Levin TR, et al. Guidelines for colonoscopy surveillance after screening and polypectomy: a consensus update by the US Multi-

Society Task Force on Colorectal Cancer. Gastroenterology. 2012;143(3):844–57.

95. Torres C, Antonioli D, Odze RD. Polypoid dysplasia and adenomas in inflammatory bowel disease: a clinical, pathologic, and follow-up study of 89 polyps from 59 patients. Am J Surg Pathol. 1998;22:275–84.
96. Engelsgjerd M, Farraye FA, Odze RD. Polypectomy may be adequate treatment for adenoma-like dysplastic lesions in chronic ulcerative colitis. Gastroenterology. 1999;117:1288–94.
97. Odze RD, Farraye FA, Hecht JL, Hornick JL. Long-term follow-up after polypectomy treatment for adenoma-like dysplastic lesions in ulcerative colitis. Clin Gastroenterol Hepatol. 2004;2(7):534–41.
98. Rubin PH, Friedman S, Harpaz N, Goldstein E, Weiser J, Schiller J, et al. Colonoscopic polypectomy in chronic colitis: conservative management after endoscopic resection of dysplastic polyps. Gastroenterology. 1999;117(6):1295–300.
99. Vieth M, Behrens H, Stolte M. Sporadic adenoma in ulcerative colitis: endoscopic resection is an adequate treatment. Gut. 2006;55:1151–5.
100. Quinn AM, Farraye FA, Naini BV, Cerda S, Coukos J, Li Y, et al. Polypectomy is adequate treatment for adenoma-like dysplastic lesions (DALMs) in Crohn's disease. Inflamm Bowel Dis. 2013;19(6):1186–93.
101. Wanders LK, Dekker E, Pullens B, Bassett P, Travis SP, East JE. Cancer risk after resection of polypoid dysplasia in patients with longstanding ulcerative colitis: a meta-analysis. Clin Gastroenterol Hepatol. 2014;12(5):756–64.
102. Smith LA, Baraza W, Tiffin N, Cross SS, Hurlstone DP. Endoscopic resection of adenoma-like mass in chronic ulcerative colitis using a combined endoscopic mucosal resection and cap assisted submucosal dissection technique. Inflamm Bowel Dis. 2008;14(10):1380–6.
103. Blonski W, Kundu R, Furth EF, Lewis J, Aberra F, Lichtenstein GR. High-grade dysplastic adenoma-like mass lesions are not an indication for colectomy in patients with ulcerative colitis. Scand J Gastroenterol. 2008;43(7):817–20.
104. Thomas T, Abrams KA, Robinson RJ, Mayberry JF. Meta-analysis: cancer risk of low-grade dysplasia in chronic ulcerative colitis. Aliment Pharmacol Ther. 2007;25(6):657–68.
105. Befrits R, Ljung T, Jaramillo E, Rubio C. Low-grade dysplasia in extensive, long-standing inflammatory bowel disease: a follow-up study. Dis Colon Rectum. 2002;45(5):615–20.
106. Hata K, Watanabe T, Kazama S, Suzuki K, Shinozaki M, Yokoyama T, et al. Earlier surveillance colonoscopy programme improves survival in patients with ulcerative colitis associated colorectal cancer: results of a 23-year surveillance programme in the Japanese population. Br J Cancer. 2003;89(7):1232–6.
107. Lim CH, Dixon MF, Vail A, Forman D, Lynch DA, Axon AT. Ten year follow up of ulcerative colitis patients with and without low grade dysplasia. Gut. 2003;52(8):1127–32.
108. Velayos FS, Terdiman JP, Walsh JM. Effect of 5-aminosalicylate use on colorectal cancer and dysplasia risk: a systematic review and metaanalysis of observational studies. Am J Gastroenterol. 2005;100(6):1345–53.
109. Subramanian V, Logan RF. Chemoprevention of colorectal cancer in inflammatory bowel disease. Best Pract Res Clin Gastroenterol. 2011;25(4–5):593–606.
110. Beaugerie L, Svrcek M, Seksik P, Bouvier AM, Simon T, Allez M, et al. Risk of colorectal high-grade dysplasia and cancer in a prospective observational cohort of patients with inflammatory bowel disease. Gastroenterology. 2013;145(1):166–75.e8.
111. Lashner BA, Heidenreich PA, Su GL, Kane SV, Hanauer SB. Effect of folate supplementation on the incidence of dysplasia and cancer in chronic ulcerative colitis. A case-control study. Gastroenterology. 1989;97(2):255–9.
112. Lashner BA, Provencher KS, Seidner DL, Knesebeck A, Brzezinski A. The effect of folic acid supplementation on the risk for cancer or dysplasia in ulcerative colitis. Gastroenterology. 1997;112(1):29–32.
113. Sebastian S, Hernández V, Myrelid P, Kariv R, Tsianos E, Toruner M, et al. Colorectal cancer in inflammatory bowel disease: results of the 3rd ECCO pathogenesis scientific workshop (I). J Crohns Colitis. 2014;8(1):5–18.
114. Tung BY, Emond MJ, Haggitt RC, Bronner MP, Kimmey MB, Kowdley KV, et al. Ursodiol use is associated with lower prevalence of colonic neoplasia in patients with ulcerative colitis and primary sclerosing cholangitis. Ann Intern Med. 2001;134(2):89–95.
115. Pardi DS, Loftus Jr EV, Kremers WK, Keach J, Lindor KD. Ursodeoxycholic acid as a chemo preventive agent in patients with ulcerative colitis and primary sclerosing cholangitis. Gastroenterology. 2003;124(4):889–93.
116. Eaton JE, Silveira MG, Pardi DS, Sinakos E, Kowdley KV, Luketic VA, et al. High-dose ursodeoxycholic acid is associated with the development of colorectal neoplasia in patients with ulcerative colitis and primary sclerosing cholangitis. Am J Gastroenterol. 2011;106(9):1638–45.
117. Chapman R, Fevery J, Kalloo A, Nagorney DM, Boberg KM, Shneider B, et al. Diagnosis and management of primary sclerosing cholangitis. Hepatology. 2010;51(2):660–78.

Inflammatory Bowel Diseases: How to Identify High-Risk Patients

61

Jacques Cosnes and Harry Sokol

Crohn's disease (CD) and ulcerative colitis (UC) are chronic conditions with progressive anatomical damage, frequent complications, and possible requirement of surgical procedures. Both involve young people and have a great impact on patient's quality of life. Medical management of IBD was revolutionized in the late nineties by the advent of increasingly effective medical therapies: immunosuppressants and biologics.

These therapies when given early in the course of the disease may prevent the development of an irreversible digestive damage unresponsive to medical therapy and requiring surgery [1, 2]. However, first the effect of these therapies is not sustained, and they should be used for a very long time, perhaps indefinitely, and second their use is associated with significant side effects, with increased risk of serious infections and/or cancers.

It is thus mandatory to identify patients most at risk of developing a disabling or complicated course who could be targeted for aggressive therapy. This should be discussed at different times during the disease course, in particular at presentation and after first surgery.

Predictive Factors

Numerous studies have tried to recognize demographic, clinical, and anatomical characteristics associated with a worse prognosis of IBD. Some characteristics do not seem to play a significant or important role and will not be examined in this review. It is the case of gender, ethnicity, state of residency, educational level, and body weight. Other characteristics may be used to identify subgroups of IBD patients who differ in their natural history and complications.

J. Cosnes, M.D. (✉) • H. Sokol, M.D., Ph.D.
Service de Gastroentérologie et Nutrition, Hôpital St-Antoine (APHP) and Pierre-et-Marie Curie University (Paris VI), 184 rue du Faubourg St-Antoine, 75571 Paris, France
e-mail: jacques.cosnes@sat.aphp.fr

Age

IBD may develop at any age, from less than 2 years to more than 90 years. In CD, it is well established that the disease course is more severe in children than in adults. Comparative studies are few, but they demonstrate that, compared to adult-onset CD, childhood-onset CD patients experience a more severe disease regarding both disease activity and medical therapy requirements [3]. This increased severity exists independently of the disease location, whereas the disease tends to be more extensive and jejunal lesions more prevalent in children [4]. These data together suggest that childhood-onset CD shares a particular severe phenotype. Moreover, due to the differences of age, complications and surgery occur at an age 15–20 years earlier than in adult-onset CD, and thus, these patients are exposed early in their life to major sequelae. These findings support an aggressive therapeutic approach in most of children diagnosed with CD [5]. Similarly, UC is often severe in children with widespread localization at diagnosis, frequent occurrence of flares unresponsive to medical treatment, a high rate of disease extension and an increased need for surgery [6, 7]. In the EPIMAD study, 20 % of children had their colon removed after 5 years [7].

In adults with CD, we found that age under 40 was associated with a more frequent disabling course during the 5-year period following diagnosis [8]. This negative effect of young age was not confirmed in another similar study from Belgium [9]. Moreover, clinical course is usually mild in elderly-onset IBD patients [10]. The risk of surgery for nonneoplastic bowel disease decreases with increasing age at diagnosis [11]. In population-based studies from Norway [12] and Maastricht [13], young age was associated with an increased risk for surgery. After surgery, the risk of postoperative recurrence does not seem dependent on age at first resection [14] but increased in young patients at disease onset [15]. On the other hand, according to European multinational population based study, CD patients above 40 years at diagnosis have an increased mortality risk compared to a background population of same age [16]. In other terms, although as a

D.C. Baumgart (ed.), *Crohn's Disease and Ulcerative Colitis*, DOI 10.1007/978-3-319-33703-6_61

whole CD may be less active in older people, the risk of death from CD is particularly elevated in this age group.

The effect of age on disease severity in UC is less clear. In a population-based study from Maastricht, it was found that in UC, older age at diagnosis initially increased recurrence risk but was subsequently protective [13]. The risk of surgery for non-neoplastic bowel disease is unrelated to age at diagnosis [11]. Finally, after proctocolectomy and IPAA, the risk of developing subsequent CD is increased in younger patients [17].

Another important point to consider is the fact that side effects of immunosuppressants and biologics are increased in patients older than 65 [18], particularly regarding the risk of lymphoma [19]. This should be kept in mind when discussing such therapies in these patients.

Severity of the First Flare

In CD, the need for steroids to treat the first flare was found to be an important predictor of disabling disease during the five following years in two independent studies including patients in the last nineties [8, 9]. Need for steroids should be regarded as a marker of a severe clinical presentation. In the IBSEN study from Norway, it was found that, in patients with ileal CD, a high C-reactive protein value was associated with an increased risk of surgery during the next 5 years [20]. A similar observation was made in children [21]. In UC, the severity of the first attack is not per se an indicator of a poor prognosis. In the Copenhagen study, patients with a severe presentation who required intensive intravenous therapy but avoided colectomy tended to have a more benign course during the following years [22]. However, high CRP at diagnosis is associated with colectomy [23].

Disease Location

Development of complications in CD is highly related to disease location. Ileal involvement may be complicated at diagnosis or during the very first years by an abscess/fistula or by a stricture followed by a fistula formation [8, 23], whereas a colonic disease may remain « uncomplicated », inflammatory, for many years [24]. Upper gastrointestinal disease at diagnosis is associated with an excess risk of flares during the first 10 years of the disease [25] and jejunal disease is more prone to strictures formation. The disease tends also to be more severe when the lesions are extensive, when compared to involvement of a short segment of small bowel or colon. This is the case in patients with diffuse jejunoileitis, or extensive ileocolitis, or pancolitis. The role of disease extent—in other terms, the length of the resection—for predicting early postoperative recurrence is more debated [26–28].

Perianal location is another important predictor in CD [29]. At presentation, about 30 % of patients share perianal lesions and 20 % have or have had a fistula [30]. Perianal location is associated with a disabling course [8, 9] and is recognized by most authors as having a negative impact on prognosis both through occurrence of local complications and its association with a more severe luminal course [31–33]. Its role in postoperative recurrence is less clear [26, 33]. Perianal lesions may worsen and require a permanent stoma, notably when there is an associated rectal disease [34]. More than 10 % of CD patients eventually require permanent fecal diversion [35].

In UC, the initial extent of the lesions is not associated with an increased risk of flares but with a higher clinical severity [13, 36–38]. Moreover in both colonic CD and UC, the risk of colorectal cancer increases in proportion of the extent of the inflammatory process within the mucosa and is maximum in pancolitis. The risk of pouchitis after proctocolectomy and ileal pouch anal anastomosis (IPAA) is also increased in case of pancolitis [39, 40].

Disease Behavior

It is not surprising that CD patients presenting at diagnosis with a stricture or a fistula are more at risk to come to surgery. Actually those patients are diagnosed too late, while the anatomical damage has become irreversible [41], complications respond poorly to medical therapy, and surgery cannot be avoided in most cases. In the Copenhagen cohort, the 20-year cumulative risk of intestinal resection was 82 % [42]. Other series from 1970 to 2000 showed rather similar rates [32, 43], and in the most recent population-based study the 7-years cumulative risk was still 28.5 % [44]. In the IBSEN study stricturing and penetrating behavior at diagnosis were independent risk factors for subsequent surgery [12], and most other studies made similar conclusions [9, 13, 45, 46]. More importantly, patients operated on for a penetrating complication (abscess, fistula, or peritonitis) have an increased risk to develop a surgical recurrence from a similar penetrating complication. Conversely, patients with a stricture tend to recur again in a stricturing mode [47]. Greenstein et al. suggested that the postoperative recurrence develops earlier in the former than in the latter [47], and some studies also found an increased risk of postoperative recurrence in patients operated on for a penetrating complication [14, 48, 49]. However, some other studies did not find such a difference [26, 50, 51]. Thus, it is not clear that perforating disease is a risk factor for recurrence.

Extraintestinal Manifestations

There is no indication that IBD patients presenting with joint, skin, or eye involvement have a more severe luminal disease than those without extraintestinal manifestations [52, 53]. In patients with extraintestinal manifestations, one study found an increased risk of surgical recurrence after first surgery in CD [14] in CD and another an increased risk of colectomy in UC [54]. In UC patients, an increased risk of pouchitis after IPAA in such patients is well documented [55–59].

Primary sclerosing cholangitis (PSC) prevalence in IBD is about 5 % in UC and 2 % in CD. IBD associated with PSC is more frequently a pancolitis, often with backwash ileitis and rectal sparing [60]. The intestinal disease activity is usually low. However, there is a higher risk of colorectal neoplasia and cancer than in IBD without PSC [60]. This higher risk is unrelated to disease location or extent [61]. Moreover, after IPAA, pouchitis is more frequent. Finally prognosis is embedded by the risk of evolution of the hepatobiliary disease which may require orthotopic liver transplantation. The risk of cholangiocarcinoma (and/or gallbladder carcinoma) is about 1 % every year.

Endoscopy and Histopathological Factors

In both acute CD [62] and UC [63], the presence of deep ulcerations at colonoscopy is associated with a worse prognosis and an increased risk of colectomy. In inactive UC, persistence of ulcers [64] and in the subset of patients with mucosal healing, basal plasmocytosis [65, 66], are associated with an increased risk of clinical relapse.

Environmental Factors

In CD, current smoking increases by more than 50 % the risk of flare-up as compared to never-smokers [45, 67], and is associated with more frequent intestinal penetrating complications. The risk of being operated on at least once during disease course is increased in smokers vs. nonsmokers in most studies [13, 43, 68].

After surgery, the cumulative rates of clinical and surgical recurrence, respectively, were found consistently more elevated in smokers than in nonsmokers, and actually smoking is the factor the most determinant for postoperative recurrence in CD [28, 69–71]. By contrast, in UC, smokers run a more benign disease course when compared to nonsmokers: flare-up and hospitalization rates are less frequent and colectomy rate is lower [72–76]. After colectomy and IPAA, current smoking is associated with an increased risk of subsequent CD [77]. It has been claimed that current smokers have a lower incidence of pouchitis [78], but this observation was not confirmed in most recent series [55, 58, 79].

Prior appendectomy, although more frequent in CD compared to a background population, has no clear effect on evolution of the disease [80]. In UC, appendectomy is associated with a less severe course and a lower colectomy rate [81, 82].

Genetic Factors

The severity of CD is unaffected by family history [83], nor that of UC [72, 84].

Despite a growing number of identified susceptibility loci in both CD and UC [85], only very few have been associated with disease outcome. The presence of NOD2 polymorphism has been associated with a more aggressive clinical course of Crohn's disease with higher risk of intestinal stenoses and earlier need for first surgery [86–88]. Genetic factors also play a major role in the response to therapies: MDR1 (multidrug resistance) predict response to steroids and cyclosporine [89], TNF (tumor necrosis factor) and MIF (migration inhibitory factor) predict response to steroids [90–92], and apoptosis genes predict response to infliximab therapy [93]. However, genetic markers will probably never be able to fully predict IBD behavior and complications, notably because of the major role of environmental factors in the disease pathogenesis. On the other hand, they can be easily associated with other types of factors, such as clinical or microbiological data to build more powerful composite predicting tools.

Serologic Markers

Many studies have been performed to assess the predictive value of specific antibodies as perinuclear anti-neutrophil antibody (pANCA) associated with UC or UC-like CD, and anti-*Saccharomyces cerevisiae* antibody (ASCA, glycan antibody) is mostly associated with CD [94, 95]. Reactivity to ASCA, OmpC anti-I2, and CBir1 have been associated with early disease onset CD, fibrostenosing and penetrating disease, and need for early small bowel surgery [96–100]. In pediatric CD patients, baseline ASCA reactivity has been associated with earlier complications, relapsing disease, and need for an additional surgery [101]. The frequency of disease complications increases with reactivity to increasing numbers of antigens (ASCA, anti-I2, anti-OmpC, and anti-CBir1) [102]. pANCA has been shown to be associated with less severe disease, UC-like disease and negatively associated with small bowel complication [97, 103]. Autoantibodies against granulocyte-macrophage colony-stimulating factor have also been associated with complications of CD [104]. On the other hand, the risk of chronic pouchitis is increased in UC patients with high pre-colectomy levels of pANCA [105]. Conversely, ASCA positivity has been associated with CD of the pouch after IPAA [106].

High-Risk Patients

From this review of the possible different predictors of the disease course, some emerged as more important: age at disease onset, severity of the first flare and perianal location in CD; young age and disease extent in UC [107]. Smoking is an important factor in CD but it may be corrected, and quitters have a course which becomes similar to that of never-smokers [70, 108]. The role of disease location and behavior is important; however, it is partly redundant and concerns mainly the

Table 61.1 Factors collected at presentation associated with a more severe course in CD

	Relative importance	References
Age < 17 years	+++	[3, 110]
Perianal disease	++	[8, 9]
Need for steroids	++	[8, 9, 111]
Ileocolonic location	+	[9, 112]
Age <40 years	+	[8]
Current smoking	+	[45, 67]
High CRP	+	[113]
Stricture	+	[9]
Disease extent	+	[114]

Table 61.2 Factors collected at surgery associated with late complications following IPAA

	Relative importance	References
Chronic pouchitis		
Pancolitis	++	[39, 40]
Associated PSC	++	[115, 116]
Younger age	+	[17]
Extraintestinal manifestations	+	[55] [57, 117] [58, 59]
High pANCA	+	[58, 105]
Nonsmoking	+	[78] [58]
	–	[79]
Crohn's disease		
Current smoking	++	[77]
Family history of Crohn's	++	[106, 118]
Younger age	+	[17]
ASCA	+	[106, 119]
CBir antibodies	+	[119]

need for surgery. Genetic and serologic markers are promising and interesting at the epidemiological level, but to date, only ASCA is accurate enough to predict disease course, in association with clinical data [109]. Now early intestinal surgery may be associated with a non severe disease, for example a short stricturing ileitis, which many physicians would refer to the surgeon. Therefore the increased risk for surgery should not be considered per se as a marker of a more severe disease. Finally it is important to note that we are not able to predict the disease course in the long term, and that prediction should be considered only as indicative. One patient with a very quiescent disease for years may suddenly develop a severe acute flare or complication leading to surgery.

The most relevant predictors are indicated in Tables 61.1–61.5: at presentation, regarding the risk of a 5-year disabling course in CD (Table 61.1), the risk of early intestinal resection in CD (Table 61.2), and the risk of colectomy in UC (Table 61.3). In addition, factors associated with an increased risk of postoperative recurrence in CD and of late complications after IPAA for UC are given in Tables 61.4 and 61.5, respectively. The relative importance of each factor is indicated, based on the data of the literature and our clinical experience.

Table 61.3 Factors collected at presentation associated with earlier surgery in CD

	Relative importance	References
Fistula or abscess	+++	[12]
Stricture	++	[12]
Jejunal location	++	[120, 121]
Ileal location	++	[43]
Younger age	++	[11–13]
Current smoking	+	[13, 43]
High C-reactive protein	+	[20]
ASCA	+	[98, 99, 122]
NOD2 polymorphism	+	[86, 87]

Table 61.4 Factors collected at presentation associated with a higher risk of colectomy in UC

	Relative importance	References
Very young age	++	[6, 7]
Extensive disease	++	[13, 36–38, 123]
No response to steroids	++	[124]
Increased C-reactive protein or ESR	++	[23, 125]
Severe endoscopic lesions	++	[63, 126]
Hospitalization soon after diagnosis	+	[127]
Low hemoglobin	+	[128]
Increased fecal calprotectin	+	[129]
Non smoking	+	[76, 123]
No appendectomy	+	[81, 130]

ESR erythrocyte sedimentation rate

Table 61.5 Factors collected at surgery and pathology associated with a higher risk of postoperative recurrence in CD

	Relative importance	References
Current smoking	+++	[28, 49, 131–134]
Short disease duration	+	[69]
Prior surgery	+	[135]
Disease extent	+	[26, 28, 136]
Jejunal disease	+	[120]
Colonic disease	+	[137]
Plexitis	+	[138, 139]
NOD2 polymorphism	+	[87]
Fistula, abscess or peritonitis	+	[48, 49, 132, 140]
	–	[50, 51, 141]
Associated perianal disease	+	[26, 33, 142]
	–	[143]

Conclusion

In patients most at risk to have a disabling disease or to require surgery, active treatment with immunosuppressants or biologics should be discussed in balance with the goal of therapy, which may be different in a young adult searching for work and a retired individual. For example, ileocecal resection may be the preferred option in a young nonsmoker patient with a limited stricturing disease, because if unoperated on he will have a disabling course whereas surgery will probably give him several years of remission. On the other hand, in one CD patient with a severe clinical presentation, an ileocolonic location, a perianal disease, and current smoking, early surgery must be avoided and to achieve this, immunosuppressants and biologics should be started within the few weeks following diagnosis. In patients operated on but at high risk of postoperative recurrence, particularly in those with prior extensive or multiple resection, postoperative anti-TNF should be considered [144]. Moreover, during the disease course, high-risk patients should be checked regularly for the presence of intestinal ulcerations and thickening, using noninvasive techniques (CRP, ferritin, fecal calprotectin, video capsule, and MRI) and treated as early as possible with the goal to heal lesions before the disease expresses clinically.

References

1. Rutgeerts P, Vermeire S, Van Assche G. Biological therapies for inflammatory bowel diseases. Gastroenterology. 2009;136: 1182–97.
2. Cosnes J, Cattan S, Blain A, Beaugerie L, Carbonnel F, Parc R, et al. Long-term evolution of disease behavior of Crohn's disease. Inflamm Bowel Dis. 2002;8:244–50.
3. Pigneur B, Seksik P, Viola S, Viala J, Beaugerie L, Girardet JP, et al. Natural history of Crohn's disease: comparison between childhood- and adult-onset disease. Inflamm Bowel Dis. 2010;16:953–61.
4. Heyman MB, Kirschner BS, Gold BD, Ferry G, Baldassano R, Cohen SA, et al. Children with early-onset inflammatory bowel disease (IBD): analysis of a pediatric IBD consortium registry. J Pediatr. 2005;146:35–40.
5. Markowitz J, Grancher K, Kohn N, Lesser M, Daum F. A multicenter trial of 6-mercaptopurine and prednisone in children with newly diagnosed Crohn's disease. Gastroenterology. 2000;119:895–902.
6. Turner D, Walsh CM, Benchimol EI, Mann EH, Thomas KE, Chow C, et al. Severe paediatric ulcerative colitis: incidence, outcomes and optimal timing for second-line therapy. Gut. 2008;57:331–8.
7. Gower-Rousseau C, Dauchet L, Vernier-Massouille G, Tilloy E, Brazier F, Merle V, et al. The natural history of pediatric ulcerative colitis: a population-based cohort study. Am J Gastroenterol. 2009;104:2080–8.
8. Beaugerie L, Seksik P, Nion-Larmurier I, Gendre JP, Cosnes J. Predictors of Crohn's disease. Gastroenterology. 2006;130:650–6.
9. Loly C, Belaiche J, Louis E. Predictors of severe Crohn's disease. Scand J Gastroenterol. 2008;43:948–54.
10. Charpentier C, Salleron J, Savoye G, Fumery M, Merle V, Laberenne JE, et al. Natural history of elderly-onset inflammatory bowel disease: a population-based cohort study. Gut. 2014;63:423–32.
11. Tremaine WJ, Timmons LJ, Loftus Jr EV, Pardi DS, Sandborn WJ, Harmsen WS, et al. Age at onset of inflammatory bowel disease and the risk of surgery for non-neoplastic bowel disease. Aliment Pharmacol Ther. 2007;25:1435–41.
12. Solberg IC, Vatn MH, Hoie O, Stray N, Sauar J, Jahnsen J, et al. Clinical course in Crohn's disease: results of a Norwegian population-based ten-year follow-up study. Clin Gastroenterol Hepatol. 2007;5:1430–8.
13. Romberg-Camps MJ, Dagnelie PC, Kester AD, Hesselink-van de Kruijs MA, Cilissen M, Engels LG, et al. Influence of phenotype at diagnosis and of other potential prognostic factors on the course of inflammatory bowel disease. Am J Gastroenterol. 2009;104:371–83.
14. Hofer B, Bottger T, Hernandez-Richter T, Seifert JK, Junginger T. The impact of clinical types of disease manifestation on the risk of early postoperative recurrence in Crohn's disease. Hepatogastroenterology. 2001;48:152–5.
15. Scarpa M, Ruffolo C, Bertin E, Polese L, Filosa T, Prando D, et al. Surgical predictors of recurrence of Crohn's disease after ileocolonic resection. Int J Colorectal Dis. 2007;22:1061–9.
16. Wolters FL, Russel MG, Sijbrandij J, Schouten LJ, Odes S, Riis L, et al. Crohn's disease: increased mortality 10 years after diagnosis in a Europe-wide population based cohort. Gut. 2006;55:510–8.
17. Melton GB, Kiran RP, Fazio VW, He J, Shen B, Goldblum JR, et al. Do preoperative factors predict subsequent diagnosis of Crohn's disease after ileal pouch-anal anastomosis for ulcerative or indeterminate colitis? Colorectal Dis. 2010;12(10):1026–32. doi:10.1111/j.1463-1318.2009.02014.x.
18. Cottone M, Kohn A, Daperno M, Armuzzi A, Guidi L, D'Inca R, et al. Age is a risk factor for severe infections and mortality in patients given anti-tumor necrosis factor therapy for inflammatory bowel disease. Clin Gastroenterol Hepatol. 2011;17:758–66.
19. Beaugerie L, Brousse N, Bouvier AM, Colombel JF, Lemann M, Cosnes J, et al. Lymphoproliferative disorders in patients receiving thiopurines for inflammatory bowel disease: a prospective observational cohort study. Lancet. 2009;374:1617–25.
20. Henriksen M, Jahnsen J, Lygren I, Stray N, Sauar J, Vatn MH, et al. C-reactive protein: a predictive factor and marker of inflammation in inflammatory bowel disease. Results from a prospective population-based study. Gut. 2008;57:1518–23.
21. Henderson P, Kennedy NA, Van Limbergen JE, Cameron FL, Satsangi J, Russell RK, et al. Serum C-reactive protein and CRP genotype in pediatric inflammatory bowel disease: influence on phenotype, natural history, and response to therapy. Inflamm Bowel Dis. 2015;21:596–605.
22. Langholz E, Munkholm P, Davidsen M, Nielsen OH, Binder V. Changes in extent of ulcerative colitis: a study on the course and prognostic factors. Scand J Gastroenterol. 1996;31:260–6.
23. Niewiadomski O, Studd C, Hair C, Wilson J, Ding NS, Heerasing N, et al. A prospective population based cohort of inflammatory bowel disease in the biologics era—Disease course and predictors of severity. J Gastroenterol Hepatol. 2015;30:1346–53.
24. Zabana Y, Garcia-Planella E, van Domselaar M, Manosa M, Gordillo J, Lopez-Sanroman A, et al. Predictors of favourable outcome in inflammatory Crohn's disease. A retrospective observational study. Gastroenterol Hepatol. 2013;36:616–23.
25. Wolters FL, Russel MG, Sijbrandij J, Ambergen T, Odes S, Riis L, et al. Phenotype at diagnosis predicts recurrence rates in Crohn's disease. Gut. 2006;55:1124–30.
26. Bernell O, Lapidus A, Hellers G. Risk factors for surgery and recurrence in 907 patients with primary ileocaecal Crohn's disease. Br J Surg. 2000;87:1697–701.
27. Baldassano RN, Han PD, Jeshion WC, Berlin JA, Piccoli DA, Lautenbach E, et al. Pediatric Crohn's disease: risk factors for postoperative recurrence. Am J Gastroenterol. 2001;96:2169–76.
28. Cottone M, Rosselli M, Orlando A, Oliva L, Puleo A, Cappello M, et al. Smoking habits and recurrence in Crohn's disease. Gastroenterology. 1994;106:643–8.
29. Vermeire S, Van Assche G, Rutgeerts P. Perianal Crohn's disease: classification and clinical evaluation. Dig Liver Dis. 2007;39:959–62.
30. Schwartz DA, Loftus Jr EV, Tremaine WJ, Panaccione R, Harmsen WS, Zinsmeister AR, et al. The natural history of fistulizing Crohn's disease in Olmsted County, Minnesota. Gastroenterology. 2002;122:875–80.
31. Veloso FT, Ferreira JT, Barros L, Almeida S. Clinical outcome of Crohn's disease: analysis according to the vienna classification and clinical activity. Inflamm Bowel Dis. 2001;7:306–13.

32. Mekhjian HS, Switz DM, Melnyk CS, Rankin GB, Brooks RK. Clinical features and natural history of Crohn's disease. Gastroenterology. 1979;77:898–906.
33. Bernell O, Lapidus A, Hellers G. Risk factors for surgery and postoperative recurrence in Crohn's disease. Ann Surg. 2000;231:38–45.
34. Cosnes J, Bourrier A, Nion-Larmurier I, Sokol H, Beaugerie L, Seksik P. Factors affecting outcomes in Crohn's disease over 15 years. Gut. 2012;61:1140–5.
35. Galandiuk S, Kimberling J, Al-Mishlab TG, Stromberg AJ. Perianal Crohn disease: predictors of need for permanent diversion. Ann Surg. 2005;241:796–801. discussion 801-2.
36. Solberg IC, Lygren I, Jahnsen J, Aadland E, Hoie O, Cvancarova M, et al. Clinical course during the first 10 years of ulcerative colitis: results from a population-based inception cohort (IBSEN Study). Scand J Gastroenterol. 2009;44:431–40.
37. Langholz E, Munkholm P, Davidsen M, Binder V. Colorectal cancer risk and mortality in patients with ulcerative colitis. Gastroenterology. 1992;103:1444–51.
38. Ekbom A, Helmick CG, Zack M, Holmberg L, Adami HO. Survival and causes of death in patients with inflammatory bowel disease: a population-based study. Gastroenterology. 1992;103:954–60.
39. Achkar JP, Al-Haddad M, Lashner B, Remzi FH, Brzezinski A, Shen B, et al. Differentiating risk factors for acute and chronic pouchitis. Clin Gastroenterol Hepatol. 2005;3:60–6.
40. Schmidt CM, Lazenby AJ, Hendrickson RJ, Sitzmann JV. Preoperative terminal ileal and colonic resection histopathology predicts risk of pouchitis in patients after ileoanal pull-through procedure. Ann Surg. 1998;227:654–62. discussion 663-5.
41. Pariente B, Mary JY, Danese S, Chowers Y, De Cruz P, D'Haens G, et al. Development of the Lemann Index to assess digestive tract damage in patients with Crohn's disease. Gastroenterology. 2015;148:52–63.
42. Munkholm P, Langholz E, Davidsen M, Binder V. Disease activity courses in a regional cohort of Crohn's disease patients. Scand J Gastroenterol. 1995;30:699–706.
43. Sands BE, Arsenault JE, Rosen MJ, Alsahli M, Bailen L, Banks P, et al. Risk of early surgery for Crohn's disease: implications for early treatment strategies. Am J Gastroenterol. 2003;98:2712–8.
44. Vester-Andersen MK, Prosberg MV, Jess T, Andersson M, Bengtsson BG, Blixt T, et al. Disease course and surgery rates in inflammatory bowel disease: a population-based, 7-year follow-up study in the era of immunomodulating therapy. Am J Gastroenterol. 2014;109:705–14.
45. Wolters FL, Joling C, Russel MG, Sijbrandij J, De Bruin M, Odes S, et al. Treatment inferred disease severity in Crohn's disease: evidence for a European gradient of disease course. Scand J Gastroenterol. 2007;42:333–44.
46. Henckaerts L, Van Steen K, Verstreken I, Cleynen I, Franke A, Schreiber S, et al. Genetic risk profiling and prediction of disease course in Crohn's disease patients. Clin Gastroenterol Hepatol. 2009;7:972–80. e2.
47. Greenstein AJ, Lachman P, Sachar DB, Springhorn J, Heimann T, Janowitz HD, et al. Perforating and nonperforating indications for repeated operations in Crohn's disease: evidence for two clinical forms. Gut. 1988;29:588–92.
48. Aeberhard P, Berchtold W, Riedtmann HJ, Stadelmann G. Surgical recurrence of perforating and nonperforating Crohn's disease. A study of 101 surgically treated patients. Dis Colon Rectum. 1996;39:80–7.
49. Avidan B, Sakhnini E, Lahat A, Lang A, Koler M, Zmora O, et al. Risk factors regarding the need for a second operation in patients with Crohn's disease. Digestion. 2005;72:248–53.
50. Hamon JF, Carbonnel F, Beaugerie L, Sezeur A, Gallot D, Malafosse M, et al. Comparison of long-term course of perforating and non-perforating Crohn disease. Gastroenterol Clin Biol. 1998;22:601–6.
51. Yamamoto T, Allan RN, Keighley MR. Perforating ileocecal Crohn's disease does not carry a high risk of recurrence but usually re-presents as perforating disease. Dis Colon Rectum. 1999;42:519–24.
52. Farhi D, Cosnes J, Zizi N, Chosidow O, Seksik P, Beaugerie L, et al. Significance of erythema nodosum and pyoderma gangrenosum in inflammatory bowel diseases: a cohort study of 2402 patients. Medicine (Baltimore). 2008;87:281–93.
53. Bardazzi G, Mannoni A, d'Albasio G, Bonanomi AG, Trallori G, Benucci M, et al. Spondyloarthritis in patients with ulcerative colitis. Ital J Gastroenterol Hepatol. 1997;29:520–4.
54. Canas-Ventura A, Marquez L, Ricart E, Domenech E, Gisbert JP, Garcia-Sanchez V, et al. Risk of colectomy in patients with ulcerative colitis under thiopurine treatment. J Crohns Colitis. 2014;8:1287–93.
55. Fleshner P, Ippoliti A, Dubinsky M, Ognibene S, Vasiliauskas E, Chelly M, et al. A prospective multivariate analysis of clinical factors associated with pouchitis after ileal pouch-anal anastomosis. Clin Gastroenterol Hepatol. 2007;5:952–8. quiz 887.
56. Shen B, Fazio VW, Remzi FH, Brzezinski A, Bennett AE, Lopez R, et al. Risk factors for diseases of ileal pouch-anal anastomosis after restorative proctocolectomy for ulcerative colitis. Clin Gastroenterol Hepatol. 2006;4:81–9. quiz 2-3.
57. Hoda KM, Collins JF, Knigge KL, Deveney KE. Predictors of pouchitis after ileal pouch-anal anastomosis: a retrospective review. Dis Colon Rectum. 2008;51:554–60.
58. Kuisma J, Jarvinen H, Kahri A, Farkkila M. Factors associated with disease activity of pouchitis after surgery for ulcerative colitis. Scand J Gastroenterol. 2004;39:544–8.
59. Hata K, Watanabe T, Shinozaki M, Nagawa H. Patients with extraintestinal manifestations have a higher risk of developing pouchitis in ulcerative colitis: multivariate analysis. Scand J Gastroenterol. 2003;38:1055–8.
60. Loftus Jr EV, Harewood GC, Loftus CG, Tremaine WJ, Harmsen WS, Zinsmeister AR, et al. PSC-IBD: a unique form of inflammatory bowel disease associated with primary sclerosing cholangitis. Gut. 2005;54:91–6.
61. Sokol H, Cosnes J, Chazouilleres O, Beaugerie L, Tiret E, Poupon R, et al. Disease activity and cancer risk in inflammatory bowel disease associated with primary sclerosing cholangitis. World J Gastroenterol. 2008;14:3497–503.
62. Allez M, Lemann M, Bonnet J, Cattan P, Jian R, Modigliani R. Long term outcome of patients with active Crohn's disease exhibiting extensive and deep ulcerations at colonoscopy. Am J Gastroenterol. 2002;97:947–53.
63. Carbonnel F, Lavergne A, Lemann M, Bitoun A, Valleur P, Hautefeuille P, et al. Colonoscopy of acute colitis. A safe and reliable tool for assessment of severity. Dig Dis Sci. 1994;39:1550–7.
64. Froslie KF, Jahnsen J, Moum BA, Vatn MH. Mucosal healing in inflammatory bowel disease: results from a Norwegian population-based cohort. Gastroenterology. 2007;133:412–22.
65. Bessissow T, Lemmens B, Ferrante M, Bisschops R, Van Steen K, Geboes K, et al. Prognostic value of serologic and histologic markers on clinical relapse in ulcerative colitis patients with mucosal healing. Am J Gastroenterol. 2012;107:1684–92.
66. Feagins LA, Melton SD, Iqbal R, Dunbar KB, Spechler SJ. Clinical implications of histologic abnormalities in colonic biopsy specimens from patients with ulcerative colitis in clinical remission. Inflamm Bowel Dis. 2013;19:1477–82.
67. Cosnes J, Carbonnel F, Beaugerie L, Le Quintrec Y, Gendre JP. Effects of cigarette smoking on the long-term course of Crohn's disease. Gastroenterology. 1996;110:424–31.
68. Moon CM, Park DI, Kim ER, Kim YH, Lee CK, Lee SH, et al. Clinical features and predictors of clinical outcomes in Korean patients with Crohn's disease: a Korean association for the study of intestinal diseases multicenter study. J Gastroenterol Hepatol. 2014;29:74–82.

69. Yamamoto T. Factors affecting recurrence after surgery for Crohn's disease. World J Gastroenterol. 2005;11:3971–9.
70. Ryan WR, Allan RN, Yamamoto T, Keighley MR. Crohn's disease patients who quit smoking have a reduced risk of reoperation for recurrence. Am J Surg. 2004;187:219–25.
71. Unkart JT, Anderson L, Li E, Miller C, Yan Y, Gu CC, et al. Risk factors for surgical recurrence after ileocolic resection of Crohn's disease. Dis Colon Rectum. 2008;51:1211–6.
72. Roth LS, Chande N, Ponich T, Roth ML, Gregor J. Predictors of disease severity in ulcerative colitis patients from Southwestern Ontario. World J Gastroenterol. 2010;16:232–6.
73. Boyko EJ, Perera DR, Koepsell TD, Keane EM, Inui TS. Effects of cigarette smoking on the clinical course of ulcerative colitis. Scand J Gastroenterol. 1988;23:1147–52.
74. Beaugerie L, Massot N, Carbonnel F, Cattan S, Gendre JP, Cosnes J. Impact of cessation of smoking on the course of ulcerative colitis. Am J Gastroenterol. 2001;96:2113–6.
75. Szamosi T, Banai J, Lakatos L, Czegledi Z, David G, Zsigmond F, et al. Early azathioprine/biological therapy is associated with decreased risk for first surgery and delays time to surgery but not reoperation in both smokers and nonsmokers with Crohn's disease, while smoking decreases the risk of colectomy in ulcerative colitis. Eur J Gastroenterol Hepatol. 2010;22:872–9.
76. Cosnes J. Tobacco and IBD: relevance in the understanding of disease mechanisms and clinical practice. Best Pract Res Clin Gastroenterol. 2004;18:481–96.
77. Shen B, Fazio VW, Remzi FH, Bennett AE, Brzezinski A, Lopez R, et al. Risk factors for clinical phenotypes of Crohn's disease of the ileal pouch. Am J Gastroenterol. 2006;101:2760–8.
78. Merrett MN, Mortensen N, Kettlewell M, Jewell DO. Smoking may prevent pouchitis in patients with restorative proctocolectomy for ulcerative colitis. Gut. 1996;38:362–4.
79. Joelsson M, Benoni C, Oresland T. Does smoking influence the risk of pouchitis following ileal pouch anal anastomosis for ulcerative colitis? Scand J Gastroenterol. 2006;41:929–33.
80. Cosnes J, Seksik P, Nion-Larmurier I, Beaugerie L, Gendre JP. Prior appendectomy and the phenotype and course of Crohn's disease. World J Gastroenterol. 2006;12:1235–42.
81. Cosnes J, Carbonnel F, Beaugerie L, Blain A, Reijasse D, Gendre JP. Effects of appendicectomy on the course of ulcerative colitis. Gut. 2002;51:803–7.
82. Radford-Smith GL, Edwards JE, Purdie DM, Pandeya N, Watson M, Martin NG, et al. Protective role of appendicectomy on onset and severity of ulcerative colitis and Crohn's disease. Gut. 2002;51:808–13.
83. Carbonnel F, Macaigne G, Beaugerie L, Gendre JP, Cosnes J. Crohn's disease severity in familial and sporadic cases. Gut. 1999;44:91–5.
84. Henriksen M, Jahnsen J, Lygren I, Vatn MH, Moum B. Are there any differences in phenotype or disease course between familial and sporadic cases of inflammatory bowel disease? Results of a population-based follow-up study. Am J Gastroenterol. 2007;102:1955–63.
85. Barrett JC, Hansoul S, Nicolae DL, Cho JH, Duerr RH, Rioux JD, et al. Genome-wide association defines more than 30 distinct susceptibility loci for Crohn's disease. Nat Genet. 2008;40:955–62.
86. Abreu MT, Taylor KD, Lin YC, Hang T, Gaiennie J, Landers CJ, et al. Mutations in NOD2 are associated with fibrostenosing disease in patients with Crohn's disease. Gastroenterology. 2002;123:679–88.
87. Alvarez-Lobos M, Arostegui JI, Sans M, Tassies D, Plaza S, Delgado S, et al. Crohn's disease patients carrying Nod2/CARD15 gene variants have an increased and early need for first surgery due to stricturing disease and higher rate of surgical recurrence. Ann Surg. 2005;242:693–700.
88. Cleynen I, Gonzalez JR, Figueroa C, Franke A, McGovern D, Bortlik M, et al. Genetic factors conferring an increased susceptibility to develop Crohn's disease also influence disease phenotype: results from the IBDchip European Project. Gut. 2013;62:1556–65.
89. Daniel F, Loriot MA, Seksik P, Cosnes J, Gornet JM, Lemann M, et al. Multidrug resistance gene-1 polymorphisms and resistance to cyclosporine A in patients with steroid resistant ulcerative colitis. Inflamm Bowel Dis. 2007;13:19–23.
90. Potocnik U, Ferkolj I, Glavac D, Dean M. Polymorphisms in multidrug resistance 1 (MDR1) gene are associated with refractory Crohn disease and ulcerative colitis. Genes Immun. 2004;5:530–9.
91. Farrell RJ, Kelleher D. Glucocorticoid resistance in inflammatory bowel disease. J Endocrinol. 2003;178:339–46.
92. Cucchiara S, Latiano A, Palmieri O, Canani RB, D'Inca R, Guariso G, et al. Polymorphisms of tumor necrosis factor-alpha but not MDR1 influence response to medical therapy in pediatric-onset inflammatory bowel disease. J Pediatr Gastroenterol Nutr. 2007;44:171–9.
93. Hlavaty T, Pierik M, Henckaerts L, Ferrante M, Joossens S, van Schuerbeek N, et al. Polymorphisms in apoptosis genes predict response to infliximab therapy in luminal and fistulizing Crohn's disease. Aliment Pharmacol Ther. 2005;22:613–26.
94. Ruemmele FM, Targan SR, Levy G, Dubinsky M, Braun J, Seidman EG. Diagnostic accuracy of serological assays in pediatric inflammatory bowel disease. Gastroenterology. 1998;115:822–9.
95. Quinton JF, Sendid B, Reumaux D, Duthilleul P, Cortot A, Grandbastien B, et al. Anti-Saccharomyces cerevisiae mannan antibodies combined with antineutrophil cytoplasmic autoantibodies in inflammatory bowel disease: prevalence and diagnostic role. Gut. 1998;42:788–91.
96. Targan SR, Landers CJ, Yang H, Lodes MJ, Cong Y, Papadakis KA, et al. Antibodies to CBir1 flagellin define a unique response that is associated independently with complicated Crohn's disease. Gastroenterology. 2005;128:2020–8.
97. Vasiliauskas EA, Kam LY, Karp LC, Gaiennie J, Yang H, Targan SR. Marker antibody expression stratifies Crohn's disease into immunologically homogeneous subgroups with distinct clinical characteristics. Gut. 2000;47:487–96.
98. Arnott ID, Landers CJ, Nimmo EJ, Drummond HE, Smith BK, Targan SR, et al. Sero-reactivity to microbial components in Crohn's disease is associated with disease severity and progression, but not NOD2/CARD15 genotype. Am J Gastroenterol. 2004;99:2376–84.
99. Adler J, Rangwalla SC, Dwamena BA, Higgins PD. The prognostic power of the NOD2 genotype for complicated Crohn's disease: a meta-analysis. Am J Gastroenterol. 2011;106:699–712.
100. Ryan JD, Silverberg MS, Xu W, Graff LA, Targownik LE, Walker JR, et al. Predicting complicated Crohn's disease and surgery: phenotypes, genetics, serology and psychological characteristics of a population-based cohort. Aliment Pharmacol Ther. 2013;38:274–83.
101. Amre DK, Lu SE, Costea F, Seidman EG. Utility of serological markers in predicting the early occurrence of complications and surgery in pediatric Crohn's disease patients. Am J Gastroenterol. 2006;101:645–52.
102. Dubinsky M. What is the role of serological markers in IBD? Pediatric and adult data. Dig Dis. 2009;27:259–68.
103. Vasiliauskas EA, Plevy SE, Landers CJ, Binder SW, Ferguson DM, Yang H, et al. Perinuclear antineutrophil cytoplasmic antibodies in patients with Crohn's disease define a clinical subgroup. Gastroenterology. 1996;110:1810–9.
104. Gathungu G, Kim MO, Ferguson JP, Sharma Y, Zhang W, Ng SM, et al. Granulocyte-macrophage colonystimulating factor autoantibodies: a marker of aggressive Crohn's disease. Inflamm Bowel Dis. 2013;19:1671–80.
105. Fleshner PR, Vasiliauskas EA, Kam LY, Fleshner NE, Gaiennie J, Abreu-Martin MT, et al. High level perinuclear antineutrophil cytoplasmic antibody (pANCA) in ulcerative colitis patients before colectomy predicts the development of chronic pouchitis after ileal pouch-anal anastomosis. Gut. 2001;49:671–7.
106. Melmed GY, Fleshner PR, Bardakcioglu O, Ippoliti A, Vasiliauskas EA, Papadakis KA, et al. Family history and serology predict Crohn's disease after ileal pouch-anal anastomosis for ulcerative colitis. Dis Colon Rectum. 2008;51:100–8.

107. Reinisch W, Reinink AR, Higgins PD. Factors associated with poor outcomes in adults with newly diagnosed ulcerative colitis. Clin Gastroenterol Hepatol. 2015;13:635–42.
108. Cosnes J, Beaugerie L, Carbonnel F, Gendre JP. Smoking cessation and the course of Crohn's disease: an intervention study. Gastroenterology. 2001;120:1093–9.
109. Solberg IC, Cvancarova M, Vatn MH, Moum B. Risk matrix for prediction of advanced disease in a population-based study of patients with Crohn's Disease (the IBSEN Study). Inflamm Bowel Dis. 2014;20:60–8.
110. Vernier-Massouille G, Balde M, Salleron J, Turck D, Dupas JL, Mouterde O, et al. Natural history of pediatric Crohn's disease: a population-based cohort study. Gastroenterology. 2008;135:1106–13.
111. Wenger S, Nikolaus S, Howaldt S, Bokemeyer B, Sturm A, Preiss JC, et al. Predictors for subsequent need for immunosuppressive therapy in early Crohn's disease. J Crohns Colitis. 2012;6:21–8.
112. Wright JP. Factors influencing first relapse in patients with Crohn's disease. J Clin Gastroenterol. 1992;15:12–6.
113. Kruis W, Katalinic A, Klugmann T, Franke GR, Weismuller J, Leifeld L, et al. Predictive factors for an uncomplicated long-term course of Crohn's disease: a retrospective analysis. J Crohns Colitis. 2013;7:e263–70.
114. Tan WC, Allan RN. Diffuse jejunoileitis of Crohn's disease. Gut. 1993;34:1374–8.
115. Keh C, Shatari T, Yamamoto T, Menon A, Clark MA, Keighley MR. Jejunal Crohn's disease is associated with a higher postoperative recurrence rate than ileocaecal Crohn's disease. Colorectal Dis. 2005;7:366–8.
116. Park SK, Yang SK, Park SH, Kim JW, Yang DH, Jung KW, et al. Long-term prognosis of the jejunal involvement of Crohn's disease. J Clin Gastroenterol. 2013;47:400–8.
117. Dubinsky MC, Lin YC, Dutridge D, Picornell Y, Landers CJ, Farrior S, et al. Serum immune responses predict rapid disease progression among children with Crohn's disease: immune responses predict disease progression. Am J Gastroenterol. 2006;101:360–7.
118. Dias CC, Rodrigues PP, Costa-Pereira AD, Magro F. Clinical predictors of colectomy in patients with ulcerative colitis: systematic review and meta-analysis of cohort studies. J Crohns Colitis. 2015;9(2):156–63.
119. Travis SP, Farrant JM, Ricketts C, Nolan DJ, Mortensen NM, Kettlewell MG, et al. Predicting outcome in severe ulcerative colitis. Gut. 1996;38:905–10.
120. Kumar S, Ghoshal UC, Aggarwal R, Saraswat VA, Choudhuri G. Severe ulcerative colitis: prospective study of parameters determining outcome. J Gastroenterol Hepatol. 2004;19:1247–52.
121. Cacheux W, Seksik P, Lemann M, Marteau P, Nion-Larmurier I, Afchain P, et al. Predictive factors of response to cyclosporine in steroid-refractory ulcerative colitis. Am J Gastroenterol. 2008;103:637–42.
122. Ananthakrishnan AN, Issa M, Beaulieu DB, Skaros S, Knox JF, Lemke K, et al. History of medical hospitalization predicts future need for colectomy in patients with ulcerative colitis. Inflamm Bowel Dis. 2009;15:176–81.
123. Jeon HH, Lee HJ, Jang HW, Yoon JY, Jung YS, Park SJ, et al. Clinical outcomes and predictive factors in oral corticosteroid-refractory active ulcerative colitis. World J Gastroenterol. 2013;19:265–73.
124. Ho GT, Lee HM, Brydon G, Ting T, Hare N, Drummond H, et al. Fecal calprotectin predicts the clinical course of acute severe ulcerative colitis. Am J Gastroenterol. 2009;104:673–8.
125. Radford-Smith GL. What is the importance of appendectomy in the natural history of IBD? Inflamm Bowel Dis. 2008;14 Suppl 2:S72–4.
126. Sutherland LR, Ramcharan S, Bryant H, Fick G. Effect of cigarette smoking on recurrence of Crohn's disease. Gastroenterology. 1990;98:1123–8.
127. Li Y, Zhu W, Zuo L, Zhang W, Gong J, Gu L, et al. Frequency and risk factors of postoperative recurrence of Crohn's disease after intestinal resection in the Chinese population. J Gastrointest Surg. 2012;16:1539–47.
128. Reese GE, Nanidis T, Borysiewicz C, Yamamoto T, Orchard T, Tekkis PP. The effect of smoking after surgery for Crohn's disease: a meta-analysis of observational studies. Int J Colorectal Dis. 2008;23:1213–21.
129. Yamamoto T, Allan RN, Keighley MR. Smoking is a predictive factor for outcome after colectomy and ileorectal anastomosis in patients with Crohn's colitis. Br J Surg. 1999;86:1069–70.
130. Pascua M, Su C, Lewis JD, Brensinger C, Lichtenstein GR. Meta-analysis: factors predicting post-operative recurrence with placebo therapy in patients with Crohn's disease. Aliment Pharmacol Ther. 2008;28:545–56.
131. Hamilton SR. Pathologic features of Crohn's disease associated with recrudescence after resection. Pathol Annu. 1983;18(Pt 1):191–203.
132. van Loo ES, Vosseberg NW, van der Heide F, Pierie JP, van der Linde K, Ploeg RJ, et al. Thiopurines are associated with a reduction in surgical re-resections in patients with Crohn's disease: a long-term follow-up study in a regional and academic cohort. Inflamm Bowel Dis. 2013;19:2801–8.
133. Ferrante M, de Hertogh G, Hlavaty T, D'Haens G, Penninckx F, D'Hoore A, et al. The value of myenteric plexitis to predict early postoperative Crohn's disease recurrence. Gastroenterology. 2006;130:1595–606.
134. Sokol H, Polin V, Lavergne-Slove A, Panis Y, Treton X, Dray X, et al. Plexitis as a predictive factor of early postoperative clinical recurrence in Crohn's disease. Gut. 2009;58:1218–25.
135. Lautenbach E, Berlin JA, Lichtenstein GR. Risk factors for early postoperative recurrence of Crohn's disease. Gastroenterology. 1998;115:259–67.
136. McDonald PJ, Fazio VW, Farmer RG, Jagelman DG, Lavery IC, Ruderman WB, et al. Perforating and nonperforating Crohn's disease. An unpredictable guide to recurrence after surgery. Dis Colon Rectum. 1989;32:117–20.
137. Gao X, Yang RP, Chen MH, Xiao YL, He Y, Chen BL, et al. Risk factors for surgery and postoperative recurrence: analysis of a south China cohort with Crohn's disease. Scand J Gastroenterol. 2012;47:1181–91.
138. Platell C, Mackay J, Woods R. A multivariate analysis of risk factors associated with recurrence following surgery for Crohn's disease. Colorectal Dis. 2001;3:100–6.
139. Penna C, Dozois R, Tremaine W, Sandborn W, LaRusso N, Schleck C, et al. Pouchitis after ileal pouch-anal anastomosis for ulcerative colitis occurs with increased frequency in patients with associated primary sclerosing cholangitis. Gut. 1996;38:234–9.
140. Abdelrazeq AS, Kandiyil N, Botterill ID, Lund JN, Reynolds JR, Holdsworth PJ, et al. Predictors for acute and chronic pouchitis following restorative proctocolectomy for ulcerative colitis. Colorectal Dis. 2008;10:805–13.
141. Shen B, Remzi FH, Brzezinski A, Lopez R, Bennett AE, Lavery IC, et al. Risk factors for pouch failure in patients with different phenotypes of Crohn's disease of the pouch. Inflamm Bowel Dis. 2008;14:942–8.
142. Shen B, Remzi FH, Hammel JP, Lashner BA, Bevins CL, Lavery IC, et al. Family history of Crohn's disease is associated with an increased risk for Crohn's disease of the pouch. Inflamm Bowel Dis. 2009;15:163–70.
143. Coukos JA, Howard LA, Weinberg JM, Becker JM, Stucchi AF, Farraye FA. ASCA IgG and CBir antibodies are associated with the development of Crohn's disease and fistulae following ileal pouch-anal anastomosis. Dig Dis Sci. 2012;57:1544–53.
144. Regueiro M, Schraut W, Baidoo L, Kip KE, Sepulveda AR, Pesci M, et al. Infliximab prevents Crohn's disease recurrence after ileal resection. Gastroenterology. 2009;136:441–50. e1; quiz 716.

Part X

Patient Perspective and Resources

Patient Perspective on Inflammatory Bowel Disease

62

Ayesha Williams and Marjorie Merrick

Approximately 1.6 million Americans have Crohn's disease and ulcerative colitis and as many as 70,000 new cases of inflammatory bowel disease (IBD) are diagnosed in the USA each year [1]. Although most people are diagnosed after the age of 15, studies estimate that approximately 5 % of all IBD patients in the USA are under the age of 20 [2]. All are seeking answers to a variety of questions about their disease.

For the newly diagnosed patient, life has just taken a much unexpected turn. The initial reaction can be shock, fear, disbelief, or even relief to finally be able to put a name to why they or their loved one has been so sick. The realization that they will have to deal with a disease that may be managed but never cured is very difficult for most patients and their families to accept. For many patients, the next step is to gather information about the immediate aspects of their illness. When first diagnosed, there are many initial general questions, which are then followed by more specific practical questions, as illustrated in the chart below.

Initial questions may include:	Practical questions may include:
What is Crohn's disease or ulcerative colitis?	Where is the nearest bathroom and will I have access to it?
Is it contagious?	How do I tell my boss (or teacher or loved one) about my disease?
Is there a cure?	What will they think about me after they know I have a "bathroom" problem?
Did I do something to make me get sick?	Will I be able to keep my job? Stay in school? How can I get accommodations?
Was it something I ate (or didn't eat)?	What can I eat that won't make me feel worse?
What diet should I follow?	How do I avoid embarrassing "accidents" that soil my clothes?
I'm under a lot of stress—did that cause me to get sick?	Why am I having problems with anger and depression?
What are the medicines used to treat this disease and which will I need? How long will I need to take the medicine? Are there side effects to the medicine?	Will my health insurance cover my medical costs? Can I get financial assistance to cover the costs of the copays of my medication?
Will I ever need surgery?	Can I qualify for Social Security Disability?
Will I get cancer?	I think I need another opinion. Who is the best doctor or hospital to treat IBD?
Why am I always tired?	Does IBD affect a woman's menstrual cycle?
Will I ever feel good again—in this lifetime?	Can I be sexually intimate with the symptoms of the disease? Can I be sexually intimate if I have an ostomy?
What research and advocacy is being done in IBD? Are we close to having a cure in my lifetime?	When should I tell someone I am dating that I have IBD?
Are there diagnostic/monitoring tests that I will need every time I see my gastroenterologist?	Can I get the necessary vaccines, such as the flu shot, if I have IBD?
How can I manage the symptoms of pain, diarrhea, and rectal pain?	Can I continue to smoke or have alcoholic beverages now that I have IBD?
Will I be able to have children?	Are there any complementary or alternative therapies that I can try?
Will my children get this disease?	Where can I find support to cope with how I am feeling?

In 2003, CCFA conducted an Internet-based survey which was completed by more than 4000 members. The study revealed a number of interesting facts about persons newly diagnosed with IBD, including their experiences in being

A. Williams, M.P.A.
IBD Help Center, Crohn's & Colitis Foundation of America, 733 Third Avenue, Suite 510, New York, NY 10017, USA

M. Merrick, M.A. (✉)
Research and Scientific Programs, Crohn's & Colitis Foundation of America, 733 Third Avenue, Suite 510, New York, NY 10017, USA
e-mail: MMerrick@ccfa.org

D.C. Baumgart (ed.), *Crohn's Disease and Ulcerative Colitis*, DOI 10.1007/978-3-319-33703-6_62

diagnosed, anxieties about their diseases, attitudes about treatment, and other aspects of living with IBD. These interesting facts have also been expressed in a 2012 study based on the Internet cohort of 7141 adults with IBD utilizing the Crohn's & Colitis Foundation of America (CCFA) Partners program. The study found, compared to the general population, IBD patients in this cohort reported more anxiety, depression, fatigue, and sleep disturbance and less social satisfaction [3]. These concerns have remained constant over the past 8 years as shared by over 100,000 patients who have contacted CCFA's Irwin M. and Suzanne R. Rosenthal IBD Resource Center (IBD Help Center) by phone, e-mail, or live chat. The IBD Help Center is a free service for all members of the IBD community. Each year, the IBD Help Center is equipped to answer questions in 170 different languages and responds to nearly 13,000 requests from patients, their families, health care professionals, and the general public. A few of the common trends are discussed below.

The average patient is fairly knowledgeable about their disease because the unpredictability and severity of IBD drives them to educate themselves about their disease. This is particularly true of parents whose young child has just been diagnosed. However, they tend to not be as knowledgeable about treatments or side effects.

Patients are very consistent in how they find educational materials. Physicians are the primary source of information. Secondary sources include CCFA's website, Internet sites, and books. The Internet has no shortage of sites purporting to be about IBD but, unfortunately, only a modest percentage of sites offer peer-reviewed, scientifically valid information. The challenge is to direct patients and families from the time of diagnosis toward reputable websites or materials for their educational needs.

Quality of life is a major concern. Patients report that they tend to spend more time at home and reduce their social activities, particularly when their disease is active. Many patients are very much afraid of not having easy access to a bathroom. They may not eat anything for several hours before a social event and consume nothing during the event to minimize the chance of embarrassing flatulence or uncontrollable diarrhea. Many patients will not venture more than a few miles so that they can return home quickly if they feel sick or have soiled their clothes. When they do go out, they may carry an extra set of clothing, "just in case," but are then embarrassed and worry that unwelcome questions will be asked if they go into the bathroom and reappear in different clothes.

Communication between physicians and patients is a key ingredient to patient satisfaction. Patients want to feel that they and their physician are partners and that treatment decisions are being made collaboratively. It is also interesting to note that quite often the physician's idea of a successful treatment is very different from the patient's evaluation. For instance, the physician may feel that the treatment that reduced the number of bowel movements from 15–20 per day to 5–7 per day is not a total success, but the patient may think that having *only* 5–7 bowel movements per day is a huge improvement that allows them to have a fuller life. Open communication—with both physician and patient asking the right questions—will help create a successful physician–patient relationship. Accordingly, one of the goals of the IBD Help Center is to equip both patients and caregivers with the most appropriate questions for the physician to help them make informed decisions about their medical care. In a 2013 IBD Help Center survey, close to 75 % of responders noted that the Center's information empowered them to feel more comfortable discussing their disease and treatment options with their gastroenterologist.

IBD patients tend to be up-to-date on what new drugs are in the pharmaceutical pipelines; in fact, it is not unusual for patients to know that a new drug has been released before their physician knows. They want to know about potential side effects, clinical trial data, and the costs of the drug. Those who need surgery want to know details about the procedure, how long it will take to recover, if they will need surgery again in the future, and what will be their functional status after the surgery. Here again, physicians need to be aware that the patient viewpoint may be very different from their own, and should take patient concerns into account and involve them in creating the treatment plan.

One of the most frequently asked questions relates to diet and nutrition. Every IBD patient has a list of foods that they do not tolerate well, especially when in an IBD flare. Patients often believe their disease is caused by and can be cured by diet. They will investigate, and likely try, any fad diet, usually without consulting their physician. Nutrition is a common discussion among the pediatric IBD community to help encourage proper growth but, unfortunately, adult patients report that diet and nutrition are not discussed as frequently with physicians. Again, a strong physician–patient partnership, along with the possible help of a dietitian or nutritionist, can ensure the best possible nutritional outcomes.

Having IBD can be emotionally burdensome, and IBD patients may experience a wide range of emotions. Anxiety and depression may be an IBD patient's daily companions, but symptoms are often downplayed to not only loved ones but also to their doctor. Family, friends, the patient's physician, a trained IBD nurse, and a mental health counselor can be very helpful, as can patient support groups and community Internet forums like those offered by CCFA.

Research confirms that Crohn's disease and ulcerative colitis are extremely expensive diseases. Direct medical costs include expenses for hospitalizations, physician services, prescription drugs, over-the-counter drugs, skilled nursing care, diagnostic procedures, and other health care services. Indirect costs are the value of lost earnings, productivity, and leisure time. Extrapolating from study data, total annual direct costs for all patients with IBD in the USA are estimated to be between $11 billion and $28 billion [1]. Total indirect costs are estimated to be $3.6 billion [4]. Based on a national health survey in 1999, nearly 32 % of symptomatic IBD patients reported being out of the work force in a 1-year period [4]. Patients and their families worry about how to pay all of their medical costs even when they have jobs, and worry about losing those jobs because they have to miss significant amounts of time when in a full flare. Even if they have adequate insurance, co-pays can be very burdensome and getting Social Security Disability benefits can be very difficult. It is estimated that the annual financial burden (adding direct and indirect costs) of IBD in the USA may be between $14.6 billion and $31.6 billion [1].

All of these are serious concerns, but there are tools available to help both physician and patient. A wealth of materials for patients, caregivers, and health care professionals can be found on CCFA's website at www.ccfa.org. These materials include brochures, fact sheets, webcasts, IBD phone apps, newsletters, and links to online community forums and support groups. Physicians will also find a series of template letters they can use to advocate for their patients to insurance companies, Social Security Administration, and others. These templates may be found at http://www.ccfa.org/science-and-professionals/programs-materials/appeal-letters.

Patients may also speak to an IBD Help Center specialist by calling 888.MY.GUT.PAIN (888-694-8872). All information and printed materials are free of charge.

References

1. The facts about inflammatory bowel disease. Crohn's & Colitis Foundation of America, November 2014. p. 16–7.
2. Kappelman MD, Moore KR, Allen JK, Cook SF. Recent trends in the prevalence of Crohn's disease and ulcerative colitis in a commercially insured US population. Dig Dis Sci. 2013;58:519–25.
3. Kappelman MD. Evaluation of the Patient Reported Outcomes Measurement Information System (PROMIS) in a large cohort of patients with inflammatory bowel diseases. In: Digestive Diseases Week Conference, May 2012.
4. Longobardi T, Jacobs P, Bernstein CN. Work losses related to inflammatory bowel disease in the United States: results from the National Health Interview Survey. Am J Gastroenterol. 2003; 98:1064–72.

Additional Resources

Crohn's & Colitis Foundation of America (www.ccfa.org).

CCFA's Irwin M. and Suzanne R. Rosenthal IBD Resource Center (IBD Help Center) (888-694-8872).

CCFA Educational Brochures (online.ccfa.org/brochures):

Living with Crohn's Disease

Living with Ulcerative Colitis

Crohn's Disease and Ulcerative Colitis: A Guide for Parents

Crohn's Disease and Ulcerative Colitis: A Guide for Teachers and Other School Personnel

Managing Flares and Other IBD Symptoms

Understanding IBD Medications and Side Effects

Surgery for Crohn's Disease and Ulcerative Colitis

IBD Fact Book

Selected Books

Kane SV. IBD self-management: the AGA guide to Crohn's disease and ulcerative colitis. 2nd ed. Bethesda, MD: American Gastroenterological Association Institute; 2014.

Saibil F. Crohn's disease and ulcerative colitis: everything you need to know the complete practical guide. 3rd ed. Canada: Firefly Books; 2011.

Warner AS, Barto AE. 100 questions and answers about Crohn's disease and ulcerative colitis: a Lahey clinic guide. Burlington: MA. Jones and Bartlett Publishers; 2010.

Farraye FA. Questions and answers about ulcerative colitis. Sudbury, MA: Jones and Bartlett Learning, LLC; 2011.

Oliva-Hemker M, Ziring D, Bousvaros A, editors. Your child with inflammatory bowel disease: a family guide for caregiving (A Johns Hopkins Press Health Book). Baltimore, MD: North American Society for Pediatric Gastroenterology, Hepatology and Nutrition; 2010.

Patient Resources in Inflammatory Bowel Disease

63

Sanna Lönnfors and Marco Greco

The Resourceful Patient

It is now recognized that patients need, and have a right, to knowledge about their condition and its treatment; however, this was not always the case. In the twenty-first century, the balance of power has shifted significantly from the traditional "paternalistic" role of the doctor, to a more egalitarian approach. In particular, the rise of "shared decision-making"[1] has, in some fortunate cases, transformed the patient experience of health care; from the patient visiting an authoritative health care professional who simply issued directions which were received with faith alone, to a situation where "treatment decisions (are) made through dialogue and discussion of evidence-based treatment options, and the values and expectations of the patient" [1]. This revolution depends on the provision of high-quality, reliable resources for people with IBD. In a survey of 1067 patients with inflammatory bowel disease (617 Crohn's disease, 450 ulcerative colitis), 81 % of the respondents reported it to be "very important" that they could be actively involved in the decision-making process, and another 17 % reported it to be "quite important" [2], and a large panel of international IBD experts recommends that in best practice support in an IBD unit, there should be shared decision-making involving the gastroenterologist (and multidisciplinary team if necessary) and the patient [3]. Governments across Europe have enshrined the principle of patient choice and shared decision-making in national policy and even law. However, despite this commitment to approaches that have high-quality information provision as prerequisites, lack of information is still considered to be a grand challenge, and an urgent need for people with IBD, particularly those who have been recently diagnosed. The empowering principles of shared decision-making and patient choice are sound, but people with IBD are not yet being provided with the resources needed to achieve these goals.

Patient Attitudes to IBD and Knowledge

As knowledge in a person with IBD increases, fear of the unknown, and the anxiety brought about by lack of control decreases; choice, and more importantly, hope, increase; this brings about true empowerment. People with IBD are engaged in a life-long fight to overcome daily symptoms of this chronic disease, which can be disabling, embarrassing, and humiliating [4]. Despite this, people with IBD are often resilient in the face of their illness, they dislike being defined through it, and they are keen to take control over their illness through acquiring knowledge. EFCCA (European Federation of Crohn's and Ulcerative Colitis Associations) believes that people with IBD have a right to clear, unbiased, and high-quality knowledge about their condition, its management, and lifestyle factors, and that IBD patients should be assisted in accessing a range of resources applicable to us by health care professionals.

The impact of IBD on quality of life ranges well beyond a narrow medical definition of the disease. There is a spectrum of complications, comorbidities, and related extraintestinal diseases. This may be why there are differing attitudes and approaches in how people with IBD perceive and tackle their illness. Desire for information about IBD is dependent on these attitudes:

[1]Shared decision-making: where patients are supported to deliberate about the possible attributes and consequences of options, to arrive at informed preferences [16].

S. Lönnfors, M.Sc.P.H., M.A.
European Federation of Crohn's and Ulcerative Colitis Associations (EFCCA), Rue des Chartreux 33-35, B-1000, Brussels, Belgium

M. Greco, LL.MM., Ph.D. (✉)
European Federation of Crohn's and Ulcerative Colitis Associations (EFCCA), Rue des Chartreux 33-35, B-1000, Brussels, Belgium

European Patients' Forum (EPF), Rue du commerce 31, B-1000, Brussels, Belgium
e-mail: marco.greco@efcca.org

D.C. Baumgart (ed.), *Crohn's Disease and Ulcerative Colitis*, DOI 10.1007/978-3-319-33703-6_63

- *Denial*. Unfortunately, a long diagnostic process, or misdiagnosis, is common in IBD. Some patients are diagnosed after a distressing emergency admission, or an acute flare-up. This may lead to intense anxiety and fear. This patient may not be interested in learning about their condition, and may seek to avoid information for a considerable time. This patient may not opt for shared decision-making processes.
- *Acceptance—the search for answers*. Patients who are more gradually exposed to the possibility of diagnosis with IBD, allowing them to come to terms with their situation, often have very specific questions and learning needs related to their condition, its management, or everyday life. This patient may approach the wealth of information available on a "question and answer" basis—ranging through multiple resources, seeking a specific answer to satisfy a particular need. Shared decision-making is important to this patient, but based around clinical issues of particular value to them.
- *Expert patients*. Many patients, after satisfying immediate information needs, may find the learning process grants control and empowerment. This patient is interested in wider background learning, and discovering new knowledge. A patient immersed in high-quality clinical knowledge may converse fluently with health care professionals, and may desire full shared decision-making.
- Gray [1] discusses the phenomenon known as "le maladie de petit papier." Patients attending a consultation with a written list of questions. Rather than scorned, this technique is now encouraged as a consulting aid, and has sometimes become "le maladie de grand print-out."

Patient Empowerment

Empowerment can be defined as a process, where a person who lacks power sets a personally meaningful goal to increase power, takes action towards this goal, and observes and reflects on the impact of this action, drawing on his or her evolving self-efficacy, knowledge, and competence related to the goal [5].

Patients may have to make behavioral changes in order to reach their goals. A five-step model for empowerment for diabetes patients developed by Funnell and Anderson [6] can be adapted to IBD as well. The first step is to deal with the past and explore the problem or issue by thinking what the hardest thing about caring for the IBD is for the patient. The second step is to deal with the present by clarifying the patient's feeling and thoughts and their meanings. The third step is developing a plan for the future taking into consideration questions like what the patient wants, how the situation would have to change so the patient can feel better about it, what are the options and the barriers as well as costs and benefits of each choice. Step four is committing the patient to action: is the patient willing to do what is needed to solve the problem, what is the patient going to do and when, and how will the patient know when he or she has succeeded. Step five is evaluating how the process when, what the patient learned, what barriers were met, and what could be done differently next time.

Classifying Patient Resources

There is no official classification of "patient's resources," neither a clear listing of them. Resources are many, and vary according to disease type, severity, and acute or chronic nature. People with IBD are familiar with several classes of resources, often depending on the time since diagnosis. Classes include but are not limited to: information resources, community-based resources, resources for health care choice, the patient medical record, and social security. Many are designed by various health care professionals, but increasingly, patient associations (such as EFCCA's 29 member associations covering 28 European countries) are developing their own high-quality resources that are truly patient-centered.

Information Resources in the Digital Age

Before the "digital age," and the emergence of the World Wide Web, patients derived information from their community—friends, family, home medical encyclopedias, or public libraries [1]. Many prefer the sense of "ownership" that holding printed information provides; however, in the digital age, printed information carries the disadvantage that it becomes out-of-date the moment it is printed. Even so, in a hospital setting where access to communications may be difficult, printed information offers advantages. The power of digital information is in personalization—the volume, and flexible format of information ensures that most patients can find a resource that is well matched to their level of literacy, interpretive skills, online expertise, cultural sensitivities, and time constraints—these factors, together with the accessibility and exclusivity of the resource, will determine an individual's resource of choice.

However, there is some evidence of the emergence of a "digital divide"—differing levels of patient empowerment between those who have technology and internet fluency, and those without, who may be from certain socioeconomic backgrounds [7]. Digital information is powerful and vast, but not available to everyone. To truly empower patients, accessibility is required.

Traditional Online Resources

In the digital age, patients are now able to access a vast wealth of information online. This includes online versions of traditional patient information "leaflets" published by for example various patient organizations, insurance companies, governmental institutions, and pharmaceutical companies. Increased patient knowledge through the use of online sources may facilitate the shared decision-making process; however, inaccurate information may cause confusion and mislead patients to poor choices. Internet resources—the online encyclopedia Wikipedia for example—may be quickly updated and therefore more up-to-date than traditional printed resources, but they may also be poorly or not at all referenced and the medical information provided in them may not be fully accurate [8]. It may therefore be beneficial for the physician to direct patients to reliable websites.

Innovative Online Resources

Whereas structured navigation helps information seekers to more quickly locate information of relevance, personalized resources may make the resources more effective in practice. Online platforms with more structured, modular information on IBD, which can be presented according to a person's specific disease, age, and topic, can work in this way. Furthermore, rather than static information content, many resources now encourage users to store personal information for later retrieval, or to submit data for processing, thus offering tools to help people with IBD gather, manage and control personal health information.

This innovation is not limited to web browsing—the emergence of mobile devices means that users can carry resources and applications with them which help track or manage diseases, or offer a specific service. Various applications for mobile devices may, for example, allow users to record daily symptoms, pain, appetite, and trips to the bathroom for discussion in the consultation, keep track of their medications or doctor appointments, locate toilet facilities quickly on satellite view, or prepare for a colonoscopy by getting reminders of when to drink bowel-clearing substance. There are also applications with real-time symptom tracking that may be able to find links between dietary or lifestyle choices and symptoms and various calorie trackers and diet applications that help figuring out the ingredients of foods, and often the data collected with the applications can be synced across multiple platforms or printed out.

Users of services providing collection of personal or medical data need of course to be aware of security and confidentiality issues, which may not always be assured or apparent, given the variance in the reputability of different publishers. Patients also need to be made fully aware that although an application may be helpful in managing the illness, it cannot replace a doctor consultation. Many of the applications available were not developed in cooperation with IBD experts and may therefore not be reliable or research-validated [8].

Peer-to-Peer Resources—Patient Experiences as a Success Factor

Rather than resources constructed by authorities to "educate" patients, some resources encourage a peer-to-peer exchange of experiences. The realization that more effective patient information includes the patient's perspective, directly through quotes, stories, and case-studies, has now gained widespread acceptance. Education and medical knowledge may be the primary goal of resources, but this learning process may be more effective, and people more empowered, through inclusion of qualitative experience [9]. People with IBD often report that health care professionals and even family members cannot truly understand the perspective of battling with this chronic disease, so in many national patient associations, discussion forums have been developed to enable people with IBD to share thoughts and reflections, ask questions and find answers, and perhaps above all, to find a sense of community and solidarity with those who share first-hand experience of IBD. Issues such as moderation need careful consideration, but must not pose a barrier to the huge potential positive impact of these resources, recognizing that uncensored and free discussion can be of good value. Static information resources which seek to educate often have a limited lifespan, but dynamic information resources which offer a first-person perspective inspire users to return, and to contribute. The sharing of the patient experience is paramount if a resource for people with IBD is to be successful, and peer-to-peer information is the cornerstone of this approach. A survey of 249 IBD patients, recruited from 35 IBD online communities, showed that participation was helpful in terms of accepting the illness and learning to manage it, and the online communities also helped members to see the illness in a more positive way and to improve subjective well-being. Furthermore online communities provide an anonymous way to interact and a way to socialize even when the illness prevents going out into the community [10].

Social Media

The emergence of social media (Facebook, Twitter, Instagram, etc.) means that patients need no longer passively consume information; they can now author and share information for others to respond to, and actively connect and network with communities through social networking. Facebook groups, for example, offer an easy mechanism for patient organizations to raise awareness, create a sense of community, and allow the sharing of information across and between communities. The notion of "critical mass" is important here—social network and community initiatives can only succeed if they capture the imagination of large numbers of users, to make the online community viable [11]. This is perhaps why Facebook itself continues to dominate, while attempts at bespoke medical or patient group social networking remain small-scale to date. It must be noted that also in social media, there are plenty of pages and groups promoting self-care and various health advice. These are often non-evidence-based and may contain links to commercial websites [8]. Patients should be advised to approach such resources with caution.

The easy online sharing of video and audio as well as blogging has made it possible for people with IBD to directly reach out to one another, without editorial constraint or regulation. The volume of material available has greatly increased, and some viewers and readers find candid information of great value. However, views are often subjective, not quality assured or evidence-based, and can occasionally even be distressing, despite community-based editorial controls. However, some national IBD patient associations have demonstrated that editorial review processes, and careful management, can ensure that first-hand, experience-based video resources are robust, without censoring, and ensuring free contribution.

Resources for Patients and for Health Care Professionals Need Not Be Separate

A fundamental dichotomy between resources for health care professionals, and resources for patients, is a misconception. In some situations, information specifically for patients is of clear benefit; however, the objectives and content are often identical for both audiences. Furthermore, expert patients are often familiar with the "hierarchy of evidence" proposed by Haynes [12], and engage with it at every level.

Resources that should be equally accessible health care professionals and patients alike include:

- *Clinical practice guidelines*. These may be international or national. Patient associations are also motivated and skilled to produce guidelines. When access to treatment, and varying treatment quality, are common issues throughout many European countries, people with IBD are found to be highly motivated to interpret treatment standards, and examine guidelines.
- *High-quality randomized controlled trials*. National IBD patient associations and EFCCA are committed to supporting research, and IBD patients are highly interested in new developments in IBD research.
- *Systematic reviews* (for example, those from the Cochrane collaboration). People with IBD understand that one trial may contradict another, and are increasingly turning to high-quality secondary evidence such as systematic reviews to provide a better answer to their information need.

Once patients becomes fluent in the language of their condition, they may become "expert patients" discerningly seeking high-quality, reputable publications that have high status in the hierarchy of evidence. Gray [1] states that equity of access to resources is important because 5 % of the public are as well educated as clinicians, most health care information is relatively simple, and a patient can spend a large amount of time learning about their condition, whereas a general practitioner has hundreds of conditions to cover, and concludes that "it makes no sense to separate knowledge resources for patients and clinicians."

The Information Revolution and the Need to Appraise Resources

In the twenty-first century, there is a vast ocean of information at a patient's fingertips. However, the majority of the information available electronically is not evidence-based. It may be tainted by subjective opinion, lack of evidence, and even outright bias—making it misleading, wrong, or even harmful. Furthermore, information must be correctly applied. Gray [1] states that "knowledge alone will not create the resourceful patient. Patients also need skills."

Patients can be forced to make a trade-off between accessibility and quality; to find a specific answer that fulfills their needs, quality must be sacrificed, and in the process of learning to live with a chronic condition like IBD, finding this specific answer might be vital to a patient's quality of life, and perhaps even the efficacy of their care.

As it is inevitable in the modern era that patients willing to learn more about their illness will be faced with huge amounts of information and have access to much of the data available, they should be guided into the right direction of high-quality, evidence-based research. It would be beneficial for both the patient and the physician if the patient possessed basic skills to critically appraise the information he or she faces. Patient-friendly appraisal tools or evaluation methods should be developed and their use promoted. Patients should be assisted in developing critical appraisal and interpretive skills.

Communities for People with IBD—EFCCA's Core Resource

The most crucial and valuable resource for an IBD patient is other IBD patients. IBD can be an isolating condition, and where people with IBD can come together in a free environment, they can be greatly empowered by sharing experience and knowledge in a community of mutual support. The first experience of freely socializing with others who also have IBD can be life changing, and this positive impact is one of the most rewarding aspects of the work of EFCCA's 29 national IBD associations around Europe, and EFCCA itself. The benefits of community-based mobilization are well documented, and part of EFCCA's core philosophy; the whole is greater than the sum of its parts. The community groups of EFCCA and its members are flourishing, using online technology to bridge distances, cross borders, and demonstrate a universal commonality in overcoming IBD.

Wherever possible, people with IBD should be supported in finding and accessing communities and groups, and this can be facilitated at the level of specific clinics, or even individual clinicians. Community-based support is not only immensely rewarding for those who take part, but it also offers a wealth of benefits for family members and friends, who may not be present at medical consultations. A large European online patient survey carried out by EFCCA showed that 63 % of those IBD patients who had engaged in patient association activities felt that it had improved their life as someone with IBD [13]. Projects such as EFCCA's summer camps for young people and children with IBD have been proven in efficacy: an online survey for participants of summer camps organized by EFCCA and its member associations showed that most of the participants felt that attending the camp improved their confidence in dealing with IBD, their acceptance of their IBD and their overall quality of life. The majority of the respondents reported that out of all camp experiences, meeting the fellow campers was the most supportive aspect [14]. EFCCA offers national IBD patient associations with resources and knowledge to establish these communities and to organize events.

Resources to Enable Choice—Health Care and Treatment Quality

Increasingly, patient choice of health service, health care provider, and treatment, is being advocated in several European countries and also internationally within the European Union. Patient choice has gained importance for reasons such as reducing waiting times and encouraging competition between providers in order to make care more responsive to patients and improve efficiency [15].

EFCCA supports informed, evidence-based patient choice, except where this fine notion may be used as an opportunity to transfer responsibility for health service quality from government, to the choice of individuals.

One's Own Resource—Owning the Medical Record

Many patients are not aware that European law gives them a legal right to access their own patient data. One's own medical records are also a valuable resource, and ownership of them can often be the beginning in a journey of understanding more about IBD, and can also be vitally useful when transferring between clinicians (particularly internationally), when traveling, or in medical emergencies. Electronic medical record projects often drawn controversy, but also offers the potential of significant rewards.

Patients' Rights as the Foundation Resource

Upholding patients' rights is one of the key challenges that any legislation has to face. Although recognizing the importance of the notion of the "patient as a consumer," the priorities for people with IBD are, at the moment, different.

It is not only difficult to diagnose and differentiate ulcerative colitis and Crohn's disease, but even more difficult to stipulate when a person's IBD meets the requirements of a formal definition of a "disability." This is not helped by the fact that IBD is still often classified as a "rare disease," even though its incidence and prevalence is greater than many more well-known conditions. These circumstances have a clear cascade-effect on people with IBD; they sustain the isolating nature of IBD on patients, and distance patients from their right to health.

A united, focused voice amongst health care professionals, together with patients, can help to overcome this situation. People with IBD must also join with people who have diseases similar in terms of characteristics or social consequences. This approach can offer a realistic chance of success, and the importance of patient-centered organizations is vast—at the national level in EFCCA's 29 member associations, at the international level with EFCCA itself, and reaching on into umbrella organizations of which EFCCA is part, such as the European Patients' Forum, the European Disability Forum and the International Alliance of Patients' Organizations.

Conclusions: Patients' Group as "trait d'union" for Describing a New Conception of Resource

This chapter demonstrates the difficulty of defining "resources for patients," but also how many and varied they are, especially in terms of quality and access.

Organizations such as EFCCA are a source of resources, a source of assistance for patients who seek help in accessing or interpreting resources, and also a beacon of equilibrium and solidarity amongst the difficult conditions in which people with IBD live each day.

References

1. Gray JAM. The resourceful patient. Oxford: eRositta Press; 2002.
2. Baars JE, Markus T, Kuipers EJ, van der Woude CJ. Patients' preferences regarding shared decision-making in the treatment of inflammatory bowel disease: results from a patient-empowerment study. Digestion. 2010;81:113–9.
3. Louis E, Dotan I, Ghosh S. Mlynarsky L, Reenaers C, Schreiber S. Optimising the inflammatory bowel disease unit to improve quality of care: expert recommendations. J Crohns Colitis. 2015. doi:10.1093/ecco-jcc/jjv085.

4. Carter MJ, Lobo AJ, Travis SPL. Guidelines for the management of inflammatory bowel disease in adults. Gut. 2004;53 Suppl 5:V1–16.
5. Cattaneo LB, Chapman AR. The process of empowerment: a model for use in research and practice. Am Psychol. 2010;65: 646–59.
6. Funnell MM, Anderson RM. Empowerment and self-management of diabetes. Clin Diabetes. 2004;22:123–7.
7. Hsu J, Huang J, Kinsman J, Fireman B, Miller R, Selby J, et al. Use of e-Health services between 1999 and 2002: a growing digital divide. J Am Med Inform Assoc. 2005;12:164–71.
8. Fortinsky KJ, Fournier MR, Benchimol EI. Internet and electronic resources for inflammatory bowel disease: a primer for providers and patients. Inflamm Bowel Dis. 2012;18:1156–63.
9. Dixon-Woods M. Writing wrongs? An analysis of published discourses about the use of patient information leaflets. Soc Sci Med. 2001;52:1417–32.
10. Coulson NS. How do online patient support communities affect the experience of inflammatory bowel disease? An online survey. J R Soc Med Sh Rep. 2013;4:1–8.
11. Sledgianowski D, Kulviwat S. Using social network sites: the effects of playfulness, critical mass and trust in a hedonic context. J Comput Inform Syst. 2009;49:74.
12. Haynes RB. Of studies, summaries, synopses and systems: the "4S" evolution of services for finding current best evidence. Evid Based Ment Health. 2001;4:37–9.
13. Lönnfors S, Vermeire S, Greco M, Hommes D, Bell C, Avedano L. IBD and health-related quality of life—discovering the true impact. J Crohns Colitis. 2014;8:1281–6.
14. Lönnfors S, McCombie A. "Now I know I'm not alone": participating in a disease-specific summer camp improves the quality of life of young people with inflammatory bowel disease. Poster session presented at: 10th congress of ECCO—inflammatory bowel diseases 2015; 18–21 2015 Feb; Barcelona, Spain.
15. Victoor A, Delnoij DMJ, Friele RD, Rademakers JJDJM. Determinants of patient choice of healthcare providers: a scoping review. BMC Health Serv Res. 2012;12:272.
16. Edwards A, Elwyn G. Shared decision-making in health care: achieving evidence-based patient choice. 2nd ed. Oxford: Oxford University Press; 2009.

Index

D.C. Baumgart (ed.), *Crohn's Disease and Ulcerative Colitis*, DOI 10.1007/978-3-319-33703-6

Q

R

T

U